Children
with
Disabilities

6TH
EDITION

Children with Disabilities

6TH EDITION

edited by

Mark L. Batshaw, M.D.

Children's National Medical Center
The George Washington University
School of Medicine and Health Sciences
Washington, D.C.

Louis Pellegrino, M.D.

SUNY Upstate Medical University
Syracuse, New York

Nancy J. Roizen, M.D.

Rainbow Babies and Children's Hospital/
Case Western Reserve School of Medicine
Cleveland, Ohio

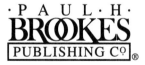

·P·A·U·L·H·
BROOKES
PUBLISHING CO®

Baltimore • London • Sydney

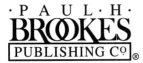

Paul H. Brookes Publishing Co.
Post Office Box 10624
Baltimore, Maryland 21285-0624

www.brookespublishing.com

Typeset by Integrated Publishing Solutions, Grand Rapids, Michigan.
Manufactured in the United States of America by
The Maple-Vail Book Manufacturing Group, York, Pennsylvania.

Illustrations, as listed, copyright © 2007 by Mark L. Batshaw. All rights reserved.
Figures 1.1–1.3, 1.5–1.8, 1.10–1.17, 2.3, 2.4, 3.1, 3.2, 4.1, 7.2, 9.3, 9.4, 9.6, 11.1–11.5, 11.8, 11.9, 12.1,
12.3–12.8, 12.11, 12.12, 13.1a, 13.1c, 13.2–13.4, 13.7–13.9, 18.1, 20.1–20.3, 26.2 (drawings only), 26.3,
26.5–26.11, 26.12 (drawing only), 28.1–28.7, 29.1, 29.2, 31.1–31.3, 31.6, 31.8–31.10, and 32.1–32.3.

Illustrations, as listed, copyright © by Lynn Reynolds. All rights reserved.
Figures 2.1, 6.1, 7.3, 7.5, 7.6, 11.7, 14.1, 14.2, 31.11, 35.3, and 35.5.

Appendix C, Commonly Used Medications, which appears on pages 699–718, provides information
about numerous drugs frequently used to treat children with disabilities. This appendix is in no way
meant to substitute for a physician's advice or expert opinion; readers should consult a medical
practitioner if they are interested in more information.

The publisher and the authors have made every effort to ensure that all of the information and
instructions given in this book are accurate and safe, but they cannot accept liability for any resulting
injury, damage, or loss to either person or property, whether direct or consequential and however it
occurs. Medical advice should only be provided under the direction of a qualified health care
professional.

The vignettes presented in this book are composite accounts that do not represent the lives or
experiences of specific individuals, and no implications should be inferred. In all instances,
names and identifying details have been changed to protect confidentiality.

Second printing, December 2008.

Library of Congress Cataloging-in-Publication Data

Children with disabilities / edited by Mark L. Batshaw, Louis Pellegrino, and
Nancy J. Roizen.—6th ed.
    p.   cm.
   Includes bibliographical references and index.
   ISBN-13: 978-1-55766-858-5 (hardcover)
   ISBN-10: 1-55766-858-2 (hardcover)
   1. Developmental disabilities.   2. Developmentally disabled children—Care.
3. Children with disabilities—Care.   I. Batshaw, Mark L., 1945–   II. Pellegrino, Louis.
III. Roizen, Nancy J.
[DNLM: 1. Disabled Children. WS 368 C537 2007]
RJ135.B38 2007
618.92—dc22   2007012613

British Library Cataloguing in Publication data are available from the British Library.

Contents

I   As Life Begins

List of Tables and Figures

About the Editors

Mark L. Batshaw, M.D., is the "Fight for Children" Chair of Academic Medicine and Chief Academic Officer at the Children's National Medical Center (CNMC) in Washington, D.C., and Professor and Chairman of Pediatrics and Associate Dean for Academic Affairs at The George Washington University School of Medicine and Health Sciences in Washington, D.C.

Dr. Batshaw is a board-certified neurodevelopmental pediatrician who has treated children with developmental disabilities for more than 30 years. In 2006, Dr. Batshaw received both the Capute Award for notable contributions to the field of children with disabilities by the American Academy of Pediatrics and the Distinguished Research Award from The Arc.

Before moving to Washington in 1998, he was Physician-in-Chief of Children's Seashore House, the child development and rehabilitation institute of The Children's Hospital of Philadelphia. Dr. Batshaw is a graduate of the University of Pennsylvania and of the University of Chicago Pritzker School of Medicine. Following pediatric residency at the Hospital for Sick Children in Toronto, he completed a fellowship in developmental pediatrics at the Kennedy Krieger Institute at The Johns Hopkins Medical Institutions.

Dr. Batshaw is director of the National Institutes of Health (NIH)–funded Mental Retardation and Developmental Disabilities Research Center at CNMC and continues to pursue his research on innovative treatments for inborn errors of metabolism, including gene therapy. He has published more than 150 articles, chapters, and reviews on his research interests and on the medical aspects of the care of children with disabilities. Dr. Batshaw was the founding editor-in-chief (1995–2001) of the journal *Mental Retardation and Developmental Disabilities Research Reviews*. He is also the editor of *When Your Child Has a Disability: The Complete Sourcebook of Daily and Medical Care, Revised Edition* (Paul H. Brookes Publishing Co., 2001).

Dr. Batshaw lives in Washington, D.C. He and his wife Karen have three children and four grandchildren.

Louis Pellegrino, M.D., is Clinical Assistant Professor of Pediatrics at SUNY Upstate Medical University in Syracuse, New York. He received his medical degree at the University of Connecticut and completed his training in pediatrics and neurodevelopmental pediatrics at Upstate Medical University and the University of Rochester. He has had the pleasure and privilege of working with both Dr. Batshaw and Dr. Roizen in the past. While at The Children's Hospital of Philadelphia/Children's Seashore House in Philadelphia, and with Dr. Batshaw's mentorship and encouragement, Dr. Pellegrino co-edited (with Dr. John P. Dormans) the book *Caring for Children with Cerebral Palsy: A Team Approach* (Paul H. Brookes Publishing Co., 1998). Dr. Pellegrino has subsequently written numerous chapters and reviews on the subject of cerebral palsy.

More recently, Dr. Pellegrino has been closely involved with children on the autism spectrum, and in addition to his clinical work, he serves on the board of directors for the central New York chapter of the Autism Society of America. He also has been closely involved with early intervention services in the central New York region and is currently working to promote the involvement of the local medical community with the goals of early intervention in general and of newborn hearing screening in particular.

Dr. Pellegrino lives in a suburb of Syracuse, New York, with his wife Dr. Joan E. Pellegrino (author of Chapter 8) and his two children, Elizabeth and Nicholas. Elizabeth is currently in the fifth grade, plays the harp, and has a brown belt in karate. Nicholas is in the first grade, plays piano, and has an orange belt. Dr. Pellegrino plays guitar and enjoys training in karate with his children; he hopes to earn his black belt in 2008.

Nancy J. Roizen, M.D., is Chief of the Division of Developmental—Behavioral Pediatrics and Psychology at Rainbow Babies and Children's Hospital, and Professor of Pediatrics at Case Western University School of Medicine in

Cleveland, Ohio. She is board certified in neurodevelopmental disabilities and in developmental and behavioral pediatrics. Dr. Roizen received her B.S. and M.D. degrees from Tufts University. After completing an internship in pediatrics at Massachusetts General Hospital, she did a residency in pediatrics at The Johns Hopkins Hospital. Her fellowships were in neurodevelopmental disabilities at the Kennedy Krieger Institute and in developmental and behavioral pediatrics at University of California, San Francisco. She then was a staff physician at the Child Development Center at Oakland Children's Hospital for 8 years, followed by 16 years as Chief of the Section of Developmental Pediatrics at the University of Chicago. Then, at SUNY Upstate Medical University, she was Vice Chair of Pediatrics, Professor of Pediatrics, and Chief of the Division of Neurosciences for 4 years. She joined the Cleveland Clinic Staff as the Chief of the Department of Developmental and Rehabilitation Pediatrics in 2005.

Dr. Roizen has published more than 90 articles, chapters, and reviews on her clinical and research interests in Down syndrome and hearing loss and on collaborations in congenital toxoplasmosis and velocardiofacial syndrome. She lives in Shaker Heights, Ohio, with her husband. They have a daughter in graduate school and a son who is in the pediatric training program at Children's Hospital of Philadelphia.

Contributors

George Acs, D.M.D., M.P.H.
Dentist

Terry Adirim, M.D., M.P.H.
Office of Health Affairs
U.S. Department of Homeland Security
Washington, D.C. 20528

Karen Batshaw, M.S.W.
Consultant
International Adoptions
Washington, D.C.

Michael Batshaw, L.C.S.W.
Licensed Social Worker
NYS Board Certified Psychotherapist
920 Broadway, 8th Floor, Suite #8
New York, NY 10010

Stephen Baumgart, M.D.
Associate Professor of Pediatrics
The George Washington University School of
    Medicine and Health Sciences
Division of Neonatology
Children's National Medical Center
111 Michigan Avenue NW
Washington, D.C. 20010

Michael J. Bell, M.D.
Associate Professor of Pediatrics
The George Washington University School of
    Medicine and Health Sciences
Children's National Medical Center
111 Michigan Avenue NW
Washington, D.C. 20010

Nathan J. Blum, M.D.
Associate Professor of Pediatrics
University of Pennsylvania School of Medicine
The Children's Hospital of Philadelphia
34th and Civic Circle Boulevard
Philadelphia, PA 19104

Jill E. Brown, M.D., M.P.H.
Staff Obstetrician/Gynecologist
National Naval Medical Center Bethesda
8901 Wisconsin Avenue
Bethesda, MD 20814

W. Bryan Burnette, M.D., M.S.
Fellow in Neuromuscular Medicine
Department of Neurology
The Johns Hopkins Hospital
600 North Wolfe Street
Baltimore, MD 21287

Seth Canion, D.D.C.
Dentist

Marilyn Cataldo, M.A.
Director of Behavioral Programming for Schools
Kennedy Krieger Institute
707 North Broadway
Baltimore, MD 21205

Michael F. Cataldo, Ph.D.
Professor of Behavioral Biology
The Johns Hopkins University School of Medicine
Director of Behavioral Psychology
Kennedy Krieger Institute
707 North Broadway
Baltimore, MD 21205

Taeun Chang, M.D.
Assistant Professor of Neurology and Pediatrics
The George Washington University School of
    Medicine and Health Sciences
Division of Child Neurology
Children's National Medical Center
111 Michigan Avenue NW
Washington, D.C. 20010

Robin P. Church, Ed.D.
Associate Professor of Education
The Johns Hopkins University
Vice President for Education
Kennedy Krieger Institute
3825 Greenspring Avenue
Baltimore, MD 21211

Elissa Batshaw Clair, M.Ed.
Teacher
Special School District of St. Louis County
12110 Clayton Road
St. Louis, MO 63131

Charles J. Conlon, M.D.
Director
Developmental Pediatrics Program
Children's National Medical Center
111 Michigan Avenue NW
Washington, D.C. 20010

Philip W. Davidson, Ph.D.
Professor of Pediatrics
University of Rochester School of Medicine and
    Dentistry
Box 671
601 Elmwood Avenue
Rochester, NY 14642

Iser G. DeLeon, Ph.D.
Assistant Professor of Psychiatry
The Johns Hopkins University School of Medicine
Kennedy Krieger Institute
707 North Broadway
Baltimore, MD 21205

Larry W. Desch, M.D.
Director
Developmental Pediatrics
Associate Clinical Professor
Advocate Hope Children's Hospital
University of Illinois at Chicago Medical School
4440 West 95th Street
Oak Lawn, IL 60453

Nienke P. Dosa, M.D., M.P.H.
Assistant Professor of Pediatrics
SUNY Upstate Medical University
750 East Adams Street
Syracuse, NY 13210

Carolyn Drews-Botsch, Ph.D., M.P.H.
Associate Professor and Director of Graduate Studies
Department of Epidemiology
Rollins School of Public Health
1518 Clifton Road NE
Atlanta, GA 30322

Ann-Christine Duhaime, M.D.
Professor of Surgery (Neurosurgery) and Pediatrics
Director of Pediatric Neurosurgery and Neuroscience
    Program
Children's Hospital at Dartmouth
Dartmouth Medical School
One Medical Center Drive
Lebanon, NH 03756

Peggy S. Eicher, M.D.
Medical Director
Center for Pediatric Feeding and Swallowing Disorders
St. Joseph's Hospital and Medical Center
703 Main Street
Paterson, NJ 07503

Diana M. Escolar, M.D.
Associate Professor of Neurology and Pediatrics
The George Washington University School of
    Medicine and Health Sciences
Children's National Medical Center
111 Michigan Avenue NW
Washington, D.C. 20010

Sarah Helen Evans, M.D.
Division Chief
Pediatric Rehabilitation
Children's National Medical Center
111 Michigan Avenue NW
Washington, D.C. 20010

Michaela L.Z. Farber, Ph.D., M.S.W., L.C.S.W.-C.
Assistant Professor
National Catholic School of Social Service
The Catholic University of America
Shahan Hall #112
620 Michigan Avenue NE
Washington, D.C. 20064

Patrick C. Friman, Ph.D.
Director of Clinical Services
Father Flanagan's Girls and Boys Home
Clinical Services and Research
Youthcare Building
13603 Flanagan Boulevard
Boys Town, NE 68010

William Davis Gaillard, M.D.
Professor of Neurology and Pediatrics
The George Washington University School of
    Medicine and Health Sciences
Director
Comprehensive Epilepsy Program
Children's National Medical Center
111 Michigan Avenue NW
Washington, D.C. 20010

Chrysanthe Gaitatzes, M.D., Ph.D.
Fellow in Neonatal/Perinatal Medicine
Children's National Medical Center
111 Michigan Avenue NW
Washington, D.C. 20010

Angelo P. Giardino, M.D., Ph.D., M.P.H.
Medical Director
Texas Children's Health Plan
Clinical Associate Professor
Baylor College of Medicine
2450 Holcombe
Houston, TX 77021

Marianne M. Glanzman, M.D.
Clinical Associate Professor of Pediatrics
University of Pennsylvania School of Medicine
Children's Seashore House
The Children's Hospital of Philadelphia
3405 Civic Center Boulevard
Philadelphia, PA 19104

Erynn S. Gordon, M.S.
Genetic Counselor
University of Maryland School of Medicine
Department of Pediatric Genetics
737 West Lombard Street
Baltimore, MD 21201

Karl F. Gumpper, R.Ph., BCNSP, BCPS, FASHP
Director
Section of Pharmacy Informatics and Technology
American Society of Health-System Pharmacists
7272 Wisconsin Avenue
Bethesda, MD 20814

Michael J. Guralnick, Ph.D.
Director
Center of Human Development and Disability
Professor of Psychology and Pediatrics
University of Washington
1701 Columbia Road
Seattle, WA 98195

William H.J. Haffner, M.D.
Professor
Obstetrics and Gynecology
Uniformed Services University of the Health Sciences
4301 Jones Bridge Road
Bethesda, MD 20814

Mark L. Helpin, D.M.D.
Director of Pediatric Dentistry
Maurice H. Kornberg School of Dentistry
Temple University
3223 North Broad Street
Philadelphia, PA 19140

Gilbert R. Herer, Ph.D.
Director Emeritus
Children's Hearing and Speech Center
Children's National Medical Center
Professor of Pediatrics
The George Washington University School
   of Medicine and Health Sciences
111 Michigan Avenue NW
Washington, D.C. 20010

Susan L. Hyman, M.D.
Associate Professor of Pediatrics
University of Rochester
Box 671
601 Elmwood Avenue
Rochester, NY 14642

Janet S. Isaacs, Ph.D.
Metabolic Dietician
Division of Genetics and Metabolism
Children's National Medical Center
111 Michigan Avenue NW
Washington, D.C. 20010

Dorothy O. Jones, M.Ed.
School Intervention Coordinator
Division of Pediatric Rehabilitation
Cincinnati Children's Hospital Medical Center
3333 Burnet Avenue
MLC 4009
Cincinnati, OH 45229

SungWoo Kahng, Ph.D.
Assistant Professor
Department of Psychiatry and Behavioral Sciences
Kennedy Krieger Institute
707 North Broadway
Baltimore, MD 21205

Robert Keating, M.D.
Associate Professor of Neurosurgery and Pediatrics
The George Washington University School of
   Medicine and Health Sciences
Chief
Division of Neurosurgery
Children's National Medical Center
111 Michigan Avenue NW
Washington, D.C. 20010

Annie Kennedy, B.S.
National Director
ALS Division
Muscular Dystrophy Association
3300 East Sunrise Drive
Tucson, AZ 85718

Carol A. Knightly, Au.D., CCC-A
Director of Clinical Operations
Center for Childhood Communication
The Children's Hospital of Philadelphia
3405 Civic Center Boulevard
Philadelphia, PA 19104

Alan E. Kohrt, M.D.
Attending Physician
Diagnostic Center
The Children's Hospital of Philadelphia
34th Street and Civic Center Boulevard
Philadelphia, PA 19104

Lisa A. Kurtz, M.Ed., OTR/L, FAOTA
Occupational Therapist
Jameson School
20 Jameson Hill Road
Old Orchard Beach, ME 04064

Mary F. Lazar, Psy.D.
Pediatric Neuropsychologist
Director
Neuropsychology Assessment Center
Clinical Assistant Professor
Institute for Graduate Clinical Psychology
Widener University
Chester, PA 19013

M.E.B. Lewis, Ed.D.
Faculty Member
School of Education
The Johns Hopkins University
Director
External Education Projects
Kennedy Krieger Institute
3825 Greenspring Avenue
Baltimore, MD 21211

Gregory S. Liptak, M.D., M.P.H.
Professor of Pediatrics
SUNY Upstate Medical University
750 East Adams Street
Syracuse, NY 13210

Gaetano R. Lotrecchiano, Ph.D.
Assistant Professor of Pediatrics
The George Washington University School
   of Medicine and Health Sciences
Program Coordinator, LEND
Children's National Medical Center
111 Michigan Avenue NW
Washington, D.C. 20010

Brian K. Martens, Ph.D.
Professor and Director of Training for the School
   Psychology Program
Syracuse University
Department of Psychology
430 Huntington Hall
Syracuse, NY 13244

Sheryl J. Menacker, M.D.
Clinical Associate
Department of Ophthalmology
University of Pennsylvania School of Medicine
319 Second Street Pike
Southampton, PA 18966

Gretchen A. Meyer, M.D.
Neurodevelopmental Pediatrician

Linda J. Michaud, M.D., M.Ed.
Aaron W. Perlman Professor of Pediatric Physical
    Medicine and Rehabilitation
Associate Professor of Clinical Physical Medicine and
    Rehabilitation and Clinical Pediatrics
Director of Pediatric Rehabilitation
Cincinnati Children's Hospital Medical Center
University of Cincinnati College of Medicine
MLC 4009
3333 Burnet Avenue
Cincinnati, OH 45339

Marijean M. Miller, M.D.
Attending Physician
Children's National Medical Center
Associate Professor of Ophthalmology and Pediatrics
The George Washington University School of
    Medicine and Health Sciences
111 Michigan Avenue NW
Washington, D.C. 20010

Gary J. Myers, M.D.
Professor of Neurology
Pediatrics and Environmental Medicine
University of Rochester School of Medicine and
    Dentistry
601 Elmwood Avenue
Box 631
Rochester, NY 14642

Man Wai Ng, D.D.S., M.P.H.
Dentist-in-Chief
Children's Hospital Boston
Lecturer in Oral and Developmental Biology
Harvard University

Joan E. Pellegrino, M.D.
Medical Geneticist
Associate Professor of Pediatrics
SUNY Upstate Medical University
750 East Adams Street
Syracuse, NY 13210

Jeffrey P. Rabin, D.O.
Associate Professor of Pediatrics
The George Washington University School of
    Medicine and Health Sciences
Physical Medicine and Rehabilitation
Children's National Medical Center
111 Michigan Avenue NW
Washington, D.C. 20010

Khodayar Rais-Bahrami, M.D.
Professor of Pediatrics
The George Washington University School of
    Medicine and Health Sciences
Children's National Medical Center
111 Michigan Avenue NW
Washington, D.C. 20010

Mark Reber, M.D.
Director of Psychiatry
Woods Services, Inc.
Route 213
Langhorne, PA 19047

Adelaide Robb, M.D.
Associate Professor of Psychiatry and Pediatrics
The George Washington University School of
    Medicine and Health Sciences
Division of Psychiatry and Behavior Medicine
Children's National Medical Center
111 Michigan Avenue NW
Washington, D.C. 20010

Howard M. Rosenberg, D.D.S., M.S.D., M.Ed.
Associate Professor of Pediatric Dentistry
University of Pennsylvania School of Dental Medicine
240 South 40 Street
Philadelphia, PA 19104

Andrew J. Satin, M.D.
Professor and Chair
Department of Obstetrics and Gynecology
Uniformed Services University of the Health Sciences
4301 Jones Bridge Road
Bethesda, MD 20814

Rhonda L. Schonberg, M.S.
Coordinator, Center for Prenatal Evaluation
Children's National Medical Center
111 Michigan Avenue NW
Washington, D.C. 20010

Vincent Schuyler, B.S.W., A.B.D.A.
Program Director
Adolescent Employment Readiness Center
Children's National Medical Center
111 Michigan Avenue NW
Washington, D.C. 20010

Bruce Shapiro, M.D.
Associate Professor of Pediatrics
The Johns Hopkins University School of Medicine
Vice President, Training
Kennedy Krieger Institute
707 North Broadway
Baltimore, MD 21205

Billie Lou Short, M.D.
Professor of Pediatrics
The George Washington University School of
    Medicine and Health Sciences
Chief
Division of Neonatology
Children's National Medical Center
111 Michigan Avenue NW
Washington, D.C. 20010

Tomas Jose Silber, M.D., M.A.S.S.
Director
Office of Ethics
Children's National Medical Center
Professor of Pediatrics
The George Washington University School
   of Medicine and Health Sciences
111 Michigan Avenue NW
Washington, D.C. 20010

Harvey S. Singer, M.D.
Haller Professor of Pediatric Neurology
The Johns Hopkins University School of Medicine
Harriet Lane Children's Health Building
200 North Wolfe Street, Suite 2157
Baltimore, MD 21287

Annie G. Steinberg, M.D.
Clinical Associate Professor
Department of Psychiatry and Pediatrics
University of Pennsylvania School of Medicine
424 Grove Place
Narberth, PA 19092

Sheela Stuart, Ph.D.
Director
Children's Hearing and Speech Center
Children's National Medical Center
111 Michigan Avenue NW
Washington, D.C. 20010

Ana Carolina Tesi Rocha, M.D.
Children's National Medical Center
111 Michigan Avenue, NW
Washington, DC 20010

Cynthia J. Tifft, M.D., Ph.D.
Chief
Division of Genetics and Metabolism
Children's National Medical Center
111 Michigan Avenue NW
Washington, D.C. 20010

Laura L. Tosi, M.D.
Director
Bone Health Program
Children's National Medical Center
111 Michigan Avenue NW
Washington, D.C. 20010

Kenneth E. Towbin, M.D.
Chief
Clinical Child and Adolescent Psychiatry, Mood and
   Anxiety Disorders Program
National Institute of Mental Health-Intramural
   Research Program
Clinical Professor, Department of Psychiatry and
   Behavioral Sciences
The George Washington University School of
   Medicine
9000 Rockville Pike
Bethesda, MD 20892

Symme Wilson Trachtenberg, M.S.W.
Clinical Associate in Pediatrics
University of Pennsylvania School of Medicine
Director
Community Education
The Children's Hospital of Philadelphia
34th and Civic Center Boulevard
Philadelphia, PA 19104

Mendel Tuchman, M.D.
Professor of Pediatrics, Biochemistry, and Molecular
   Biology
The George Washington University School of
   Medicine and Health Sciences
Children's National Medical Center
111 Michigan Avenue NW
Washington, D.C. 20010

Renee M. Turchi, M.D., M.P.H.
Assistant Professor of Pediatrics
St. Christopher's Hospital for Children
Erie Avenue at Front Street
Philadelphia, PA 19134

Kim Van Naarden Braun, Ph.D.
Epidemiologist
Centers for Disease Control and Prevention
National Center on Birth Defects and Developmental
   Disabilities
1600 Clifton Road
MS-E86
Atlanta, GA 30333

Shari L. Wade, Ph.D.
Professor of Pediatrics
Director of Research
Division of Pediatric Rehabilitation
Cincinnati Children's Hospital Medical Center
University of Cincinnati College of Medicine
3333 Brunet Avenue
MLC 4009
Cincinnati, OH 45229

Steven L. Weinstein, M.D.
Professor of Neurology and Pediatrics
The George Washington University School of
   Medicine and Health Sciences
Division of Neurology
Children's National Medical Center
111 Michigan Avenue NW
Washington, D.C. 20010

Patience H. White, M.D.
Chief Public Health Officer
Arthritis Foundation
Professor of Medicine and Pediatrics
Division of Rheumatology
Department of Medicine
The George Washington University
2150 Pennsylvania Avenue NW
Washington, D.C. 20037

Amanda L. Yaun, M.D.
Pediatric Neurosurgeon
Assistant Professor of Neurology and Pediatrics
The George Washington University School of
   Medicine and Health Sciences
Division of Neurosurgery
Children's National Medical Center
111 Michigan Avenue NW
Washington, D.C. 20010

Marshalyn Yeargin-Allsopp, M.D.
Medical Epidemiologist
Centers for Disease Control and Prevention
MS E-86
1600 Clifton Road
Atlanta, GA 30333

A Personal Note to the Reader

As it enters its sixth edition, *Children with Disabilities* has continued to evolve. The first edition was derived from lectures I gave for a special education course I taught at The Johns Hopkins University in Baltimore. The book contained 23 chapters, and I authored or co-authored virtually all of them. When I started writing the first edition I was 3 years out of my neurodevelopmental disabilities fellowship training program, and I thought I knew everything about developmental disabilities! I also considered myself an expert in my own children's development, having just welcomed into our family our third child, Andrew.

With this edition of the book the number of chapters and pages has basically doubled since its inception, and I have authored but a few chapters. I have recognized the need for additional help and counsel and have brought on two valued colleagues, Dr. Louis Pellegrino and Dr. Nancy J. Roizen, to co-edit the book with me. Lou was one of my finest neurodevelopmental disabilities fellows at the Children's Seashore House in Philadelphia, and my friendship with Nancy dates back to our training at Hopkins. Based on our areas of expertise we divided the book up, with Lou taking the sections As Life Begins and The Developing Child, Nancy taking Developmental Disabilities, and me taking Interventions, Families, and Outcomes.

The book has also become somewhat of a family affair. My son Michael, a psychotherapist, and my wife Karen, a social worker, co-authored the chapter "Caring and Coping." My daughter Elissa, a special education teacher, co-authored the chapter "Special Education Services." And Andrew has continued his autobiographical letters concerning the effect of attention-deficit/hyperactivity disorder on his life. Finally, Lou's wife, Joan, has authored the new chapter "Newborn Screening."

It has been both personally and professionally very rewarding to develop this book over a quarter century. Many of those rewards have come from the students, colleagues, and parents who have shared with me their thoughts and advice about the book. It is my hope that *Children with Disabilities* will continue to fill the needs of its diverse users for many years to come.

Mark L. Batshaw

Preface

One of the first questions asked about a subsequent edition of a textbook is "What's new?" The challenge of determining what to revise, what to add, and, in some cases, what to delete is always significant in preparing a new edition in a field changing as rapidly as developmental disabilities. Since the publication of the fifth edition in 2002, advances in the fields of neuroscience and genetics have greatly enhanced our understanding of the brain and inheritance, bringing forth opportunities for treatments previously not thought possible for children with developmental disabilities. The human genome has been mapped and the brain probed by functional imaging techniques. The need to examine and explain this increased knowledge and its significance for children with disabilities has necessitated an increase in the depth and breadth of the subjects covered in the book. Yet, while the book is now more expansive and has several new chapters, we have worked hard to ensure that it retains its clarity and cohesion. Its mission continues to be to provide the individual working with and caring for children with disabilities the necessary background to understand different disabilities and their treatments, thereby enabling affected children to reach their full potential.

THE AUDIENCE

Since it was originally published, *Children with Disabilities* has been used by students in a wide range of disciplines as a medical textbook addressing the impact of disabilities on child development and function. It has also served as a professional reference for special educators, general educators, physical therapists, occupational therapists, speech-language pathologists, psychologists, child life specialists, social workers, nurses, physicians, advocates, and others providing care for children with disabilities. Finally, as a family resource, parents, grandparents, siblings, and other family members and friends have found useful information on the medical and (re)habilitative aspects of care for the child with developmental disabilities.

FEATURES FOR THE READER

We have been told that the strengths of previous editions of this book have been the accessible writing style, the clear illustrations, and the up-to-date information and references. We have dedicated our efforts to retaining these strengths. Some of the features you will find include the following:

- *Teaching goals*—Each chapter begins with learning objectives to orient you to the content of that particular chapter.

- *Situational examples*—Most chapters include one or more stories, or case studies, to help bring alive the conditions and issues discussed in the chapter.

- *Key terms*—As medical terms are introduced in the text, they appear in boldface type at their first use; definitions for these terms appear in the Glossary (Appendix A).

- *Illustrations and tables*—More than 200 drawings, photographs, X rays, imaging scans, and tables reinforce the points of the text and provide ways for you to more easily understand and remember the material you are reading.

- *Summary*—Each chapter closes with a final section that reviews its key elements and provides you with an abstract of the covered material.

- *References*—The reference list accompanying each chapter can be thought of as more than just a list of the literature cited in the chapter. These citations include review articles, reports of study findings and research discoveries, and other key references that can help you find additional information.

- *Appendices*—In addition to the Glossary, there are four other helpful appendices: 1) Syndromes and Inborn Errors of Metabolism, a mini-reference of pertinent information on more than 110 inherited disorders causing disabilities; 2) Commonly Used Medications, to describe indications and side effects of medications often prescribed for children with disabilities; 3) Childhood Disabilities Resources, Services, and Organizations, a directory of a wide range of national organizations, federal agencies, information sources, self-advocacy and accessibility programs, and support groups that can provide assistance to families and professionals; and 4) Cognitive Testing and Screening Testing, to outline commonly used instruments.

CONTENT

In developing this sixth edition, we have aimed for a balance between consistency with the text that many of you have come to know so well in its previous editions and innovation in exploring the new topics that demand our attention. All of the chapters from the fifth edition have been rewritten to include an expanded focus on psychosocial, (re)habilitative, and educational interventions as well as to provide information discovered through educational, medical, and scientific advances since 2002. In addition, five new chapters have been added to address the following topics: environmental toxins, infections and the fetus, newborn screening, patterns of development and disability, and epidemiology. They focus on recently gained knowledge that is transforming our understanding of the causes of developmental disabilities.

The chapters are grouped in sections and have been organized to help guide readers through the breadth of content. The book starts with a section titled As Life Begins, which addresses what happens before, during, or shortly after birth to cause a child at risk to have a developmental disability. The concepts and consequences of genetics, embryology, infections and fetal development, the birth process, and prematurity are explained. The next section of the book, The Developing Child, covers environmental causes of developmental disabilities and examines the various organ systems—how they develop and work and what can go wrong. Nutrition, vision, hearing, language, patterns of development, and the brain and musculoskeletal systems are discussed in individual chapters. As its title implies, the third section, Developmental Disabilities, provides comprehensive descriptions of various developmental disabilities and genetic syndromes causing disabilities and includes chapters on intellectual disability, Down syndrome, fragile X syndrome, inborn errors of metabolism, psychiatric disorders in

developmental disabilities, autism spectrum disorders, attention-deficit/hyperactivity disorder, specific learning disabilities, cerebral palsy, neural tube defects, epilepsy, and traumatic brain injury. The final section, Interventions, Families, and Outcomes, contains chapters that focus on various interventions including early intervention and special education services, feeding, dental care, behavioral assessment and support, assistive technology, and physical and occupational therapy. This section also concentrates on the ethical, legal, emotional, and transition-to-adulthood issues that are common to most families of children with disabilities and to professionals who work with them. The book closes with a discussion of the prospects for providing health care in the 21st century.

THE AUTHORS AND EDITORS

Louis Pellegrino and Nancy J. Roizen have jointed me as editors for this edition of the text. Like me, Lou and Nancy are neurodevelomental pediatricians, and they have been contributors to prior editions of the book. We have chosen physicians and other health care professionals who are experts in the areas they write about as authors of *Children with Disabilities*. Many are colleagues from Children's National Medical Center and Children's Seashore House of The Children's Hospital of Philadelphia. Each chapter in the book has undergone editing at Paul H. Brookes Publishing Co. to ensure consistency in style and accessibility of content. Once the initial drafts were completed, each chapter was sent for peer review by two or three major clinical and academic leaders in the field and was revised according to their input.

A FEW NOTES ABOUT TERMINOLOGY AND STYLE

As is the case with any book of this scope, the editor or author faces decisions about the use of particular words or the presentation style of information. We would like to share with you some of the decisions we have made for this book.

- *Reference style*—In general, the citation style of the American Psychological Association has been followed, with one particular exception. To conserve space, given the number of co-authors so often listed on primary source material, we have elected to use the "et al." format for all references with more than three names.

- *Categories of intellectual disability*—This book uses the American Psychiatric Association's categories according to the term *mental retardation* (i.e., mild, moderate, severe, profound) when discussing medical diagnosis and treatment and uses the categories that the American Association on Intellectual and Developmental Disabilities (formerly the American Association on Mental Retardation) established in 1992 (i.e., requiring limited, intermittent, extensive, or pervasive support) when discussing educational and other interventions, thus emphasizing the capabilities rather than the impairments of individuals with intellectual disability.

- *"Typical" and "normal"*—Recognizing diversity and the fact that no one type of person or lifestyle is inherently "normal," we have chosen to refer to the general population of children as "typical" or "typically developing," meaning that they follow the natural continuum of development.

- *Person-first language*—We have tried to preserve the dignity and personhood of all individuals with disabilities by consistently using person-first language, speaking, for example, of "a child with autism," instead of "an autistic child." In this way, we are able to emphasize the person, not define him or her by the condition.

As you read this sixth edition of *Children with Disabilities*, we hope you will find that the text continues to address the frequently asked question "Why this child?" and to provide the medical background you need to care for children with developmental disabilities.

For our children and grandchildren: Benjamin, Julian, Rebecca,
Sophia, Elizabeth, Nicolas, Jeff and Jennifer

Acknowledgments

We gratefully acknowledge Gaetano R. Lotrecchiano, Ph.D., who organized the project as well as contributed to the book's appendices. For this edition, we had the opportunity to include user input from our fellows and trainees who participate in the Maternal and Child Health Bureau–funded Leadership Education in Neurodevelopmental Disabilities (LEND) program at Children's National Medical Center. Their contributions greatly affected the layout of the volume.

A book such as *Children with Disabilities* is best understood with illustrations that help to explain medical concepts. An expert medical illustrator is crucial in this effort. Lynn Reynolds has contributed to this endeavor in both past editions and with new additions in this volume. We deeply acknowledge her important contribution.

We also thank our colleagues at Paul H. Brookes Publishing Co. for their great help. Heather Shrestha provided developmental oversight of the project. Tara Gebhardt, Sara Shepke, and Nicole Schmidl served as editors for the text. Finally, many of our colleagues reviewed and edited the manuscript for content and accuracy, and we would like to acknowledge their efforts.

Why me?
Why me?
Why do I have to do so much more than others?
Why am I so forgetful?
Why am I so hyperactive?
And why can't I spell?
Why me? O'why me?

I remember when I almost failed first grade because I couldn't read. I would cry hour after hour because my mother would try to make me read. Now I love to read. I couldn't write in cursive but my mother helped me and now I can. I don't have as bad a learning disability as others. At lest I can go to a normal school. I am trying as hard as I can (I just hope it is enough). My worst nightmare is to go to a special school because I don't want to be treated differently.

I am getting to like working. I guess since my dad is so successful and has a learning disability, it helps make me not want to give up. Many people say that I am smart, but sometimes I doubt it. I am very good at math, but sometimes I read a number like 169 as 196, so that messes things up. I also hear things incorrectly, for instants entrepreneur as horse manure (that really happened). I guess the reason why a lot of people don't like me is because I say the wrong answer a lot of times.

I had to take medication, but then I got off the medication and did well. Then in 7th grade I wasn't doing well but I didn't tell my parents because I thought they would just scream at me. My dad talked to the guidance counselor and found out. It wasn't till a week ago that I started on the medication again; I have been doing fine since than. As I have been getting more organized, I have had more free time. I guess I feel good when I succeed in things that take hard work.

This is my true story. . .

Andrew Batshaw

Andrew Batshaw
1989

In applying to colleges during my senior year of high school, I found that most had as an essay topic, "Tell us something about yourself." I decided to write about my ADHD and learning disability as it is a big part of who I am. I wrote "I have found that while a disability inherently leaves you with a weakness, adapting to that disability can provide rewards. I feel that from coping with my disability, I have gained pride, determination, and a strength that will be with me all of my life." I guess Vassar College agreed; they admitted me.

When it came time for high school graduation, we had a problem. My sister was graduating from the University of Chicago on the same day that I graduated from high school in Philadelphia. The only solution was for one parent to attend my graduation while the other one was with my sister in Chicago. The decision as to who would go to which graduation was easy. My mother insisted that she attend my graduation because it was a product of her hard work as well as my own. I remember she said to me that day, "When I think of the boy who cried himself to sleep because he could not remember how to spell the word 'who,' it makes me so happy to see you now."

My parents expressed themselves in different ways about my leaving for college. My mother and I found ourselves getting into many arguments over simple things (the old severing of the umbilical cord; I am the baby of the family). My father, however, made sure to remind me to start my stimulant medication 2 weeks before classes began!

The first semester I took four courses: Poetry, Linear Algebra, Computer Science, and Music Theory. As the semester continued, I developed an increasing interest in computer science, until finally I decided to become a computer science major. I was very flattered, however, when during a meeting with my English professor, she asked if I planned to be an English major. To think that someone who could not read until the end of second grade would become a member of the Vassar English department seemed almost unbelievable. Well, I might have been proud but not that proud. I stuck with computer science.

On the whole, I would say that my freshman year was a good one. I learned a great deal, both inside and outside of classes, about myself and others. What will I do after college? What will I end up doing with my life? These are questions that continually run through my mind. I have no clear answers, but there is one thing of which I am sure: My disability will not keep me from doing anything. I will not let it.

Andrew Batshaw

Andrew Batshaw
June 1996

As a college graduate, I find that my ADHD and learning disabilities are much less of an issue; however, that was not the case during my early college years. In my second year of college, I took a year-long introductory German class that fulfilled my language requirement. Forgetting that languages don't come easily to me, I chose the intensive German class that met an extra day a week and moved faster than the regular class. I watched my exam grades slowly slide into the C range during the first semester and decided to switch to the regular class for the rest of the year. While this was happening, some medical warnings were issued concerning the stimulant medication I was taking, so I decided to discontinue its use.

In the new German class, we had exams every other week, so I received regular feedback on how I was doing. Unfortunately, it was not positive feedback. After receiving an F on the first quiz, I decided that I needed to work harder in the class. I started studying more and was less than relieved when on my next exam my grade rose to a D! Again, I studied even more and still received a D on the test that followed. At this point, I began to doubt myself. I felt like I was doing everything I could, and still I wasn't improving. I said to myself, "I know you have always told yourself that you could do anything you really gave your all to, but maybe there are just some things you can't do." I was disheartened, but felt that I had no choice but to just keep working. I received a C and then a C+ on my next two exams, but my overall class grade was still very low. My professor spoke to me and said that as long as I received at least a C+ on the final exam, he would pass me. I did all I could to prepare for the test and took the exam without reservation, simply willing to accept the results, whatever they might be. I ran into my professor a week after the final exam and was told that not only had I passed the final exam, but that I had received an A, one of the highest grades in the class. As you might expect, I was ecstatic. I looked back on the day when I had thought, "Maybe there really are things that I just can't do," and smiled, because I proved myself wrong. On top of that, I had accomplished it without the help of medication. That was when I truly felt that I had overcome my ADHD and learning disabilities.

In fact, some of the most important activities in my life are things that at first glance you wouldn't think someone with ADHD would find attractive. I meditate every day, which involves sitting in one place and not moving for long periods of time. When I meditate, I am actually watching how my mind works. I see how easily I am distracted from simply sitting by thinking about all kinds of things, like what I did yesterday or what I am going to do later. Nevertheless, I keep bringing myself back, over and over again, and sometimes my mind becomes very quiet and clear. I find that this has had a positive impact on all aspects of my life. I was talking with my older brother, Michael, after attending my first 3-day meditation retreat, and he told me how proud he was of me. He said that after seeing me bounce off the walls and have such difficulty concentrating while growing up, he was amazed that I could sit still and meditate for 3 days.

After 4 years, including 6 months at the University of York in England, I graduated from Vassar College with a B.A. in Computer Science in May 1999. After graduation, I worked for a year as a software engineer and then started my own company with my brother and a friend. Unfortunately, after developing the company for a year, we became one of the many casualties of the dot-com collapse. Naturally, I was very disappointed, but it was an incredible experience that I will always value. It sparked in me a passion for entrepreneurship that led to my decision to attend business school.

Throughout the process of applying to business school, it became clear to me how my learning disability had been transformed from a hindrance to an asset. The work habits I had developed to overcome my disability allowed me to stick to a rigorous preparation program for my business school entrance exams. As a result, I scored in the 98th percentile. In addition, when preparing my applications, I chose to include an essay about how overcoming a disability had taught me to treat failure as a natural and necessary part of important accomplishments. Furthermore, it instilled in me a drive to achieve and to take calculated risks that are essential to being successful in business. I will be attending the University of Southern California Business School with a full scholarship.

Drew Batshaw
April 2002

Five eventful years have passed since I wrote my foreword to the fifth edition of this text. I graduated from business school, fell in love and married an amazing woman, and have been pursuing a career in business. Through all of these experiences, my ADHD and learning disability continue to impact my life in both subtle and not-so-subtle ways.

At the end of my last letter, I spoke about pursuing an MBA at the University of Southern California. My experience in business school was positive, both academically and socially. I'd come a long way from my childhood struggles; my ADHD and learning deficits had little effect on my performance. I excelled, my teachers respected me, and other students regularly sought me out to work on projects with them.

For me, business school was easier than college for a number of reasons. The subject matter was generally more engaging and played to my strengths: thinking on my feet, presenting ideas orally, and using analytical reasoning. In addition, much of the learning took place in an interactive and experiential environment that kept my interest and attention. For example, we discussed real situations that companies have had in the past and how we would have managed them, and we role-played as consultants with 90 minutes to prepare a thorough presentation for the class. Another significant factor was that writing (which historically has been my most challenging form of communication) is different and easier for me in a business setting than an academic one. In business writing, lengthy discourse is discouraged and traditional writing rules are far less important than presenting information in a clear and concise way; plus, of course, I'd had many years to hone my writing skills since I entered Vassar. Finally, I'd learned to manage my disability and identify environments like business school where I would be most successful.

After graduating with my MBA, I launched a company that provided coaching services for young executives and business owners. My job as a coach was to assist clients in their effectively working through problems, as opposed to the traditional consultant model of doing the work for them. After about 18 months, I realized that my heart was no longer in building the business; I missed managing tangible projects and found coaching to be lonely. I had many clients but no peers to interact with on a daily basis. I then moved to my current job, where I run the operations and technology of an education technology company that helps low-income children improve their reading skills. It is very satisfying to be involved in a business that helps children who have reading difficulties like I had. In contrast to the coaching work, this job allows me to manage many different projects and work with a great team.

I have also found that I reap unexpected benefits from my ADHD. Professionally, I am known for my ability to effectively problem-solve with limited information. Unlike others who are intimidated by their lack of knowledge or information, I delight in jumping right into the problem and figuring it out as I go (much like how I used to raise my hand all the time in grade school even though I didn't know the answer). In addition, I juggle many different projects and priorities with finesse. I thrive in environments that offer variety, allow me to wear many different hats, and require the use of a broad set of skills throughout the course of each day. Perhaps because of this I have changed jobs every 1 to 2 years since graduating from college (7 years ago): I have been a software developer, a dot-com founder, a business school student, and an executive coach, and now I am a manager of technology and finance. When I first start a job, I'm very excited and engaged in the work, but after I become proficient, I start to itch to do something different. Does my ADHD cause me to need a certain kind of sustained and varied stimulation that I have not yet found? I'm not sure, but I do know that I require a high level of change and stimulation to stay engaged and productive.

My ADHD impacted my early adulthood in other ways. For many years, no matter how much I achieved or how well I succeeded, I was still left with the shame of not being good enough during my formative years. As a child, my disability affected my self-image as well as my academic performance. Despite my mother telling me, "You are intelligent. It's just your learning disability that affects how you do in school," I still measured my worth in comparison to everyone else—for example, how far I got in a spelling bee, how long it took me to read a book, or what grade I received on a writing assignment. Through much of my twenties, when something didn't go well in my life—professionally, personally, or sometimes even when I was just sick—I would feel like that little boy again who just couldn't do anything right. I can see now that no amount of achievement would have transformed those feelings of inadequacy.

What has helped me most in dealing with this legacy is counseling and rewarding intimate relationships. Counseling has helped me to recognize when this old shame is triggered and how to notice it and move on. Through intimate relationships, I've come to understand and own my worth in a greater sense—how I offer so much more than just what I can achieve. For example, I have a positive impact on others by just being in their lives, and I can move people with my emotions and words. These things are all effortless. I don't have to try or work hard to make them happen. They simply occur as a natural result of who I am inherently.

My greatest teacher in this has been my wife, Amy. We were married in August 2005 after dating for 2 years. Her capacity for love, joy, and compassion amazes me. While preparing this letter, I asked her how my disability impacts our relationship. She smiled and said, "Well, you don't like to wash the dishes or go clothes shopping with me!" Much as I'd like to blame that on ADHD, I'm not sure that would be fair. What I *have* noticed are some of Amy's qualities that make her an especially good match for someone like me with ADHD. Professionally, she is a coach and organizing consultant, and, as a result, naturally provides structure and organization to our lives. In addition, she gives me a lot of space and honors the transition time I need between being by myself and being with her. Finally, she is very accepting and offers me constant appreciation and encouragement. I am a lucky man!

In sum, I lead an extraordinarily blissful life. I have a wonderful wife, my current work is stimulating and meaningful, and my relationships with family and friends are warm and fulfilling. I am immensely grateful for all I have been given and all I have been able to accomplish—in spite of and *because of* my disability.

Andrew Batshaw
2007

I As Life Begins

1 Genetics and Developmental Disabilities

Mark L. Batshaw

Upon completion of this chapter, the reader will

- Know about the human genome and its implication for the origins of developmental disabilities

- Be able to explain errors in mitosis and meiosis, including nondisjunction, translocation, and deletion

- Know the differences and similarities among autosomal recessive, autosomal dominant, and X-linked genetic disorders

- Understand the concepts of genomic imprinting, anticipation, and mitochondrial inheritance

- Understand the ways in which environment and heredity contribute to the development of multifactorial disorders

---

KATY

Katy was developing typically until she was 2 years old, when she started to have episodes of vomiting and lethargy after high-protein meals. Her parents became very concerned because their older son, Andrew, had died in infancy of coma, although no specific diagnosis had been made. With extensive testing by a genetic metabolic specialist, Katy was discovered to have an error (mutation) in the gene that codes for ornithine transcarbamylase (OTC), an **enzyme** that prevents the accumulation of ammonia in body and brain that can lead to coma. The OTC gene is located on the X chromosome so its deficiency is inherited as an X-linked disorder. Girls are therefore less likely to be affected than boys and, when affected, they generally have less severe manifestations. It turns out that Andrew also carried this mutation. Katy was placed on a low-protein diet and given medication to provide an alternate pathway to rid the body of ammonia, and she has done well. Now age 7, it looks like she may have a mild nonverbal learning disability; if Katy had been left untreated, she would probably not be alive.

Whether we have brown or blue eyes is determined by genes passed on to us from our parents. Other traits, such as height and weight, are affected by genes and by our environment both before and after birth. In a similar manner, genes alone or in combination with environmental factors can place us at increased risk for many disorders, including birth defects such as spina bifida (see Chapter 7). The spectrum ranges from purely genetic disorders, such as OTC deficiency and muscular dystrophy (see Chapter 20), which result from a **single-gene defect,** and Down syndrome (see Chapter 18), which results from an extra chromosome, to purely environmentally induced conditions, including infectious diseases such as cytomegalovirus (see Chapter 6).

As an introduction to the discussion in the chapters that follow, this chapter describes the human cell and explains what chromosomes and genes are. It also reviews and provides some illustrations of the errors that can occur in the processes of **mitosis** and **meiosis** and discusses inheritance patterns of single-gene disorders. As you progress through this book, bear in mind that the purpose of this discussion is to focus on the abnormalities that can occur in human development; however, few infants are affected by these disorders.

GENETIC DISORDERS

Our bodies are composed of approximately 100 trillion cells. There are many cell types, including nerve cells, muscle cells, white blood cells, and skin cells, to name a few. Each cell is divided into two compartments: 1) a central, enclosed core—the nucleus; and 2) an outer area—the **cytoplasm** (Figure 1.1), except for the red blood cell, which does not have a nucleus. The nucleus houses **chromosomes,** structures that contain the genetic code (**deoxyribonucleic acid [DNA]**), organized into hundreds of units of heredity, termed **genes.** These genes are responsible for our physical attributes and biological functions. Under the direction of the genes, the products that are needed for the growth and functioning of the organism, including waste disposal and the release of energy, are made in the cytoplasm. The nucleus, then, contains the blueprint for an individual's development, and the cytoplasm manufactures the products needed to complete the task.

When there is a defect within this system, the result may be a genetic disorder. There is a continuum of genetic disorders ranging from the addition (e.g., Down syndrome) or loss (e.g., Turner syndrome) of an entire chromosome in each cell, to the loss of a significant part of a chromosome (e.g., cri-du-chat syndrome), to a **microdeletion** of a number of contiguous genes within a chromosome (e.g., 22q11.2 deletion syndrome or velocardiofacial syndrome [VCFS]), to a defect within a single gene (e.g., phenylketonuria). This chapter discusses each of these types of genetic defects, beginning with chromosomes and problems in their division.

CHROMOSOMES

Each organism has a fixed number of chromosomes that direct the cell's activities. In humans, in each cell there are 46 chromosomes. Each chromosome contains hundreds of genes, but some chromosomes have more (e.g., 500–800 gene loci in chromosomes 1, 19, and X) and others less (50–120 in chromosomes 13, 18, 21, and Y). The 46 chromosomes are organized into 23 pairs of complementary chromosomes. Normally, one chromosome from each pair comes from the mother and one from the father; the one exception is uniparental disomy (found in certain cases of Prader-Willi syndrome, in which both chromosome 15s come from the father [Gingsburg, Fokstuen, & Schinzel, 2000]). Egg and sperm cells, however, each contain only 23 chromosomes. During conception, these **germ cells** fuse to produce a fertilized egg with the full complement of 46 chromosomes.

Among the 23 pairs of chromosomes, 22 are termed **autosomes.** The 23rd pair consists of the X and Y chromosomes, or the **sex chromosomes.** The Y chromosome, which determines "maleness," is one third to one half as long as the X chromosome, has a different shape, and has far fewer genes. Two X chromosomes determine the child to be female; an X and a Y chromosome determine the child to be male.

CELL DIVISION AND ITS DISORDERS

Cells have the ability to divide into daughter cells that contain identical genetic information. The prenatal development of a human being is

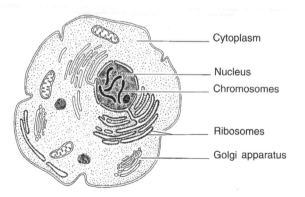

Figure 1.1. An idealized cell. The genes within chromosomes direct the creation of a product on the ribosomes. The product is then packaged in the Golgi apparatus and released from the cell.

accomplished through cell division, differentiation into different cell types, and movement to different locations in the body. There are two kinds of cell division: mitosis and meiosis. In mitosis, or nonreductive division, two daughter cells, each containing 46 chromosomes, are formed from one parent cell. In meiosis, or reductive division, four daughter cells, each containing only 23 chromosomes, are formed from one parent cell. Although mitosis occurs in all cells, meiosis takes place only in the germ cells and creates sperm and eggs (Turnpenny & Ellard, 2005).

The ability of cells to continue to undergo mitosis throughout the life span is essential for proper bodily functioning. Cells divide at different rates, however, ranging from once every 10 hours for skin cells to once a year for liver cells. This is why a skin abrasion heals in a few days, but the liver may take a year to recover from hepatitis. By adulthood, some cells, including neurons and muscle cells, appear to have a significantly decreased ability to divide. This limits the body's capacity to recover after a stroke or sports injury.

One of the primary differences between mitosis and meiosis can be seen during the first of the two meiotic divisions. During this phase, the corresponding chromosomes line up beside each other in pairs (e.g., both copies of chromosome 1 line up together). Unlike in mitosis, however, they intertwine and may "cross over," exchanging genetic material (Figure 1.2). Although this crossing over (or recombination) of the chromosomes may result in disorders, it also allows for the mutual transfer of genetic information, reducing the chance that siblings end up as exact copies (clones) of each other. Some of the variability among siblings can also be attributed to the random assortment of maternal and paternal chromosomes during the first of two meiotic divisions.

Throughout the life span of the male, meiosis of the immature sperm produces **spermatocytes** with 23 chromosomes each. These cells will lose most of their cytoplasm, sprout tails, and become mature sperm. In the female, meiosis forms oocytes that will ultimately become mature eggs. By the time a girl is born, her body has produced all of the approximately 2 million eggs she will ever have. A number of events that adversely affect a child's development can occur during meiosis. When chromosomes divide unequally, a process known as **nondisjunction,** the result is that one daughter egg or sperm contains 24 chromosomes and the other 22

chromosomes. Usually, these cells do not survive, but on occasion they do and lead to the child being born with too many (e.g., Down syndrome) or too few (e.g., Turner syndrome) chromosomes. It is interesting to note that the most commonly found **trisomy** in miscarriages is trisomy 16, but embryos with trisomy 16 are never carried to term (Nagaishi, Yamamoto, & Iinuma, 2004). The reason is probably that the chromosome 16 contains so many genes important to development that its disruption is incompatible with life. Conversely, trisomies 13, 18, and 21 are the most commonly observed chromosomal disorders at birth, probably because these chromosomes contain a relatively small number of gene loci and their disruption is compatible with life (Parker et al., 2003). Even so, the majority of fetuses carrying chromosomal abnormalities are spontaneously aborted. Among those children who survive these genetic missteps, **intellectual disability,** unusual (dysmorphic) facial appearances, and various **congenital** malformations are common. In the general population, chromosomal errors causing disorders occur in 6–9 per 1,000 of all live

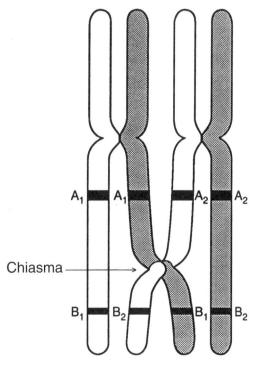

Figure 1.2. The process of crossing over, or recombination, at a chiasma permits exchange of genetic material among chromosomes and accounts for much of the genetic variability of human traits. In this illustration, there is an exchange on the banding area labeled B between two chromosomes. (*Source:* Jorde et al., 2001.)

births. In children who have intellectual disability, however, this prevalence increases 10- to 40-fold (Flint et al., 1995).

Chromosomal Gain: Down Syndrome

The most frequent chromosomal abnormality is nondisjunction of autosomes, and the most common clinical consequence is trisomy 21, or Down syndrome (see Chapter 18). Nondisjunction can occur during either mitosis or meiosis but is more common in meiosis (Figure 1.3). When nondisjunction occurs during the first meiotic division, both copies of chromosome 21 end up in one cell. Instead of an equal distribution of chromosomes among cells (23 each), one daughter cell receives 24 chromosomes, whereas the other receives only 22. The cell containing 22 chromosomes is unable to survive. However, the egg (or sperm) with 24 chromosomes occasionally can survive. After fertilization with

a sperm (or egg) containing 23 chromosomes, the resulting embryo contains three copies of chromosome 21, or trisomy 21. The child will be born with 47 rather than 46 chromsomes in each cell and have Down syndrome (Figure 1.4).

A majority of individuals with Down syndrome (approximately 90%) acquire it as a result of a nondisjunction during meiosis of the egg; only 5% acquire Down syndrome from nondisjunction of the sperm (Soares et al., 2001). Another 3%–4% of individuals acquire Down syndrome as a result of **translocation** (discussed later) and 1%–2% from **mosaicism** (some cells being affected and others not; this is also discussed later).

Other nonsex chromosomes that seem particularly susceptible to nondisjunction are chromosomes 13 and 18. The resulting trisomy 13 and trisomy 18 are associated with even more severe cognitive impairments than Down syndrome and often with early death (Parker et al., 2003).

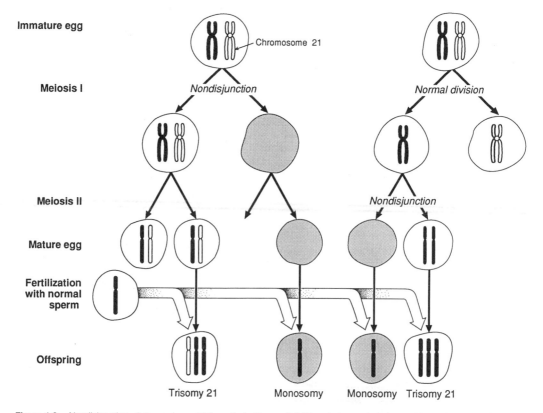

Figure 1.3. Nondisjunction of chromosome 21 in meiosis. Unequal division during meiosis I or meiosis II can result in trisomy or monosomy.

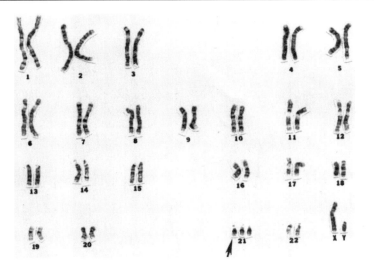

Figure 1.4. Karyotype of a boy with Down syndrome (47, XY). Note that the child has 47 chromosomes; the extra one is a chromosome 21.

Chromosomal Loss: Turner Syndrome

Turner syndrome (45, X), which affects girls, is the only disorder in which a fetus can survive despite the loss of an entire chromosome. Even so, more than 99% of the 45, X conceptions appear to be miscarried (Hall, 1992). Females with Turner syndrome (1 in every 5,000 live births) have only a single X chromosome and no second X or Y chromosome, for a total of 45, rather than 46, chromosomes. In contrast to Down syndrome, 80% of individuals with **monosomy** X conditions are affected by meiotic errors in sperm production; these children usually receive an X chromosome from their mothers but no sex chromosome from their fathers.

Girls with Turner syndrome have short stature, a webbed neck, a broad "shield-like" chest with widely spaced nipples, and nonfunctional ovaries. Twenty percent have obstruction of the left side of the heart, most commonly caused by a **coarctation** of the **aorta**. Unlike children with Down syndrome, most girls with Turner syndrome have typical intelligence. They do, however, have visual–perceptual impairments that predispose them to develop nonverbal learning disabilities (Rovet, 2004). Human growth hormone injections have been effective in increasing height in girls with Turner syndrome, and **estrogen** supplementation can lead to the emergence of secondary sexual characteristics; however, these girls remain infertile (Sybert & McCauley, 2004).

Mosaicism

In mosaicism, different cells have a different genetic makeup (Chen et al., 2004). For example, a child with the mosaic form of Down syndrome may have trisomy 21 in blood cells but not in skin cells or in some, but not all, brain cells. Children with mosaicism often appear as if they have the condition (in this case, Down syndrome), although the physical abnormalities and cognitive impairments may be less severe. Usually mosaicism occurs when some cells in a trisomy conception lose the extra chromosome via nondisjunction during mitosis. Mosaicism also can occur if some cells lose a chromosome after a normal conception (e.g., some cells lose an X chromosome in mosaic Turner syndrome). Mosaicism is rare and accounts for only 5%–10% of all children with chromosomal abnormalities (Delatycki & Gardner, 1997).

Translocations

A relatively common dysfunction in cell division, translocation, can occur during mitosis and meiosis when the chromosomes break and lose or exchange parts with other chromosomes. Translocation involves the transfer of a portion of one chromosome to a completely different chromosome. For example, a portion of chromosome 21 might attach itself to chromosome 14 (Figure 1.5). If this occurs during meiosis, one daughter cell will then have 23 chromosomes but will have both a chromosome 21 and

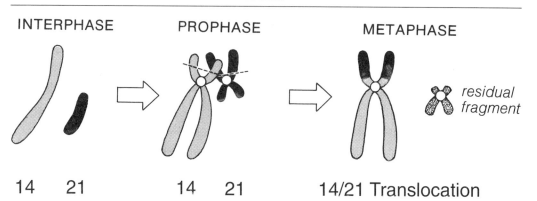

Figure 1.5. Translocation. During **prophase** of meiosis in a parent, there may be a transfer of a portion of one chromosome to another. In this figure, the long arm of chromosome 21 is translocated to chromosome 14, and the residual fragments are lost.

a chromosome 14/21 translocation. Fertilization of this egg or sperm with a cell containing the normal complement of 23 chromosomes will result in a child with 46 chromosomes, including two copies of chromosome 21, one chromosome 14/21, and one chromosome 14. This child will have Down syndrome because of the trisomy 21 caused by the translocation.

Deletions

Another somewhat common dysfunction in cell division is deletion. Here, part, but not all of a chromosome is lost. Chromosomal deletions occur in two forms, visible deletions and microdeletions. Those that are large enough to be seen through the microscope are called visible deletions. Those that are so small that they can only be detected at the molecular level are called microdeletions.

Cri-du-chat ("cat cry") syndrome is an example of a visible chromosomal deletion in which a portion of the short arm of chromosome 5 is lost. Cri-du-chat syndrome affects 1 in 50,000 children, causing microcephaly and an unusual facial appearance with a round face, widely spaced eyes, **epicanthal folds,** and low-set ears. Individuals with the syndrome have a high-pitched cry and intellectual disability (Cornish & Bramble, 2002).

Examples of **microdeletion syndromes** include Williams syndrome and VCFS (Yamagishi & Srivastava, 2003). The former is due to a deletion in the long arm of chromosome 7 and the latter to a deletion in the long arm of chromosome 22. Children with VCFS syndrome may have a cleft palate, a congenital heart defect, a characteristic facial appearance, and a nonverbal learning disability (Greenhalgh et al., 2003). Children with Williams syndrome have

intellectual disability with a distinctive facial appearance, cardiac defects, and a unique cognitive profile with unexpected eloquence (Tassabehji, 2003).

Microdeletion syndromes are also called **contiguous gene syndromes** because they involve the deletion of a number of adjacent genes. A number of microdeletion syndromes can now be diagnosed using a novel technique with the whimsical acronym **FISH (fluorescent in situ hybridization;** Irons, 2003). These include Miller-Dieker syndrome, Williams syndrome, Angelman syndrome and Prader-Willi syndrome. FISH employs a fluorescently labeled compound that binds with and identifies a specific gene sequence on the chromosome. In the future, targeted genomic microarray analysis will be used for identification of chromosome abnormalities (Shaffer et al., 2006).

Frequency of Chromosomal Abnormalities

In total, approximately 25% of eggs and 3%–4% of sperm have an extra or missing chromosome, and an additional 1% and 5%, respectively, have a structural chromosomal abnormality (Nicolaidis & Petersen, 1998). As a result, 10%–15% of all conceptions have a chromosomal abnormality. Somewhat more than 50% of these abnormalities are trisomies, 20% are monosomies, and 15% are **triploids** (69 chromosomes). The remainder is composed of structural abnormalities and **tetraploids** (92 chromosomes). It may therefore seem surprising that more children are not born with chromosomal abnormalities. The explanation is that more than 95% of fetuses with chromosomal abnormalities do not survive to term.

GENES AND THEIR DISORDERS

The underlying problem with the previously mentioned chromosomal disorders is the presence of too many or too few genes, resulting from extra or deleted chromosomal material. Genetic disorders can also result from an abnormality in a single gene. The Human Genome Project, a public–private partnership developed to unravel the genetic makeup of mankind, established that the human **genome** contains approximately 20,000–25,000 genes (Dennis & Gallagher, 2002; Watson & Berry, 2003). This is quite remarkable given that the fruit fly has approximately 13,000 genes, the round worm 19,000 genes, and a simple plant 26,000 genes. Before the project started it was projected that humans would have more than 100,000 genes. How is this possible given that genes are responsible for producing specific protein products (e.g., hormones, enzymes, blood-type proteins) as well as regulating the development and function of the body? It was previously thought that each gene regulated the production of a single protein. Now it is known that it is much more complicated than this; single genes in humans code for multiple proteins, giving humans the combinational diversity that lower organisms lack. Humans can produce approximately 100,000 proteins from one quarter that many genes. However, it must be acknowledged that the chimp shares 99% of the human genome. Having examined the genome of more than 80 organisms up to 2006, the minimum number of genes necessary for life is approximately 300, and all living organisms share these 300 genes.

The study of the formation of proteins is called proteomics, just as the study of the genome is termed genomics. The mechanism by which genes act as blueprints for producing specific proteins needed for body functions is as follows. Genes are composed of various lengths of DNA that together with intervening DNA sequences form the chromosome. DNA is formed as a **double helix,** a structure that resembles a twisted ladder (Figure 1.6). The sides of the ladder are composed of sugar and phosphate molecules, whereas the "rungs" are made up of four chemicals called **nucleotide bases: cytosine** (C), **guanine** (G), **adenine** (A), and **thymine** (T). Pairs of nucleotides bases interlock to form each rung: cytosine bonds with guanine, and adenine with thymine. The sequence of nucleotide bases on a segment of DNA (spelled out by the 4–letter alphabet C, G, A, T) make up one's genetic code. Genes range in size, containing from 1,500 to more than 2 million nucleotide base pairs. Overall there are approximately 3.3 billion base pairs in the human genome, but less than 3% encode genes that serve as a blueprint for protein production. It should also be noted that all genes are not "turned on" at all times. Some are only active during fetal life (e.g., fetal hemoglobin gene), and it is hoped that some never are turned on (e.g., oncogenes causing specific cancers). This turning on and off plays a particularly important role during fetal development; as a result, problems in the on–off switching can be devastating at this time.

Transcription

The production of a specific protein begins when the DNA comprising that gene unwinds, and the two strands, or sides of the ladder, unzip to expose the code (Jorde et al., 2001). The ex-

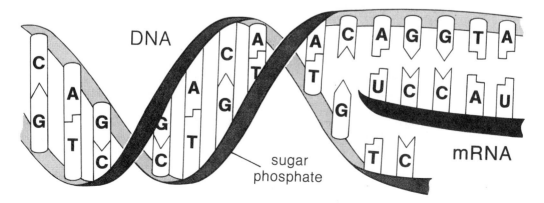

Figure 1.6. DNA. Four nucleotides (C, cytosine; G, guanine; A, adenosine; T, thymine) form the genetic code. On the mRNA molecule, uracil (U) substitutes for thymine. The DNA unzips to transcribe its message as mRNA.

posed DNA sequence then serves as a template for the formation, or **transcription,** of a similar nucleotide sequence called **messenger ribonucleic acid (mRNA)** (Figure 1.7). In all RNA, the nucleotides are the same as in DNA except that uracil (U) substitutes for thymine (T). As might be expected, errors or mutations may occur during transcription; however, a proofreading enzyme generally catches and repairs these errors. If not corrected, the transcription error can lead to the production of a disordered protein and a disease state.

Translation

Once transcribed, the single-stranded mRNA detaches, and the double-stranded DNA zips back together. The mRNA then moves out of the nucleus into the cytoplasm, where it provides instructions for the production of a protein, a process termed **translation** (Figure 1.8). Once in the cytoplasm, the mRNA attaches itself to a **ribosome.** The ribosome moves along the mRNA strand, reading the message like a videocassette recorder (VCR) in three-letter "words," or **codons,** such as GCU, CUA, and UAG. Most of these triplets code for specific **amino acids,** the building blocks of proteins. As these triplets are read, another type of RNA, transfer RNA (tRNA), carries the requisite amino acids to the ribosome, where they are linked to form a protein. Certain triplets, termed stop codons, instruct the ribosome to terminate the sequence. The stop codon indicates that all

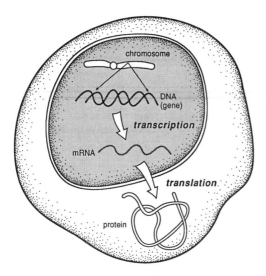

Figure 1.7. A summary of the steps leading from gene to protein formation. Transcription of the DNA (gene) onto mRNA occurs in the cell nucleus. The mRNA is then transported to the cytoplasm, where translation into protein occurs.

of the correct amino acids are in place to form the complete protein.

Once the protein is complete, the mRNA, ribosome, and protein separate, and the protein is released into the cytoplasm. The protein is either used by the cytoplasm or prepared for release into the bloodstream. If the protein is to be secreted, it is transferred to the **Golgi apparatus** (Figure 1.1), which packages it in a form that can be released through the cell membrane and carried throughout the body.

Mutations

An abnormality at any step in this translation process can cause the body to produce a structurally abnormal protein, reduced amounts of a protein, or no protein at all. When the error occurs in the gene itself, thus disrupting the subsequent steps, that mistake is called a mutation. The likelihood of mutations occurring increases with the size of the gene. In egg and sperm cells, the mutation rate also increases with parental age, especially in males (Figure 1.9; Green et al., 1999). Although most mutations occur spontaneously, they can be induced by radiation, toxins, and viruses. Once they occur, mutations become part of a person's genetic code and can be passed on from one generation to the next.

Point Mutations The most common type of mutation is a single base pair substitution (Jorde, 2003), also called a **point mutation.** Because there is redundancy in human DNA, many of these mutations have no adverse consequences. Depending on where in the gene they occur, however, point mutations are capable of causing a **missense mutation** or a **nonsense mutation** (Figure 1.10). A missense mutation results in a change in the triplet code that substitutes a different amino acid in the protein chain. For example, in the **inborn error of metabolism phenylketonuria (PKU),** a single base substitution causes an error in the production of phenylalanine hydroxylase, the enzyme necessary to metabolize the amino acid **phenylalanine.** The result is an accumulation of phenylalanine in blood and brain that can cause brain damage (see Chapter 20). In a nonsense mutation, the single base pair substitution produces a stop codon that prematurely terminates the protein formation. In this case, no useful protein is formed. Neurofibromatosis is an example of a disorder commonly caused by a nonsense mutation. Here, neurofibromin, a tumor suppressor, is not formed. As a result, multiple benign neurofibroma tumors form on the body

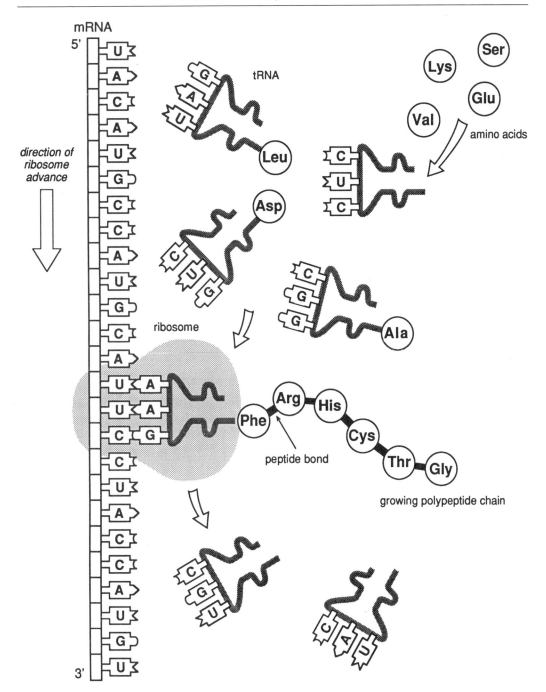

Figure 1.8. Translation of mRNA into protein. The ribosome moves along the mRNA strand assembling a growing polypeptide chain using tRNA–amino acid complexes. In this example, it has already assembled six amino acids (phenylalanine [Phe], arginine [Arg], histidine [His], cystine [Cys], threonine [Thr], and glycine [Gly]) into a polypeptide chain that will become a protein.

and in the brain. Children with the disorder also have a high incidence of attention-deficit/hyperactivity disorder (Listernick & Charrow, 2004).

Insertions and Deletions Mutations may also involve the insertion or deletion of one

or more nucleotide bases. The most common mutation in individuals with spinal muscular atrophy involves an insertion in the survival motor neuron gene, rendering it defective and resulting in a polio-like disorder (Iannaccone, Smith, & Simard, 2004). In contrast, a common muta-

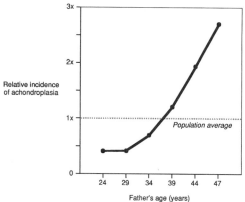

Figure 1.9. The risk of producing a child with the single-gene autosomal dominant disease achondroplasia (y-axis) increases with the father's age (x-axis). (From Vogel, F., & Rathenberg, R. [1975]. Spontaneous mutation in man. *Advances in Human Genetics, 5,* 267; reprinted by permission.)

tion in Duchenne muscular dystrophy involves a deletion (see Chapter 14). Base additions or subtractions may also lead to a **frame shift** in which the three base pair reading frame is shifted. All subsequent triplets are misread, often leading to the production of a stop codon and a nonfunctional protein. Certain children with Tay-Sachs disease (discussed later) have this type of mutation.

Other mutations can affect regions of the gene that regulate transcription but that do not actually code for an amino acid. These areas are called promoter and enhancer areas. They help turn other genes on and off and are very im-

portant in the normal development of the fetus. A mutation in a transcription gene leads to Rubinstein-Taybi syndrome, which is associated with multiple congenital malformations and severe intellectual disability (Wiley et al., 2003). Mutations in a transcription gene also may result in a normal protein being formed but at a much slower rate than usual, leading to an enzyme or other protein deficiency.

Triplet Repeat Expansion Another type of mutation involves a **triplet repeat expansion.** For reasons not fully understood, some nucleotide triplets (codons) are repeated multiple times in certain regions of normal genes. However, if the number of triplet copies is expanded markedly, usually during defective meiosis, a gene can be turned off, leading to conditions such as Huntington disease or fragile X syndrome (Everett & Wood, 2004; Willemsen et al., 2004). Triplet repeats are further described in the discussion of fragile X syndrome in Chapter 19.

Selective Advantage

The **incidence** of a genetic disease in a population depends on the difference between the rate of mutation production and that of mutation removal. Typically, genetic diseases enter populations through mutation errors. Natural selection, the process by which individuals with a selective advantage survive and pass on their genes, works to remove these errors. For instance, be-

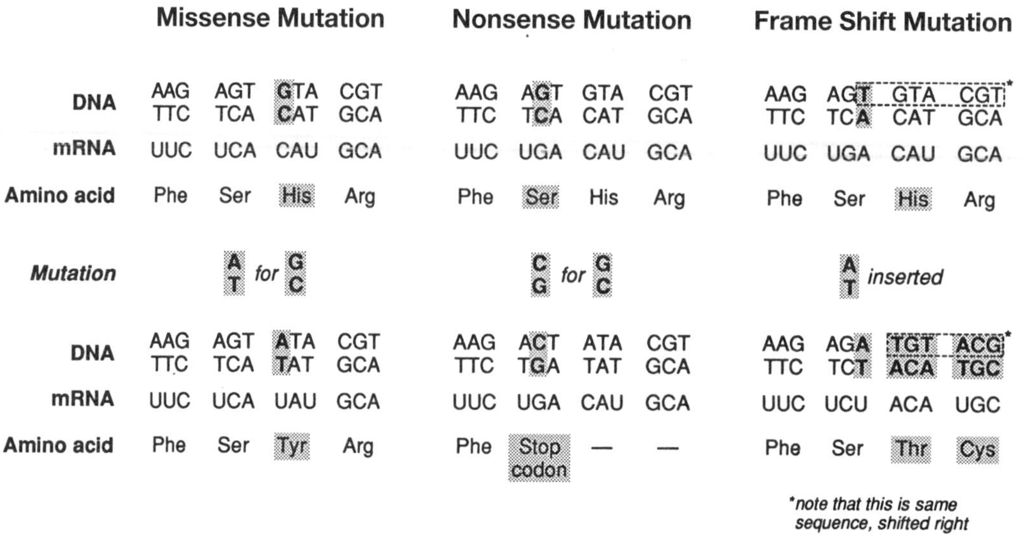

	Missense Mutation				**Nonsense Mutation**				**Frame Shift Mutation**			
DNA	AAG TTC	AGT TCA	GTA CAT	CGT GCA	AAG TTC	AGT TCA	GTA CAT	CGT GCA	AAG TTC	AGT TCA	GTA CAT	CGT GCA*
mRNA	UUC	UCA	CAU	GCA	UUC	UGA	CAU	GCA	UUC	UGA	CAU	GCA
Amino acid	Phe	Ser	His	Arg	Phe	Ser	His	Arg	Phe	Ser	His	Arg
Mutation		A/T *for* G/C			C/G *for* G/C				A/T *inserted*			
DNA	AAG TTC	AGT TCA	ATA TAT	CGT GCA	AAG TTC	ACT TGA	ATA TAT	CGT GCA	AAG TTC	AGA TCT	TGT ACA	ACG* TGC
mRNA	UUC	UCA	UAU	GCA	UUC	UGA	CAU	GCA	UUC	UCU	ACA	UGC
Amino acid	Phe	Ser	Tyr	Arg	Phe	Stop codon	—	—	Phe	Ser	Thr	Cys

*note that this is same sequence, shifted right

Figure 1.10. Examples of single-gene mutations: Missense mutation, nonsense mutation, and frame shift mutation. The shaded areas mark the point of mutation.

cause individuals with sickle cell anemia, an **autosomal recessive** inherited blood disorder, often have a decreased life span, the gene that causes the disorder would be expected to be gradually removed from the gene pool. Sometimes natural selection, however, favors the individual who carries one copy of a mutated recessive gene. In the case of sickle cell anemia, unaffected carriers, who appear clinically healthy, actually have minor differences in their hemoglobin structure that make it more resistant to a malarial parasite (Feng et al., 2004). In Africa, where malaria is endemic, this gives the carriers a selective advantage. This selection has maintained the sickle cell trait among Africans. Northern Europeans, for whom malaria is not an issue, rarely carry the sickle cell gene at all; this mutation has presumably died out via natural selection (Jorde et al., 2001).

Single Nucleotide Polymorphisms (SNPs)

Of the more than 3 billion base pair genetic code, people of all races and geography share 99.9% genetic identity (Dennis & Gallagher, 2002). Although this is quite remarkable, that 0.1% difference means there are about 3 million DNA sequence variations, also called **single nucleotide polymorphisms (SNPs).** This genetic variation is the basis of evolution, but it can also contribute to health, unique traits, and disease. One SNP involved in muscle formation, if present, makes individuals much more likely to become "buff" if they weight lift, and another is associated with perfect musical pitch. There is a SNP that makes individuals more susceptible to adverse effects from medication, as it leads to slower metabolism of drugs. There also is a SNP that places people at greater risk for developing Alzheimer's disease or Crohn's disease (an inflammatory bowel disorder) (Li et al., 2004; Russell, Nimmo, & Satsangi, 2004). It is likely that at some time in the not too distant future, doctors will take blood samples to test for various SNPs associated with health or disease to practice preventive medicine (Glazier, Nadeau, & Aitman, 2002).

Single Gene (Mendelian) Disorders

Gregor Mendel (1822–1884), an Austrian monk, pioneered our understanding of single-gene defects. While cultivating pea plants, he noted that when he bred two differently colored plants— yellow and green—the **hybrid** offspring all were green rather than mixed in color. Mendel concluded that the green trait was **dominant,** whereas the yellow trait was **recessive** (from the Latin word for "hidden"). Yet, this yellow trait sometimes appeared in subsequent generations. Later, scientists determined that many human traits, including some birth defects, are also inherited in this fashion. They are referred to as **Mendelian traits.**

Table 1.1 indicates the prevalence of some of the more common genetic disorders. Approximately 1% of the population has a Mendelian, or single-gene, disorder. These disorders can be transmitted to offspring on the autosomes or on the X chromosome. Mendelian traits may be either dominant or recessive. Thus, Mendelian disorders are characterized as being autosomal recessive, **autosomal dominant,** or X-linked.

Autosomal Recessive Disorders
Among the Mendelian disorders, approxi-

Table 1.1. Prevalence of genetic disorders

Disease	Approximate prevalence
Chromosomal disorders	
Down syndrome	1/700–1/1,000
Klinefelter syndrome	1/1,000 males
Trisomy 13	1/10,000
Trisomy 18	1/6,000
Turner syndrome	1/2,500–1/10,000
Single-gene disorders	
Duchenne muscular dystrophy	1/3,500 males
Fragile X syndrome	1/1,500 males; 1/2,500 females
Neurofibromatosis	1/3,000–1/3,500
Phenylketonuria	1/14,000
Tay-Sachs disease	1/3,000 in Ashkenazi Jews
Multifactorial inheritance	
Cleft lip/palate	1/500–1/1,000
Club foot	1/1,000
Neural tube defects	1/1,000
Pyloric stenosis	3/1,000
Mitochondrial inheritance	
Leber hereditary optic neuropathy	Rare
MELAS and MERRF	Rare
Mitochondrial encephalopathy	Rare

Source: Jorde et al. (2001).

Key: MELAS, **m**itochondrial **e**ncephalomyelopathy, **l**actic **a**cidosis, and **s**troke-like episodes; MERRF, **m**yoclonic **e**pilepsy and **r**agged **r**ed **f**ibers.

mately 1,700 are inherited as autosomal recessive traits (McKusick et al., 2005). For a child to inherit a disorder that is autosomal recessive, he or she must receive an abnormal gene from both the mother and father.

Tay-Sachs disease is an example of an autosomal recessive, progressive neurological disorder. It is caused by the absence of an enzyme, hexosaminidase A, that normally metabolizes a potentially toxic product of nerve cell metabolism (Sutton, 2002). In individuals with Tay-Sachs disease, this product cannot be broken down and is stored in the brain, leading to brain damage and early death.

Alternate forms of the gene for hexosaminidase A are known to exist. The different forms of a gene, called **alleles,** include the normal gene, which can be symbolized by a capital *A* as it is dominant, and the mutated allele

(in this example, carrying Tay-Sachs disease), which can be symbolized by the lowercase *a* as it is recessive (Figure 1.11). Upon fertilization, the embryo receives two genes for hexosaminidase A, one from the father and one from the mother. The following combinations of alleles could theoretically occur: **homozygous** (carrying the same allele) combinations, AA and aa; or **heterozygous** (carrying alternate allele) combinations, aA and Aa. Because Tay-Sachs disease is a recessive disorder, two abnormal recessive genes (aa) are needed to produce a child who has the disease. Therefore, a child with aa would be homozygous for the Tay-Sachs gene (i.e., have two copies of the mutated gene and manifest the disease), a child with aA or Aa would be heterozygous and a healthy carrier of the Tay-Sachs gene, and a child with AA would be a healthy noncarrier.

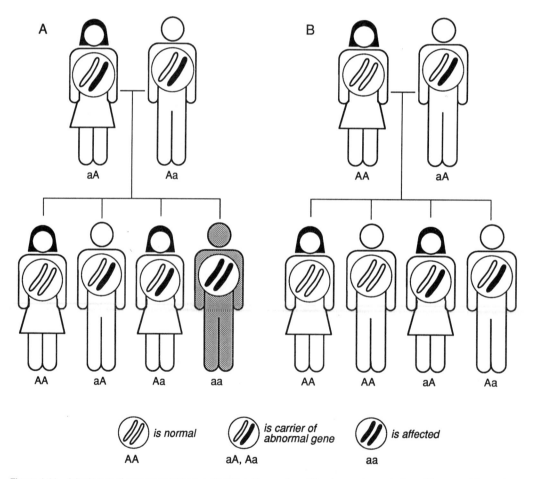

Figure 1.11. Inheritance of autosomal recessive disorders. Two copies of the abnormal gene (aa) must be present to produce the disease state. A) Two carriers mating, will result, on average, in 25% of the children being affected, 50% being carriers, and 25% not being affected. B) A carrier and a noncarrier mating, will result in 50% noncarriers and 50% carriers. No children will be affected.

If two heterozygotes (carrying alternate alleles) were to have children (aA x Aa or Aa x aA), the following combinations could occur: AA, aA or Aa, or aa (Figure 1.11). According to the law of probability, each pregnancy would carry a 1 in 4 chance of the child being a noncarrier (AA), a 1 in 2 chance of the child being a carrier (aA or Aa), and a 1 in 4 risk of the child having Tay-Sachs disease (aa). If a carrier has children with a noncarrier (aA x AA), each pregnancy carries a 1 in 2 chance of the child being a carrier (aA, Aa) and a 1 in 2 chance of the child being a noncarrier (AA); no child would be at risk for having Tay-Sachs disease (Figure 1.11). The significance is that siblings of affected children, even if they are carriers, are unlikely to produce children with the disease. This can only occur if they have children with another carrier, an unlikely occurrence in these rare diseases.

The 1 in 4 risk when two carriers have children is a probability risk. This does not mean that if a family has one affected child, the next three will be unaffected. Each new pregnancy carries the same 1 in 4 risk; the parents could by chance have three affected children in a row or five unaffected ones. In the case of Tay-Sachs disease, carrier screening and prenatal diagnosis are available to help alter these odds (see Chapter 8).

Because it is unlikely for a carrier of an unusual disease to have children with another carrier of the same disease, these types of disorders are quite rare in the general population, ranging from 1 in 2,000 to 1 in 200,000 births (McKusick et al., 2005). When intermarriage within an extended family or among ethnically, religiously, or geographically isolated populations occurs, however, the incidence of these disorders increases markedly (Figure 1.12), which probably underlies the biblical proscription against marrying one's immediate relatives. For example, Tay-Sachs disease tends to occur among Jewish children, and another inborn error of metabolism, glutaric acidemia, tends to occur disproportionately among the Amish.

Like Tay-Sachs disease, many autosomal recessive disorders are caused by mutations that lead to an enzyme deficiency of some kind. In most cases, there are a number of different mutations within the gene that can produce the same disease. Because these enzyme deficiencies generally lead to biochemical abnormalities involving either the insufficient production of a needed product or the buildup of toxic materials, **developmental disabilities** or early death

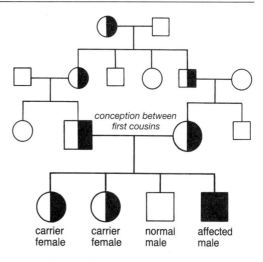

Figure 1.12. A family tree illustrating the effect of consanguinity (in this case, a marriage between first cousins) on the risk of inheriting an autosomal recessive disorder. The chance of both parents being carriers is usually less than 1 in 300. When first cousins conceive a child, however, the chance of both parents being carriers rises to 1 in 8. The risk, then, of having an affected child increases almost 40-fold.

may result (see Chapter 20). These disorders affect males and females equally, and there tends to be clustering in families (i.e., more than one affected child per family). Yet, a history of the disease in past generations rarely exists unless blood relatives have had children together (**consanguinity**).

Autosomal Dominant Disorders

Approximately 4,500 autosomal dominant disorders have been identified, the most common ones having a frequency of 1 in 500 births (Table 1.2) (McKusick et al., 2005). Autosomal dominant disorders are quite different from autosomal recessive disorders in mechanism, incidence, and clinical characteristics. Because autosomal dominant disorders are caused by a single abnormal allele, individuals with the **genotypes** AA, Aa, or aA are all affected.

To better understand this, consider neurofibromatosis, the neurological disorder discussed previously. Suppose a represents the normal recessive gene and A indicates the mutated dominant gene for neurofibromatosis. If a person with neurofibromatosis (aA or Aa) has a child with an unaffected individual (aa) there is a 1 in 2 risk, statistically speaking, that the child will have the disorder (aA or Aa), and a 1 in 2 chance he or she will be unaffected (aa; Figure 1.13). An unaffected child will not carry the abnormal allele and, therefore, cannot pass it on to his or her children.

Table 1.2. Comparison of autosomal recessive, autosomal dominant, and X-linked inheritance patterns

	Autosomal recessive	Autosomal dominant	X-linked
Type of disorder	Enzyme deficiency	Structural abnormalities	Mixed
Examples of disorder	Tay-Sachs disease	Achondroplasia	Fragile X syndrome
	Phenylketonuria (PKU)	Neurofibromatosis	Muscular dystrophy
Carrier expresses disorder	No	Yes	Sometimes
Increased risk in other family members from consanguinity	Yes	No	No

Autosomal dominant disorders affect men and women with equal frequency. They tend to involve structural (physical) abnormalities rather than enzymatic defects. In affected individuals, there is often a family history of the disease, but approximately half of affected individuals represent a new mutation. Although individuals with a new mutation will risk passing the mutated gene to their offspring, their parents are unaffected and at no greater risk than the general population of having a second affected child.

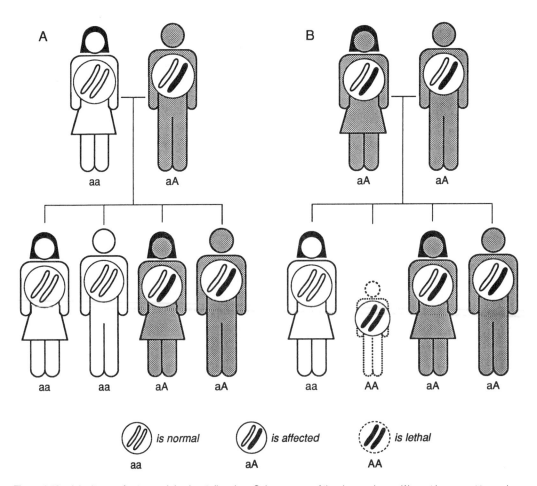

Figure 1.13. Inheritance of autosomal dominant disorders. Only one copy of the abnormal gene (A) must be present to produce the disease state. A) If an affected person conceives a child with an unaffected person, statistically speaking, 50% of the children will be affected and 50% will be unaffected. B) If two affected people have children, 25% of the children will be unaffected, 50% will have the disorder, and 25% will have an often fatal, severe form of the disorder as a result of a double dose of the abnormal gene.

X-Linked Disorders Unlike autosomal recessive and autosomal dominant disorders, which involve genes located on the 22 non-sex chromosomes, X-linked (previously called sex-linked) recessive disorders involve mutant genes located on the X chromosome. X-linked disorders primarily affect males (Ropers & Hamel, 2005). Because males have only one X chromosome, a single dose of the abnormal recessive gene still causes disease. As females have two X chromosomes, a single recessive allele should not cause disease, provided there is a normal allele on the second X chromosome. Approximately 900 X-linked disorders have been described, including Duchenne muscular dystrophy and hemophilia (McKusick et al., 2005; Figure 1.14). These disorders are passed on from one generation to the next by carrier mothers.

As an example, children with Duchenne muscular dystrophy develop a progressive muscle weakness, typically requiring the use of a wheelchair by adolescence (Tidball & Wehling-Henricks, 2004). The disease results from a mutation in the dystrophin gene, located on the X chromosome, the function of which is to ensure stability of the muscle cell membrane. Because the disease affects all muscles, eventually the heart muscle and the diaphragmatic muscles needed for circulation and breathing are impaired, leading to early death. Dystrophin is also required for typical brain development and function, so affected boys often have cognitive impairments.

In fact, approximately 25% of males with intellectual disability and 10% of females with learning disabilities are affected by X-linked conditions (see Chapter 19). The most common of these is fragile X syndrome. The finding that males are more likely to have intellectual disability than females is attributable for the most

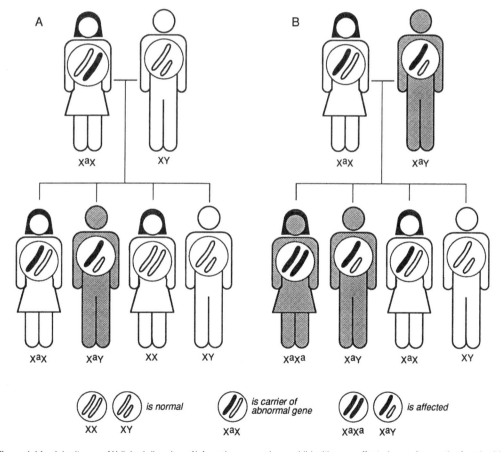

Figure 1.14. Inheritance of X-linked disorders. A) A carrier woman has a child with an unaffected man. Among the female children, statistically speaking, 50% will be carriers and 50% will be unaffected; among the male children, 50% will be affected and 50% will be unaffected. B) A carrier woman has a child with an affected man. Of the female children, 50% will be carriers and 50% will be affected. Of the male children, statistically speaking, 50% will be unaffected and 50% will be affected.

part to X-linked disorders affecting males disproportionately more than females.

The mechanism for passing an X-linked recessive trait to the next generation is as follows: Women who have a recessive mutation (Xa) on one of their X chromosomes are designated carriers of the gene. Although usually clinically unaffected, they can pass on the abnormal gene to their children. Assuming the father is unaffected, each female child born to a carrier mother has a 1 in 2 chance of being a carrier (i.e., inheriting the mutant Xa allele from her mother and the normal X allele from her father; Figure 1.14). A male child (who has only one X chromosome), however, has a 1 in 2 risk of having the disorder. This occurs if he inherits the X chromosome containing the mutated gene (XaY) instead of the normal one (XY). A family tree frequently reveals that some maternal uncles and male siblings have the disease.

Occasionally, females are affected by X-linked diseases. This can occur if the woman has adverse lyonization (inactivation of one of the X chromosomes) or if the disorder is X-linked dominant. Regarding the former mechanism, geneticist Mary Lyon questioned why women have the same amount of X-chromosome-directed gene product as men instead of twice as much, as would be predicted from their genetic makeup. Dr. Lyon postulated that early in embryogenesis, one of the two X chromosomes in each cell was inactivated, making every female fetus a mosaic. This implied that some cells would contain an active X chromosome derived from the father, whereas others would contain an active X chromosome derived from the mother. This lyonization hypothesis was later proved to be correct. In most instances, the cells in a woman's body have a fairly equal division between maternally and paternally derived active X chromosomes. In a minority of women, however, the distribution is very unequal. If the normal X chromosome is inactivated preferentially in cells of a carrier of an X-linked disorder, the woman will manifest the disease, although usually in a less severe form than the male. An example is OTC deficiency, the disorder Katy had in this chapter's opening case study (see also Chapter 20).

The second mechanism for a female to manifest an X-linked disorder is if the disorder is transmitted as X-linked dominant. Although most X-linked disorders are recessive, a few appear to be dominant. One example is Rett syndrome (Percy & Lane, 2004). It appears that in this disorder, the presence of the mutated transcription gene, MECP2, on the X chromosome of a male embryo leads to lethality. When it occurs in one of the X chromosomes of the female, however, it is compatible with survival but results in a syndrome marked by microcephaly, intellectual disability, and autism-like behaviors (Christodoulou & Weaving, 2003).

REVISING MENDELIAN GENETICS

Genomic Imprinting

According to Mendelian genetics, the **phenotype,** or appearance, of an individual should be the same whether the given gene is inherited from the mother or the father. This is not always the case, however, because of a phenomenon called **genomic imprinting** (da Rocha & Ferguson-Smith, 2004; Vogels & Fryns, 2002). Researchers have found that certain genes passed on from the mother, although containing the identical DNA sequence as in the father, differ in their effect on the fetus. For instance, if a particular deletion occurs on the long arm of the chromosome 15 derived from the father, the child will have Prader-Willi syndrome (Zipf, 2004). If the same deletion occurs on the chromosome 15 derived from the mother, however, the child will develop Angelman syndrome (Clayton-Smith & Laag, 2003; Guerrini et al., 2003). Prader-Willi syndrome is associated with short stature, obesity, and intellectual disability; children with Angelman syndrome also have intellectual disability but are not obese and have epilepsy and a gait abnormality (Jiang et al., 2004). The exact mechanism for genomic imprinting remains unclear.

Anticipation

Mendel also predicted that an inherited trait should look the same from one generation to the next in a given family. In a few disorders associated with expanded triplet repeats, however, the manifestations actually increase in severity with each subsequent generation—a phenomenon called **anticipation** (see Chapter 19). For example, the expanded triplet repeat (CAG) that causes Huntington disease—an autosomal dominant, progressive neurological disease associated with a movement disorder (chorea), cognitive impairment, and behavior disturbances (Bonelli & Hofmann, 2004)—increases in each generation (Figure 1.15). The greater the expansion of triplet repeats, the more severe the manifestations of the disorder.

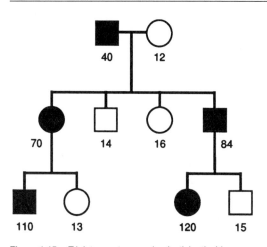

Figure 1.15. Triplet repeat expansion (anticipation) in an extended family with Huntington disease. This disorder is inherited as an autosomal dominant trait. Numbers indicate the number of CAG triplet repeats. Normal range is 11–34, affected 37–121. In subsequent generations, the number of triplet repeats increases in affected individuals. Shading indicates affected members of the family. Squares represent males, circles females.

The same is true of fragile X syndrome (Willemsen et al., 2004).

Mitochondrial Inheritance

Each cell contains several hundred mitochondria in its cytoplasm (Figure 1.1). Mitochondria produce the energy needed for cellular function through a complex process termed **oxidative phosphorylation.** It has been proposed that mitochondria were originally independent microorganisms that invaded our bodies during the process of human evolution and then developed a symbiotic relationship with the cells in the human body. They are unique among cellular organelles (the specialized parts of a cell) in that they possess their own DNA, which is in a circular pattern rather than the double-helical pattern of nuclear DNA and contains genes different from those contained in nuclear DNA (Figure 1.16). A mutation in a mitochondrial gene can result in defective energy production and a disease state (Thorburn, 2004). An example of a mitochondrial disorder is MELAS (*m*itochondrial *e*ncephalomyelopathy, *l*actic *a*cidosis, and *s*troke-like episodes), a progressive neurological disorder marked by episodes of stroke and dementia. Other mitochondrial disorders can lead to blindness, deafness, or muscle weakness (Scaglia et al., 2004). Over 60 mitochondrial disorders have been described (McKusick et al., 2005).

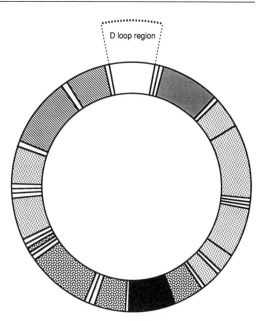

Figure 1.16. Mitochondrial DNA genome. The genes code for various enzyme complexes involved in energy production in the cell. The displacement loop (D loop) is not involved in energy production. (*Key:* Complex I genes [NADH dehydrogenase], Complex III genes [ubiquinol: cytochrome *c* oxidoreductase], tRNA genes, Complex IV genes [cytochrome *c* oxidase], Complex V genes [ATP synthase], ribosomal RNA genes.) (From Jorde, L.B., Carey, J.C., Bamshad, M.J., et al. [2001]. *Medical genetics* [Rev. 2nd ed., p. 105]. St. Louis: Mosby; adapted by permission.)

Because eggs, but not sperm, contain cytoplasm, mitochondria are inherited from one's mother. As a result, mitochondrial DNA disorders are passed on from generally unaffected mothers to their children, both male and female. As expected, men affected by these mitochondrial disorders cannot pass the trait to their children (Figure 1.17).

ENVIRONMENTAL INFLUENCES ON HEREDITY

The particular genes that a person possesses determine that person's genotype, whereas the manner in which those genes are expressed is called the phenotype. For some traits and clinical disorders, the same genotype can produce quite different phenotypes, depending on environmental influences. In terms of traits, although bright parents tend to have bright children and tall parents tend to have tall children, the interaction of genetics with the pre- and postnatal environments allows for many possible outcomes. For example, it has been found that as a result of an increased protein intake

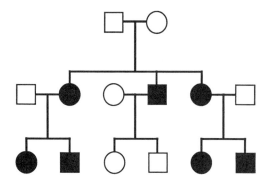

Figure 1.17. Mitochondrial inheritance. As mitochondria are inherited exclusively from the mother, defects in mitochondrial disease will be passed on from the mother to her children, as illustrated in this pedigree. Shading indicates affected individuals. Squares are males, circles females.

during childhood, second-generation Asians who grow up in the United States are significantly taller than their parents who grew up in Asia. Diabetes, meningomyelocele, cleft palate, and pyloric stenosis are examples of disorders that have both genetic and environmental influences (Clark, 2003; Glazier et al., 2002). Taking the example of PKU, an affected child will develop intellectual disability if the PKU is not treated early but will have typical development if it is treated with a diet low in phenylalanine from infancy (see Chapter 20); newborn screening now makes it possible to know when such a diet is necessary.

SUMMARY

Each human cell contains a full complement of genetic information encoded in genes contained in 46 chromosomes. Not only does this genetic code determine our physical appearance and biochemical makeup, but it is also the legacy we pass on to our children. The unequal division of the reproductive cells, the deletion of a part of a chromosome, or the mutation in a single gene can each have significant consequences. Yet, despite these and other potential problems that can occur during the development of the embryo and fetus, approximately 95% of infants are born without birth defects.

REFERENCES

Bonelli, R.M., & Hofmann, P. (2004). A review of the treatment options for Huntington's disease. *Expert Opinion in Pharmacotherapy, 5*(4), 767–776.

Chen, C.P., Lee, C.C., Chang, T.Y., et al. (2004). Prenatal diagnosis of mosaic distal 5p deletion and review of the literature. *Prenatal Diagnosis, 24,* 50–57.

Christodoulou, J., & Weaving, L.S. (2003). MECP2 and beyond: Phenotype–genotype correlations in Rett syndrome. *Journal of Child Neurology, 18*(10), 669–674.

Clark, A.G. (2003). Finding genes underlying risk of complex disease by linkage disequilibrium mapping. *Current Opinion in Genetics and Development, 13*(3), 296–302.

Clayton-Smith, J., & Laan, L. (2003). Angelman syndrome: A review of the clinical and genetic aspects. *Journal of Medical Genetics, 40*(2), 87–95.

Cornish, K., & Bramble, D. (2002). Cri du chat syndrome: Genotype-phenotype correlations and recommendations for clinical management. *Developmental Medicine and Child Neurology, 44*(7), 494–497.

da Rocha, S.T., & Ferguson-Smith, A.C. (2004). Genomic imprinting. *Current Biology, 14*(16), R646–R649.

Delatycki, M., & Gardner, R.J. (1997). Three cases of trisomy 13 mosaicism and a review of the literature. *Clinical Genetics, 51,* 403–407.

Dennis, C., & Gallagher, R. (Eds.). (2002). *The human genome.* New York: Palgrave Macmillan.

Everett, C.M., & Wood, N.W. (2004). Trinucleotide repeats and neurodegenerative disease. *Brain, 127*(Pt. 11), 2385–2405.

Feng, Z., Smith D.L., McKenzie, F.E., et al. (2004). Coupling ecology and evolution: malaria and the S-gene across time scales. *Mathematical Biosciences, 189* (1), 1–19.

Flint, J., Wilkie, A.O., Buckle V.J., et al. (1995). The detection of subtelomeric chromosomal rearrangements in idiopathic intellectual disability. *Nature Genetics, 9,* 132–140.

Ginsburg, C., Fokstuen, S., & Schinzel, A. (2000). The contribution of uniparental disomy to congenital development defects in children born to mothers at advanced childbearing age. *American Journal of Medical Genetics, 95*(5), 454–460.

Glazier, A.M., Nadeau, J.H., & Aitman, T.J. (2002). Finding genes that underlie complex traits. *Science, 298,* 2345–2349.

Green, P.M., Saad, S., Lewis, C.M., et al. (1999). Mutation rates in humans, I: Overall and sex-specific rates obtained from a population study of hemophilia B. *American Journal of Human Genetics, 65,* 1572–1579.

Greenhalgh, K.L., Aligianis, I.A., Bromilow, G., et al. (2003). 22q11 deletion: A multisystem disorder requiring multidisciplinary input. *Archives of Disease in Childhood, 88*(6), 523–524.

Guerrini, R., Carrozzo, R., Rinaldi, R., et al. (2003). Angelman syndrome: Etiology, clinical features, diagnosis, and management of symptoms. *Paediatric Drugs, 5*(10), 647–661.

Hall, J.C. (1992). Turner syndrome. In R.A. King, J.I. Rotter, & A.G. Motulsky (Eds.), *The genetic basis of common disease* (pp. 895–914). New York: Oxford University Press.

Iannaccone, S.T., Smith, S.A., & Simard, L.R. (2004). Spinal muscular atrophy. *Current Neurology and Neuroscience Reports, 4*(1), 74–80.

Irons, M. (2003). Use of subtelomeric fluorescence in situ hybridization in cytogenetic diagnosis. *Current Opinion in Pediatrics, 15*(6), 594–597.

Jiang, Y.H., Bressler, J., & Beaudet, A.L. (2004). Epigenetics and human disease. *Annual Review of Genomics and Human Genetics, 5,* 479–510.

Jorde, L.B. (2003). *Medical genetics* (3rd ed.). St. Louis: Mosby.

Jorde, L.B., Carey, J.C., Bamshad, M.J., et al. (2001). *Medical genetics* (Rev. 2nd ed.). St. Louis: Mosby.

Li, Y., Nowotny, P., Holmans, P., et al. (2004). Association of late-onset Alzheimer's disease with genetic variation in multiple members of the GAPD gene family. *Proceedings of the National Academy of Sciences of the United States of America, 101*(44), 15688–15693.

Listernick, R., & Charrow, J. (2004). Neurofibromatosis-1 in childhood. *Advances in Dermatology, 20,* 75–115.

McKusick, V.A., et al. (2005). *Online Mendelian Inheritance in Man.* Retrieved October 10, 2006, from http://www.ncbi.nlm.nih.gov/omim

Nagaishi, M., Yamamoto, T., & Iinuma, K., et al. (2004). Chromosome abnormalities identified in 347 spontaneous abortions collected in Japan. *Journal of Obstetrics and Gynaecology Research, 30*(3), 237–241.

Nicolaidis, P., & Petersen, M.B. (1998). Origin and mechanisms of non-disjunction in human autosomal trisomies. *Human Reproduction, 13,* 313–319.

Parker, M.J., Budd, J.L., Draper, E.S., et al. (2003). Trisomy 13 and trisomy 18 in a defined population: Epidemiological, genetic and prenatal observations. *Prenatal Diagnosis, 23*(10), 856–860.

Percy, A.K., & Lane, J.B. (2004). Rett syndrome: Clinical and molecular update. *Current Opinion in Pediatrics, 16*(6), 670–677.

Ropers, H.H., & Hamel, B.C. (2005). X-linked intellectual disability. *Nature Reviews Genetics, 6*(1), 46–57.

Rovet, J. (2004). Turner syndrome: A review of genetic and hormonal influences on neuropsychological functioning. *Neuropsychology, Development, and Cognition. Section C: Child Neuropsychology, 10*(4), 262–279.

Russell, R.K., Nimmo, E.R., & Satsangi, J. (2004). Molecular genetics of Crohn's disease. *Current Opinion in Genetics and Development, 14*(3), 264–270.

Scaglia, F., Towbin, J.A., Craigen, W.J., (2004). Clinical spectrum, morbidity, and mortality in 113 pediatric patients with mitochondrial disease. *Pediatrics, 114*(4), 925–931.

Shaffer, L.G., Kashork, C.D., Saleki, R., et al. (2006). Targeted genomic microarray analysis for identification of chromosome abnormalities in 1500 consecutive clinical cases. *The Journal of Pediatrics, 149,* 98–102.

Soares, S.R., Templado, C., Blanco, J., et al. (2001). Numerical chromosome abnormalities in the spermatozoa of the fathers of children with trisomy 21 of paternal origin: Generalised tendency to meiotic non-disjunction. *Human Genetics, 108*(2), 134–139.

Sutton, V.R. (2002). Tay-Sachs disease screening and counseling families at risk for metabolic disease. *Obstetrics and Gynecology Clinics of North America, 29*(2), 287–296.

Sybert, V.P., & McCauley, E. (2004). Turner's syndrome. *The New England Journal of Medicine, 351*(12), 1227–1238.

Tassabehji, M. (2003). Williams-Beuren syndrome: A challenge for genotype-phenotype correlations. *Human Molecular Genetics, 12*(Spec. No. 2), R229—R237.

Thorburn, D.R. (2004). Mitochondrial disorders: Prevalence, myths and advances. *Journal of Inherited Metabolic Disease, 27*(3), 349–362.

Tidball, J.G. & Wehling-Henricks, M. (2004). Evolving therapeutic strategies for Duchenne muscular dystrophy: Targeting downstream events. *Pediatric Research, 56*(6), 831–841.

Turnpenny, P.D., & Ellard, S. (Ed.). (2005). *Emery's elements of medical genetics* (12th ed.). New York: Churchill Livingstone.

Vogel, F., & Rathenberg, R. (1975). Spontaneous mutation in man. *Advances in Human Genetics, 5,* 223–318.

Vogels, A., & Fryns, J.P. (2002). The Prader-Willi syndrome and the Angelman syndrome. *Genetic Counseling, 13*(4), 385–396.

Watson, J.D., & Berry, A. (2003). *DNA: The secret of life.* New York: Knopf.

Wiley, S., Swayne, S., Rubinstein, J.H., et al. (2003). Rubinstein-Taybi syndrome medical guidelines. *American Journal of Medical Genetics Part A., 119*(2), 101–110.

Willemsen, R., Oostra, B.A., Bassell, G.J., et al. (2004). The fragile X syndrome: From molecular genetics to neurobiology. *Mental Retardation and Developmental Disabilities Research Reviews, 10*(1), 60–67.

Yamagishi, H., & Srivastava, D. (2003). Unraveling the genetic and developmental mysteries of 22q11 deletion syndrome. *Trends in Molecular Medicine, 9*(9), 383–389.

Zipf, W.B. (2004). Prader-Willi syndrome: The care and treatment of infants, children, and adults. *Advances in Pediatrics, 51,* 409–434.

2 Development Before Birth

William H.J. Haffner

Upon completion of this chapter, the reader will

- Understand the fertilization and implantation process
- Be aware of the various stages of prenatal development
- Be able to describe the early development of the central nervous system
- Be able to discuss the effects of maternal nutrition on fetal development

---

The greatest risk for severe developmental disabilities occurs in the period between conception/**implantation** and birth (Decoufle et al., 2001). Both genetic and environmental influences can adversely affect the developing organism, and there can be interactions between the two. Environmental agents that can affect fetal development are called **teratogens** (see Chapter 5). These range from heavy metals (see Chapter 5) and radiation to medications and drugs of abuse, from infectious agents (see Chapter 6) to chronic maternal illnesses. The susceptibility of the fetus to these influences depends on his or her genetic sensitivity in combination with the timing, magnitude, and duration of exposure to the teratogen and its ability to cross the placenta. This chapter discusses principles of fetal development and introduces several factors that can lead to abnormalities in fetal growth and development.

FERTILIZATION

If sexual intercourse occurs near the time of ovulation, when the mature ovum (egg) is released, conception can occur. During ejaculation, 300 million sperm or more are released and deposited in the vagina; however, only about 200 reach the fallopian tubes. The sperm travel through the cervix and uterus into the fallopian tubes and can remain viable in the tubes for up to 2–3 days (Figure 2.1). In contrast, the egg can be fertilized only for 12–24 hours after ovulation. Once it is released from the ovary, the egg is actively moved by the finger-like fimbria from the opening of the fallopian tube inward to the junction of the outer two thirds of the tube. There, if a sperm successfully penetrates the ovum, fertilization occurs. The fertilized egg becomes a **zygote,** a diploid cell containing 46 chromosomes, 23 each contributed by the egg and sperm. While still in the fallopian tube, the zygote undergoes a series of divisions (cleavage) resulting in the formation of blastomeres which continue to slowly divide. At approximately 3–4 days after fertilization a solid mulberry-like ball of compacted blastomeres is formed, called a **morula,** which then arrives in the uterine cavity (Figure 2.1). Fluid accumulates slowly between the cells within the morula over the next few days, leading to the formation of the early **blastocyst.** The blastocyst lies free in the uterine cavity for approximately 2 days before attaching, or implanting, to an inside wall of the uterus (endometrium). This marks the formal beginning of pregnancy, nearly 5–7 days after ovulation and fertilization.

At one end of the early blastocyst are cells comprising the inner cell mass, which is destined to produce the embryo. At the other end is a mass of cells that becomes the **trophoblasts** (Figure 2.1), forming part of the placenta. The trophoblasts invade the endometrium so that the blastocyst soon becomes covered. The endometrium becomes the site for subsequent development of the embryo/fetus and placenta. The embryonic stem cells differentiate into 3 types of cells that ultimately form the various body organs: the **ectoderm** (skin, **spinal cord,** teeth), **mesoderm** (blood vessels, muscle, bone), and **endoderm** (lungs and digestive and urinary systems). By week 3 after ovulation and fertil-

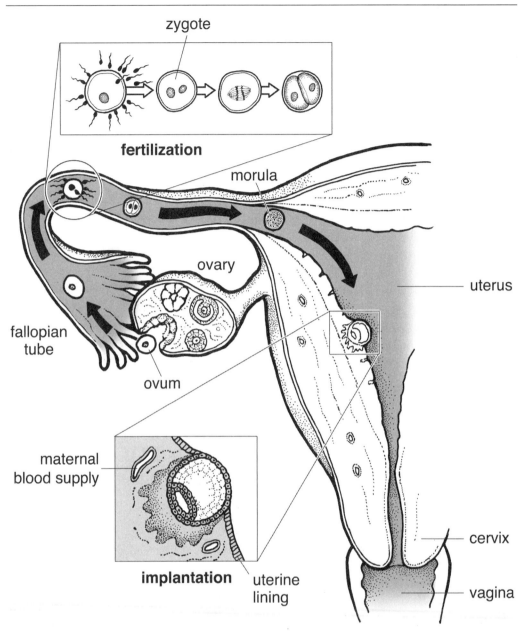

Figure 2.1. Fertilization and implantation. The ovum, or egg, is dropped from the ovary into the fallopian tube, where it is fertilized by a sperm. The fertilized egg thus gains its diploid number of chromosomes and starts dividing as it travels toward the uterus. It reaches the uterus after 5–7 days, and implantation of the embryo (trophoblast) then takes place.

ization, the placenta has formed and is becoming the principal site of nutrient transfer between the embryo and the mother.

The blastocyst sometimes can become implanted in an abnormal location such as a fallopian tube, an ovary, the cervix, or even in the abdominal cavity. This is referred to as an **ectopic pregnancy,** a pregnancy which is almost always nonviable. Such a condition is very important to recognize as early as possible because it can be associated with significant bleeding, pain, and even death of the mother if left untreated.

EMBRYONIC AND FETAL DEVELOPMENT

In utero development can be divided into two periods, embryonic and fetal. The **embryonic**

period of in utero development lasts from week 3 to week 8 after ovulation and fertilization or from week 5 to week 10 after the first day of the last menstrual period (Figure 2.2). Organs form during the embryonic time period. Exposure to teratogens may lead to structural abnormalities or fetal death. In contrast, exposure to a teratogen prior to this time will usually lead to either a spontaneous abortion (miscarriage) or to an unaffected fetus. This is true because so few cells exist at this stage of development that irreparable damage to some cells tends to be lethal to all. If the embryo survives, however, there is generally no organ damage because repair or replacement occurs.

As the embryo grows, it becomes surrounded by a cavity of **amniotic fluid.** Early in the pregnancy, most of the amniotic fluid is formed in the fetal compartment; later in pregnancy, much of the fluid is derived from fetal urine. Abnormalities of amniotic fluid volume in the fetal period can occur from obstruction of the fetal urinary tract, which can lead to a diminished amount of amniotic fluid, a condition called **oligohydramnios.** Conversely, an inability of the fetus to swallow or absorb the amniotic fluid will result in excessive amniotic fluid in the uterine cavity, a condition called **polyhydramnios.** Thus, too little or too much amniotic fluid can serve as a marker for certain congenital malformations.

The head and tail folds of the embryo are distinctly developed by days 24–27 after ovulation and fertilization. At this time, the optic vesicles and lens form the embryonic eye; the limb buds are present; and the heart, liver, lungs, and thyroid gland appear. The cardiovascular system is the first fetal system to reach a functional state, beginning to contract by day 22 (Figure 2.2). An ebb and flow circulation occurs. Placental transfer of substances is usually established by the fifth week after ovulation and fertilization. Blood from the placenta carries oxygen and other nutrients from the mother, traveling to the fetus through the umbilical vein.

Formation of the **palate** begins with the projecting of two processes vertically downward on either side of the tongue which then subsequently meet in the mid-line and fuse. If mid-line fusion fails, the nasal cavity and mouth are not separated normally and a cleft lip or palate results. The timing of this event is pre-

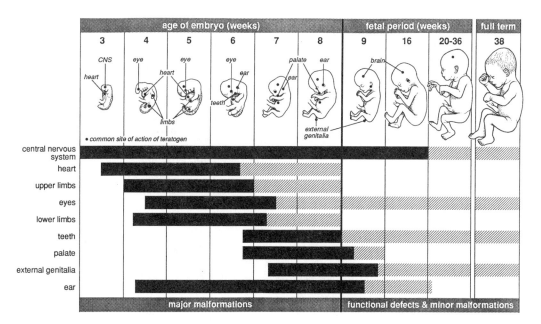

Figure 2.2. Embryogenesis and fetal development. The changes that take place during embryogenesis, between 3 and 8 weeks after fertilization, are enormous. All body systems are formed, and the embryo takes on a human form. Length increases 20-fold during this time. The fetal period lasts from 9 weeks to birth. Teratogens cause malformations if acting during the time a specific organ or group of organs are being formed. Damage to an organ during the time represented by a solid bar will lead to a major malformation, and damage during the time represented by the hatched bar will lead to functional defects or minor morphological abnormalities. (From Moore, K.L., & Persaud, T.V.N. [1993]. *Before we are born: Essentials of embryology and birth defects* [4th ed., inside back cover]. Philadelphia: W.B. Saunders. Copyright © Elsevier; adapted by permission.)

cise; cleft lip and cleft palate are known to occur between 7 and 8 weeks after ovulation and fertilization.

The four **branchial arches** (destined to form structures of the **pharynx** and throat) are present by days 27–29 after ovulation and fertilization. The first branchial arch is known as the mandibular arch and is divided into two processes. The first forms the **mandible** and the second forms the **maxilla,** the lower and upper jawbones, respectively. Problems at this stage lead to abnormal development of the jaw.

The **fetal period** of in utero development period begins 8 weeks after ovulation and fertilization. Most pregnancy tests are positive by this time. Development during this period consists of growth and maturation of structures that were formed during the embryonic period. Teratogen exposure at this time is more likely to lead to placental functional deficits or fetal growth restriction rather than to the types of birth defects that occur during the embryonic period.

The placenta continues to grow and supply nutrients to the fetus. By the end of the 12th week after ovulation and fertilization the fetus is 6–7 centimeters (2½ inches) in length and weighs approximately 100 grams (3 ounces). Individual fingers and toes become evident and the external genitalia show signs of male or female differentiation. In the absence of TDF (testis-determining factor), which is coded on the short arm of the Y chromosome, ovaries develop during weeks 11–12.

The embryonic and fetal development processes are directly under complex genetic control. Chapter 1 introduced a variety of conditions related to chromosome disorders and gene mutations that can lead to structural and developmental abnormalities. Since the late 1990s, the central role of a group of regulatory genes known as **homeobox (HOX) genes** has been elucidated. These genes act by making proteins in the developing embryo, which then work through their target genes to produce new messenger proteins, thus establishing a pattern for controlling the development of the basic body plan. Such developmental molecules are expressed in very specific concentrations in a gradient across regions of the embryo, letting every cell know what type of cell it is to become and where it is in relationship to its neighbors. In this way, the HOX genes create a chemical blueprint for the developing embryo. Subtle changes in such concentrations or in timing or gene specificity can cause major mutations, or they may even have no consequences at all for the developing embryo and fetus (Brady, 2000).

Other genetic mechanisms also contribute to the formation of specific embryonic tissues. For example, genes can be turned on or off by a process known as **methylation** (Nussbaum, McInnes, & Willard, 2001). It is now known that every human cell contains the entire genome, but not all of the complement of genes is active in any given cell. Chemical modification of specific genes by methylation inactivates some genes, resulting in differential expression of the genetic code in different tissues and organs. Increased knowledge of processes such as methylation is likely to markedly enhance our understanding of the mechanisms of developmental malformations in the embryo and fetus and in seemingly unrelated processes such as genetic roles in cancer and other diseases in adults. A large-scale study of the proteins that package DNA in humans and mice resulted in the mapping of such switches that turn genes on and off (Bernstein et al., 2005). Thus, factors that regulate the genome may be as important as gene mutations in the **etiology** of diseases such as cancer.

DEVELOPMENT OF THE CENTRAL NERVOUS SYSTEM

The **central nervous system (CNS)** starts to form in the embryo from its thin plate of ectoderm (the outer cell layer of the embryo) by the third week after ovulation and fertilization. As the ectodermal cells proliferate, they differentiate into outer and inner cell layers. These cell layers form the **neural folds** that then rise and fuse to form a **neural tube,** the fusion starting in the midbrain region. Fusion proceeds both anteriorly and posteriorly, leaving both ends open (Figure 2.3). The head portion of the neural tube will form the fetal brain, with the hollow tube in the head portion persisting as the **ventricular system** of the mature brain. The tail portion of the neural tube will form the **spinal cord.** Disruptions in the closure of the neural tube (neural tube defects, or NTDs) are most common in the lower lumbosacral portion, resulting in formation of a **meningomyelocele,** and much less commonly in the upper or head portion, resulting in **anencephaly** (see Chapter 28; Botto et al., 1999).

As the forward region of the neural tube continues its development, three distinct bulges

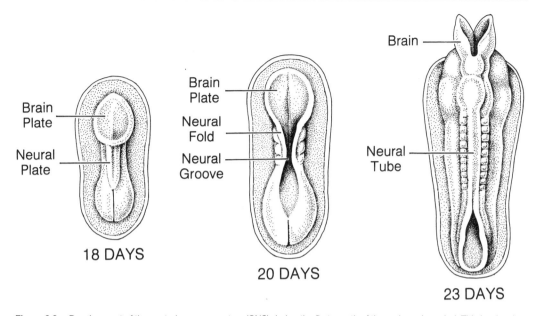

Figure 2.3. Development of the central nervous system (CNS) during the first month of the embryonic period. This is a longitudinal view showing the gradual closure of the neural tube to form the spinal column and the rounding up of the head region to form the primitive brain.

form, becoming the **prosencephalon (fore-brain,** including the cerebral hemispheres, **basal ganglia,** and **thalamus**), the **mesenecephalon** (midbrain), and the **rhombencephalon** (hindbrain, including cerebellum and **brainstem**) (ten Donkelaar, 2000; Figure 2.4). At five weeks after ovulation/fertilization, these parts of the early brain begin to curve into their more adult shape. The cerebral hemispheres will eventually rest on top of the brainstem. However, the cerebellum is the last part of the CNS to develop, and it is still immature at birth (Figure 2.4). As a result of the extended time of formation and completion of the development, the CNS is sensitive to the adverse effects of teratogens throughout the entire embryonic and fetal development periods (Institute of Medicine, 1996).

MATERNAL FACTORS IN FETAL DEVELOPMENT

Knowledge is steadily increasing about causes of congenital malformations. Even so, among children born in the United States with congenital malformations, approximately two thirds of the malformations are caused by unknown sources (Beckman & Brent, 1986). Of the remaining one third with identifiable causes, approximately 55% are single-gene defects, 25% are chromosomal disorders, and 20% are cases

of genetic etiology in which the mechanism was not identified (Baird et al., 1988). Developmental issues related to single-gene defects, chromosomal disorders, environmental exposure to toxins, and maternal infections are discussed elsewhere (Chapters 1, 5, and 6). This chapter addresses several of the other known maternal causes of congenital malformations, including nutrition problems, prescription drugs and substances of abuse, and several chronic maternal illnesses.

Discussion of the numerous and often complex maternal factors leading to **low birth weight (LBW)** infants and to infants who are born **small for gestational age (SGA)** is beyond the scope of this chapter. Clearly, however, many of the maternal factors discussed next can and frequently do contribute to either LBW or SGA status. The long-term childhood impact of being born too early or too small is a subject of active study. For example, adolescents who were born prematurely (at or earlier than 37 weeks' gestation) and were extremely SGA (at or below the third percentile for birth weight) were more likely to experience learning difficulties, and girls who were extremely SGA were found to be more likely to have attentional problems and low reading scores (O'Keeffe et al., 2003). Thus, preventing or appropriately treating maternal risk factors for LBW and SGA through proper nutrition, avoiding medications

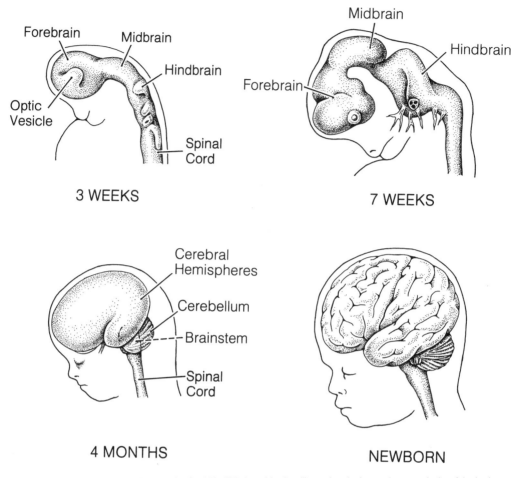

Figure 2.4. Development of the brain during fetal life. This is a side view illustrating the increasing complexity of the brain over time. The forebrain, or prosencephalon, develops into the cerebral hemispheres; the midbrain, or mesencephalon, develops into the brainstem; and the hindbrain, or rhombencephalon, develops into the cerebellum. Although all brain structures are formed by 4 months, the brain grows greatly in size and complexity during the final months of prenatal development.

and drugs known to potentially have an adverse impact on the developing fetus, and optimizing maternal health status (including management of chronic illnesses) will improve the intrauterine environment for the fetus and optimize the likelihood for the birth of a healthy infant.

Nutrition

The growth and development of the fetus requires a continuous supply of nutrients, which are transported across the placental membrane and absorbed by the fetus. A typical pregnancy requires a woman to consume approximately 300 additional calories per day. Most healthy women who eat a well-balanced diet with a caloric balance of approximately 50%–60% from complex carbohydrates, 10%–20% from proteins, and

20%–30% from fats satisfactorily meet the daily nutritional requirements during pregnancy. There is no evidence that a high-protein diet is beneficial (Hay et al., 1997).

Women with poor weight gain during pregnancy, however, are at increased risk for having newborns with LBW (Abrams & Selvin, 1995; Smith et al., 1998). To prevent this and other fetal complications, it is recommended that most women gain at least 15 pounds during pregnancy. If the mother is below ideal body weight prior to pregnancy, she should gain even more weight. Women who are classified as obese are encouraged to gain no more than 15 pounds. Greater weight gain in obese women is associated with an increased risk for stillbirth, among other problems in pregnancy (Institute of Medicine, 1990).

There has been considerable interest about the potential impact of vitamin supplementation during pregnancy on the health of the newborn. Most healthy women who consume a well-balanced diet and gain an appropriate amount of weight during pregnancy will only need to take typical prenatal vitamins. In order to significantly reduce the risk for neural tube defects (see Chapter 28), however, the American College of Obstetricians and Gynecologists (ACOG, 2003) recommends that all women take 0.4 **milligrams** (mg) of **folic acid** daily prior to conception and that this supplement be continued at least through the first 12 weeks of gestation. Because the neural tube is already forming at the time of the first missed menstrual period, initiating folic acid supplementation at that time is inadequate. Furthermore, women who have had a prior child with an NTD should take a much higher dosage (4 mg per day), thus reducing the risk for recurrence by 70% (MRC Vitamin Study Research Group, 1991). This higher level of folic acid supplementation is also recommended for women who have multiple gestations, those who have hemoglobinopathies (e.g., sickle cell anemia), and those who are taking antiepileptic medication (Hernandez-Diaz et al., 2000).

The recommended daily allowance of vitamin A is 2,700 international units (IU) per day. Although vitamin A is required for normal fetal growth and tissue differentiation, vitamin A deficiency is unusual in the United States because this recommended amount is contained in most diets. Thus, supplementation is not recommended. In fact, studies have shown that intake of more than 10,000 IU per day of vitamin A is associated with an increased incidence of NTDs (Azais-Braesco & Pascal, 2000; Rothman et al., 1995). Therefore, the acne medication isotretinoin (Accutane), an isomer or derivative of vitamin A, should not be used by a woman who is pregnant or who is considering a pregnancy.

Medications and Drugs of Abuse

Most medications taken in pregnancy, whether prescription or nonprescription, have no adverse effect on fetal development. Some, however, are known to cause significant problems and should be avoided if at all possible.

A classic example is thalidomide, which was commonly used in Europe (but not approved for sale in the United States) in the late 1950s as an agent to control nausea and vomiting during the first trimester of pregnancy. It was discovered, however, that at least 20% of the children whose mothers had used thalidomide between 35 and 50 days after ovulation and fertilization demonstrated significant teratogenic effects (Newman, 1985; Taussig, 1962). Thalidomide was removed from the market in Europe. In 1998, however, thalidomide was approved in the United States for the treatment of leprosy under extremely restrictive circumstances and only by specially registered physicians and pharmacists. According to the U.S. Food and Drug Administration (FDA; 2006), even a single dose taken by a pregnant woman can cause severe birth defects.

Seizure disorders in pregnant women are associated with an increase in congenital malformations (Holmes, Harvey, & Coull, 2001). It is not clear whether the disease process leading to the seizures, the antiepileptic drugs used to treat them, or both cause the observed increase in birth defects. It is clear, however, that during pregnancy a single antiepileptic drug should be used whenever possible and at the lowest dosage needed for seizure control. Certain antiepileptic drugs interfere with folic acid metabolism, and their use in pregnancy can lead to fetal NTDs (Centers for Disease Control and Prevention, 1992). Overall, there is an approximately 8% chance that a fetus will develop birth defects if exposed to one of the following antiepileptics: phenytoin (Dilantin), phenobarbital (Luminal), carbamazepine (Carbatrol, Tegretol), and valproic acid (Depakene, Depakote) (Kaneko et al., 1988; Nakane et al., 1980). Carbamazepine, when used alone in the first trimester, carries a 1%–2% risk of NTD, mostly in the lumbosacral region (Rosa, 1991). It is also associated with microcephaly, growth restriction, and developmental delay. The phenytoin syndrome, characterized by limb defects, growth restriction, intellectual disability, microcephaly, heart defects, and unusual **craniofacial** features, is seen in fewer than 10% of fetuses exposed to phenytoin in utero. The effects depend on whether the fetus inherits a mutant gene that decreases the production of an enzyme that is needed to break down phenytoin. Phenytoin, phenobarbital, carbamazepine, and valproic acid are all listed as FDA Pregnancy Category D, meaning there is positive evidence of human fetal risk but benefit may outweigh fetal risk in serious situations (U.S. FDA, 2006). Newer antiepileptic agents such as topiramate (Topamax), lamotrigene (Lamictal), levetiracetam (Keppra), oxcarbazepine (Trileptal), and zonisamide (Zonegran) are all FDA Pregnancy Category C, meaning that animal studies have shown fetal effects but no adequate controlled human studies have been reported yet. In addition, oxycarbezepine is closely linked to carbamazepine, such that human fetal effects are expected to be reported in the future (U.S. FDA, 2006).

Like radiation therapy, **chemotherapy** used to treat cancer during pregnancy places the fetus at risk. The risk of exposure must be balanced against the risk of the malignant disease process that is being treated. The first 12 weeks of gestation are the most critical. The use of chemotherapeutic agents during this period can potentially cause congenital malformations, fetal death, or growth restriction (Gililland & Weinstein, 1983). If chemotherapy is needed during pregnancy, it should be delayed whenever possible until after the first 12 weeks of gestation. If such a delay is not possible, then termination of the pregnancy is often considered. Of the drugs used to treat cancer, those most commonly associated with teratogenic effects are folic acid antagonists such as methotrexate. Methotrexate has been shown to cause delayed skull formation, limb deformities, and cerebral anomalies.

Pregnant women who have chronic **hypertension** or develop hypertension as part of preeclampsia (a medical condition of pregnancy that includes hypertension, protein in the urine, and edema) may require antihypertensive medication during pregnancy. Most of the drugs are safe for the fetus but a few require caution. The use of an angiotensin-converting enzyme (ACE) inhibitor medication, such as captopril, during pregnancy has been associated with fetal kidney abnormalities. Pregnant women taking ACE inhibitors should be advised to discontinue them, especially because safer alternatives are available. Alpha-methyldopa (Aldomet) is considered the first-line antihypertensive agent for use during pregnancy because it is the only drug for which safety has been demonstrated in long-term follow-up studies. Labetolol (Normodyne) and atenolol (Tenormin) are acceptable alternatives. In terms of the use of diuretics such as furosemide (Lasix) or chlorothiazide (Diuril) for blood pressure control, there are no data demonstrating an increased perinatal mortality rate or decreased birth weight when maternal diuretic therapy is begun before 24 weeks of gestation. Although there is a theoretical risk of dehydration when diuretics are used later in pregnancy, they may be continued as long as there is no clinical evidence of growth restriction or reduced uterine or placental blood flow.

Alcohol freely crosses the placenta, and its fetal toxicity is known to be dose related. The greatest risk of exposure is during the first 12 weeks of gestation, but the risk to the fetus of maternal alcohol use continues throughout pregnancy. It is difficult to calculate an exact risk because of the frequent presence of confounders such as multiple drug use (both legal and illicit) and cigarette smoking. In the United States, however, 12% of pregnant women admit to drinking some alcohol during the previous month (Substance Abuse and Mental Health Services Administration, 2002). Alcohol use during pregnancy is the most commonly identified preventable cause of intellectual disability in the United States (National Institute on Alcohol Abuse and Alcoholism, 2000). Thus, the ACOG (2004) recommended the use of universal screening questions, brief interventions, and referral to treatment when necessary in pregnancy.

Heroin use during pregnancy can cause growth restriction, preterm labor and delivery, stillbirth, and neonatal mortality. Furthermore, affected newborns are at risk for narcotic withdrawal syndrome in the first days of life that can be potentially fatal. A high-pitched cry, tremors, irritability, and occasional seizures characterize this withdrawal syndrome. Treatment of the mother with methadone improves pregnancy outcome, but neonatal narcotic withdrawal syndrome for methadone can be more severe and prolonged than for heroin due to the longer half-life of methadone.

Exposure to cocaine in the first trimester is associated with an increased risk of spontaneous abortion, fetal death, growth restriction, and separation of the placenta (placental abruption, or abruptio placenta). It is also associated with congenital malformations of the heart, limbs, face, and genitourinary tract. The exact risk of exposure is difficult to establish because of the frequent concurrent abuse of other substances. (See Chapter 5 for further discussion of the effects of prenatal exposure to alcohol and environmental toxins.)

Maternal Chronic Illness

Studies have shown that several maternal chronic illnesses, including hypertension, thyroid disease, diabetes, and autoimmune disorders, can result in impaired intrauterine fetal growth and development.

Hypertensive disorders occur in approximately 1%–5% of all pregnancies in the United States and in a higher percentage among older pregnant women (Sibai, 1996). These disorders are a significant cause of perinatal **morbidity** (complications) and mortality. The direct fetal effects seen with hypertensive disorders include growth restriction and decreased volume of amniotic fluid. These are thought to result from decreased maternal blood flow to the uterus, placenta, and kidneys. Other maternal and fetal risks include preeclampsia, abruptio placenta, and preterm delivery. If antihypertensive medication is initiated during pregnancy, it is important to observe the fetus for further growth restriction (Butler, Kennedy, & Rubin, 1990).

Because thyroid insufficiency is commonly associated with infertility, most pregnancies are not complicated by overt **hypothyroidism.** For the most part, infants of mothers with hypothyroidism are healthy and show no evidence of thyroid dysfunction. Nevertheless, there is an increased incidence of pregnancy-induced hypertension and placental abruption in women with thyroid deficiency who are untreated. Depending upon the degree of untreated thyroid deficiency, children of mothers with hypothyroidism may have lower IQ scores (Haddow et al., 1999). Levothyroxine (Synthroid) is in FDA Category A, meaning that it is appropriate for treatment of hypothyroidism in pregnancy (U.S. FDA, 2006).

Most medications commonly used to treat **thyrotoxicosis** or **hyperthyroidism** (overactive thyroid) in nonpregnant women can be safely used during pregnancy (Mulder, 1998). Propylthiouracil (PTU), the drug of choice for treatment of thyrotoxicosis, however, crosses the placenta and can potentially cause hypothyroidism in the fetus as well as a fetal **goiter.** Another drug used for hyperthyroidism, methimazole (Tapazole), also crosses the placenta, leading to an increased risk for development of an unusual scalp defect. There is no consistent evidence, however, that suggests that either PTU or methimazole is teratogenic. Fetuses of mothers who are exposed to increased amounts of iodide for long periods of time are at increased risk of developing hypothyroidism and a fetal goiter because iodide easily crosses the placenta and is absorbed by the fetal thyroid. Therefore, radioiodine studies are not generally recommended during pregnancy unless the mother has severe thyrotoxicosis; thyroidectomy, however, can be safely carried out. Women who continue to have hyperthyroidism despite medical therapy and those whose disease remains untreated are at increased risk for developing pregnancy-induced hypertension and congestive heart failure, leading to an increased incidence of fetal death and preterm labor and delivery.

Diabetes is one of the most common medical complications of pregnancy. Gestational diabetes accounts for approximately 90% of all patients with diabetes during pregnancy. This diagnosis is made in a pregnant woman who was not diabetic before becoming pregnant but who has abnormally elevated blood glucose levels after consuming a specific amount of an oral glucose solution. In these patients, the disorder is usually well controlled with the American Diabetes Association diet (i.e., medical nutrition therapy) for gestational diabetes (ACOG, 2001).

Poorly treated maternal diabetes, both gestational and pregestational, however, is associated with increased incidences of fetal anomalies (accounting for approximately half of perinatal deaths in diabetic pregnancies), preterm birth, delayed fetal lung maturity, large fetal body size (**macrosomia**), and otherwise unexplained fetal death. Preconceptional counseling (Willhoite et al., 1993) and maintenance of tight metabolic control of the mother's glucose levels throughout the pregnancy can decrease the risk of these complications (ACOG, 2001).

Women with autoimmune conditions such as antiphospholipid antibody syndrome or systemic lupus erythematosus (SLE), or lupus, are at increased risk for recurrent pregnancy losses. Antiphospholipid antibody syndrome is associated with pregnancy loss, thrombosis (stroke), and decreased platelet count. Mothers with SLE, a severe multisystem chronic illness associated with skin rash, hypertension, kidney disease, and potentially **encephalopathy,** may have infants born with lupus, skin lesions, a number of systemic problems, and occasionally heart block (Peaceman & Ramsey-Goldman, 2001). Thus, close antepartum surveillance is necessary to reduce the risk for adverse maternal or fetal outcomes.

SUMMARY

Although this chapter has focused on the many complications that can occur during pregnancy, it is important to emphasize that the vast majority of all children are born well. There are certain proactive steps that a woman can take to decrease the risk of fetal developmental complications in pregnancy. These include eating a nutritious and well-balanced diet, seeking early prenatal care, taking only medically recommended dosages of vitamin supplements, and avoiding environmental agents that can potentially harm the developing fetus. If there is exposure to a potentially teratogenic agent, the risk to the fetus depends on the specific teratogen; the extent, duration, and timing of exposure; the ability of the teratogen to cross the placenta; and genetic predisposition. Teratogenic agents include radiation, certain medications, legal and illegal drugs of abuse, bacteria, protozoa, and viruses. Adverse effects of teratogens can range from growth restriction, to malformations, to fetal death. In addition, certain chronic maternal illnesses such as hypertension, diabetes, thyroid disease, and lupus can place the fetus at risk. The best protection from most of the known factors leading to problems in pregnancy is prevention or early detection and, whenever possible, appropriate intervention. Preconceptional counseling and optimizing of a woman's health status prior to pregnancy are important steps in reaching the objectives of prevention or early detection.

REFERENCES

Abrams, B., & Selvin, S. (1995). Maternal weight gain pattern and birth weight. *Obstetrics and Gynecology, 86,* 163–169.

American College of Obstetricians and Gynecologists. (2001). Gestational diabetes (ACOG Practice Bulletin 30). *Obstetrics and Gynecology, 98,* 525–538.

American College of Obstetricians and Gynecologists. (2003). Neural tube defects (ACOG Practice Bulletin 44). *International Journal of Gynecology and Obstetrics, 83,* 123–133.

American College of Obstetricians and Gynecologists. (2004). At-risk drinking and illicit drug use: Ethical issues in obstetric and gynecologic practice (ACOG Committee Opinion 294). *Obstetrics and Gynecology, 103,* 1021–1031.

Azais-Braesco, V., & Pascal, G. (2000). Vitamin A in pregnancy: Requirements and safety limits. *American Journal of Clinical Nutrition, 71*(5, Suppl.), 1325S–1333S.

Baird, P.A., Anderson, T.W., Newcombe, H.B., et al. (1988). Genetic disorders in children and young adults: A population study. *American Journal of Human Genetics, 42*(5), 677–693.

Beckman, A.A., & Brent, R.L. (1986). Mechanisms of known environmental teratogens: Drugs and chemicals. *Clinics in Perinatology, 13,* 649–687.

Bernstein, B.E., Kamal, M., Lindblad-Toh, K., et al. (2005). Genomic maps and comparative analysis of histone modifications in human and mouse. *Cell, 120,* 169–181.

Botto, L.D., Moore, C.A., Khoury, M.J., et al. (1999). Neural-tube defects. *The New England Journal of Medicine, 341,* 1509–1519.

Brady, G. (2000). Hox genes: "The molecular architects." *The Irish Scientist Yearbook,* 8.

Butler, L., Kennedy, S., & Rubin, P.C. (1990). Atenolol in essential hypertension during pregnancy. *British Medical Journal, 301,* 587–590.

Centers for Disease Control and Prevention. (1992). Recommendations for the use of folic acid to reduce the number of cases of spina bifida and other neural tube defects. *Morbidity and Mortality Weekly Report, 41MO*(RR-14), 1–7.

Decoufle, P., Boyle, C.A., Paulozzi, L.J., et al. (2001). Increased risk for developmental disabilities in children who have major birth defects: A population-based study. *Pediatrics, 108,* 728–734.

Gililland, J., & Weinstein, L. (1983). The effects of cancer chemotherapeutic agents on the developing fetus. *Obstetrical and Gynecological Survey, 38,* 6–13.

Haddow, J.E., Palomaki, G.E., Allan, W.C., et al. (1999). Maternal thyroid deficiency during pregnancy and subsequent neuropsychological development of the child. *The New England Journal of Medicine, 341,* 549–555.

Hay, W.W., Catz, C.S., Grave, G.D., et al. (1997). Workshop summary: Fetal growth. Its regulation and disorders. *Journal of Pediatrics, 99,* 585–592.

Hernandez-Diaz, S., Werler, M.M., Walker, A.M., et al. (2000). Folic acid antagonists during pregnancy and the risk of birth defects. *The New England Journal of Medicine, 343,* 1608–1614.

Holmes, L.B., Harvey, E.A., & Coull, B.A. (2001). The teratogenicity of anticonvulsant drugs. *The New England Journal of Medicine, 344,* 1132–1138.

Institute of Medicine. (1990). *Nutrition during pregnancy.* Washington, DC: National Academies Press.

Institute of Medicine. (1996). *Fetal alcohol syndrome: Diagnosis, epidemiology, prevention, and treatment.* Washington, DC: National Academies Press, 2, 33–37.

Kaneko, S., Otani, K., Fukushima, Y., et al. (1988). Teratogenicity of anti-epileptic drugs: Analysis of possible risk factors. *Epilepsia, 29,* 459–467.

Moore, K.L., & Persaud, T.V.N. (1993). *Before we are born: Essentials of embryology and birth defects.* Philadelphia: W.B. Saunders.

MRC Vitamin Research Group. (1991). Prevention of neural tube defects: results of the Medical Research Council Vitamin Study. *The Lancet, 338,* 131–137.

Mulder, J.E. (1998). Thyroid disease in women. *Medical Clinics of North America, 82,* 104–125.

Nakane, Y., Okuma, T., Takahashi, R., et al. (1980). Multi-institutional study on the teratogenicity and fetal toxicity of anti-epileptic drugs: A report of collaborative study group in Japan. *Epilepsia, 21,* 663–380.

National Institute on Alcohol Abuse and Alcoholism. (2000). Fetal alcohol exposure and the brain. *Alcohol Alert, 50,* 1–6.

Newman, C.G. (1985). Teratogen update: Clinical aspects of thalidomide embryopathy. A continuing preoccupation. *Teratology, 32,* 133–144.

Nussbaum, R.L., McInnes, R.R., & Willard, H.F. (2001). *Thompson and Thompson genetics in medicine* (6th ed.). Philadelphia: W.B. Saunders.

O'Keeffe, M.J., O'Callaghan, M., Williams, G.M., et al. (2003). Learning, cognitive, and attentional problems in adolescents born small for gestational age. *Pediatrics, 112*(2), 301–307.

Peaceman, A.M., & Ramsey-Goldman, R. (2001). Autoimmune connective tissue disease in pregnancy. *Sciarra's Obstetrics and Gynecology, 3*(20), 1–5.

Rosa, F.W. (1991). Spina bifida in infants of women treated with carbamazepine during pregnancy. *The New England Journal of Medicine, 324,* 674–677.

Rothman, K.J., Moore, L.L., Singer, M.R., et al. (1995). Teratogenicity of high vitamin A intake. *The New England Journal of Medicine, 333*, 1369.

Sibai, B. (1996). Treatment of hypertension in pregnant women. *The New England Journal of Medicine, 335*, 257–265.

Smith, G., Smith, M., McNay, M.B., et al. (1998). First trimester growth and the risk of low birth weight. *The New England Journal of Medicine, 339*, 1817–1822.

Substance Abuse and Mental Health Services Administration. (2002). *Results from the 2001 National Household Survey on Drug Abuse: Volume I. Summary of national findings: SAMHSA.* Rockville, MD: Author.

Taussig, H.B. (1962). Thalidomide: A lesson in remote effects of drugs. *American Journal of Diseases of Children, 104*, 111–113.

ten Donkelaar, H.J. (2000). Major events in the development of the forebrain. *European Journal of Morphology, 38*, 301–308.

U.S. Food and Drug Administration. (2006). *FDA prescription drug package inserts.* Washington, DC: Author.

Willhoite, M.B., Benvert, H.W., Palomaki, G.E., et al. (1993). The impact of preconception counseling on pregnancy outcomes: The experience of the Maine Diabetes in Pregnancy Program. *Diabetes Care, 16*, 450–455.

3

Having a Baby

The Birth Process

Jill E. Brown and Andrew J. Satin

Upon completion of this chapter, the reader will

- Be able to describe the stages of labor and techniques for monitoring labor
- Be able to identify causes of abnormal labor or dystocia
- Be aware of pregnancy complications that influence the condition of the newborn
- Be aware of special pregnancy conditions that are associated with increased risk to mother and fetus

---

It is a common misconception that many developmental disabilities result from complications that occur during labor and delivery. In fact, scientific evidence suggests that complications during this period account for fewer that 10% of all cases of severe disabilities in childhood. The overall incidence of neonatal encephalopathy attributable to intrapartum hypoxia, in the absence of any other preconceptional or antepartum abnormality, is 1.6 per 10,000 births. (Hankins et al., 2003). It is now understood that problems during labor and delivery are often secondary to an underlying condition or problem that occurred prenatally and are not themselves the cause of subsequent disability. This chapter focuses on the process of labor and delivery and the technology that is being employed to prevent brain injury.

DATING A PREGNANCY

One of the most crucial steps in antepartum (prenatal) care is to date the pregnancy. Several different terms are used to define the duration of the pregnancy. Estimated gestational age (EGA) or menstrual age is the time from the first day of the last menstrual period (LMP). It should be noted that gestational age is 14 days longer than conceptional age because of the time between the LMP and ovulation and implantation of the embryo (see Chapter 2). The average duration of a pregnancy is 280 days, or 40 weeks EGA. Obstetricians typically refer to the EGA during prenatal care. The estimated due date (EDD) and **estimated date of confinement (EDC)** are terms used interchangeably. A quick estimate of the EDD can be made by adding 7 days to the first day of the LMP and subtracting 3 months. For example, if the first day of a woman's LMP is October 15, her due date will be July 22. A pregnancy is considered term between 38 and 42 weeks EGA. **Preterm birth** is delivery prior to 38 weeks. **Postterm birth** is delivery with an EGA greater then 42 weeks.

DECIDING WHEN TO DELIVER THE BABY

The most important decision an obstetrician makes is if and when to influence labor. **Tocolysis** is the prescribing of medicines in an effort to prevent preterm labor. Labor augmentation and induction are efforts to stimulate the uterus to contract. Obstetric decision analysis balances the risk of delivery versus pregnancy continuation for both mother and fetus. These decisions can be particularly difficult when the decision to deliver may be medically beneficial to the mother but clearly disadvantageous to the fetus. Knowledge of gestational age is central to these treatment decisions.

PERINATAL MORTALITY

Since the mid-20th century, both perinatal and maternal mortality rates have declined dramatically. Improvements in the quality of care during pregnancy and labor have contributed to the decline in the stillbirth rate, and improved intensive care of newborns has resulted in a decline in neonatal deaths. Fetal and neonatal deaths may arise from difficulties originating antepartum, during labor, or at birth. Perinatal mortality, which is defined as the number of stillbirths (intrauterine death occurring after 20 weeks' gestation but prior to delivery) plus neonatal deaths (deaths which occur in the first 28 days of life), has been falling steadily since the 1970s. Perinatal mortality in high-risk pregnancies has been reduced fourfold since 1984 (Creasy, Resnik, & Iams, 2004). The perinatal mortality rate in 2002 in the United States was steady at 2.3 deaths per 1,000 live births. The infant mortality rate (IMR) however, rose in 2002 to 7.0 per 1,000 live births from an all-time low of 6.8 deaths per 1,000 in 2001, the first increase in more than 40 years (Table 3.1). The neonatal mortality rate also rose from 4.5 to 4.7 per 1,000 from 2001 to 2002. This increase is thought to be due to a shift in birth weight distribution toward extremely low birth weight (LBW) infants (Martin et al., 2005). In fact, the most common cause of neonatal death is LBW, usually as a result of preterm delivery. Preterm delivery accounts for 85% of all perinatal complications (Norwitz, Robinson, & Challis 1999).

LABOR

Labor is defined by the presence of regular uterine contractions leading to progressive effacement (thinning) and dilation of the cervix and expulsion of the fetus. Labor is divided into three stages. The first stage of labor begins

Table 3.1. Infant mortality rates in 2002 in the United States for leading causes per 100,000 live births

Cause	Death rate
Congenital malformation	140
Preterm birth and low birth weight	115
Sudden infant death syndrome	57
Maternal complications or pregnancy	43
Delivery complications or pregnancy	26
Accidents and adverse effects	24
Respiratory distress syndrome	23
Infections	19
Intrauterine hypoxia or birth asphyxia	15

Source: Martin et al. (2005).

when uterine contractions bring about effacement and progressive dilatation of the cervix. This stage ends when the cervix is fully effaced, or paper-thin, and completely dilated, typically 10 centimeters (cm). The first stage of labor is divided into a latent and an active phase. The latent phase is characterized by infrequent and irregular contractions, which typically result in only modest discomfort. The active phase is characterized by regular, intense, and typically painful contractions. This phase typically begins when the cervix is 3–4 cm dilated and concludes when the cervix is 10 cm dilated. The second stage of labor, or pushing stage, begins when dilation of the cervix is complete and ends with expulsion of the fetus. The third stage of labor begins immediately after delivery of the fetus and ends with the delivery of the placenta.

MONITORING LABOR

Once labor begins, the **fetal heart rate (FHR)** and uterine contractions are monitored. Continuous electronic fetal monitoring (EFM) has been used routinely in obstetrics since the 1960s. The EFM may be done with either external or internal monitors. External monitors employ Doppler ultrasound technology to monitor the FHR and tocodynamometer to measure contraction activity. Internal monitors include a fetal scalp electrode and an intrauterine pressure catheter, which have the advantage of providing exact measurements of the FHR and contraction strength, respectively.

Evaluation of a fetal heart tracing should include analysis of rate, variability, and periodic changes. A normal baseline heart rate is between 120 and 160 beats per minute (bpm) (Freeman, Garite, & Nageotte, 1991). Fetal **bradycardia** (slowed heart rate) is present if the baseline heart rate remains less than 110 bpm. Causes of fetal bradycardia may include uterine hypertonus (excessive tone), epidural-induced **hypotension, placental abruption** (discussed later in this chapter), and any other problems that decrease blood flow to the fetus. Treatment of fetal bradycardia involves determining the cause and correcting it to restore adequate blood flow to the fetus. If bradycardia does not resolve in a timely manner, then delivery is accomplished either by cesarean delivery or forceps or vacuum extraction, depending on which can be accomplished more quickly and safely.

Fetal **tachycardia** (rapid heart rate) is diagnosed when there is a sustained FHR of greater than 160 bpm. Intra-amniotic infection may cause a maternal fever, which in turn causes fetal tachycardia. Other causes include fetal arrhythmia and administration of certain medications to the mother. Although mild tachycardia (160–180 bpm) in the absence of other concerning findings may be monitored, severe tachycardia (>200 bpm) often requires delivery. Accelerations, or an increase in the FHR of as much as 15 bpm for 15 seconds, should not be confused with sustained tachycardia. The presence of accelerations is similar to fetal rate variability in that when present, fetal compromise is rare.

It is normal for FHR to be variable. Short-term variability refers to the beat-to-beat changes of the FHR and long-term variability changes that occur over 1-minute intervals. Decreased short- and long-term variability may be observed during normal sleep cycles or after administration of narcotics during labor. Nevertheless, severely diminished or absent variability in the presence of decelerations can be an ominous sign of a compromised fetus. Decelerations, or periodic decreases in the FHR, should be evaluated in relation to contractions, as the cause and treatment of different types of decelerations may vary.

Alterations in FHR related to contractions are referred to as periodic changes. With each uterine contraction, the fetus experiences significant physiologic changes. Contractions decrease placental blood flow, which in turn decreases oxygen delivery to the fetus for short periods of time. Although a healthy fetus does well and can compensate for this stress, fetuses who are affected by **preeclampsia** (discussed later in this chapter), **intrauterine growth restriction (IUGR)**, genetic syndromes, or are extremely premature may become **hypoxic** (deprived of oxygen) during labor and develop abnormal FHR patterns. Contractions may also compress the umbilical cord or the fetal head, which also cause characteristic changes in the fetal heart tracing.

When the fetal head is compressed by contractions, which usually occurs during the second stage of labor, the FHR may be seen to drop in a manner that mirrors the contraction. This form of deceleration is termed an early deceleration and is not a sign of distress. In contrast, when the umbilical cord is compressed during a uterine contraction, the fetal heart decelerations are not uniform in nature and do not occur exactly with contractions (Figure 3.1a). Variable decelerations may be treated with maternal position changes, with amnioinfusion (infusion of 250–500 cubic centimeters of fluid into the uterine cavity after the amniotic sac has broken), or with one of a group of drugs referred to as tocolytics, which are designed to stop contractions for a short period of time. These measures are designed to relieve compression on the umbilical cord. When variable decelerations are persistently below 60 bpm for more than 60 seconds and demonstrate slow return to baseline or decreased variability, or when tachycardia is present between contractions, there is a correlation with fetal jeopardy.

Late decelerations are symmetric in appearance, much like early decelerations, but they do not begin until after the peak of a contraction and do not return to baseline until after the contraction has ended. Late decelerations are not usually as obvious as variable decelerations and may involve only a slight decrease in the FHR below the baseline. Late decelerations are of great concern as they are indicative of uteroplacental insufficiency and fetal jeopardy (Figure 3.1b). Late decelerations may be seen with maternal hypotension from **epidural anesthesia** or uterine hyperactivity but may also be present with preeclampsia, diabetes, or placental abruption. If late decelerations are repetitive and associated with decreased variability, then immediate delivery is indicated.

DELIVERY

Most deliveries occur spontaneously, and are referred to as spontaneous vaginal deliveries (SVDs). The infant's head is delivered and the nose and mouth are bulb-suctioned to clear the airway. When the umbilical cord is wrapped around the neck, as it is in approximately one quarter of births, it is called a nuchal cord and is either manually released or clamped and cut. Following delivery of the shoulders, the cord is clamped and cut and the infant is placed on the mother's abdomen or under a warmer to be cleaned and resuscitated if needed.

Operative deliveries include the use of forceps and vacuum devices to assist or expedite delivery. These are used only when the cervix is fully dilated, fetal head position is known, and the infant is sufficiently far enough down in the pelvis to be reached without difficulty. Indications for operative delivery include fetal distress, maternal exhaustion, and the need to avoid pushing for maternal factors (e.g., maternal cardiac conditions that might be exacerbated by cardiovascular stress). There do not appear to be any long-term adverse developmental consequences associated with the ap-

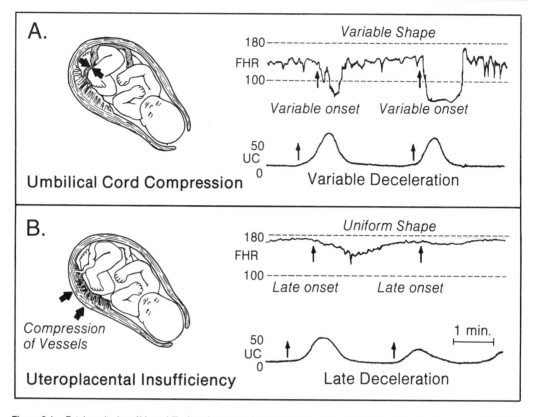

Figure 3.1. Fetal monitoring. A) In umbilical cord compression, there is a variable deceleration of the fetal heart rate (FHR). This abnormal finding of early, mid-, and late deceleration suggests compression and obstruction of the umbilical cord circulation during labor. B) In uteroplacental insufficiency, late deceleration of FHR occurs if the placental blood vessels are abnormally pressed together during the end of the uterine contraction (UC; see arrows). (From Hon, E. [1968]. *An atlas of fetal heart rate patterns.* New Haven, CT: Harty; adapted by permission.)

propriate use of forceps or vacuum devices (Wesley et al., 1993).

CESAREAN SECTION

Cesarean deliveries, which involve delivering the baby through an incision in the abdomen and uterus, may be performed for fetal jeopardy; if necessary, the infant can be delivered within minutes. Cesareans are also performed when the fetus is too large or the pelvis is too small for vaginal delivery. Cesareans may also be used in case of malpresentation (e.g., footling breech presentation) or for high-order multiple pregnancies (e.g., triplets or more). Cesarean delivery is usually performed under either epidural or spinal anesthesia with the mother awake, with general anesthesia being used only in emergency cases or when contraindications to epidural/spinal anesthesia are present.

Cesareans have become much more common in the United States since the mid-1960s, increasing from 5% of deliveries in 1965 to 27.6% to 2003, a record high (Eskew et al., 1994; Martin et al., 2005). After declines in the cesarean delivery rate from 1989–1996, the rate has risen each year; the current rate is one third higher than that for 1996 (20.7%) (DiMarco et al., 2000). The reasons for this are many but may include the use of continuous fetal monitoring with increased diagnosis of fetal distress, a decrease in the number of vaginal breech deliveries, an increase in the primary cesarean rate (percent of cesareans among women with no previous cesarean delivery), and an increase in elective repeat cesareans. It was initially believed that all patients who had a cesarean needed a repeat cesarean with subsequent pregnancies, but now many women are encouraged to attempt a vaginal birth after cesarean (VBAC). VBAC success rates range for 60%–80%

(Flamm, 1995; Rosen, Dickinson, & Westhoff, 1991). Contraindications to a VBAC include a previous classical cesarean (in which the uterine incision was vertical rather than horizontal and entered into the upper, contractile portion of the uterus), previous uterine surgery in which the endometrial cavity was entered, or a previous uterine rupture.

ABNORMAL LABOR OR DYSTOCIA

Dystocia is defined as difficult labor or childbirth. Typically, labor abnormalities are characterized as slower than normal (protraction disorders) or complete cessation of progress (arrest disorders). Identification of the potential cause of dystocia involves assessment of the three Ps: *p*ower (uterine contraction intensity), *p*assenger (fetus), and *p*assage (maternal anatomy). Uterine hypocontractility (decreased power of contraction) is a common cause of dystocia. It may be treated with a carefully administered intravenous infusion of oxytocin. Oxytocin stimulates the uterus to contract. The size, presentation, and position of the fetus may contribute to dystocia. Fetal anomalies such as hydrocephalus and spina bifida may obstruct labor. Infrequently, the maternal bony pelvis may contribute to dystocia. This may be seen after trauma or with severe **malnutrition.**

PREGNANCY COMPLICATIONS

Pregnancy and labor complications undoubtedly influence the condition of the newborn. Although a definitive discussion of all complications of pregnancies is beyond the scope of this chapter, several problems merit review. Diabetes, **hypertension,** and trauma are maternal conditions that can influence newborn status. Preterm labor, preterm rupture of membranes, and placental abruption are obstetric conditions that may result in preterm birth. Perinatal viral, parasitic, and bacterial infections may affect both mother and child.

Maternal Conditions

Diabetes Approximately 2%–3% of pregnancies are affected by diabetes, with 90% of these being gestational diabetes, or diabetes diagnosed in pregnancy (American College of Obstetricians and Gynecologists [ACOG], 2001). Mothers with type 1 diabetes (those requiring insulin) are at a 3% risk for developing diabetic ketoacidosis (DKA) during pregnancy. Ten percent of pregnancies in women with DKA result in intrauterine fetal death (Chauhan et al., 1996). Women with type 1 diabetes who have poor glucose control during the period of fetal organogenesis have a four-fold increase in the likelihood of having a baby with major congenital anomalies (ACOG, 2001). Women with well-controlled diabetes during organogenesis have rates of anomalies approaching the general population (Crowther et al., 2005).

Uncontrolled diabetes in pregnancy also places the fetus at increased risk for preterm delivery, polyhydramnios (increased amniotic fluid), IUGR, preeclampsia, fetal macrosomia (large body size, which may necessitate cesarean delivery if the infant is too large to fit through the pelvis), and stillbirth. (Dunne, 1999). Poor glucose control during labor and delivery can result in maternal **hyperglycemia,** which can cause severe **hypoglycemia** in the infant soon after birth as the maternal glucose is removed and the infant's own excess insulin remains.

Most pregnant women are screened for diabetes between 24 and 28 weeks of gestation, with a 50-gram glucose load and a serum glucose 1 hour later. If the test result is abnormal, then gestational diabetes is diagnosed and a diabetic diet with close monitoring is prescribed. If dietary management does not maintain glucose levels in the appropriate range, then either oral hypoglycemic therapy or insulin therapy is started, and a treatment plan is implemented in the same manner as for pregestational diabetes.

Hypertensive Disorders of Pregnancy The National Institutes of Health (NIH) working group on hypertension has classified hypertensive disorders during pregnancy into four groups: 1) chronic hypertension (CHTN), 2) preeclampsia–eclampsia, 3) preeclampsia superimposed on chronic hypertension, and 4) transient hypertension.

CHTN occurs in 1%–5% of pregnancies (Sibai, 1996). It is defined as elevated blood pressure (greater than 140/90 mm Hg) that occurs either before pregnancy or prior to 20 weeks' gestation. Ninety percent of women with chronic hypertension have essential (i.e., unknown cause) hypertension, with the other

10% having underlying medical problems, such as kidney, collagen vascular (e.g., lupus), endocrine, or vascular diseases. Risk factors for CHTN include obesity, heredity, race, and diabetes (Mroz, 1999). Pregnant women with CHTN must be monitored closely for development of IUGR (weight less than 10th percentile for gestational age) and superimposed preeclampsia–eclampsia during their pregnancy. They are also at increased risk for placental abruption.

Preeclampsia is hypertension occurring after the 20th week of gestation, accompanied by either proteinuria (protein in the urine) or edema (the accumulation of fluid in tissue). Preeclampsia complicates 7% of pregnancies (Creasy et al., 2004). It is a disease that most commonly affects women having their first baby. Other risk factors include extremes of childbearing age, multiple gestation, and certain medical disorders (e.g., CHTN, renal disease, diabetes; see Table 3.2). The cause of preeclampsia is not known; however, several physiologic changes are evident that result in decreased placental **perfusion** (Napolitano et al., 1997). Because of these changes, the fetus is at risk for developing IUGR.

Eclampsia, or seizures, may develop in a small number of patients with preeclampsia. Thus, whenever a woman develops signs of impending eclampsia, emergency delivery is usually indicated, even in the case of prematurity. In addition to induction of labor, magnesium sulfate is administered to prevent seizures during both labor and postpartum. In patients with eclampsia, the perinatal mortality rate has been reported to be between 130 to 300 per 1,000 cases, and eclampsia recurs in approximately 5% of subsequent pregnancies (Cunningham et al., 2005).

Table 3.2. Risk factors for developing preeclampsia

Extremes of childbearing age
Family history of preeclampsia
Underlying medical disorders:
Chronic hypertension
Renal disease
Diabetes mellitus
Systemic lupus erythematosus
Multiple gestation
Hydatidiform mole
Fetal hydrops
First pregnancy

Trauma and Abuse   It has been reported that 10%–20% of women will suffer some form of trauma during pregnancy (Cunningham, 2005). Trauma in pregnancy can be divided into blunt and penetrating abdominal trauma. Motor vehicle accidents are the most common type of blunt abdominal trauma seen, with falls and assaults being seen with approximately equal lesser frequency (Connolly et al., 1997). Some data suggest that patterns of domestic violence may escalate during pregnancy (ACOG, 2006b). The most common complication seen with blunt abdominal trauma in pregnancy is preterm labor, which occurs in up to 28% of cases. A more serious complication of blunt abdominal trauma is placental abruption, which can progress rapidly and be life threatening for both the mother and the fetus. Penetrating abdominal trauma is less common than blunt trauma in pregnancy. The pregnant uterus is actually protective of the mother's internal organs; the incidence of organ injury in pregnant women who suffer penetrating abdominal trauma, usually form gunshot or stab wounds, is between 16% and 38%, compared with 80%–90% injury rate in the general population (Stone, 1999).

Obstetric Conditions

Preterm Labor   Preterm labor puts the fetus at significant risk; 85% of all neonatal deaths that are not associated with congenital anomalies can be attributed to preterm delivery. One third of preterm deliveries are associated with placental hemorrhage or maternal hypertension. It is important to note that two thirds are due to spontaneous preterm labor with or without rupture of membranes (Meis et al., 1995). Many factors may increase the risk of preterm delivery. Prior preterm delivery is most predictive of recurrent preterm birth, with a rate of 20%–30%. Other contributing causes include an overdistended uterus (e.g., from multiple gestations), uterine or **cervical** abnormalities, low socioeconomic status, sexually transmitted diseases, intrauterine infections, and substance abuse.

Preterm Membrane Rupture   Preterm membrane rupture between 24–34 weeks' EGA occurs in less than 2% of pregnancies but contributes to 20% of all prenatal deaths during that period. (Cox, Williams, & Leveno, 1988; Parry & Straus, 1998). Preterm membrane rupture is associated with other obstetric complications, including multifetal gestation, **chorioamnionitis** (infection of the amniotic membranes), FHR abnormalities, and abruption. Tocolytics have not been effective in delaying delivery in the presence of rupture of membranes. Although a NIH Consensus Conference concluded the use of corticosteroids to promote fetal lung maturation in the presence of rupture of membranes is controversial, they are often given. Antibiotics are prescribed to these women, as antibiotics prolong the interval between rupture of membranes and delivery (Mercer & Arheart, 1995). Delivery is indicated if intrauterine infection develops.

Abruption   Placental abruption, or abruptio placenta, is premature separation of the placenta from the uterus (Figure 3.2). It is a significant cause of both maternal and fetal mortality and occurs in approximately 1% of pregnancies in the United States (Saftlas et al., 1991). The usual presentation of an abruption includes bleeding, uterine contractions, and FHR abnormalities. The uterine contractions are painful

and often very close together, resulting in rapid delivery. The fetus may develop distress rapidly and then may deteriorate quickly due to the significant and ongoing blood loss. A cesarean delivery is often necessary because of fetal distress. Perinatal mortality rates associated with placental abruption range from 20%–40%. Risk factors for abruption include ruptured membranes, chorioamnionitis, preeclampsia, maternal age greater than 35 years, and cocaine abuse (Kramer et al., 1997; see Table 3.3). The risk of recurrence is reported to be between 4% and 12%. Cigarette smoking also is associated with placental abruptions, with each pack per day smoked increasing the risk by 40%, and the perinatal mortality rate when placental abruption occurs is also significantly increased (Raymond & Mills, 1993). Trauma is also a significant cause of placental abruption.

Umbilical Cord Prolapse   **Umbilical cord prolapse** occurs when the umbilical cord descends through the birth canal in advance of the infant during labor. The incidence of the condition is approximately 0.4%, and it occurs more often when the infant has an abnormal presentation (see the Abnormal Presentations

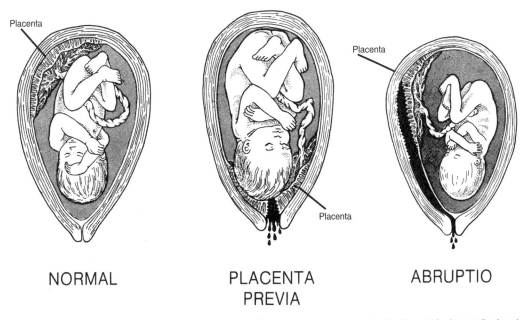

NORMAL   PLACENTA   ABRUPTIO
                PREVIA

Figure 3.2.   A normal placenta is located in the upper third of the uterus. In placenta pervia, the placenta is abnormally placed so that it lies over the cervical opening. During labor, as the cervix dilates, the placenta may tear and bleeding may occur. In abruptio placenta, a normally placed placenta becomes partially separated from the uterine wall in the second or third trimester, and bleeding results.

Table 3.3. Risk factors for abruption

Chorioamnionitis

Ruptured membranes > 24 hours prior to delivery

Low socioeconomic status

Preeclampsia/hypertension

Previous abruptio

Maternal age greater than 35 years

Cigarette smoking

Cocaine abuse

Male fetus

Trauma

discussion under the Special Conditions heading) or LBW. A prolapsed umbilical cord is prone to compressive forces which may compromise blood flow to the fetus, placing the infant at risk, and is therefore considered an obstetrical emergency (Kahana et al., 2004).

Perinatal Infections Cytomegalovirus (CMV), **parvovirus** B19, varicella zoster virus (chicken pox), and toxoplasmosis may be acquired by the mother and lead to adverse perinatal consequences. Typically, perinatal infections have more severe fetal consequences when acquired early in pregnancy. (See Chapter 6 for a discussion of the effect of infections on prenatal development.)

Although viral infections are usually contracted prior to or during delivery, most bacterial infections develop after birth, with the exception of Group B streptococcal (GBS) infection. GBS is the most common cause of neonatal meningitis and **sepsis** (McKenna & Iams, 1998). Approximately 8,000 cases of neonatal GBS infections occur yearly, with an incidence of 1.8 cases per 1,000 live births. Although maternal GBS infections are fairly benign, neonatal GBS infections carry a high risk of morbidity and mortality. Therefore, penicillin G (Bicillin) is recommended in labor for women colonized with GBS or those at high risk. Risk factors indicating antibiotic **prophylaxis** include prematurity, preterm rupture of membranes, membrane rupture greater than 18 hours before delivery, previous birth of a child with GBS infection, or maternal fever during labor greater than or equal to 100.4° F (38.0° C). Maternal GBS colonization is diagnosed by lower vaginal or rectal culture or presence in maternal urine. ACOG concurs with recommendations of the Centers for Disease Control and Prevention to culture all pregnant women at

35–37 weeks' gestation or to adopt a strategy for selective screening based on clinical risk factors.

Special Conditions

Abnormal Placentation Usually, the placenta is attached to the upper third of the uterus. Approximately one in every 200 pregnancies, however, is complicated by **placenta previa,** in which the placenta is implanted low in the uterus and lies over the cervical opening (Love & Wallace, 1996; Figure 3.2). The more extensive the overlay, the greater the risk of bleeding when the cervix dilates during labor. Even before labor begins, the effacement of the cervix or uterine contractions can cause bleeding. Significant hemorrhage may endanger both the fetus and the mother.

With improvement in obstetric care, including the performance of cesarean sections and administration of blood transfusion, maternal mortality is rare. Perinatal infant mortality remains a concern, however, primarily as a result of preterm birth in women with placenta previa. Placenta previa is more common in women who are older than 35 years of age or who have had multiple abortions. In addition, maternal smoking and a past history of a cesarean place women at increase risk for a placenta previa. Women with placenta previa are often prescribed decreased activity and pelvic rest (i.e., no intercourse) in an attempt to prolong pregnancy and avoid bleeding. A cesarean is frequently performed in an attempt to avoid life-threatening hemorrhage once it is has been determined that the fetus is mature enough to survive outside the uterus. At the time of cesarean delivery, individuals with placenta previa have a 5%–10% likelihood of requiring a hysterectomy. The recurrence rate for placenta previa is approximately 2.5% (Rasmussen, Albrechtsen, & Dalaker, 1996).

Another type of abnormal implantation is called **placenta accreta,** which results when the placenta abnormally attaches itself directly to the muscular wall of the uterus. Placenta accreta is usually associated with significant hemorrhage when the placenta is removed after delivery. Risk factors for developing an accreta include placenta previa, prior cesarean delivery, prior uterine curettage, and advanced maternal age (older than 35 years at delivery). Women with placenta previa and one previous cesarean delivery have a 25% risk of having placenta accreta. The risk of placenta accreta rises to 50%–

60% when there is a history of multiple cesarean births. These cases often result in such significant hemorrhage that transfusion and hysterectomy are required.

Multiple Gestations With the widespread use of assisted reproductive technologies, the incidence of multiple gestation pregnancies has increased dramatically. Between 1980 and 2002, the rate of twins increased from 1 per 53 to 1 per 32 and triplets from 1 per 2,703 to 1 per 543 (Martin et al., 2005), which are 65% and 497% increases, respectively. Multiple gestations accounted for 3.3% of all births in 2002. This is important because multiple gestations are at significantly increased risk for LBW and preterm labor and birth. Given that the two strongest factors influencing perinatal survival are gestational age at delivery and relative birth weight, it is easy to see that multiple gestations are at special risk for both short- and long-term complications.

Abnormal Presentations A breech presentation is one in which either the fetal buttocks or lower extremities are the presenting part or parts. A frank breech presentation means the infant's legs are flexed at the hip and extended at the knees so that the feet are close to the infant's head and the buttocks present first. An incomplete breech presentation occurs when a foot or knee is the presenting part, and the risk of umbilical cord prolapse is increased in this case. The incidence of breech presentation at term is approximately 3%. Some factors that increase the likelihood of a breech presentation include multiple gestation, uterine anomalies, polyhydramnios, and pelvic tumors. There has been significant controversy as to the safety of delivering breech infants vaginally. There is some data to suggest that performing a planned cesarean delivery is safer than a planned vaginal delivery for breech infants delivered at term (Hannah et al., 2000). As result of this data, ACOG recommended cesarean delivery for persistent breech presentation at term (ACOG, 2006a). Consequently, the rate of cesarean delivery for breech infants at term increased from 12% in 1970 to 87% in 2001.

An alternative to cesarean delivery for breech infants is external cephalic version (ECV). In an ECV, an attempt is made to turn the fetus to the cephalic (head down) position by manipulating the maternal abdomen. It is usually attempted at 37 weeks' gestation and has a success rate of approximately 60%. The rate of conversion back to a breech position is very low. Thus, most fetuses that are successfully turned will deliver vaginally, allowing the mother to avoid a cesarean.

A transverse presentation of the fetus at term occurs in approximately 1 in 360 deliveries. It is often initially suspected by inspection of the maternal abdomen that appears unusually wide. Common causes and associated anomalies in transverse lies include multiple previous gestations, excessive amniotic fluid, prematurity, and placenta previa. If the fetus remains in a transverse position, vaginal delivery is impossible. If the amniotic sac breaks, the fetus is at risk for prolapsing the umbilical cord through the cervix, necessitating emergency cesarean delivery.

Face presentations, in which the neck of the fetus is hyperextended and the chin is the presenting part, occur in only 2 per 1,000 pregnancies. These are diagnosed by vaginal exam. Risk factors include multiple previous pregnancies, and anencephalic fetus (see Chapter 28), and a large fetus. With normal labor, face presentations will often convert to the normal vertex position and can be delivered vaginally.

Birth Injuries and Defects Birth injuries occur in 2–7 per 1,000 of deliveries (Creasy et al., 2004). Some of the most common injuries include facial nerve palsy, fracture of the clavicle, and brachial plexus injuries. The facial nerve may be injured during delivery by compression. Although often attributed to forceps delivery, the majority of cases are encountered after either cesarean or spontaneous vaginal deliveries. Nearly all of these injuries resolve quickly within the first few days of life.

Fractured clavicles occur in approximately 4 per 1,000 of vaginal births (Roberts et al., 1995). Although these may occur during deliveries complicated by shoulder dystocia (in which the shoulder becomes lodged in the mother's pelvic opening after delivery of the baby's head), they often occur during uncomplicated births. A large study of more that 65,000 deliveries looked at the occurrence of clavicular fractures in an attempt to determine what factors may be associated and therefore avoided. The researchers concluded that this injury appears to be unpredictable, but fortunately it does not cause long-term problems (Roberts et al., 1995).

Brachial plexus injuries are reported to occur in approximately 1–2 per 1,000 deliveries

(Gilbert, Thomas, & Beate, 1999). There are multiple factors associated with brachial plexus injuries, but none of them have been found to be predictive enough to permit prevention. It is known, however, that women with gestational diabetes who undergo a forceps delivery or vacuum extraction or who experience shoulder dystocia are at increased risk for delivering a baby with a brachial plexus injury. The most common types of brachial plexus injuries are Erb's palsy and Klumpke's palsy. In Erb's palsy, the infant's affected arm lies limp at his or her side and the grasp reflex is intact. In Klumpke's palsy, the hand is paralyzed, and the grasp reflex is absent. Fortunately, more than 90% of all brachial plexus injuries resolve within 6 months with no sequelae (Nocon et al., 1993).

Certain malformations of the fetus may make labor and delivery difficult or may necessitate a cesarean delivery. For example, fetuses with hydrocephalus may have such an enlarged head that vaginal delivery is impossible. Fetuses with enlarged bladders or renal or hepatic tumors may also not be candidates for vaginal delivery because of the enlarged fetal abdomen.

SUMMARY

The period of late pregnancy, labor, and delivery is a critical one for the live birth and normal development of the infant. Complications can result from such different sources as preexisting maternal disease, preeclampsia, preterm labor and delivery, premature rupture of membranes, perinatal maternal illness, abnormal placentation, breech presentation, multiple gestation, and birth injuries. The impact of such complications can be severe and long lasting. Fortunately, the vast majority of babies are born well, and improved prenatal care and surveillance have improved outcomes in high-risk pregnancies. Nevertheless, additional public health measures, including improved prenatal care of teenagers and women with limited resources, are needed to ensure the health of pregnant women and their infants.

REFERENCES

American College of Obstetricians and Gynecologists. (2001). Gestational diabetes (ACOG Practice Bulletin 30). *Obstetrics and Gynecology, 98*, 525–538.

American College of Obstetricians and Gynecologists. (2002). Perinatal viral and parasitic infections (ACOG Practice Bulletin 20). *International Journal of Gynecology and Obstetrics, 76*, 95–107.

American College of Obstetricians and Gynecologists. (2003). Dystocia and the augmentation of labor (ACOG Technical Bulletin 218). *Obstetrics and Gynecology, 102*, 1445–1454.

American College of Obstetricians and Gynecologists. (2006a). Mode of term singleton breech delivery (ACOG Committee on Obstetric Practice Committee Opinion 340). *Obstetrics and Gynecology, 108*, 235–237.

American College of Obstetricians and Gynecologists. (2006b). Psychosocial risk factors: Perinatal screening and intervention (ACOG Committee on Obstetric Practice Committee Opinion 343). *Obstetrics and Gynecology, 108*, 469–477.

Chauhan, S.P., Perry, K.G., Jr., McLaughlin, B.N., et al. (1996). Diabetic ketoacidosis complicating pregnancy. *Journal of Perinatology, 16*(3), 173–175.

Connolly, A., Katz, V.L., Bash, K.L., et al. (1997). Trauma and pregnancy. *American Journal of Perinatology, 14*(6), 331–336.

Cox, S., Williams, M.L., & Leveno K.J. (1988). The natural history of preterm ruptured membranes: What to expect from expectant management. *Obstetrics and Gynecology, 71*, 558.

Creasy, R.K., Resnik, R., & Iams, J. (2004). *Maternal-fetal medicine: Principles and practice* (5th ed.). Philadelphia: W.B. Saunders.

Crowther, C.A., Hiller, J.E., Moss, J.R., et al. (2005). Effect of treatment of gestational diabetes mellitus on pregnancy outcomes. *The New England Journal of Medicine, 352*, 2477–2486.

Cunningham, F.G., Leveno, K.J., Boom, S.L., et al. (2005). *Williams obstetrics* (22nd ed). New York: McGraw-Hill.

DiMarco, C.S., Ramsey, P.S., Williams, L.H., et al. (2000). Temporal trends in operative obstetric delivery: 1992–1999. *Obstetrics and Gynecology, 95*(4, Suppl. 1), S39.

Dunne, F.P. (1999). Pregestational diabetes mellitus and pregnancy. *Trends in Endocrinology and Metabolism, 10*(5), 179–182.

Eskew, P.N., Jr., Saywell, R.M. Jr., et al. (1994). Trends in the frequency of cesarean delivery: A 21-year experience, 1970–1990. *The Journal of Reproductive Medicine, 39*(10), 809–817.

Flamm, B.L. (1995). Vaginal birth after cesarean section. In B.L. Flamm & E.J. Quilligan (Eds.). *Cesarean section: Guidelines for appropriate utilization* (pp. 51–64). New York: Springer-Verlag.

Freeman, R.K., Garite, T.H., & Nageotte, M.P. (1991). *Fetal heart rate monitoring* (2nd ed.). Philadelphia: Lippincott, Williams & Wilkins.

Gilbert, W.M., Thomas, N.S., & Beate, D. (1999). Associated factors in 1611 cases of brachial plexus injuries. *Obstetrics and Gynecology, 93*(4), 536–540.

Hankins, G.D.V., D'Alton, M., Depp, R., et al. (2003). *Neonatal encephalopathy and cerebral palsy: Defining the pathogenesis and pathophysiology.* Washington, DC: The American College of Obstetricians and Gynecologists & The American Academy of Pediatrics.

Hannah, M.E., Hannah, W.J., Hewson, S.A., et al. (2000). Planned caesarean section versus planned vaginal birth for breech presentation at term: A randomized multicenter trial. *The Lancet, 356*, 1375–1783.

Hon, E. (1968). *An atlas of fetal heart rate patterns.* New Haven, CT: Harty.

Kahana, B., Sheiner, E., Levy, A., et al. (2004). Umbilical cord prolapse and perinatal outcomes. *International Journal of Gynaecology and Obstetrics, 84*(2), 127–132.

Kramer, M.S., Usher, R.H., Pollack, R., et al. (1997). Etiologic determinants of abruptio placentae. *Obstetrics and Gynecology, 89*(2), 221–226.

Love, C.D., & Wallace, E.M. (1996). Pregnancies complicated by placenta previa: What is appropriate management? *British Journal of Obstetrics and Gynaecology, 103*, 864–867.

Martin, J.A., Kochanek, K.D., Strobino, D.M., et al. (2005). Annual summary of vital statistics: 2003. *Pediatrics, 115*(3), 619–634.

McKenna, D.S., & Iams, J.D. (1998). Group B streptococcal infections. *Seminars in Perinatology, 22*(4), 267–276.

Meis, P.T., Michielutte, R., Peters, T.J., et al. (1995). Factors associated with preterm birth in Cardiff, Wales. *American Journal of Obstetrics and Gynecology, 173*, 590.

Mercer, B.M., & Arheart, K.L. (1995). Antimicrobial therapy in expectant management of preterm premature rupture of membranes. *The Lancet, 346*, 1271–1279.

Mroz, L.A. (1999). Hypertensive disorders of pregnancy. *Anesthesiology Clinics of North America, 17*(3), 679–691.

Nocon, J.J., McKenzie, D.K., Thomas, L.J., et al. (1993). Shoulder dystocia: An analysis of risks and obstetric maneuvers. *American Journal of Obstetrics and Gynecology, 168*(6, Pt. 1), 1732–1737; discussion, 1737–1739.

Napolitano, P.G., Hoeldtke, N., Moore, K., et al. (1997). The fetoplacental pressor effects of low-dose acetylsalicylic acid and angiotensin II in the ex vivo cotyledon model. *American Journal of Obstetrics and Gynecology, 177*, 1093–1096.

Norwitz, E., Robinson, J., & Challis, J. (1999). The control of labor. *The New England Journal of Medicine, 341*(9), 660–666.

Parry, S., & Strauss, J.F. (1998). Premature rupture of fetal membranes. *The New England Journal of Medicine, 338*(10), 663–670.

Rasmussen, S., Albrechtsen, S., & Dalaker, D. (1996). Obstetric history and the risk of placenta previa. *Acta Obstetrica et Gynecologica Scandinavia, 79*(6), 502–507.

Raymond, E.G., & Mills, J.L. (1993). Placental abruption: Maternal risk factors and associated fetal conditions. *Acta Obstetrica et Gynecologica Scandinavia, 72*(8), 633–639.

Roberts, S.W., Hernandez, C., Maberry, M.C., et al. (1995). Obstetric clavicular fracture: The enigma of normal birth. *Obstetrics and Gynecology, 86*, 978.

Rosen, M.G., Dickinson, J.C., & Westhoff, C.L. (1991). Vaginal birth after cesarean: A meta-analysis of morbidity and mortality. *Obstetrics and Gynecology, 77*, 465–470.

Saftlas, A.F., Olson, D.R., Atrash, H.K., et al. (1991). National trends in the incidence of abruptio placentae, 1979–1987. *Obstetrics and Gynecology, 78*(6), 1081–1086.

Sibai, B. (1996). Treatment of hypertension in pregnant women. *The New England Journal of Medicine, 335*(4), 257–265.

Stone, I.K. (1999). Trauma in the obstetric patient. *Obstetrics and Gynecology Clinics of North America, 26*(3), 459–467.

Wesley, B., Van den Berg, B., & Reece, E.A. (1993). The effect of forceps delivery on cognitive development. *American Journal of Obstetrics and Gynecology, 169*(5), 1091–1095.

4

The First Weeks of Life

Chrysanthe Gaitatzes, Taeun Chang, and Stephen Baumgart

> Upon completion of this chapter the reader will
> - Have a basic understanding of the events taking place during transition from fetal to extrauterine life
> - Have a basic understanding of neonatal problems associated with long-term disability, such as persistent pulmonary hypertension, hypoxic ischemic encephalopathy, neonatal seizures, hypoglycemia and other metabolic disturbances, neonatal stroke, neonatal infection, and neonatal hyperbilirubinemia

Given that most infants are born into the world without any special difficulty, it is easy to take for granted the astonishing complexity of the birth process. Several events have to take place in a precise and well-timed sequence for the newborn to have a healthy beginning. Understanding the basic principles of normal fetal physiology is key to understanding the normal transition to the extrauterine environment that occurs at the time of birth.

JUSTIN

Justin was born at 39 weeks' gestation to a 26 year-old mother. This was her third pregnancy; she had previously delivered two healthy full-term infants. Justin's mother developed insulin-dependent diabetes during her pregnancy (a blood sugar high enough to require treatment). Other prenatal laboratory screening tests were unremarkable. She presented to the hospital in active labor (uterine contractions occurring every few minutes). Fetal heart rate monitoring (fetal heart sounds detected by ultrasound) revealed fetal distress with long periods of abnormally low heart rate during and between labor contractions, indicating a poor oxygen supply to the baby's heart muscle and other vital organs. Justin was therefore delivered by emergency cesarean section (a surgical delivery of the fetus), with anesthesia and surgery performed within 20 minutes of detecting his dis-

tress. The obstetric doctor noted that Justin had passed thick **meconium** (first bowel movement, usually passed after birth) into the amniotic fluid before his delivery. Because of his mother's diabetes, he was **large for gestational age (LGA)**, weighing more than 4 kilograms (or more than 9 pounds). This made his delivery somewhat difficult mechanically through the small cesarean incision.

THE FETUS BEFORE BIRTH

The Fetal Circulation

The fetal heart begins to develop during the third week of gestation. It starts to beat during the fourth week, and soon after that blood circulation is established. Blood carrying oxygen and nutrients circulates from the placenta through the umbilical cord via a single umbilical vein. The umbilical vein then passes through the ductus venosus near the baby's liver into the inferior vena cava (the main vein feeding into the baby's heart). The vena cava blood flows into the right atrium and then the right ventricle of the heart. In our adult circulation, blood exits the right ventricle via the **pulmonary** artery into the lungs. In the fetus, only 10% of the blood volume ejected out of the right ventricle goes through the pulmonary blood vessels that pass into the lungs. The rest (90%) is shunted away from the right and into the left side of the fetal heart through the foramen ovale (a tiny window between the right atrium and the left atrium) and through the ductus arteriosus (a fetal blood vessel that bypasses the main pulmonary artery and lungs). This way, oxygenated blood from the placenta flows into the aorta to enter the systemic circulation, perfusing the entire body and its major organs (Figure 4.1). After the vital organs extract oxygen and nutrients from the arterial blood circulation, venous blood returns to the placenta via two umbilical arteries that pass out of the umbilical cord to get replenished with oxygen and nutrients derived from the mother's circulation and to have carbon dioxide (CO_2), heat, and other metabolic waste products (e.g., acids) removed (placental circulation; Figure 4.1).

The fetal lungs play no role in oxygenation (transfer of O_2 into the baby) or ventilation (removal of CO_2 from the baby) prior to birth. They receive only a small percentage of the fetal circulating blood volume. Instead, the fetal lungs are filled with a clear fluid secreted by the lung cells, which act like a gland during prenatal life. Some of this fluid, in combination with the fetus' urine, comprises the amniotic fluid.

Amniotic Fluid, Kidneys, and Gastrointestinal Tract

Amniotic fluid is important for cushioning the infant within the mother's uterus, for allowing free movement of developing limbs and muscles, and for promoting symmetric unrestricted body growth. Amniotic fluid is also essential for normal lung development, as the fetus practices breathing movements before birth. An appropriate amount of amniotic fluid is therefore critically important to normal lung exercise and development. The presence of too little fluid (oligohydramnios) is associated with hypoplastic lungs (small, underdeveloped lungs). The presence of too much amniotic fluid (polyhydramnios) may be associated with certain malformations that obstruct the amniotic fluid circulation through the gastrointestinal system (fetal swallowing), kidneys, and the fetal heart.

Before birth, the fetal kidneys produce sterile urine, which comprises the majority of the amniotic fluid volume. The fetus urinates regularly while in utero. If the kidneys do not function properly, the mother develops oligohydramnios. The genitourinary tract continues to develop even after birth, as urine volume increases during rapid postnatal body growth.

The gastrointestinal tract is also very active during fetal development. The fetus swallows and absorbs amniotic fluid regularly. Meconium (fetal stool that is not normally passed until after birth) consists mostly of swallowed amniotic fluid debris, gastrointestinal mucous, green bile secretions from the liver, and sloughed off gastrointestinal lining cells. Meconium begins to form during the first trimester of pregnancy. Under normal nonstress conditions, the fetus does not pass meconium in utero. Meconium-stained amniotic fluid is a sign of intrauterine fetal distress, usually caused by lack of oxygen from the placenta, which stimulates early bowel movement. Meconium can be irritating and dangerous to the baby if aspirated into the lungs at the time of delivery.

The Nervous System

Fetal brain development represents a very delicate sequence of events (see Chapter 2). Disruptions of these events can lead to subtle or serious brain malformations. The fetal brain has been shown to be active prenatally. Functional imaging techniques (e.g., **positron emission tomography [PET]** scans, **magnetic resonance spectroscopy [MRS]**) are used to elucidate the activity level of various areas of the brain at different stages during fetal development. Many fetal reflexes have been identified, such as swallowing and sucking, which provide a crucial foundation of skills needed for the infant to survive the early days and weeks of postnatal life.

In the sections that follow, the typical fetal-to-neonatal transition process is described, presuming that fetal development has otherwise progressed normally until the full term of human gestation (37–40 weeks). Departures from the typical birthing processes are also described, highlighting some of the most commonly encountered early life problems that result in a serious risk for future impairment.

THE BIRTH PROCESS

JUSTIN

After the obstetrician delivered Justin's head but before delivering his body, she suctioned his nostrils and throat with a bulb syringe, to clear as much of the meconium out of his airways as possible prior to his first breath. After Justin was delivered, he was quickly placed under a radiant heating lamp. He was apneic (not breathing on his own) and had poor muscle tone (i.e., he was as flaccid as a rag doll). The pediatrician in atten-

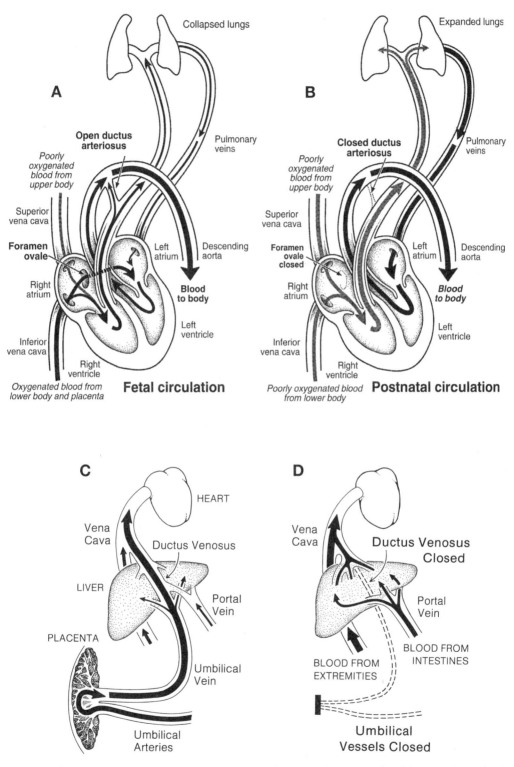

Figure 4.1. Circulation. Top half of figure: A) Fetal circulation. The foramen ovale and patent (open) ductus arteriosus allow the blood flow to bypass the unexpanded lungs. B) Postnatal circulation. The fetal bypasses close off with expansion of the lungs. Bottom half of figure: C) Fetal-placental circulation. The blood from the umbilical vein bypasses the liver through the ductus venosus. D) Postnatal circulation. The umbilical vein ceases to function and the ductus venosus closes. Now blood from the body passes through the liver, where it is cleansed.

dance for this high-risk delivery placed a plastic tube into his airway (intubation), and suction was applied. Thick, tar-like meconium was aspirated out of the trachea. The procedure was repeated three times, until no more meconium was cleared. By then, the baby was 80 seconds old and had not taken his first breath (persisting apnea). His heart rate was about 60 beats per minute (bpm; normal heart rate is above 100 bpm). On the basis of the **Apgar scoring system,** the first-minute Apgar score (see Table 4.1) was assigned, giving Justin only 1 point (for the presence of a slow heart rate under 100 bpm). Justin was vigorously stimulated by rubbing his chest and abdomen with a warm, dry towel, and **positive pressure ventilation** (PPV, or artificial breathing) was provided with a rubber facemask and bag, connected to 100% oxygen. After 30 seconds of PPV, Justin continued to have no respiratory effort, and his heart rate was now less than 60 bpm. The pediatrician started chest compressions of the sternum over the baby's heart while a nurse continued PPV, and after 30 seconds, Justin's heart began to beat at a normal rate of approximately 120–140 bpm. The medical team continued to stimulate Justin, but his breathing effort remained very erratic. A tube was once again placed into his trachea, but this time it was taped into place to allow Justin to receive mechanical ventilation. His Apgar score at 5 minutes was 3 (2 points for heart rate above 100 per minute and 1 point awarded for attempted but poor respirations). Justin remained completely flaccid, with no muscle tone or spontaneous movement.

The First Breath

Under normal circumstances, the fetal lungs are filled with fluid. Although they receive a small portion of the cardiac output before birth, they are not responsible for exchange of respiratory gases (oxygen and carbon dioxide). The process of clearing the fluid from the alveoli (the tiny air sacks where gases are exchanged) is stimulated by the initiation of labor (Bland, 1992; Welty, Hansen, & Corbet, 2005). The mechanical compression of the infant's chest as it passes through the narrow birth canal contributes to the fluid's evacuation out of the **alveoli.**

The first breath for any newborn baby is the hardest to take. The pressure that the newborn has to generate against the lung fluid (or surface tension) approaches an incredible 60 centimeters (cm) of water, whereas normal adult respirations at rest only generate 2–3 cm of water pressure. This amount of initial force is very difficult to generate and is like blowing air through a 2- to 3-foot long straw or snorkel under water. After the first few breaths, the majority of the fluid is pushed out of the alveoli and is absorbed into the pulmonary capillaries and lymphatic vessels by this forceful breathing effort. Thereafter, breathing becomes much easier (Nelson, 2005; Figure 4.2), and normal gas exchange (oxygen for carbon dioxide) takes place. The effort required to breath is also reduced when the first breath into the alveolar spaces stimulates the secretion of **surfactant** from gland-like cells in the lung. Surfactant is a lipoprotein that acts like a soap bubble, allowing for a significant decrease in the alveolar membrane's surface tension, making breathing much easier and the lungs much more flexible.

Aeration also improves **PaO_2** (a measurement of the pressure of oxygen in the infant's blood), increases pH (blood acidity), and decreases the $PaCO_2$ (the pressure of carbon dioxide, a waste by-product of the infant's metabolism). These changes enhance **pulmonary vasodilation** (relaxation and dilation of blood vessels within the lung) in response to gas entry,

Table 4.1.   Apgar scoring system for the newborn's transition to normal breathing and activity during the first five minutes of life after birth

	Sign	0 Points	1 Point	2 Points
A	Activity (Muscle tone)	Absent, flaccid	Arms and legs flexed	Vigorous movements
P	Pulse	Absent	< 100 bpm	> 100 bpm
G	Grimace (reflex irritability)	No response	Grimacing only	Sneezing, coughing, crying
A	Appearance (skin color)	Blue-gray, pale despite oxygen administration	Normally pink, except for extremities, may require oxygen to become pink	Normally pink over entire body without giving extra oxygen
R	Respiration	Absent (i.e., apnea)	Slow, irregular, or gasping	Good, vigorous, crying

Key: bpm, beats per minute.

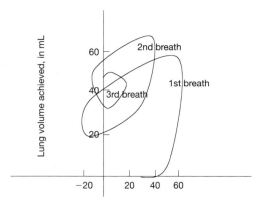

Transpulmonary pressure generated, in cm H$_2$O

Figure 4.2. The first three breaths of neonatal life, indicating that the most pressure (on the horizontal axis) is required for the first breath while the lung volume (on the vertical axis) fills with air, making the second and third breaths much easier to achieve full lung volume (i.e., requiring less and less pressure successively). (From Nelson, N.M. [2005]. The onset of respiration. In G.B. Avery, M.A. Fletcher, & M.G. MacDonald [Eds.], *Neonatology: Pathophysiology and management of the newborn* [5th ed., p. 265]. Philadelphia: Lippincott, Williams & Wilkins; Copyright © 2005 Lippincott, Williams & Wilkins; adapted by permission.) (*Key:* mL, milliliter; cm, centimeter.)

allowing blood to circulate more freely through the lungs. The flow of blood to the lungs stimulates the closure of the ductus arteriosus and the foramen ovale, completing the transition from fetal circulation to the postnatal adult-like circulation.

Apgar Score

Virginia Apgar (1909–1974) was a physician and humanitarian who is best known for the scoring system she devised in 1952 for systematically assessing the well-being of newborns. This scoring system is still in routine use today and consists of a total of 10 points that are given for the infant's color appearance, heart rate, respirations, reflex irritability when stimulated, and muscle tone at rest (Table 4.1). The Apgar score is usually assigned at 1 and at 5 minutes of life. When resuscitation is required, as for baby Justin, a 10-minute Apgar score is added. The 1-minute Apgar primarily reflects the baby's condition resulting from the intrauterine experience immediately prior to birth; the 5- and 10-minute scores reflect the baby's condition in the immediate postnatal period. Apgar scores are most helpful in allowing health care professionals to communicate their impression of a new-

born's condition with other health care professionals; Apgar scores are not intended to determine decisions regarding resuscitation and generally are not predictive of long-term developmental outcomes.

JUSTIN

While Justin was in the delivery room and after the umbilical cord was cut by the delivering obstetrician, a central (deep vein) intravenous catheter was placed via Justin's umbilical cord stump. Through that line, Justin received an infusion of normal saline (a salt solution used to improve circulatory perfusion and to correct low blood pressure). Initial measurement of his serum glucose level showed significant hypoglycemia (a dangerously low blood sugar level, probably due to the mother's poor blood sugar regulation as a result of her diabetes). He was then given a bolus of intravenous dextrose (a simple sugar similar to glucose to correct his blood sugar) and was transferred to the **neonatal intensive care unit (NICU)** for further management.

In the NICU, Justin's endotracheal tube was connected to a mechanical **ventilator** to assist his breathing. He was started on a continuous infusion of dopamine (an adrenaline-like drug) to increase his falling blood pressure and to promote recirculation to his brain. He continued to require 100% oxygen to stay pink (instead of the 21% oxygen found in room air). That high oxygen requirement, in combination with the history of meconium aspiration in the delivery room, suggested the possibility that Justin had developed the condition known as **persistent pulmonary hypertension of the newborn (PPHN).**

Persistent Pulmonary Hypertension of the Newborn (Persistent Fetal Circulation)

In the fetus, the pulmonary blood vessels offer high resistance to blood flow from the heart, allowing blood oxygenated in the placenta to bypass the nonfunctioning fetal lungs and to enter the rest of the body. At birth, the **pulmonary vascular resistance** must drop (the blood vessels of the lungs must dilate) to allow the lungs to take over the function of delivering oxygen to the blood. For reasons that are not fully understood, this drop in pulmonary vascular resistance does not occur in a timely manner in some infants. The first spontaneous breath facilitates vasodilation by causing alterations in the blood (improved pH, oxygen, and carbon dioxide content), so lack of this first breath may hamper the changeover process. Persistent pulmonary blood vessel constriction causes decreased circulation through the lungs and blue (deoxygenated) blood to be shunted from the right side of the heart to the left side of the heart through the **patent ductus arteriosus (PDA)** and/or through the foramen ovale, without first going through the lungs to get oxygenated and to exhale carbon dioxide (Figure 4.1a). This causes a significant strain to the heart (from both hypoxia and high blood pressure in the lungs) and can possibly cause heart failure (resulting in shock for the rest of the body).

In addition to meconium aspiration, pneumonia, sepsis (bacterial infection in the blood or in the lungs), aspiration of amniotic fluid or blood, and lung hypoplasia (insufficient development of the lungs) can cause PPHN. Most infants with PPHN respond in time to administered oxygen with mechanical ventilation, or to **inhaled nitric oxide (iNO),** a new therapeutic gas mixed with the baby's oxygen supply. For infants that do not respond to iNO, the only remaining life-saving therapy is a procedure known as **extracorporeal membrane oxygenation,** or ECMO. ECMO is an invasive life-support system that passes blood through an artificial membrane lung oxygenator by placement of large catheters in blood vessels in the infant's neck (the right jugular vein and right internal carotid artery directly feeding into the brain). The baby's circulating blood is redirected by a mechanical pump through the artificial membrane lung oxygenator, thus bypassing the baby's native lungs and/or the heart (if the baby's heart has also failed); ECMO is, in effect, a heart-lung bypass machine. ECMO is administered until the infant's lung blood vessels are able to relax on their own.

JUSTIN

Justin responded well to iNO, and within a few days his oxygen level was weaned from 100% oxygen back to room air; by 2 weeks of life, he was able to breathe on his own. A head **computed tomography (CT)** scan that was obtained when he was 4 days old, however, revealed evidence of diffuse hypoxic injury to his brain. Just before going home, Justin had a **magnetic resonance imaging (MRI)** scan of the brain that confirmed global, severe cerebral injury involving multiple cortical and subcortical areas of the brain.

By his third week of life, Justin was off of intravenous nutrition. He was able to tolerate formula provided through a feeding tube, but he showed no evidence of a suck reflex or a protective gag reflex, raising concerns that he might not be able to recover the oral-motor skills necessary to feed on his own. At the time of his discharge from the NICU, Justin was receiving his feedings through a nasogastric tube, with the understanding that if he was unable to recover oral feeding skills, he might eventually require a permanent gastrostomy feeding tube (see Chapter 31). Justin's parents also understood that he was at high risk for cerebral palsy, intellectual disability, and hearing and vision problems; appropriate early intervention therapy and a medical follow-up were scheduled accordingly.

Hypoxic Ischemic Encephalopathy

Hypoxic (low oxygen) ischemic (low blood pressure and low blood flow) encephalopathy, or HIE, is caused by changes in the blood flow and the oxygen supply to the brain. It is now widely accepted that HIE can occur prenatally due to placental insufficiency that is often associated with maternal problems (e.g., the gestational diabetes that Justin's mother had), or it can occur postnatally due to cardiorespiratory failure at birth, which produces disturbances to the cerebral blood flow. HIE is much less likely to be the product of poor obstetrical management. In Justin's case, the mother presented in labor with signs of fetal distress already evident, and a cesarean was preformed promptly within 20 minutes of recognizing the low fetal heart rate. When HIE develops, the body responds by redistributing blood away from "nonvital organs" (e.g., kidneys, liver, lungs, intestines, skeletal muscles) in order to maintain the perfusion of the "vital organs" (i.e., the heart, brain, and adrenal glands). This is why kidney and liver failure often occur concurrently with severe HIE .

Full-term infants with HIE have abnormal neurological function from birth, including decreased activity level, poor suck and feeding difficulty, respiratory difficulty with retained mucous secretions in the lungs, temperature instability (hypothermia, and/or fevers in early infancy), and **neonatal seizures.** Prenatal risk factors are those that compromise placental blood supply to the fetus, such as maternal diabetes (as in Justin's case), or maternal hypertension (also termed preeclampsia or toxemia of pregnancy), placental abruption (early separation of the placenta from the uterine wall interrupting oxygen supply), maternal shock, severe maternal bleeding (often resulting from an abruption), umbilical cord prolapse (delivery of the cord prior to the baby, resulting in compression of the infant's blood flow during labor), and intrauterine growth restriction (IUGR; often resulting from retarded placental development).

The most popular system for grading the severity of HIE in neonates is known as the **Sarnat neurological score** (Sarnat & Sarnat, 1976). This system includes several clinical findings as well as electroencephalography (EEG) testing. HIE is graded into three stages, with Stage 3 being the most severe (Table 4.2). Unlike the Apgar score, the Sarnat neurological score has demonstrated an ability to predict subsequent delays in neurological development. A baby with a Sarnat score of 1 may be hyper-alert and jittery for a day or so after birth but is likely to recover completely before going home in 2–3 days. He or she is at low risk for cerebral palsy or intellectual disability. A baby with a Sarnat score of 3 (like Justin) is much more likely to either die shortly after birth or to go on to develop cerebral palsy and global developmental delay by 1–2 years of age (in almost 70% of cases).

Neuroimaging is very helpful in assessing the extent of the hypoxic-ischemic injury. A severely abnormal CT or MRI scan performed shortly after birth showing involvement of both cerebral hemispheres and deep structural abnormalities, as in Justin's case, is strongly correlated with a poor neurodevelopmental outcome in survivors (Bianioni et al., 2001; Rutherford et al., 2004). A specific MRI technique known as **diffusion-weighted imaging (DWI)** is currently the gold standard for identifying early ischemic injury. Five pathology distinct patterns of brain injury caused by HIE have been noted and may correlate with specific functional outcomes (Volpe, 2001).

The medical management of infants with HIE is mostly life-supportive care. Hypoxemia (low oxygen), hypercarbia (high carbon dioxide), acidosis, hypotension (low blood pressure; i.e., shock), hypoglycemia (low blood glucose), seizures, and other metabolic disturbances are corrected with the use of oxygen, mechanical ventilation, intravenous medications, seizure medications, control of brain edema, and thermoregulation support. Antiepileptic medications are often necessary. Other medications such as excitatory amino acid (glutamine) **antagonists,** anti-inflammatory **steroids** (e.g., dexamethasone), nitric oxide synthase inhibitors, antioxidants, calcium channel blockers, or magnesium, along with barbiturates in very high doses are currently being studied to determine if they can slow the neuronal **necrosis** process (Whitelaw & Thoresen, 2002). Brain cooling or hypothermia (decrease of brain temperature and therefore decrease of metabolic activity) is now an area of intense research, with promising results in animal and early human neonatal studies (Bruno et al., 1994; Gluckman et al., 2005; Gunn & Gunn, 1998).

Long-term follow-up with neurologists and developmental specialists is vitally necessary for infants like Justin. Outcome is difficult to predict. It varies from learning disabilities when children reach school age (Chapter 25), to

Table 4.2. Sarnat examination for scoring neonatal encephalopathy

Factor	Stage 1	Stage 2	Stage 3
Level of consciousness	Hyper-alert appearance	Obtunded/lethargic	Stuporous/coma
Neuromuscular tone	Normal, vigorous	Hypotonia, looseness	Flaccid or fixed stiffness (decerebrate posturing)
Reflexes	Hyperactive Moro reflex	Weak primitive reflexes	Absent reflexes
Autonomic (vital signs)	Fast heart rate (tachycardia)	Slow heart rate (bradycardia), pupils constricted	Slower heart rate, pupils dilated/unreactive
Seizures	None	Multifocal	Brainstem reflex only
Electroencephalogram (EEG)	Normal, organized rhythms, sleep cycles present	Epileptic threshold (delta waves seen)	Depressed or absent voltages, flat EEG, electrographic seizures present

Source: Sarnat and Sarnat (1976).

Stage 1: Mild encephalopathy that lasts for less than 24 hours: child is likely to have typical developmental outcome.

Stage 2: Moderate encephalopathy that lasts for less than 5 days: child is likely to have a typical development outcome; if it lasts for more than 7 days: child is likely to have a poor outcome.

Stage 3: Severe encephalopathy results in severe impairment or death (likely in 70% of cases).

visual and hearing impairment (Chapters 11 and 12), to intellectual disability (Chapter 17), to cerebral palsy (Chapter 26) (Hardy, 2003). According to the National Collaborative Perinatal Project (NCPP; Hardy, 2003), factors that were found to be associated with increased morbidity in follow-up visits include decreased activity after the first day of life, temperature instability past the first 3 days of life, poor feeding, and breathing difficulties.

Neonatal Seizures

Possible causes of neonatal seizures are very broad. They may occur as a consequence of HIE but are also seen associated with metabolic disturbances such as **hypoglycemia, hypocalcemia** (low blood calcium), hyper- or hyponatremia (high or low sodium most often caused by incorrect mixing of infant formulas), and other electrolyte imbalances. Other causes of neonatal seizures include traumatic brain injury from forceps or vacuum-assisted deliveries; maternal trauma with in utero injury to the fetus; thrombosis (clot) or brain hemorrhage (bleed), also called a cerebrovascular accident (CVA; stroke); infections such as **meningitis** (inflammation and/or infection of the meninges) or encephalitis (infection of the brain itself); inborn errors of metabolism (genetically inherited enzymatic problems of amino acid or protein regulation); and maternal substance abuse (e.g., heroin, cocaine, methamphetamine, diazepam abuse).

Neonatal seizures can present clinically (physically evident) or electrographically (without any external signs or symptoms of seizure activity). Clinical seizures often manifest as stiffening (tonic) or jerking (clonic) movements of the arms or legs or as bicycling or rowing movements of the extremities. They can also be very subtle, such as orolingual movements like spasmodic lip smacking or tongue thrusting, ocular movements like excessive blinking or prolonged eye opening/staring, or as apneas and bradycardia (no breathing, with a resultant slowing of the heart rate).

EEG is the standard tool for assessing clinically observed seizures for brain injury, the presence of epileptiform brain activity (electrically hyperactive cortical activity), and electrographic seizures (Figure 4.3). Background electrical activity of the brain, reactivity in response to varying external stimuli, changes with mental alertness, **focal** or general electrical irritability or excitability, and seizures are examined during the EEG recording. Modern methods of continuous bedside monitoring of brain activity such as by video EEG (continuous EEG recording in conjunction with video camera monitoring of baby movements) and amplitude-integrated electroencephalography (aEEG; Toet et al., 2002) are also available in some institutions. Neonatal EEGs provide both diagnostic and prognostic information. Poor background organization or reactivity to stimuli suggests a diffuse **insult** to the brain, whereas focal irritability or seizures suggest an underlying focus for the process suggesting an acute brain injury. Subtle seizures or electrographic seizures can also be distinguished and monitored in response to medical treatment. The prognostic value of the EEG is increased if performed within the first 48 hours of life (or injury), and if repeated frequently (every 24–48 hours) to evaluate recovery. For example, an EEG pattern failing to improve, or becoming progressively more abnormal during the first few days of life, is associated with long-term neurological sequelae.

The use of antiepileptic drugs for control of seizures in neonates is an area of active debate. The most common seizure medications used in newborns are phenobarbital and phenytoin (Dilantin). Traditionally, antiepileptic drugs were prescribed for prolonged periods of time to prevent seizure recurrence (for up to 2 years). The current approach attempts to avoid the potentially deleterious effects of long-term antiepileptic drug therapy on the developing neonatal brain. Once the cause of the seizure is identified and adequately treated, a trial period off medications is instituted before hospital discharge. If there is no recurrence of seizure activity, the infant is discharged home without antiepileptic drugs and with a plan for close neurological follow-up and monitoring.

Hypoglycemia and Other Metabolic Disturbances

Newborns are vulnerable to hypoglycemia because access liver glycogen stores (the main form of glucose energy storage present at the time of birth) is poorly regulated and immature. Hypoglycemia, when severe or prolonged, is just as harmful as lack of oxygen, because the neonatal brain is completely dependent on glucose for generating energy to live and to interact. Hypoglycemia in the newborn is not strictly defined. The levels of serum glucose that are considered to be pathologic (usually

Montage: DOUBLE DISTANCE II   High Cut: 70 Hz   Low Cut: 1.00 Hz   Sensitivity: 3 µV/mm   Speed: 20 s/page

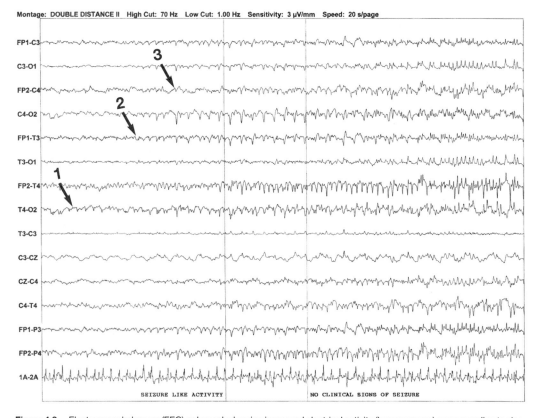

Figure 4.3. Electroencephalogram (EEG) polygraph showing increased electrical activity (bumpy waves) corresponding to electrographic seizures recorded from wires taped to the scalp over the right side of the brain and resulting in left-sided seizure movements clinically, as noted at the bottom. The first arrow (1) indicates seizure activity beginning in the right frontal-temporal region. Seizures quickly spread to involve the entire right hemisphere (shown by the second arrow [2]) and then the entire brain (shown by the third arrow [3]). Note that clinical seizure activity is not noted until the first vertical event marker at the bottom of this figure and that clinical seizure activity is no longer seen after the second vertical event marker despite the fact that there are generalized electrographic seizures on the EEG, which continue for another 20–30 seconds beyond what is shown here. Cortical seizures may be present even in the absence of abnormal movements in an infant with brain injury.

below a concentration of 40 milligrams/100 milliliter blood level for a period of time) depend on the age of the infant. Young newborns younger than 12 hours old normally have lower levels of circulating glucose when compared with older newborns. Neonatal hypoglycemia can be completely asymptomatic but may also present with seizures or other nonspecific symptoms, such as jitteriness, tremors, apneic spells, weak or high-pitched cry, limpness, lethargy, or difficulty feeding. Hypoglycemia is common in infants of mothers with diabetes (as in Justin's case). These infants need close periodic monitoring of blood glucose testing (every 30 minutes to 2 hours) for the first 48–72 hours of life. Other full-term neonates at high risk for developing hypoglycemia are infants who are small for gestational age or have had IUGR, asphyxia, hypoxia, or sepsis (blood infection). Severe or prolonged hypoglycemia can cause serious neu-

rodevelopmental deficits. Prevention of hypoglycemic encephalopathy is relatively simple. A continuous intravenous infusion of dextrose is provided for a few days until the infant is feeding and the blood tests become consistently normal.

Other metabolic disturbances that may present during the first few weeks of life include electrolyte abnormalities such as hypocalcemia, hypo- or hypernatremia, or hypomagnesemia. In addition, rare congenital enzyme deficiencies can cause elevated levels of metabolites (particularly amino acids or other organic acids) that can be toxic to the developing brain (see Chapter 20).

Neonatal Stroke

Stroke (or brain injury secondary to lack of blood flow to a region of the brain) in the neonate is an important cause of cerebral palsy. It occurs in approximately 2–9 per 10,000 live births (Boardman et al., 2005; Mercuri et al., 2004). It is most often arterial in origin (Figure 4.4), although sinus vein thrombosis (clots) also accounts for as many as 30% of neonatal strokes (Ferriero, 2004; de Veber et al., 2001). Seizures in the first few days of life are the most common clinical presenting sign of a neonatal stroke. However, other infants may present with late onset of seizures in the first weeks of life or even later or may develop a motor deficit. Risk factors implicated in neonatal stroke include an inherited or acquired thrombophilia (tendency for one's blood to clot more than normal) or a structural vascular abnormality within the brain (**arterial-venous malformation [AVM],** which is often associated also with a disastrous post-thrombotic hemorrhage into the brain substance itself). Preeclampsia and IUGR have also been associated with an increased occurrence of neonatal stroke (Wu et al., 2004). Unlike strokes due to hardening of the arteries (atherosclerosis) in aging adults, the risk of recurrence for neonatal stroke after presenting with one at birth is minimal. Only infants with congenital heart disease and clots emanating from abnormal cardiac structures are at increased risk of stroke recurrence. There is no specific medical treatment for neonatal stroke except when a clotting disorder is identified (antiplatelet or anticoagulation medications may be used in these cases). Early physical therapy is important

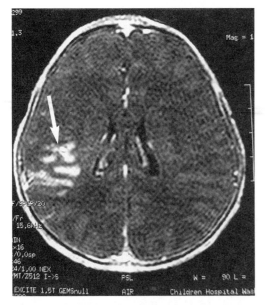

Figure 4.4. Magnetic resonance imaging (MRI) showing a right-side middle cerebral artery (MCA) infarction (white areas, arrow).

for improving functional outcome and to help avoid muscle weakness and joint contractures in the stroke-affected areas. Cognitive impairments may also occur (Mercuri et al., 2004).

Neonatal Sepsis

The newborn's immunity to bacterial and viral pathogens is immature at birth. Fewer and less aggressive white blood cells, as well as lower concentrations of specific immunoglobulin antibodies (antibodies acquired passively from the mother in utero gradually wane after birth), make the infant relatively vulnerable to infection. The newborn infant's neutrophils, or white blood cells that are responsible for primary defense against bacteria, exhibit poor chemotaxis (migration toward the area of infectious infiltration by the pathogen). The T cell lymphocyte population (white blood cells responsible for recognizing and chemically encoding into immunologic memory any foreign bacterial substances, or antigens) is also not as effective in infants younger than 6 months of age. Although fetal immunoglobulins begin to form during the fourth month of gestation, their number at birth is still minimal compared with their number after 6 months of age. Therefore, the presentation of any bacterial antigen in a newborn at birth does not stimulate as rapid an antibody formation response as in an older child. Also, the neonate's physical barriers to infection—such as the skin and the mucous membranes lining the upper respiratory passages, lungs, intestines, and urinary tract—are not as robust a defense barrier as they will be later in life. This is particularly true in premature infants, for whom bacterial infections are generally more common and devastating. These and other factors make any newborn particularly vulnerable to acquiring an infection.

Neonatal sepsis can be categorized into two epidemiologic time frames: 1) early onset (presenting in the first 7 days of life) or 2) late onset (presenting after the first week of life). Early-onset sepsis is usually caused by maternal microorganisms that infect the newborn either during passage through the colonized vaginal canal or transplacentally. The most common bacteria that cause early onset neonatal sepsis are **group B *Streptococcus* (GBS),** *Escherichia coli, Haemophilus influenzae,* and *Listeria monocytogenes.* In some cases, GBS infection results from direct aspiration of the bacteria into the infant's mouth, throat, and lungs during the birth process, with subsequent passage of the bacteria directly into the blood stream. Late-onset sepsis is more often due to bacteria acquired from the environment with passage onto the skin or from the young infant's gastrointestinal tract. The most common late-onset pathogens include *Staphylococcus aureus* (now becoming disturbingly resistant to the usual first-line antibiotics), *Escherichia coli, Klebsiella pneumoniae, Pseudomonas, Enterobacter, Candida*, and GBS. Pneumonia is the most common presentation for early-onset sepsis, whereas meningitis is most common with late-onset sepsis. Viruses such as adenovirus, enterovirus, coxsackie virus, or herpes virus can also be the causative agents of neonatal sepsis and particularly of meningoencephalitis (generalized and often devastating infections of the brain and central nervous system).

The mortality from neonatal sepsis can be greater than 50% in the untreated or late-treated infant. As a result, physicians need to be suspicious of sepsis and aggressive in managing infants with suspected sepsis (involving immediate hospitalization for intravenous antibiotics therapy). The American Academy of Obstetrics and Gynecology (2002) recommends screening all pregnant women for GBS colonization at 36 weeks' gestation.

Presentation of infection in the neonate can be vague and nonspecific. Infants can develop poor feeding (probably the first and most sensitive sign of an unwell infant), become excessively sleepy and difficult to arouse, become irritable and inconsolable, have hypo- or hyperthermia, have increased respiratory rate, or become seriously hypoglycemic. They can also appear well until the sepsis becomes overwhelming, in which case they may deteriorate very quickly and even die within 12–24 hours despite beginning antibiotics emergently. Blood, cerebrospinal fluid, and urine must be sampled and sent for microscopic analysis and cultures for the most likely organisms known to infect newborns in the first 2 months of life. Any fever, therefore, is considered a medical emergency in this age-group infant. Neuroimaging with brain CT or MRI can be useful in identifying focal areas of discrete infection (e.g., brain abscess), **meningeal** inflammation (meningitis), brain swelling (cerebral edema), cerebrospinal fluid (CSF) accumulation due to obstruction (hydrocephalus), hemorrhage from leaky blood vessels, and infarction (from septic emboli or septic shock). Repeat scans can also be useful in assessing response to therapy and delineating injury to determine prognosis for neurodevelopment if the infant survives.

Broad-spectrum antibiotics should be started as soon as neonatal sepsis is suspected, even if it means a delay in obtaining diagnostic cultures. As soon as a pathogen has been identified, antibiotic coverage needs to be focused and appropriately directed to penetrate and kill the specific bacteria identified (simple penicillin is still best against GBS). IVIG (intravenous immune globulin) has been proposed as an additional means of immunological therapy for serious infections, although no study has shown consistently improved survival (Stiehm, 1990). If hydrocephalus is seen on imaging studies, a neurosurgeon may be consulted to determine the need for relief of increasing intracranial pressure by tapping the fontanelle (soft spot on the skull) with a needle or by performing a **lumbar puncture.** If severe persistent hydrocephalus is present, the infant may need the surgical placement of a **ventriculoperitoneal shunt (VP shunt)** that relieves chronically elevated intracranial pressure by shunting CSF away from the brain's ventricular cavities, where it accumulates after damage caused by an infection, and directly into the abdominal cavity, where it may be reabsorbed readily and safely. Outcomes of neonatal sepsis and meningitis vary and depend on the organ systems most involved. CSF bacterial infection can be devastating, with cognitive impairment and hearing loss among the most common complications. Up to 25% of newborns with bacterial or viral meningitis will have some degree of serious, lifelong neurological impairment (Grimwood et al., 1995). Behavioral audiometry and vision testing should also be planned, since the risk for sensorineural hearing loss is particularly high with meningitis infections.

Neonatal Jaundice, Bilirubin Encephalopathy, and Kernicturus

Jaundice is a condition that commonly affects near-term and full-term infants. The name comes from the French word *jaune*, which means "yellow." The skin and the whites of the eyes of jaundiced infants appear yellow, especially when viewed under bright sunlight. Jaundice is caused by high blood levels of a pigment called bilirubin. Bilirubin pigment is the toxic waste product of the normal metabolism of hemoglobin, the molecule that carries oxygen inside the red blood cells. Bilirubin is normally removed from the circulation when passing through the liver; it is then excreted into the normal digestive green bile flow coming out of the liver and into the gastrointestinal tract to eventually exit the body as colored pigments in the stools (the first baby stools are also called breast milk or "transitional stools" and are normally intensely yellow-green because they are stained by the bile and conjugated bilirubin mixture). Infant feedings accelerate the removal of bilirubin from the gastrointestinal tract. Normal newborn jaundice in the absence of harmful maternal antibodies (tested for routinely prenatally) is called physiologic jaundice. Breast-feeding jaundice, an exaggerated form of physiologic jaundice, occurs in infants who are exclusively breast-fed and receive insufficient amounts of breast milk for the first few days of life until their mother's milk fully "comes in." Infants born slightly premature at near term (i.e., at between 35 and 37 weeks of gestation), are also at higher risk of developing jaundice compared with infants born at full term (Sarici et al., 2004).

Hyperbilirubinemia refers to abnormally elevated blood levels of bilirubin. If the level of bilirubin exceeds a certain threshold, it may cross out of the blood stream and into the newborn infant's brain, acting as a direct neurotoxin. The earliest symptoms of this are termed acute bilirubin encephalopathy and include poor feeding and decreased muscle tone and lethargy. The later symptoms are seizures, high-pitched cry, opisthotonus (abnormal posturing with hyperextension of the neck and back), and possibly even death in extreme cases; however, the majority of symptomatic babies recover from acute bilirubin encephalopathy. *Kernicterus* is a pathologist's term referring to the yellow staining of particular parts of the brain tissue (basal ganglia, cerebellum, and hippocampus) that is seen after death from severe acute bilirubin encephalopathy. Chronic bilirubin encephalopathy is a constellation of symptoms that occurs much later as the result of acute bilirubin toxicity occurring in the first weeks of life. The manifestations of chronic bilirubin encephalopathy include hearing and language acquisition problems, visual impairment, dental enamel abnormalities, and, rarely, choreoathetoid cerebral palsy (see Chapter 26; Shapiro, 2005).

Treatment goals for neonatal jaundice include early recognition and aggressive monitoring, and provision, when necessary, of specific therapies to accelerate the removal of bilirubin from the bloodstream. Neonatal physiologic jaundice is a common, usually benign condition, and in most instances resolves without the need for specific therapy. In cases where blood levels of bilirubin exceed a specific level (based on an infant's birth weight, gestational age, and postnatal age in hours; American Academy of Pediatrics Subcommittee on Hyperbilirubinemia, 2004), intravenous hydration and phototherapy may be used to lower bilirubin levels. Phototherapy uses a special blue fluorescent light exposed to the infant's skin, which promotes the chemical conversion of bilirubin to a compound that is more easily removed from the body by the kidneys and liver. If intravenous hydration and phototherapy are insufficient to avoid potentially neurotoxic levels of bilirubin, then exchange transfusion may be required. This involves exchanging some of the infant's bilirubin-contaminated blood with transfused blood, allowing for a more rapid decrease in bilirubin levels.

SUMMARY

Although the vast majority of infants make the transition from intrauterine to extrauterine life without difficulty, the complexities of the birth process and subsequent hazards in the weeks immediately following birth present challenges for some infants. Persistent pulmonary hypertension, **hypoxic ischemic encephalopathy,** neonatal seizures, metabolic disturbances, neonatal stroke, neonatal infection, and neonatal hyperbilirubinemia can result in long-term neurodevelopmental disability and require aggressive medical intervention. Advances in perinatal and neonatal care provide hope that progress will continue toward reducing these adverse outcomes.

REFERENCES

American Academy of Pediatrics Subcommittee on Hyperbilirubinemia. (2004). Management of hyperbilirubinemia in the newborn infant 35 or more weeks of gestation. *Pediatrics, 114,* 297–316.

American College of Obstetricians and Gynecology. (2002). Prevention of early-onset group B streptococcal disease in newborns (ACOG Committee Opinion number 279). *Obstetrics and Gynecology, 100*(6), 1405–1412.

Bianioni, E., Mercuri, E., Rutherford, M.A., et al. (2001). Combined use of EEG and MRI in full-term neonates with acute encephalopathy. *Pediatrics, 107*(3), 461–468.

Bland, R.D. (1992). Developmental changes in lung epithelial ion transport and liquid movement. *Annual Review of Physiology, 54,* 373.

Boardman, J.P., Ganesan, V., Rutherford, M.A., et al. (2005). Magnetic resonance image correlates of hemiparesis after neonatal and childhood middle cerebral artery stroke. *Pediatrics, 115,* 321–326.

Bruno, V.M.G., Goldberg, M.P., Dugan, L.L., et al.

(1994). Neuroprotective effect of hypothermia in cortical cultures exposed to oxygen-glucose deprivation or excitatory amino acids. *Journal of Neurochemistry, 63*, 1398–1406.

de Veber, G., Andrew, M., Adams, C., et al. (2001). Cerebral sinovenous thrombosis in children. *The New England Journal of Medicine, 345*, 417–423.

Ferriero, D.M. (2004). Medical progress: Neonatal brain injury. *The New England Journal of Medicine, 351*, 1985–1995.

Gluckman, P.D., Wyatt, J.S., Azzopardi, D., et al. (2005). Selective head cooling with mild systemic hypothermia after neonatal encephalopathy: Multicentre randomized trial. *The Lancet, 365*, 663–670.

Grimwood, K., Anderson, V.A., Bond, L., et al. (1995). Adverse outcomes of bacterial meningitis in school-age survivors. *Pediatrics, 95*, 646–656.

Gunn, A.J., & Gunn, T.R. (1998). The 'pharmacology' of neuronal rescue with cerebral hypothermia. *Early Human Development, 53*, 19–35.

Hardy, J.B. (2003). The Collaborative Perinatal Project: Lessons and legacy. *Annals of Epidemiology, 13*(5), 303–311.

Mercuri, E., Barnett, A., Rutherford, M., (2004). Neonatal cerebral infarction and neuromotor outcome at school age. *Pediatrics, 113*, 95–100.

Nelson, N.M. (2005). The onset of respiration. In G.B. Avery, M.A. Fletcher, & M.G MacDonald (Eds.), *Neonatology: Pathophysiology and management of the newborn* (5th ed., p. 265). Philadelphia: Lippincott, Williams & Wilkins.

Rutherford, M., Counsell, S., Allsop, J., et al. (2004). Diffusion-weighted magnetic resonance imaging in term perinatal brain injury: A comparison with site of lesion and time from birth. *Pediatrics, 114*, 1004–1014.

Sarici, S.U., Serdar, M.A., Korkmaz, A., et al. (2004). Incidence, course and prediction of hyperbilirubinemia in near-term and term newborns. *Pediatrics, 113*, 775–780.

Sarnat, H.B., & Sarnat, M.S. (1976). Neonatal encephalopathy following fetal distress. *Archives of Neurology, 33*, 696–705.

Shapiro, S.M. (2005). Definition of the clinical spectrum of kernicterus and bilirubin-induced neurologic dysfunction (BIND). *Journal of Perinatolology, 25*, 54-59.

Stiehm, E.R. (1990). Role of immunoglobulin therapy in neonatal infections: Where we stand today. *Reviews of Infectious Diseases, 12*(Suppl. 4), S349-42.

Toet, M.C., van der Meij, W., deVries, L.S., et al. (2002). Comparison between simultaneously recorded amplitude integrated electroencephalogram (cerebral function monitor) and standard electroencephalogram in neonates. *Pediatrics, 109*, 772–779.

Volpe, J.J. (2001). Unit III: Hypoxic-ischemic encephalopathy. In *Neurology of the newborn* (4th ed., pp. 217–397). Philadelphia: W.B. Saunders Co.

Welty, S., Hansen, T.N., & Corbet, A. (2005). Respiratory distress in the preterm infant. In H.W. Taeusch, R.A. Ballard RA, & C.A. Gleason (Eds.), *Avery's diseases of the newborn* (8th ed.). Philadelphia: Elsevier/Saunders.

Whitelaw, A., & Thoresen, M. (2002). Clinical trials of treatments after perinatal asphyxia. *Current Opinion in Pediatrics, 14*, 664–668.

Wu, Y.W., March, W.M., Croen, L.A., et al. (2004). Perinatal stroke in children with motor impairment: A population-based study. *Pediatrics, 114*, 612–619.

5   Environmental Toxins

Philip W. Davidson and Gary J. Myers

Upon completion of this chapter, the reader will

- Recognize the wide array of toxins present in the environment
- Be aware of the known and suspected effects of environmental toxins on the developing nervous system
- Understand the adverse neurodevelopmental outcomes that may result from exposure to environmental toxins

---

The United States annually produces more than 85,000 chemicals, approximately 3,000 of these in quantities exceeding 1,000,000 tons per year. More than 75% of these chemicals have not been put through any developmental toxicology screening. There is the possibility that many may have neurotoxic properties; that is, they are directly or indirectly associated with neurological dysfunction. **Neurotoxicants** include naturally occurring substances—such as metals including lead, mercury, cadmium, and manganese—and man-made chemicals—such as pesticides (organophosphates), persistent organic pollutants (e.g., **polychlorinated biphenyls [PCBs]**, dioxin), solvents (e.g., methanol, ethanol), and cigarette smoke. Many extrinsic agents may act as human developmental neurotoxicants and be associated with adverse effects, including intellectual disability, autism spectrum phenotypic behaviors, attention-deficit/hyperactivity disorder (ADHD), learning disabilities, sensory and motor deficits, memory deficits, and social and behavioral abnormalities.Cataloguing the neurotoxic effects of various chemicals is critical to establishing public health and environmental regulatory policies that are well grounded scientifically. The intent of this chapter is to review scientific evidence for or against the association between exposures to some common environmental contaminants and the occurrence of developmental disabilities. All of the substances considered are, in one form or another, found in the environments frequented by pregnant women and young children and, therefore, have the potential to adversely affect early brain development.

TOXICOLOGICAL AND EPIDEMIOLOGICAL ISSUES

Health Effects versus Developmental-Behavioral Effects

Environmental contaminants are present in the air, soil, and water. Human exposure may occur through direct contact with the contaminant (e.g., inhaling a **pesticide**) or through indirect contact (e.g., eating fish containing high levels of methylmercury). Some chemicals can cause health effects, such as respiratory disease or cancer, but have no impact on neurodevelopment. Contaminants that affect prenatal development, however, typically have an adverse impact on the central nervous system (CNS) and are called neurotoxicants. Some neurotoxicants have adverse health effects as well as adverse effects on development, such as exposure to tobacco smoke. Some forms of the same chemical may have neurotoxic effects whereas other forms may not, and different compounds involving the same chemical may have different neurotoxic effects. Furthermore, the neurotoxic effects of some chemical contaminants may be enhanced by the presence of other neurotoxicants. For example, fish containing both methylmercury and PCBs may be more neurotoxic than fish that contains only methylmercury (Stewart et al., 2003).

Timing and Magnitude of the Dose

Many variables influence neurodevelopmental outcome following exposures to neurotoxicants including the total amount, or "dose," of the neurotoxicant and the timing of the exposure. For example, the fetal brain is especially sensitive to some contaminants, so in utero exposure to these substances may be more neurotoxic than postnatal exposure. Other substances appear to be more dangerous if the exposure occurs postnatally, and still others are equally neurotoxic pre- and postnatally. The way in which an exposure takes place (whether it is chronic or acute, whether it is high or low dose) may influence the presence and severity of developmental effects. Complicating things further, exposures rarely occur in isolation. Soil, air, and bodies of water can and are often contaminated with numerous chemicals that act as neurotoxicants, making it difficult to scientifically untangle the specific contributions of a particular chemical to developmental outcomes. It is also possible that some constituents of an exposure medium may be acting to modify the exposure effects of one or more co-constituents. Such outcomes include genetic or social factors that predispose a child to exposure effects or modulate such effects. This is called effect modification (Bellinger, 2000). The presence of a preexisting developmental disability is typically an exclusion criterion in most of the research literature addressing the consequences of neurotoxic exposures. There is little research to document the consequences of exposures to neurotoxicants among people who already have a developmental disability.

Dose Response

Prenatal or postnatal exposures to high doses of some neurotoxicants have been associated with major CNS damage. Such outcomes are uncommon and typically result from acute poisonings. More commonly, there is exposure over a prolonged period of time to lower dosages of a neurotoxicant that is more widespread in the environment, such as lead. Such exposures may be associated with mild clinical consequences for any individual who is exposed but might affect the distribution of affected traits such as IQ scores in a population (Bellinger, 2006). In the case of PCBs and methylmercury, the deficits may change over the course of the exposure from mild deficits in specific functions to more global deficits later in life (Jacobson & Jacobson, 1996; Spyker, 1975).

Paucity of Neurotoxicity Data

Developmental neurotoxicity data have been accumulated sporadically and only on a very small number of well-known compounds, such as lead, mercury, PCBs, and ethanol. Data are limited and incomplete (especially in human studies) concerning many other ubiquitous environmental substances, such as phthalates, methanol, pesticides, and tobacco smoke. Moreover, the available data is typically restricted to one chemical effect at a time, despite the recognition that the environment contains multiple contaminants to which humans and animals are exposed simultaneously.

Human epidemiological studies are very expensive, time-consuming, and subject to many limitations. Complicating matters further is the observation that care must be taken when attempting to draw parallels between human exposures and the results of animal studies because of limited correspondence between human and animal dose effects and a lack of comparable outcome measures (Rice, 2006).

EVIDENCE FOR DEVELOPMENTAL NEUROTOXICITY

The remainder of this chapter is devoted to review of research on the neurotoxicity of the several environmental contaminants for which credible data exist.

Heavy Metals

Heavy metals occur naturally and are ubiquitous in the environment; some level of exposure is present for everyone. Excessive amounts of these metals cause adverse human health effects, but neurotoxicity has been documented for only a few. The two metals with the greatest neurotoxicity, lead and mercury, are present throughout the environment, and children are commonly exposed to them.

Heavy metals usually exist in multiple chemical forms, each with distinct biological effects. The consequences of exposure also differ depending on whether the exposure is prenatal or postnatal. Most heavy metals enter the body either through inhalation (e.g., of inorganic mercury vapor) or through ingestion (e.g., of paint chips containing lead).

Mercury Human exposure to mercury stems from eating fish (methylmercury); receiving vaccines that include **thimerosal** (merthiolate, also known as sodium eythlmercuithiosalicylate), which was mainly used in the past as a preservative for vaccines; and dental amalgams (vaporized elemental mercury). The exposure risk varies with each type of exposure (Clarkson, 2002).

Methylmercury The fetal brain is known to be especially susceptible to damage from exposure to methylmercury (Rodier, 1995). Evidence from nonhuman primates additionally indicates that neurobehavioral effects of low exposures to methylmercury during postnatal development may not emerge until later in life (Rice, 1996a). Outbreaks of methylmercury poisonings in Minamata and Niigata, Japan, in the 1950s and 1960s (Harada, 1968) and in Iraq in the 1970s (Bakir et al., 1973) confirmed the sensitivity of the fetal brain to this chemical. A study of 83 children exposed prenatally in Iraq (see Marsh, 1994, for a summary) suggested a dose–response relationship. There was delayed achievement of developmental milestones in response to exposures as low as 10 to 20 parts per million (ppm) in maternal hair. Subsequent studies of prenatal and postnatal effects of dietary exposure to methylmercury were conducted in a number of countries (Cordier et al., 2002; Grandjean et al., 2004 Marsh et al., 1995; Ramirez, Cruz, et al., 2000; Ramirez, Pagulayan, et al., 2003). The data taken together suggested that adverse associations should be expected from both prenatal and postnatal exposure. However, diversity in sample size, age of subjects, time of exposure, and degree of experimental control across studies has limited confidence in these conclusions.

In the mid-1980s, two large cohort studies were initiated to confirm earlier findings of neurotoxic developmental effects stemming from prenatal exposure to methylmercury, one in the Republic of Seychelles (Seychelles Child Development Study [SCDS]; Myers et al., 2003) and the other in the Faeroe Islands (cf., Grandjean et al., 1997). These studies yielded complex and, in some respects, contrasting results that are still being analyzed. Possible effects of prenatal exposure to methylmercury on neurodevelopmental functions included memory, attention, language, visual spatial skills, and auditory processing impairments (Crump et al., 2000; Debes et al., 2006; Grandjean, Murata, et al., 2004; Grandjean, White, et al.; 2003; Huang et al., 2005; Murata et al., 2004; Myers & Davidson, 2006). There is also evidence that nutrients in seafood may mitigate the potential adverse effects of methylmercury exposure on the brain, but the details of this effect are not understood yet.

There has been a great deal of interest and speculation surrounding the notion that either prenatal or postnatal exposure to mercury compounds might be causally associated with autism spectrum disorders (ASDs). Investigators in Texas (Palmer et al., 2006) and California (Windham et al., 2005) reported a possible link between ASDs and exposure to methylmercury, but they relied on indirect estimates rather than direct assessment of exposure to methylmercury. Another study (Fombonne et al., 2005) included direct measures of methylmercury exposure and found no association with ASDs. However, the sample was small, methylmercury was measured only at entry into the study, and no data on prenatal and early postnatal exposure were available. Nelson and Bauman (2003) noted that although the Faeroese and Seychelles studies were large enough to detect a link between ASDs and prenatal methylmercury exposure, neither study focused on behavioral phenotypes that would have been recognized as ASDs. Without augmentation of one or both of these studies, the question of ASD following prenatal exposure to methylmercury cannot be answered easily. The Institute of Medicine (2004) reviewed this issue and concluded that although it is biologically plausible, there is presently insufficient evidence to support or refute the hypothesis that mercury and ASDs are associated.

Thimerosal (merthiolate, also known as sodium eythlmercuithiosalicylate) was previously used as a preservative in vaccines, although it has been removed from most vaccines, especially those used in children. There is continuing parental concern that postnatal mercury exposure from immunizations may be associated with an increase in the incidence of ASDs. Much of this worry has arisen from a publication by Bernard and colleagues in 2000 that postnatal exposure to vaccines containing thimerosal may be associated with ASDs symptoms. Subsequent studies, however, have not provided scientific support for such an association (Parker et al., 2004; Andrews et al., 2004). For example, a study conducted by the Centers for Disease Control and Prevention (CDC; Verstraeten et al., 2003) found no significant associations between thimerosal-containing vaccines and neurodevelopmental outcomes, including ASDs. As with many studies of this type, this one relied on retrospective data gleaned from medical record reviews to establish exposures and developmental diagnoses. One conclusion from a review of the Vaccine Datalink Database studies by an expert panel commissioned by the National Institute of Environmental Health Sciences (2006) was that the question of a link between ASDs and prenatal exposure to methylmercury has not been addressed. Given the fact that existing evidence does not support the theory that thimerosal is causatively associated with autism, there is a strong consensus in the scientific and medical community that current immunization practices should be maintained (Institute of Medicine, 2004; Parker et al., 2004).

Dental Amalgams Dental fillings are amalgamated with inorganic mercury. During filling placement and afterward (during chewing), small amounts of mercury vapor escape into the mouth and enter the bloodstream. If the dental patient is a pregnant woman, the exposure could theoretically affect the fetus. In addition, postnatally multiple exposures to mercury vapor might result from routine dental **prophylaxis.** As yet, however, there is no behavioral or biochemical evidence that such exposures are associated with adverse neurodevelopmental outcomes in children (Clarkson, 2002).

Lead Food and excess environmental exposures to airborne lead deposits in dirt and dust are the principle sources of human exposure to inorganic lead. Other sources of lead exposure that were once common are slowly being eliminated. These include lead water pipes or copper pipes soldered with lead, lead-based paints, industrial emissions, lead-glazed pottery, and lead additives in gasoline. Unfortunately, children from urban settings in developing countries, especially those who live near vehicular traffic, continue to have high lead exposures (Romieu et al., 1992).

High dose lead exposures resulting in blood levels above 80 micrograms per deciliter can result in an acute encephalopathy with increased intracranial pressure, resulting in death or severe brain damage if untreated. Fortunately, this occurrence is now very rare in developed countries. Since the 1970s, a large number of cross sectional and longitudinal studies in children have focused on the association between lower dose lead exposures, IQ scores, and behavioral outcomes (Bellinger et al., 1992; Dietrich et al., 1991; McMichael et al., 1992). There is now strong evidence that lead levels as low as 10 micrograms per deciliter are associated with a decrease in IQ score. Additional

studies suggest that effects on IQ score, cognitive processes, and learning may occur at exposures levels below this level, calling into question whether there is any "safe" level of lead exposure for children (Canfield et al., 2004; Chiodo et al., 2004; Lanphear et al., 2000).

Polychlorinated •Biphenyls (PCBs) and Dioxins

PCBs are chemicals used in a wide variety of industrial applications, and dioxins are the by-products of a number of industrial manufacturing processes. There are more than 400 different compounds classified as either PCBs or dioxins. When in widespread use (prior to the 1980s), they were released into the environment and will remain there indefinitely. Most countries, including the United States, have banned their use; however, as they are still present in the environment, human exposure continues, primarily through consumption of foods from contaminated soil or water.

Prenatal and postnatal exposure to some but not all PCB and dioxin-containing compounds has been associated with neurotoxic effects in both animal models and humans. As with heavy metals, single high dose prenatal exposure, stemming from poisonings, lead to neurodevelopmental effects and abnormalities in auditory processing in the offspring. These deficits are more likely to occur in males, leading to the suggestion that PCBs and dioxins have gender-related disrupting effects on the developing endocrine system (Vreugdenhil & Weisglas-Kuperus, 2006).

Most of the evidence for human neurotoxic effects of both prenatal and postnatal PCB and dioxin exposures derives from several longitudinal cohort studies from different parts of the world (Jacobson & Jacobson, 1996; Koopman-Esseboom et al., 1996; Lonky et al., 1996; Winnike et al., 1998). In all of these studies, the medium of exposure was consumption of PCB-contaminated fish or sea mammals. These studies showed adverse effects of prenatal PCB exposure on neonatal and infant muscle tone and reflexes, although these abnormalities improved as the children grew older. Neurocognitive problems, including effects on attention, memory, verbal abilities, and auditory processing ability were also reported, and these persisted into at least early to middle childhood (Jacobson & Jacobson, 1996; Patandin et al., 1999; Walkowiak et al., 2001). Persistent adverse effects in older school-age children were reported for some of the cohorts (Vreugdenhil, Mulder, et al., 2004; Vreugdenhil, Van Zanten, et al., 2004).

Adverse effects of postnatal exposure to PCBs and dioxins have not been widely studied but have been reported in Dutch (Koopman-Esseboom et al., 1996) and German studies (Walkowiak et al., 2001). The Dutch cohort was also studied in school-age children, and adverse effects on a number of neurocognitive, motor, sensory, and neurophysiologic endpoints were reported for both prenatal and postnatal exposure. These effects were more pronounced in children who lived in homes with low socioeconomic status and in those who had younger mothers, a finding reminiscent of the effect modification found with lead exposure (Bellinger, 2000). Vreugdenhil and colleagues (2002) also reported an association between gender-specific play behaviors and PCB exposure, which they attributed to endocrine disruption effects.

Pesticides, Herbicides, and Fungicides

A variety of organic compounds have been used for centuries to protect agricultural produce from contamination and destruction from insects and microscopic organisms. Human and animal exposure to some of these compounds in high enough dosages can lead to severe neurotoxic effects, including paralysis, abnormal brain function, and death. Lower dose exposures, both acute and chronic, have been shown to produce milder but adverse neurological behavioral, cognitive, and emotional effects.

Human exposure to pesticides is widespread, given the ubiquitous use of these substances worldwide. They can be inhaled or consumed with the foods they are intended to protect. The mechanism of neurotoxicity varies with the compound, and the list of compounds approved for use as pesticides by governmental regulators has undergone substantial changes since their introduction into the commercial market in the 19th century. The older compounds, whether natural chemicals such as lead, arsenic, or sulfur, or synthetic compounds like DDT (chlorophenothane), have been replaced by organophosphates (OPs). According to a review by Needleman (2006), more than 34,000 pesticides are registered by the Environmental Protection Agency, and more than 1 billion pounds of conventional pesticides are used annually in the United States.

Most of the literature concerning neurotoxic exposure effects of pesticides derives from animal studies or studies of children or adults who experience exposures in occupational or school settings (Alarcon et al., 2005). To date, there have been no epidemiological neurodevelopmental studies of infants or children exposed prenatally or postnatally to pesticides. There has been research with animals focusing on exposure to OPs, with a few studies addressing carbamate and pyrathroid exposure. These studies suggest that OP exposure can also impair cell development, which has been linked to deficits in the ability for rodents to learn to solve a maze, activity level (Levin et al., 2001), immune function (Navarro et al., 2001), synaptic development (Dam et al., 1999), and DNA synthesis (Dam et al., 1998).

The principal mechanism of toxicity appears to be decreased production of acetyl cholinesterase, an enzyme in the CNS that regulates the levels on the neurotransmitter acetylcholine. Increased availability of this neurotransmitter results in overstimulation of acetylcholine-mediated synaptic transmission (Slotkin, 1999). Postnatal exposure to OPs at high dosages in humans can result in a variety of central and peripheral neuropathies (Abdiou-Donia & Lapadula, 1990). Mood symptoms and minor effects on attention and eye–hand coordination occur at lower doses (Metcalf & Holmes, 1969).

Alcohol

Both methanol (wood alcohol) and ethanol (found in alcoholic beverages) have neurotoxic effects. Although ethanol is not usually considered an environmental toxin, it is discussed here because of its importance as a fetal toxin and because it is paradigmatic of the effects of the alcohol group of organic solvents on the fetus. Prenatal exposure to ethanol through maternal consumption of alcoholic beverages in sufficient dosages has been linked to fetal alcohol syndrome (FAS) and, in lower exposures, to **alcohol-related neurodevelopmental disorder (ARND).**

Ethanol passes easily through the placenta and can result in characteristic congenital abnormalities and neurodevelopmental impairments, including craniofacial and limb anomalies, delays in physical growth, behavioral problems and developmental deficits in cognition, language, and memory (American Academy of Pediatrics, 2000). Sometimes, prenatal exposure results in developmental effects without the characteristic FAS facial dysmorphology, and this outcome is referred to as ARND. Barr and Streissguth (2001) recommended the term *fetal alcohol spectrum disorder (FASD)* to unify the description of these conditions as a single disorder varying along a teratogenic continuum. The prevalence of FASD is approximately 1 in 100 live births (Burbacher & Grant, 2006).

The exposure effects of ethanol are dose dependent and are related to the timing and pattern of exposure. The most severe effects on cognition seem to be related to material binge drinking (four or more drinks) that produces an acute marked increase in blood alcohol level (Jacobson et al., 1998; Streissguth, Barr, Olson, et al., 1994).

A number of well designed large-scale longitudinal epidemiological studies of fetal alcohol exposure have been conducted (Baer et al., 2003; Coles et al., 2002, Goldschmidt et al., 2004; Riley et al., 2003; Streissguth, Barr, Olson, et al., 1994; Streissguth, Barr, Sampson, et al., 1994; Wilford et al., 2004). These projects followed children to middle school, documenting consistent early appearing impairments in cognition and language, followed by later appearing learning, behavioral, and social problems. These effects were more likely in children whose exposure occurred early in pregnancy and whose mothers engaged in binge drinking (Burbacher & Grant, 2006).

Methanol, or wood alcohol, is an industrial solvent used in the synthesis of a number of consumer products. Occupational exposure effects are dose dependent. High-dosage exposure can result in a severe movement disorder or death. Fetal exposure in utero however, has been only recently studied. This has become important as methanol has emerged as a potential alternative fuel source for automobiles, increasing the potential for widespread prenatal exposure through inhalation. Although there are no studies of human neurodevelopmental outcomes after prenatal exposure to methanol, this exposure has been shown to effect later motor activity and operant learning in laboratory rodents (Weiss et al., 1996). Burbacher and colleagues (Burbacher, Grant, et al., 2004; Burbacher, Shen, et al., 2004) conducted the first controlled study of prenatal exposure to inhaled methanol among nonhuman primates, in which the dosage was designed to mimic environmental effects of emissions from automobile exhausts. The results indicated that relatively low dose maternal exposure was associated with significant decre-

ments in two measures of infant perception and cognition, visually directed reaching, and visual recognition memory.

Tobacco Smoke

Exposure to tobacco smoke during brain development can occur in two ways: by active in utero exposure through maternal smoking and by passive postnatal exposure through inhalation of ambient smoke. The prevalence of maternal smoking remains high in North America; about one quarter of pregnant women smoke by self-report (Fried et al., 2003).

Animal studies have confirmed that nicotine in tobacco smoke may compromise brain growth (Hellstrom-Lindahl & Norberg, 2002), disrupt neuronal migration (Wessler, Kirkpatrick, & Racke, 1998), and cause prematurity and low birth weight in offspring (Miller et al., 1995). Little is known about the effects on neurodevelopment of other potential neurotoxicants in smoke, including aromatic hydrocarbons and cadmium. Postnatally, tobacco smoke exposed animals show increased activity level, as well as attention, memory, and learning impairments (Levin et al., 1993).

Although human research has not directly linked neurodevelopmental deficits to an objective biomarker of tobacco, there is a considerable literature documenting adverse effects of in utero exposure to smoking. In one comprehensive longitudinal epidemiological study maternal cigarette smoking during pregnancy was associated with altered newborn neurobehavior (Law et al., 2003), lower scores on measures of global cognition seen as early as 12 months of age and persisting through ages 9 to 12 years (Fried & Watkinson, 2000; Fried et al., 1998). Other studies have reported associations between prenatal exposure and behavioral impairments (Day et al., 2000), ADHD (Kahn et al., 2003; Mick et al., 2002; Wakschlag et al., 2006), and school learning problems (Byrd & Weitzman, 1994).

There is really no way to effectively separate these in utero exposure effects from postnatal passive exposure to tobacco smoke in the child's environment. Weitzman Kananaugh, and Florin (2006) argued that ambient tobacco smoke contains twice the number of chemicals as inhaled smoke and may be more dangerous to the developing brain than in utero exposure. It is also difficult to separate in utero exposure to tobacco smoke from coincident and correlated exposures to alcohol (Jacobson et al., 2002) and to other toxins that may influence fetal development.

Endocrine Disrupters

Weiss (2006) defined *endocrine disrupters* as contaminants that interfere with the biological functions of hormones. Some pesticides, PCBs, and dioxins may act as endocrine disrupters, but many other compounds may also disrupt endocrine function, including phthalates, cadmium, lead, methylmercury, and nicotine. The specific effects on the endocrine system of exposures to such compounds are not well understood.

FROM SCIENCE TO POLICY

At the outset of this chapter, we described a disparity between the large number of chemicals that are bioavailable in the environment and the small number of such contaminants for which there is adequate scientific evidence either for or against their potential for neurotoxicity. This forces regulators and health policy makers to use what data they have to make critical judgments about relative risks. Some substances, such as methylmercury, are obviously neurotoxic at high dosages, but human exposure occurs mainly through maternal consumption of fish and seafood, which is a plentiful and an important source of many essential nutrients. Restrictions in consumption to reduce mercury exposure could have unintended adverse affects on fetal development.

This dilemma underscores the somewhat tenuous relationship between science and policy. Gordis (1996) commented that the role of science is quite limited in defining the association between science and public policy as it relates to exposures to disease. As it applies to the field of neurotoxicology, risk assessment, not epidemiological studies, is the major vehicle for translating scientific findings into policy recommendations.

Klerman (1987) described the Ideal model for public policy. The model depends on a balance between knowledge and social and political forces. It can break down when the zeal for policy based on current assumptions or perceptions is not consonant with the scientific data (Levine & Lilienfield, 1987). Governmental agencies establishing research funding priorities must accelerate the growth of scientific data and press research scientists in this field to bring those data to policy makers as rapidly as possible.

SUMMARY

This chapter reviewed the documented and hypothesized influences on child development of a variety of environmental contaminants. The resulting picture is very complex and not comprehensively researched. The available literature suggests that many contaminants have adverse effects on brain development that may not be reversible. The conditions of exposure that lead to these outcomes vary considerably from neurotoxin to neurotoxin. Consequently, giving advice to consumers and their families may be less than straightforward. More data are also required to aid in setting public policies designed to limit exposures.

REFERENCES

Abdiou-Donia, M.B., & Lapadula, D.M. (1990). Mechanisms of organophosphorus ester-induced delayed neurotoxicity Type I and II. *Annual Review of Pharmacology and Toxicology, 30,* 405–440.

Alarcon, W.A., Calvert, G.M., Blondell, J.M., et al. (2005). Acute illnesses associated with pesticide exposure at schools. *Journal of the American Medical Association, 294*(4), 455–465.

American Academy of Pediatrics, Committee on Substance Abuse and Committee on Children with Disabilities. (2000). Fetal alcohol syndrome and alcohol–related neurodevelopmental disorders. *Pediatrics, 106,* 358–361.

Andrews, N., Miller, E., Grant, A., et al. (2004). Trimerosal exposure in infants and developmental disorders: A retrospective cohort study in the United Kingdom does not support a causal association. *Pediatrics, 114,* 584–591.

Baer, J.S., Sampson, P.D., Barr, H.M., et al. (2003). A 21-year longitudinal analysis of the effects of prenatal alcohol exposure on young adult drinking. *Archives of General Psychiatry, 60,* 377–385.

Bakir, F., Damluji, S.F., Amin-Zaki, L., et al. (1973). Methylmercury poisoning in Iraq. *Science, 181,* 230–241.

Barr, H.M., & Streissguth, A.P. (2001). Identifying maternal self-reported alcohol use associated with fetal alcohol spectrum disorders. *Alcoholism: Clinical and Experimental Research, 25*(2), 283–287.

Bellinger, D.C. (2000). Effect modification in epidemiologic studies of low-level neurotoxicant exposures and health outcomes. *Neurotoxicology and Teratology, 22,* 133–140.

Bellinger, D.C. (2006). Neurobehavioral assessment in studies of exposures to neurotoxicants. In P.W. Davidson, G.J. Myers, & B. Weiss (Eds.), *International review of mental retardation research: Vol. 30.* Neurotoxicology and developmental disabilities (pp. 263–300). San Diego: Elsevier Academic Press.

Bellinger, D.C., Stiles, K.M., & Needleman, H.L. (1992). Low-level lead exposure, intelligence and academic achievement: A long-term follow-up study. *Pediatrics, 90,* 855–861.

Bernard, S., Enayati, A., Redwood, L., Roger, H., & Binstock, T. (2000). Autism: A novel form of mercury poisoning. *Medical Hypotheses, 56*(4), 452–471.

Burbacher, T.M., & Grant, K.S. (2006) Neurodevelopmental Effects of Alcohol. In P.W. Davidson, G.J. Myers, & B. Weiss (Eds.), *International review of mental retardation research: Vol. 30. Neurotoxicology and developmental disabilities* (pp. 1–46). San Diego: Elsevier Academic Press.

Burbacher, T.M., Grant, K.S., Shen, D.D., et al. (2004). Chronic maternal methanol inhalation in nonhuman primates (Macaca fascicularis): Reproductive performance and birth outcome. *Neurotoxicology and Teratology, 26*, 639–650.

Burbacher, T.M., Shen, D.D., Lalovic, B., et al. (2004). Chronic maternal methanol inhalation in nonhuman primates (Macaca fascicularis): Exposure and toxicokinetics prior to and during pregnancy. *Neurotoxicology and Teratology, 26*(2), 201–221.

Byrd, R., & Weitzman, M. (1994). Predictors of early grade retention among children in the United States. *Pediatrics, 93*, 481–487.

Canfield, R.L., Gendle, M.H., & Cory-Slechta, D.A. (2004). Impaired neuropsychological functioning in lead-exposed children. *Developmental Neuropsychology, 26*, 513–540.

Chen, Y.C., Guo, Y.L., Hsu, C.C., et al. (1992). Cognitive development of Yu-Cheng ("oil disease") children prenatally exposed to heat-degraded PCBs. *Journal of the American Medical Association, 268*, 3213–3218.

Chen, Y.J., & Hsu, C.C. (1994). Effects of prenatal exposure to PCBs on the neurological function of children: A neuropsychological and neurophysiological study. *Developmental Medicine and Child Neurology, 36*, 312–320.

Chiodo, L.M., Jacobson, J.L., & Jacobson, S.W. (2004). Neurodevelopmental effects of postnatal lead exposure at very low levels. *Neurotoxicology and Teratology, 26*(3), 359–371.

Clarkson, T.W. (2002). The three modern faces of mercury. *Environmental Health Perspectives, 110*(Suppl. 1), 11–23.

Coles, C.D., Platzman, K.A., Lynch, M.E., et al. (2002). Auditory and visual sustained attention in adolescents prenatally exposed to alcohol. *Alcoholism: Clinical and Experimental Research, 26*, 263–271.

Cordier, S., Garel, M., Manderau, L., et al. (2002). Neurodevelopmental investigations among methylmercury-exposed children in French Guiana. *Environmental Research, 89*, 1–11.

Cory-Slechta, D. (2006). Interactions of lead exposure and stress: Implications for cognitive dysfunction. In P.W. Davidson, G.J. Myers, & B. Weiss (Eds.), *International review of mental retardation research: Vol. 30. Neurotoxicology and developmental disabilities* (pp. 87–140). San Diego: Elsevier Academic Press.

Cory-Slechta, D.A., Virgolini, M.B., Thiruchelvam, M., et al. (2004). Maternal stress modulates effects of developmental lead exposure. *Environmental Health Perspectives, 112*(6), 717–730.

Crump, K.S., Landingham, V., Shamlaye, C.F., et al. (2000). Benchmark concentrations for methylmercury obtained from the Seychelles Child Development Study. *Environmental Health Perspectives, 108*(3), 257–263.

Dam, K., Garcia, S., Seidler, F., et al. (1999). Neonatal chlopyrifos alters synaptic development and neuronal activity in cholinergic and chatacholaminergic pathways. *Brain Research and Developmental Brain Research, 116*, 9–20.

Dam, K., Seidler, F.J., & Slotkin, T.A. (1998) Developmental neurotoxicity of chlorpyrifos: Delayed targeting of DNA synthesis after repeated administration. *Brain Research and Developmental Brain Research, 108* (1–2), 39–45.

Day, N., Richardson, G., Goldschmidt, L., et al. (2000). Effects of prenatal tobacco exposure on preschoolers' behavior. *Journal of Developmental and Behavioral Pediatrics, 21*, 180–188.

Debes, F., Budtz-Jøgensen, E., Weihe, P., et al. (2006). Impact of prenatal methylmercury exposure on neurobehavioral function at age 14 years. *Neurotoxicology and Teratology. 28*, 363–375.

Dietrich, K.N., Succop, P.A., Berger, O.G., et al. (1991). Lead exposure and the cognitive development of urban preschool children: The Cincinnati Lead Study cohort at age 4 years. *Neurotoxicology and Teratology, 13*, 203–211.

Fergusson, D., Horwood, L., & Lynskey, M. (1993). Maternal smoking before and after pregnancy: Effects on behavioral outcomes in middle childhood. *Pediatrics, 92*, 815–822.

Fischer, L.J., Seegal, R.F., Ganey, P.E., et al. (1998). Symposium overview: Toxicity of non-coplanar PCBs. *Toxicological Science, 41*, 49–61.

Fombonne, E., Zakarian, R., Assouad, P., et al. (2005, May 5–7). *Genetics, environment, nutrition. Exploring autism in children: The gene-A study.* Paper presented at the International Meeting for Autism Research, Boston.

Fried, P., Watkinson, B., & Gray, R. (1998). Differential effects on cognitive functioning in 9- to 12-year olds prenatally exposed to cigarettes and marihuana. *Neurotoxicology and Teratology, 20*, 293–306.

Fried, P., & Watkinson, B. (2000). Visuoperceptual functioning differs in 9- to 12-year olds prenatally exposed to cigarettes and marijuana. *Neurotoxicology and Teratology, 22*, 11–20.

Fried, V., Prager, K., MacKay, A., et al. (2003). *Chartbook on the trends in the health of Americans.* Hyattsville, MD: National Center for Health Statistics.

Goldschmidt, L., Richardson, G.A., Cornelius, M.D., et al. (2004). Prenatal marijuana and alcohol exposure and academic achievement at age 10. *Neurotoxicology and Teratology, 26*, 521–532.

Gordis, L. (1996). *Epidemiology.* Philadelphia: W.B. Saunders.

Grandjean, P., Murata, K., Budtz-Jorgensen, E., et al. (2004). Cardiac autonomic activity in methylmercury neurotoxicity: 14-year follow-up of a Faroese birth cohort. *Journal of Pediatrics, 144*, 169–176.

Grandjean, P., Weihe, P., White, R.F., et al. (1997). Cognitive deficit in 7-year-old children with prenatal exposure to methylmercury. *Neurotoxicology and Teratology, 19*(6), 417–428.

Grandjean, P., White, R.F., Weihe, P., et al. (2003). Neurotoxic risk caused by stable and variable exposure to methylmercury from seafood. *Ambulatory Pediatrics, 3*(1), 18–23.

Harada, Y. (1968). Congenital (or fetal) Minamata disease (Study Group of Minamata Disease). In *Japan* (pp. 93–118). Kumamoto, Japan: Kumamoto University.

Hellstrom-Lindahl, E., & Norberg, A. (2002). Smoking during pregnancy: A way to transfer the addiction to the next generation. *Respiration, 69*, 289–293.

Huang, L.S., Cox, C., Myers, G.J., et al. (2005). Exploring nonlinear association between prenatal methylmercury exposure from fish consumption and child development: Evaluation of the Seychelles Child Development Study nine-year data using semiparametric additive models. *Environmental Research, 97,* 100–108.

Institute of Medicine, Immunization Safety Review Committee. (2004). *Immunization safety review: Vaccines and autism.* Washington, DC: National Academies Press.

Jacobson, J.L., & Jacobson, S.W. (1996). Intellectual impairment in children exposed to polychorinated biphenyls in utero. *The New England Journal of Medicine, 335,* 783–789.

Jacobson, S.W., Chiodo, L.M., Sokol, R.J., et al. (2002). Validity of maternal report of prenatal alcohol, cocaine, and smoking in relation to neurobehavioral outcome. *Pediatrics, 109*(5), 815–825.

Jacobson, S.W., Jacobson, J.L., Sokol, R.J., et al. (1998). Preliminary evidence of working memory and attention deficits in 7-year-olds prenatally exposed to alcohol. *Alcoholism: Clinical and Experimental Research, 22,* 61A.

Kahn, R.S., Khoury, J., Nichols, W.C., et al. (2003). Effects of prenatal alcohol exposure on infant visual acuity. *The Journal of Pediatrics, 147,* 473–479.

Klerman, G. (1987). Psychiatric epidemiology and mental health policy. In S. Levine & A. Lilienfield (Eds.), *Epidemiology and health policy* (pp. 227–264). New York: Tavistock.

Koopman-Esseboom, C., Weisglas-Kuperus, N., de Ridder, M.A., et al. (1996). Effects of polychlorinated biphenyl/dioxin exposure and feeding type on infants' mental and psychomotor development. *Pediatrics, 97,* 700–706.

Lanphear, B.P., Dietrich, K., Auinger, P., et al. (2000). Cognitive deficits associated with blood lead concentrations <10 microg/dL in US children and adolescents. *Public Health Reports, 115*(6), 521–529.

Law, K.L., Stroud, L.R., LaGasse, L.L., et al. (2003). Smoking during pregnancy and newborn neurobehavior. *Pediatrics, 111,* 1318–1323.

Levin, E., Briggs, S., Christopher, N., & Rose, J. (1993). Prenatal nicotine exposure and cognitive performance in rats. *Neurotoxicology and Teratology, 15,* 251–260.

Levin, E., Nakajima, A., Christopher, N., et al. (2001). Persistent behavioural consequences of neonatal chlorpyrifos exposure in rats. *Brain Research and Developmental Brain Research, 130,* 83–89.

Levine, S., & Lilienfield, A. (1987). Introduction. In S. Levine & A. Lilienfield (Eds.), *Epidemiology and health policy* (pp. 1–14). New York: Tavistock.

Lonky, E., Reihman, J., Darvill, T., et al. (1996). Neonatal Behavioral Assessment Scale performance in humans influenced by maternal consumption of environmentally contaminated Lake Ontario fish. *Journal of Great Lakes 22,* 198–212.

Marsh, D.O. (1994). Organic mercury: Clinical and neurotoxicological aspects. *Handbook of Clinical Neurology, 20,* 413–429.

Marsh, D.O., Turner, M.D., Smith, J.C., et al. (1995). Fetal methylmercury study in a Peruvian fish-eating population. *NeuroToxicology, 16,* 717–726.

McMichael, A.J., Baghurst, P.A., Vimpani, G., et al. (1992). Sociodemographic factors modifying the effect of environmental lead on neuropsychological development in early childhood. *Neurotoxicology and Teratology, 14,* 321–327.

Metcalf, D.R., & Holmes, J.H. (1969). EEG, psychological, and neurological alternations in humans with organophosphorus exposure. *Annals New York Academy of Sciences, 160,* 357–365.

Mick, E., Biederman, J., Faraone, S., et al. (2002). Case-control study of attention-deficit hyperactivity disorder and maternal smoking, alcohol use, and drug use during pregnancy. *Journal of the American Academy of Child and Adolescent Psychiatry, 41,* 378–385.

Miller, J., Boudreaux, M., & Regan, F. (1995). A case-control study of cocaine use in pregnancy. *American Journal of Obstetrics and Gynecology, 172*(1), 180–185.

Murata, K., Weihe, P., Budtz-Jorgensen, E., et al. (2004). Delayed brainstem auditory evoked potential latencies in 14-year-old children exposed to methylmercury. *Journal of Pediatrics, 144,* 177–183.

Myers, G.J., & Davidson, P.W. (2006). Developmental disabilities following fetal exposure to methylmercury from maternal fish consumption: A review of the evidence. In P.W. Davidson, G.J. Myers, & B. Weiss (Eds.), *International review of mental retardation research: Vol. 30. Neurotoxicology and developmental disabilities* (pp. 141–170). San Diego: Elsevier Academic Press.

Myers, G.J., Davidson, P.W., Cox, C., et al. (2003). Prenatal methylmercury exposure from ocean fish consumption in the Seychelles child development study. *The Lancet, 361,* 1686–1692.

Navarro, H., Basta, P., Seidler, F., et al. (2001). Neonatal chloropyrifos administration elicits deficits in immune function in adulthood: A neural effect? *Brain Research and Developmental Brain Research, 130,* 249–252.

Needleman, H.L. (2006). The neurotoxic properties of pesticides. In P.W. Davidson, G.J. Myers, & B. Weiss (Eds.), *International review of mental retardation research: Vol. 30. Neurotoxicology and developmental disabilities* (pp. 225–236). San Diego: Elsevier Academic Press.

Nelson, K.B., & Bauman, M.L. (2003). Thimerosal and autism? *Pediatrics, 111,* 674–679.

National Institute of Environmental Health Sciences. (2006). *Thimerosal exposure in pediatric vaccines: Feasibility of studies using the Vaccine Safety Datalink. Report of the Expert Panel.* Retrieved January 19, 2007, from http://www.safeminds.org/pressroom/pres_releases/Thimerosal_Pediatric_Vaccines.pdf

Palmer, R.F., Blanchard, S., Stein, Z., et al. (2006). Environmental mercury release, special education rates, and autism disorder: An ecological study of Texas. *Health Place, 12,* 203–209.

Parker, S.K., Schwartz, B., Todd, J., et al. (2004). Thimerosal-containing vaccines and autistic spectrum disorder: A critical review of published original data. *Pediatrics, 114,* 793–804.

Patandin, S., Dagnelie, P.C., Mulder, P.G., et al. (1999). Dietary exposure to polychlorinated biphenyls and dioxins from infancy until adulthood. A comparison between breast-feeding, toddler, and long- term exposure. *Environmental Health Perspectives, 107,* 45–51.

Ramirez, G.B., Cruz, M.C., Pagulayan, O., et al. (2000). The Tagum study I: analysis and clinical correlates of mercury in maternal and cord blood, breast milk, meconium, and infants' hair. *Pediatrics, 106,* 774–781.

Ramirez, G.B., Pagulayan, O., Akagi, H., et al. (2003). Tagum study II: Follow-up study at two years of age after prenatal exposure to mercury. *Pediatrics, 111*(3), 289–295.

Rice, D.C. (1996a). Evidence for delayed neurotoxicity produced by methylmercury. *NeuroToxicology, 17,* 583–596.

Rice, D.C. (1996b). Behavioral effects of lead: Commonalities between experimental and epidemiological data. *Environmental Health Perspectives, 104,* 337–351.

Rice, D.C. (2006). From animals to humans: Models and

constructs. In P.W. Davidson, G.J. Myers, & B. Weiss (Eds.), *International review of mental retardation research: Vol. 30. Neurotoxicology and developmental disabilities* (pp. 301–338). San Diego: Elsevier Academic Press.

Riley, E.P., Mattson, S.N., Li, T.K., et al. (2003). Neurobehavioral consequences of prenatal alcohol exposure: An international perspective. *Alcoholism: Clinical and Experimental Research, 27,* 362–373.

Rodier, P. (1995). Developing brain as a target for toxicity. *Environmental Health Perspectives, 103*(Suppl. 6), 73–76.

Romieu, I., Palazuelos, E., Meneses, F., et al. (1992). Vehicular traffic as a determinant of blood-lead levels in children: A pilot study in Mexico City. *Archives of Environmental Health, 47*(4), 246–249.

Shain, W., Bush, B., & Seegal, R. (1991). Neurotoxicity of polychlorinated biphenyls: Structure–activity relationship of individual congeners. *Toxicology and Applied Pharmacology, 111,* 33–42.

Slotkin, T.A. (1999). Developmental cholinotoxicants: Nicotine and chlopyrifos. *Environmental Health Perspectives, 107*(Suppl. 1), 71–80.

Spyker, J.M. (1975) Assessing the impact of low level chemicals on development: Behavioral and latent effects. *Federation Proceedings, 34*(9), 1835–1844.

Stewart, P.W., Reihman, J., Lonky, E., et al. (2003). Cognitive development in preschool children prenatally exposed to PCBs and MeHg. *Neurotoxicology and Teratology, 25,* 11–22.

Streissguth, A.P., Barr, H.M., Olson, H.C., et al. (1994). Drinking during pregnancy decreases word attack and arithmetic scores on standardized tests: Adolescent data from a population-based prospective study. *Alcoholism: Clinical and Experimental Research, 18,* 248–254.

Streissguth, A.P., Barr, H.M., Sampson, P.D., et al. (1994). Prenatal alcohol and offspring development: The first fourteen years. *Drug and Alcohol Dependence, 36,* 89–99.

Verstraeten, T., Davis, R.L., DeStefano, F., et al. (2003). Safety of thimerosal-containing vaccines: A two-phased study of computerized health maintenance organization databases. *Pediatrics, 112*(5), 1039–1048.

Vreugdenhil, H.J., Slijper, F.M., Mulder, P.G., et al. (2002). Effects of perinatal exposure to PCBs and dioxins on play behavior in Dutch children at school age. *Environmental Health Perspectives, 110,* A593–A598.

Vreugdenhil, H.J.I., Mulder, P.G., Emmen, H.H., et al. (2004). Effects of perinatal exposure to PCBs on neuropsychological functions in the Rotterdam cohort at 9 years of age. *Neuropsychology 18,* 185–193.

Vreugdenhil, H.J.I., Van Zanten, G.A., Brocaar, M.P., et al. (2004). Prenatal PCB exposure and breast-feeding

affect auditory P300 latencies in 9 year-old Dutch children. *Developmental Medicine and Child Neurology 46,* 398–405.

Vreugdenhil, H.J.I., & Weisglas-Kuperus, N. (2006). PCBs and Dioxins. In P.W. Davidson, G.J. Myers, & B. Weiss (Eds.), *International review of mental retardation research: Vol. 30. Neurotoxicology and developmental disabilities* (pp. 47–86). San Diego: Elsevier Academic Press.

Wakschlag, L.S., Pickett, K.E., Kasza, K.E., & et al. (2006). Is prenatal smoking associated with a developmental pattern of conduct problems in young boys? *Journal of the American Academy of Child and Adolescent Psychiatry, 45*(4), 461–467.

Walkowiak, J., Wiener, J.A., Fastabend, A.,et al. (2001). Environmental exposure to polychlorinated biphenyls and quality of the home environment: Effects on psychodevelopment in early childhood. *The Lancet, 358,* 1602–1607.

Weiss, B. (2006). Endocrine disrupters as a factor in mental retardation. In P.W. Davidson, G.J. Myers, & B. Weiss (Eds.), *International review of mental retardation research: Vol. 30. Neurotoxicology and developmental disabilities* (pp. 195–224). San Diego: Elsevier Academic Press.

Weiss, B., Stern, S., Soderholm, S.C., et al. (1996). Developmental neurotoxicity of methanol exposure by inhalation in rats. *Health Effects Institute Research Report, 73,* 1–70.

Wessler, I., Kirkpatrick, C., & Racke, K. (1998). Non-neuronal acetylcholine, a locally acting molecule, widely distributed in biological systems: Expression and function in humans. *Pharmacology & Therapeutics, 77,* 59–79.

Weitzman, M., Kananaugh, M., & Florin, T.A. (2006). Parental smoking and children's behavioral and cognitive functioning. In P.W. Davidson, G.J. Myers, & B. Weiss (Eds.), *International review of mental retardation research: Vol. 30. Neurotoxicology and developmental disabilities* (pp. 237–261). San Diego: Elsevier Academic Press.

Willford, J.A., Richardson, G.A., Leech, S.L., et al. (2004). Verbal and visuospatial learning and memory function in children with moderate prenatal alcohol exposure. *Alcoholism: Clinical and Experimental Research, 28,* 497–507.

Windham, G., Zhang, L., Gunier, R., et al. (2005, May 5–7). *Autism spectrum disorders in relation to distribution of hazardous air pollutants.* Paper presented at the International Meeting For Autism Research, Boston.

Winneke, G., Bucholski, A., Heinzow, B., et al. (1998). Developmental neurotoxicity of polychlorinated biphenyls (PCBS): Cognitive and psychomotor functions in 7-month old children. *Toxicology Letters, 102–103,* 423–428.

6 Infections and the Fetus

Michael J. Bell

Upon completion of this chapter, the reader will

- Know about specific agents that commonly cause fetal and neonatal infections that lead to disabilities
- Be able to discuss the most common pathogens responsible for direct brain injury
- Understand the relationship between nonspecific intrauterine infections and subsequent developmental brain injuries

---

During normal brain development, neural stem cells expand and differentiate into the cells required for reading, speaking, ambulating, regulating body functions, envisioning the future, and countless other complex biological processes. These few cells in early embryogenesis must 1) multiply to more than 100 billion in the adult, 2) migrate to the correct position, 3) establish the proper connections, and 4) execute dozens of intra- and intercellular reactions for proper functioning. Processes that alter these events can have grave consequences on the development of the infant, child, and, eventually, adult (see Chapter 13).

Infections during the fetal period can lead to critical alterations in this brain development process. Infectious agents can directly damage developing neural structures in early fetal life, altering their function forever. Overwhelming infections of the fetus can affect brain development by diminishing nutrient supply to the

brain or other mechanisms. Most recently, it has been proposed that the fetal inflammatory response to a subclinical infection can also lead to maldevelopment of the nervous system (Bell & Hallenbeck, 2002). This chapter first reviews specific agents that commonly cause fetal and neonatal infections that lead to disabilities. The number of pathogens responsible for direct brain injury continues to grow and the most common ones are discussed (see Table 6.1). Then, the relationship between nonspecific intrauterine infections and subsequent developmental brain injuries is discussed, with evidence from human and animal studies presented. A thorough understanding of these processes is essential to develop and implement preventative strategies in the future.

JEROME

Jerome is a 7-year-old who was found, in retrospect, to have been infected with **human immunodeficiency virus (HIV)** at birth. His mother had been using intravenous drugs of abuse but had not been tested for HIV. At the time of Jerome's birth, prenatal screening and perinatal treatment for HIV infection were not well established. His initial evaluation for HIV occurred at 6 months of age as a result of recurrent infections, diarrhea, and **failure to thrive.** At that time Jerome had a severely suppressed immune system. His CD4 T-cell count (the cell in the immune system that is destroyed by the HIV infection) was only 40

Table 6.1. Pathogens responsible for fetal or neonatal brain injuries

Bacteria	Group B *Streptococcus*
	Treponema Pallidum
Parasites	*Toxoplasma gondii*
Viruses	Rubella
	Cytomegalovirus (CMV)
	Herpes simplex viruses (HSV)
	Human immunodeficiency virus (HIV)
	Lymphocytic choriomeningitis virus (LCMV)

cells per cubic millimeter, rather than the normal count for his age of greater than 1,500 cells per cubic millimeter). In addition, only 3% of total lymphocytes were CD4, instead of the normal finding of greater than 35%. His plasma HIV viral load was very high: 240,000 copies per milliliter.

Jerome was enrolled in an experimental multidrug protocol supported by the Pediatric AIDS Clinical Trials Group of the National Institutes of Health. He was initially placed on the reverse transcriptase inhibitors zidovudine (ZDV) and lamivudine. He tolerated these well, and 2 weeks later a protease inhibitor, nelfinavir, was added to the drug regimen. On this therapy Jerome showed a reduction in the plasma HIV viral load to below the limits of detection (less than 400 copies per milliliter). After 5 months of therapy, his CD4 lymphocyte count had increased to 1,490 cells per cubic millimeter, equaling 40% of his T-cells. Over the following years, his viral load has remained undetectable at almost every measurement, and he has remained clinically healthy. When he entered first grade, he was found to have some learning impairments but has done well in a general education classroom with special education supports.

Jerome's mother, who was HIV positive but did not have clinical symptoms, entered a drug abuse treatment program and began antiretroviral therapy at the same time as her son. She is now working as a teacher's aide in a preschool program. She had another child 4 years after having Jerome. Because Jerome's mother took **antiretroviral agents (ARVs),** her daughter, Tanya, received intrauterine exposure to them, was delivered by cesarean section, and received 6 weeks of postnatal treatment with ZDV. Tanya had two negative virologic HIV tests at 1 and 4 months of age. At her 18-month checkup, she had a negative HIV enzyme-linked immunosorbent assay (ELISA). Now 3 years old, Tanya's development has been entirely typical.

SPECIFIC PATHOGENS

A number of perinatal infections have long been known to cause brain damage in children. These infections are colloquially grouped as TORCH infections, so named for *t*oxoplasmosis, *o*ther (HIV, **syphilis,** and others), *r*ubella, *c*ytomegalovirus, and *h*erpes family infections. This classification scheme may be useful in forming differential diagnoses in children with perinatal brain injuries; however, each of these teratogenic infections has characteristic patterns of infection and damage to the developing nervous system that are outlined next (see also Table 6.2).

Group B Streptococcus

Although it is not one of the TORCH infections, *Streptococcus agalactiae* or group B *Streptococcus* (GBS), is a major cause of sepsis and **men-**

Table 6.2. Common complications of intrauterine infections

Types of complication	*Treponema pallidum*	*Toxoplasma gondii*	Rubella virus	Cyto-megalo-virus	Herpes simplex viruses	Lymphocytic chorio-meningitis virus
Systemic complications						
Premature birth	Yes	Yes	No	No	Yes	No
Intrauterine growth restriction	Yes	Yes	Yes	Yes	Yes	No
Hepatosplenomegaly	Yes	Yes	Yes	Yes	No	No
Jaundice	Yes	Yes	Yes	Yes	No	No
Lymphadenopathy	Yes	Yes	Yes	No	No	No
Central nervous system complications						
Meningoencephalitis	Yes	Yes	Yes	Yes	Yes	Yes
Microcephaly	No	Yes	No	Yes	Yes	Yes
Hydrocephaly	No	Yes	Yes	Yes	Yes	Yes
Intracranial calcifications	No	Yes	No	Yes	Yes	Yes
Hearing deficits	Yes	Yes	Yes	Yes	No	Yes
Chorioretinitis	Yes	Yes	Yes	Yes	Yes	Yes
Hydrancephaly	No	No	No	No	Yes	No

ingitis in the perinatal period (during the first 30 days of life). GBS is bacterium that can cause vertical transmission (from pregnant mothers to the delivering fetus) and lead to significant brain injury. The relationship between maternal colonization with GBS and the development of perinatal infection was established in the 1970s and 1980s. In 1996, the Centers for Disease Control and Prevention (CDC) issued guidelines recommending antimicrobial prophylaxis of colonized pregnant women in order to diminish perinatal morbidity and mortality. Before these prevention efforts, up to 7,500 cases of perinatal GBS disease were reported yearly, with a fatality rate of up to 20%. Despite these efforts, at the time of publication of this text GBS remains the most important bacterial pathogen causing central nervous system (CNS) and systemic infections in the neonatal period (Berner, 2002; Platt & O'Brien, 2003).

Pathogenesis of GBS begins with colonization of the vaginal wall. The lower gastrointestinal tract is the reservoir for GBS in women, and isolation of GBS from urinary specimens is indicative of heavy colonization. Diabetes, young age, fewer pregnancies, and African American race are independent risk factors for vaginal colonization. The intensity of maternal colonization, premature rupture of fetal amniotic membranes, or fetal descent through an infected vaginal canal all lead to an increased risk for perinatal GBS disease. Horizontal GBS infection (from hospital personnel or other environmental sources) has been reported but fortunately is relatively rare (Berner, 2002).

Neonatal illness with GBS manifests as early onset (occurring within the first 6–7 days of life) or late onset (occurring up to 3 months after birth). Early onset illness is routinely associated with systemic infection, an increased severity of disease, and increased mortality (up to 60% in some series). Late onset disease manifests primarily as meningitis and has a more limited mortality and severity of illness at presentation. The signs and symptoms of early-onset GBS illness are relatively nonspecific, with the classical findings of meningitis (bulging fontanelle and nuchal rigidity) only rarely observed. Fever, poor activity level, poor skin color, and seizures are common symptoms in full-term infants with GBS sepsis or meningitis. In preterm infants, respiratory distress alone may be the only presenting symptom. Definitive diagnosis of GBS meningitis or sepsis requires isolation of the organism from the spinal fluid or blood, respectively. Identification of white blood cells within the CSF or latex-agglutination assays (identifying GBS protein) can be used as presumptive evidence of GBS disease when cultures are unavailable or impractical. DNA assays (polymerase chain reaction [PCR]) have been developed that detect GBS within 2 hours of birth with good sensitivity and specificity. Therapy for GBS disease includes supportive intensive care and antibiotics. Significant resistance of GBS to conventional antibiotics has not been observed to date. Therefore, therapy with either ampicillin or penicillin alone or with a combination of ampicillin and gentamicin is currently recommended to eradicate the infection.

Although the infection is relatively easy to eradicate, the sequelae can be quite severe. In a series of children with neonatal meningitis, 26% of children died and another 27% sustained significant neurological injuries, including cerebral palsy, seizures, and learning disability (Hristeva et al., 1993). Abnormalities on electroencephalograms in the acute stage of disease were predictive of severe neurological injury. Currently, the most effective treatment strategy to prevent neurological disease after early onset GBS infection in children remains GBS prophylaxis through the effective use of antibiotics in pregnant mothers (Platt & O'Brien, 2003). Unfortunately, there is no prophylaxis regimen that is proven to prevent late-onset disease.

Treponema Pallidum

The spirochete *Treponema pallidum*, or *T. pallidum*, is the infectious agent responsible for syphilis (Genc & Ledger, 2000). The incidence of syphilis during pregnancy varies greatly between different populations, from 30 cases per 100,000 in the United States, to 175 cases per 100,000 in Russia, to 3,000 per 100,000 in some areas of sub-Saharan Africa. Transmission of *T. pallidum* occurs via transmission from an infected lesion in the genital region. Transmission from an infected mother to the fetus can occur either transplacentally or as a result of contact with a genital lesion during birth. Transplacental infection can occur as early as 9 weeks' gestation and results in the most severe sequelae of infection (stillbirth, spontaneous abortion, intrauterine growth restriction [IUGR], premature delivery, and severe neurological sequelae of surviving infants). *T. pallidum* infects all organs, including the developing central nervous system. A vigorous inflammatory response is activated at the onset of infection that may be responsible for some or most of the injury to the developing brain. As an indication of the severity of untreated syphilis, up to 60% of children infected in the era prior to penicillin were stillborn, died in the first month of life, or had severe brain damage (Golden, Marra, & Holmes, 2003).

Clinical diagnosis of congenital syphilis is challenging because many of the symptoms are nonspecific (Wicher & Wicher, 2001). The stereotypical sign of profound rhinorrhea and cough termed *snuffles* is specific to syphilis but is only present in approximately 20% of cases. **Hepatosplenomegaly** (enlarged liver and spleen), **petechiae** (minute skin hemorrhages), **anemia, lymphadenopathy** (enlarged lymph nodes), and **jaundice** are all common early signs that should raise suspicion. Later physical findings, including (deafness, interstitial keratitis, deformities of the teeth, and Caskin disorder), sensory neural hearing loss and bossing of the forehead indicate that extensive damage to the child has already occurred. The diagnosis of syphilis is dependent on blood tests. Treatment of maternal syphilis as early as possible is the best therapy to prevent congenital syphilis. *T. pallidum* remains exquisitely sensitive to penicillin, and a single injection during an acute infection in mothers can prevent up to 98% of congenital cases. The Jarisch-Herxheimer reaction (consisting of fever, chills, muscle pain, headache, hypotension, and tachycardia) occurs after treatment in approximately 50% of pregnant women with active syphilis and should be anticipated. Some have advocated for multiple doses of benzathine penicillin because of an increased incidence of IUGR and premature delivery in infants infected with syphilis who were treated with less aggressive regimens (Genc & Ledger, 2000) To date, no other studies have validated this finding. Despite treatment, long term neurological sequelae from congenital syphilis can still be severe including intellectual disability, deafness, retinal scarring, and seizures (Michelow et al., 2002). Although treatment will not undo damage that has already occurred, early identification and treatment can prevent subsequent abnormalities.

Toxoplasma Gondii

Toxoplasma gondii, or *T. gondii,* is a protozoan that has been known to cause fetal brain injury for decades. Humans are infected with *T. gondii* by ingestion of infected meat or protozoan eggs from feces of infected cats. Congenital trans-mission of *T. gondii* to the fetus can occur by placental transfer of the parasite from recently infected mothers. Paradoxically, frequency of congenital infection and severity of disease at birth are inversely related. When maternal infection occurs within the first trimester, congenital infection is least likely (less than 10%), yet the degree of brain injury is most severe. In contrast, transmission of *T. gondii* to fetuses is very frequent in late pregnancy yet leads to few clinical sequelae unless untreated. An estimated 4,000 cases of congenital **toxoplasmosis** occur in the United States each year (Montoya & Liesenfeld, 2004).

Transmission of specific stages of the protozoan's life cycle (the sporozoite) across the placenta leads to congenital toxoplasmosis. In nonpregnant adults, this infection causes a robust immune response. This immune response has not been studied in pregnant women or in fetuses, but it seems likely to take place in these circumstances as well. Within 2 weeks of infection, immunoglobulins are readily produced within the lymphatic system. Inflamed lymph glands are the distinctive systemic clinical feature of toxoplasmosis in cases acquired after birth. Within the fetal and newborn brain, damage is characterized by discrete areas of necrosis that can enlarge as the process evolves. Microglial cells are localized within these areas, further implicating a role for inflammatory cytokines. These necrotic regions can calcify or expand into regions that may obstruct the flow of cerebrospinal fluid, leading to hydrocephalous. Infected fetuses have areas of necrosis throughout the cortex with a predilection for the basal ganglia and periventricular regions (Jones et al., 2001).

Diagnosis of congenital toxoplasmosis can be made by clinical criteria, radiological assessment, and serological tests. In utero, ultrasonographic evidence of intracranial calcifications, ventricular dilatation, hepatic enlargement and increased placental thickness can suggest congenital toxoplasmosis. Postnatal signs of infection are myriad but include microcephaly, chorioretinitis (inflammation of the back of the eye involving the choroid and retina), strabismus, blindness, seizures, intellectual disability, low platelet count, and anemia. The classic triad of cerebral calcifications, hydrocephalous, and chorioretinitis, although rarely observed, is highly suggestive of toxoplasmosis. Blood testing has evolved significantly over the past years. The detection of immunoglobulin G (IgG) antibodies in pregnant women suggests infection within the past 3 months. Direct detection of DNA in body fluids by PCR has revolutionized prenatal diagnosis of toxoplasmosis. This assessment can be made from amniotic fluid, fetal blood, spinal fluid, or urine. Diagnosis of the infected newborn is often difficult due to the high rate of false negative and false positive results seen using serology tests performed by commercial laboratories. Therefore diagnosis is best pursued with the input of a reference laboratory using a combination of antibody tests.

At the time of this text's publication, spiramycin is the recommended treatment from the time of diagnosis until delivery. Findings from several studies, however have suggested that this regimen may not reduce the rate of affected children. Postnatally and for the first year of life, combination therapy with pyrimethamine and sulfonamides is recommended for children with congenital toxoplasmosis. Despite these efforts, congenital toxoplasmosis continues to cause a wide variety of sequelae including learning impairment, visual disturbances, cerebral palsy, intellectual disability, seizures, and many other developmental injuries.

Rubella Virus

Rubella virus is a Toga virus that has been recognized as a fetal teratogen since the 1940s. There is only one type of rubella virus, and humans are the only hosts. The virus circulates throughout a nonimmune population year-round, but endemic infections are more common in late winter and spring. Along with constant and low-level endemic transmission of the virus, there are worldwide epidemics every 6–9 years in many areas. During a 2-year period in the 1960s, there were 11,000 estimated fetal deaths and approximately 20,000 infants born with birth defects from **rubella.** Fortunately, since the institution of vaccination and surveillance programs in the early 1970s, fewer than 20 infants are born each year in the United States with a congenital rubella syndrome (Atreya, Mohan, & Kulkarni, 2004; Danovara-Holliday, Gordon, & Woernle, 2003).

Congenital rubella syndrome occurs as a result of a maternal viral infection during pregnancy. In mothers with the virus, placental infection (50%–70%) and fetal infection (20%–30%) are relatively common. Placental or fetal infection can lead to stillbirth, spontaneous abortion, or congenital abnormalities of the developing fetus. Maternal immunity to rubella fully protects fetuses from any such complications and is the mainstay of prevention. As with other prenatal infections, the most severe injuries occur when infections occur during the first trimester (up to 80% of fetuses of infected mothers are infected, and 90% of these infants have severe complications). Rubella has been isolated from brain, bone marrow, and circulating white blood cells in fetuses during pregnancy, and inflammatory reactions have been noted in virtually all organs at autopsy.

The classical clinical findings of congenital rubella syndrome are cataracts, deafness, and congenital heart disease. A wide range of other symptoms including microcephaly, developmental problems (delayed motor, intellectual, and language development), intellectual disability, and progressive encephalopathy can be manifested in the first years of life. Unilateral or bilateral deafness occurs in 80% of cases and is often the only discernable symptom of illness. CNS malformations may occur when maternal infection occurs before week 8, but the auditory nerve is vulnerable up to weeks 16–20 of pregnancy. Late effects of congenital rubella syndrome include **insulin-dependent diabetes mellitus** and hypothyroidism. Diagnosis of congenital rubella infection is routinely performed by detecting rubella-specific **immunoglobulin M (IgM)** antibody in the serum, along with the previously listed common clinical signs and symptoms. There is no effective treatment for congenital rubella syndrome once the fetus is infected; full immunization of women of childbearing age is the only effective strategy to prevent these lifelong disabilities.

Cytomegalovirus

Cytomegalovirus (CMV) is a member of the herpes family and contains a double-stranded DNA genome of more than 200 genes. It shares many features with the other herpes viruses, including the ability to cause persistent and latent (hidden inactive) infection. Unlike other teratogenic infections, a majority of adults are latently infected with CMV (approximately 50%–80% of the population). This virus infrequently causes disease except in the immunocompromised and fetuses in utero. Approximately 1% of all newborns worldwide are infected with CMV in utero and excrete virus at birth. Fortunately, fewer than 1 in 1000 of these infants have congenital CMV disease or develop postnatal sequelae. Children born to women who acquire primary CMV infection *during* pregnancy appear at greatest risk for developing symptomatic CMV disease, particularly if the infection occurs in the first half of the pregnancy (Revello & Gerna, 2002).

CMV appears to be transmitted to the fetus transplacentally, leading to an active viral infection in the fetus at critical developmental stages. CMV has been localized in all fetal organs and tissues, thereby explaining the myriad of injuries recognized in symptomatic children. The CNS is one of the most frequently involved sites, with microcephaly and intracranial calcifications being the most common manifestations of disease. As with other prenatal infections, hepatosplenomegaly, hepatitis, jaundice, anemia, and low platelet count are often observed. Approximately 15% of infants who have no symptoms at birth develop significant intellectual disability or hearing deficit within the first 5 years of life. Children with symptomatic infections often have viremia (virus that can be isolated from the blood) at birth, which may persist for the first few months of life. Both symptomatic and asymptomatic children excrete CMV in urine typically for up to 6 years and for 4 years in the saliva postnatally.

Although hearing deficit may be mild or absent at birth, progressive hearing loss may develop over the first several years of life, perhaps as a result of the chronic CMV infection. The severity of intellectual disability and developmental delay, which are the most serious neurological sequelae of this infection, is difficult to predict at birth. Therefore, children with congenital infection, including those without symptoms, should not be given a firm prognosis at birth.

Diagnosis and treatment of congenital CMV infection are quite different from other viral pathogens. Growth of CMV from urinary samples obtained within the first 2–3 weeks of life is diagnostic of congenital CMV infection, and the viral assay will accurately identify shed virus within 48 to 72 hours. However, the identification of shed virus has little predictive value of further injury for previously stated reasons (up to 90% of infants shedding virus at birth will develop typically). Therefore, performing this test in children with symptoms consistent with CMV infection is most likely to yield meaningful clinical information. Antibody screening for CMV, a mainstay in several other infections, is only useful in mothers known to be seronegative for CMV, as this would rule out congenital infection. Ganciclovir, an antiviral agent, is effective in treating and preventing shedding of CMV. In congenital CMV disease,

a randomized trial has demonstrated that 6 weeks of ganciclovir therapy mitigates hearing impairment at 1 year of age. In this study, the treated infants did have low white blood cell count as a side effect that required dosage adjustments and an increased risk of sepsis (Kimberlin et al., 2003). Ultimately, the development of a CMV vaccine may be the best way to minimize the effects of this virus on the developing nervous system (Gellin & Modlin, 2004).

Herpes Simplex Viruses

The **herpes simplex virus (HSV),** a member of the Herpesviridae family of viruses, has a double-stranded DNA genome of 150,000 base pairs. There are 2 types—HSV-1 and HSV-2—which differ in their antigenic and biologic properties. As with other herpes viruses, they commonly cause latent infection and recurrences. Only 5% of all neonatal infections with HSV are acquired in utero with 85% occurring as a result of contact during the birth process with infected maternal lesions or asymptomatic cervical shedding of HSV. The remainder is presumably acquired from environmental sources, such as persons with oral HSV infections. In utero infection during the first 20 weeks of pregnancy is associated with the highest infant morbidity and mortality, including stillbirths and spontaneous abortions. Although the exact route by which infants acquire intrauterine HSV infections is not known, several observations suggest that most infants become infected by the virus ascending from the vagina and entering the fetus through the placental membrane rather than from passage of HSV from the maternal bloodstream to the fetus. Thus, delivery via cesarean-section greatly reduces the incidence of infection (Schleiss, 2003; Whitley, 2002).

Diagnosis of intrauterine HSV infection requires clinical evidence of HSV infection at birth and virologic confirmation by recovery of the virus from the newborn within the first 48 hours of life. The classic triad of symptoms is skin lesions, hydranencephaly (complete or almost complete absence of the cerebral hemispheres), and chorioretinitis. Dissemination with multisystem involvement usually involves the liver, kidneys, and hematologic and central nervous systems. Within the brain, hydranencephaly, microcephaly, intracranial calcifications, hydrocephalus, porencephaly (deficient development of the cerebral cortex and gray matter so that cystic cavities communicate with the brain surface), and subdural or epidural cysts may occur, with subsequent development of blindness, deafness, and intellectual disability. Involvement of the eye, particularly chorioretinitis with a concomitant strabismus, is common. This occurs more frequently with intrauterine HSV infection than with HSV infection acquired during or after birth. Intrauterine HSV infection often leads to disseminated disease, resulting in spontaneous abortion or stillbirth. Infants born alive with intrauterine HSV infection are likely to have a localized skin infection. The morbidity and mortality of children with intrauterine HSV infections is similar to rates in children with infection at birth or shortly after. If the infection is untreated, the mortality is about 70%; treatment with the antiviral agent acyclovir reduces it to about 30%. The effect of antiviral therapy on morbidity is unknown, and many treated infants, particularly those with CNS involvement, will have blindness, deafness, or profound intellectual disability.

Diagnosis of intrauterine HSV infections is made by recovery of virus from the infant within the first 48 hours of life (Enright & Prober, 2002). HSV isolation within 48 hours of birth from infants who have none of the manifestations of intrauterine HSV infection may merely reflect perinatal HSV colonization. HSV should be recoverable from skin lesions or vesicles, if present at birth. A Tzanck test of epithelial cells scraped from skin lesions may reveal multinucleated giant cells. PCR analysis of cerebrospinal fluid has been developed to diagnose herpetic encephalitis. Antiviral therapy with acyclovir should be initiated promptly for newborns with suspected intrauterine HSV infection. There is a high incidence of recurrence of HSV after therapy, particularly of skin lesions, and these children should be monitored carefully.

Human Immunodeficiency Virus

HIV is a **retrovirus** that infects cells of the immune system, rendering the affected individual incapable of mounting sufficient immunological responses to a host of infections. It is the cause of acquired immunodeficiency syndrome (AIDS) and has a complex life cycle linked to CD4 cells in the bloodstream (see Figure 6.1). Approximately 25% of infants born to mothers with HIV infection will become infected if no intervention occurs. In some infants, transmission of the virus appears to occur in utero be-

cause the virus is detectable in their blood at birth. In others, transmission appears to occur in the perinatal period because these infants demonstrate viremia as early as the second day of life up to 2 months of age. Transmission via breast milk also occurs and may be important in disease transmission in undiagnosed mothers and those in developing countries (Berk et al., 2005; Newell et al., 2004).

As many as half of infected children manifest signs or symptoms of infections within the first year of life, and severity of symptomatology can be grouped into several categories (see Table 6.3). A group of rapid progressors (those who exhibit symptoms of HIV at much earlier time periods) was long believed to consist predominantly of children who were infected in utero. More recent evidence suggests that the viral load is more predictive of disease progression (750,000 copies of virus per milliliter of blood in the rapid progressors at 1 month of age, compared to less than 300,000 in other in-

Table 6.3. Pediatric human immunodeficiency virus (HIV) classification

Immunological categories	Clinical categories			
1: No evidence of immunosuppression	N1	A1	B1	C1
2: Evidence of moderate immunosuppression	N2	A2	B2	C2
3: Severe immunosuppression	N3	A3	B3	C3

Adapted from Centers for Disease Control and Prevention. (1994). 1994 revised classification system for human immunodeficiency virus infection in children less than 13 years of age. *Morbidity and Mortality Weekly Report, 43* (No. RR-12), 2.

Key: N, no signs; A, mild signs; B, moderate signs; C, severe signs or symptoms or symptoms.

Note: Children whose HIV infection status is not confirmed are classified by using the above classifications with the letter E (for perinatally exposed) before the appropriate classification code (e.g., EN2 for perinatally exposed with no signs/symptoms and evidence of moderate immunosuppression).

Clinical Category N characterizes children who are infected with HIV but remain asymptomatic.

Clinical Category A includes mildly symptomatic children who have enlargement of lymph nodes, liver, and spleen and recurrent infections of the middle ear and sinus cavities.

Clinical Category B includes moderately symptomatic children. Symptoms include but are not limited to low counts of various blood cell types (anemia, thrombocytopenia, or neutropenia), a single episode of serious bacterial infection (bacterial pneumonia, bone or joint infection, meningitis, bacteremia), chickenpox, herpes simplex oral infection, cardiomyopathy (abnormality of the heart muscle, leading to its relative weakness and widening of its chambers), and other conditions.

Clinical Category C includes children with severe symptoms such as multiple system bacterial infections or opportunistic infections that are considered to be acquired immunodeficiency syndrome (AIDS) indicator diseases, including tuberculosis, *Candida* infection of the esophagus, cryptococcal infection, *Pneumocystis carinii* pneumonia, B-cell lymphoma, and others.

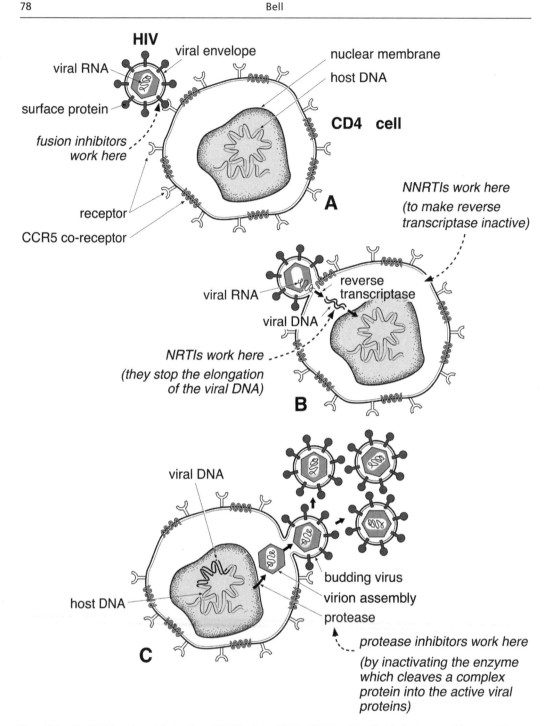

Figure 6.1. The HIV life cycle and destruction of CD4 T-cells by HIV. The CD4 T-cell is critical to the immune defense, and its destruction is the major cause of the progressive immunodeficiency disorder that is the hallmark of HIV infection. One mechanism of destruction involves HIV a) entering and b) replicating in the CD4 cell and then c) budding from and damaging the cell membrane. (*Key:* NNRTIs, non-nucleoside reverse transcriptase inhibitors; NRTIs, nucleoside reverse transcriptase inhibitors.)

fants). Initial signs or symptoms of HIV infection can present acutely or gradually. Recurrent or difficult-to-eradicate oral candidiasis (yeast infection), generalized lymphadenopathy, and hepatosplenomegaly are common early signs of infection, and children infected in utero may be born already manifesting signs of disease. Conditions that are common in the general pediatric population, including ear infections, upper respiratory tract infections, gastroenteritis, and pneumonia, occur more frequently in children with HIV than in other children. AIDS-defining conditions are uncommon in children with normally functioning immune systems and can be the earliest indicators of HIV infection. Poor weight gain, lymphadenopathy, or recurrent oral candidiasis often present before the AIDS-defining condition, although their significance may not be appreciated. *Pneumocystis carinii* pneumonia (PCP) is the most common AIDS-defining condition presenting in infancy, although CMV disease and toxoplasmosis are commonly seen in such infants as well. With successful treatment, however, these conditions are rarely seen.

Diagnosis of HIV in infants requires isolation of virus or viral particles as well as serological analysis. Infants born to women with HIV acquire HIV antibodies passively from their mothers. Preterm infants can rarely be born before transfer of maternal antibody and have negative serology at birth. Therefore, virtually all infants of women with HIV possess antibody against HIV at birth, yet only about one fourth are actually infected. Maternal HIV antibodies typically persist for 9–12 months, with virtually 100% of uninfected infants losing antibodies by 18 months of age. It is desirable to identify children with HIV early, and improved diagnostic methods allow most children to be identified in the first weeks or months of life as having HIV. Although serological tests can be used as screening tools in children younger than 18 months old, the diagnosis of HIV infection is best confirmed by a molecular assay. This HIV DNA PCR method has a sensitivity and specificity of greater than 99%. HIV PCR testing at birth (within 48 hours), at 1–2 months of age, and at 4–6 months of age in suspected children is recommended. PCR for HIV DNA will be negative in approximately 60% of infected children at birth because the viral load is below the level of detection of the assay. When PCR is positive, a second confirmatory test should be performed. The confirmatory test can be a second PCR, an HIV culture, or a viral load test. The latter has the advantage of both confirming the result and serving as a baseline before initiation of therapy. If all PCR results remain negative by 4–6 months of age, the infant has a greater than 99% chance of not being infected with HIV.

Treatment for congenital HIV infection has become more and more aggressive because this approach has been shown to lead to a marked decrease in the transmission of virus to fetuses and children. As of 2006, ZDV is the pharmacologic agent in use to reduce perinatal HIV transmission. Treatment consists of three separate phases: 1) oral ZDV as part of a minimum three-drug regimen for the infected mother beginning at the fourteenth week of pregnancy if the pregnant woman was not already receiving treatment at the time of conception, 2) intravenous ZDV during labor, and 3) oral ZDV for the infant during the first 6 weeks of life. Multidrug regimens are almost always prescribed for the pregnant woman based on the most current guidelines.

Since the early 1990s, guidelines addressing the complex issues of treatment of pediatric HIV disease have been developed. In general, antiretroviral agents should be used in combination in the treatment of all children with HIV. Single drug therapy has been shown to be inferior, presumably because HIV can develop mutations that render the virus resistant to individual agents. The availability of different drugs with different actions has led to combination therapy referred to as highly active antiretroviral therapy (HAART). These regimens routinely involve the use of three or more drugs, including a protease inhibitor. Another principal that has been adopted for care of HIV infected children is the measurement of viral load. This can assess the adequacy of medical therapies with the goal being suppression of viral number below limits of detection of the assay. Adjustments of dosages of medications for weight are an ongoing part of good clinical care because underdosing of medications can lead to development of viral resistance. For newly diagnosed cases in infants, therapy should be started as soon as a confirmed diagnosis is established.

HIV enters the CNS in the early stages of the infection, and the brain is thought to be a reservoir for HIV sequestration for several reasons. The blood–brain barrier protects HIV from the actions of many antiretroviral therapies and endogenous immune mechanisms that can lead to reduction of viral load. Microglial cells, which normally respond to infections, possess the HIV receptor (CD4) and are the likely site for HIV latent infection. Neurons and glial cells are damaged by HIV either through direct actions of the virus or by releasing neurotoxic compounds. Moreover, children with HIV are susceptible to opportunistic infections of the central nervous system, including toxoplasma encephalitis, cryptococcal meningitis, cytomegalovirus encephalitis, and progressive multifocal leukoencephalopathy. In sum, children with congenital HIV infection are uniquely susceptible to developmental brain injuries for a myriad of reasons.

Lymphocytic Choriomeningitis Virus

Lymphocytic choriomeningitis virus (LCMV), an Arena virus first isolated in 1933, has been recently discovered as a fetal infection that can lead to serious neurological sequelae (Barton & Mets, 2001). The principal reservoir for LCMV infection is chronically infected mice and hamsters, with humans acquiring infection after inhalation or contact with infected fomites (inanimate particles via which pathogenic organisms may be transferred). Primary infection causes CNS symptoms in over half of the cases, predominantly clinical symptoms consistent with aseptic (viral) meningitis. Classic LCMV infection in adults is a biphasic illness characterized by fever, malaise, headache, and photophobia (visual discomfort with bright light) preceding a variety of neurological complications (transverse myelitis, auditory nerve deafness, **Guillain Barré syndrome,** and hydrocephalous). Congenital LCMV infection is believed to occur via transplacental passage of the virus in the first and second trimester of pregnancy. Only several dozen cases of proven congenital LCMV infection have been documented, but the serological diagnosis of infection has only recently been made available. The predominant neurological impairments noted in children with congenital LCMV infection are chorioretinitis (over 90%), retinal scarring, optic atrophy, nystagmus, microcephaly, and periventricular calcifications. Of surviving infants, most manifest severe developmental injury including cerebral palsy, intellectual disability, seizures and diminished visual acuity. Experimental infection of mice with LCMV results in initial viral replication within the ependyma (membranous web lining the ventricle) and subsequent hydrocephalous, whereas infection of the virus in neonatal rats leads to retinitis. Although definitive therapy for LCMV has not been attempted, the antiviral agent ribavirin has shown efficacy in vitro (Bechtel, Haught, & Mets, 1997; Larsen et al., 1993).

Infection with LCMV likely activates the immune system, and brains of affected children show inflammatory changes. Because of this pattern of immune activation, serological diagnosis of LCMV is now possible. An immunofluorescent antibody test specific for LCMV has been developed with a high degree of specificity and sensitivity. More recently, a more rapid enzyme-linked immunosorbent assay (ELISA) has shown promise at the CDC.

INTRAUTERINE INFLAMMATION AND DEVELOPMENTAL DISABILITIES

In addition to the neurological and developmental brain injuries caused by these specific pathogens that either invade the CNS or the meninges, evidence is accumulating that many nonspecific infections and inflammation at critical times during brain formation can lead to injuries to the fetus. Damage to the developing white matter, the pathological condition called **periventricular leukomalacia (PVL),** has been linked to intrauterine inflammation as well as the development of cerebral palsy. The root cause of this association is not clear. However, investigations suggest that mediators of inflammation may damage developing cells of the white matter as outlined next.

Since the mid-1990s, there have been several epidemiological studies implicating intrauterine inflammation and infections within the placental tissues as causes of cerebral palsy and other white matter disorders. Chorioamnionitis is the infection of the amniotic sac with invading organisms and is generally defined by clinical assessment (maternal fever after birth, foul smelling amniotic fluid) or laboratory (evidence of invading organisms within pathology specimens). In one of the most comprehensive studies, Grether and Nelson found that mothers with clinical chorioamnionitis were over nine times more likely to deliver a child who developed cerebral palsy than those without infection (Grether & Nelson, 1997). There have been at least 12 studies confirming the association between clinical chorioamnionitis and cerebral palsy, and 7 other studies have found the association with cystic PVL (Wu, 2002). A total of 11 studies demonstrated the association between histological chorioamnionitis and either of these conditions. In the most comprehensive study to date, Wu and colleagues performed a meta-analysis of these studies and demonstrated that chorioamnionitis is associated with approximately a two-fold increase in risk of developing cerebral palsy or PVL (Wu & Colford, 2000).

Detection of cytokines in pathological specimens provides further evidence for a link between developmental brain injuries and intrauterine inflammation. Cytokines mediate the response of the body to inflammatory stimuli by recruiting immune cells to the site of infection and aiding in eradicating the invading microorganisms. However, in many disease states, the actions of cytokines result in damage to organs and deaths of developing cells. In intrauterine inflammation and infection, four cytokines (tumor necrosis factor [TNF], interferon-gamma [IFN-γ], interleukin-1 [IL-1] and inter-leukin-6 [IL6]) have been detected in fetal blood, placenta or amniotic fluid in children ultimately found to have cerebral palsy or similar brain injury (Arntzen et al., 1998; Fortunato et al., 1996; Grether et al., 1999; Nelson et al., 2003; Yoon, Jun, Romero, et al., 1997; Yoon, Kim, Romero, et al., 1997; Yoon et al., 1996). More directly, TNF and IL-2 have been localized to periventricular lesions in autopsy specimens, suggesting a direct role of these cytokines in brain injury in children (Deguchi, Mizuguchi, & Takashima, 1996; Iida et al., 1993; Kadhim et al., 2002). In tissue culture, combinations of the cytokines TNF and IFN-γ kill progenitor (stem) cells of the oligodendrocyte lineage. It is these cells that are responsible for effective myelin production during development and are uniquely susceptible to injury in children with cerebral palsy (Andrews, Zhang, & Bhat, 1998; Back et al., 2001; Pouly et al., 2000). These associations have been studied in many animal models with the hope that mechanisms of injuries can be better understood, leading to prevention of these injuries in children (Bell & Hallenbeck, 2002; Cai et al., 2000; Duncan et al., 2002; Gilles, Leviton, & Kerr, 1976; Lenhardt et al., 2002; Yoon, Kim, Romero, et al., 1997).

SUMMARY

In conclusion, fetal infection can have profound effects on brain development. Many specific agents are known to cause injuries, and newer evidence suggests that infections within the amnion-placental unit can also be detrimental. The mechanisms responsible for injuries to the developing brain are still not clear. It is likely that continued efforts at determining the effects of specific pathogens and other stimuli may lead to a better understanding of the processes responsible for cellular damage, ultimately leading to improved therapeutic options for affected children and mothers.

REFERENCES

Andrews, G., Zhang, P., & Bhat, N. (1998). TNF potentiates INF-induced cell death in oligodendrocyte progenitors. *Journal of Neuroscience Research, 54*, 574–583.

Arntzen, K.J., Kjollesdal, A.M., Halgunset, J., et al. (1998). TNF, IL-1, IL-6, IL-8 and soluble TNF receptors in relation to chorioamnionitis and premature labor. *Journal of Perinatal Medicine, 26*, 17–26.

Atreya, C., Mohan, K., & Kulkarni, S. (2004). Rubella virus and birth defects: Molecular insights into the viral teratogenesis at the cellular level. *Birth Defects Research, 70*, 431–437.

Back, S., Luo, N., Borenstein, N., et al. (2001). Late oligodendrocyte progenitors coincide with the developmental window of vulnerability for human perinatal white matter injury. *Journal of Neuroscience, 21*, 1302–1312.

Barton, L., & Mets, M. (2001). Congenital lymphocytic choriomeningitis virus infection: Decade of rediscovery. *Clinical Infectious Diseases, 33*, 370–374.

Bechtel, R., Haught, K., & Mets, M. (1997). Lymphocytic choriomeningitis virus: A new addition to the TORCH evaluation. *Archives of Opthalmology, 115*, 680–681.

Bell, M., & Hallenbeck, J. (2002). Effects of intrauterine inflammation on developing rat brain. *Journal of Neuroscience Research, 70*(4), 570–579.

Berk, D., Falkovitz-Halpern, M., Hill, D., et al. (2005). Temporal trends in early clinical manifestations of perinatal HIV infection in a population based cohort. *Journal of the American Medical Association, 293*, 2221–2231.

Berner, R. (2002). Group B streptococci during pregnancy and infancy. *Current Opinion in Infectious Diseases, 15*, 307–313.

Cai, Z., Pan, Z.-L., Pang, Y., et al. (2000). Cytokine induction in fetal rat brains and brain injury in neonatal rats after maternal lipopolysaccharide administration. *Pediatric Research, 47*, 64–72.

Centers for Disease Control and Prevention. (1994). 1994 revised classification system for human immunodeficiency virus infection in children less than 13 years of age. *Morbidity and Mortality Weekly Report, 43*(RR-12), 2.

Centers for Disease Control and Prevention. (1996). Prevention of perinatal group B streptococcal disease: A public health perspective. *Morbidity and Mortality Weekly Report, 45*(RR-7), 1–24.

Danovara-Holliday, C., Gordon, E., & Woernle, C. (2003). Identifying risk factors for rubella susceptibility in a population at risk in the United States. *American Journal of Public Health, 93*, 289–291.

Deguchi, K., Mizuguchi, M., & Takashima, S. (1996). Immunohistochemical expression of TNF in neonatal leukomalacia. *Pediatric Neurology, 14*, 13–16.

Duncan, J., Cock, M., Scheerlinck, J., et al. (2002). White matter injury after repeated endotoxin exposure in the preterm ovine fetus. *Pediatric Research, 52*, 941–949.

Enright, A., & Prober, C. (2002). Neonatal herpes infection: Diagnosis, treatment and prevention. *Seminars in Neonatology, 7*, 283–291.

Fortunato, S.J., Menon, R.P., Swan, K.F., et al. (1996). Inflammatory cytokine (interleukin 1, 6, 8 and tumor necrosis factor a) release from cultured human fetal membranes in response to endotoxic lipopolysaccharide mirrors amniotic fluid concentrations. *American Journal of Obstetrics and Gynecology, 174*, 1855–1862.

Gellin, B., & Modlin, J. (2004). Vaccine development to prevent cytomegalovirus disease: Report from the National Vaccine Advisory Committee. *Clinical Infectious Diseases, 39*, 233–239.

Genc, M., & Ledger, W. (2000). Syphilis in pregnancy. *Sexually Transmitted Infections, 76*, 73–79.

Gilles, F.H., Leviton, A., & Kerr, C.S. (1976). Endotoxin leucoencephalopathy in the telencephalon of the newborn kitten. *Journal of Neurological Sciences, 27*, 183–191.

Golden, M., Marra, C., & Holmes, K. (2003). Update on syphilis. *Journal of the American Medical Association, 290,* 1510–1514.

Grether, J., & Nelson, K. (1997). Maternal infection and cerebral palsy in infants of normal birth weight. *Journal of the American Medical Association, 278,* 207–211.

Grether, J., Nelson, K., Dambrosia, J., et al. (1999). Interferons and cerebral palsy. *Journal of Pediatrics, 134,* 324–332.

Hristeva, L., Booy, R., Bowler, I. et al. (1993). Prospective surveillance of neonatal meningitis. *Archives of Disease in Childhood, 69*(1, Spec. No.), 14–18.

Iida, K., Takashima, S., Takeuchi, Y., et al. (1993). Neuropathological study of newborns with prenatal-onset leukomalacia. *Pediatric Neurology, 9,* 45–48.

Jones, J., Lopez, A., Wilson, M., et al. (2001). Congenital toxoplasmosis: A review. *Obstetrical & Gynecological Survey, 56,* 296–305.

Kadhim, H., Tabarki, B., De Prez, C., et al. (2002). Interleukin-2 in the pathogenesis of perinatal white matter damage. *Neurology, 58,* 1125–1128.

Kimberlin, D.W., Lin, C.Y., Sanchez, P.J., et al. (2003). Effect of ganciclovir therapy on hearing in symptomatic congenital cytomegalovirus disease involving the central nervous system: A randomized, controlled trial. *The Journal of Pediatrics, 143*(1), 16–25.

Larsen, P., Chartrand, S., Tomashek, K., (1993). Hydrocephalous complicating lymphocytic choriomeningitis virus infection. *Pediatric Infectious Disease Journal, 12,* 528–531.

Lenhardt, S., Lachance, C., Patrizi, S., et al. (2002). The Toll-like receptor TLR4 is necessary for lipopolysaccharide-induced oligodendrocyte injury in the central nervous system. *Journal of Neuroscience, 22,* 2478–2486.

Michelow, I., Wendel, G., Norgard, M., et al. (2002). Central nervous system infection in congenital syphilis. *The New England Journal of Medicine, 346,* 1792–1798.

Montoya, J., & Liesenfeld, O. (2004). Toxoplasmosis. *The Lancet, 363,* 1965–1976.

Nelson, K.B., Grether, J.K., Dambrosia, J.M., et al. (2003). Neonatal cytokines and cerebral palsy in very preterm infants. *Pediatric Research, 53*(4), 600–607.

Newell, M.-L., Hoosen, C., Cortina-Borja, M., et al. (2004). Mortality of infected and uninfected infants born to HIV-infected mothers in Africa: A pooled analysis. *The Lancet, 364,* 1236–1243.

Platt, J., & O'Brien, W. (2003). Group B streptococcus: Prevention of early onset neonatal sepsis. *Obstetrical & Gynecological Survey, 58,* 191–196.

Pouly, S., Becher, B., Blain, M., et al. (2000). Interferon gamma modulates human oligodendrocyte susceptibility to Fas-mediated apoptosis. *Journal of Neuropathy and Experimental Neurology, 59,* 280–286.

Revello, M., & Gerna, G. (2002). Diagnosis and management of human cytomegalovirus infection in the mother, fetus and newborn infant. *Clinical Microbiology Reviews, 15,* 680–715.

Schleiss, M. (2003). Vertically transmitted herpes virus infections. *Herpes, 10,* 4–11.

Whitley, R. (2002). Herpes simplex virus infection. *Seminars in Pediatrics, 13,* 6–11.

Wicher, V., & Wicher, K. (2001). Pathogenesis of maternal-fetal syphilis revisited. *Clinical Infectious Diseases, 33,* 354–363.

Wu, Y. (2002). Systematic review of chorioamnionitis and cerebral palsy. *Mental Retardation and Developmental Disabilities Research Reviews, 8,* 25–29.

Wu, Y., & Colford, J. (2000). Chorioamnionitis as a risk factor for cerebral palsy: A meta-analysis. *Journal of the American Medical Association, 284,* 1417–1424.

Yoon, B.-H., Jun, J. K., Romero, R., et al. (1997). Amniotic fluid inflammatory cytokines (interleukin-6, interleukin-1B, and tumor necrosis factor-a), neonatal brain white matter lesions and cerebral palsy. *American Journal of Obstetrics and Gynecology, 177,* 19–26.

Yoon, B.-H., Kim, C. J., Romero, R., et al. (1997). Experimentally induced intrauterine infection causes fetal brain white matter lesions in rabbits. *American Journal of Obstetrics and Gynecology, 177,* 797–802.

Yoon, B.-H., Romero, R., Tang, S.H., et al. (1996). Interleukin-6 concentrations in umbilical cord plasma are elevated in neonates with white matter lesions associated with periventricular leukomalacia. *American Journal of Obstetrics and Gynecology, 174,* 1433–1440.

7 Birth Defects and Prenatal Diagnosis

Rhonda L. Schonberg and Cynthia J. Tifft

Upon completion of this chapter, the reader will

- Be knowledgeable about the indications for and limitations of first and second trimester screening for birth defects, ultrasonography, fetal magnetic resonance imaging, and echocardiography

- Understand noninvasive prenatal screening and the techniques of amniocentesis and chorionic villus sampling and be able to determine when invasive diagnostic testing is indicated

- Be familiar with alternative reproductive techniques and realize in what circumstances couples might benefit from such technologies

- Become familiar with some of the current approaches to fetal therapy

- Understand the psychosocial needs of families who are at increased risk for bearing children with genetic disorders or birth defects

---

The birth of a child with disabilities can have a devastating impact on parents and extended family members. As couples grieve the loss of their expected "normal" child and work to accept the child they have, they look to the future to understand what happened to them and why. Although most infants are born without complications, in the United States 3% of births result in a child who has a birth defect or a genetic disorder (Centers for Disease Control and Prevention, 2006). These events can affect any couple regardless of age or ethnicity. Although we know of circumstances that can increase the risk, some of which are discussed in this chapter, most newborns with a birth defect/genetic disorder will be born to couples who are unaware they are at risk and have no family history of similarly affected children. When this occurs, genetic evaluation can help determine a diagnosis and/or mode of inheritance (discussed in Chapter 1). Advances in prenatal diagnosis have provided couples the opportunity to gain information about their pregnancy, including birth defects or genetic disorders that may affect their child, and to examine a range of family planning alternatives.

This chapter discusses genetic screening available prior to and during pregnancy, diagnostic testing available for pregnancies determined to be at an increased risk for specific genetic disorders, recent advances in fetal therapy, and alternative reproductive choices.

CHELSEA

Susan, a 31-year-old who had previously miscarried, was enjoying her second pregnancy. Her fears were raised in the second trimester when a maternal serum screening test revealed an elevated **alpha-fetoprotein (AFP)** level. Her obstetrician recommended a detailed fetal ultrasound, which showed a fetal abdominal wall defect (**gastroschisis**). Susan and her husband Rick met with the genetics staff, who explained that gastroschisis is usually an isolated malformation not associated with a chromosomal abnormality, additional medical problems, or learning disabilities. After considering the information provided and weighing the risks, the couple decided not to undergo amniocentesis. They met with a pediatric surgeon to discuss the management of an infant with gastroschisis and visited the high-risk nursery where their baby would be treated after birth. On the basis of the information they received, Susan and Rick decided to continue the pregnancy and prepared for the birth of their child. Susan had ultrasounds every 3–4 weeks throughout the remainder of the pregnancy to monitor fetal growth and **amniotic fluid** volume. When delivery came, the family and the surgical team were prepared. Surgery was performed on baby Chelsea's first day of life with an uneventful recovery. At 1 year of age, Chelsea is a growing, thriving, healthy child.

GENETIC ASSESSMENT

Many individuals wonder what their risk of having a child with a birth defect or genetic disorder might be. Genetic counselors can help in this area (National Society of Genetic Counselors, 1983):

> Genetic counselors are health professionals with specialized graduate degrees and experience in the area of medical genetics and counseling. . . . as members of a health care team . . . They identify families at risk, investigate the problem present in the family, interpret information about the disorder, analyze inheritance patterns and risks of recurrence and review available options with the family.

Throughout the United States, many centers offer the skills of a genetic counselor combined with the medical expertise of physicians trained in genetics. (An updated listing of these centers can be found at http://www.GeneClinics.org.) Assessing reproductive risk generally involves reviewing an individual's medical history and obtaining an extended family history, including birth defects, genetic disorders, unexplained infant deaths, and recurrent pregnancy losses. Information on maternal medication use and occupational or other exposures can also provide clues to possible reproductive risks. Many perinatologists and obstetricians also receive specialized training in genetics and can offer information about the management and potential outcome of pregnancies known to be complicated by a fetal birth defect or a genetic disorder.

Knowing an individual's ethnic background can be one of the initial steps in assessing risk. Individuals from defined ethnic backgrounds have a higher chance of carrying a gene known to be associated with a particular genetic disorder (Table 7.1). Most of the disorders amenable to carrier screening are autosomal recessive, meaning two parents would have to be identified as carriers to be at increased risk of having an affected child (see Chapter 1) and have high morbidity and mortality. Advanced knowledge of this risk provides couples the opportunity to consider alternative reproductive options or undergo prenatal diagnostic testing. Couples of mixed ethnicity may also decide to meet with a genetic counselor to discuss their individual situation.

A couple may also be at increased risk for having a child with a genetic disorder if a previous child or other family member has been di-

Table 7.1. Disorders with increased carrier frequencies in particular ethnic groups (carrier testing and prenatal diagnosis is available for each of these disorders)

Ethnic group	Disorder at risk	Estimated carrier frequency
African American or West African	Sickle cell anemia	1 in 12
Ashkenazi Jewish (Eastern European Jewish)	Gaucher disease (type 1)	1 in 15
	Cystic fibrosis	1 in 25
	Tay-Sachs disease	1 in 27
	Familial dysautonomia	1 in 36
	Canavan disease	1 in 40
	Fanconi anemia	1 in 90
	Niemann-Pick disease (type A)	1 in 90
	Bloom syndrome	1 in 100
Asian	Alpha thalassemia	1 in 8 to 1 in 20
European and North American (Caucasian)	Cystic fibrosis	1 in 25
French Canadian	Tay-Sachs disease	1 in 27
Mediterranean	Beta thalassemia	1 in 15 to 1 in 20

From Seashore, M.R. (1999). Clinical genetics. In B.N. Burrow & T.P. Duffy (Eds.), *Medical complications during pregnancy* (5th ed., p. 216). Philadelphia: W.B. Saunders; adapted by permission.

agnosed with the disorder. A detailed review of the family history, pregnancy history, and medical records (if available), as well as examination of the affected individual to verify or establish the diagnosis, can be extremely helpful in discussing reproductive risks and prenatal testing options.

As of December 2006, specific genetic testing was available for nearly 1,340 genetic disorders, and the number continues to grow. Medical centers that provide genetic services have the most up-to-date information on the availability and limitations of genetic testing. The genetic services staff can also help locate appropriate resources and support groups for families. Three such resources are the Genetics Home Reference, a National Library of Medicine supported database of information about genetic conditions, genes and chromosomes, and patient resources for the general public (http://ghr.nlm.nih.gov); the Genetic Alliance, a clearinghouse for information and support groups for genetic disorders (http://www.geneticalliance.org); and the National Organization for Rare Disorders (http://www.rarediseases.org).

Women who will be 35 years old or older at the birth of their child have an increased risk to have a baby with Down syndrome or another chromosomal abnormality (Hook, 1981; Morris et al., 2003; see Figure 7.1). Additional indications for prenatal diagnosis are noted in Table 7.2.

SCREENING EVALUATIONS DURING PREGNANCY

It is now considered standard of care for prenatal service providers in developed countries to offer indicated screening evaluations and genetic diagnostic testing during pregnancy. The following sections describe particular screenings conducted during the first and second trimesters.

First Trimester

Screening in the first trimester of pregnancy can allow for earlier assessments, diagnosis, and genetic counseling. Such evaluations can take the form of first-trimester ultrasonography and maternal serum screening. Although there have been continued advances in first trimester screening, the American College of Obstetrics and Gynecology continues to recommend that all women age 35 or greater also be offered di-

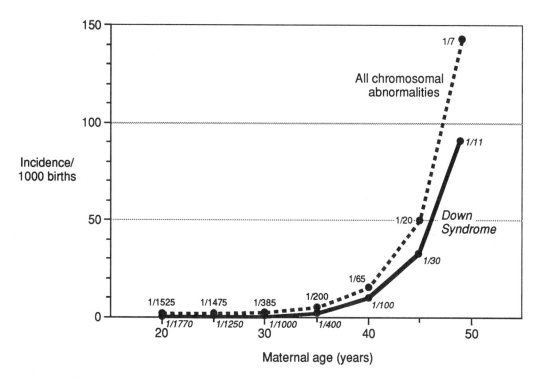

Figure 7.1. Risk of trisomy 21 and all chromosome abnormalities in pregnant women of various ages. Risk increases markedly after 35 years of age. (*Source:* Hook, 1981.)

Table 7.2. Common indications for chorionic villus sampling (CVS) and amniocentesis

Indication	CVS	Amniocentesis
Maternal age 35 or older	X	X
Previous offspring with a chromosome abnormality	X	X
Increased risk to have a child with a genetic disorder (e.g., previous affected child, positive carrier testing, carrier of X-linked disorder)	X	X
Previous offspring with a neural tube defect (e.g., spina bifida, anencephaly)		X
Increased nuchal translucency and screen positive first trimester maternal serum screening	X	X
Increased risk for having a child with a chromosome abnormality or neural tube defect based on a second trimester maternal serum screening test		X
Anatomic abnormality identified via ultrasound		X

agnostic testing using chorionic villus sampling (CVS; performed in the first trimester) or **amniocentesis** (performed in the second trimester).

First-Trimester Ultrasound Ultrasound can establish fetal viability, determine the number of fetuses (useful when a patient has had in vitro fertilization), and locate placental position. It can also measure the nuchal translucency (the transparency of the fluid-filled cavity at the nape of the neck), which may indicate an increased risk for Down syndrome (Nicolaides, 2004).

First-Trimester Maternal Serum Screening Testing of maternal serum free beta human chorionic gonadotropin (free beta-hCG) and pregnancy-associated plasma protein A (PAPP-A) at 10–14 weeks' gestation add to the risk assessment. For instance, elevations in PAPP-A and free beta-hCG combined with an ultrasound finding of increased nuchal translucency have been found to correctly identify 87% of fetuses with Down syndrome (Orlandi et al., 1997). When maternal age is included in the analysis, the sensitivity for identifying a

Down syndrome pregnancy is 90%, with a false positive rate of 5% (Nicolaides, 2004).

Increased nuchal translucency in the absence of a chromosomal abnormality is associated with adverse outcome including a greater incidence of congenital heart disease (CHD), other fetal anomalies (and therefore warrants a recommendation for further ultrasound studies and a fetal echocardiogram later in the pregnancy), and fetal death (Hafner et al., 2003; Souka et al., 2005). Extreme variations in the maternal serum analytes free beta-hCG or PAPP-A can also indicate adverse outcome of pregnancy including low birth weight, stillbirth, fetal loss, and early delivery (Dugoff et al., 2004; Krantz et al., 2004).

Chorionic Villus Sampling CVS is a minute biopsy of the **chorion,** the outermost membrane surrounding the embryo. Chorionic **villi,** consisting of rapidly dividing cells of fetal origin, can be analyzed directly or grown in culture prior to testing (Blakemore, 1988). CVS can be used for chromosome analysis, enzyme assay, or molecular DNA analysis.

CVS is performed at 10–12 weeks' gestation, before a woman may appear pregnant and prior to "quickening" (the detection of fetal movement by the mother). Using ultrasound guidance, a chorionic villus biopsy is performed either by suction through a small catheter passed through the cervix or by aspiration via a needle inserted through the abdominal wall and uterus (Figure 7.2). CVS increases the risk of first trimester pregnancy loss by 1% (Goldberg, Porter, & Golbus, 1990). Limb reduction defects (foreshortened fingers, arms, or legs), possibly the result of placental bleeding or hypoxia caused by the procedure, have been reported in fewer than 1 in 1,000 procedures. Limb reduction abnormalities were reported more often when the CVS was performed prior to 10 weeks' gestation or by an operator not fully experienced with the technique (Burton, Schultz, & Burd, 1992). For that reason, CVS is now routinely offered after 10 weeks' gestation, and referral to a high-volume center is encouraged.

Second Trimester

Two primary screening tests—maternal serum screening and ultrasonography—are also offered in the second trimester. Magnetic resonance imaging (MRI) and fetal echocardiography can add important information in select circumstances.

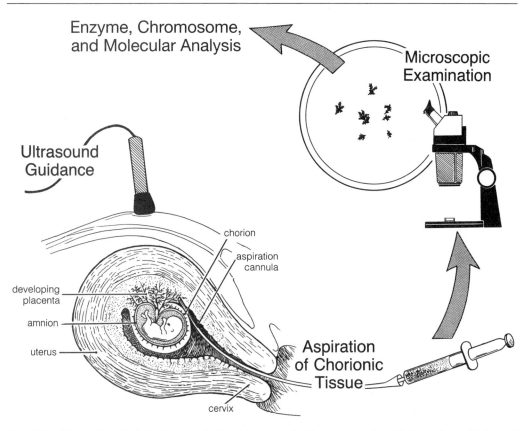

Figure 7.2. Transcervical chorionic villus sampling is performed at 10–12 weeks' gestation. A hollow instrument is inserted through the vagina and passed into the uterus, guided by ultrasound. A small amount of chorionic tissue is removed by suction. The tissue is then examined under a microscope to make sure it is sufficient. Chromosome, enzyme, and/or DNA analyses can be performed without first growing the cells, although cell culture is needed for most analyses. Results are available in a few days in select situations; more often they are ready in 10–14 days.

Second-Trimester Maternal Serum Screening Approximately 70% of women in the United States have a maternal serum screening test and/or detailed ultrasound study to detect or indicate an increased risk for common birth defects. Women 35 years and older are also offered diagnostic testing for chromosome disorders. Although screening sensitivity is improving, it is not diagnostic; if screening results are abnormal, additional studies are needed.

Typically a blood specimen can be drawn at approximately 16 weeks' gestation and analyzed for AFP, hCG, and unconjugated serum estriol (uE3). A fourth marker, Inhibin A, has been added to improve the detection rate for Down syndrome in the second trimester to 80%, with a 5% false positive rate (Canick & Macrae, 2005). The level of these analytes combined with other indicators, including maternal age, weight, race, diabetes status, and number of fetuses, is used to assess the likelihood that a fetus has an increased risk for neural tube defects (e.g., **spina bifida, anencephaly**; see Chapter 28), abdominal wall defects (gastroschisis or an **omphalocele**), Down syndrome (see Chapter 18); or trisomy 18 syndrome (see Appendix B) (Haddow et al., 1992).

Screening tests are designed to maximize the number of affected fetuses correctly identified while limiting the number of false positive results. For example, increased levels of AFP suggest a fetus with a neural tube defect, an abdominal wall defect, or a rare kidney disorder. High AFP levels can also be associated with a multiple gestation; gestational age greater than anticipated (Milunsky, 1998); or a pregnancy at a higher risk for preterm delivery, stillbirth, or intrauterine loss (Waller et al., 1991; Waller et al., 1996). Adverse pregnancy outcome has also been associated with extreme variations of the other second trimester serum analytes (Dugoff et al., 2004).

If the maternal serum screen in the second trimester suggests an increased risk for Down syndrome or trisomy 18, diagnostic testing by amniocentesis and a detailed ultrasound evaluation are recommended. (Correct gestational age is important for an accurate interpretation of the screening results.) Some physicians choose to offer maternal serum screening to women 35 and older to modify their age-related risks. Many women who are screen positive may chose not to have invasive testing. Limitations of screening versus diagnostic testing must be carefully presented because these women may decline amniocentesis based on their serum screen result, and pregnancies with Down syndrome or other chromosome anomalies may thus go undetected.

Second trimester screening, with appropriate follow-up, can lead to a diagnosis of an abnormal (or normal) outcome at 18–20 weeks' gestation. Studies are in progress to identify additional biochemical or sonographic markers that will improve the sensitivity and specificity of screening tests with a goal of reducing the number of invasive procedures.

Second-Trimester Ultrasonography

Approximately two thirds of pregnant women undergo **real-time ultrasonography** during their pregnancy. Ultrasound can identify structures of varying density such as the heart, liver, bone, or fluid-filled spaces. Advances in ultrasound technology and practitioners' clinical experience have improved, resulting in the ability to identify subtle findings that can be associated with chromosomal abnormalities or other genetic disorders including echogenic bowel, pyelectasis and intracardiac echogenic focus (Benacerraf, Nadel, & Bromley, 1994; Stewart, 2004; Filkins & Koos, 2005). In addition to neural tube defects and abdominal wall defects, facial clefts, renal anomalies, skeletal anomalies, hydrocephalus, heart defects, and other malformations can be diagnosed. Three-dimensional ultrasound is also being used in some centers to enhance the ability of physicians to detect variations such as facial clefts (Johnson et al., 2000). Although the identification of structural abnormalities by ultrasound is improving, it cannot replace definitive diagnostic testing for chromosomal abnormalities, genetic mutations, and biochemical analyses that are possible using amniocentesis or CVS. Often ultrasound and other diagnostic testing complement each other for a diagnosis.

Amniocentesis

Amniocentesis Amniocentesis is traditionally performed between 15 and 18 weeks after the last menstrual period. Under ultrasound guidance in a sterile field, a needle is inserted just below the umbilicus through the abdominal and uterine walls. It enters the amniotic sac and 1–2 ounces of amniotic fluid are aspirated (Figure 7.3). Through natural processes (mostly fetal urination), the fluid is replaced within 24 hours. Often, the amniocentesis is performed at the time of a detailed ultrasound. The risk of pregnancy loss following a genetic amniocentesis at 15+ weeks ranges from 0.5% to 1.1% (Wilson, 2000). Early amniocentesis, performed before 14 weeks' gestation, has been implemented in some centers as an alternative to CVS in the first trimester. A multi-center, randomized trial, however, found an increased risk of pregnancy loss, a higher incidence of musculoskeletal (most often clubfoot) deformities, and a greater chance of amniotic fluid leakage (Delisle & Wilson, 1999; Wilson et al., 1998). For this reason, CVS continues to be the preferred procedure for first trimester diagnosis (Jenkins & Wapner, 1999).

One advantage of amniocentesis is the ability to assay the amniotic fluid directly for abnormal levels of biochemical compounds such as AFP. Although ultrasound evaluations have improved in specificity and accuracy, an elevated amniotic fluid AFP of greater than 2.0 multiples of the median with a positive acetylcholinesterase test is diagnostic for a neural tube defect in greater than 98% of cases (Rose & Mennutti, 1993). Abdominal wall defects and some kidney disorders can also be diagnosed based on elevations in the amniotic fluid AFP (Milunsky, 1998; Nyberg, Mahoney, & Pretorius, 1990). Individuals should carefully consider their reason for having an amniocentesis or CVS and how they would utilize the information (e.g., preparation for birth, termination consideration).

Magnetic Resonance Imaging

High-resolution ultrasound has revolutionized the ability to identify fetal anatomic abnormalities; however, the technology has limitations. In selected circumstances, MRI can add to the clinical understanding of an ultrasound variation at approximately 17 weeks' gestation or later (Levine et al., 1997). Because MRI uses ultra-fast imaging sequences, neither mother nor fetus requires sedation for a detailed study. Although there have been no known risks associated with the use of MRI to date, the long-term effects are unknown (De Wilde, Rivers & Price, 2005). MRI of the central nervous system can demonstrate the presence or absence of the corpus callosum (the band of tissue connecting

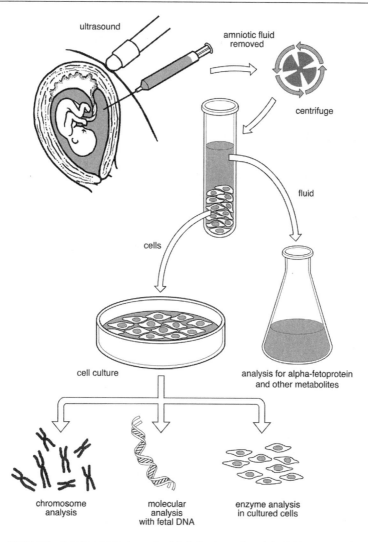

Figure 7.3. Amniocentesis. Approximately 1–2 ounces of amniotic fluid are removed at 16–18 weeks' gestation. The sample is spun in a centrifuge to separate the fluid from the fetal cells. The alpha-fetoprotein in the fluid is measured to test for a neural tube defect. The fluid can also be used to check for metabolites associated with inborn errors of metabolism when indicated. The cells are grown for a week, and then chromosome, enzyme, or DNA analyses can be performed. Most results are available in 10–14 days. (*Source:* Rose & Mennuti, 1993).

the two cerebral hemispheres), Chiari malformations of the brain (seen in spina bifida), and the cause of enlarged ventricles (hydrocephalus) (Levine et al., 1997). Another ultrasound finding that may be clarified by MRI is the amount of normal lung tissue present in a fetus with a diaphragmatic hernia (an incompletely formed diaphragm, which allows the stomach and intestines to herniate into the fetal chest, compromising lung development; Figure 7.4). The additional information gleaned from MRI can assist obstetricians, surgeons, and neonatologists in preparing for delivery of a baby in need

of immediate assistance, such as a fetus with a large neck mass who may present with an occluded airway (Kathary et al., 2001). Alternatively, MRI can also confirm normal anatomy when an abnormality has been suspected by ultrasound.

Fetal Echocardiography Echocardiography has become a valuable tool in the assessment of a fetus with CHD. This targeted ultrasound is performed at 18–20 weeks' gestation, when the fetal heart is approximately the size of an adult's thumbnail. With fetal echocar-

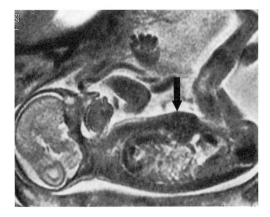

Figure 7.4. Magnetic resonance image of fetus with a diaphragmatic hernia demonstrating bowel loops (intestine) in the chest area. (Courtesy of Dorothy I. Bulas, M.D., Department of Diagnostic Imaging, Children's National Medical Center, Washington, D.C.)

Table 7.3. Ultrasound findings in certain chromosomal abnormalities

Syndrome	Findings
Trisomy 13	Cleft lip and palate
	Congenital heart defect
	Cystic kidneys
	Extra finger or toe
	Mid-line facial defect
Trisomy 18	Clenched hands with overlapping fingers
	Congenital heart defect
	Excessive amniotic fluid
	Growth retardation
	Rocker-bottom feet
Trisomy 21	Abnormal gastrointestinal tract
	Congenital heart defect
	Excess neck skin/ increased nuchal translucency
	Absent nasal bone

Sources: D'Alton & DeCherney (1993); Nicolaides (2004); and Viora, Errante, Sciarrone, et al. (2005).

diography, it is possible to evaluate the structure and function of the fetal heart and monitor fetal blood flow. Three- and four-dimensional studies offer the opportunity for multiple views of normal and complex anatomy (Devore, 2005). A family history of CHD, increased nuchal translucency in the first trimester (Hafner et al., 2003; Souka et al., 2005), maternal diabetes, a fetal diagnosis of Down syndrome or velocardiofacial syndrome (VCFS; see Appendix B), or other birth defects noted by ultrasound increase the likelihood that a congenital heart defect will be identified. Because fetal circulation differs from that of the newborn, coarctation (severe narrowing) of the aorta, interrupted aortic arch, and small atrial or ventricular septal defects (ASD or VSD) may not be accurately diagnosed using fetal echocardiography. A careful cardiac evaluation should also be performed postnatally in infants known to be at increased risk for CHD. An increase in the prenatal diagnosis of congenital heart defects result in earlier postnatal diagnosis and a redirection toward care in a tertiary care setting (Mohan, Kleinman, & Kern, 2005).

When a heart defect is identified in utero, a detailed ultrasound study is indicated to screen for other malformations. Approximately 10%–15% of infants with CHD have an underlying chromosomal abnormality and will often have additional anomalies, developmental delay, or intellectual disability (Table 7.3; Brown, 2000). When a fetus is identified with a CHD, genetic counseling and diagnostic testing via amniocentesis are warranted because the long-term outcome for a child with an isolated CHD can be much different from the expected outcome for a child with a chromosomal abnormality or genetic disorder.

Diagnostic Testing of Fetal Cells

The leading indication for invasive diagnostic testing is chromosome analysis for advanced maternal age. The fetal cells obtained by amniocentesis or CVS can also be used for molecular analysis of fetal DNA and biochemical analysis by enzyme determination (Thompson, McInnes, & Willard, 2004).

Both CVS and amniocentesis are well-established techniques for obtaining fetal cells. The most common test requested is chromosomal analysis; however, biochemical analysis for inborn errors of metabolism such as Tay-Sachs disease or DNA analysis for disorders such as fragile X syndrome or cystic fibrosis can be performed on the cells. Indeed, any genetic disorder for which a familial DNA mutation has been identified can be analyzed using DNA isolated from the fetal cells (Figure 7.5).

Fluorescent *in situ* hybridization (FISH) is a technique that utilizes short pieces of DNA of known sequence (called a DNA probe) that can hybridize, or attach, to a unique region on a chromosome. The probe contains a fluorescent tag, making it visible under a fluorescent microscope. FISH is used to identify chromosomes or to indicate small deletions of a defined region of a specific chromosome. When a rapid

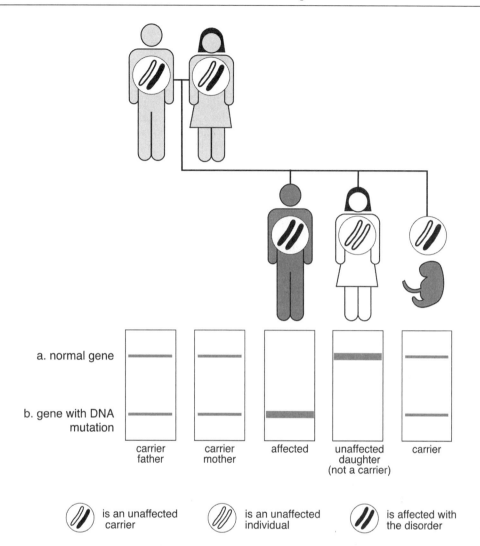

Figure 7.5. Prenatal diagnosis by DNA analysis in a family at risk for a child with a recessive disorder. The top of the figure illustrates the members of the family. This couple's first son was diagnosed with an autosomal recessive disorder. Blood samples from the child and his parents were obtained and DNA was extracted. The DNA was digested with enzymes that broke it into different lengths depending on whether a genetic change (mutation) was present or not. The samples were then applied to a special gel and separated by size using an electric current. The upper band (a) is associated with the functional gene, whereas the lower band (b) is associated with the gene that contains a mutation rendering it nonfunctional. Genes are present in pairs and as expected, each carrier parent was found to carry one gene containing the DNA mutation associated with this disease and one functional gene (represented by two bands on the gel). Their son with the autosomal recessive disorder had a single (b) band of greater intensity representing two copies of the nonfunctional gene. On the basis of this information, the next pregnancy was monitored with prenatal diagnosis and the couple learned that their daughter would not be affected—after DNA analysis on amniotic fluid cells only an (a) band was found. The couple are again pregnant and have decided to have prenatal testing. This time the fetus was found to be a carrier with two bands identified (a and b). The family can feel reassured that the new baby will not have the disorder.

result is required for prenatal diagnosis, this technique can be used to test for trisomies 13, 18, and 21 and variations in the number of X or Y chromosomes (Ward et al., 1993). In addition, FISH can be used to diagnose some genetic syndromes caused by chromosome deletions or variations that are too small to be detected by conventional analysis. For example, the discovery of certain CHDs by fetal ultra-

sound or echocardiography should prompt consideration of using FISH analysis to detect the 22q11.2 deletion that occurs in 1 in 4,000 live births and is associated with VCFS (see Appendix B).

Array comparative genomic hybridization is a new technology allowing the evaluation of small, submicroscopic genomic deletions and duplications that are responsible for approximately 15% of known genetic disorders (Vissers et al., 2005). Advances in this technology have enabled high-resolution examination of genetic alterations that are not otherwise identifiable. As the technology improves, its application to prenatal diagnosis and assisted reproductive technology (ART) will expand (Van den Veyver & Beaudet, 2006). DNA microarray analysis can be offered as a prenatal service when multiple anomalies are identified via ultrasound and conventional chromosomal analysis is normal.

Percutaneous Umbilical Blood Sampling

Percutaneous umbilical blood sampling (PUBS), also referred to as cordocentesis, is performed after 20 weeks' gestation. Under ultrasound guidance, a needle is inserted through the abdominal and uterine walls and directed to the umbilical vein to obtain a small sample of fetal blood. With a risk of pregnancy loss approaching 2%, and the increase in availability of molecular diagnosis by amniocentesis or CVS, the use of PUBS has diminished (Hickock & Mills, 1992).

As technology improves the indications for prenatal diagnosis will increase. Unfortunately, even the most sophisticated technology cannot guarantee the birth of a typical child. Most of the disorders that cause developmental disabilities in the absence of structural malformations are not currently amenable to prenatal diagnosis. Prenatal testing, however, has offered some parents at high risk for having a child with a severe genetic disorder the opportunity of having healthy children who otherwise would not have been conceived or may have been terminated. For other families, it gives the time to prepare for immediate surgical or medical intervention following a timed delivery or plan for a special farewell for a child who may not survive.

PREVENTION, FETAL THERAPY, AND ALTERNATIVE REPRODUCTIVE CHOICES

Prevention

Although birth defects cannot be prevented, attention to a number of factors can contribute to a favorable outcome. Recommendations such as receiving early prenatal care, avoiding alcoholic beverages and smoking, and minimizing unnecessary medication are familiar to most women.

In addition, ingestion of 0.4 mg of folic acid (found in most multivitamins) by all women of childbearing age starting 3 months before attempted conception is now recommended to reduce the risk of neural tube defects. Recent evidence indicates that folic acid may also reduce the incidence of other birth defects, including cardiac malformations and facial clefts (Desposito et al., 1999).

A number of maternal conditions can predispose an infant to birth defects or developmental delay. For example, a woman with phenylketonuria (PKU) is at risk of having a child with microcephaly and mental retardation if she does not maintain a phenylalanine-restricted diet during pregnancy (see Chapter 20). Other maternal disorders, such as diabetes, or certain medications taken to control illness, such as **anticonvulsants** for a seizure disorder, also increase the risk of birth defects (see Chapter 2).

Fetal Therapy

When a fetal abnormality is identified, questions about prognosis and treatment immediately arise. In utero transplantation of human stem cells shows promise to treat a large number of diseases by transplanting healthy cells into a fetus with a birth defect. At least 45 transplants have been performed for a variety of diseases, and success has been achieved for severe combined immune deficiency (Muench, 2005).

Some birth defects can be repaired soon after birth and have a very good outcome: isolated cleft lip/palate, gastroschisis, and some forms of CHD, for example. With other birth defects, the fetal condition can worsen as the pregnancy continues, compromising the ability of the child to survive after birth and/or his or her quality of life. In these extreme circumstances, fetal surgery has been explored. Surgery has been performed for obstructive uropathy (Crombleholme, 1994); diaphragmatic hernia; cystic adenomatoid malformations, sacrococcygeal teratomas (Adzick & Kitano, 2003); and, most recently, spina bifida (Tulipan, 2004). In utero cardiac catheterization has also been attempted with success (Tworetzky & Marshall, 2004). A clinical trial to evaluate in utero surgery for menigomyelocele is ongoing (Tulipan, 2004).

Families considering fetal therapy should be provided accurate information about the procedures, limitations, risks, and prognosis following birth. Multidisciplinary teams comprised of surgeons, obstetricians, and neonatologists are available at some major medical centers to advise couples regarding their particular situation. Fetal surgery remains controversial due to maternal and fetal complications; however, as tocolytic therapy and neonatal intensive care improve, the use of fetal therapy will expand (Cortes & Farmer, 2004).

Alternative Reproductive Choices

In Vitro Fertilization When a couple has an increased risk to have a child with a serious genetic disorder and they prefer not to face the decision of interrupting an affected pregnancy, other reproductive options may be available. Mendelian genetic disorders may be inherited as autosomal recessive (with two carrier parents), X-linked recessive (with a carrier mother), or autosomal dominant (with one parent being affected), as described in Chapter 1. Techniques such as artificial insemination using donor sperm or in vitro fertilization (IVF) with a donor egg may be appropriate considerations under these circumstances. Couples considering these options should assess how donors are chosen: what carrier testing is performed to make sure the donor is not a carrier for an identifiable genetic disease, the ethnic/racial background of the donor, and the donor's family history. Families should also inquire about the rate of successful pregnancies, the risk for multiple gestation (e.g., twins, triplets), and the increased risk of birth defects (Hansen et al., 2005) when ART is considered.

Intracytoplasmic sperm injection (ICSI) is a technology available to infertile males who have low sperm count or poor sperm motility (Palermo et al., 1998). Sperm from the prospective father are harvested, and the cytoplasmic portions of the sperm are removed. A sperm nucleus is then introduced into a harvested egg by microinjection, and the developing blastocyst is subsequently transferred into the uterus. Genetic causes of male infertility, including microdeletion within fertility-associated regions of the Y chromosome, carriers for certain cystic fibrosis mutations, and Klinefelter syndrome, may be indications for ICSI. For approximately 1% of conceptions accomplished through ICSI, sex chromosome aneuploidy (e.g., an extra X or Y chromosome) has been reported; therefore, genetic counseling is recommended prior to initiating ICSI (Pauer et al., 1997).

Preimplantation Genetic Diagnosis Preimplantation genetic diagnosis (PGD) is available for couples who are at high risk of having a child with a known genetic disorder, who wish to conceive an unaffected child that is biologically their own, and who want to avoid the risk of pregnancy termination. Originally introduced in 1990 for couples at risk of having a child with an X-linked disorder, PGD has expanded with the development of FISH technology to identify common trisomies (13, 18, and 21) in women of advanced age (Kuliev & Verlinsky, 2004).

There are two approaches to PGD, as described in Figure 7.6. The first involves polar body testing of the woman's eggs to establish the presence or absence of the mutation in question. Only embryos from fertilized eggs determined to contain the normal gene are transferred to the mother's uterus to establish a pregnancy.

The second approach is to perform in vitro fertilization on harvested eggs and allow them to develop in culture to the blastomere, or eight-cell stage. A single cell is then microdissected from each blastomere and analyzed for the presence of mutations or aneuploidy. Only unaffected embryos are subsequently transferred to the uterus. Approximately 20% of implanted embryos will survive to birth. Pregnancies utilizing these methods have been successful for couples at high risk for bearing a child with a number of genetic disorders or common trisomies (Verlinsky et al., 2004).

ARTs are costly in terms of physical, emotional, and financial resources, and at present these services are rarely covered by health insurance plans. The risk of multiple gestations is also a concern, particularly if fetal reduction (i.e., abortion of one or more fetuses) is not a consideration. As with IVF, couples should request detailed information regarding techniques that are used, risk of error in diagnosis, cost per attempt, rate of successful pregnancies, and risk of multiple gestation.

PSYCHOSOCIAL IMPLICATIONS

With advances in prenatal screening technology and testing, choices can be overwhelming for a family. A preliminary discussion that is difficult and often avoided is an exploration of how a couple would respond to the diagnosis of an abnormality or, if they already have a child with a disability, how they would respond to a recurrence of the genetic problem in their next child. For some couples, having advanced knowledge allows for preparation prior to birth; for others, it may mean not continuing a pregnancy.

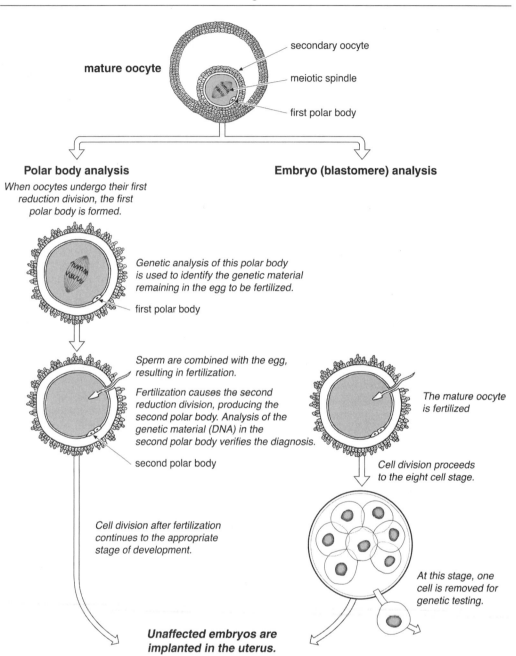

mature oocyte

secondary oocyte

meiotic spindle

first polar body

Polar body analysis

When oocytes undergo their first reduction division, the first polar body is formed.

Embryo (blastomere) analysis

Genetic analysis of this polar body is used to identify the genetic material remaining in the egg to be fertilized.

first polar body

Sperm are combined with the egg, resulting in fertilization.

Fertilization causes the second reduction division, producing the second polar body. Analysis of the genetic material (DNA) in the second polar body verifies the diagnosis.

second polar body

The mature oocyte is fertilized

Cell division proceeds to the eight cell stage.

Cell division after fertilization continues to the appropriate stage of development.

At this stage, one cell is removed for genetic testing.

Unaffected embryos are implanted in the uterus.

Figure 7.6. Preimplantation genetic diagnosis (PGD). Individuals who undergo PGD begin the process as they would for in vitro fertilization. The ovary is stimulated to produce mature oocytes, which are then harvested for fertilization outside of the woman's body. These mature oocytes can be used for polar body analysis, or they can be fertilized and processed for a blastomere biopsy. This figure describes the path toward the preimplantation diagnosis using both methods. Polar body analysis is limited to those disorders or variations that would be present in the maternal genetic material, whereas an embryo biopsy can analyze both maternal and paternal genetic contributions. As with in vitro fertilization, not all pregnancies will progress to term. Prenatal diagnosis at a later stage of gestation by chorionic villus sampling or amniocentesis is recommended to confirm the preimplantation diagnosis.

Many of these issues are best addressed prior to attempting pregnancy so that prenatal diagnostic techniques, genetic screening, and other specialized tests can be investigated. Exploring each individual's reproductive choices and options is time consuming but necessary. It is imperative that health care professionals focus on the family's psychosocial needs as well as the clinical information the couple is requesting.

When a woman gives birth to a child with special needs or a child who does not survive, the experience can be devastating for the family. Each family is unique, and assumptions by health care providers as to what a family should or should not do in a given situation must be avoided. Genetic counselors and medical geneticists who are trained in nondirective counseling can often help families understand their options and choose a course of action that is consistent with the family's own values and resources. Often, support groups or individual counseling can be beneficial.

SUMMARY

A wealth of information exists for couples considering a pregnancy. This is particularly true for couples who have an increased risk for conceiving a child with a specific genetic disorder or who have previously conceived a child with a birth defect or genetic disorder. The array of screening and diagnostic tests can be both overwhelming and reassuring. Health care providers working together with genetics professionals are in a unique position to help families carefully consider and understand their reproductive options and the effects that prenatal diagnosis or genetic screening will have on them physically, emotionally, and financially.

REFERENCES

Adzick, N.S., & Kitano, Y. (2003). Fetal surgery for lung lesions, congenital diaphragmatic hernia, and sacrococcygeal teratoma. *Seminars in Pediatric Surgery, 12,* 154–167

Benacerraf, B.R., Nadel, A., & Bromley, B. (1994). Identification of second-trimester fetuses with autosomal trisomy by use of a sonographic scoring index. *Radiology, 193,* 135–140.

Blakemore, K.J. (1988). Prenatal diagnosis by chorionic villus sampling. *Obstetrics and Gynecology Clinics of North America, 15,* 179–213.

Brown, D.L. (2000). Family history of congenital heart disease. In C.B. Benson, P.H. Arger, & E.I. Bluth (Eds.), *Ultrasonography in obstetrics and gynecology: A practical approach* (pp. 155–166). New York: Thieme Medical Publishers.

Burton, B.K., Schultz, C.J., & Burd, L.I. (1992). Limb abnormalities associated with chorionic villus sampling. *Obstetrics and Gynecology, 79,* 726–730.

Canick, J., & Macrae, A. (2005). Second trimester serum markers. *Seminars in Perinatology, 29*(4), 203–208.

Centers for Disease Control and Prevention. *(2006). Improved national prevalence estimates for 18 selected major birth defects—United States, 1999–2001.* Morbidity and Mortality Weekly Report, 54(51 & 52), 1301—1305.

Cortes, R., & Farmer, D. (2004). Recent advances in fetal surgery. *Seminars in Perinatology, 28*(3), 199–211.

Crombleholme, T.M. (1994). Invasive fetal therapy:

Current status and future directions. *Seminars in Perinatology, 18,* 385–397.

D'Alton, M.E., & DeCherney, A.H. (1993). Prenatal diagnosis. *The New England Journal of Medicine, 328,* 114–119.

Delisle, M., & Wilson, R.D. (1999). First trimester prenatal diagnosis. *Seminars in Perinatology, 23,* 414–423.

Desposito, F., Cuniff, C., Frias, J.L., et al. (1999). Folic acid for the prevention of neural tube defects. *Pediatrics, 104,* 325–327.

Devore, G. (2005). Three-dimensional and four-dimensional fetal echocardiography: A new frontier. *Current Opinion Pediatrics, 17*(5), 592–604.

De Wilde, J.P., Rivers, A. W., & Price, D.L. (2005). A review of the current use of magnetic resonance imaging in pregnancy and safety implications for the fetus. *Progress in Biophysics and Molecular Biology, 87,* 335–353

Dugoff, L., Hobbins, J., Malone, F., et al. (2004). First-trimester maternal serum PAPP-A and free-beta subunit human chorionic gonadotropin concentrations and nuchal translucency are associated with obstetric complications: A population-based screening study (The FASTER Trial). *American Journal of Obstetrics and Gynecology, 191,* 1446–1451.

Filkins, K., & Koos, B.J. (2005). Ultrasound and fetal diagnosis. *Current Opinion in Obstetrics and Gynecology, 17,* 185–195

Goldberg, J.D., Porter, A.E., & Golbus, M.S. (1990). Current assessment of fetal losses as a direct consequence of chorionic villus sampling. *American Journal of Medical Genetics, 35,* 174–177.

Haddow, J.E., Palomaki, G.E., Knight, G.J., et al. (1992). Prenatal screening for Down's syndrome with use of maternal serum markers. *The New England Journal of Medicine, 327,* 588–593.

Hafner, L., Schuller T., Metzenbauer M., et al. (2003). Increased nuchal translucency and congenital heart defects in a low-risk population. *Prenatal Diagnosis, 23,* 985–989.

Hansen, M., Bower, C., Milne, E., et al. (2005). Assisted reproductive technologies and the risk of birth defects: A systematic review. *Human Reproduction, 20,* 328–338.

Hickock, D.E., & Mills, M. (1992). Percutaneous umbilical blood sampling: Results from a multicenter collaborative registry. *American Journal of Obstetrics and Gynecology, 166,* 1614–1617.

Hook, E.B. (1981). Rates of chromosomal abnormalities at different maternal ages. *Obstetrics and Gynecology, 58,* 282–285.

Jenkins, T.J., & Wapner, R.J. (1999). First trimester prenatal diagnosis: Chorionic villus sampling. *Seminars in Perinatology, 223,* 403–413.

Johnson, D.D., Pretorius, D.H., Budorick, N.E., et al. (2000). Fetal lip and primary palate: Three-dimensional versus two-dimensional US. *Radiology, 217,* 236–239.

Kathary, N., Bulas, D.I., Newman, K.D., et al. (2001). MRI imaging and fetal neck masses with airway compromise: Utility in delivery planning. *Pediatric Radiology, 31,* 727–731.

Krantz, D., Goetzl L., Simpson J., et al. (2004). Association of extreme first-trimester free human chorionic gonadotropin-ß, pregnancy-associated plasma protein A, and nuchal translucency with intrauterine growth restriction and other adverse pregnancy outcomes. *American Journal of Obstetrics and Gynecology, 191,* 1452–1458.

Kuliev A., & Verlinsky, Y. (2004). Meiotic and Mitotic nondisjunction: Lessons from preimplantation genetic diagnosis. *Human Reproduction Update, 10,* 401–407.

Levine, D., Barnes, P.D., Madsen, J.R., et al. (1997). Fetal central nervous system anomalies: MR imaging augments sonographic diagnosis. *Radiology, 204,* 635–642.

Milunsky, A. (1998). Maternal serum screening for neural tube defects. In A. Milunsky (Ed.), *Genetic disorders and the fetus: Diagnosis, prevention, and treatment* (4th ed., pp. 507–511). Baltimore: The Johns Hopkins University Press.

Mohan, U., Kleinman, C., & Kern J. (2005). Fetal echocardiography and its evolving impact 1992–2002. *American Journal of Cardiology, 96*(1), 134–136.

Morris, J.K., Wald, N.J., Mutton, D.E. et al. (2003). Comparison models of maternal age-specific risk for Down syndrome live births. *Prenatal Diagnosis, 23,* 252–258

Muench, M. (2005). In utero transplantation: Baby steps towards an effective therapy. *Bone Marrow Transplant, 35*(6), 537–547.

National Society of Genetic Counselors. (1983). *Genetic counseling as a profession.* Retrieved January 16, 2007, from http://www.nsgc.org/career

Nicolaides, K.H. (2004). Nuchal translucency and other first-trimester sonographic markers of chromosomal abnormalities. *American Journal of Obstetrics and Gynecology, 191,* 45–67.

Nyberg, D.A., Mahoney, B.S., & Pretorius, D.H. (Eds.). (1990). *Diagnostic ultrasound of fetal anomalies: Text and atlas.* St. Louis: Mosby.

Orlandi, F., Damaini, G., Hallahan, T.W., et al. (1997). First-trimester screening for fetal aneuploidy: Biochemistry and nuchal translucency. *Ultrasound in Obstetrics and Gynecology, 10,* 381–386.

Palermo, G.D., Schlegel, P.N., Sills, E.S., et al. (1998). Births after intracytoplasmic injection of sperm obtained by testicular extraction from men with nonmosaic Klinefelter's syndrome. *The New England Journal of Medicine, 338,* 588–590.

Pauer, H.U., Hinney, B., Michelmann, H.W., et al. (1997). Relevance of genetic counseling in couples prior to intracytoplasmic sperm injection. *Human Reproduction, 12,* 1909–1912.

Rose, N.C., & Mennutti, M.T. (1993). Alpha-fetoprotein and neural tube defects. In J.J. Sciarra & P.V. Dilts, Jr. (Eds.), *Gynecology and obstetrics* (Rev. ed., pp. 1–14). New York: HarperCollins.

Seashore, M.R. (1999). Clinical genetics. In B.N. Burrow & T.P. Duffy (Eds.), *Medical complications during pregnancy* (5th ed., pp. 197–223). Philadelphia: W.B. Saunders.

Souka, A., von Kaisenberg C., Hyetts J., et al. (2005). Increased nuchal translucency with normal karyotype. *American Journal of Obstetrics and Gynecology, 192,* 1005–1021.

Stewart, T.L. (2004). Screening for aneuploidy: The genetic sonogram. *Obstetrics and Gynecology Clinic of North America, 31,* 21–33.

Thompson, M.W., McInnes, R.R., & Willard, H.F. (Eds.). (2004). *Thompson & Thompson genetics in medicine* (6th ed.). Philadelphia: W.B. Saunders.

Tulipan, N. (2004). *Intrauterine closure of myelomeningocele: An update.* Neurosurgery Focus, 16(2), E2.

Tworetzky, W., & Marshall, A.C. (2004). Fetal interventions for cardiac defects. *Pediatric Clinics of North America, 51*(6), 1503–1513.

Van den Veyver, I.B., & Beaudet, A.L. (2006). Comparative genomic hybridization and prenatal diagnosis. *Current Opinion in Obstetrics and Gynecology, 18,* 185–191.

Verlinsky, Y., Cohen, J., Munne, S., et al. (2004). Over a decade of experience with preimplantation genetic diagnosis: A multicenter report. *Fertility and Sterility, 82,* 292–294.

Viora, E., Errante, G., Sciarrone, A., et al. (2005). Fetal nasal bone and trisomy 21 in the second trimester. *Prenatal Diagnosis, 25,* 511–515.

Vissers, L.E., Veltman, J.A., van Kessel, A.G., et al. (2005). Identification of disease genes by whole genome CGH arrays. *Human Molecular Genetics, 14* (Spec. No. 2), R215–R223.

Waller, D.K., Lustig, L.S., Cunningham, G.C., et al. (1991). Second-trimester maternal serum alpha-fetoprotein levels and the risk of subsequent fetal death. *The New England Journal of Medicine, 325,* 6–10.

Waller, D.K., Lustig, L.S., Cunningham, G.C., et al. (1996). The association between maternal serum alpha-fetoprotein and preterm birth, small for gestational age infants, preeclampsia and placental complications. *Obstetrics and Gynecology, 88,* 816–822.

Ward, B.E., Gersen, S.L., Carelli, M.P., et al. (1993). Rapid prenatal diagnosis of chromosomal aneuploidies by fluorescence in situ hybridization: Clinical experience with 4,500 specimens. *American Journal of Medical Genetics, 52,* 854–865.

Wilson, R.D. (2000). Amniocentesis and chorionic villus sampling. *Current Opinion in Obstetrics and Gynecology, 12,* 81–86.

Wilson, R.D., Johnson, J.M., Dansereau, J., et al. (1998). Randomized trial to assess safety and fetal outcome of early and midtrimester amniocentesis. *The Lancet, 351,* 242–247.

8 Newborn Screening

Opportunities for Prevention of Developmental Disabilities

Joan E. Pellegrino

Upon completion of the chapter the reader will

- Understand the rationale for newborn screening
- Understand the difference between a screening test and diagnostic test
- Be familiar with the types of screening tests available
- Understand the limitations and pitfalls of screening

ASHLEY

Denise, a 32-year-old healthy female, was pregnant with her second child. The pregnancy was uncomplicated, and she had a normal maternal serum screening test in the second trimester and normal prenatal ultrasounds. The delivery was uncomplicated, and she and her daughter Ashley were discharged home from the hospital when Ashley was 3 days old. Ashley's parents were therefore upset and confused to receive a telephone call that Ashley had screened positive for medium chain acyl-CoA-dehydrogenase deficiency (MCAD). They did not know what this disease was, and they did not understand why Ashley should screen positive for an "inherited" condition when they already had a healthy 2-year-old daughter at home. Denise did recall reading that her state had expanded newborn screening, but she was unsure what this meant. Ashley was seen by her pediatrician and underwent diagnostic testing for MCAD. The diagnosis was confirmed, and Ashley was treated with a frequent, regular feeding schedule. Her sister had not been tested for MCAD, as this test was not part of the newborn screen in her state at the time of her birth. She was subsequently tested and found to be affected as well.

The birth of a new baby is a joyous time, but for some families a shadow is cast on their first hopes by the worrisome results of a newborn screening test. The baby's mother will have undergone a number of screening procedures during the pregnancy (see Chapter 7), but she may be unaware that her newborn will also have several screening tests performed. This chapter describes the rationale for newborn screening, summarizes the types of disorders for which screening is conducted, and reviews the methods for assuring proper follow-up on the results of newborn screening.

WHAT IS A SCREENING TEST?

A **screening test,** as the name implies, is a test designed to screen for, but not definitively diagnose, a particular condition. When applied to a group of individuals, a screening test separates those who are at risk for a condition from those who are not. The ideal screening test would perform this operation with perfect accuracy, but in reality, all screening tests produce false positive results (normal individuals identified as being at risk) and some produce false negative results (affected individuals identified as not being at risk). Because the goal of newborn screening is to identify *all* truly affected individuals, interpretive methods and screening algorithms are devised to eliminate false negative results while still trying to minimize false positives. In some cases, this is accomplished by setting a numerical cut-off for a test that favors the identification of truly affected individuals, at the expense of overidentifying some unaffected individuals as being at risk for the tested condition (Figure 8.1). Because any particular condition tested for by newborn screening is relatively rare, the number of individuals affected by that condition will be much smaller than the number of unaffected individuals. Depending on the technology used, this means that the majority of positive screens may turn out to be false positives. For some conditions, retesting a child using the same or alternative screening tests will improve the efficiency of the screening process, but ultimately, a final group of individuals with positive screening results must undergo diagnostic testing. A **diagnostic test** is designed to definitively confirm or exclude the presence of a disease or condition in a particular individual. Diagnostic tests, in theory, should produce no false positive or false negative results, so they would actually represent the ideal "screening test." In practice, diagnostic tests are generally either too cumbersome or too expensive to perform on large numbers of individuals, hence the need for screening tests.

WHY SCREEN NEWBORNS?

Of the hundreds of diseases and conditions that may potentially affect infants and young children, a limited number will be appropriate for inclusion in a newborn screening program. The American Academy of Pediatrics (AAP) convened a national task force on newborn screening and issued a report addressing this issue (AAP Task Force, 2000). They recommended the following inclusion criteria:

1. The condition to be tested for should be an important health problem that occurs frequently enough to justify screening an entire population.

2. The treatment for the condition should be effective when initiated early, accepted among health care professionals, and available to all screened newborns.

3. The test for the condition should be simple, safe, precise, validated, and acceptable.

In other words, the condition screened for must be serious, identifiable, and treatable. In this context, being treatable does not necessarily mean that the condition is curable; it means that interventions should result in significant amelioration of the expected consequences of that

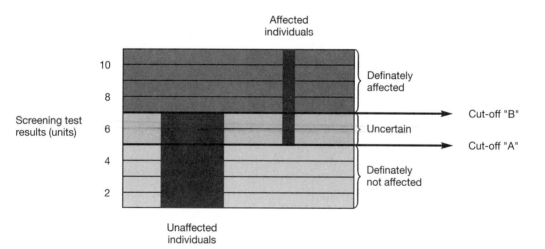

Figure 8.1. Setting a cut-off level for a screening test. In this example, a hypothetical screening test is applied with the ultimate goal of identifying individuals who are affected by a particular disease or condition. Individuals who ultimately prove to be unaffected show test results from 0 to 7 units; individuals who prove to be affected show test results ranging from 5 to 11 units. Individuals with test results above 7 or below 5 will be definitely identified by the screen as be affected or unaffected; individuals testing between 5 and 7 may or may not be affected. If cut-off "A" is selected, all affected individuals will be correctly identified, but some unaffected individuals will be incorrectly identified as having disease (false positives). Because the number of unaffected individuals is so much larger than the number with disease, the majority of individuals testing positive will turn out to be unaffected. If cut-off "B" is selected, all unaffected individuals will be correctly identified, but some individuals with disease will be missed (false negatives). Selecting a cut-off level between "A" and "B" will result in a mix of false positives and false negatives.

condition. Historically, there has been a great deal of variability in the interpretation of these criteria and in the implementation of newborn screening programs across the United States and in other parts of the world. In general, the types of diseases and disorders usually screened for fall into the following categories: endocrine disorders, lung disorders, blood disorders, infectious diseases, and metabolic disorders. In addition, hearing loss is screened for in the newborn period (see Chapter 12). This chapter focuses on medical conditions that can be identified by newborn screening and that place the child at significant risk for developmental disabilities. It should be noted, however, that screenings are conducted in the newborn period for additional conditions that carry significant medical and related emotional issues (i.e., congenital adrenal hyperplasia, cystic fibrosis, and sickle cell anemia).

Endocrine Disorders

The endocrine system produces and regulates a variety of hormones that are critical to maintaining the body in a normal and balanced physiological state, called homeostasis. Several specific hormones are critical to the early growth and development of the central nervous system. Congenital hypothyroidism is a condition in which the newborn produces inadequate thyroid hormone; 1 in 3,000 infants is born with the condition, making it relatively common compared with other disorders screened for in the newborn period. Early identification of this condition allows for early treatment with thyroid hormone replacement. Untreated infants have severe growth problems and abnormal brain development, resulting in serious lifelong cognitive disability (Delange, 1997).

Infectious Diseases

Currently, two states require screening for human immunodeficiency virus (HIV), and another two screen for *Toxoplasmosis gondii*. These are potentially serious infections in newborns (see Chapter 6). A positive screen for either of these organisms would require consultation with an infectious disease specialist for confirmation and treatment. A positive HIV screen in the newborn indicates that the mother is infected and the newborn needs to be followed for the increased risk of disease. The goal of treatment for affected newborns with HIV is long-term suppression of viral replication in order to prevent clinical symptoms of acquired immunodeficiency virus (AIDS) and preserve the immune system. Guidelines for treatment are available (see http://www.hivatis.org). Untreated congenital toxoplasmosis results in multisystem disease including neurologic complications such as seizures, visual impairments, and intellectual disability. The incidence of congenital toxoplasmosis is 1 in 1,000 to 1 in 8,000 live births. Newborns identified through newborn screening require treatment with medication to reduce the incidence of the sequelae (Guerina et al., 1994).

Metabolic Disorders

Metabolic disorders, also known as inborn errors of metabolism, represent a diverse group of genetic conditions that manifest as abnormalities of body "chemistry" at the cellular level (see Chapter 20). These conditions are often associated with the accumulation of abnormal substances, or metabolites, in body fluids and tissues as a consequence of abnormal functioning of proteins known as enzymes. Phenylketonuria (PKU) is a classic example of a screenable metabolic condition. In the United States, the incidence of PKU is 1 in 10,000 and is increased in Caucasians of European descent. The disorder belongs to a group of metabolic conditions known as **amino acid disorders.** In PKU, a genetic mutation results in deficiency of an enzyme needed to process phenylalanine, an amino acid common to most protein-laden foods, including meat and dairy products. Early identification of PKU by newborn screening allows implementation of a protein-restricted diet. Lack of treatment results in accumulation of phenylalanine in blood and body tissues, with particularly severe consequences for the developing central nervous system. Another relatively common metabolic disorder (with an incidence of 1 in 15,000) is Ashley's disorder, MCAD. This disorder is the most common example of a group of metabolic conditions called **fatty acid oxidation disorders.** Normally, the body processes fat in order to release energy through oxidation. This is especially important during periods of fasting, when fat becomes the main source of energy for the body. Children with MCAD may become seriously ill after a period of fasting, and may suffer permanent brain damage as a consequence. Careful monitoring and frequent feedings are essential, especially during infancy. Several other categories of metabolic disease, including **organic acidemias** (organic acid disorders), **disorders of carbohydrate metabolism** (e.g., **galactosemia**), and several miscellaneous enzyme deficiencies (e.g., **biotinidase deficiency**) are amenable to dietary intervention or to specific medical treatments. As a group, the metabolic disorders now represent the largest number of potentially treatable conditions that may be identified through newborn screening and are the primary target of the newest screening technologies.

HOW IS NEWBORN SCREENING DONE?

Most newborn screening tests rely on blood samples obtained during the first few days after birth. Testing begins by collecting a blood sample from a heel prick and blotting this onto a special filter paper collection device. The sample is collected before the newborn is discharged from the birthing facility but after the

Table 8.1. Disorders detectable in newborns by tandem mass spectroscopy

Amino acid disorders	5-oxoprolinuria
	Argininemia
	Argininosuccinate lyase deficiency (ASL)
	Citrullinemia
	Citrullinemia II
	Defects of biopterin cofactor biosynthesis
	Defects of biopterin cofactor regeneration
	Homocystinuria
	Hyperammonemia, hyperornithinemia, homocitrullinemia (HHH)
	Hypermethioninemia
	Maple syrup urine disease (MSUD)
	Nonketotic hyperglycinemia
	Phenylketonuria (PKU)
	Tyrosinemia type I, II, and III
Organic acid disorders	2-methyl-3-hydroxybutyryl CoA dehydrogenase (2M3HBA)
	2-methylbutyrl CoA dehydrogenase deficiency (2MBG)
	3-hydroxy-3-methylglutaryl-CoA lyase deficiency (HMG)
	3-methylcrotonyl-CoA carboxylase deficiency (3-MCC)
	3-methylglutaconyl-CoA hydratase deficiency (3MGA)
	Beta-ketothiolase deficiency (BKT)
	Glutaric acidemia type 1 (GA1)
	Isobutyryl-CoA dehydrogenase deficiency (IBG)
	Isovaleric acidemia (IVA)
	Malonic aciduria (MAL)
	Methylmalonic acidemia–Cbl A, B
	Methylmalonic acidemia–Cbl C, D
	Methylmalonic acidemia–mutase deficiency (MUT)
	Multiple carboxylase deficiency (MCD)
	Propionic acidemia (PA)
Fatty acid oxidation disorders	2,4, dienoyl-CoA reductase deficiency (DE RED)
	3-hydroxy long chain acyl-CoA dehydrogenase deficiency (LCHAD)
	Carnitine palmitoyltransferase I and II (CPT I and II)
	Carnitine uptake defects (CUD)
	Carnitine/acylcarnitine translocase deficiency (CACT)
	Medium chain acyl-CoA dehydrogenase deficiency (MCAD)
	Medium chain ketoacyl-CoA thiolase deficiency (MCKAT)
	Medium/short chain hydroxy Acyl-CoA dehydrogenase deficiency (M/SCHAD)
	Multiple acyl-CoA dehydrogenase deficiency (glutaric acidemia Type II)
	Short chain Acyl-CoA dehydrogenase deficiency (SCAD)
	Trifunctional protein deficiency (TFP)
	Very long chain acyl-CoA dehydrogenase deficiency (VLCAD)

infant has had an opportunity to feed, ideally after 24 hours of age. This is done because certain metabolic disorders cannot be detected until the body is challenged to metabolize the substances present in breast milk or formula. The paper is dried and sent to a newborn screening laboratory. The specimen is then divided into multiple samples so that a variety of tests can be run looking for specific diseases. In the past, a different test was required for each disease. With the advent of **tandem mass spectroscopy,** the number of tests possible has increased exponentially.

The mass spectrometer is a device that separates and quantifies ions based on their mass-to-charge ratio (American College of Medical Genetics & American Society of Human Genetics, 2000). The **tandem mass spectrometer (MS/MS)** consists of two of these devices separated by a reaction chamber such that accurate measurements of many different types of metabolites can be obtained at once (Chace et al., 1999). This is a very rapid and sensitive method for mass screening, because a single sample can be screened in 1–2 minutes for numerous disorders (Table 8.1) (Chace et al., 2003). This technology can also improve the detection rate (lower the number of false positives) for other diseases such as PKU (Chace et al., 1998; Marsden, Larson, & Levy, 2006). It is important to note that not all of the currently mandated disorders can be screened in this way, so other methods will continue to be needed (Table 8.2).

The use of tandem mass spectroscopy has increased the number of diagnoses of inborn errors of metabolism. In one study, the detection rate using this method to screen for 12 diseases (excluding PKU) was 10.6 in 100,000 (Waisbren et al., 2003). Among this group, 40% of in-

fants had MCAD. In another study the detection rate was increased from the previous rate of 9 in 100,000 births to 15.7 in 100,000 births over a 4-year period when 31 diseases (again excluding PKU) were screened for using MS/MS (Wilcken et al., 2003). In this study, the most commonly diagnosed disorder was also MCAD.

WHAT SHOULD BE DONE WHEN A CHILD HAS A POSITIVE NEWBORN SCREEN?

In practice, each state decides how to handle positive screening results and how to follow up, although national guidelines for some conditions are available (Pass et al., 2000). In general, there should be prompt notification of the physician of record (usually the primary care pediatrician or family practitioner) and the infant's family. Treatment should be initiated if appropriate, and the infant should be evaluated further. Definitive testing should confirm the diagnosis. If the diagnosis is confirmed, a treatment plan specific to that disorder should be initiated. The family is typically referred to a specialty consultant or program, and genetic counseling is offered.

Even when follow-up on a positive newborn screen operates efficiently and effectively, families may still experience significant stress related to the process. As previously mentioned, many positive screens turn out to be false positives. In many conditions, for every 10 infants with a positive screen, only 1 will be found to have the disease. Even though these other 9 children will ultimately prove to be without disease, the process leading to this conclusion can be difficult for families. Mothers of false-positive infants have significantly increased stress level scores compared to mothers of screen-negative infants, and they score higher on measures of parent–child dysfunction. Having the child seen through a specialty center (e.g., a metabolic program) or communicating repeat screening results in person seems to improve this situation (Waisbren et al., 2003). On the one hand, it is important for families to understand that a positive newborn screen does not automatically mean that their infant has a problem. On the other hand, it is obviously important that appropriate follow-up is pursued in a timely fashion to allow identification of truly affected infants.

When a child screens positive for a particular disorder, follow-up testing methods and algorithms will differ depending on the charac-

Table 8.2. Disorders detected in newborns by technologies other than tandem mass spectroscopy

Arginase deficiency
Biotinidase deficiency
Congenital adrenal hyperplasia
Congenital hypothyroidism
Congenital toxoplasmosis
Cystic fibrosis
Galactokinase deficiency
Galactose epimerase deficiency
Galactose-1-phosphate uridyltransferase deficiency
Glucose-6-phosphate dehydrogenase deficiency
Hemoglobinopathies: S/S; S/C; S/ßTh variants
Human immunodeficiency virus (HIV)
Hearing loss

teristics of the specific disorder and the methods used for the initial screen. For example, genetic testing may be part of the second tier of the newborn screening process or may be requested once a screen is positive in order to help confirm the diagnosis. Second-tier testing is usually performed by the same laboratory that performed the initial screen and occurs automatically as part of the screening algorithm. Under this method, a sample is tested and flagged as abnormal relative to an expected range for the test. The sample is then sent for a second-tier test that aids in the interpretation of the initial screening result. Only abnormal samples have second-tier tests. For example, a specimen might be abnormal for immunoreactive trypsinogen (IRT), a test for cystic fibrosis. That sample is then tested for some of the more common DNA mutations associated with cystic fibrosis. If two mutations are found, the sample may be coded as "positive." If no mutation, or only one mutation is found, then the sample may be coded as negative or positive depending on the level of IRT. By adding second-tier DNA testing for multiple mutations, the sensitivity of the test is increased, but an increased number of carriers (individuals with a single copy of the mutated gene who do not have cystic fibrosis) are also identified, creating another layer of complexity from a genetic counseling perspective (Comeau et al., 2004).

WHAT HAPPENS TO CHILDREN WITH CONFIRMED DISEASE?

Infants with a positive newborn screen are often referred to a center where they are seen by a physician with expertise in the condition for which screening occurred. This may be a hematologist, a pulmonologist, an endocrinologist, or a geneticist. In some states, families may have access to multidisciplinary programs that include nurses, genetic counselors, social workers, and nutritionists in addition to specialty physicians. Additional testing is then obtained to confirm the specific diagnosis or to aid in genetic counseling. Once the diagnosis is established, the child will require ongoing (and often lifelong) care for that condition. The specific interventions employed will depend on the diagnosis obtained (e.g., see Chapter 20 to learn about interventions for metabolic disorders). In general, the goal is to provide long-term therapy for the child and ongoing counseling to the family, with the ultimate goal of improving medical, neurodevelopmental, and psychosocial outcomes. Some disorders are relatively easy to

manage with medications or supplements (e.g., thyroid hormone replacement therapy for congenital hypothyroidism, or biotin therapy [a B vitamin] for biotinidase deficiency). Other disorders are more complex and may require a combination of medications, supplements, and dietary changes. For example, the treatment of PKU requires protein restriction and replacement of normal food items with synthetic, non-phenylalanine-containing substitutes. This is usually achieved using special formulas in children or supplemental nutrition bars in adults. Although this sounds quite simple, it is for most individuals and families a very burdensome diet and is complicated by the fact that these specialized foods are costly.

Because most of these disorders are genetic, genetic testing may be recommended to confirm the diagnosis or to provide additional prognostic information. Once a specific mutation is identified, prenatal diagnosis may be available in the next pregnancy, if the family chooses to pursue this. Recurrence risk (risk that another child will be born with the same condition in the future) is an appropriate concern. Because most metabolic disorders are inherited as an autosomal recessive trait (see Chapter 1), the risk of recurrence is 25%. By comparison, an individual actually diagnosed with a metabolic disorder is at much lower risk for having a child with the same condition. There are additional issues to consider, however, when a woman with a metabolic disorder becomes pregnant herself. Her disease may have an impact on the developing fetus, even though the fetus does not have the disease itself (e.g., see description of maternal PKU in Chapter 20). Although the teratogenic effects of phenylalanine on the fetus have been well described, this is not the case for many other metabolic disorders. With increasing numbers of individuals being identified with severe metabolic disorders earlier and treated sooner, it is expected that more affected women will survive into childbearing age and the effects of these disorders on the developing fetus will be further elucidated.

WHAT IS THE RISK OF DEVELOPMENTAL DISABILITY IN CHILDREN WITH CONFIRMED DISEASE?

The neurodevelopmental and functional sequelae of a particular disorder identified through newborn screening is specific to that disorder. A few studies have addressed the issue of developmental outcomes in children who have an underlying metabolic disorder. A population-based surveillance study of children with severe developmental disabilities (intellectual disability, cerebral palsy, hearing loss, and vision impairment) who had a true-positive newborn screen revealed that only 3 of 147 infants showed signs of these disorders (Van Naarden et al., 2003). Two of the infants had maple syrup urine disease (MSUD) and one had galactosemia. All three children had intellectual disability that was attributable to their metabolic disorder. However, when this study was expanded to look for children with positive newborn screen who were receiving special education services, there were 9 children out of 216 who had a less severe form of developmental disability (developmental delay, speech-language impairment, learning disability). Seven children had a form of galactosemia, and two had congenital hypothyroidism. One child with classic galactosemia had developmental delays, another child had a specific learning disability, and the remaining seven had speech-language impairments. In the Waisbren study (2003), the children identified by newborn screening had fewer developmental and health problems and functioned better (as evidenced by developmental testing) compared with those children diagnosed at a later age based on clinical symptoms. The children identified through screening had fewer hospitalizations, shorter hospital stays, and 60% fewer medical problems, and they scored significantly higher on developmental testing. Despite the positive outlook in these studies, many of these diseases are still associated with severe developmental disabilities.

HOW CAN SCREENING FAIL?

There are a number of steps during which newborn screening can fail. It is important to keep in mind that a newborn may not have been screened at the hospital. Many states allow for exemptions from newborn screening based on religious or other reasons. Other possibilities are that the newborn may have been born at home, the newborn may have been transferred to another hospital, or the specimen could have been lost or misidentified. There are also reasons why an infant could screen negative but still have a disease (i.e., a false negative result). For example, it is possible that the specimen was obtained at the wrong time. As previously noted, for some of the metabolic disorders, the infant needs to be at least 24 hours old and must have been fed an adequate amount of formula or

breast milk before a screening test can be valid. If the infant has not eaten, then the metabolites for some of the diseases will not accumulate and the test will yield a false negative result. For some disorders, the test is not accurate if the infant has had a blood transfusion. Things as simple as how much blood is collected, how long the sample is dried, how long it took to get to the lab, and even the weather conditions during shipment can result in abnormal test results. In addition, infants are sometimes "lost" to follow-up. It may be difficult to actually locate a specific infant due to a name change for the baby, family relocations, inadequate information provided with the sample (e.g., wrong address or telephone number), or a new physician of record.

The purpose of newborn screening is to identify affected infants, but as previously noted, a certain number of unaffected infants will be identified as being at risk. For some conditions, these false positive cases turn out to represent individuals who are carriers for the condition. With the advent of DNA testing, an increasing number of carrier infants have been identified. These infants do not have the disease but are carrying one DNA mutation for the screened disease. In many cases, the families of these newborns will be referred to a specialty center for further testing and counseling. If it is determined that the infant is a carrier, then genetic counseling will be offered to the parents so that they can better understand the risk of recurrence for themselves, for their child (and his or her future children), and for the child's siblings (who may also be carriers for the condition).

THE PAST, PRESENT, AND FUTURE OF NEWBORN SCREENING

The first successful newborn screening program was started in Massachusetts in 1962 with screening for PKU (MacCready, 1963). Preventive screening was mandated by the state and subsequently adopted by other states over a period of several years. Expansion of newborn screening began in earnest in 1975 when a test was developed to screen for congenital hypothyroidism (Dussault et al., 1975). The success of newborn screening for this disorder led to the addition of an increasing number of disorders., There are approximately 4,000,000 infants screened each year in the United States for a variety of disorders (Council of Regional Networks, 1995; see also http://genes-r-us.uthscsa.edu). Each state decides which disorders will be screened for, resulting in significant variability in screening programs from state to state (U.S. General Accounting Office, 2003) (see Table 8.3). All states must provide newborn screening. Whereas the majority of states have mandatory screening (all infants must be screened), some have voluntary screening (parents may choose whether their child is screened). Some states require written informed consent; others have an implied consent but require written informed dissent (the parents must sign if they choose not to participate). Some states have a single designated laboratory that performs all screening testing; others contract with regional centers,

university laboratories, or private laboratories. Each state must decide how the screening process is to be conducted, how to notify the parents and professionals of the results, and how to follow up on abnormal results. Each state may make a different decision depending on a number of factors including its resources, population mix, and birth rate. There is a movement to get all states to follow a uniform practice for performing and following up on newborn screening.

Further expansion of screening programs has been driven by consumer activism and new technologies (especially tandem mass spec-

Table 8.3.   Recommended newborn screening core panel

Disorder	Number of states mandated[a]
Amino acid disorders	
Argininosuccinate lyase deficiency (ASA)	36
Citrullinemia	36
Homocystinuria	41
Maple syrup urine disease (MSUD)	43
Phenylketonuria (PKU)	51
Tyrosinemia type I	32
Organic acid disorders	
3-hydroxy-3-methylglutaryl-CoA lyase deficiency (HMG)	34
3-methylcrotonyl-CoA carboxylase deficiency (3-MCC)	35
Beta-ketothiolase deficiency	32
Glutaric acidemia type 1 (GA1)	35
Isovaleric acidemia (IVA)	35
Multiple carboxylase deficiency	29
Methylmalonic acidemia (Cbl A,B)	35
Methylmalonic acidemia (mutase deficiency)	35
Propionic acidemia (PA)	36
Fatty acid oxidation disorders	
3-hydroxy long chain acyl-CoA dehydrogenase deficiency (LCHAD)	34
Carnitine uptake defect	24
Medium chain acyl-CoA dehydrogenase deficiency (MCAD)	44
Trifunctional protein deficiency (TFP)	31
Very long chain acyl-CoA dehydrogenase deficiency (VLCAD)	35
Hemoglobinopathies	
Hb S/S; Hb S/ßTh; Hb S/C	51
Other	
Biotinidase deficiency	41
Congenital adrenal hyperplasia	45
Congenital hypothyroidism	51
Cystic fibrosis	22
Galactose-1-phosphate uridyltransferase deficiency	51
Hearing loss	28[b]

Based on data from National Newborn Screening and Genetics Resource Center (NNSGRC). Data retrieved April 25, 2006, from http://genes-r-us.uthscsa.edu, from material updated by NNSGRC as of April 11, 2006. Please see http://genes-r-us.uthscsa.edu for most updated list.

[a]Only states that universally require a screening by law are counted (other states have universally offered screening but do not require it universally or for selected populations); Washington, D.C., is counted for "51 states."

[b]Twenty-three additional states universally offer but do not universally require hearing screening.

troscopy). Many states are considering revising their criteria. In 2005, the number of disorders screened for in the 50 states ranged from 4 to 41 (National Newborn Screening and Genetics Resource Center, 2007). All states screen for PKU, congenital hypothyroidism galactosemia, and sickle cell disease. The American College of Medical Genetics has convened a group of experts to develop recommendations regarding the disorders that all states should consider screening for when revising their programs. Consensus guidelines were developed through the Genetic Disease Branch of the federal Maternal and Child Health Bureau of the Health Resources and Services Administration in collaboration with the American Academy of Pediatrics and the American College of Medical Genetics to address the issue of inclusion criteria for newborn screening (Newborn Screening Expert Group, 2005). As previously noted, the technologies of tandem mass spectroscopy and DNA analysis have dramatically increased the number of possible diseases and disorders for which screening is possible. This group considered 84 diseases and recommended a core group of 29 diseases and disorders for newborn screening based on a number of factors, including disease or disorder frequency and availability of treatment (Table 8.3). Another 25 diseases were considered to be secondary targets for newborn screening and were named because they will be identified incidentally using certain technologies (e.g., full-scan MS/MS) that identify the core group. Twenty-seven disorders were deemed not appropriate for newborn screening, and three were deferred for later consideration. This expert panel recommended that all states mandate screening for the 29 core diseases and disorders and report abnormal results on the secondary targets. They also recommended the use of tandem mass spectrometry (23 of the 29 core diseases are diagnosed by this method). As of 2006, 88% of states are using this technology (National Newborn Screening and Genetics Resource Center, 2007). Recommendations were also made for evaluation of the newborn screening system, long-term data collection, and surveillance and oversight of the programs. As new technologies are developed and therapeutic advances are made, the list of conditions recommended for newborn screening is likely to expand. As an example, with the completion of the Human Genome Project, the discovery of hundreds of mutations causing disorders being screened for opens the possibility of using expression microarray technology to screen for these mutations in the newborn period rather than to screen for metabolic abnormalities resulting from the mutations (the MS/MS method).

PRENATAL SCREENING

Complementary to newborn screening is **prenatal screening** (screening during pregnancy to identify conditions that affected the fetus). As with newborn screening, numerous prenatal screening tests are now available (see Chapter 7). One can choose first-trimester screening tests, consisting of a blood test with a fetal ultrasound examination, or a second-trimester maternal serum screening. In addition, screening can be done before pregnancies in at-risk populations (e.g., carrier detection for Tay-Sachs disease in the Ashkenazi Jewish population, screening for cystic fibrosis in Caucasians) or in at-risk families (e.g., mutation analysis for fragile X syndrome in an extended family in which one family member has the disorder). Prenatal screening tests are particularly relevant in instances where increased risk is recognized on the basis of advanced maternal age, ethnicity, or a positive family history for a particular inherited disorder. Positive results from screening tests may prompt more involved diagnostic testing, including high-resolution fetal imaging, amniocentesis, chorionic villus sampling, and even percutaneous umbilical blood sampling. These are considered diagnostic tests because they are performed to look for a specific diagnosis. Chromosomal analysis, enzymatic assays, and molecular testing can all be done on fetal tissue that is obtained through diagnostic testing in order to confirm a diagnosis or to rule it out.

SUMMARY

Screening tests are important tools used to help define increased risk for significant medical and genetic conditions. These tests can be used for mass screening of newborns, and they are also useful for prenatal screening and targeted screening of specific at-risk populations and ethnic groups. Newborn screening is one of the most important and effective public health measures. Many infants have been identified through this early screening and have been successfully treated with improved outcomes. However, some of the metabolic disorders can have lifelong complications despite therapy. The number of diseases and disorders screened for has grown over time and will likely continue to increase. As more infants are identified with more diseases and disorders, future research should be aimed at developing innovative therapies to further improve outcomes.

REFERENCES

American Academy of Pediatrics Newborn Screening Task Force. (2000). Serving the family from birth to the medical home, newborn screening: A blueprint for the future, a call for a national agenda on state newborn screening programs. *Pediatrics, 389,* 389–427.

American College of Medical Genetics & American Society of Human Genetics Test and Technology Transfer Committee Working Group. (2000). Tandem mass spectroscopy in newborn screening. *Genetics in Medicine, 2,* 267–269.

Chace, D.H., Sherwin, J.E., Hillman, S.L., et al. (1998). Use of phenylalanine-to-tyrosine ratio determined by tandem mass spectroscopy to improve newborn screening for phenylketonuria of early discharge specimens in the first 24 hours. *Clinical Chemistry, 44,* 2405–2409.

Chace, D.H., DiPerna, J.C. & Naylor, E.W. (1999). Laboratory integration and utilization of tandem mass spectroscopy in neonatal screening: a model for clinical mass spectroscopy in the next millennium. *Acta Paediatric Supplement, 88,* 45–47.

Chace, D.H., Kalas, T.A. & Naylor, E.W. (2003). Use of tandem mass spectrometry for multianalyte screening of dried blood specimens from newborns. *Clinical Chemistry, 49,* 1797–1817.

Comeau, A.M., Parad, R.B., Dorkin, H.L., et al. (2004). Population-based newborn screening for genetic disorders when multiple mutation DNA testing is incorporated: A cystic fibrosis newborn screening model demonstrating increased sensitivity but more carrier detections. *Pediatrics, 113,* 1573–1581.

Council of Regional Networks for Genetic Services (CORN) Newborn Screening Committee. (1995). *National Newborn Screening Report–1995.* Atlanta, GA. Council of Regional Network s for Genetic Services.

Delange, F. (1997). Neonatal screening for congenital hypothyroidism: Results and perspectives. *Hormone Research, 48,* 51–61.

Dussault, J.H., Coulombe, P., Laberge, C., et al. (1975). Preliminary report on a mass screening program for neonatal hypothyroidism. *Journal of Pediatrics, 86,* 670–674.

Guerina, N.G., Hsu, H.W., Meissner, H.C., et al. (1994). Neonatal serologic screening and early treatment for congenital toxoplasma gondii infection. *The New England Journal of Medicine, 330*(26), 1858–1863.

MacCready, R. (1963). Phenylketonuria screening program. *The New England Journal of Medicine 269,* 52–56.

Marsden, D., Larson, C., & Levy, H.L. (2006). Newborn screening for metabolic disorders. *Journal of Pediatrics, 148,* 577–584

National Newborn Screeninig and Genetics Resource Center. (2007). *National newborn screening status report.* Retrieved January 16, 2007, from http://genes-r-us .uthscsa.edu/nbsdisorders.htm

Newborn Screening Expert Group. (2005). Newborn screening: Towards a uniform screening panel and system. *Federal Register 70,* 44. Retrieved March 8, 2005, from http://mchb.hrsa.gov/screening

Pass, K.A., Lane, P.A., Fernhoff, P.M. et al. (2000). U.S. newborn screening system guidelines II: Follow-up of children, diagnosis, management, and evaluation: Statement of the Council of Regional Networks for Genetic Services. *Journal of Pediatrics, 137,* S1–S46.

U.S. General Accounting Office. (2003). *Newborn screening characteristics of state programs* Retrieved April 25, 2006, from http://www.gao.gov/new.items/d03449.pdf

Van Naarden Braun, K., Yeargin-Allsopp, M., Schendel, D. et al. (2003). Long-term developmental outcomes of children identified through a newborn screening program with a metabolic or endocrine disorder: A population-based approach. *Journal of Pediatrics, 143,* 236–242.

Waisbren, S.E., Albers, S., Amato, S., et al. (2003). Effect of expanded newborn screening for biochemical genetic disorders on child outcomes and parental stress. *Journal of the American Medical Association 290,* 2564–2572.

Wilcken, B., Wiley, V., Hammond, J. et al. (2003). Screening newborns for inborn errors of metabolism by tandem mass spectroscopy. *The New England Journal of Medicine, 348,* 2304–312.

9 Premature and Small-for-Dates Infants

Khodayar Rais-Bahrami and Billie Lou Short

Upon completion of this chapter, the reader will

- Recognize some of the causes of prematurity and being small for gestational age
- Be able to identify physical characteristics of the premature infant
- Understand the complications and illnesses associated with preterm birth
- Be aware of the methods used to care for low birth weight infants
- Know the results of outcome studies

The preterm infant is at an immediate disadvantage compared with the full-term infant. In addition to facing all of the usual challenges of making the transition from intrauterine to extrauterine life (see Chapter 5), the preterm infant must make these changes using organs that are not ready to perform the task. Almost every organ is immature. Decreased production of a substance called surfactant in the lungs can lead to respiratory distress syndrome (RDS); immaturity of the central nervous system places the preterm infant at increased risk for an **intraventricular hemorrhage (IVH), periventricular leukomalacia (PVL),** and **hydrocephalus;** and inadequate kidney function makes fluid and metabolic management difficult. An immature gastrointestinal tract impairs the infant's ability to digest and absorb certain nutrients and places the gut at risk for developing a life-threatening disorder called **necrotizing enterocolitis (NEC)** that results from inadequate blood supply. Finally, the preterm infant's eyes are more susceptible to the damaging effects of the oxygen that is used to treat respiratory distress. This may result in retinopathy of prematurity (ROP) and subsequent vision loss. Given these risks, it is remarkable that most preterm infants overcome these acute problems with little residual effects. A minority, however, do sustain long-term medical and neurodevelopmental complications. A

discussion of these complications and their prevention is the focus of this chapter.

ERIN

Erin was born prematurely, at 23 weeks' gestation, and weighed less than 500 grams (less than 1.5 pounds). During Erin's first day of life, she needed artificial ventilation and surfactant therapy to keep the air passages in her lungs open. By 2 months of age, she was doing well enough to receive a pressurized oxygen–air mixture through a high flow **nasal cannula** (HFNC- Vapotherm), but she had brief breathing arrests (apnea) associated with a slowed heart rate (bradycardia). This was treated successfully with caffeine and frequent physical stimulation. In addition, she developed NEC, leading to bowel perforation that required two major abdominal surgeries 10 weeks apart.

Meeting Erin's nutritional requirements was also a problem. Initially, Erin needed intravenous nutrition. Gradually, she was able to accept increasing amounts of elemental infant formula by a nasogastric tube, and by 3 months, she was strong enough to receive some of her feedings by bottle. At her 168th day of life (postconceptional age of 45 weeks), weighing 3,760 grams (8 pounds, 4½ ounces), Erin went home on oxygen and caffeine and was hooked up to an apnea monitor. Her parents had been instructed how to administer oxygen therapy, how to use the monitor, and how to administer cardiopulmonary resuscitation (CPR), if needed. Although her prognosis is good, Erin will need continued medical and neurodevelopmental monitoring until she is school age.

DEFINITIONS OF PREMATURITY AND LOW BIRTH WEIGHT

A preterm or premature infant is one born before the 37th week of gestation. Although there is no universal system for birth weight classification, it is commonly accepted that an infant with a birth weight less than 2,500 grams (5½ pounds) is **low birth weight (LBW);** an infant born weighing less than 1,500 grams (3⅓ pounds) is **very low birth weight (VLBW);** and an infant with a birth weight lower than 1,000 grams (2¼ pounds) is **extremely low birth weight (ELBW).** An infant weighing less than 800 grams (1¾ pounds) is sometimes called a **micropreemie.** Assessment of gestational age is also important, as infants of low birth weight may represent prematurely born infants or those who are small for gestational age (SGA).

Small-for-Gestational-Age Infants

SGA infants can be either full term or premature. In either case, they have a birth weight below the 10th percentile for a population-specific birth weight verses gestational age plot (Figure 9.1). SGA infants are also referred to as dysmature, or small for dates. In addition to being small, these infants also appear malnourished, usually because of intrauterine growth restriction. About one half of SGA births are attributable to maternal illness, smoking, or malnutrition. These infants tend to be underweight but have normal length and head circumference; they are said to have asymmetric SGA because of this discrepancy in growth pattern. The other half of SGA births are said to have symmetric SGA (equally deviant in length, weight, and head circumference). These infants may have been exposed in utero to alcohol or to infections such as cytomegalovirus (see Chapter 3). Infants with certain chromosomal and other genetic disorders also present as symmetrical SGA infants (Suresh et al., 2001). SGA infants, whether full term or preterm, are recognized as having an increased risk for many complications in the newborn period (e.g., hypoxia, hy-

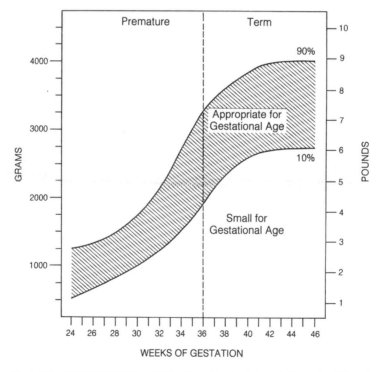

Figure 9.1. Newborn weight by gestational age. The shaded area between the 10th and 90th percentiles represents infants who are appropriate for gestational age. Weight below the 10th percentile makes an infant small for gestational age (SGA). Prematurity is defined as being born before 36 weeks' gestation. (From Lubchenco, L.O. [1976]. *The high risk infant.* Philadelphia: W.B. Saunders. Copyright © Elsevier; reprinted by permission.)

pothermia, hypoglycemia), long-term growth impairments, developmental disabilities, and increased perinatal and neonatal mortality (Aucott et al., 2004; Brandt et al., 2005).

Assessment of Gestational Age

Assessment of gestational age helps distinguish an appropriate-for-gestational-age infant from a SGA infant. In addition, it will influence treatment approaches, neurodevelopmental assess-

ment, and outcome. The gestational age is calculated from the projected birth date, or estimated date of confinement (EDC). This can be obtained using the Nägele rule: Add 7 days and subtract 3 months from the date of the last menstrual period. The accuracy of menstrual dating, however, is quite variable, especially in anticipated preterm deliveries. In most cases, uterine size is an accurate predictor of gestational age and can be measured by clinical and ultrasound examination. Another way of estimating gesta-

Neuromuscular Maturity

	-1	0	1	2	3	4	5
Posture							
Square Window (wrist)	>90°	90°	60°	45°	30°	0°	
Arm Recoil		180°	140°-180°	110°-140°	90-110°	<90°	
Popliteal Angle	180°	160°	140°	120°	100°	90°	<90°
Scarf Sign							
Heel to Ear							

Physical Maturity

									Maturity Rating	
									score	weeks
Skin	sticky friable transparent	gelatinous red, translucent	smooth pink, visible veins	superficial peeling &/or rash. few veins	cracking pale areas rare veins	parchment deep cracking no vessels	leathery cracked wrinkled		-10	20
									-5	22
Lanugo	none	sparse	abundant	thinning	bald areas	mostly bald			0	24
Plantar Surface	heel-toe 40-50 mm:-1 <40 mm:-2	>50mm no crease	faint red marks	anterior transverse crease only	creases ant. 2/3	creases over entire sole			5	26
									10	28
Breast	imperceptible	barely perceptible	flat areola no bud	stippled areola 1-2mm bud	raised areola 3-4mm bud	full areola 5-10mm bud			15	30
									20	32
Eye/Ear	lids fused loosely:-1 tightly:-2	lids open pinna flat stays folded	sl. curved pinna; soft; slow recoil	well-curved pinna; soft but ready recoil	formed & firm instant recoil	thick cartilage ear stiff			25	34
									30	36
Genitals male	scrotum flat, smooth	scrotum empty faint rugae	testes in upper canal rare rugae	testes descending few rugae	testes down good rugae	testes pendulous deep rugae			35	38
									40	40
Genitals female	clitoris prominent labia flat	prominent clitoris small labia minora	prominent clitoris enlarging minora	majora & minora equally prominent	majora large minora small	majora cover clitoris & minora			45	42
									50	44

Figure 9.2. Scoring system to assess newborn infants. The score for each of the neuromuscular and physical signs is added together to obtain a score called the total maturity score. Gestational age is determined from this score. (This figure was published in *Journal of Pediatrics, 119,* 418, Ballard, J.L., Khoury, J.C., Wedig, K., et al. New Ballard score, expanded to include extremely premature infants, Copyright © Elsevier, 1991; reprinted by permission.)

tional age is by noting when fetal activity first develops. **Quickening** is first felt by the mother at approximately 16–18 weeks' gestation, and fetal heart sounds can be first detected at approximately 10–12 weeks by ultrasound and at 20 weeks by fetoscope (similar to a stethoscope). Following birth, the gestational age can be assessed using a clinical scoring system called the modified Dubowitz examination (discussed next). Another technique allows for estimating the degree of prematurity by examining the maturity of the lens of the eye in the first 24–48 hours of life (Nagpal, Kumar, & Ramji, 2004). Using a combination of these methods increases the accuracy of gestational age assessment.

Physical and Behavioral Characteristics of the Premature Infant

Several physical and developmental characteristics distinguish the premature infant from the full-term infant. A scoring system developed by Dubowitz, Dubowitz, and Goldberg (1970) and updated by Ballard et al. (1991; Figure 9.2) takes these characteristics into account and enables the physician to estimate the infant's gestational age with some accuracy. The limitation of this scoring system is the postnatal age of the infant. If the scoring is not performed within the first 24 hours of birth, neurological and some physical features (e.g., skin texture) can change and make the infant appear more mature than is the case. Also, any severely ill infant can be difficult to evaluate due to altered neurological status.

The main physical characteristics that distinguish a premature from a full-term infant are the presence in the premature infant of fine body hair (**lanugo**); smooth, reddish skin; and the absence of skin creases, ear cartilage, and breast buds (Figure 9.3). In addition to the physical appearance, premature infants display distinctive neurological and behavioral characteristics, including reduced muscle tone and activity and increased joint mobility (Constantine et al., 1987). Low muscle tone is particularly evident in the infant born before 28 weeks' gestation; it gradually improves with advancing gestational age, starting with the legs and moving up to the arms by 32 weeks. Thus, although the premature infant lies in a floppy, extended position, the full-term infant rests in a semi-flexed position. As flexion tone improves over the weeks after birth, increased joint mobility disappears. Finally, as compared with the full-term infant, the premature infant may appear

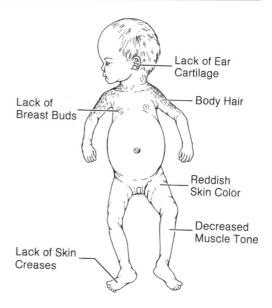

Figure 9.3. Typical physical features of a premature infant.

behaviorally passive and disorganized in the first weeks of life (Mandrich et al., 1994).

INCIDENCE OF PRETERM BIRTHS

Preterm birth occurs in only 12.3% of all pregnancies. Yet, it is responsible for the majority of neonatal deaths and nearly one half of all cases of neonatal-onset neurodevelopmental disabilities, including cerebral palsy (Martin et al., 2005). This risk is highest in those infants born before 32 weeks' gestation, representing 2% of all births. The incidence of preterm births has risen since the early 1990s, and preterm births occur twice as frequently in African Americans as in Caucasians. Of LBW infants weighing less than 2,500 grams, 70% are preterm and 30% are full-term infants who are SGA. The preterm birth rate is up 16% since 1990, and the percentage of children born at low birth weight rose slightly in 2003 to the highest level reported since 1970 (7.9%) (Martin et al., 2005).

CAUSES OF PREMATURE BIRTH

The rise in reported rates of preterm delivery is certainly a cause for concern and has been attributed to many co-factors, including increased obstetric intervention, use of assisted reproduction techniques, high number of multiple pregnancies, increased prevalence of substance abuse in urban areas, and a rise in idiopathic preterm delivery rates due to the adverse effect of low socioeconomic factors (Slattery &

Morrison 2002). Other common causes of preterm delivery are maternal infections and adolescence, and these often occur together. Although less than 5% of all pregnancies occur in adolescents, these pregnancies account for 20% of all preterm births (Cooper, Leland, & Alexander, 1995). In addition, up to 80% of early preterm births (births before 30 weeks' gestation) are associated with an intrauterine infection that precedes the rupture of membranes (Klein & Gibbs, 2005). Other risk factors include inadequate prenatal care, poverty, acute and chronic maternal illness, multiple-gestation births, a history of previous premature pregnancies, placental bleeding, preeclampsia, smoking, and substance abuse (Adams et al., 2000). Congenital anomalies or injuries to the fetus may also lead to premature birth. Certain fetal conditions such as **Rh incompatibility** and poor fetal growth may require early delivery.

COMPLICATIONS OF PREMATURITY

The premature infant must undergo the same physiologic transitions to extrauterine life as the full-term infant (see Chapter 5). The preterm infant, however, must accomplish this difficult task using immature body organs. The result is a significant risk of complications in virtually every organ system in the body. This risk increases with the degree of prematurity.

Respiratory Problems

Hyaline Membrane Disease Hyaline membrane disease (HMD), also called RDS, is a disorder characterized by respiratory distress in the newborn period. The underlying abnormality is decreased production of surfactant that normally keeps the alveoli (the terminal airway passages) stable, permitting the exchange of oxygen and carbon dioxide (Figure 9.4). A chest X ray can clinically confirm HMD, showing a "ground glass" appearance of the lungs. This results from the collapsed alveoli appearing dense and hazy in comparison with the translucent, air-filled lung of a typical full-term newborn, which appears black (Figure 9.5). The clinical course of HMD involves peak severity between 24 and 48 hours after birth, followed by improvement over the next 24–48 hours. In uncomplicated cases, HMD will resolve within 72–96 hours after birth. This classical course of HMD has fortunately been modified by the administration of exogenous surfactant replacement. Improvement in pulmonary function usually begins within minutes after the first dose of surfactant, and effective gas exchange can be achieved with a significantly lower level of oxygen and ventilatory support after one or two doses. Except in severe cases of HMD, it is unusual for an infant to require more than two doses of surfactant.

Inflated Alveolus in Full-term Infant

Collapsed Alveolus in Premature with RDS

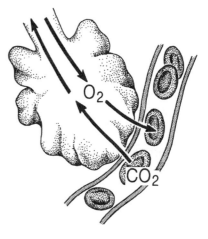

Figure 9.4. Schematic drawing of alveoli in a normal newborn and in a premature infant with respiratory distress syndrome (RDS). Note that the inflated alveolus is kept open by surfactant. Oxygen (O_2) moves from the alveolus to the red blood cells in the pulmonary capillary. Carbon dioxide (CO_2) moves in the opposite direction. This exchange is much less efficient when the alveolus is collapsed. The result is hypoxia.

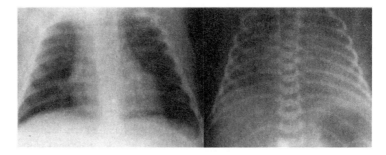

Figure 9.5.   Chest X rays of a normal newborn (left) and of a premature infant with respiratory distress syndrome (RDS; right), which shows a "white out" of the lungs due to surfactant deficiency.

Infants with mild HMD generally do well with supplemental oxygen alone or in combination with continuous positive airway pressure (CPAP). CPAP involves providing a mixture of oxygen and air under continuous pressure; this prevents the alveoli from collapsing between breaths. More severely affected infants may require the placement of an endotracheal tube for mechanical ventilatory support as well as administration of exogenous surfactant. Although surfactant therapy has significantly reduced mortality in ELBW premature infants, there has been no appreciable change in long-term pulmonary and neurodevelopmental complications in these infants (D'Angio et al., 2002; Horbar et al., 2002). Therefore, close follow-up to school entry is important.

A related approach to treating surfactant deficiency is to stimulate its production. There is evidence that administration of steroids to mothers 24–36 hours before delivery stimulates surfactant production and pulmonary maturation in the fetus. This lessens the likelihood and/or severity of HMD. The effect of antenatal steroids is additive to surfactant replacement therapy in reducing respiratory distress and mortality. It is therefore recommended that **steroids** be given prior to birth for potential preterm delivery of fetuses between 24 and 34 weeks' gestational age (NIH Consensus Development Panel, 1995).

Bronchopulmonary Dysplasia   The improved survival of ELBW newborns has increased the number of infants at risk for various forms of respiratory morbidity associated with mechanical ventilation, including **bronchopulmonary dysplasia (BPD).** This term is generally used to describe infants who require supplemental oxygen and/or mechanical ventilation beyond 28 days postnatal age and/or corrected gestational age of 36 weeks and who have persistently abnormal chest X rays and respiratory

examinations (e.g., rapid breathing, wheezing). BPD primarily occurs in infants who are born at less than 32 weeks' gestation and require mechanical ventilation during the first week of life for treatment of HMD (Farrell & Fiascone, 1997; Walsh et al., 2005).

The development of BPD has been attributed to lung injury from a combination of barotrauma (pressure damage from prolonged mechanical ventilation), oxygen toxicity, infection, and inflammation; the exact mechanism of BPD remains poorly understood. Since the 1970s, newer methods of respiratory support, including high-frequency ventilation and surfactant therapy, have increased the survival rate of smaller and less mature infants, but the total number of infants who develop BPD has not decreased. BPD remains the most common chronic lung disease of infancy in the United States, with some 7,000 new cases being diagnosed each year. Long-term studies of pulmonary function in this population indicate that as these infants grow, there is clinical improvement. Abnormalities in airway resistance and pulmonary compliance, however, persist into adulthood, resulting in a high risk of asthma (Kennedy et al., 2000).

Approaches to postnatal prevention and treatment of BPD have included corticosteroid therapy, supplemental vitamin A, high-frequency ventilation, use of bronchodilators (asthma medication), and administration of diuretics to increase urinary excretion. The use of postnatal corticosteroid medication such as dexamethasone (Decadron) for prevention and treatment of BPD has been a matter of controversy. There is evidence that early treatment with dexamethasone reduces pulmonary inflammation and decreases the need for supplemental oxygen and mechanical ventilation (Tapia et al., 1998). Although its potential for adverse long-term effects on physical growth and neurodevelopment has been of concern (Papile et al., 1998), a more recent study has shown that a 42-day course of dexamethasone therapy beginning at 2 weeks of age in preterm infants who were at high risk for severe chronic lung disease was associated with improved long-term neurodevelopmental outcome (Gross, Abner, & Mettelman, 2005). It is not unusual for infants with BPD to require prolonged support with supplemental oxygen, diuretics, and bronchodilators after discharge from the hospital. Even with supportive care and treatment, infants with BPD continue to have long-term problems, including limited tolerance of physical exercise, feeding difficulties that contribute to poor physical growth, excessive caloric requirement, and an increased risk of developmental disabilities (Valleur-Masson et al., 1993).

Neurologic Problems

Intraventricular Hemorrhage IVH is an important neurological complication of extremely premature infants. The risk of IVH correlates directly with the degree of prematurity. Fortunately, its incidence appears to be declining. About 50% of IVH occurs during the first day of life and 90% by the third day of life (Owens, 2005). Ultrasound of the head is the most reliable and safest technique for diagnosis of IVH. It is commonly graded by severity into four levels (Volpe, 2001). Grade I is defined by bleeding into the germinal matrix, a network of blood vessels in the roof of the lateral ventricles. If the hemorrhage expands beyond the germinal matrix into the ventricular system, it is Grade II. Grade I and II account for the majority of IVH, and significant neurological impairment is fortunately rare with these types of IVH. About 20% of hemorrhages, however, are severe enough to dilate the ventricle (Grade III) or invade the brain substance (Grade IV). Grade IV is often called periventricular hemorrhagic infarction. These hemorrhages can lead to PVL, or damage of the white matter surrounding the ventricles (Volpe, 2001). The long-term neurological outcome is related to the severity of the hemorrhage, with cerebral palsy and/or intellectual disability seen in 30% of the patients with Grade III hemorrhages and in 75% of those with Grade IV hemorrhages (Pleacher et al., 2004).

Avoidance of hypoxic-ischemic events that lead to fluctuations in cerebral blood pressure, expert delivery room stabilization, effective resuscitation and ventilation, gentle handling, and use of muscle relaxants during mechanical ventilation have all been associated with a reduction in the incidence and severity of IVH (Volpe, 2001). A number of medications have been studied for preventing or treating IVH, with varied results. These include antenatal use of steroids and postnatal use of phenobarbital (Luminal), vitamin K, vitamin E, and indomethacin (Greer, 1995; Leviton et al., 1993). Indomethacin, given soon after birth, appears to significantly reduce the incidence and severity of IVH, but the other medications do not appear to benefit the infant (Ment et al., 2000).

Periventricular Leukomalacia The periventricular white matter is the region of the brain closest to the ventricles. It is especially vulnerable to injury in the premature infant. In addition, the glial cells, a major constituent of white matter, undergo rapid growth by the end of the second trimester and are more susceptible to injury caused by fluctuations in cerebral blood pressure during this period. Finally, there is evidence that maternal infection involving the membranes surrounding the fetus (chorioamnionitis) increases the risk of injury. PVL results when this area sustains damage either due to low oxygen or low blood flow (Blumenthal, 2004; Volpe, 2005).

PVL has been reported to occur in 4%–15% of premature infants (Perlman, Risser, & Broyles, 1996). It may occur in association with IVH or independently (Figure 9.6). The diagnosis of PVL is best made by serial cranial (head) ultrasounds that may show the development of cystic lesions in the white matter. Serial cranial ultrasounds or a magnetic resonance imaging (MRI) at near term gestation in VLBW neonates also have been shown to be important predictors of the subsequent development of **spastic diplegia** (a form of cerebral palsy that impairs lower extremity function) and **hemiplegia** (a form of cerebral palsy that affects one side of the body) (Mirmiran et al., 2004; see Chapter 23). Large cysts (greater than 3 millimeters in diameter) place the child at increased risk of developing **spastic quadriplegia** (a form of cerebral palsy that affects all four limbs), visual impairment, intellectual disability, and seizures in early childhood (Okumura et al., 2003).

Hearing Impairment

ELBW infants are at increased risk for hearing loss because of multisystem illness and the frequent use of medications, such as aminoglycoside antibiotics and diuretics, that can be toxic to the auditory system. The overall prevalence of sensorineural hearing impairment is about 4 per 10,000 in full-term infants. This increases

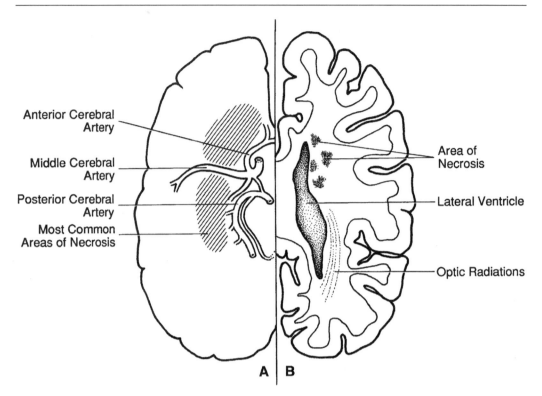

Figure 9.6. Periventricular leukomalacia (PVL). A) The blood vessel supply to the brain, and B) the brain structures. The area of the white matter surrounding the lateral ventricle (particularly the top part) is especially susceptible to hypoxic-ischemic damage because it is not well supplied by blood vessels. It lies in a watershed area between the anterior, middle, and posterior cerebral arteries. In premature infants, poor oxygenation and decreased blood flow associated with respiratory distress syndrome (RDS) may lead to necrosis of this brain tissue, a condition termed *periventricular leukomalacia*. When the posterior portion is affected, the optic radiations may be damaged, resulting in cortical blindness.

to 13 per 10,000 in LBW infants and to 51 per 10,000 among VLBW infants (Van Naarden & Decoufle, 1999). In 1994, the Joint Committee on Infant Hearing recommended that all VLBW infants undergo auditory screening (Joint Committee on Infant Hearing, 1995). The committee further expanded this statement in 2000 to advocate testing for all newborns (Joint Committee on Infant Hearing, 2000). The most commonly performed tests are brainstem auditory evoked response (BAER) and **otoacoustic emission (OAE)** (Johnson et al., 2005).

Apnea and Bradycardia

Apnea is clinically defined as a respiratory pause lasting 15–20 seconds associated with a decrease in heart rate to below 80–100 beats per minute. It is the most common disorder of respiratory control found in the neonatal intensive care unit (NICU) and is related to immaturity of the central nervous system. About 10% of all LBW infants and more than 40% of VLBW

infants experience clinically significant apnea (Baird, 2004).

Apnea that occurs with sustained bradycardia (very low heart rate) may be a symptom of an underlying medical condition. If all serious underlying causes have been ruled out, the infant is said to have apnea of prematurity. Medications such as caffeine and theophylline can stimulate respiration and are commonly used to treat apnea of prematurity (Larsen et al., 1995). Caffeine and theophylline appear to have comparable therapeutic efficacy, but the frequency of reported side effects is greater with theophylline. Therefore, caffeine is usually employed in centers that can measure caffeine levels in blood to ensure that therapeutic levels are maintained. Theophylline is used, however, in the infant who has both apnea and reactive airway disease (asthma) because it is a known bronchodilator, whereas caffeine is not.

The risk of apnea of prematurity declines with advancing postnatal maturation. Developmental immaturity of respiratory control underlies the pathogenesis of neonatal apnea. Even after apparent resolution, however, apnea can recur in certain clinical situations, particularly with respiratory syncytial virus infection and severe anemia.

Sudden Infant Death Syndrome

Sudden infant death syndrome (SIDS) occurs more than twice as frequently in premature infants as in full-term infants, usually between 2 and 5 months of life. Contrary to earlier beliefs, apnea of prematurity is not a major predisposing factor for SIDS (Hodgman, 1998). Because of the increased incidence of SIDS, however, the extremely premature infant who is having significant apneic spells in the 2 weeks before discharge may be sent home with an apnea monitor (Committee on Fetus and Newborn, 2003). Although these monitors emit an alarm if the infant stops breathing, studies on their use have not shown effectiveness in reducing the incidence of SIDS. The monitors do, however, provide reassurance to parents and physicians about the status of the infant (Abendroth et al., 1999). Parents of such high-risk infants should be trained in neonatal CPR prior to taking their infant home on an apnea monitor. The monitor is generally not required for more than a few months.

In order to prevent SIDS, in 1992 the American Academy of Pediatrics, through its Task Force on Infant Position and SIDS, began recommending that infants be placed on their back for sleep. In addition, fluffy blankets and toys should not be placed in the crib during sleep times and the home environment should be smoke free. These changes have resulted in a 40% reduction in the incidence of SIDS (Gibson et al., 2000).

Cardiovascular Problems

The most common cardiovascular problem in LBW infants is a **patent ductus arteriosus (PDA)**. The ductus arteriosis is the fetal vessel that diverts blood flow from the lungs. It normally closes at birth, allowing blood to flow to the lungs and be oxygenated. About 30% of all premature infants, and more than 50% of those born weighing less than 1,000 grams, will have a patent (open) ductus arteriosis diagnosed during the first few days of life. This is especially true in premature infants who have RDS. In these children, a PDA will divert blood from the lungs and further decrease oxygenation to the body and brain, increasing the work of the heart. This can lead to hypoxia, decreased blood flow to specific organs, and heart failure. The presence of a PDA can be detected by echocardiography, a form of ultrasound of the heart. Its management involves medical and supportive measures, including fluid restriction, diuresis (stimulation of urination), and the use of CPAP. If this fails, closure is possible using medications such as indomethacin or ibuprofen (Van Overmeire et al., 2000). In a small percentage of infants, surgical closure is required.

Gastrointestinal Problems

Although premature infants may be born with a suck-and-swallow response, it is immature and poorly coordinated until approximately 32 to 34 weeks' gestation. Thus, most premature infants require nasogastric or nasojejunal tube feedings until they can make the transition to oral feeds (Premji & Chessell, 2001). The nutritional needs of the premature infant are also different from those of the full-term infant and require the use of specialty formulas. In addition to physiological problems, premature infants are at increased risk for two major gastrointestinal disorders, NEC and **gastroesophageal reflux (GER),** that can inhibit growth and be life threatening.

Necrotizing Enterocolitis NEC is the most commonly acquired life-threatening intestinal disease in premature infants (Horton, 2005). It involves severe injury to a portion of the bowel wall. The exact cause of NEC is unknown, but prematurity appears to be the most common predisposing factor. Approximately 80% of infants with NEC are born at less than 38 weeks' gestation and weigh less than 2,500 grams at birth. Other predisposing factors include fetal distress, premature rupture of membranes, low Apgar scores, and exchange transfusion. The incidence of NEC is 1–2 per 1,000 live births, and the overall mortality rate for infants with NEC is 20%. The mortality rate of ELBW infants with NEC, however, is greater than 40% (Snyder et al., 1997).

Medical management of NEC involves withholding feedings combined with nasogastric suction to decrease pressure on the bowel wall, antibiotics to fight the suspected underlying infection, and intravenous fluids and nutrition to prevent dehydration and weight loss. Although medical treatment can be successful in many infants with NEC, approximately half require surgery to remove the diseased section of the bowel (Chandler & Hebra, 2000). Survivors of NEC may experience a variety of postoperative complications related to the disease, the operation, or treatment measures. For example, surgery for NEC is the leading cause of short bowel syndrome in infancy (Horwitz et al., 1995). The removal of a large portion of the bowel leads to decreased absorption of nutrients. This occurs in up to 11% of postsurgical NEC survivors and results in chronic diarrhea, malabsorption, nutritional deficiencies, impaired growth, and the long-term need for intravenous nutrition (an intravenous infusion of nutrients such as fats, carbohydrates, and amino acids).

Gastroesophageal Reflux The immaturity of gastric sphincter muscular control and delayed stomach emptying in premature infants may result in GER, a syndrome in which the contents of the stomach are regurgitated back into the **esophagus** (Dhillon & Ewer, 2004). Infants with severe GER are at increased risk for vomiting and **aspiration pneumonia** (an infection precipitated by the **aspiration** of food into the lung). This may be worsened by nasogastric tube feedings. Signs of GER include refusal of oral feeding, apnea, and back arching. Treatment is targeted toward special positioning techniques and medications (see Chapter 27).

Ophthalmologic Problems

Abnormalities in retinal vascular development after preterm birth lead to retinopathy of prematurity (ROP), formerly called retrolental fibroplasia. ELBW infants are at the greatest risk for developing ROP (Darlow et al., 2005; Tasman et al., 2006). An examination by a pediatric **ophthalmologist** should be performed at 4–6 weeks after birth or at 32–33 weeks' gestation (whichever comes first) for early detection of ROP. Follow-up examinations should be done until retinal vascularization is complete, around term gestation (see Chapter 10). Preventive therapy with vitamin E may decrease the severity of ROP in susceptible infants (Raju et al., 1997). Severe ROP is treated by laser to prevent permanent retinal detachment.

Immunologic Problems

The premature infant is born with an immature immune system. As a result, the infant is at increased risk for infection in the first months of life (Klein & Gibbs, 2005). Generalized bacter-

ial and fungal infections, occurring in approximately 30% of extremely premature infants, are major life-threatening illnesses and can lead to a poor neurodevelopmental outcome (Wheater & Renie, 2000). Premature infants who remain in the hospital for prolonged periods should receive routine immunizations based on their chronological age.

Other Physiologic Abnormalities

Premature infants are at increased risk for many of the same transient physiological abnormalities that occur in full-term infants (see Chapter 5). These include hyperbilirubinemia, anemia, hypo- and hyperglycemia, hypocalcemia, and hypothermia. In addition, some develop transient hypothyroidism that is not seen in full-term infants (Van Wassenaer et al., 2002). These problems place the premature infant at increased risk for brain damage.

Acidosis and hypoxia can increase the permeability of the blood–brain barrier to bilirubin, making preterm infants more susceptible to kernicterus (see Chapter 5). Thus, the bilirubin level that is used to determine whether phototherapy or an exchange transfusion should be performed is lower for the preterm infant than for the full-term infant (Watchko & Claassen, 1994). **Glucose** and **electrolyte** instability are also common in premature infants, especially the micropreemie.

Anemia is also more of a problem for the premature infant as it decreases the oxygen-carrying capacity of the red blood cells and can lead to hypoxic-ischemic brain damage. In severe cases, correction of anemia with blood transfusion and/or treatment with erythropoietin, to stimulate the bone marrow to produce red blood cells, may be necessary (Obladen & Maier, 1995). Since the late 1990s, studies have shown that changes in transfusion practices have significantly reduced the need for transfusion in the LBW premature infant and reduced the need for erythropoietin, which is very costly and does not affect the transfusion requirement in VLBW infants (Ohls et al., 2001).

Finally, premature infants often have a transient deficiency of thyroid hormone production. In severe cases, it may be associated with neurodevelopmental impairments; however, in most cases, the hypothyroidism resolves without the need for thyroid hormone replacement therapy which may not impact their long-term outcome (Van Wassenaer et al., 2002).

MEDICAL AND DEVELOPMENTAL CARE OF LOW BIRTH WEIGHT INFANTS

The best treatment for LBW infants is prevention of preterm births. This starts with identifying women at risk and providing them with education and prenatal health care; detecting preterm labor early; and using labor-arresting agents and antenatal steroids (Joffe et al., 1995). Prenatal care has improved appreciably since the 1970s, but the incidence of preterm delivery remains high and might even be rising (Martin et al., 2005). Preterm and SGA infants are best managed and cared for in high-risk obstetrical centers with NICUs.

Increased survival rate of preterm infants in the 1990s has been associated with an increased risk of significant neurodevelopmental impairment (Wilson-Costello et al., 2005). As survival rates of preterm infants have improved, the focus of care is now including a consideration of the optimal environment within the NICU for the premature infant to develop. Traditional NICU care has focused on medical protocols and procedures. A newer approach uses a more relationship-based, individualized, developmentally supportive model. This approach recognizes that the usual NICU setting is not optimal for the premature infant's developmental progress. Typical NICU care has involved the infant experiencing prolonged diffuse sleep states, unattended crying, a high ambient noise level, a lack of opportunity for sucking, and poorly timed social and caregiving interactions.

The newer approach seeks to observe the infant's behavior and respond to it appropriately by providing individualized neurodevelopmental care and actively involving the parents in their infant's care (Als et al., 2005). It involves documenting infant behavior, including breathing pattern, color fluctuations, startles, posture, and sleep state. This then leads to caregiving suggestions and environmental modifications. One of the techniques involving the parent in caregiving is termed continuous skin-to-skin or "kangaroo" care. Once the premature infant has reached physiologic stability and does not require major respiratory support, he or she is placed on the parent's chest.

These developmental approaches have been associated with improved functioning in the NICU, including reduced number of apnea events, improved oxygenation, faster weight gain, and improved motor maturity and state organization (Feldman & Eidelman, 1998). Research is ongoing to determine whether this approach carries long-term benefits.

In addition to environmental modifications to stimulate development, early intervention services can be provided even before the child is discharged from the NICU. Once the infant is medically stable, a team consisting of a physical and/or an occupational therapist, a developmental psychologist, and/or a developmental pediatrician should evaluate the child. Care plans should be developed for the ongoing developmental needs of the child leading to referral to an early intervention program prior to discharge (see Chapter 33).

SURVIVAL OF LOW BIRTH WEIGHT INFANTS

Advances in the technology of newborn intensive care and their application to the premature infant have been very successful in reducing mortality. Since 1960, survival of LBW infants has increased from 50% to more than 90% (Table 9.1). This improvement has been even more remarkable in ELBW and micropremie infants; in one study comparing the 1980s with the 1990s, the survival among preterm infants born with birth weight of 500 to 999 grams has increased from 49% to 67% (Wilson-Costello et al., 2005).

CARE AFTER DISCHARGE FROM THE HOSPITAL

The medical cost of the hospitalization and care of the preterm infant who requires a prolonged NICU stay is extraordinarily high, often measured in hundreds of thousands of dollars. Length of stay is a major factor in this cost. Because of this, many centers are developing care pathways, that allow the medical team to consider earlier discharge of the stable premature

Table 9.1. Improvement in survival rate of premature infants

	Survival (%)	
Birth weight	1960	1990
0.5–0.75 kilograms (kg)	10	30
0.75–1.0 kg	20	70
1.0–1.5 kg	30	90
1.5–2.0 kg	50	90

Sources: Emsley et al. (1998); O'Shea et al. (1997); and O'Shea et al. (1998).

infant than previously practiced. This new approach needs to be monitored closely to ensure that earlier discharge does not compromise the health of the child and result in an increased risk of readmission to the hospital for treatment of medical complications.

Clinical criteria for discharging preterm LBW infants are based on the achievement of sufficient weight and maturity of body organ function to ensure medical stability and continued growth in a home environment. This generally involves the infant being able to feed well by mouth, continue to gain weight, maintain a stable body temperature outside of an isolette, and no longer experience episodes of apnea and bradycardia. Most preterm LBW infants meet these eligibility criteria at a postconceptional age of 35–37 weeks. For ELBW infants, discharge at a postconceptional age of 37–42 weeks is a more realistic goal (Rawlings & Scott, 1996). At the time of discharge, most infants weight between 1,800 and 2,000 grams (4–4½ pounds).

When the child comes home, the parents may be faced with the stress and difficulty of caring for an infant with many special needs. In addition, the infant may be more irritable, cry more often, and have a poorer sleep–wake cycle compared with a full-term infant. Because of an immature sucking pattern, the infant also requires more frequent feedings. There is now specialized formula and/or breast milk supplementation with a human milk fortifier available to meet caloric needs of the premature infant post discharge. The prolonged duration of hospitalization and separation from parents also may have interfered with the usual mother–infant bonding.

As a result of these stresses, it is important to provide adequate support for the family after discharge, including close medical supervision and home care visits by nursing and/or social work staff (Broedsgaard & Wagner, 2005). Parental education and understanding of the needs of a growing preterm infant are also extremely important. Ideally the infant should be discharged to a home environment that is free of smoke and any other potential respiratory irritants such as kerosene heaters, fresh paint, and people with respiratory-related viral illness. Each of these factors plays a crucial role in causing subsequent respiratory illnesses or in exacerbating the underlying lung disease.

To prepare for discharge, most centers provide rooming-in services for the parents. This allows the parents to take over the care of their infant under the supervision of the NICU staff who determine whether there are unforeseen problems. The parents also learn about the care of their infant, thereby reducing the stress and anxiety of taking a preterm infant home.

EARLY INTERVENTION PROGRAMS

Early intervention programs have been shown to have a beneficial effect on the neurodevelopment of most premature infants through 3 years of age, although longer-term effects are still debated (Ramey, Ramey, & Friedlander, 1999). In many premature infants, these programs should start at discharge from the hospital and continue until 36 months corrected age. Corrected age is calculated by subtracting the number of weeks earlier than 40 weeks' gestation that the infant was born from the infant's current chronological age (e.g., corrected age of an 8-month-old born at 28 weeks' gestation is 5 months). The intervention strategy incorporates parent group meetings; home visits; and, after 24 months chronological age, attendance at a multidisciplinary child development center with a low teacher–infant ratio (1:3–1:4; see Chapter 29). It is important to recognize that even after completion of the early intervention program, many of these children continue to need special education services, including speech-language therapy, special education, behavior therapy, and treatment of emotional problems. If these children do not receive these services, the benefits of early intervention may be lost over time (Guralnick, 2005).

NEURODEVELOPMENTAL OUTCOME

Most infants born prematurely can be viewed during infancy as developing at a typical rate when their corrected or adjusted age is determined from their expected date of birth rather than from their actual birth date. There are, however, differences between full-term and preterm infants, even when gestational age is taken into account. In terms of motor skills, although few premature infants develop cerebral palsy, they often lack the smooth, rhythmic movement patterns of full-term infants. Devices such as walkers and jumpers should be avoided because they encourage the infant to stand on tiptoe and walk in an abnormal pattern. In later infancy, visual-motor tasks that require the planned use of arms and hand are also more difficult. Coordinating reach and grasp, scooping with a spoon, managing a standard cup, copying block constructions, and completing crayon/paper tasks can be more difficult (Glass, 2001).

By school age the developmental status of preterm children who had birth weights above 1,500 grams is not very different from full-term infants. Below this birth weight, however, there is an increased risk for developmental disabilities. School-age children who were born in the 1990s and were very preterm or had ELBW are at greater risk of developing executive dysfunction and require ongoing neuropsychological follow-up through middle childhood (Anderson & Doyle, 2004; Hintz et al., 2005; Mikkola et al., 2005; Vohr et al., 2005; Wilson-Costello et al., 2007). In terms of behavior issues, children born prematurely are at risk for lower levels of social competence, are less adaptable, less regular in their habits, less persistent, and more withdrawn. Attention-deficit/hyperactivity disorder (ADHD) is also more common in this group (Hack et al., 2004). Signs of ADHD may appear as early as 2 years of age as hyperactivity and difficulty following verbal directions and listening to a story in a small group. In addition, there may be behavior differences such as sleep disturbances, feeding difficulties, tantrums, or resistance to limit setting (Gray, Indurkhya, & McCormick, 2004). Learning problems may be anticipated in children whose language is delayed and who demonstrate poor visual-motor coordination (Breslau et al., 2004). Family factors have also been found to be strong predictors of future school performance (Gross et al., 2001). Optimal school outcome has been significantly associated with increased parental education, child rearing by two parents, and stability in family composition and geographic residence.

In studies of children with birth weight less than 1,000 grams (ELBW and micropreemies), major developmental disabilities have been found in about one quarter of children. This includes cerebral palsy (15%), hearing impairment (9%–11%), and visual impairment (1%–9%) (Hack et al., 2000). At 18–22 months corrected age, the mean Bayley Mental Developmental Index (Bayley, 1993) was 75, and 29% of the children had a score less than 70. Although cerebral palsy, especially spastic diplegia, is not uncommon in children who were VLBW, many "outgrow" this diagnosis by school age and simply appear to lack coordination.

In terms of predicting future neurodevelopmental disabilities, in one study nearly 30% of ELBW infants with a normal cranial ultrasound were later found to have either cerebral

palsy or intellectual disability. Neonatal brain MRI before discharge appears to be a better predictor of severe neurodevelopmental disorders (Mirmiran et al, 2004). Sensorineural impairments were correlated with neonatal sepsis and jaundice. Neurological, developmental, neurosensory, and functional morbidities increased with decreasing birth weight, and overall, males were more at risk for disabilities than were females.

SUMMARY

When compared with full-term infants, LBW infants are at greater risk for many problems in the newborn period that may lead to long-term complications. Physiologic immaturity of organ systems leads to RDS, hyperbilirubinemia, hypoglycemia, and hypocalcemia. Fortunately, the infants usually recover from these complications without major long-term sequelae. Other problems, however, such as IVH, PVL, sepsis, and persistent apnea and bradycardia are associated with poor neurodevelopmental outcome. With increased public awareness, improved prenatal care, and advanced neonatal intensive care, and early intervention services, the outcome of premature and SGA infants is likely to continue to improve.

REFERENCES

Abendroth, D., Moser, D.K., Dracup, K., et al. (1999). Do apnea monitors decrease emotional distress in parents of infants at high risk for cardiopulmonary arrest? *Journal of Pediatric Health Care, 13,* 50–57.

Adams, M.M., Elam-Evans, L.D., Wilson, H.G., et al. (2000). Rates of and factors associated with recurrence of preterm delivery. *Journal of the American Medical Association, 283,* 1591–1596.

Als, H., Duffy, F.H., McAnulty, G.B., et al. (2005). Early experience alters brain function and structure. *Pediatrics, 113,* 846–857.

American Academy of Pediatrics Task Force on Infant Position and SIDS. (1992). Position and SIDS. *Pediatrics, 89,* 1120–1126.

Anderson, P.J., & Doyle, L. W. (2004). Executive functioning in school-aged children who were born very preterm or with extremely low birth weight in the 1990s. *Pediatrics, 114,* 50–57.

Aucott, S.W., Donohue, P.K., & Northington, F.J. (2004). Increased morbidity in severe early intrauterine growth restriction. *Journal of Perinatology, 24,* 435–440.

Baird, T.M. (2004). Clinical correlates, natural history and outcome of neonatal apnoea. *Seminars in Neonatology, 9,* 205–211.

Ballard, J.L., Khoury, J.C., Wedig, K., et al. (1991). New Ballard score, expanded to include extremely premature infants. *The Journal of Pediatrics, 119,* 417–423.

Bayley, N. (1993). *Bayley Scales of Infant Development—*

Second Edition. San Antonio, TX: Harcourt Assessment.

Blumenthal, I. (2004). Periventricular leucomalacia: A review. *European Journal of Pediatrics, 163,* 435–442.

Brandt, I., Sticker, E.J., Gausche, R., et al. (2005). Catchup growth of supine length/height of very low birth weight, small for gestational age preterm infants to adulthood. *The Journal of Pediatrics, 147,* 662–668.

Breslau, N., Paneth, N.S., & Lucia, V.C. (2004). *Pediatrics, 114,* 1035–1040.

Broedsgaard, A., & Wagner, L. (2005). How to facilitate parents and their premature infant for the transition home. *International Nursing Review, 52,* 196–203

Chandler, J.C., & Hebra, A. (2000). Necrotizing enterocolitis in infants with very low birth weight. *Seminars in Pediatric Surgery, 9,* 63–72.

Committee on Fetus and Newborn, American Academy of Pediatrics. (2003). Apnea, sudden infant death syndrome, and home monitoring. *Pediatrics, 111,* 914–917.

Constantine, N.A., Kraemer, H.C., Kendall-Tackett, K.A., et al. (1987). Use of physical and neurologic observations in assessment of gestational age in low-birth-weight infants. *The Journal of Pediatrics, 110,* 921–928.

Cooper, L.G., Leland, N.L., & Alexander, G. (1995). Effect of maternal age on birth outcomes among young adolescents. *Social Biology, 42,* 22–35.

D'Angio, C.T., Sinkin, R.A., Stevens, T.P., et al. (2002). Longitudinal, 15-year follow-up of children born at less than 29 weeks' gestation after introduction of surfactant therapy into a region: Neurologic, cognitive, and educational outcomes. *Pediatrics, 110,* 1094–1102

Darlow, B.A., Hutchinson, J.L., Henderson-Smart, D.J., et. al. (2005). Prenatal risk factors for severe retinopathy of prematurity among very preterm infants of the Australian and New Zealand Neonatal Network. *Pediatrics, 115,* 990–996.

Dhillon, A.S., & Ewer A.K. (2004). Diagnosis and management of gastro-oesophageal reflux in preterm infants in neonatal intensive care units. *Acta Paediatrica, 93,* 88–93.

Dubowitz, L.M., Dubowitz, V., & Goldberg, C. (1970). Clinical assessment of gestational age in the newborn infant. *The Journal of Pediatrics, 77,* 1–10.

Emsley, H.C.A., Wardle, S.P., Sims, D.G., et al. (1998). Increased survival and deteriorating developmental outcome in 23 to 25 week old gestation infants, 1990–4 compared with 1984–9. *Archives of Disease in Childhood, Fetal and Neonatal Edition, 78,*F99–F104.

Farrell, P.A., & Fiascone, J.M. (1997). Bronchopulmonary dysplasia in the 1990s: A review for the pediatrician. *Current Problems in Pediatrics, 27,* 129–163.

Feldman, R., & Eidelman, A.I. (1998). Intervention programs for premature infants. *Clinics in Perinatology, 25,* 613–626.

Gibson, E., Dembofsky, C.A., Rubin, S., et al. (2000). Infant sleep position practices 2 years into the "Back to Sleep" campaign. *Clinical Pediatrics, 39,* 285–289.

Glass, P. (2001). Your baby was born prematurely. In M.L. Batshaw (Ed.), *When your child has a disability: The complete sourcebook of daily and medical care* (Rev. ed., pp. 59–71). Baltimore: Paul H. Brookes Publishing Co.

Gray, R.F., Indurkhya, A., & McCormick, M.C. (2004). Prevalence, stability, and predictors of clinically significant behavior problems in low birth weight children at 3, 5, and 8 years of age. *Pediatrics, 114,* 736–743.

Greer, F.R. (1995). Vitamin K deficiency and hemorrhage in infancy. *Clinics in Perinatology, 22,* 759–777.

Gross, S.J., Abner, R.D., & Mettelman, B.B. (2005). Follow-up at 15 years of preterm infants from a controlled trial of moderately early dexamethasone for the prevention of chronic lung disease. *Pediatrics, 115,* 681–687.

Gross, S.J., Mettelman, B.B., Dye, T.D., et al. (2001). Impact of family structure and stability on academic outcome in preterm children at 10 years of age. *The Journal of Pediatrics, 138,* 16–75.

Guralnick, M.J. (Ed.). (2005). *The developmental systems approach to early intervention.* Baltimore: Paul H. Brookes Publishing Co.

Hack, M., Wilson-Costello, D., Friedman, H., et al. (2000). Neurodevelopment and predictors of outcome of children with birth weights of less than 1000g: 1992–1995. *Archives of Pediatric and Adolescent Medicine, 154,* 725–731.

Hack, M., Youngstrom, E.A., Cartar, L., et al. (2004). Behavioral outcomes and evidence of psychopathology among very low birth weight infants at age 20 years. *Pediatrics, 114,* 932–940.

Hintz, S.R., Kendrick, D.E., Vohr, B.R., et al. (2005). Changes in neurodevelopmenal outcomes at 18 to 22 months' corrected age among infants of less than 25 weeks' gestational age born in 1993–1999. *Pediatrics, 115,* 1645–1651.

Hodgman, J.E. (1998). Apnea of prematurity and the risk for SIDS. *Pediatrics, 102,* 969–971.

Horbar, J.D., Badger, G.J., Carpenter, J.H., et al. (2002). Trends in mortality and morbidity for very low birth weight infants, 1991–1999. *Pediatrics, 110,* 143–151.

Horton, K.K. (2005). Pathophysiology and current management of necrotizing enterocolitis. *Neonatal Network, 24,* 37–46.

Horwitz, J.R., Lally, K.P., Cheu, H.W., et al. (1995). Complications after surgical intervention for necrotizing enterocolitis: A multicenter review. *Journal of Pediatric Surgery, 30,* 994–998.

Joffe, G.M., Symonds, R., Alverson, D., et al. (1995). The effect of a comprehensive prematurity prevention program on the number of admissions to the neonatal intensive care unit. *Journal of Perinatology, 15,* 305–309.

Johnson, J.L., White, K.R., Widen, J.E., et al. (2005). A multicenter evaluation of how many infants with permanent hearing loss pass a two-stage otoacoustic emissions/automated auditory brainstem response newborn hearing screening protocol. *Pediatrics, 116,* 663–672.

Joint Committee on Infant Hearing. (1995). *Joint Committee on Infant Hearing 1994 Position Statement. Pediatrics, 95*(1), 152–156.

Joint Committee on Infant Hearing. (2000). Year 2000 position statement: Principles and guidelines for early hearing detection and intervention programs. *Pediatrics, 106,* 798–817.

Kennedy, J.D., Edward, L.J., Bates, D.J., et al. (2000). Effects of birthweight and oxygen supplementation on lung function in late childhood in children of very low birth weight. *Pediatric Pulmonology, 30,* 32–40.

Klein, L.L., & Gibbs, R.S. (2005). Infection and preterm birth. *Obstetrics and Gynecology Clinics of North America, 32,* 397–410.

Larsen, P.B., Brendstrup, L., Skov, L., et al. (1995). Aminophylline versus caffeine citrate for apnea and bradycardia prophylaxis in premature neonates. *Acta Paediatrica, 84,* 360–364.

Leviton, A., Kuban, K., Bagano, M., et al. (1993). Antenatal corticosteroids appear to reduce the risk of postnatal germinal matrix hemorrhage in intubated low birth weight newborns. *Pediatrics, 81,* 1083–1088.

Lubchenco, L.O. (1976). *The high risk infant.* Philadelphia: W.B. Saunders.

Mandrich, M., Simons, C.J., Ritchie, S., et al. (1994). Motor development, infantile reactions and postural responses of preterm, at-risk infants. *Developmental Medicine and Child Neurology, 36,* 397–405.

Martin, J.A., Kochanek, K.D., Strobino, D.M., et al. (2005). Annual summary of vital statistics: 2003. *Pediatrics, 115,* 619–634.

Ment, L.R., Vohr, B., Allan, W., et al. (2000). Outcome of children in the indomethacin intraventricular hemorrhage trial. *Pediatrics, 105,* 485–491.

Mikkola, K., Ritari, N., Tommiska, V., et al. (2005). Neurodevelopmental outcome at 5 years of age of a national cohort of extremely low birth weight infants who were born in 1996–1997. *Pediatrics, 116,* 1391–1400.

Mirmiran, M., Barnes, P.D., & Keller, K. (2004). Neonatal brain magnetic resonance imaging before discharge is better than serial ultrasound in predicting cerebral palsy in very low birth weight preterm infants. *Pediatrics, 114,* 992–998

Nagpal, J., Kumar, A., & Ramji, S. (2004). Anterior lens capsule vascularity in evaluating gestation in small for gestation neonates. *Indian Pediatrics, 41,* 817–821.

NIH Consensus Development Panel on the Effect of Corticosteroids for Fetal Maturation on Perinatal Outcomes. (1995). Effect of corticosteroids for fetal maturation on perinatal outcomes. *Journal of the American Medical Association, 273,* 413–418.

Obladen, M., & Maier, R.F. (1995). Recombinant erythropoietin for "prevention" of anemia in preterm infants. *Journal of Perinatal Medicine, 23,* 119–126.

Ohls, R.K., Ehrenkarnz, R.A., Wright, L.L., et al. (2001). Effect of early erythropoetin therapy on the transfusion requirements of preterm infants below 1250 grams birth weight: A muticenter, randomized, controlled trial. *Pediatrics, 108,* 934–942.

Okumura, A., Hayakawa, F., Kato, T., et al. (2003). Abnormal sharp transients on electroencephalograms in preterm infants with periventricular leukomalacia. *The Journal of Pediatrics, 143,* 26–30.

O'Shea, T.M., Klinepeter, K.L., Goldstein, D.J., et al. (1997). Survival and developmental disability in infants with birth weights of 501 to 800 grams, born between 1979 and 1994. *Pediatrics, 100,* 982–986.

O'Shea, T.M., Preisser, J.S., Klinepeter, K.L., et al. (1998). Trends in mortality and cerebral palsy in a geographically based cohort of very low birth weight neonates born between 1982 and 1994. *Pediatrics, 101,* 642–647.

Owens, R. (2005). Intraventricular hemorrhage in the premature neonate. *Neonatal Network, 24,* 55–71.

Papile, L., Tyson, J.E., Stoll, B.J., et al. (1998). A multicenter trial of two dexamethasone regimens in ventilator-dependent premature infants. *The New England Journal of Medicine, 338,* 1112–1118.

Perlman, J.M., Risser, R., & Broyles, R.S. (1996). Bilateral cystic periventricular leukomalacia in premature infants: Associated risk factors. *Pediatrics, 97,* 822–827.

Pleacher, M.D., Vohr, B.R., Katz, K.H., et al. (2004). An evidence-based approach to predicting low IQ in very preterm infants from the neurological examination: Outcome data from the indomethacin Indomethacin Intraventricular Hemorrhage Prevention Trial. *Pediatrics, 113,* 416–419.

Premji, S., & Chessell, L. (2001). Continuous nasogastric milk feeding versus intermittent bolus milk feeding for premature infants less than 1500 grams. *Cochrane Database of Systematic Reviews,* CD001819.

Raju, T.N.K., Langenberg, P., Bhutani, V., et al. (1997). Vitamin E prophylaxis to reduce retinopathy of prematurity: A reappraisal of published trials. *The Journal of Pediatrics, 131,* 844–850.

Ramey, S.L., Ramey, C.T., & Friedlander, M.J. (1999). Early experience and early intervention. *Mental Retardation and Developmental Disabilities Research Reviews, 5,* 1–99.

Rawlings, J.S., & Scott, J.S. (1996). Postconceptional age of surviving preterm low-birth-weight infants at hospital discharge. *Archives of Pediatrics and Adolescent Medicine, 150,* 260–262.

Slattery, M.M., & Morrison, J.J. (2002). Preterm delivery. *The Lancet, 360,* 1489-1497.

Snyder, C.L., Gittes, G.K., Murphy, J.P., et al. (1997). Survival after necrotizing enterocolitis in infants weighing less than 1000 g: 25 years' experience at a single institution. *Journal of Pediatric Surgery, 32,* 434–437.

Suresh, G.K., Horbar, J.D., Kenny, M., et al. (2001). Major birth defects in very low birth weight infants in the Vermont Oxford Network. *The Journal of Pediatrics, 139,* 366–373.

Tapia, J.L., Ramirez, R., Cifuentes, J., et al. (1998). The effect of early dexamethasone administration on bronchopulmonary dysplasia in preterm infants with respiratory distress syndrome. *The Journal of Pediatrics, 132,* 48–52.

Tasman, W., Patz, A., McNamara, J.A., et al. (2006). Retinopathy of prematurity: The life of a lifetime disease. *American Journal of Ophthalmology, 141,* 167–174.

Valleur-Masson, D., Vodovar, M., Zeller, J., et al. (1993). Bronchopulmonary dysplasia: Course over 3 years in 88 children born between 1984 and 1988. *Archives of Pediatrics, 50,* 553–559.

Van Naarden, K., & Decoufle, P. (1999). Relative and attributable risks for moderate to profound bilateral sensorineural hearing impairment associated with lower birth weight in children 3 to 10 years old. *Pediatrics, 104,* 905–910.

Van Overmeire, B., Smets, K., Lecoutere, D., et al. (2000). A comparison of ibuprofen and indomethacin for closure of patent ductus arteriosus. *The New England Journal of Medicine, 343,* 674–681.

Van Wassenaer, A.G., Briet, J.M., & Van Baar, A. (2002). Free thyroxine levels during the first week of life and neurodevelopmental outcome until the age of 5 years in very preterm infants. *Pediatrics, 109,* 534–539.

Vohr, B.R., Wright, L.L., Poole, W.K., et al. (2005). Neurodevelopmental outcomes of extremely low birth weight infants <32 weeks' gestation between 1993–1998. *Pediatrics, 116,* 635–643.

Volpe, J.J. (2001). *Neurology of the newborn* (4th ed.). Philadelphia: W.B. Saunders.

Volpe, J.J. (2005). Encephalopathy of prematurity includes neuronal abnormalities. *Pediatrics, 116,* 221–225.

Walsh, M.C., Morris, B.H., Wrage, L.A., et al. (2005). Extremely low birthweight neonates with protracted ventilation: Mortality and 18-month neurodevelopmental outcomes. *The Journal of Pediatrics, 146,* 798–804.

Watchko, J.F., & Claassen, D. (1994). Kernicterus in premature infants: Current prevalence and relationship to NICHD Phototherapy Study exchange criteria. *Pediatrics, 93,* 996–999.

Wheater, M., & Renie, J.M. (2000). Perinatal infection is an important risk factor for cerebral palsy in very-low-birth-weight infants. *Developmental Medicine and Child Neurology, 42,* 364–367.

Wilson-Costello D., Friedman H., Minich N., et al. (2005). Improved survival with increased neurodevelopmental disability for extremely low birth weight infants in the 1990s. *Pediatrics, 115,* 997–1003.

Wilson-Costello, D., Friedman, H., Minich, N., et al. (2007). Improved neurodevelopmental outcomes for extremely low birth weight infants in 2000–2002. *Pediatrics, 119,* 37–45.

II The Developing Child

10 Nutrition and Children with Disabilities

Janet S. Isaacs

Upon completion of this chapter, the reader will

- Understand nutritional requirements and their assessment in children
- Identify how disabilities modify nutritional requirements
- Understand the fundamental role of nutrition in the growth and development of children
- Understand how nutritional interventions are included in a child's care plan

---

Nutrition is the study of foods, their nutrients and other components of the diet that affect biological processes and health (Brown, 2005). Human requirements for protein, fats, carbohydrates, vitamins and minerals vary with age, activity level, medical diagnosis, genetic heritage and physiological state (Institute of Medicine, 2002). A typical diet provides all of the nutrients, minerals, and vitamins needed for normal growth and development. In children with disabilities, however, this may not be the case. As a result of motor impairments, a child with cerebral palsy may have difficulty ingesting sufficient food. A child with an autism spectrum disorder (ASD) may have food selectivity that results in nutritional deficiencies. Conversely, a child with Prader-Willi syndrome often engages in hyperphagia (pathological eating), and the child with spina bifida may become obese through inactivity. Typically, the impact of nutrition is greatest during infancy and childhood when the body is actively growing. For children with disabilities, the need for medical nutritional therapy may be lifelong. This term, medical nutrition therapy, is defined as the manipulation of nutrients and dietary components to affect a disease or condition (American Dietetic Association, 2006). This therapy also takes into account the psychosocial environment in which the child lives. Food selection and preparation are major cultural characteristics of all societies, and within the context of home and family, providing and preparing food for children expresses parental love and concern. This chapter focuses on the nutritional needs of children with disabilities and emphasizes medical nutrition therapy as part of a comprehensive care plan.

ALYSSA

Alyssa's parents were notified at 7 days of age that she had an abnormal newborn screening test. She was seen in the metabolism clinic of the local children's hospital, where studies confirmed the diagnosis of phenylketonuria (PKU), and her parents met with a geneticist and nutritionist. The geneticist explained this metabolic disorder, its genetics, and laboratory test results (see Chapter 20). The parents came to understand that the basic problem in PKU was the inability to metabolize a specific essential amino acid, phenylalanine. The nutritionist explained that Alyssa would need to be on a special diet and that this would be a lifelong requirement. The parents learned how to follow the prescribed diet that substituted most, but not all, of the protein usually consumed. They had to learn how much phenylalanine was in various foods. The nutritionist had them make up a formula to provide the missing protein she could not tolerate. Each time Alyssa and her parents came into the metabolism clinic they would meet with the nutritionist who would measure her growth, review her diet, educate the parents, answer their questions, and adjust her formula and food intake as needed. At the age when Alyssa started walking, the nutritionist instructed the family on low-protein substitutes for pasta, as well as rice that could be ordered on the Internet to vary the diet. By age 7, Alyssa was selecting most of her foods. Her liquid formula was replaced with low-volume versions and bars so that her diet was more appropriate for her age. She started "owning" the responsibility for treating her disorder. At age 9, her blood test results showed Alyssa was eating too much "regular" food. She rebelled sometimes about finishing her phenylalanine-free formula. The nutritionist worked with the parents to give Alyssa more choices and recommended a therapist who worked with the whole family. Routine blood phenylalanine test results were used by the nutritionist to adjust the diet, along with growth measurements, Alyssa's likes and dislikes, and her parent's concerns. Alyssa wanted to be just like everyone else, and the physician, nutritionist, and family worked together to find solutions to her problems in living with a strict diet. Her parents were encouraged to let Alyssa attend a PKU camp next summer when she would be 10 years old.

TYPICAL GROWTH DURING CHILDHOOD

Nutritional requirements for infants and children are determined based on what is needed to produce typical patterns of growth and development. The average full-term infant weighs 3.4 kilograms (about 7½ pounds) at birth, and gains 20–30 grams (about an ounce) each day for several months. By 4–6 months of age, the infant's birth weight has doubled, and by 12 months, it has tripled (National Center for Health Statistics, 2000). As the child becomes more active and is walking, weight gain slows to about 5 pounds per year until approximately 9–10 years of age, when the adolescent growth spurt begins. Length advances at a slower pace than weight, increasing by 50% during the first year of life (from an average of 50 centimeters or about 19½ inches at birth), doubling by 4 years of age, and tripling by 13 years of age. Increase in head circumference parallels brain growth. Head circumference increases by 3 inches during the first year of life, and brain weight doubles by 2 years of age (National Center for Health Statistics, 2000).

In addition to the basic measures of growth—weight, length, and head circumference—a number of useful growth indices have been developed that provide a more nuanced and clinically relevant way of assessing a child's nutritional status. Among these, the **body mass index (BMI)** is especially important. The BMI is a measure of the relationship between stature (length) and weight across ages that was developed by the Centers for Disease Control and Prevention (Speiser et al., 2005; see Table 10.1). By placing weight into the context of a child's overall size and body habitus, the BMI allows for a more accurate assessment of whether a child is over- or underweight. Direct measures of body fat utilizing specialized equipment and

Table 10.1. Growth parameters and nutrition assessment

Growth parameter	Utility in nutrition assessment
Weight for age (pounds or kilograms)	Provides direct comparison to established norms for age; key parameter for monitoring short- and long-term changes in nutritional status
Length for age (inches or centimeters)	Provides direct comparison to established norms for age; key measure of linear growth
Head circumference for age (inches or centimeters)	Provides direct comparison to established norms for age; key proxy for brain growth
Height-to-weight proportionality	Provides a rough estimate of nutritional status by relating weight to stature
Body mass index (weight in pounds × 703 / height in inches × height in inches)	Provides an estimate of body fat relative to weight and height
Rate of weight and length accretion (change in weight or length over a given time interval)	Precise method of tracking patterns and rates of growth
Body fat indices	Direct measures of body fat using reliable, specialized equipment and techniques

techniques are not as widely available but offer an even more accurate way of assessing this critical aspect of a child's nutritional status.

NUTRITIONAL GUIDELINES

Research-based nutrition guidelines published by the National Academies of Sciences recommend daily intake of specific vitamins and minerals based on age and gender (Institute of Medicine, 1997, 2002). Energy and protein intake recommendations were updated in 2002 (Institute of Medicine, 2002) and have been incorporated into the nutrients included in food labels. They are also reflected in the standard growth charts commonly used by health care professionals (National Centers for Health Statistics, 2000). The concept of a "balanced diet" derives from standard nutritional guidelines, and is based on the notion that typical children will require specific amounts and proportions of specific nutrients. Although these guidelines are a good starting point for determining the nutrition requirements for children with disabilities, adjustments are often required, and in some cases an apparently "unbalanced" diet is most appropriate for a specific child or specific condition. For example, a typical 10-year-old girl who is normally active needs about 2,000 calories daily. In contrast, a 10-year-old girl with spina bifida may need many fewer calories daily, whereas a child with choreoathetoid cere-

bral palsy may need more (Sleigh & Brockle-hurst, 2004). An all-liquid diet or a diet of a only few different foods may be recommended for a child with limited oral-motor skills. For a child like Alyssa with a special metabolic condition, it is critically important that certain elements of the diet be reduced, eliminated, or enhanced to avoid the build-up of toxic metabolites. Table 10.2 provides other examples of how specific dietary components and calorie content can be manipulated to address the special needs of specific medical conditions and disabilities.

NUTRITIONAL ISSUES IN CHILDREN WITH DISABILITIES

Children with disabilities have many of the same nutrition problems as children without disabilities. These include being over- or underweight, refusing to eat or drink a variety of foods and beverages, and fighting for control with parents at mealtimes. Children with disabilities, however, are prone to more serious and varied problems that are especially related to impaired oral motor skills (e.g., swallowing incoordination among children with cerebral palsy), medical problems (e.g., prolonged gastroesophageal reflux [GER] among children who were former premature infants), and food refusal (e.g., dislike of certain food textures among children with ASDs) (Sandritter, 2003; Schwarz et al., 2001). As a result, common nu-

Table 10.2. Dietary adjustments for specific medical conditions and disabilities

Dietary Element	Condition	Specific adjustment required
Fats	Smith-Lemli-Opitz syndrome	Cholesterol (purified form) increased
	Long chain fatty acid oxidation disorders	Fat decreased, greater than 75% of nutrition from fat-free foods
	Uncontrollable seizures	Ketogenic diet, fat increased
Proteins	Phenylketonuria, maple syrup urine disease	Protein decreased by more than 80%, addition of vitamins and minerals
	Glycogen storage disease	Protein increased, fat decreased, fruits and sugars severely restricted
Carbohydrates	Galactosemia, lactose intolerance	Specific types of sugar (e.g., galactose, lactose) decreased
	Hereditary fructose intolerance	Specific types of sugar (e.g., fructose) decreased
Vitamins and minerals	Vitamin B_{12} disorders	Vitamin B_{12} increased, often protein content decreased
	Iron-deficiency anemia	Foods rich in iron increased or supplement iron added
	Rickets	Foods rich in calcium and vitamin D increased or supplements added
Energy (calories)	Obesity and overweight	Calories decreased 10%–30% (fats, proteins, and carbohydrates), activity level increased
	Hypotonia in Down syndrome or Prader-Willi syndrome	Calories decreased 30%–40% (fats, proteins, and carbohydrates)

tritional advice for typically developing children may not be appropriate for children with disabilities (see Table 10.3). Instead, diets must be targeted to specific conditions and disabilities, as illustrated in Table 10.2.

Obesity

Intake of food energy, or kilocalories (more commonly referred to simply as calories), is a critical aspect of nutrition, and disorders involving excess or insufficient energy intake are of great importance for children with disabilities (Bandini et al., 2005; Taylor & Rogers, 2005). Obesity is caused by excessive energy intake relative to energy expenditure and is typically defined by an elevated BMI (see Table 10.1). Obesity and overweight are increasing worldwide, but there is still controversy about the ideal way to assess the risks of obesity in children and adolescents (Speiser et al., 2005). BMI includes underlying assumptions about stature and body composition that may not apply to children with disabilities. For example, scoliosis may interfere with accurate height measurements, which in turn can affect the calculation of the BMI. Other disorders that may not be well described by the BMI criteria are Prader-Willi syndrome, spina bifida, and Down syndrome (Bandini et al., 2005).

Undernutrition

Concern about the adequacy of energy intake is more common in children with disabilities than in typical children. Increased energy needs are commonly observed in children who 1) are born prematurely, 2) are acutely ill, 3) are recovering from surgery, or 4) have experienced specific medication side effects (Vohr & McKinley, 2003). Certain disorders, such as cystic fibrosis (Borowitz, Baker, & Stallings, 2002), choreoathetoid cerebral palsy, and Rett syndrome (Isaacs et al., 2003; Percy & Lane, 2004) are also associated with increased energy needs. In these cases, the goal of medical nutrition therapy is to provide extra calories as food or nutritional supplements.

When Disabilities Affect Stature

Extra calories and nutrients may not normalize growth in many disabilities that are known to be associated with short stature, such as translocation chromosomal disorders, Turner syndrome, Down syndrome, Williams syndrome, chromosome 22q11 microdeletion syndromes (e.g., velocardiofacial syndrome, DiGeorge syndrome), spina bifida, and fetal alcohol syndrome (Chudley et al., 2005). Providing extra calories in these conditions may simply result in obesity. There may be a role for growth hormone therapy in some of these conditions to increase linear growth (The Canadian Growth Hormone Advisory Committee, 2005). Diagnosis-specific growth reports are based on smaller population groups than the standard growth charts for typical children (Arvay et al., 2005). They are helpful in setting realistic expectations for growth after the diagnosis is made. Conditions in which

Table 10.3.   Common nutrition advice that may not apply to children with disabilities

Common nutrition advice	How this advice may not apply to children with disabilities
"If she won't eat now, don't worry; she will eat when she is hungry."	The child may not respond to hunger cues.
	Hunger may be masked by fatigue, medications, or specific medical conditions.
"Don't worry. Others in the family are small."	Genetic and hereditary factors are important to identify, but many "small" children with disabilities are often undernourished due to lack of sufficient intake.
"He's just picky."	Behaviorally based feeding problems are common in children with disabilities.
	Some food refusals are key symptoms of an underlying medical problem.
"He's failing to thrive."	Many disabilities are associated with atypical growth patterns (disability-specific growth charts allow for more accurate interpretation of growth patterns).
"He eats the same foods all the time. He should eat a variety of foods."	Monotonous self-restricted eating patterns are common in children with developmental disabilities, especially those who have autism spectrum disorders.
	Some medical conditions (especially metabolic disorders) require a limited range of food types to prevent complications.

excess growth is unrelated to nutritional intake also are known, including genetic conditions as Sotos syndrome, Marfan syndrome, and types of gigantism that result from growth hormone overproduction. Typically, an important measure of sufficient nutrition is adequate growth. Yet, many developmental disabilities are associated with these atypical patterns of growth. As a result, it may be difficult to determine whether a child with a developmental disability who has apparent inadequate growth is truly undernourished (Pedersen, Parsons, & Dewey, 2004).

When Disabilities Limit Eating

The child with a developmental disability may not want to eat or may have physical difficulties in eating. Rather than being a pleasure, mealtime becomes an aversive experience for both the child and parents. It is imperative to identify the root causes of the feeding disorder in these children and to design a therapy program appropriate for the problem. A child who is unable to eat because of fatigue and weakness caused by a neuromuscular disability is approached differently than a child who refuses to eat as a result of behavioral or cognitive issues. Children with dyskinetic cerebral palsy may have such severe difficulty in chewing and swallowing that it places them at risk for aspiration as well as undernutrition. In this case, nutritional therapy might be directed at providing alternative routes for nutrition (e.g., **gastrostomy** tube formula feedings). In contrast, although typical toddlers go on "food jags" in which they prefer the same food for several days in a row, children with ASDs may have such severe and persistent restricted food preferences that it affects their growth (Field, Garland, & Williams, 2003). The goal of nutrition therapy under these circumstances is to use behavior management techniques to gradually add new food items to the child's menu. A reward system for trying a new food and encouraging the child to participate in preparing food may be a part of behavior management at home.

Recognizing undernutrition and malnutrition is also difficult because nutrient needs and activity levels may be higher or lower in children with disabilities (Taylor & Rogers, 2005). For example, short stature in usually not a sign of limited nutrition in children with Down syndrome, but it can reflect long-term inadequate nutrition in PKU (Borowitz et al., 2002). Thin appearance is common in spastic quadriplegia (a severe form of cerebral palsy; see Chapter 26)

(Isaacs et al., 2004), and although it can be the result of **undernutrition,** it may instead be the result of muscle atrophy due to central nervous system damage. In the former instance, nutritional intake should be increased; in the latter, added nutrition will result in added fat but will not improve muscle bulk and may actually contribute to obesity.

MEDICAL NUTRITIONAL THERAPY

The overall goal of medical nutrition therapy is to improve a child's health and nutritional status while promoting a family's enjoyment of their child at mealtimes. Examples of good outcomes include encouraging success with self-feeding, meeting general nutritional needs, and correcting energy imbalances.

Nutrition Assessment and Nutrition Care Plan

The tools of medical nutrition therapy are the nutritional assessment and the nutritional care plan that is customized to the needs of each child. A nutritional assessment usually answers the following three questions:

1. Is the child being fed a diet that meets his or her nutritional requirements?

2. Is the child growing as expected for his or her age, gender, and condition?

3. Is there a feeding or eating problem interfering with growth or meeting nutritional requirements?

The nutrition assessment is the first step in the process of documenting a child's nutritional status. This involves the steps outlined in Table 10.4; the measurement and interpretation of

Table 10.4.   Elements of a nutrition assessment

Review the child's medical history (including diagnoses, laboratory findings, medications used, and developmental levels).

Assess and interpret the child's growth parameters (see Table 10.1).

Obtain the child's dietary history from caregivers (including intake patterns for food and drink, portion sizes, meal duration, and use of supplements).

Analyze and interpret the dietary intake information, based on the child's age and gender, for macronutrients (protein, fats, and carbohydrates), micronutrients (vitamins and minerals), fluids, and other dietary components (e.g., dietary fiber); computer dietary analysis programs are generally used.

Summarize impressions of the child's nutritional status and the adequacy of his or her diet; make recommendations and referrals.

growth parameters are defined in Table 10.1. If a child is not in a good nutritional state, recommendations are made to improve the diet and feeding or eating practices.

The nutrition care plan articulates these recommendations and spells out monitoring and follow-up needs. Common activities in a nutrition care plan are shown in Table 10.5. In addition to offering general dietary and feeding recommendations, a well-developed nutrition care plan addresses the role of food in the family and in the family's culture, including meal and snack patterns, food choices, and food preparation. Take the example of a child with Down syndrome who is significantly overweight. If obesity is a family problem, the weight loss plan should involve changing eating patterns of the entire family. If the family culture involves the ingestion of fatty and fried foods, different cooking patterns must be taught. When providing food is equated by the parent to providing love, emotional needs are interfering with nutri-

Table 10.5. Sample activities from a nutrition care plan

Recommend meal and snack schedules or timing.

Counter side effects from medications (e.g., increased appetite, effect on taste).

Prevent overweight or underweight.

Monitor planned weight gain, weight loss, or catch-up growth.

Apply specialty (disease-specific) growth charts for growth assessment.

Estimate fat stores and body composition for in-depth growth assessment.

Analyze and interpret home intake diet record.

Modify diets for specific nutrients, such as low protein, high calorie, or low fat.

Reinforce breast feeding, infant formula, or formula preparation steps.

Select foods to address food texture problems or avoid choking.

Plan a menu based on food composition.

Manage food refusals, food jags, or other food behaviors.

Demonstrate how to determine portion sizes and measure foods.

Order special formulas or supplements.

Reinforce signs of hunger, fullness, and right pace of eating or feeding.

Document food insecurity and refer the family to community food banks.

Coordinate with other health care providers and educators.

Complete referrals for WIC (Special Supplemental Nutrition Program for Women, Infants and Children), early intervention services, or other providers.

tional requirements. If food is used as a behavioral reinforcer, another equally effective reinforcer must be identified.

Nutrition Support for Children Who Cannot Eat

Nutrition support provides nutrients at high enough levels to meet nutrition requirements when the child is unable to eat or drink in the usual manner. It separates the delivery of nutrients from the act of eating by providing complete nutritional supplements and nutrients enterally—that is, directly to the gastrointestinal (GI) tract—or parenterally—that is, directly into the blood stream. Enteral feeding involves a gastric tube or **gastrostomy** placement surgery, resulting in feeding directly into the stomach (Ellett, 2004). Complications from placement of gastrostomy tubes include infection, GER, and aspiration (Sleigh & Brocklehurst, 2004). Successful placement, however, not only improves nutrition but also decreases the family's psychological stress around feeding issues (Heyman et al., 2004). When it is important for feeding to bypass the GI tract, **parenteral feeding** is used. This involves administering nutrients directly into the blood stream. Usually parenteral feeding is administered in a hospital setting on a short-term basis. The most common developmental disabilities that require nutrition support include cerebral palsy (spastic quadriplegia), progressive neurologic disorders (e.g., Tay-Sachs disease), uncontrolled seizures (e.g., Lennox-Gastaut syndrome), and certain inborn errors of metabolism (Ellett, 2004, Fung et al., 2002; Isaacs et al., 2004; Sleigh & Brocklehurst, 2004). Table 10.6 illustrates a sample dietary intake for a child with spastic quadriplegia. Although nutritional support can correct the signs and symptoms of undernourishment, no special nutritional interventions have been identified to correct the short stature and low weight that is typical in severe cerebral palsy (Krick et al., 1996). These issues are discussed further in Chapter 31.

Nutrition Support Formulas

A wide range of formulas are available as food replacements, as food supplements, and for nutrition support as described in Table 10.7. These differ from infant formulas in terms of energy content, osmolarity (the concentration of dissolved particles in a liquid), and the level of supplemented vitamins and minerals. Nutrition

Table 10.6. Sample intake and feeding schedule for a child with a gastrostomy tube and limited ability to eat by mouth

6:30 A.M.	Stop night feeding pump
9:30 A.M.	Oral snack at school: milk in a cup and spoon-fed applesauce
11:45 A.M.	School lunch: modified soft texture, 30% self-feeding
1:00 P.M.	Gastrostomy feeding of 8 fluid ounces of complete nutritional supplement
3:30 P.M.	After-school snack at home: self-fed cookie and milk in a cup
6:00 P.M.	Supper with family: mashed potato with gravy on a spoon and juice in a cup
8:30 P.M.	Start night feeding of 60 cubic centimeters per hour complete nutritional supplement, providing 40% of calories and 70% of protein

support formulas differ from one another in specific nutrients, caloric density, intended use, and mode of administration (Nevin-Folino, 2003). Infants older than 1 year of age who require nutritional supplementation may be transitioned to pediatric formulas (intended for children up to 10 years of age) that provide 30 calories per fluid ounce (as compared with regular infant formulas that provide 20 calories per fluid ounce), or to formulas used for adults, such as Ensure (Nevin-Folino, 2003). Products such as protein-free or carbohydrate-free formulas employed in inborn errors of metabolism (see Chapter 20) are not used alone, as they create a nutritional deficiency if not mixed with other formulas or foods. The goal of maintaining regular foods in the diet and minimizing reliance

on complete nutritional supplements is common for children with oral-motor feeding problems, such as those with Rett syndrome and certain forms of cerebral palsy (Percy & Lane, 2004).

SPECIAL NUTRITIONAL CONCERNS IN CHILDREN WITH DISABILITIES

Some of the nutritional concerns associated with specific developmental disabilities are listed in Table 10.8. In most cases, families of children with specialized diets benefit from the involvement of a registered dietitian, who can help monitor the diets, and who can provide consultative support to schools and other agencies to assure appropriate implementation of dietary recommendations.

Therapeutic Diets

Diets for inborn errors of metabolism, such as PKU, and the **ketogenic diet** used in some children with intractable epilepsy provide examples of customized diets that differ in composition and goals. Both diets are similar in requiring close monitoring and in causing behavior problems around food at home, in school, and at restaurants. Table 10.9 shows a sample daily nutritional intake for a 10-year-old with PKU who is maintaining good compliance with a low-protein diet. With the rapid expansion of newborn screening for a variety of genetic and metabolic conditions (Chapter 8), a parallel expansion will be necessary to address the special nutritional requirements of children identified as having such disorders (Association of State and Territorial Health Officials, 2004; Milling-

Table 10.7. Selected formulas for children with disabilities

Formulas and their components	Use based on diagnosis or condition
Standard infant formulas; 20 calories per fluid ounce	Full-term newborns up to 1 year
	Preterm infants with a corrected age of 40 weeks
Modified infant formula; 22 or 24 calories per fluid ounce	Preterm infants at 32 weeks of gestation or later
	Infants with higher energy, protein, calcium, and phosphorus requirements
Complete nutritional supplements (e.g., Pediasure, Boost); 30 calories per fluid ounce	Meal or snack substitutes
	Increase calories
	Ensure intake of specific nutrients (e.g., protein)
Formulas modified in the balance of nutrients; these are not used alone	Protein free: protein-restricted diets
	High protein: diet for glycogen storage disease
	Carbohydrate free: ketogenic diet
	Fat free: diets for gastrointestinal disorders or long chain fatty acid oxidation disorders
	Specific amino acids removed: phenylketonuria

Table 10.8. Common nutrition concerns of particular developmental disabilities

Prematurity-related nutrition problems likely in the first 3 years	Formula changes to accommodate medical problems
	Delayed self-feeding
	Rate of growth corrected for preterm birth
	Difficulty with setting feeding schedules
	Variable appetite, especially with illness
	Gastrointestinal problems (constipation, gastroesophageal reflux) reducing appetite
Neuromuscular disorders (cerebral palsy)	Difficulty gaining weight, particularly with frequent illness
	Underweight with small muscle mass
	Short stature
	Constipation and lack of response to dietary fiber
	Feeding problems/swallowing incoordination limiting food types
	Need to consider supplementation or gastrostomy
Developmental delays/intellectual disabilities (e.g., Down syndrome, Prader-Willi syndrome)	Unusual growth patterns
	Underweight or overweight
	Unusual level of activity, either higher or lower
	Delayed self-feeding skills
	Self-restricted diet
	Difficulty identifying hunger and fullness
	Constipation that is not responsive to dietary fiber
Attention-deficit/hyperactivity disorder	Inability to sit long enough to eat a meal
	Distractibility interfering with eating and meals
	Lack of a structured meal and snack patterns
	Possible decreased appetite as medication side effect
	Difficulty with socializing at meals
Epilepsy	A growth plateau is likely, even if eating well
	Possible changes in appetite as medication side effect
	A post-seizure state is likely to interfere with meals and energy intake
	Unusual growth patterns in children with poorly controlled seizures
	Ketogenic diet may result in overweight (see Table 10.10)

ton & Koeberl, 2003). Because the effectiveness of early dietary treatment has been demonstrated for PKU, the list of disorders that can be treated by diet early in life has increased markedly (American College of Medical Genetics, 2006; Millington & Koeberl, 2003). Treatment and follow-up of these rare genetic conditions has provided a model of customized nutrition therapy that may have broader applications in creating nutritional interventions tailored to the genetic characteristics of specific individuals (American College of Medical Genetics, 2006; Comuzzie, 2004; Olson, 2003).

Table 10.10 shows a sample dietary intake for an older child on a ketogenic diet. A ketogenic diet is deliberately designed to be very high in fat content and very low in carbohydrates. This results in the accumulation of ketones in the body, which is thought to be the mechanism of improved seizure control (see Chapter 29). The sample diet shown is for an older child used to eating regular foods. Specific fat-modified formulas and dietary components are used when a child who is fed through a gastrostomy needs a ketogenic diet.

Food Allergies

There is increasing public concern about links between various types of food allergies and chronic illnesses (e.g., asthma) and disabilities affecting behavior. The evidence for a causative relationship, however, is very weak (Collier, Fulhan, & Duggan, 2004; Mcgough et al., 2005). For example, there have been attempts to use **lactose** and gluten restrictions to treat individuals with disabilities (especially those with ASDs) who may or may not have had confirmatory allergy testing performed. In addition, there are "hypoallergenic" infant formulas. More research needs to be done in this area.

Table 10.9. Sample diet for a 10-year-old with phenylketonuria (PKU)

Breakfast	Snack bag of Fritos
	One honey-oats granola bar
	12 fluid ounces of Pepsi
	8 fluid ounces of PKU formula
Lunch	Medium garden salad with ranch dressing
	Baked apple slices with brown sugar and cinnamon
	16 fluid ounces of Sprite
After-school snack	Skittles
	8 fluid ounces of PKU formula
Dinner	Single-serving size box of Rice Krispies cereal with liquid Coffeemate
	Hot dog bun with mayonnaise, mustard, ketchup, and pickles
	Banana
	6 fluid ounces of PKU formula

Table 10.10. Sample ketogenic diet intake for an older child

Breakfast	4 fluid ounces of heavy whipping cream
	Scrambled egg with two slices bacon and 1 tablespoon fresh mushrooms
Lunch	4 fluid ounces of heavy whipping cream
	Hard-boiled egg mixed with 1 tablespoon mayonnaise
	2 tablespoons green beans with butter
After-school snack	Carbohydrate-free multivitamin and mineral pill
	Sugar-free popsicle
	Diet soda
Dinner	4 fluid ounces of heavy whipping cream
	Black olives (3)
	Sugar-free gelatin topped with whipped cream
	Slice of full-fat ham
	Slice of tomato
Snack	Walnuts (3)
	Diet soda

Constipation

Gastrointestinal dysfunction is a frequent concern for children with disabilities. Substituting whole wheat bread for white bread and fresh apples with the peel for apple juice are typical suggestions for families dealing with a toddler who has spina bifida or Down syndrome. However, constipation that is refractory to routine dietary interventions (i.e., increasing fiber in the diet) is common in children with cerebral palsy and Rett syndrome (Benninga, Voskuijl, & Taminiau, 2004). A variety of laxatives at small daily doses have been found to be effective in preventing impaction, discomfort, and **anorexia** from constipation (Benninga et al., 2004).

Celiac Disease

Celiac disease involves a permanent sensitivity to gluten, the protein fraction of wheat and rye. Some with celiac disease also have to avoid oats. Children with a number of conditions associated with developmental disabilities have a higher incidence of celiac disease than children in the typically developing population; these conditions include ASDs, Down syndrome, Turner syndrome, and Williams syndrome (Goldberg, 2004; Hill et al., 2005). In affected children, a gluten-free diet has to be followed strictly, even when children are asymptomatic. Many processed foods, from both grocery stores and restaurants, must be avoided because they use wheat and other flours for fillers and binding agents. Potato-, soy-, and rice-based products can be substituted for regular breads and pastas, although these specialized foods may be prohibitively expensive for many families.

Dietary Self-Restriction

Dietary self-restriction is a common problem in children with developmental disabilities. These problems include food refusal, selectivity by type of food or food texture, oral-motor delay, and dysphagia (Field et al., 2003; see also Chapter 31). ASDs (see Chapter 23) are especially associated with a self-imposed eating style. Over 60% of children with ASDs are selective eaters by type of food (Arnold et al., 2003). Sensitivities to the food colors, textures, and temperature are often reported. In such a case, a child refuses to eat many foods and is rigid in what he or she will eat. When not given preferred foods, the child completely refuses to eat and may have temper tantrums. The child also prefers to drink rather than to eat foods; so a high proportion of total calories come from one type of drink. Interventions to improve the child's diet might include providing a complete vitamin and mineral supplement and adding new foods one at a time by offering them many times (15–20 times) over 1–2 months paired with positive reinforcers (i.e., foods the child likes) (see

Chapter 35). Usually children with ASDs have normal growth despite their unusual eating habits. One study of 36 children with ASDs reported that their amino acid profiles were suggestive of poor protein intake, but no amino acid pattern specific to ASDs was identified (Arnold et al., 2003).

Issues Specific to Premature Infants

The nutrition problems related to preterm birth are emphasized in Table 10.8. Nutritional interventions for preterm infants represent the frontier of nutrition science. Premature infants have behaviorally based feeding problems complicated by medical and growth concerns and are an increasing proportion of children with disabilities (Cooke, Ainsworth, & Fenton, 2004). In one study, children born at 25 weeks of gestation age and assessed 3 years later were shown to have continued feeding difficulties as well as slower growth (Wood et al., 2003). The immaturity of the gastrointestinal system is one of the limiting factors in meeting nutrition requirements in premature infants, and this results in the need to supplement human breast milk with increased calories, specific fats, protein, vitamins, and minerals (Brandt, Sticker, Lentze, 2003, Diehl-Jones & Askin, 2004; Vohr & McKinley, 2003). Recommendations about specific vitamin and mineral requirements and long chain fatty acids supplements after preterm birth are evolving (Collier, Fulhan, & Duggan, 2004). Supplemental vitamin D from dietary sources and from exposure to sunlight is now recommended because of the recognition of an increased risk of **rickets** among preterm children (American Academy of Pediatrics, 2003; Meyer, 2004). It should be noted that persistent feeding problems may be an early sign of cerebral palsy (Fung et al., 2002).

NUTRITION WITHIN COMPLEMENTARY AND ALTERNATIVE MEDICAL CARE

Products claiming to boost energy or correct nutritional deficiencies are attractive to parents of children with disabilities. A survey of families with children with special needs found that 64% used some form of complementary and alternative medical therapy, or "CAM" (Sanders et al., 2003). CAM includes **megavitamin therapy,** amino acid and mineral supplements, and herbal remedies. Although CAM approaches are often presumed to be harmless, the safety of the

various forms of CAM is not well documented, and no CAM nutritional therapy has been proven effective by scientific methods. Furthermore, some CAM is clearly unsafe—for example, ingesting high doses of specific vitamins and amino acids to improve the cognitive abilities of children with Down syndrome and behavior in children with ASDs (American Dietetic Association, 2002b; Lewith & Chan, 2002). CAM in the form of nutritional supplements can also lead to an increased risk for or new side effects of medication received to control the underlying disability (e.g., antiepileptic medication). Thus, a child's medical/nutrition history should include a comprehensive list of supplements (Pediatric Desk Reference for Herbal Medicines, 2000; Pediatric Desk Reference for Nutritional Supplements, 2001).

SUMMARY

Underweight, overweight, constipation, food allergies, feeding difficulties, and other GI disturbances that interfere with appetite are more common in children with developmental disabilities than in typically developing children. Typical dietary guidelines for Americans (U.S. Department of Agriculture, 2005) and the MyPyramid Plan (U.S. Department of Agriculture, n.d.) are not sufficient resources for customizing nutrition recommendations for many children with developmental disabilities). Thus, medical nutrition therapy that includes a nutrition assessment and care plan should be part of the comprehensive care for children with disabilities. Pediatric nutrition experts work in a variety of care settings (e.g., schools, clinics, hospitals) to ensure that children with disabilities receive good nutrition services and that the children's parents are supported in their efforts to make feeding and nutrition a positive aspect of parenting and family life.

REFERENCES

American Academy of Pediatrics. (2003). Prevention of rickets and vitamin D deficiency: New guidelines for vitamin D intake. *Pediatrics, 111*, 908–910.

American College of Medical Genetics. (2006). Newborn screening: Toward a uniform screening panel and system: Final report. *ACMG Medical Geneticist 8*, (5, Suppl.), 12–252.

American Dietetic Association. (2002a). Position of the American Dietetic Association: Ethical and legal issues in nutrition, hydration and feeding. *Journal of the American Dietetic Association, 102*, 716–725.

American Dietetic Association. (2002b). Position of the American Dietetic Association: Food and nutrition misinformation. *Journal of the American Dietetic Association,102*, 260–266.

American Dietetic Association. (2006). Retrieved December 15, 2006 from http://www.eatright.org/cps/rde/xchg/ada/hs.xsl/nutrition_mntdoc_ENU_HTML.htm

Arnold, G.L., Hyman, S.L., Mooney, R.A., et al. (2003). Plasma Amino acids profiles in children with autism: Potential risk of nutritional deficiencies. *Journal of Autism and Developmental Disorders, 33*, 449–454.

Arvay, J., Zemel, B.S., Gallagher, P.R., et al. (2005). Body composition of children Aged 1 to 12 years with biliary atresia or Alagille Syndrome. *Journal of Pediatric Gastroenterology and Nutrition, 40*, 146–150.

Association of State and Territorial Health Officials. (2004). *Issue brief: State strategies to promote coordination of the newborn screening system.* Washington, DC: Author.

Bandini, L.G., Curtin, C., Hamad, C., et al. (2005). Prevalence of overweight in children with developmental disorders in the continuous national health and nutrition examination survey (NHANES) 1999–2002. *The Journal of Pediatrics, 146*(6), 738–743.

Benninga, M.A., Voskuijl, W.P., & Taminiau, J.A. (2004). Childhood constipation: Is there new light in the tunnel? *Journal of Pediatric Gastroenterology and Nutrition, 39*, 448–464.

Borowitz, D., Baker, R.D., & Stallings, V. (2002). Consensus report on nutrition for pediatric patients with cystic fibrosis. *Journal of Pediatric Gastroenterology and Nutrition, 35*, 246–259.

Brandt, I., Sticker, E.J., & Lentze, M.J. (2003). Catch-up growth of head circumference of very low birth weight, small for gestational age preterm infants and mental development to adulthood. *The Journal of Pediatrics, 142*, 463–470.

Brown, J.E. (Ed.). (2005). *Nutrition through the life cycle* (2nd ed.). Belmont, CA: Wadsworth.

The Canadian Growth Hormone Advisory Committee. (2005). Impact of growth hormone supplementation on adult height in Turner syndrome: Results of the Canadian Randomized Controlled Trial. *Journal of Clinical Endocrinology and Metabolism, 90*, 3360–3366.

Chudley, A.E., Conry, J., Cook, J.L., et al. (2005). Fetal alcohol spectrum disorder: Canadian guidelines for diagnosis. *Canadian Medical Association Journal, 172*(5, Suppl.), S1–S21.

Collier, S., Fulhan, J., & Duggan, C. (2004) Nutrition for the pediatric office: Update on vitamins, infant feeding and food allergies. *Current Opinion in Pediatrics, 16*, 314–320.

Comuzzie, A.G. (2004). Nutrient selection and the genetics of complex phenotypes. *American Journal of Clinical Nutrition, 79*, 715–716.

Cooke, R.J., Ainsworth, S.B., & Fenton, A.C. (2004). Postnatal growth retardation: A universal problem in preterm infants. *Archives of Disease in Childhood: Fetal and Neonatal Edition, 89*, F428–F430.

Diehl-Jones, W.L., & Askin, D.F. (2004). Nutritional modulation of neonatal outcomes. *AACN Clinical Issues: Advanced Practice in Acute and Critical Care. Biological Mediators, 15*, 83–96.

Ellett, M.L.C. (2004). What is known about methods of correctly placing gastric tubes in adults and children. *Gastroenterology Nursing, 27*, 253–259.

Field, D., Garland, M., & Williams, K. (2003). Correlates of specific childhood feeding problems. *Journal of Paediatrics and Child Health, 39*, 299–304.

Fung, E.B., Samson-Fang L., Stallings, V.A., et al. (2002). Feeding dysfunction is associated with poor growth and health status in children with cerebral palsy. *Journal of the American Dietetic Association, 102*, 361–673.

Goldberg, E.A. (2004). The link between gastroenterology and autism. *Gastroenterology Nursing, 27*, 16–19.

Heyman, M.B., Harmatz, P., Acree, M., et al. (2004). Economic And psychologic costs for maternal caregivers of gastrostomy-dependent children. *The Journal of Pediatrics, 145*, 511–516.

Hill, I.D., Dirks, M.H., Liptak, G.S., et al. (2005). Guideline for the diagnosis and treatment of celiac disease in children: Recommendations of the North American Society for Pediatric Gastroenterology, Hepatology and Nutrition. *Journal of Pediatric Gastroenterology and Nutrition, 40*, 1–19.

Institute of Medicine, Food and Nutrition Board. (1997). *Dietary reference intakes for calcium, phorphorus, magnesium, vitamin D, and fluoride.* Washington DC: National Academies Press.

Institute of Medicine, Food and Nutrition Board. (2001). *Dietary reference intakes for vitamin A, vitamin K, arsenic, boron, chromium, copper, iodine, iron. molybdenum, nickel, silicon, vanadium, and zinc.* Washington, DC: National Academies Press.

Institute of Medicine, Food and Nutrition Board. (2002). *Dietary reference intakes for energy, carbohydrate, fiber, fat, fatty acids, cholesterol, protein, and amino acids.* Retrieved July 13, 2006, from http:/www/nap/edu

Isaacs, D., Kilham, H., Somerville, H., et al. (2004). Nutrition in cerebral palsy. *Journal of Paediatrics and Child Health, 40*, 308–310.

Isaacs, J.S., Murdock, M., Lane, J., et al. (2003). Eating difficulties in girls with Rett syndrome compared with other developmental disabilities. *Journal of the American Dietetic Association,103*(2), 224–230.

Krick, J., Murphy-Miller, P., Zeger, S., et al. (1996). Pattern of growth in children with cerebral palsy. *Journal of the American Dietetic Association, 96*, 680–685.

Lewith, G.T., & Chan, J. (2002). An exploratory qualitative study to investigate how patients evaluate complementary and conventional medicine. *Complementary Therapies in Medicine, 10*, 69–77.

Mcgough, J.J., Biederman, J., Wigal, S.B., et al. (2005). Long-term tolerability and effectiveness of once-daily mixed amphetamine salts (Adderall XR) in children with ADHD. *Journal of the American Academy of Child & Adolescent Psychiatry, 44*, 530–538.

Meyer C. (2004). Scientists probe role of vitamin D: Deficiency a significant problem. *Journal of the American Medical Association, 292*, 1416–1418.

Millington, D., & Koeberl, D. (2003). Metabolic screening in the newborn. *Genetics & Hormones, 19*, 33–38.

National Center for Health Statistics. (2000). *NCHS growth curves for children 0–19 years.* Washington, DC: U.S. Government Printing Office.

Nevin-Folino, N. (Ed.). (2003). *Pediatric manual of clinical dietetics* (2nd ed.). Chicago: American Dietetic Association.

Olson, R.E. (2003). Nutrition and genetics: an expanding frontier. *American Journal of Clinical Nutrition, 78*, 201–208.

Pedersen, S.D., Parsons, H.G., & Dewey, D. (2004). Stress levels experienced by the parents of enterally fed children. *Child: Care, Health & Development, 30*, 507–513.

Pediatric Desk Reference (PDR) for herbal medicines (2nd ed.). (2000). Montvale, NJ: Medical Economics Company.

Pediatric Desk Reference(PDR) for nutritional supplements. (2001). Montvale, NJ: Medical Economics Company.

Percy, A.K., & Lane, J.B. (2004). Rett syndrome: Clinical and molecular update *Current Opinion in Pediatrics, 16,* 670–677.

Sanders, H., Davis, M.F., Duncan, B., et al. (2003). Use of complementary and alternative medical therapies among children with special health care needs in southern Arizona. *Pediatrics,111,* 584–587.

Sandritter, T. (2003). Gastroesophageal reflux disease in infants and children. *Journal of Pediatric Health Care, 17*(4), 198–205.

Schwarz, S.M., Corredor, J., Fisher-Medina, J., et al. (2001). Diagnosis and treatment of feeding disorders in children with developmental disabilities. *Pediatrics, 108,* 671–676.

Sleigh, G., & Brocklehurst, P. (2004). Gastrostomy feeding in cerebral palsy: A systematic review. *Archives of Disease in Childhood, 89,* 534–539.

Speiser, P.W., Rudolf, M.C.J., Anhalt, H. et al. (2005). *Consensus statement: Childhood obesity.* Journal of Clinical Endocrinology & Metabolism, 90, 1871–1887.

Taylor, E.,& Rogers, J.W. (2005). Practitioner review: Early adversity and developmental disorders. *Journal of Child Psychology and Psychiatry, 46,* 451–467.

U.S. Department of Agriculture. (n.d.). *MyPyramid plan.* Retrieved November 29, 2006, from http://www .mypyramid.gov

U.S. Department of Agriculture. (2005). *Dietary guidelines for Americans.* Retrieved July 13, 2006, from http://www.health/gov/dietary guidelines

Vohr, B.R., & McKinley, L.T. (2003). The challenge pays off: Early enhanced nutritional intake for VLBW small-for-gestation neonates improves long-term outcome. *Journal of Pediatrics, 142,* 459–461

Wood, N.S., Costeloe, K., Gibson, A.T., et al. (2003). The EPICure study: Growth and associated problems in children born at 25 weeks of gestational age or less. *Archives of Disease in Childhood: Fetal and Neonatal Edition, 88,* F492–F500.

11 Vision

Our Window to the World

Marijean M. Miller and Sheryl J. Menacker

Upon completion of this chapter, the reader will

- Be able to describe the anatomy and function of the eye
- Know about common eye problems in children
- Be aware of the tests used to determine visual acuity
- Understand how a child typically develops visual skills
- Know the definition and major causes of visual impairment in children
- Recognize some of the ways in which the development of a child with visual impairment differs from that of a sighted child and some approaches to intervention

Impairment of sight in childhood can have detrimental effects on physical, neurological, cognitive, and emotional development. A severe visual impairment causes delays in walking and talking and affects behavior and socialization. Although it may occur as an isolated disability, visual impairment is often associated with other developmental disabilities, including intellectual disability and cerebral palsy.

If visual loss is identified early, effective interventions can be instituted. With this goal in mind, this chapter explores the embryonic development of the eye and its normal structure and function. It also examines ocular disorders and common visual problems of the child with disabilities. Finally, the effects of blindness on a child's development are discussed and relevant educational resources are introduced.

MARY

Mary is a 12-year-old who has cerebral palsy and poor vision with nystagmus. She has optic atrophy from hydrocephalus, so her reading materials need to be in darker and larger print. From prematurity, her retinas have developed myopic degeneration. She requires extremely thick glasses (−18.50 right eye and −24.00 left eye), which shrink the image she sees and compress the image into a tunnel.

Mary wrote an essay to describe her disabilities and adaptations at school:

"One thing I don't like about homework is that sometimes I can't see the print. I have retinopathy of prematurity and degenerative **myopia** and **nystagmus.** I have a slant board to use for my ergonomic posture which brings my work closer so I won't have to bend over. My areas of need are being shy and not asking to move closer to the board if I can't see. Also, I have to ask for extended time for assignments and tests. I sometimes use a speaking dictionary. I also do use a magnifier and telescope, when I need to. I have trouble in remembering to scan and go back and check my work."

In her ophthalmologist's office Mary's binocular vision measures 20/50. However, with her compounded disabilities of optic atrophy, nystagmus, myopic degeneration, and tunnel vision from her glasses, she requires many adaptations to function in her classroom.

STRUCTURE OF THE EYE

In many ways, the structure of the eye is similar to that of a camera (Figure 11.1). In the eye, the

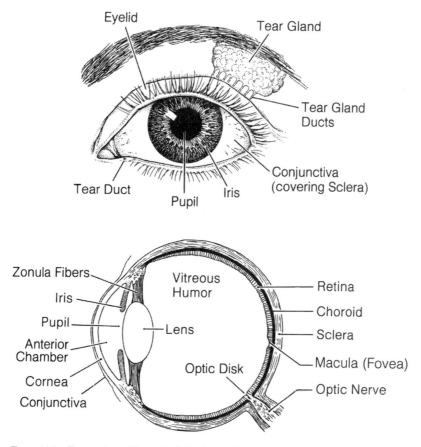

Figure 11.1. The structure of the eye is similar to that of a camera.

thick, white fibrous covering called the **sclera** functions as the camera body. Like a shutter, the colored region, called the **iris,** responds to changes in light conditions by opening and closing. The **pupil** is the aperture in the center of the iris. Light rays entering the eye through the pupil are focused first by the **cornea,** the clear dome that covers and protects the iris, and then by the **lens,** which lies behind the pupil. The cornea is the most important refracting surface of the eye. The lens further focuses light rays toward the retina, the photographic film of the eye, which lines its inner surface. The retina records the image in an upside-down, reversed format and sends the image via the optic nerve to the brain for interpretation.

The round shape of the eye is maintained by two substances: the **aqueous humor,** a watery liquid in the **anterior** chamber (the space between the cornea and lens), and the translucent, jelly-like **vitreous humor** that fills the **posterior** space between the lens and retina. The eye itself sits in a bony socket of the skull,

the orbit, which provides support and protection. This space also is occupied by blood vessels, muscles that move the eye, a lacrimal gland that produces tears, and the optic nerve, which sends images from the eye to the brain. Additional protection for the eyeball is provided by the eyelids, eyelashes, and **conjunctiva.** Blinking the eyelids wipes dust and other foreign bodies from the surface of the eye. Eyelashes help to protect the eye from airborne debris. The conjunctiva, a thin, transparent layer covering the sclera, contains tiny nutritive blood vessels that give a "bloodshot" appearance to the eye when it is inflamed or infected (called conjunctivitis).

OCULAR DEVELOPMENT

In the human embryo, the structures that will develop into eyes first appear at 4 weeks' gestation as two spherical bulbs at the side of the head (Figure 11.2). These bulbs gradually indent to form the optic cups. Three specialized

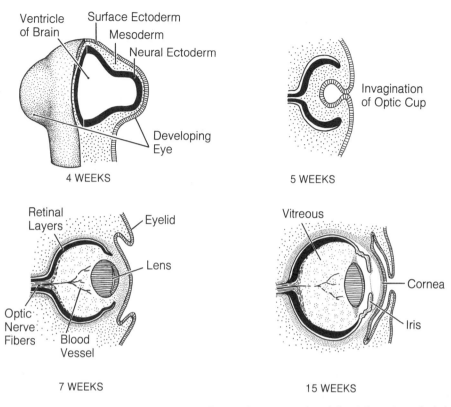

Figure 11.2. Embryonic development of the eye. The eyes first appear at 4 weeks' gestation as two spherical bulges at the side of the head. They indent in the next week to form the optic cups. By 7 weeks, the eyes have already assumed their basic form. The eye is completely formed by 15 weeks.

cell layers in these cups subsequently develop into the various parts of the eye. By 7 weeks' gestation, when the embryo is only 1 inch long, the eyes have already assumed their basic form (Sadler, 1990). As fetal growth continues, the eyes gradually move from the side of the head to the center of the face.

Deviations from typical development can lead to a wide variety of ocular defects, ranging from **anophthalmia,** a lack of eyes, to subtle abnormalities such as irregularly shaped pupils. Ocular malformations can occur as an isolated defect or as part of a syndrome (see Table 11.1 and Appendix B). Approximately 15%–30% of children with small eyes and coloboma (a cleft-like defect in the eye), have the CHARGE syndrome (Jongmans et al., 2006); these children may exhibit a variety of congenital anomalies, and in some cases have significant vision and hearing impairments (referred to as deafblindness; see http://www.dblink.org/lib/topics/charge-articles05.htm for more information).

Abnormalities occurring later in embryogenesis, when the eyes usually migrate closer together, may lead to abnormal widely spaced eyes, called **hemihypertrophy.** Finally, intrauterine infections (see Chapters 3 and 6) can cause **cataracts, glaucoma,** and/or **chorioretinitis** (an inflammation of the **choroid** and retinal layers of the eye), depending on when the infection occurs during development and which tissues are affected (Table 11.1).

DEVELOPMENT OF VISUAL SKILLS

As in the acquisition of language and motor skills, vision has developmental milestones (Friendly, 1993). Although the eyes have good optical clarity within days of birth, the visual system remains immature in many respects (Simons, 1993). Although infants will fixate briefly on a face soon after birth, steady fixation and tracking of a small target at near range is not expected until 3 months of age in term infants (Friendly, 1993). Although variable eye misalignments can be seen soon after birth, they should diminish in frequency over time, and the eyes should be absolutely straight by 3 months.

Table 11.1. Selected genetic syndromes associated with eye abnormalities

Syndrome	Eye abnormality
Aicardi syndrome	Retinal abnormalities
CHARGE association	Coloboma, microphthalmia
Galactosemia	Cataracts
Homocystinuria	Dislocated lens, glaucoma
Hurler syndrome	Cloudy cornea
Lowe syndrome	Cataracts, glaucoma
Marfan syndrome	Dislocated lens
Osteogenesis imperfecta	Blue sclera, cataracts
Osteopetrosis	Cranial nerve palsies, optic atrophy
Stickler syndrome	Extreme myopia
Tuberous sclerosis	Retinal defects, iris depigmentation
Tay-Sachs disease	Cherry-red spot in macula, optic nerve atrophy
Trisomy 13, trisomy 18	Microphthalmia, coloboma
Zellweger syndrome	Cataracts, retinitis pigmentosa

Key: CHARGE association: *c*oloboma of the eye, congenital *h*eart defect, choanal *a*tresia, *r*etarded growth and development, *g*enital abnormalities, and *e*ar malformations with or without hearing loss.

By age 3–4 years, many children can sit and have vision objectively measured by identifying a series of pictures at a distance. The test result should be approximately 20/40 or better. (A visual acuity result of 20/40 means the child can see at 20 feet an object that a person with typical vision can see at 40 feet.) There also should be minimal vision difference between eyes, less than two test lines.

Amblyopia

Until age 8, the visual system remains immature (Gwiazda & Thorn, 1999) and susceptible to a unique type of visual regression called **amblyopia.** Here a "healthy" eye does not see well because it is "turned off" by the brain. Unless the amblyopia is identified and treated with patching, blurry eye drops or special glasses before age 8, vision could permanently decrease even to the level of legal blindness.

Visual Development in Children with Disabilities

Many of the causes of developmental disabilities can also influence the visual system (Mervis

et al., 2000). In fact, one half to two thirds of individuals with developmental disabilities have a significant ocular disorder. Processes governing eye motions, alignment, visual acuity, and visual perception may mature slowly, partially, or abnormally in these children. Refractive errors, ocular misalignment, and eye movement disorders are especially common (Simon, Calhoun, & Parks, 1998). Because of these associations, it is imperative that an examination by a pediatric ophthalmologist be included in the overall assessment for a child with a disability.

FUNCTION AND DISEASES OF THE EYE

This section describes the functions of the cornea, anterior chamber, lens, retina, optic nerves, visual cortex, and eye muscles, along with some of the common disorders that affect them.

The Cornea

The cornea focuses light on the retina, including the **fovea centralis.** When a person looks at a tree, for example, a series of parallel rays of light leave the tree and reach the dome-shaped surface of the cornea, where they are **refracted,** or bent, toward a focal point on the retina. The rays are further refracted by the lens and come into focus on the fovea centralis, resulting in a sharp image that is transmitted to the brain (Figure 11.3). If the cornea is cloudy or deformed, however, the images will be blurred and indistinct. This requires prompt evaluation and treatment to avoid amblyopia. In infants, some causes of a cloudy cornea include birth trauma from a forceps delivery, congenital glaucoma, herpes infection, and certain inborn errors of metabolism.

The Anterior Chamber

The anterior chamber is a fluid-filled space located behind the cornea and in front of the iris. This area is like a water balloon with plumbing to maintain ocular pressure. The aqueous humor is made in the ciliary body just behind the iris and drains out of the eye in the angle where the cornea meets the iris through a sponge-like meshwork to Schlemm's canal (Figure 11.4). If fluid drainage is obstructed or slowed, the pressure rises, a condition called glaucoma may develop, which can injure the optic nerve and damage vision.

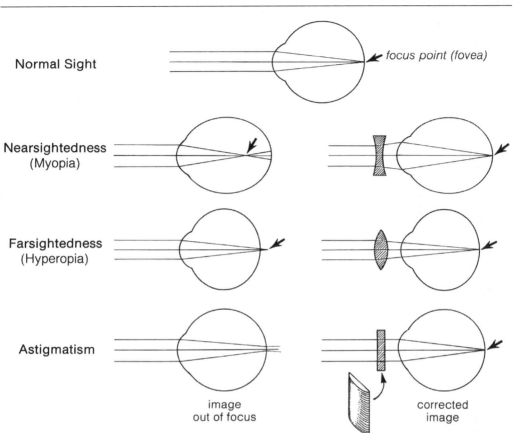

Figure 11.3. Refractive errors. If the eyeball is too long, images are focused in front of the retina (myopia). A concave lens deflects the rays, correcting the problem. If the eyeball is too short, the image focuses behind the retina and is again blurred (hyperopia). A convex lens corrects this. In astigmatism, the eyeball is the correct size, but typically the cornea is misshapen. A cylindrical lens is required to compensate.

The Lens

The lens, the second refracting surface of the eye, is a translucent, globular body located behind the iris, about one third of the way between the cornea and retina. It is convex on both sides and is attached by **ciliary muscles** to the inside of the eye. The ciliary muscle, by stretching or relaxing, changes the shape of the lens, fine-tuning the focus to accommodate changes in the distance of an object from the eye (Figure 11.5). When light comes from a distant object, the rays are close together and well focused. Because little refraction is needed, the ciliary muscles tighten, pulling the lens so that it is stretched and minimally refracts the light rays (Figure 11.5). To see a nearby object, in which the rays are more dispersed, the ciliary muscles relax so that the lens assumes a more globular shape and has greater refractive power. As a person ages, the lens becomes less flexible

and therefore less able to accommodate, causing near vision to become blurred (a condition termed **presbyopia**). Wearing bifocals or reading glasses helps to compensate for this loss of lens flexibility.

Cataracts   The major disorder affecting the lens is cataracts (Khater & Koch, 1998), which are defects in the clarity of the lens. Small cataracts often do not worsen or need to be removed. A dense central cataract larger than 3 millimeters, however, requires surgical removal. It appears as a white spot in the pupil; if untreated, it will cause amblyopia (Figure 11.6). In the newborn nursery, pediatricians screen for cataracts using an instrument called a direct **ophthalmoscope.** This permits magnification of the pupil and retroillumination to look for black spots or irregularities that could indicate a cataract. Any child with a suspected cataract should see a pediatric ophthalmologist promptly.

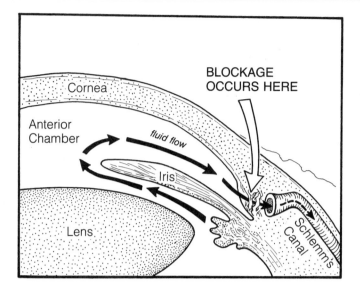

Figure 11.4. Glaucoma. Fluid normally drains from the anterior chamber through Schlemm's canal. A blockage in this passage leads to the accumulation of fluid and pressure, or glaucoma.

Although cataracts are primarily seen in adults, they also occur in about 1 in 250 infants, accounting for about 15% of blindness in children (Moore, 1994). A cataract may be an isolated abnormality or part of a syndrome or disease. For example, children with certain inborn errors of metabolism (e.g., galactosemia; see Chapter 20), congenital infections (e.g., rubella), and eye trauma may develop cataracts (Cassidy & Taylor, 1999).

In the case of a dense congenital cataract, surgery is needed soon after birth (Potter, 1993).

Studies of children with congenital cataracts indicate that **binocular vision** develops during the first 3 months after birth. Better visual outcomes for children with severe, unilateral cataracts are found in those who have cataract surgery before 6 weeks of age (Birch & Stager, 1996). Children with dense, bilateral cataracts who have surgery after 2 months of age have poorer vision (amblyopia) and unsteady eyes (nystagmus; Lambert & Drack, 1996). The surgery is a procedure in which the contents of the lens are aspirated, leaving only some of

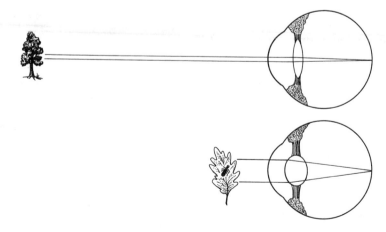

Figure 11.5. Accommodation. The lens changes shape to focus on a near or far object. The lens becomes thin and less refractive for distant objects and rounded and more refractive for near vision.

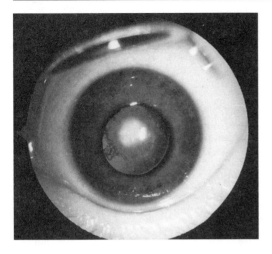

Figure 11.6. Photograph of a cataract, the white body seen through the pupil.

the outer shell of the lens intact. The surgery is safe and can be performed as an outpatient procedure.

The Retina

The retina is the light-sensitive "film" of the eye on which visual images are projected before transmission to the brain. Anatomically, the retina is like wallpaper inside the eyeball. The sclera and choroid are the tissues underlying the retina, providing support, protection, and nourishment (Figure 11.1). Within the retina are two types of **photoreceptor** cells: the **rods** and **cones.** Both respond to light by undergoing a chemical reaction.

For detailed vision, such as reading, seeing distant objects, and having color vision, cones are needed. They are located primarily in the fovea centralis, or **macula,** where central vision is processed. Each cone is sensitive to one of three distinct colors: red, green, or blue. The light from a colored object elicits a different response from each type of cone and leads to a patchwork pattern that is interpreted in the brain as shades of color. In the more peripheral or outside areas of the retina, rods predominate. Rods function in conditions of diminished light and are therefore necessary for night vision.

Nystagmus Nystagmus is an unsteady jiggling of the eyes seen by observation or by eye movement recording. Sensory **nystagmus** is an indicator of impaired vision: When the sensory input to the brain from the eye is impaired (for a variety of reasons), the eye becomes unsteady. A small optic nerve (optic nerve **hypo-**

plasia), absent macula (macular hypoplasia), or a variety of rod or cone abnormalities can result in nystagmus. Some children have idiopathic congenital nystagmus, in which there is no anatomic disorder (Neely & Sprunger, 1999).

The evaluation of children with nystagmus should include a comprehensive pediatric ophthalmologic examination. When the retina appears normal yet the vision is poor, an **electroretinogram (ERG)** may be suggested to test rod and cone function. If there is evidence of neurologic disease or if the nystagmus has atypical features such as rotatory or vertical components, then neurologic evaluation with neuroimaging should be considered (Brodsky, Baker, & Hamed, 1996).

Disorders of Photoreceptors: Color and Night Blindness A number of disorders involve abnormalities in the rods or cones in the retina. The most common is color blindness, in which one of the three types of cones is either abnormal or missing from birth. Red–green color blindness, the most common form, is typically inherited as an X-linked trait (see Chapter 1) and affects about 8% of men and 1% of women (Neitz & Neitz, 2000).

Retinopathy of Prematurity In infants, the most common cause of retinal damage is retinopathy of prematurity (ROP). Nearly one quarter of infants weighing less than 2,500 grams at birth will develop some degree of ROP (Hussain, Clive, & Bhandari, 1999). The actual number of affected infants has increased (Hameed et al., 2004), which is related in part to increased survival among VLBW infants.

ROP results from vascular damage to the retina. During the fourth month of gestation, retinal blood vessels start growing at the optic nerve in the back of the eye. By the ninth month, they have reached the furthest edges of the retina, near the front of the eye (Cook, Sulik, & Wright, 1995). In premature infants, this blood vessel growth is incomplete. In the catching-up process, a ridge can develop, with some blood vessels growing into the vitreous (toward the center of the eye) instead of along the back wall of the eye on the retinal surface. These abnormal blood vessels eventually die, and the resultant scar tissue can constrict, pulling on the retina. This pulling can lead to a retinal detachment and loss of vision. All infants weighing less than 1,500 grams at birth or with a gestational age of 32 weeks or less should be screened for ROP by an ophthalmologist with experience in ROP screening until the blood vessels are matured around 40 weeks from conception (American Academy of Pediatrics et al., 2006). Additional guidelines have been created for treating "aggressive posterior ROP," which may improve outcomes (International Committee for the Classification of ROP, 2005).

If ROP becomes severe enough to make detachment possible, it is treated with laser application to the avascular retina (Andrews, Hartnett, & Hirose, 1999). Despite treatment, many children with ROP will have significant visual impairments. These may include poor central vision, nearsightedness (myopia), **strabismus**, glaucoma, and even blindness (Figure 11.7; Ng et al., 2002). In addition, extremely low birth weight infants (those weighing less than 1,000 grams) sustain many neurologic insults, such as periventricular leukomalacia (see Chapters 9 and 26), that can worsen the impact of ROP on vision (Gosch et al., 1997; Msall et al., 2004).

Other Retinal Disorders Other disorders that damage the retina include nonaccidental injury (e.g., shaken baby syndrome) that can cause retinal hemorrhages, scarring, and detachment of the retina; toxoplasmosis and other congenital infections; and certain inborn errors of metabolism such as Tay-Sachs disease, in which abnormal cellular material is deposited in the retina. Finally, retinal tumors, such as

retinoblastoma, can lead to blindness in the affected eye.

The Optic Nerves

The surface of the retina contains more than 1 million optic nerve fibers that are connected to the rods and cones. The fibers come together at the back of the eye in an area called the optic disc (DeCarlo & Nowakowski, 1999). This region is also known as the blind spot because it contains nerve fibers but no rods or cones; therefore, no vision occurs when light rays are projected onto this area of the eye (Figure 11.1). One optic nerve emerges from behind each eye and begins its journey toward the brain. Some of the fibers from each nerve cross at a point called the optic chiasm that rests within the skull just before the nerves enter the brain (Figure 11.8). Each optic nerve (at this point called a tract) continues through the cerebral hemisphere to the occipital (back) lobe of the brain (Figure 11.8). Because some nerve fibers from each eye cross to the opposite side, each eye sends information to both the right and left sides of the brain. Therefore, damage to the right or left optic tract at any point after the optic chiasm will cause defects in the visual fields of both eyes (Figure 11.8). By identifying the part of a visual field affected, an ophthal-

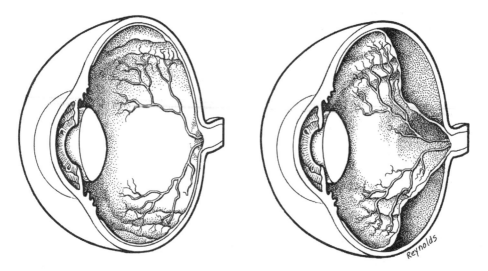

Figure 11.7.   Retinopathy of prematurity (ROP). Blood vessels in the retina proliferate (left). Eventually they stop growing, leaving a fibrous scar that contracts in the most severe cases and pulls the retina away from the back of the eye, causing blindness (right). (From Batshaw, M.L., & Schaffer, D.B. [1991]. Vision and its disorders. In M.L. Batshaw *Your child has a disability: A complete sourcebook of daily and medical care* [p. 165]. Baltimore: Paul H. Brookes Publishing Co.; reprinted by permission. Copyright © 1991 by M.L. Batshaw; illustrations copyright © 1991 by Lynn Reynolds. All rights reserved.)

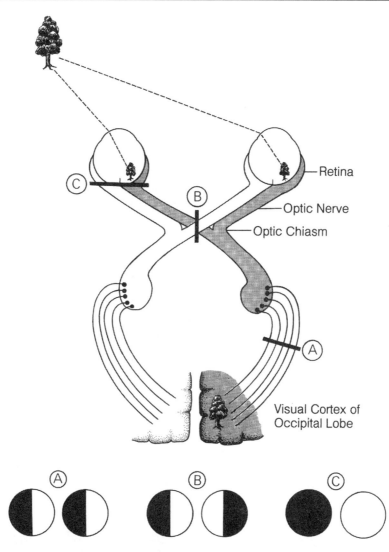

Figure 11.8. The visual pathway. One optic nerve emerges from behind each eye. A portion of the fibers from each crosses at the optic chiasm. An abnormality at various points along the route (upper figure) will lead to different patterns of visual loss (shown as black areas in the lower figures). These are illustrated: A) abnormality at the cortical pathway; B) damage to the optic chiasm; C) retinal damage.

mologist often can determine where the damage has occurred.

In optic nerve hypoplasia, a small, thin optic nerve transmits impaired information to the brain. Sensory nystagmus is observed. Midline structures in the brain can also be hypoplasic. When the pituitary gland is also small, hormone supplements may be required. Children with unilateral or bilateral optic nerve hypoplasia have neuroimaging performed, especially when there is poor growth. Optic nerve hypoplasia is a common cause of visual disability in the United States.

The Visual Cortex

The visual cortex is the region of the occipital lobe responsible for receiving and decoding information sent by the eyes. The information is subsequently relayed to the **temporal** and **parietal lobes.** Damage to these areas can result in a type of visual loss called cortical visual impairment (CVI; previously called cortical blindness), which in children is most commonly caused by oxygen deprivation (hypoxia), infections of the central nervous system (encephalitis), traumatic brain injury (see Chapter 30), and hydrocephalus (Brodsky et al., 1996; Good et al., 1994).

Cortical Visual Impairment Cortical visual impairment (CVI) is characterized by visual perceptual deficits in the setting of an ophthalmologic examination that is normal or has only minor abnormalities and is one of the most common causes of visual impairment in children in the developed world (Steinkuller et al., 1999). Children with CVI present with a variety of classic behaviors and visual attention can range from mildly impaired to absent. Early on, parents note their infant appreciates light and dark but may not look directly at the parents' faces, even at 6 months of age. The parents may be unsure what the child sees, but they are sure the child has some vision. Later, when the child is most alert, the parents observe visual tracking behavior, if brief, and the child may "look over" items but not directly at them. A full ophthalmologic examination must be performed to rule out treatable causes of visual impairment. In pure cortical visual impairment, the eye is normal yet the child sees poorly (Good et al., 1994).

Delayed Visual Maturation It is important to differentiate CVI from delayed visual maturation (DVM) in the infant with visual inattention. Both groups show no response to visual stimuli in early infancy. Children with DVM, however, have normal gestational and birth histories, normal eye examinations, no cortical abnormalities, and usually only mild to moderate developmental delays (Brodsky et al., 1996; Mercuri et al., 1997). In DVM, improvement of visual function occurs spontaneously in infancy as the overall development of the child progresses. The cause of DVM is poorly understood (Russell-Eggitt, Harris, & Kriss, 1998).

The Eye Muscles

Six muscles direct the eye toward an object and maintain binocular vision (Figure 11.9). The four recti muscles lie along the upper, lower, inner, and outer portions of the eye. The horizontal recti muscles converge the eyes toward the nose for near activities or diverge the eyes to look at distance. The horizontal recti muscles also move the eyes into right and left gaze. The recti muscles above and below the eyes serve to elevate and lower the eyes and also have some rotational functions. The oblique muscles lie obliquely above and below the eye and serve primarily a rotational function with secondary functions contributing to movement of the eyes in the horizontal and vertical plane.

Three nerves originating in the brainstem control the movement of these six eye muscles. The oculomotor, or third, cranial nerve controls the majority of eye muscles. Two muscles are controlled by their own assigned nerve: the trochlear, or fourth, cranial nerve controls the superior oblique muscle, and the abducens, or sixth, cranial nerve controls the lateral rectus muscles. The complex, coordinated movement of these eye muscles allows us to look in all directions without turning our heads and to maintain proper alignment of the eyes. The loss of this coordinated movement leads to misalignment of the eyes, or strabismus.

Strabismus Overall, strabismus occurs in about 3%–4% of children. It occurs, however, in 15% of former premature infants and in 40% of children with cerebral palsy (Olitsky & Nelson, 1998). Two main forms of strabismus exist: **esotropia** (cross-eyed), in which the eyes turn in, and *exotropia* (wall-eyed), in which the eyes turn out (Figure 11.9). Esotropia is much more common. Strabismus may be apparent all the time or only intermittently, such as when the child tires. Recall that strabismus is a cause of amblyopia in children younger than age 8.

Misalignment of the eyes can result from an abnormality in eye focusing, in the nerves supplying the eye muscles, in the eye muscles themselves, or in the brain regions controlling eye movement (Wright, 1995). With regard to eye focusing, or **accommodation,** the eyes normally converge toward the nose to read a book (near vision). Children who are farsighted must do this same sort of accommodation for both distance and near vision. In some children, this focusing effort leads to esotropia after the age of 2, which can be improved by eyeglasses that correct the farsightedness. In contrast, healthy infants who cross the eyes after 3 months of life will often need surgical correction of the esotropia. Neurologic problems such as cerebral palsy may alter the brain's signals to the eye muscles and cause strabismus which is treated with surgery. This is also true for the child with hydrocephalus who may develop strabismus as a result of nerve palsy caused by increased intracranial pressure.

Anomalous head postures can be caused by a number of ophthalmologic conditions, including strabismus and nystagmus. Thus, children with tilted or turned heads should see an ophthalmologist as part of their evaluation. Chil-

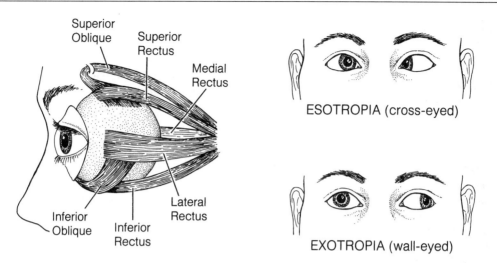

Figure 11.9. The eye muscles. Six muscles move the eyeball. A weakness of one of these muscles causes strabismus. In esotropia, the eye turns in, whereas in exotropia, the eye turns out. Esotropia and exotropia of the left eye are illustrated.

dren with nystagmus turn the head so that the eyes are placed where they "jiggle" the least and vision is most stable (the "null point") Strabismus surgery can reposition the eyes so that this null point is in the head-straight position. When vertical strabismus is present because of a congenital paralysis of the superior oblique muscle, the head tilts toward the opposite shoulder. Approximately 80% of children show good ocular alignment following strabismus surgery (Shauly, Miller, & Meyer, 1997).

REFRACTIVE ERRORS IN CHILDREN

As discussed previously, light entering the eye is focused by the cornea and lens. Under optimal conditions, the light rays are perfectly refracted onto the retina, resulting in a clearly focused image. If the eye is too long or if the refracting mechanisms of the eye are too strong, the focused image falls in front of the retina, and the picture is blurred (Figure 11.3). This is called **myopia,** or nearsightedness. If the eye is too short or the refracting mechanisms are too weak, the image is focused behind the retina, also producing a blurred image (Figure 11.3). In this instance, the person has **hyperopia,** or farsightedness. The other common refractive problem is **astigmatism** (Figure 11.3). Astigmatism typically occurs when the surface of the cornea has an elliptical rather than spherical shape. Because of this, light rays entering the eye do not focus on a single point and the image is blurred.

Farsightedness is the most common refractive error of childhood (Moore, 1997). The important difference between myopia and hyperopia is that with farsightedness, the eye can use its power of accommodation to further focus light rays onto the retina. As a result, most children with mild farsightedness require no correction and have excellent visual acuity. Hyperopia of more than 4 **diopters** often requires correction with glasses. A diopter is a unit of light-bending power of a lens; it is the reciprocal of the distance in meters to the point where the rays intersect (Cole et al., 2001). The accommodative load on the child to maintain sharp focus must be considered, especially in children with disabilities. With farsightedness greater than 4 diopters, the accommodative load may be so great that the child always has blurred vision except for those brief moments when something of exceptional interest triggers more complete accommodation effort and precise focus. Children with more than 6 diopters of hyperopia can develop both amblyopia and esotropia.

With myopia, the child sees clearly only at a near range. Severe myopia, such as that found in former premature infants who had ROP, may have a clear range of focus of only a few inches from the face. These children need eyeglass correction from infancy to expand their distance vision. Mild refractive errors, conversely, may not necessitate glasses if a child is functioning well. Both severe hyperopia and myopia, however, can impair the development of the visual system, causing amblyopia and affecting the child's interactions with the world.

In children with disabilities, even small refractive errors should be corrected to optimize performance. Furthermore, when there is a significant difference in refractive error between eyes, glasses must be prescribed to avert amblyopia in the eye more poorly in focus. In these cases, glasses ensure that the images focused on the retina of each eye are of equal clarity.

Eyeglasses can be prescribed even for the youngest infant and for the child with multiple disabilities. This is because a method exists for assessing refractive errors that relies completely on objective measures rather than on subjective input from the child. After instillation of eyedrops, which dilate the pupils and paralyze accommodation, the ophthalmologist views the child's eyes through a **retinoscope** (a magnifying, streak light source) and can determine, using lenses of varying powers, the refractive error and the required correction. Eyeglasses can then be prescribed.

VISION TESTS

Assessing the visual function of children with developmental disabilities is critical in helping to determine the best interventions. In experienced hands, vision testing can be quite informative even when the child is not able to or will not cooperate. Tests of visual function fall into two general categories: those based on direct observation of the eyes and the use of eye charts and those using higher technology.

Assessing Visual Function Through Acuity Charts and Observation

In early childhood, parental report may be the best indicator of visual function. In addition, many verbal and cooperative children can identify picture characters or symbols on an eye chart beginning at age 3–3½ years (Broderick, 1998). Several symbol tests exist: Allen pictures, LEA symbols, and the HOTV test (Hartmann et al., 2000).

Older children can identify letters at distance. In nonverbal children, a matching game can be used in which the child points to the figure on a near card to show what he or she sees at distance. Although it is easier to test visual acuity by showing characters one at a time rather than in groups, this tends to underestimate amblyopia because acuity is better for single symbols than for groups; this phenomenon is called the crowding effect (von Noorden, 1996). This problem is avoided by a method of visual acuity testing that uses a distance chart in which only the letters *H, O, T,* and *V* appear with black bars

beside the letters, allowing characters to be shown individually (Cole et al., 2001).

Assessing Visual Function Through Higher Technology

Several techniques are available for testing visual function without relying on verbal responses or character recognition (Jackson & Saunders, 1999). These techniques include **optokinetic** nystagmus (OKN), preferential looking (PL), and electrophysiological testing (Mackie & McCulloch, 1995).

Optokinetic Nystagmus The OKN response is determined by rotating a black-and-white, vertically striped drum in front of the child's eyes. Similar to the effect of watching a picket fence from a passing car, the child's eyes should jiggle back and forth as they follow the movement of one stripe and then quickly jerk back to fixate on another. OKN is an involuntary response that should be evident soon after birth (Lewis, Maurer, & Brent, 1989). It is estimated that the minimum vision necessary for an OKN response is perception of fingers held in front of the eyes (Burde, Savino, & Trobe, 1985).

Preferential Looking Techniques PL testing relies on the fact that an infant or young child will preferentially fixate on a boldly patterned striped target rather than on an equally luminous blank target (Teller et al., 1986). In PL testing, the child is shown a series of cards containing a pattern of black-and-white stripes, or gratings, on one side and a blank gray target of equal luminance on the other side (Dobson et al., 1995). The stripe widths become progressively thinner on successive cards, creating finer gratings that require better visual resolution (Figure 11.10). The tester presents the cards at a predetermined distance and watches the child's fixation through a peephole in the center of each card. The finest set of stripes for which the child reliably looks to the patterned side is called the grating visual acuity. Grating visual acuity with the Teller test is not as precise in the low vision setting as the Snellen vision chart is. Grating visual acuity done in infancy may suggest that a child has better vision than will eventually be determined by using the Snellen vision chart when the child is older and capable of reading the Snellen letter chart.

Electrophysiological Testing Electrophysiological testing includes ERGs and visual evoked potentials (VEPs) to determine

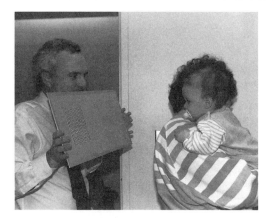

Figure 11.10. Teller preferential looking cards. The infant is held, and a card is shown with a grating pattern on one side and a gray color on the other. The infant prefers the grating to a plain color. The sides are switched to ensure that the infant is looking at the pattern. Successively smaller gratings are shown until the infant no longer shows a preference, indicating that he or she cannot differentiate the stripes from the solid color. The smallest discriminable size determines the grating visual acuity. (Courtesy of Graham Quinn, M.D., Children's Hospital of Philadelphia.)

whether the vision problem lies primarily in the eyes or in the brain (Weleber & Palmer, 1991).

Electroretinogram An ophthalmologist may decide to obtain an ERG when the retina looks normal but vision is absent or is very poor. The ERG tests retinal functioning by evaluating the quality of cone and rod response to light stimuli. It is particularly useful in demonstrating diseases of the retina and for assessing poor night vision. In ERG testing, modified contact lenses are placed on the corneas of the child after instillation of topical anesthetic drops. Depending on the type of equipment used, one to three electrodes are also affixed to the face and/or body. Lights are momentarily flashed in the child's eyes under different conditions while a computer analyzes the information received from the electrodes and from leads attached to the contact lenses.

Visual Evoked Potential VEP testing may be considered once an ERG indicates that the retina is functioning normally. Flash VEP testing is used to evaluate the pathway between the eye and the brain in children suspected of having CVI; pattern VEP testing is used to assess visual acuity in infants and children with severe disabilities Iinuma, Lombroso, & Matsumiya, 1997). Pattern VEP testing for children, however, is available only at a few research centers, and flash VEP provides limited information.

BLINDNESS

The definition of blindness from a legal and federal educational standpoint is visual acuity of 20/200 or worse in the better eye with correction or a visual field that subtends to an angle of not greater than 20 degrees instead of the usual 105 degrees (Bishop, 1991; Individuals with Disabilities Education Improvement Act of 2004, PL 108-446). Individuals with low vision (partially sighted) are defined as having a visual acuity better than 20/200 but worse than 20/70 with correction (Education for All Handicapped Children Act of 1975, PL 94-142). Both of these categories of students are considered to have visual impairments. Most people who are legally blind have considerable useful vision and may be able to distinguish light and dark or detect objects (20/500 to 20/800) or may read large-print texts (20/200 to 20/500). Other people with blindness, however, do not have light and dark perception. To provide the best services to children with multiple disabilities and some degree of visual impairment, it is important to know the extent of limitations from the visual impairment (Jan & Freeman, 1998).

Causes of Blindness

In childhood, the causes of blindness are many and varied. The three leading causes of visual impairment in the United States are CVI, ROP, and optic nerve hypoplasia (Hatton, 2001). Malformations of the visual system range from colobomas of the retina (e.g., CHARGE syndrome) to optic nerve abnormalities and cerebral malformations. Other causes of blindness include traumatic brain injury, severe eye infections, and tumors (Jacobson et al., 1998). Blindness is far more prevalent in developing countries, where nutritional disorders such as vitamin A deficiency and infections such as **trachoma,** measles, and tuberculosis are common (Foster & Johnson, 1990).

Identifying the Child with Severe Visual Impairment

Blindness can be an isolated disability or part of a condition involving multiple disabilities. For example, visual impairment caused by an inherited disorder such as albinism (in which there is a reduction in retinal pigment) may be an isolated finding, whereas CVI caused by hypoxia-ischemia in the newborn period is often associated with cerebral palsy and intellectual disability. About half of all children with severe visual impairments have other associated developmental disabilities (Ferrell, 1998; Teplin, 1995).

Several clues may indicate that an infant has a severe visual impairment. The child will not visually fixate on a parent's face or show interest in following brightly colored objects. Parents also may notice abnormalities in the movement of the child's eyes, including wandering eye motions, nystagmus, or eyes that always gaze in one particular direction. In addition, the infant may not blink or cry when a threatening gesture is made or a bright light is shined in the eyes. Any of these findings should lead to a thorough examination by an ophthalmologist.

Developmental Variations in the Child with Severe Visual Impairment

One might expect severe visual impairment to result in lags in early childhood development. Being unable to establish eye contact with parents could have an impact on the infant's attachment and socialization skills. Preverbal communication, which is dependent on visual observation and imitation, could be delayed. Hypotonia and/or fear of movement combined with parental concern about injury might affect the development of motor skills in the child who is blind. Studies that have examined these issues have in fact found developmental delays, but the delays appear to be dependent on the amount of residual vision and the presence or absence of associated developmental disabilities (Hatton et al., 1997).

The early development of children with vision better than 20/500 and with no other severe associated impairments may approximate that of sighted children, whereas that of children with less than 20/500 visual acuity (or 20/800 in some studies) has shown significant lags in early developmental milestones (Figure 11.11). Children with early developmental lags, provided that they have no associated severe developmental disabilities (e.g., cerebral palsy, intellectual disability, hearing impairment), test typically by school age (Ferrell, 1998). If there are associated impairments, however, the delays will persist (Ferrell, 1998; Teplin, 1995). The origin of the visual loss (eye, optic nerve, brain) does not seem to influence the degree of delay in milestone acquisition.

Children with visual impairments who reach most early developmental milestones at a typical age may show some delays (Cass, Sonkesen, & McConachie, 1994; Dekker & Koole, 1992). Searching for dropped objects, crawling, and walking without support are all acquired later. There are also differences in the use of words and difficulty with pragmatics and pronouns (e.g., saying "you" for "I"; Perez-Pereira & Conti-Ramsden, 1999). In the child with average intelligence, speech and language become typical by school age. Speech, however, is accompanied by less body and facial "language," and conversation skills may be less developed. In all areas, children with isolated visual disability will be capable of reaching developmental milestones (Pogrund, et al., 1992).

In addition to developmental differences, there may be behavioral mannerisms that have been termed "blindisms." These self-stimulatory behaviors include eye pressing, blinking forcefully, gazing at lights, waving fingers in front of the face, rolling the head, and swaying the body (Good & Hoyt, 1989). Eye pressing seems to occur only in children with retinal disease, in whom it produces visual stimulation. Fortunately, most children with these mannerisms learn to inhibit them as they grow older. These behaviors may persist into adulthood, however, in individuals who also have an intellectual disability (Jan, 1991).

It is interesting to note that the child with congenital blindness may be unaware of having an impairment until 4–5 years of age. In the school-age child, however, social skills impairments may be related to social isolation and poor self-image. Therefore, inclusion in a program with typically developing children should include an agenda to promote socialization (Warren, 1994; Zell Sacks, Kekelis, & Gaylord-Ross, 1992).

Most tests of infant development are based primarily on performance of visual skills, and may not be optimal in evaluating infants with severe visual impairment. Alternative non–visually based developmental scales should be used to help in educational planning (Wodrich, 1997).

Early Intervention for the Infant and Young Child with Severe Visual Impairment

As soon as an infant is diagnosed with a severe visual impairment, he or she should be entered into an early intervention program. The early intervention staff should be trained in the effects of visual impairment on a child's early development, and the team should include an ori-

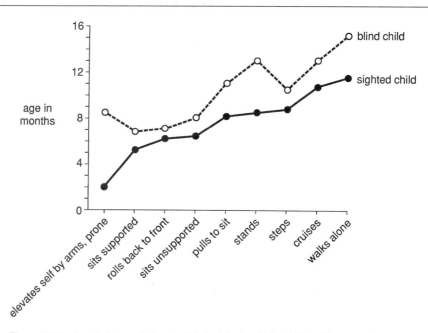

Figure 11.11. Age of attainment of motor skills in sighted and blind children. The motor development of a blind child is delayed. (From *Insights from the blind: Comparative studies of blind and sighted infants* [p. 204], by Selma Fraiberg. Reprinted by permission of Basic Books, member of Perseus Books Group.)

entation and mobility specialist and a teacher certified in the area of visual impairment. (Fiedler, Best, & Bax, 1994; Harrison, 1993). The focus should be to increase skills in other senses, to improve body concept and awareness, and to promote locomotion and active exploration of the environment (Dietz & Ferrell, 1993; Zambone, 1989).

While awake, infants should be placed on the stomach rather than on the back to strengthen neck and trunk muscles (Moller, 1993). The young child with a severe visual impairment must explore the world through touch and sound (Niemann & Jacob, 2000; Pogrund et al., 1992). Therefore, parents and therapists should place or store toys at a height the child can reach. Textured and sound-producing toys are generally favored. If there is any usable vision, the child should be encouraged to take advantage of it. Bright colors should be used, and the child's vision and attention directed verbally toward them (Holbrook, 1995). It is very important for the parents, teachers, and therapists to give verbal cuing to provide the child with information prior to being touched/handled to eliminate any resistance to touch (tactile defensiveness; Warren, 1994).

The child's name should be used frequently to encourage inclusion in conversations and to ensure that the child will respond to questions in the absence of verbal cues. There also should be a verbal explanation before, during, and after a task is performed (Ferrell, 1985). While the child is moving from one space to another, the purpose of the move and the orientation of the space should be explained.

Orientation encompasses such skills as laterality and directionality. In terms of orientation and mobility, the child is first taught by an orientation and mobility specialist to locate familiar objects within the home and then progresses to travel outdoors. The child should be urged to walk despite the risks of scrapes and bruises. Poor peripheral vision (tunnel vision) is more of a problem in walking than the loss of central vision is. Any residual vision, however, is better than total absence of vision. The use of mobility aids for walking should be encouraged, including push toys (Sonksen, Petrie, & Drew, 1991).

The educational placement for a child depends on age, extent of visual impairment, and associated disabilities (Warren, 1994; Wheeler et al., 1997). For the infant, an early intervention program usually entails a once-per-week home-based program in which the early childhood educator visits and works with the parent to set up a stimulating environment. By 2–3 years of age, the child is usually ready for a school-based program. Over the next few years, listening, concept development, conversation, and daily living skills (e.g., dressing, eating, personal hygiene) are emphasized. Literacy modality assessment can also begin at this time so that emergent literacy activities can be part of the child's educational program. Self-dressing should be encouraged by using loose clothing and Velcro straps to fasten shoes, pants, and shirts. Play and social skills training and behavior therapy for "blindisms" may also be a part of the program. It is important to create an attitude of stimulating all areas of sensory development, including visual skills in the child who has some residual vision. It is equally important that the parents and other caregivers do not perform too many tasks for the child so that he or she is encouraged to interact with the environment. Otherwise, the child will develop a distorted understanding of how the world works (Dietz & Ferrell, 1993).

Educating the School-Age Child with Severe Visual Impairment

By the time the child reaches school age, the extent of the visual loss is usually clear. A child's ability to work efficiently without excessive fatigue, reading rates over a time with a variety of materials, and the expectation in some cases for progressive visual loss will all be factors considered for school. Some children will succeed best with optical aids and devices and larger print books, whereas others may succeed best with a transition to **braille.**

Braille is a code formed from a series of raised dots on a page that are read from left to right. Visual efficiency, visual fatigue, prognosis for future visual loss or gain, and reading rates with a variety of materials are all factors to consider. Reading readiness for braille begins in kindergarten (Castellano & Kosman, 1997). Fine motor skills and tactile sensitivity are taught first. When the child is able to recognize small shapes, differentiate between rough and smooth, and follow a line of small figures across a page, the learning of the braille alphabet can begin (Swenson, 1999).

Children with severe visual impairments should also learn to type on a computer by fourth grade. No accommodations are needed, except that a computer mouse cannot be used. In addition, a wide variety of books on tape are available from Recording for the Blind & Dys-

lexic (see http://www.rfbd.org) and from bookstores and libraries. It is critical to make sure that the child has all of the appropriate equipment needed for learning and independence. With these tools, children with severe visual impairments should be able to succeed in a general academic setting. They may, however, need certain specialized assistance and training in the use of braille, low vision devices, orientation and mobility aids, and so forth.

Assistive Technology

The computer age is greatly benefiting individuals with severe visual impairment. Voice recognition software permits individuals to input instructions to computer applications verbally. Conversely, various devices from calculators to computers produce voice messages, vocalize results of calculations, and so forth. There are computers that convert print into braille (Blenkhorn, 1997) and haptic interface technology that makes digital information tactile (Fritz & Barner, 1999). In addition, there is research on producing a visual prosthesis (Arno et al., 1999; Dobelle, 2000) analogous to the cochlear implant that is used in deafness (see Chapter 12).

Communities are also becoming more accessible to individuals with visual impairment by implementing elevators that announce floors, crosswalk indicators that beep when it is safe to cross the street, ramps, and so forth. The classic mobility aid (long cane) is being replaced by devices with sophisticated laser/ultrasound wave processing and spatial hearing capacity (Bitjoka & Pourcelot, 1999; Shoval, Borenstein, & Koren, 1998). Global Positioning System (GPS) software may soon permit individuals to be guided verbally to their destination.

Intervention for Children with Multiple Disabilities

The incidence of blindness in children with multiple developmental disabilities is more than 200 times that found in the general population (Warburg, Frederiksen, & Rattleff, 1979). One third of children with partial sight and two thirds of children with blindness have other developmental disabilities, the most common being intellectual disability, hearing impairments, seizure disorders, and cerebral palsy. The majority of these children have two or more disabilities in addition to visual impairment (Curtis & Donlon, 1984; Teplin, 1995). Treatment of these children must address all the disabilities and use all the senses and abilities that remain. A multidisciplinary approach involving a range of educational and health care professionals is essential.

Outcome for Severe Visual Impairment

Outcome for the child with severe visual impairment depends on the amount of residual vision, the presence of associated disabilities, the motivation of the child and family, and the skills of the involved teachers and therapists. In general, less severe visual impairment and the absence of associated impairments predict typical development and good outcomes for independence and occupational success.

SUMMARY

Abnormalities of the visual system are among the many obstacles that children with developmental disabilities may face. The visual challenges encountered may range from minor to severe, transient to permanent, stable to progressive, and ocular to cortical. Children with developmental disabilities, as a group, are at higher risk for visual impairment than children in the general population are. Because the visual system is undergoing a process of maturation during childhood, early recognition of visual disorders is essential to ensure prompt treatment and to optimize visual outcome. Therefore, careful visual assessment is important for all children and can be performed regardless of a child's level of impairment or ability to cooperate. The outcome for children with visual impairments depends on the degree of the visual loss, developmental status, motivation of child and family, and skill of involved teachers and therapists.

REFERENCES

American Academy of Pediatrics, American Academy of Ophthalmology, & American Association for Pediatric Ophthalmology and Strabismus. (2006). Policy statement: Screening examination of the premature infants for retinopathy of prematurity. *Pediatrics, 117,* 572–576.

Andrews, A.P., Hartnett, M.E., & Hirose, T. (1999). Surgical advances in retinopathy of prematurity. *International Ophthalmology Clinics, 39,* 275–290.

Arno, P., Capelle, C., Wanet-Defalque, M.C., et al. (1999). Auditory coding of visual patterns for the blind. *Perception, 28,* 1013–1029.

Batshaw, M.L., & Schaffer, D.B. (1991). Vision and its disorders. In M.L. Batshaw *Your child has a disability: A complete sourcebook of daily and medical care* (pp. 161–177). Baltimore: Paul H. Brookes Publishing Co.

Birch, E.E., & Stager D.R. (1996). The critical period of surgical treatment of dense congenital unilateral cataract. *Investigative Ophthalmology and Visual Science, 37,* 1532–1538.

Bishop, V.E. (1991). Preschool visually impaired children: A demographic study. *Journal of Visual Impairment and Blindness, 85,* 69–74.

Bitjoka, L., & Pourcelot, L. (1999). New blind mobility aid devices based on the ultrasonic Doppler effect. *International Journal of Rehabilitation Research, 22,* 227–231.

Blenkhorn, P. (1997). A system for converting print into braille. *IEEE Transactions on Rehabilitation Engineering, 5,* 121–129.

Boyle, C.A., Yeargin-Allsopp, M. Doernberg, N.S., et al. (1996). Prevalence of selected developmental disabilities in children 3-10 years of age: The Metropolitan Atlanta Developmental Disabilities Surveillance Program, 1991. *Morbidity and Mortality Weekly Report, 45* (2), 1–14.

Broderick, P. (1998). Pediatric vision screening for the family physician. *American Family Physician, 58,* 691–700, 703–704.

Brodsky, M.C., Baker, R.S., & Hamed, L.M. (1996). *Pediatric neuro-ophthalmology.* New York: Springer-Verlag.

Burde, R.M., Savino, P.J., & Trobe, J.D. (1985). *Clinical decisions in neuro-ophthalmology.* St. Louis: Mosby.

Cass, H.D., Sonkesen, P.M., & McConachie, H.R. (1994). Developmental setback in severe visual impairment. *Archives of Disease in Childhood, 70,* 192–196.

Cassidy, L., & Taylor, D. (1999). Congenital cataract and multisystem disorders. *Eye, 13,* 464–473.

Castellano, C., & Kosman, D. (1997). *The bridge to braille: Reading and school success for the young blind child.* Baltimore: National Organization of Parents of Blind Children.

Cole, S.R., Beck, R.W., Moke, P.S., et al. (2001). The Amblyopia Treatment Index. *Journal of AAPOS, 5,* 250–254.

Cook, C.S., Sulik, K.K., & Wright, K.W. (1995). Embryology. In K.W. Wright (Ed.), *Pediatric ophthalmology and strabismus* (pp. 3–43). St. Louis: Mosby.

Curtis, W.S., & Donlon, E.T. (1984). A ten-year follow-up study of deaf-blind children. *Exceptional Child, 50,* 449–455.

DeCarlo, D.K., & Nowakowski, R. (1999). Causes of visual impairment among students at the Alabama School for the Blind. *Journal of the American Optometric Association, 70,* 647–652.

Dekker, R., & Koole, F.D. (1992). Visually impaired children's visual characteristics and intelligence. *Developmental Medicine and Child Neurology, 34,* 123–133.

Dietz, S.J., & Ferrell, K.A. (1993). Early services for young children with visual impairment: From diagnosis to comprehensive services. *Infants and Young Children, 6,* 68–76.

Dobelle, W.H. (2000). Artificial vision for the blind by connecting a television camera to the visual cortex. *ASAIO Journal, 46,* 3–9.

Dobson, V., Quinn, G.E., Saunders, R.A., et al. (1995). Grating visual acuity in eyes with retinal residua of retinopathy of prematurity. *Archives of Ophthalmology, 113,* 1172–1177.

Education for All Handicapped Children Act of 1975, PL 94-142, 20 U.S.C. §§ 1400 *et seq.*

Ferrell, K. (1998). *Project PRISM: A longitudinal study of developmental patterns of children who are visually im-*

paired (Final report). Greeley: University of Northern Colorado, Division of Special Education.

Ferrell, K.A. (1985). *Reach out and teach: Meeting the training needs of parents of visually and multiply handicapped young children.* New York: American Foundation for the Blind.

Fiedler, A., Best, A., & Bax, M.C.O. (1994). *Clinics in developmental medicine: No. 128. Management of visual impairment in childhood.* New York: Cambridge University Press.

Foster, A., & Johnson, G.J. (1990). Magnitude and causes of blindness in the developing world. *International Ophthalmology, 14,* 135–140.

Fraiberg, S., with the collaboration of Fraiberg, L. (1977). *Insights from the blind: Comparative studies of blind and sighted infants.* New York: Perseus Books Group.

Friendly, D.S. (1993). Development of vision in infants and young children. *Pediatric Clinics of North America, 40,* 693–704.

Fritz, J.P., & Barner, K.E. (1999). Design of a haptic data visualization system for people with visual impairments. *IEEE Transactions on Rehabilitation Engineering, 7,* 372–384.

Good, W.V., & Hoyt, C.S. (1989). Behavioral correlates of poor vision in children. *International Ophthalmology Clinics, 29,* 57–60.

Good, W.V., Jan, J.E., DeSa, L., et al. (1994). Cortical visual impairment in children. *Survey of Ophthalmology, 38,* 251–264.

Gosch, A., Brambring M., Gennat, H., et al. (1997). Longitudinal study of neuropsychological outcome in blind extremely-low-birthweigh children. *Developmental Medicine and Child Neurology, 39,* 295–304.

Gwiazda, J., & Thorn, F. (1999). Development of refraction and strabismus. *Current Opinion in Ophthalmology, 10,* 293–299.

Hameed B., Shyamanur K., Kotecha S., et al. (2004). Trends in the incidence of severe retinopathy of prematurity in a geographically defined population over a 10-year period. *Pediatrics, 113,* 1653–1657.

Harrison, F. (1993). *Living and learning with blind children: A guide for parents and teachers of visually impaired children.* Toronto: University of Toronto Press.

Hartmann, E.E., Dobson, V., Hainline, L., et al. (2000). Preschool vision screening: Summary of a task force report. *Pediatrics, 106,* 1105–1112.

Hatton, D.D. (2001). Model registry of early childhood visual impaired collaborative group: First year results. *Journal of Blindness and Visual Impairments, 95,* 418–433.

Hatton, D.D., Bailey, D.B., Burchinal, J.R., et al. (1997). Developmental growth curves of preschool children with vision impairments. *Child Development, 68,* 788–806.

Holbrook, M.C. (1995). *Children with visual impairments: A parents' guide.* Bethesda, MD: Woodbine House.

Hussain, N., Clive, J., & Bhandari, V. (1999). Current incidence of retinopathy of prematurity, 1989–1997. *Pediatrics, 104,* e26.

Iinuma, K., Lombroso, C.T., & Matsumiya, Y. (1997). Prognostic value of visual evoked potentials (VEP) in infants with inattentiveness. *Electroencephalography and Clinical Neurophysiology, 104,* 165–170.

Individuals with Disabilities Education Improvement Act of 2004, PL 108-446, 20 U.S.C. §§ 1400 *et seq.*

International Committee for the Classification of Retinopathy of Prematurity. (2005). The International Classification of Retinopathy of Prematurity revisited. *Archives of Ophthalmology, 123,* 991–999.

Jackson, A.J., & Saunders, K.J. (1999). The optometric assessment of the visually impaired infant and child. *Ophthalmic and Physiological Optics, 2,* S49–S62.

Jacobson, L., Fernall, E., Broberger, U., et al. (1998). Children with blindness due to retinopathy of prematurity: A population-based study. Perinatal data, neurological and ophthalmological outcome. *Developmental Medicine and Child Neurology, 40,* 155–159.

Jan, J.E. (1991). Head movements of visually impaired children. *Developmental Medicine and Child Neurology, 33,* 645–647.

Jan, J.E., & Freeman, R.D. (1998). Who is a visually impaired child? *Developmental Medicine and Child Neurology, 40,* 65–67.

Jongmans, M.C., Admiraal, R.J., van der Donk, K.P., et al. (2006). CHARGE syndrome: The phenotypic spectrum of mutations in the CHD7 gene. *Journal of Medical Genetics, 43*(4), 306–314.

Khater, T.T., & Koch, D.D. (1998). Pediatric cataracts. *Current Opinion in Ophthalmology, 9,* 26–32.

Lambert, S.R., & Drack, A.V. (1996). Infantile cataracts. *Survey of Ophthalmology, 40,* 427–458.

Lewis, T.L., Maurer, D., & Brent, H.P. (1989). Optokinetic nystagmus in normal and visually deprived children: Implications for cortical development. *Canadian Journal of Psychology, 43,* 121–140.

Mackie, R.T., & McCulloch, D.L. (1995). Assessment of visual acuity in multiply handicapped children. *British Journal of Ophthalmology, 79,* 290–296.

Mercuri, E., Atkinson, L., Braddick, O., et al. (1997). The aetiology of delayed visual maturation: Short review and personal findings in relation to magnetic resonance imaging. *European Journal of Pediatric Neurology, 1,* 31–34.

Mervis, C.A., Yeargin-Allsopp, M., Winter, S., et al. (2000). Aetiology of childhood vision impairment, Metropolitan Atlanta, 1991–93. *Paediatric and Perinatal Epidemiology, 14,* 70–77.

Moller, M.A. (1993). Working with visually impaired children and their families. *Pediatric Clinics of North America, 40,* 881–890.

Moore, B.D. (1994). Pediatric cataracts: Diagnosis and treatment. *Optometry and Vision Science, 71,* 168–173.

Moore, B.D. (1997). *Eye care for infants and young children.* Woburn, MA: Butterworth-Heinemann Medical.

Msall M.E., Phelps D.L., Hardy R.J., et al. (2004). Educational and social competencies at 8 years in children with threshold retinopathy of prematurity in the CRYO-ROP multicenter study. *Pediatrics, 113,* 790–799.

Neely, D.E., & Sprunger, D.T. (1999). Nystagmus. *Current Opinion in Ophthalmology, 11,* 320–326.

Neitz, M., & Neitz, J. (2000). Molecular genetics of color vision and color vision defects. *Archives of Ophthalmology, 118,* 691–700.

Niemann, S., & Jacob, N. (2000). *Helping children who are blind: Family and community support for children with low vision.* Berkeley, CA: Hesperian Foundation.

Ng, E.Y., Connolly, B.P., McNamara, J.A., et al. (2002). A comparison of laser photocoagulation with cryotherapy for threshold retinopathy of prematurity at 10 years: Part 1. Visual function and structural outcome. *Ophthalmology, 109*(5), 928–934.

Olitsky, S.E., & Nelson, L.B. (1998). Common ophthalmologic concerns in infants and children. *Pediatric Clinics of North America, 45,* 993–1012.

Perez-Pereira, M., & Conti-Ramsden, G. (1999). *Language development and social interaction in blind children.* Philadelphia: Psychology Press.

Pogrund, R.L., Fazzi, D.L., & Lampert, J.S. (Eds.). (1992). *Early focus: Working with young blind and visually impaired children and their families* (2nd ed.). New York: American Foundation for the Blind.

Potter, W.S. (1993). Pediatric cataracts. *Pediatric Clinics of North America, 40,* 841–854.

Russell-Eggitt, I., Harris, C.M., & Kriss, A. (1998). Delayed visual maturation: An update. *Developmental Medicine and Child Neurology, 40,* 130–136.

Sadler, T.W. (1990). *Langman's medical embryology* (6th ed.). Philadelphia: Lippincott Williams & Wilkins.

Shauly, Y., Miller, B., & Meyer, E. (1997). Clinical characteristics and long-term postoperative results of esotropia and myopia. *Journal of Pediatric Ophthalmology and Strabismus, 34,* 357–364.

Shoval, S., Borenstein, J., & Koren, Y. (1998). The NavBelt: A computerized travel aid for the blind based on mobile robotics technology. *IEEE Transactions on Biomedical Engineering, 45,* 1376–1386.

Simon, J.W., Calhoun, J.H., & Parks, M.M. (1998). *A child's eyes: A guide to pediatric primary care.* Gainesville, FL: Triad.

Simons, K. (Ed.). (1993). *Early visual development normal and abnormal.* New York: Oxford University Press.

Sonksen, P.M., Petrie, A., & Drew, K.J. (1991). Promotion of visual development of severely visually impaired babies: Evaluation of a developmentally based programme. *Developmental Medicine and Child Neurology, 33,* 320–335.

Steinkuller, P.G., Du, L., Gilbert C., et al. (1999). Childhood blindness. *Journal of AAPOS, 3,* 26–32.

Swenson, A.M. (1999). *Beginning with Braille: Firsthand experiences with a balanced approach to literacy.* New York: American Foundation for the Blind.

Teller, D.Y., McDonald, M., Preston, K., et al. (1986). Assessment of visual acuity in infants and children: The acuity card procedure. *Developmental Medicine and Child Neurology, 28,* 779.

Teplin, S. (1995). Visual impairments in infants and young children. *Infants and Young Children, 8,* 18–51.

von Noorden, G.K. (1996). *Binocular vision and ocular motility* (5th ed.). St. Louis: Mosby.

Warburg, M., Frederiksen, P., & Rattleff, J. (1979). Blindness among 7,720 mentally retarded children in Denmark. *Clinics in Developmental Medicine, 73,* 56–67.

Warren, D.H. (1994). *Blindness and children: An individual differences approach.* New York: Cambridge University Press.

Weleber, R.G., & Palmer, E.A. (1991). Electrophysiological evaluation of children with visual impairment. *Seminars in Ophthalmology, 6,* 161–168.

Wheeler, L.C., Griffin, H.D., Taylor, R.J., et al. (1997). Educational intervention strategies for children with visual impairments with emphasis on retinopathy of prematurity. *Journal of Pediatric Health Care, 11,* 275–279.

Wodrich, D.L. (1997). *Children's psychological testing: A guide for nonpsychologists* (3rd ed.). Baltimore: Paul H. Brookes Publishing Co.

Wright, K.W. (Ed.). (1995). *Pediatric ophthalmology and strabismus.* St. Louis: Mosby-Year Book.

Zambone, A.M. (1989). Serving the young child with visual impairments: An overview of disability impact and intervention needs. *Infants and Young Children, 2,* 11–23.

Zell Sacks, S., Kekelis, L.S., & Gaylord-Ross, R.J. (Eds.). (1992). *The development of social skills by blind and visually impaired students: Exploratory studies and strategies.* New York: American Foundation for the Blind.

12 Hearing

Sounds and Silences

Gilbert R. Herer, Carol A. Knightly, and Annie G. Steinberg

Upon completion of this chapter, the reader will

- Be able to describe the anatomy of the ear
- Know the different types of hearing losses, their causes, and their incidence rates
- Gain an understanding of newborn hearing screening and its outcomes
- Be aware of various hearing tests and their uses
- Understand the treatment options, including cochlear implants, for the child with a hearing loss
- Be able to discuss the educational options and potential outcomes for the child with a hearing loss

The sense of hearing is integral to one of the most fundamental of human activities: the use of language for communication. It is through hearing that children acquire a linguistic system to both transmit and receive information, express thoughts and feelings, learn, and influence the behaviors of their parents and peers. Problems with hearing can negatively affect a child in the areas of language/speech, social-emotional development, and learning in school. Therefore, early identification and intervention for children with hearing problems and their families are imperative. This chapter reviews the human auditory system, hearing loss and its effects on the development of a child's communication skills, and various approaches to treatment and education of children with hearing loss.

The following story illustrates the array of opportunities, needs, and circumstances surrounding a child born with a severe hearing loss. These issues are summarized in Table 12.1.

MATT

Matt, a healthy 8½-pound baby, failed his newborn hearing screening. He was referred for a diagnostic auditory brainstem evoked response test that revealed no measurable responses in his left ear and a mild to severe sensorineural (SN) hearing loss in his right ear. Several interventions were initiated immediately, including taking earmold impressions in preparation for hearing aid use, providing Matt's parents with information about hearing loss, and conducting a medical evaluation to explore the origin of his hearing loss. Ultimately, an intrauterine cytomegalovirus (CMV) infection was identified as the reason for Matt's hearing loss.

At 4 months of age, Matt was fitted with behind-the-ear hearing aids that included an FM system and a wireless microphone for his parents' use. This permitted them to speak directly to Matt from anywhere in a room. Matt, his mother, and his 3-year-old brother (who has normal hearing) were seen for weekly intervention sessions designed to demonstrate auditory and speech-language activities for use at home, share information about hearing/hearing loss, and provide continuing family support. Because CMV is known to cause progressive hearing loss, Matt had repeat audiological evaluations every 3 months.

Matt was enrolled in a public school early intervention program at 14 months of age and received weekly home visits by a speech-language pathologist until age 2, when he was enrolled in a local preschool program. Support services followed Matt and his family to the preschool. At age 3, he lost all hearing in his right ear because of the underlying CMV infection and was deemed an appropriate candidate for a cochlear implant in the right ear. He received the implant 3 months later. Matt entered a general education kindergarten class with his age peers, and he continued receiving support services in speech-language development.

Matt is now 9 years old and just finished the third grade. His language skills are at age level, and his speech is as intelligible and fluent as his age peers. However, Matt still experiences communication difficulties in group situations, including in his classroom. He sometimes misses key words and phrases that provide contextual meaning, and as a result, his responses are sometimes off-topic. Through his parents' advocacy and his school's cooperation, these circumstances are addressed in school through prevention/intervention services of a speech-language pathologist. Matt is a straight A student academically as he now enters the fourth grade.

DEFINING SOUND

When we hear a sound, we are actually processing and interpreting a pattern of vibrating air molecules. An initial vibration sets successive

Table 12.1. Opportunities for and needs of a child born with a severe hearing loss

1. Early detection through universal newborn hearing screening
2. Immediate audiological evaluation to identify the type, configuration, and extent of the hearing loss
3. Use of hearing aids by 4 months of age
4. Comprehensive medical assessment to search for an origin of the hearing loss and possible related medical problems
5. Parent education, support, and advocacy for their child
6. Immediate access to appropriate family-focused intervention based on the child's age and development
7. Frequent hearing, hearing aid, and speech-language assessments
8. Preliteracy experiences
9. Immediate response to any changes in a child's hearing status
10. Vigilance to even subtle communicative needs of a child during the school years
11. Close parent–school collaboration and family-centered programming to meet the unique needs of the child

rows of air molecules into motion in oscillating concentric circles, or waves. This movement of the molecules is described in terms of the **frequency** with which the oscillations occur and the amplitude of the oscillations from the resting point (Figure 12.1).

The frequency of a sound is perceived as **pitch** and is measured in cycles per second, or **hertz (Hz).** The more cycles that occur per second, the higher the frequency, or pitch, of the sound. Middle C on the musical scale is 256 Hz, whereas the ring of a cellular telephone is approximately 2,000 Hz. The human ear can detect frequencies ranging from 20 Hz to 20,000 Hz, but it is most sensitive to sounds in the 500 to 6,000 Hz range, in which most of the sounds of speech occur (Mullin et al., 2003).

The amplitude of the molecular oscillation is perceived as the loudness, or intensity, of the sound and is measured in **decibels (dB).** The softest sound an individual with normal hearing can usually detect is defined as 0 dB hearing level (HL). A whisper is about 20 dB HL, typical conversation is at about 40 dB HL, and a shout close by can be 70 dB HL. A lawn mower or chain saw is measured at about 100 dB HL (Northern & Downs, 2002).

Speech, however, does not occur at a single intensity or frequency. In general, vowel sounds are low frequency in nature and more intense, whereas consonants, particularly the voiceless consonants (e.g., /s/, /sh/, /t/, /th/ as in *thin*, /k/, /p/, /h/), are composed of higher frequencies and are the least intense (Figure 12.2). Furthermore, during a conversation, the speaker will change the intensity of speech by talking in a louder or softer voice to express emotion or emphasis. This circumstance can adversely affect an individual with a hearing loss, especially if the loss is not consistent at all frequencies. If an individual has a high-frequency hearing loss but normal hearing in the low-frequency region, that individual will be able to hear speech (because of the relative loudness of vowels) but may not be able to understand it because of the softness of voiceless consonants. The person may hear only parts of words and therefore would find it difficult to follow a conversation.

THE HEARING SYSTEM

The anatomical mechanism for hearing is a complex system (Jahn & Santos-Sacchi, 2001). It is divided into a peripheral auditory mechanism, which starts at the external ear and ends at the auditory nerve, and a central auditory sys-

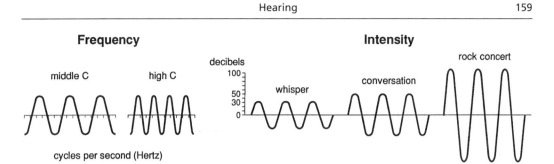

Figure 12.1. Frequency and intensity of sound waves. The frequency of a sound, or its pitch, is expressed as cycles per second, or hertz (Hz). Middle C is 256 Hz; one octave higher (high C) is 512 Hz. Intensity of sound is expressed as decibels (dB) and varies from a whisper at 20 dB to a rock concert at 100 dB or more.

tem, which extends from the auditory nerve to the brain. A disorder in the peripheral system results in a hearing loss, whereas a central auditory problem interferes with the interpretation of what is heard.

The peripheral auditory system is divided into the external, middle, and inner ear. The external ear includes the **auricle** and the ear canal (Figure 12.3). The auricle channels sound into the ear canal and thence to the middle ear. The skin of the ear canal contains glands that produce **cerumen** (ear wax).

At the end of the ear canal lies the eardrum, or tympanic membrane, which separates the external ear from the middle ear. The tympanic membrane is attached to the first of a series of three small bones of the middle ear—the **malleus, incus,** and **stapes**—which are collectively called the ossicles. The end of the ossicular chain, the stapes footplate, is attached by ligaments to the oval window, which serves as the boundary between the middle ear and the bony housing of the inner ear, the cochlea.

The **eustachian tube** is also part of the middle ear. This tube runs from the anterior wall of the middle-ear space down to the **nasopharynx.** The eustachian tube is usually closed but opens during a swallow or yawn, allowing a small amount of air to pass between the nasopharynx and the middle ear to equalize its air pressure with that in the external canal.

When sound waves strike the tympanic membrane, the membrane vibrates and thus sets the ossicular chain into motion. Because the tympanic membrane has a larger surface area than the oval window and because the ossicles act as a lever system, the incoming sound pressure is amplified by about 30 dB.

The inner ear is composed of the **vestibular system** and the **cochlea.** The vestibular system houses the sensory organ of balance, whereas the cochlea houses the sensory organ of hearing (Figure 12.4). The actual end organ of hearing, the organ of Corti, consists of multiple rows of delicate hair cells that are the receptors for the auditory nerve. Three to five rows of outer hair cells and one row of inner hair cells are present along the **organ of Corti.** The cochlea is arranged **tonotopically;** that is, hair cells located at the base of the cochlea, near the **oval window,** respond more specifically to high-frequency sounds (above 2,000 Hz), whereas those in the middle and top respond more to gradually lower-frequency sounds (Figure 12.5). The organ of Corti converts the mechanical energy arriving from the middle ear into electrical energy, or the nerve impulse. As the ossicular chain is set into motion by the vibrating tympanic membrane, the movement is transmitted through the chambers of the cochlea and results in release of neurotransmitters from the hair cells. This generates a nerve impulse that is transmitted via the ascending auditory pathway to the brain. Most of the nerve impulses from the right cochlea cross over to ascend the left central auditory pathway to the left portion of the brain, and vice versa for impulses from the left ear (Figure 12.6). Also, when stimulated, the outer hair cells produce very soft level sounds called otoacoustic emissions (OAEs) that can be measured in the outer ear canal; these are used in newborn hearing screening.

From the inner ear, sound is carried to the auditory cortex in the temporal lobe of the brain. The route from ear to cortex involves at least four neural relay stations (Figure 12.6). The final destination is the auditory cortex, where sound can be associated with other sensory information and memory to permit perception and interpretation. The auditory cortex is not needed to perceive sound, but it is needed to interpret language.

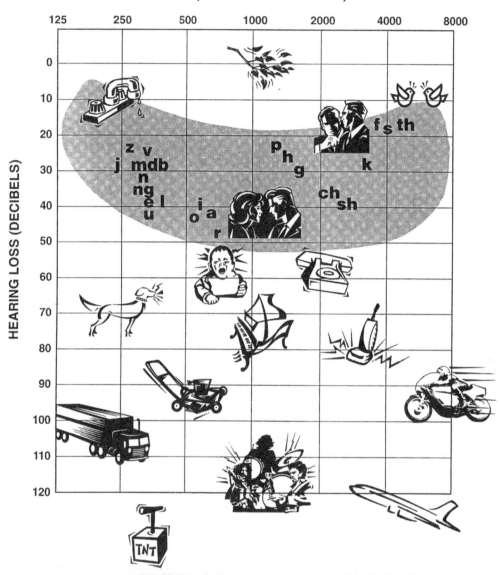

Figure 12.2. Frequency spectrum of familiar sounds plotted on a standard audiogram. The shaded area contains most of the sound elements of speech. (From Northern, J.L., & Downs, M.P. [2002]. Hearing in children [5th ed., p. 18]. Philadelphia: Lippincott, Williams & Wilkins. Copyright © Lippincott Williams & Wilkins; reprinted by permission.)

DEFINING HEARING LOSS

Terms that describe the degree of loss for a person with a bilateral loss (both ears) include *deaf* or *hard of hearing*. The former is often reserved for individuals with profound losses, greater than 70 dB HL. Using hearing aids, children with this degree of loss may hear only the rhythm of speech, their own voice, and environmental sounds (Northern & Downs, 2002).

However, using a cochlear implant, children with this degree of loss can acquire very effective oral speech-language abilities. *Hard of hearing* is a term frequently used for individuals with losses in the better ear of 25–70 dB HL. Children who are hard of hearing benefit greatly from amplification through hearing aids and communicate primarily through spoken language.

Other descriptors of degree of hearing loss are *slight*, *mild*, *moderate*, *severe*, and *profound*.

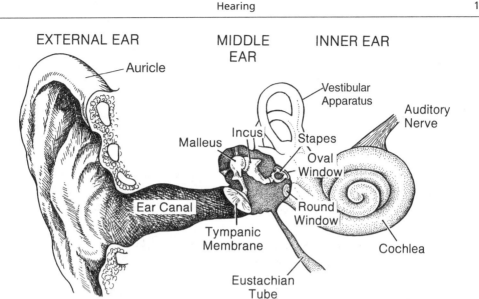

Figure 12.3. Structure of the ear. The middle ear is composed of the tympanic membrane, or eardrum, and the three ear bones: the malleus, the incus, and the stapes. The stapes footplate lies on the oval window, the gateway to the inner ear. The inner ear contains the cochlea and the vestibular (balance) apparatus, collectively called the **labyrinth.**

Each of these terms is often accompanied by specific threshold levels of loss in the frequency region for speech; that is, the average threshold loss for 500 Hz, 1,000 Hz, and 2,000 Hz (see the Degrees of Hearing Loss section for more information). These terms are meant to convey the extent of unilateral loss (loss in one ear) or bilateral loss and are useful in explaining to parents how much of speech their child can expect to hear. Each child's capacities do vary as a consequence of listening circumstances. These descriptive terms, therefore, may only partially explain the listening experiences of a particular child. For example, a child with a mild hearing

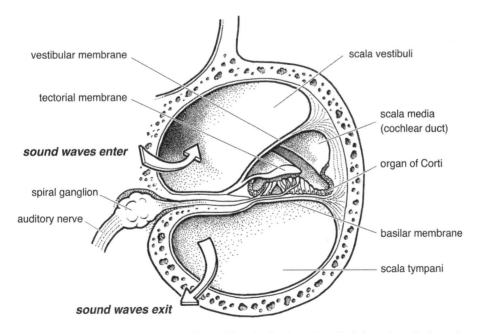

Figure 12.4. The cochlea. Cross-section of the cochlea, showing the scala vestibuli, the scala media, the scala tympani, and the organ of Corti.

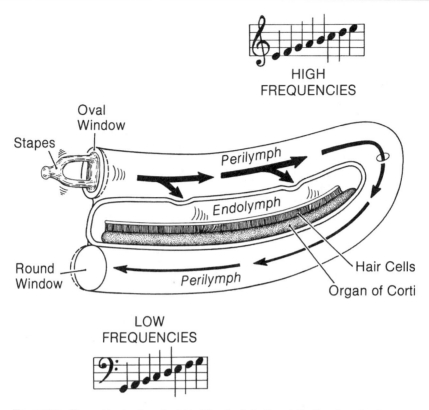

Figure 12.5. The cochlea has been "unfolded" for simplicity. Sound vibrations from the stapes are transmitted as waves in the perilymph. This leads to the displacement of hair cells in the organ of Corti. These hair cells lie above and attach to the auditory nerve, and the impulses generated are fed to the brain. High-frequency sounds stimulate hair cells close to the oval window, whereas low-frequency sounds stimulate the middle and top end of the organ. The sound wave in the perilymph is rapidly dissipated through the round window, and the cochlea is ready to accept a new set of vibrations.

loss in both ears may encounter as much difficulty in listening as a child with a moderate loss.

Types of Hearing Loss

Dysfunction of the external or middle ear causes a conductive hearing loss. If the cochlea or auditory nerve malfunctions, a SN hearing loss results. Occasionally, the term *sensorineural* is broken down further into the terms *sensory hearing loss*, implicating the cochlea, and *neural hearing loss*, implicating the auditory nerve. A mixed hearing loss indicates that there are both conductive and SN components to the loss.

The effect of a hearing loss on speech and language depends on a number of variables, including severity, age at onset, age at discovery, and age at intervention. Hearing losses acquired after language has been well established usually have less of an impact on language and speech skills and later academic achievement than do hearing losses occurring in infancy. However, there is strong evidence that infants identified

prior to 6 months of age and provided with hearing aids along with immediate family-centered intervention demonstrate remarkable language-speech development that can be close to or within normal limits by age 3 years (Yoshinaga-Itano, 2003).

As noted, hearing loss may be unilateral or bilateral. Although it is more subtle, unilateral hearing loss can have an impact on a child's communication, interpersonal relationships, and educational achievement. Progressive hearing losses can be challenging to recognize early and are often associated with genetic factors or syndromes related to hearing loss (Janecke et al., 2002; Kemperman et al., 2004).

Auditory neuropathy/dys-synchrony (AN/AD) is a recently identified auditory disorder that may be present among some children with hearing losses. Children with AN/AD have behavioral hearing test results that reflect substantial loss, as do their interactions with the world of sound, but these children show poor benefit from or dissatisfaction with hearing aid

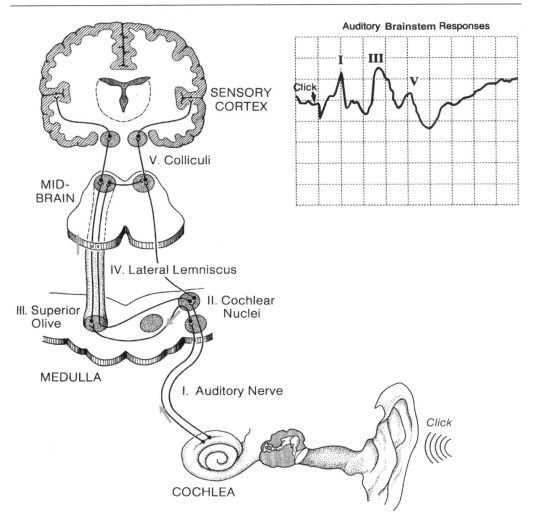

Figure 12.6. The auditory pathway and auditory brainstem responses (ABRs). The auditory nerve carries sounds to the cochlear nuclei in the medullary portion of the brainstem. Here, most impulses cross over to the superior olivary body and then ascend to the opposite inferior colliculus and ultimately the sensory cortex, where the sound is perceived. The function of this pathway can be measured by ABR testing. Each wave corresponds to a higher level of the pathway (denoted by Roman numerals in the pathway and in the reporting of ABRs). Shaded arrows indicate the direction of travel of the nerve impulse along the pathway.

amplification. They are found to have normal outer hair cell function within the cochlea by evoked otoacoustic emissions (EOAE) tests, but auditory brainstem response (ABR) testing shows poor auditory nerve function. The normal outer hair cell results may explain why some children considered to have AN/AD are dissatisfied with amplification (Berlin et al., 2003; Sininger & Starr, 2001; Zeng et al., 2005).

CAUSES OF HEARING LOSS

Hearing losses present at birth are described as congenital, regardless of causation, whereas those that develop after birth are described as acquired. The incidence and prevalence of

hearing loss is discussed in Chapter 16. SN hearing loss in children can occur as a result of hereditary factors, an event or injury in utero, perinatal circumstances, or an occurrence after birth (Smith, Bale, & White, 2005). At least half of SN hearing loss in children is caused by genetic factors (Cohn et al., 1999). For children with SN hearing loss of nongenetic origin, it is estimated that approximately one third have additional disabilities. Nongenetic hearing loss (congenital or acquired) can result from prenatal and postnatal factors related to infections, anoxic brain injury, prematurity, physical trauma, excessively loud noise, or exposure to **ototoxic** agents (e.g., certain antibiotics). Conductive hearing losses can be congenital or acquired. They can result from malformations of the outer or middle ear but are much more often due to middle-ear infections (Northern & Downs, 2002).

Genetic Causes

Genetic factors are responsible for at least half of all children with SN hearing loss (Nance, 2003). In approximately 80% of children with hereditary hearing loss, the hearing loss is inherited as an autosomal recessive trait (see Chapter 1) and is not associated with a syndrome; that is, hearing loss is the child's sole disability. About half of all affected childhood nonsyndromic autosomal recessive hearing losses are caused by mutations in the connexin 26 (Cx26) gene (GJB2/DFNB1) (Nance, 2003). Other hereditary disorders can affect the formation or function of any part of the hearing mechanism (Wolf, Spencer, & Gleason, 2002). Children with syndromic hearing loss have hearing loss as part of a genetic condition with broader physical and developmental manifestations. There are more than 70 documented inherited syndromes associated with deafness, some of which manifest later in life. Table 12.2 describes some of the most common genetic disorders associated with hearing loss.

Cleft palate, in which the roof of the mouth fails to close during embryological de-

velopment, is a malformation with associated conductive hearing loss. It has a multifactorial inheritance pattern and an incidence of about 1 in 1,600–4,000 (Witt & Rapley, 2003). It may occur alone or together with cleft lip. Of children with a cleft palate, 50%–90% are susceptible to significant and persistent middle-ear infections (Sheahan et al., 2003). Because of the absence of closure of the palate, the tensor veli palati muscle does not have a normal mid-line attachment and functions poorly in opening the eustachian tube, predisposing the child to middle-ear involvement (Witt & Rapley, 2003). Close monitoring of hearing in a child with cleft palate is important. Also, surgical **myringotomy** and pressure-equalization tube insertions are often necessary to remediate the middle-ear condition and conductive hearing loss.

Pre-, Peri-, and Postnatal Factors and Prematurity

Environmental exposures to viruses, bacteria, and other toxins such as drugs prior to or following birth can result in SN hearing loss (Roizen, 2003). During delivery or in the newborn period, a number of other complications, such as hypoxia, may cause damage to the hearing mechanism, particularly the cochlea (Morales-Angulo et al., 2004). Neonatal hyperbilirubine-

Table 12.2.   Examples of genetic disorders associated with hearing loss

Syndrome	Inheritance pattern	Type of hearing loss	Other characteristics
Treacher Collins syndrome	Autosomal dominant	Conductive or mixed	Abnormal facial appearance, deformed auricles, defects of ear canal and middle ear
Waardenburg syndrome	Autosomal dominant	Sensorineural, stable	Unusual facial appearance, irises of different colors, white forelock, absent organ of Corti
Bardet-Biedl syndrome	Autosomal recessive	Sensorineural, progressive	Retinitis pigmentosa, intellectual disability, obesity, extra fingers or toes
Usher syndrome	Autosomal recessive	Sensorineural; progressive in type III	Retinitis pigmentosa; central nervous system effects, including vertigo, loss of sense of smell, intellectual disability, epilepsy; half have psychosis
CHARGE association	Autosomal dominant (new mutation)	Mixed, progressive	Eye, gastrointestinal, and other malformations
Down syndrome	Chromosomal	Conductive; occasionally sensorineural	Small auricles, narrow ear canals, high incidence of middle-ear infections
Trisomy 13, trisomy 18	Chromosomal	Sensorineural	Central nervous system malformations
Cleft palate	Multifactorial	Conductive	Cleft lip

Key: CHARGE association: **c**oloboma, congenital **h**eart defect, choanal **a**rtesia, **r**etarded growth and development, **g**enital abnormalities, and **e**ar malformations with or without hearing loss.

mia and intracranial hemorrhage also have been associated with subsequent SN hearing loss. Premature infants, especially those born weighing less than 1,500 grams, have an increased susceptibility to all three of these problems. Children with such histories should have their hearing evaluated as soon as possible, receive intervention services as necessary, and have their hearing tested at least once a year (see Chapters 4 and 9).

Infections

Infections, both intrauterine and those acquired following birth, are common causes of SN hearing loss. If the mother contracts rubella during pregnancy, there is a risk of bearing a child with a hearing loss. Congenital rubella can be prevented by a vaccine, but there are still other infections during pregnancy, including toxoplasmosis, herpes virus, syphilis, and CMV, that may cause severe to profound SN hearing loss. Among these, CMV is the most frequent. It is estimated that congenital CMV is responsible for 40% of SN hearing loss of unknown causes and accounts for essentially all hearing loss previously attributed to all congenital infections taken together (Barbi et al., 2003).

Infections of infancy and childhood also can lead to a SN hearing loss. Bacterial meningitis carries a 7%–14% risk of bilateral hearing loss from damage to the cochlea, predominantly from *Streptococcus pneumoniae* (Koomen et al., 2003). It can cause unilateral SN hearing loss as well (Stevens et al., 2003). It is important to recognize severe bilateral SN loss early, as there is only a small window of opportunity to provide a cochlear implant for some losses, such as those due to meningitis.

Association with Conditions Causing Intellectual Disability

Children with an intellectual disability are at increased risk for hearing loss, especially when a genetic condition is the cause of the disability (see Chapter 17). Children with Down syndrome are particularly prone to conductive hearing loss, with incidences ranging from 38% to 78% (Shott, Joseph, & Heithaus, 2001). Several reports of the results of hearing screenings completed on adolescents and adults participating in Special Olympics sports events suggest that many individuals with intellectual disability have significant, undetected hearing loss (Montgomery et al., 2005; Neumann et al.,

2006). In these studies, 26%–38% of individuals failed screening tests, and a significant proportion of these participants were confirmed to have conductive, SN, or mixed hearing loss.

Middle-Ear Disease

*Otitis media with **effusion*** (OME) is the term used for middle-ear infection with fluid that may be mediated by antibiotics and tympanostomy tubes (see Figure 12.7) or left to resolve by itself. Episodic OME, acute but not chronic in nature, is most common in very young children and can cause slight-to-mild conductive hearing loss. Such losses often go undiagnosed, are transient, and do not affect communicative development and school achievement. A major reason for medical management of chronic OME has been its anticipated deleterious effects upon hearing and consequent problems in communicative development and learning. Children, especially infants and toddlers, with chronic OME (defined as more than six episodes within a 12-month period) were once thought to experience durations of fluctuating hearing that would interfere with speech-language development and learning in school. However, studies have not found a correlation between the duration of OME and speech production skills in otherwise healthy children (Campbell et al., 2003; Paradise et al., 2003). In addition, studies of OME and language development show either no relationship in children

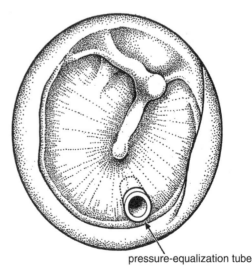

pressure-equalization tube

Figure 12.7.   The procedure of myringotomy and tube placement involves the surgical incision of the tympanic membrane. The effusion is withdrawn, and a plastic tube is then inserted through the opening to permit ongoing drainage of fluid and equilibration of air pressure.

younger than 3 years (Agency for Healthcare Research & Quality, 2002) or only a slight effect when frequency of OME (not hearing loss) is considered (Casby, 2001).

Although the range of conductive loss is large, the average hearing loss for children appears to be mild-minimal (Gravel & Wallace, 2000). A comprehensive review of current knowledge concerning the effects of OME on language and learning in the primary school grades indicates that it does not pose great risks in these areas for typically developing children (Roberts et al., 2004). However, the authors of this review recommended the following reasonable best practices: evaluate the hearing of a child after 3 months of bilateral OME or when a family member or caregiver expresses concern about a child's hearing, screen for OME and hearing loss on a regular basis in special populations of children (including those with intellectual disability, cleft palate, and other conditions that place children at risk for OME), screen a child's language when hearing loss is accompanied by a concern about language development, and encourage families of children with OME to provide an enriched language and literacy environment (Roberts et al., 2004).

Trauma

A blow to the skull, resulting in trauma to the cochlea, may lead to a sudden unilateral SN hearing loss (Ort, Beus, & Isaacson, 2004). Such a blow can also cause damage to the ossicles of the middle ear, resulting in a conductive hearing loss. Sudden, traumatically loud noises also can cause SN hearing losses. Sources of such noise include firecrackers, fireworks, and cap pistols (Segal et al., 2003). Exposure to very loud sounds over time can cause permanent hearing losses in children as well. Examples include using stereo headphones at high-intensity levels; playing in school bands; and attending rock concerts, where noise levels may exceed 100–110 dB (Haller & Montgomery, 2004).

Ototoxic Agents

Certain antibiotics, particularly aminoglycosides (i.e., kanamycin, gentamicin, vancomycin, and tobramycin), used to treat severe bacterial infections in childhood may cause irreversible bilateral SN hearing loss due to damage to the sensory cells within the cochlea. The damage is dose-dependent, and the hearing loss is usually in the high frequencies. It can also be due to ge-

netic predispositions, principally caused by an inherited mutation in the mitochondrial 12S ribosomal RNA gene (Nance, 2003). Chemotherapy drugs such as cisplatin, used to treat cancer, also can cause bilateral moderate to severe high-frequency SN hearing loss. The cumulative dose of cisplatin and the age at treatment are two important risk factors for such loss, with children younger than 5 years at greatest risk (Li, Womer, & Silber, 2004). Children given aminoglycosides or chemotherapy should receive pretreatment audiological testing to establish baseline auditory test results. They should receive frequent posttreatment testing to monitor the effects of treatment on hearing (Bergeron et al., 2005; Berlin et al., 2005; Mitchell et al., 2004).

IDENTIFICATION OF HEARING LOSS

The earliest identification of children with hearing loss in the United States is accomplished through universal newborn hearing screening programs at birthing hospitals (National Institute on Deafness and Other Communication Disorders, 1997; White & Maxon, 2005). All babies in the well-baby nursery are screened for hearing status before hospital discharge, usually within the first 24 hours of life. Babies in a hospital's neonatal intensive care unit (NICU) are screened, too, usually just before being discharged home. The objective, noninvasive electrophysiological procedures of EOAE and/or screening auditory brainstem response (SABR) technologies are used. Infants who do not pass this discharge screening are followed for postdischarge rescreens within several weeks. For those who do not pass the rescreen, audiological diagnostic evaluations are conducted immediately. As of 2006, 39 states mandate hearing screening of newborns before hospital discharge (National Center for Hearing Assessment & Management, 2006). See the Screening for Hearing Loss section for more information.

The importance of early identification of hearing loss soon after birth is analogous to the need for early detection of a vision loss. The brain pathways for both of these senses are immature at birth and develop normally only when stimulated. Evidence indicates that identifying hearing loss and providing intervention (including hearing aids) prior to 6 months of age, regardless of the degree of hearing loss, can lead to typical communicative development at ages from 1 to 5 years (Yoshinaga-Itano, 2003).

Hearing Milestones for Detecting Hearing Loss

The newborn clearly prefers to listen to speech as opposed to other environmental sounds, just as the infant prefers to fixate visually on a face rather than an object. By 2 months of age, the typically developing infant can distinguish vowel from consonant sounds, and by 4 months, the infant shows a preference for speech patterns that have varied rhythm and stress (Northern & Downs, 2002). He or she prefers listening to prolonged discourse rather than to repetitive baby talk. During this early period, an infant with normal hearing can be seen orienting its body toward a familiar sound source from its right or left.

Up to 5 months of age, the speech sounds an infant makes are not influenced by the speech sounds heard. The early vocalizations of infants from different countries sound alike. After 5 months of age, however, the infant's babbling starts to imitate the parents' speech patterns (Kuhl, 2004; Northern & Downs, 2002). Thus, the babbling of an infant with Spanish-speaking parents becomes different from that of an infant with English-speaking parents. For all hearing children, however, listening to spoken language during early life is a critical prerequisite for the typical development of speech. The same can be true for children with hearing loss who, because of detection by newborn hearing screening programs, can get access to spoken language in early life through early intervention services, including hearing aid amplification.

Signs of Hearing Impairment

An early sign of severe hearing loss is a sleeping infant who does not awaken to loud noises. Even an infant who is deaf, however, may react to vibrations, leading family members to assume that he or she has actually heard the sound. Between 3 and 4 months of age, infants who are deaf coo and laugh normally. However, their consonant-vowel babbling, which normally occurs around age 6 months, is often reduced, delayed, or absent. In children with unaffected hearing, babbling becomes more varied and eventually is attached to meanings (e.g., the babble "dadadadada" becomes the word *Dada*). The vocalizations of infants who are deaf show less variety in speech articulation and are less likely to become meaningful and recognizable words, unless the babies have benefited from early identification and intervention. Between the ages of 5 months and 17 months, hearing infants significantly increase their repertoire of consonant sounds; without intervention, their deaf peers demonstrate a reduction in consonant variety, resulting in poor speech intelligibility. It is this failure to develop comprehensible speech that leads parents to suspect a hearing loss, if it has not been identified already.

Receptive language also lags in children with hearing loss. By 4 months of age, the hearing child generally orients his or her head or body toward a parent's voice. The child with a hearing loss may or may not exhibit such sound localization behavior, depending on the severity and configuration of the loss. By 8 to 9 months, a direct head turn (right or left) to locate the parent's voice or a familiar sound can be observed in a baby with typical hearing but not in one with a severe to profound loss. At around 12 months of age, babies receive verbal instructions accompanied by gestures, such as "Wave bye-bye." The deaf child of this age may seem to understand the message because he or she can figure out the command by following gestures and understanding the context. Similarly, a toddler who is deaf may get his or her jacket when others do, whether or not he or she has understood "Get your coat." By about 16 months of age, the hearing child responds to more complex instructions by words alone. The child with an undiagnosed hearing loss, however, may have great difficulty in doing this and may stop following instructions unless they can be inferred from context or are accompanied by gestures. This failure to respond to verbal instructions may lead parents to suspect a hearing loss but also can be misperceived as oppositional behavior. Hearing children with intellectual disabilities also are delayed in achieving these language milestones. These children, however, are similarly delayed in speech, motor, and cognitive skills. The child with hearing impairment without access to early intervention has slow development of speech and language skills but usually has typical development of other abilities.

Screening for Hearing Loss

The vast majority of SN hearing loss in children is present in the newborn period (Herer, 2004). The prevalence rate for well babies is 1.2 per 1,000; it is 3.9 per 1,000 for infants requiring hospitalization in the NICU. This very early presence of permanent hearing loss highlights the need for immediate identification and intervention. Certain risk factors predispose some children to hearing loss in the neonatal period.

Screening for such factors in children's histories was recommended through the mid-1990s as the method of choice for the earliest identification of children with SN losses (Joint Committee on Infant Hearing [JCIH], 1990). However, only half of those with SN hearing losses at birth have identifiable risk-history factors (Herer, 2004). The development of effective electrophysiological hearing screening methods in the early 1990s has enabled the promotion of newborn hearing screening programs that have the potential to identify all infants with hearing loss in the neonatal period.

Early Hearing Detection and Intervention (EHDI) programs aim to screen all well babies and all those from the neonatal intensive care unit (NICU) before hospital discharge. Screening of well newborns usually occurs between 9 hours and 24 hours of life. The hearing screening protocols at birthing hospitals can vary with respect to the use of EOAE and SABR technologies. Many hospitals use EOAE as a first screen. followed by SABR for infants failing the EOAE screen. This protocol can be very efficient, resulting in a 1%–4% referral rate to follow up postdischarge rescreening or diagnostic audiological testing (Hall, Smith, & Popelka, 2004; Herer, 2004). EHDI programs have several positive outcomes, especially when intervention begins before 6 months of age. These include significant language and speech development, social-emotional growth and parental bonding (Yoshinaga-Itano, 2003).

Children with identifiable risk factors may not demonstrate hearing loss at birth but may do so later in childhood. Therefore, it is essential to provide such children with semiannual audiological evaluations through age 3 years to determine their hearing status and to monitor their developmental language milestones, with immediate hearing tests for those suspected of delays (JCIH, 2000). JCIH has identified specific risk factors for hearing loss in neonates. These include

- An illness or condition requiring admission of 48 hours or greater to a NICU

- Stigmata or other findings associated with a genetic syndrome known to include a SN hearing loss and/or conductive hearing loss

- Family history of permanent childhood SN hearing loss

- Craniofacial anomalies, including those with morphologic abnormalities of the pinna and ear canal

- In-utero infection such as CMV, herpes, toxoplasmosis, or rubella

In addition to observing the JCIH guidelines, pediatricians, other primary health care providers, and preschool educators should monitor developmental language milestones and obtain a hearing test for any child whose parents report delays in speech and/or language development. A child's hearing can be tested at any age, even within 24 hours of birth, so parental concern should prompt an immediate referral for audiological testing.

Hearing Tests

Electrophysiological Methods In addition to the screening versions being used in EHDI programs, diagnostic EOAE and ABR measures are part of the battery of audiological tests for infants, toddlers, and young children (Northern & Downs, 2002). They are also very useful in assessing children with developmental disabilities who are unable to respond to conventional behavioral audiometric testing (Berlin et al., 2005; Driscoll et al., 2002).

EOAE measures consist of transient evoked otoacoustic emissions (TEOAE) and distortion product otoacoustic emissions (DPOAE) (Robinette & Glattke, 2002). EOAE testing is ideally suited for use in very young children or those with challenging behavior because results are achieved rapidly and do not require the child's cooperation. A small probe assembly is placed at the edge of the outer ear canal. The probe contains an earphone and a microphone. The EOAE earphone introduces clicks (TEOAE) or tones of various frequencies (DPOAE) into the ear canal that are transmitted to the cochlea. If the cochlea's outer hair cells respond, it transmits signals to the brain. It also directs very low-level sounds back to the outer ear canal. The microphone in the EOAE probe assembly receives these evoked responses from the outer hair cells and transmits them to computer software for analyses. Each ear is tested individually. If there is damage to cochlear structures sufficient to cause a hearing loss of 30 dB or greater, no EOAE responses are obtained. EOAE responses also may not be recorded due to a middle-ear effusion or malformation. Because EOAE testing objectively measures the responses of the inner ear's outer hair cells, the outcome data can help differentiate sensory hearing loss from neural components of SN hearing loss. They also can monitor the status of cochlear function that could be affected by use of ototoxic drugs or by exposure to loud sounds, resulting in progressive hearing loss (Lonsbury-Martin, 2005).

Diagnostic ABR audiometry evaluates both cochlear function and the auditory neural pathway. The ABR method is a highly sensitive test for both hearing loss and neural disruption of the central auditory pathway (Sininger & Cone-Wesson, 2001). ABR procedures involve affixing electroencephalogram (EEG) sensors at various sites on a child's head and presenting sound stimuli to the child through earphones. Click and tone burst stimuli, usually in the 1,000–4,000 Hz frequency range, are used to explore threshold hearing and neural activity in the brainstem pathway. ABR responses are analyzed through computer software. Each ear is evaluated separately as with EOAE testing. Some children require a mild sedative so they will sleep during the ABR procedure. In infants, the ABR waveform is composed of three distinct waves, numbered I, III, and V (Figure 12.6), that represent successively higher levels of the ascending auditory pathway. An absence of waveform at a given intensity suggests a hearing loss, whereas the complete absence of a particular wave suggests an abnormality at a particular location of the brain pathway.

Auditory steady-state response (ASSR) methodology has been added to evoked potential testing and holds great benefits for evaluating the hearing of infants, young children, and others who are difficult to test behaviorally (Cone-Wesson et al., 2002; Picton et al., 2003). This electrophysiological method is capable of contributing refined hearing threshold data in the low-frequency (Hz) region and at very high-stimulus (dB) levels. Such outcomes are a distinct advantage when evaluating children with severe or profound losses for hearing aid use and, in particular, for cochlear implantation (Stueve & O'Rourke, 2003).

Behavioral Hearing Tests The outcome of behavioral tests is regarded as the "gold standard" for judging a child's auditory status and function in everyday life. Behavioral hearing testing is performed to 1) determine if a hearing loss exists, 2) differentiate a conductive hearing loss from a SN hearing loss, 3) determine each ear's degree of loss across a range of test frequencies, and 4) estimate the clarity with which speech can be understood. The methodology and specific techniques must be modified for the developmental age of the child (Northern & Downs, 2002).

Testing Infants up to 8 Months of Age
Both behavioral observation audiometry (BOA) and electrophysiological test methods are used to detect hearing loss in infants up to 8 months of age. BOA relies on subjective observation of a baby's reactions to a variety of sound stimuli in a structured sound environment (Northern & Downs, 2002). Observable responses usually occur to familiar sounds, such as the mother's voice and familiar toys that produce sounds. Starting at 4 months of age, infants begin to locate familiar sounds by turning their head toward the sound source, and this is the response sought when using BOA. This head-turning localization behavior becomes quicker and more precise starting at 6 months of age.

Testing Children with Developmental Ages from 8 Months to 2½ Years As a child's responses to auditory stimuli mature, visual reinforcement audiometry (VRA) can be used to assess hearing sensitivity. VRA provides objective behavioral data in head-turn response to sound stimuli using principles of operant conditioning and control trials. A well-defined VRA test protocol can determine reliable minimum response levels for pure tone, noise, and speech stimuli in each ear using insert earphones for most babies from 8 months of age. These behavioral data can validate the electrophysiological results of EOAE and ABR testing obtained with infants at earlier ages (Jayarajan et al., 2005; Parry et al., 2003).

Testing Children with Developmental Ages Greater than 2½ Years Conditioned play audiometry (CPA) can be used for testing children generally between the ages of 2½ and 4 years (Northern & Downs, 2002). The child usually wears earphones and is conditioned to perform a play task whenever a pure tone or speech stimulus is heard. For example, the child may stack blocks, put rings on a peg, or perform some other motor task in response to hearing the auditory stimulus. By about 4 years of age, the child can respond by pressing a button or raising a hand in response to the stimulus. If conditioning of the child is successful, audiometric results are as complete as those obtained from a mature child or adult (Kemaloglu et al., 2005).

When a child's hearing is assessed via loudspeakers or earphones (i.e., air conduction; Figure 12.8a) and a hearing loss is identified, it is not possible to determine whether the loss is conductive or SN. Therefore, pure tone sounds are presented through a bone conduction vibrator, usually placed on the mastoid bone behind the ear (Figure 12.8b). Whereas air conduction testing involves the contribution of the external, middle, and inner ear, bone conduction testing essentially bypasses the external and middle ear and stimulates the inner ear directly. If the child demonstrates a hearing loss by air conduction but normal hearing by bone conduction, the hearing loss is conductive in nature. Likewise, if the child evidences hearing loss of equal magnitude by air and bone conduction, the hearing loss is SN (Figure 12.9) (Bess & Humes, 2003).

Speech audiometry is another important method for assessing the auditory function of children 2½ years and older. It complements CPA by determining threshold acuity for speech stimuli, which can validate CPA's pure tone threshold results. Speech audiometry methods can also evaluate how well a child understands information at levels above threshold (e.g., at comfortable conversational levels). Such speech testing can provide insights about the effects of a hearing loss on everyday listening/understanding. Test material and methods used in speech audiometry must be consistent with a child's developmental age (i.e., vocabulary age—e.g., use of pictures of test vocabulary). The test material usually is presented to a child through an earphone or loudspeaker without any visual cues (Thibodeau, 2000).

The usual speech audiometry procedures employed with children 2½ years and older include the speech awareness threshold (the lowest level at which speech is detected), the speech reception threshold (the lowest level a child can correctly repeat two-syllable words (e.g., *cupcake*) at least half the time, and supra-threshold word recognition tests (Smoski, 2005).

Assessing Middle-Ear Function

Measurements of the physiological function of a child's middle-ear system contribute significantly to the differential diagnosis of conductive and SN hearing loss and can help monitor the course of middle-ear disease and treatment. To evaluate objectively the function of the middle-ear system, immittance measures (which assess the resistance and compliance of the system) are used. Any significant change to these characteristics of the middle-ear system can affect transmission of sound energy to the cochlea (Lilly, 2005). Immittance tests include **tympanometry** and acoustic reflex measures. Tympanometry examines middle-ear pressure, tympanic membrane compliance, mobility of the ossicles, and eustachian tube function. Acoustic

reflex measurements assess the contraction of the muscle tendon attached to the head of the stapes when a very loud sound enters the cochlea.

In tympanometry, an ear probe presenting a steady-state tone is placed in the ear canal. Varying amounts of air pressure (positive, negative, or atmospheric) are also sent through the probe to the eardrum. A microphone in the probe measures intensity differences of the tone in the ear canal as the air pressure changes. The air pressure–intensity relationships in tympanometry are plotted graphically and can show normal function in the middle-ear system or various problems within it (Figure 12.10). The presence of the acoustic stapedial tendon reflex in a child is strong indication of a healthy middle-ear system, as well as normal functioning of the inner ear hair cells and eighth nerve (Berlin et al., 2005).

Assessing Central Auditory Function

A child's brain receives, analyzes, identifies, stores, recalls, and relates auditory information to make sense of the stimuli/events of the surrounding auditory world. This dynamic process is regarded as among the highest cognitive functions of the human brain. The outcome of this process is readily seen in the rapid evolution of a child's complex speech-language system in early childhood.

For reasons that are currently unclear, some children have problems of auditory processing that are attributed to inadequate functioning of sites within the central auditory neurological system of the brain. The problems most often become apparent as a child approaches school age or enters adolescence. They manifest as difficulties with listening and understanding in noisy conditions, paying attention to or remembering spoken information, following multistep directions, carrying out instructions in a reasonable time frame, understanding language, developing vocabulary, reading (including comprehension), spelling and vocabulary, and low academic performance. Children exhibiting such difficulties are often described as having a central auditory processing disorder (CAPD) but typically have normal threshold hearing and typical intelligence. CAPD, however, is also ascribed to coexist with other conditions such as dyslexia, attention-deficit/hyperactivity disorder, autism spectrum disorders, developmental delay, or specific language impairment.

Testing for suspected CAPD involves presenting special listening tasks to the child that

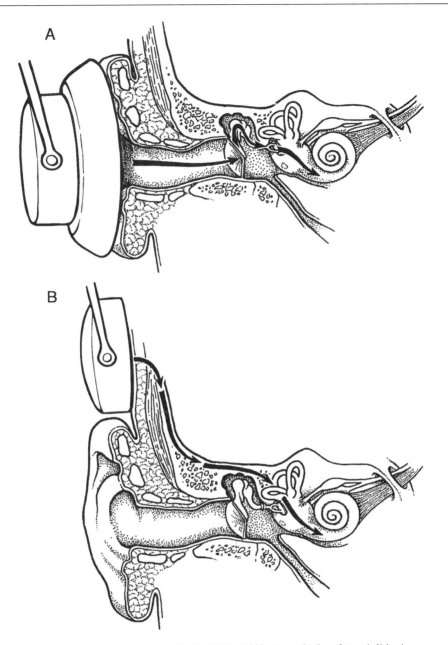

Figure 12.8a &b. Approaches to testing air and mastoid bone conduction of sound. A) In air conduction, the sound comes through the ear canal and middle ear to reach the inner ear. B) In bone conduction, the sound bypasses the external ear and for the most part the middle ear, and then goes directly to the inner ear.

tax the auditory system's ability to understand or integrate auditory information. Most of these behavioral test procedures have normative data for children starting at 7 years of age, as children at this age are capable of participating in the sophisticated listening–responding tasks. Therefore, such CAPD behavioral test procedures are not useful at this time for younger children. Electroacoustic and electro-

physiologic procedures are also used by audiologists to determine possible clues to CAPD in children, including immittance audiometry, EOAE, and ABR tests (Jerger & Musiek, 2000).

Degrees of Hearing Loss

In general, defining the degree of hearing loss is meant to predict the difficulty a child will have

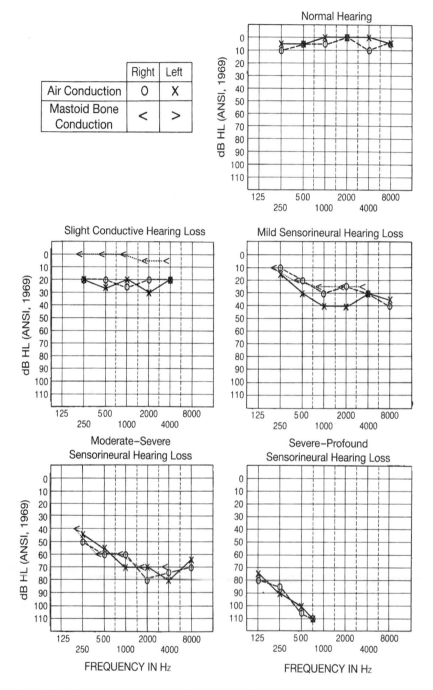

Figure 12.9. Audiograms showing normal hearing and various degrees of hearing loss. Note that in all cases shown, both ears are equally affected. In a conductive hearing loss, bone conduction is found to be better than air conduction because it bypasses the external and the middle ear where the problem exists. In sensorineural hearing loss, bone and air conduction produce similar results because the problem is within the inner ear and/or auditory nerve. The range of hearing loss is as follows: slight, 15–25 dB (decibels) HL (hearing level); mild, 25–30 dB; moderate, 30–50 dB; severe, 50–70 dB; profound, 71 dB HL and greater. (*Key:* ANSI, American National Standards Institute; Hz, hertz.) (Courtesy of Brad Friedrich, Ph.D.)

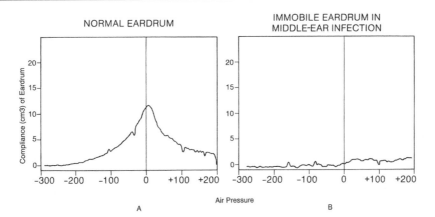

Figure 12.10. Tympanogram. The zero point represents atmospheric air pressure. The positive and negative numbers indicate that positive or negative pressures (relative to atmospheric pressure) have been applied to the eardrum. The compliance values are determined by the intensity of the probe tone at the various pressures and are influenced by the presence or absence of middle-ear pathology. A) A normal tent-shaped tympanogram. B) During otitis media (middle-ear infection), a flattened function may be obtained. (*Key:* cm3, cubic centimeters.) (Courtesy of Brad Friedrich, Ph.D.)

in understanding speech through hearing alone and, therefore, in acquiring language and information through hearing. Some believe that the more severe the bilateral hearing loss, the more the individual is apt to rely on vision for language acquisition and learning; the less severe the loss, the more effective amplification with hearing aids is likely to be. However, these are generalizations. Many variables other than the degree of hearing loss affect the way a child can acquire language, learn information, and progress educationally. These include age of onset, the threshold configuration of the hearing loss, supra-threshold speech understanding, general intelligence, and especially family support. It is therefore not possible to state definitively what language teaching method, intervention strategies, or educational format is appropriate for all children with a specific degree of hearing loss.

Degree of hearing loss is categorized from slight to profound. A slight loss ranges from 15 to 25 dB HL (at 500–2,000 Hz); a mild loss, from 25 to 30 dB HL; a moderate loss, from 30 to 50 dB HL; a severe loss, from 50 to 70 dB HL; and a profound loss, 71 dB HL and greater (Northern & Downs, 2002). As noted, the degree of hearing loss is determined frequently by measuring and averaging the minimum response levels at three test frequencies (500 Hz, 1,000 Hz, and 2,000 Hz). Generalizations of ranges of hearing levels, albeit convenient, often result in misperceptions of the consequences of the loss. For example, a so-called mild bilateral hearing loss has potentially serious implications for the language and emo-

tional development of a preverbal child, whereas a similar loss in an adolescent may have less of an impact. A description of the functional impact of the hearing loss is the best measure of the degree of hearing loss for a specific child and should accompany any interpretation of audiological testing.

A slight loss typically has no significant effect on development, especially if the loss is transitory. A child with a mild bilateral loss typically has difficulty hearing distant sounds or soft speech, missing 25%–40% of speech at typical conversational loudness. The child has difficulty perceiving the unvoiced consonants /s/, /p/, /t/, /k/, /th/ as in *thin*, /f/, and /sh/, which are soft, high-frequency sounds. As a result, the child may miss some of the content of class and home discussions and confuse forms of language that depend on these sounds (e.g., plurals, possessives). Hearing aid use is often a consideration for a child with a permanent mild loss in each ear.

Children with a moderate or severe bilateral hearing loss may hear conversational level speech as a whisper or just detect some sound when people speak. These degrees of loss affect the ability to hear even loud conversation without intervention. If the loss is permanent, hearing aid use is essential. Nonetheless, no assumptions can be made about the vocabulary, speech production, or voice quality of children with these degrees of hearing loss. Speech-language evaluations are essential in identifying these behaviors. Learning problems often result, however, from the significantly reduced auditory input associated with a moderate or severe hearing loss. Academic supports, hearing aids and classroom amplification, speech-language therapy, tutoring, and possibly special education services should be considered, based on the needs of the individual child.

Functionally, a child with a profound bilateral hearing loss may hear very loud environmental sounds nearby without amplification but not speech of typical conversational volume. Even with amplification, certain consonant sounds are likely to be missed. If the loss occurs before 2 years of age, language and speech may not develop spontaneously unless identification/intervention begins prior to 6 months of age (Yoshinaga-Itano, 2003).

Children with profound bilateral losses may receive help from powerful hearing aids to stay in contact with the auditory world. They most often benefit from cochlear implantation that provides significant opportunities for oral language communication. Spoken language, however, is not the sole language option available to children with a profound hearing loss and their families. Visual communication strategies, the most prominent example of which is sign language, can be very important to a child with this degree of loss. Many parents who are deaf opt to raise their child in a signing environment to foster the development of the family's language system. The need for visual communication is not limited to children with profound deafness. Some children with severe losses have enough difficulty in receiving and processing auditory information that they benefit from visual communication as well.

INTERVENTION FOR HEARING LOSS

Parents need to make informed decisions for their child about communication methods, hearing aid use, cochlear implantation, and education. They need to be presented with substantial information from professionals with expertise in these important areas, such as physicians, pediatric audiologists, educators, and speech-language pathologists. Other individuals and groups with knowledge about hearing loss also can be helpful to parents, including organizations concerned with hearing loss, other parents of children with hearing loss, and local school systems.

When a child has a hearing loss ranging from mild to severe, the language and speech choices usually focus on a variety of aural/oral intervention methodologies. When a child has a severe or profound loss, the child's family will want to learn about the sign language methods of learning language, as well as aural/oral methods. Parents need immediate access to complete information about the variety of approaches to communication development and education so that they can make informed choices (Davis, 1999; Li, Bain, & Steinberg, 2003).

Early Intervention

Once the diagnosis of a hearing impairment has been made, the infant or child should be referred for assessment to a multidisciplinary, family-centered comprehensive early intervention program (Moore-Brown & Montgomery, 2001). Hearing loss has been one of the categories listed in early intervention legislation since its inception (Brannen et al., 2000). Regardless of the language approach, the goals for successful intervention include family adaptation to and acceptance of the child's special communication needs and the provision of a linguistically accessible environment at home and school that enhances the child's self-esteem. Optimally, programs should be flexible in their orientation and include family supports and integration with community services. Parent education materials, support groups, and national information centers are now available to assist parents in selecting an appropriate intervention site and a language acquisition strategy.

The regulations for the Individuals with Disabilities Education Improvement Act of 2004 (PL 108-446, IDEA 2004) require that individualized education program (IEP) teams consider the following for a child who is deaf or hard of hearing. As noted in Brannen et al. (2000),

> The language and communication needs, opportunities for direct communications with peers and professional personnel in the child's language and communication mode, academic level and full range of needs, including opportunities for direct instruction in the child's language and communication mode; and whether the child needs assistive technology devices and services. (Appendix A, p. 20)

Amplification

Amplification (e.g., hearing aids, assistive listening devices) is an important part of the services required by the child with hearing loss (Scollie & Seewald, 2001). Hearing aids can be used by children of any age and should be fitted as soon as a persistent or permanent hearing loss has been identified, even if all of the information about the hearing loss is not yet available. Assistive listening devices, such as FM systems, are often used in conjunction with hearing aids in difficult listening situations, such as the classroom (Anderson & Goldstein, 2004). Recent technological advances, however, have produced hearing aids containing FM capabilities that can be used as the primary amplification option. These systems are particularly useful in fitting infants recently identified with hearing losses. A parent can wear a wireless lapel microphone and thus speak to the infant from anywhere in the room, providing constant vocal stimulation typical of parent interaction with an awake infant.

Audiologists are responsible for the appropriate fitting of amplification devices for children. The selection and utilization of amplification for children, particularly preverbal children, differs significantly from the procedures used in adult fittings (Bagatto et al., 2002; Stelmachowicz et al., 2004). First, the selection of hearing aids for a child is an ongoing process that extends far beyond the identification of hearing loss and the initial fitting of an amplification device. Second, the settings of hearing aids are subject to change as new information regarding the hearing loss and responses to amplification are obtained by frequent audiological evaluations of the child. Moreover, the degree of hearing loss is not the only consideration in determining a child's candidacy for amplification. Profiles of the child's existing speech and language skills, intellectual ability, commonly encountered listening situations, and school performance are all important factors in determining the appropriateness of hearing aid use and its specific fitting.

Hearing aids have three components: a microphone that changes the acoustic signal into electrical energy, one or more amplifiers that increase the intensity of the electrical signal, and a receiver that converts the electrical signal back to an amplified acoustical signal. The amplified sound is channeled into the ear canal through an earmold. The hearing aid is powered by a battery, and the loudness of the aid can be adjusted by its volume control. Children's hearing aids also should permit direct audio input to allow coupling to an FM system, should have tamper-resistant battery compartments to prevent swallowing of the batteries, and should have a cover for the volume dial to prevent inadvertent changing of the setting.

Four categories of hearing aids exist: behind-the-ear (BTE) aids, in-the-ear (ITE) canal aids, body aids, and bone conduction aids.

BTE hearing aids (Figure 12.11) accommodate more circuitry and controls, allowing for more fitting flexibility than the much smaller ITE hearing aids. This flexibility is especially important if the child's audiometric information is incomplete or if the possibility of progressive hearing loss exists. Also, as the child's ear canal grows, ear molds can be remade for the BTE aid without having to replace the entire aid, as is necessary with the ITE aid. Programmable hearing aids and those with digital technology permit hearing aid settings to be modified based on listening environments.

Body hearing aids are now used infrequently with children. Bone conduction hearing aids are most helpful with children who have bilateral malformations of the external and/or middle ear accompanied by conductive hearing loss or who have chronic middle-ear drainage into the external ear canal. The latter condition would prevent use of an ITE hearing aid or an earmold with a BTE instrument.

Binaural hearing aids (hearing aids in both ears) are preferred with children, unless there are contraindications to fitting both ears, such as structural abnormalities or the absence of any usable hearing in one ear. Although hearing aids are valuable tools, it is important to understand that hearing aids make speech sounds louder but not always clearer. Also, they do not selectively amplify speech from other sounds. Therefore, when SN hearing loss is present, the child may have difficulty understanding what is said, even when the hearing aids provide speech sounds that are comfortably loud. The child and family must have realistic expectations from amplification and recognize the importance of speech and language education as well as ways to modify the child's listening environment.

Cochlear Implantation for Severe or Profound Sensorineural Hearing Loss

A cochlear implant (CI) is a prosthetic device that electrically stimulates the cochlea via an electrode array surgically implanted in the inner ear. The reasoning behind the use of a CI is that many auditory nerve fibers and the central auditory neurological pathway remain functional even when the sensory hair cells in the cochlea are damaged severely or reduced in number.

The device provides auditory information via five components: a microphone, a signal processor that encodes incoming sounds, a transmitter, a receiver, and the implanted elec-

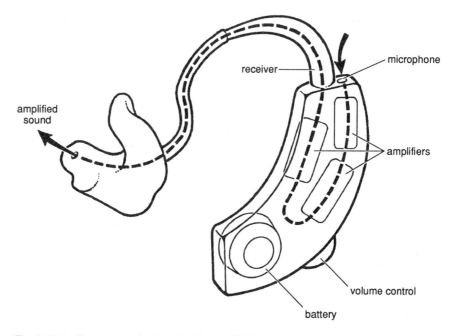

Figure 12.11. The components of a behind-the-ear (BTE) hearing aid. The aid consists of a microphone, a battery power supply, an amplifier, and a receiver that directs the amplified sound through the earmold into the ear canal.

trodes (Figure 12.12). The sound is received by the microphone and sent to the signal processor. The processor is a computer that analyzes and digitizes the sound signal into individually programmed electrical information. This information is sent to the transmitter, located on the skin surface behind the ear. The transmitter sends the coded signals to an implanted receiver just under the skin. The receiver delivers the coded electrical signals to the array of electrodes that has been surgically inserted into the cochlea. These electrodes stimulate auditory nerve fibers at different locations along the cochlea, and sound sensations progress through the central auditory system to the brain.

The scientific literature since 2000 is replete with reports of the positive benefits of multichannel CIs on language, speech, and literacy for children (Anderson et al., 2004; Manrique et al., 2004; Schauwers et al., 2004; Svirsky, Teoh, & Neuburger, 2004). A central theme of these studies is "the earlier, the better." Significant benefits with regard to speech and language development, as well as improved interactions with hearing peers, are noted when implantation occurs before 4 years of age (preferably before 2 years of age). Nevertheless, benefits can accrue for children who receive implants even after 8 years of age (Waltzman,

Roland, & Cohen, 2002). A recent trend is to implant before 2 years of age, as this provides greater benefits than implantation between 2 and 3 years. In addition, increasing numbers of children with good auditory skills before implantation and more residual hearing are receiving implants. Outcome studies also show that children in oral education programs achieve more benefit than children in total communication programs and that younger children make more effective use of oral communication than older children (Osberger et al., 2002).

CIs have been found to be safe in children as young as 7 to 12 months of age, although anesthesia considerations need to be taken into account (Young, 2002). The use of CIs improves central auditory pathway maturation (Sharma et al., 2004). Factors found to predict post-CI speech perception capabilities are the child's cognitive abilities and learning style, short duration of deafness, young age at implantation and family structure/support (Nikolopoulis, Gibbin, & Dyar, 2004). There are no long-term adverse effects of electrical CI stimulation; that is, neither a decrease in CI device performance over time nor deleterious device problems (electrode migration/extrusion) (Waltzman et al., 2002). Post-CI meningitis has occurred in some children and is related to young age at im-

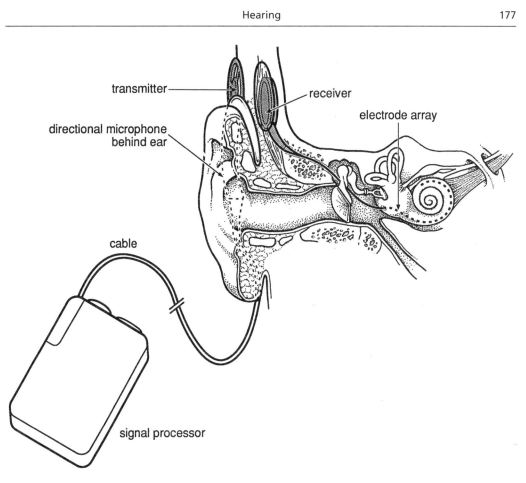

Figure 12.12. Cochlear implant. The device has four components: a microphone to capture sound, a signal processor that electronically encodes the incoming sounds, a receiver, and the electrodes that have been surgically threaded into the cochlea. The electrodes stimulate nerve fibers along the cochlea, and the child perceives sound.

plantation, malformations of the cochlea or temporal bone, and use of a two-electrode system. However, providing prospective CI users with a meningitis vaccination, considering anatomical abnormalities, and not using at-risk electrode arrays should significantly reduce the incidence of meningitis (Cohen, Roland, & Marrinan, 2004). Reimplantation of multichannel devices in children, if necessary, is possible and allows for continued improvement in auditory development (Parisier et al., 2001).

Initial and follow-up programming of a child's CI by an audiologist is critical to the child's successful use of the acoustic features of speech and language. Threshold levels, comfort levels, and the dynamic ranges with the CI do change while using the device (Dawson, Decker, & Psarros, 2004).

Studies of language, literacy, and conversational fluency of children using CIs have identified strengths and needs that frame intervention and educational recommendations. Children with CIs can demonstrate capacities close to their hearing peers in language, reading comprehension, and written accuracy. However, they have been shown to produce fewer words in written narratives and incorrect grammatical structures when creating written and oral sentences. Furthermore, children educated without signs were at a significant advantage in their use of narratives, in the extent of their vocabulary, in the length of utterances, and in the complexity of syntax used in spontaneous language (Geers, Nicholas, & Sedey, 2003; Uchanski & Geers, 2003).

Attitudes of children with CIs and their hearing parents are positive. The families of children using CIs for 4 or more years express a high degree of satisfaction with the results of their use. Parents have a favorable view about the CI's effects on family life and their child's well-being, but their satisfaction with their child's implant is significantly related to the child's speech-language achievements. Children with CIs indicate that they are successfully managing the demands of social and educational activities, regardless of postimplant speech-language capabilities (Nicholas & Geers, 2003). There is some evidence, too, that the Deaf community is becoming more accepting of cochlear implantation, regarding it as one of a continuum of intervention strategies for parents to consider. Deaf parents of some children with CIs have great interest in their children's spoken language development but support the use of signing before and after implantation (Christiansen & Leigh, 2004).

Current research into CI surgical methods and device hardware include studies of bilateral implantation, a totally implantable device, behind-the-ear speech processors and short electrode arrays coupled with hearing aid use (Cohen, 2004). These endeavors, coupled with "the earlier, the better" CI approach, provide an exciting future for children with severe or profound SN hearing losses.

Education and Communication

Education and communication are inextricably linked for the child with a hearing loss because educational curricula are language based. Without adequate language skills, a child who is deaf or hard of hearing is at a functional disadvantage in all academic areas. The goal of educators of the Deaf/Hard of Hearing, speech-language pathologists, educational audiologists, and teachers/special educators should be the facilitation of optimal communication, utilizing whatever is most beneficial for the individual child based on his or her cognitive, attentional, and sensory profile and other related variables, including family preferences (Luetke-Stahlman & Neilson, 2004). The two factors most predictive of the educational achievement of people with deafness are language development and educational opportunities (Kuder, 1997).

To improve communication for a child with hearing loss, education and intervention should focus on developing listening skills and all aspects of language, including syntax and grammar, increasing speech or sign language production, and expanding vocabulary. The educational achievement of students with deafness is weakest in the areas of reading and writing (Kuder, 1997). Good practice specifies that literacy experiences be an intrinsic component of education and intervention and that preliter-

acy experiences must begin with infants and toddlers (Moore-Brown & Montgomery, 2001).

The roles of interventionists will vary depending on the context of the service provision. Some speech-language pathologists, teachers of students who are deaf or hard of hearing, and educational audiologists, for example, work in the classroom alongside a teacher or special educator. Some work in conjunction with preschool programs for children with hearing loss; still others work as independent contractors either in school-linked consultations or as providers of education/therapy sessions at the homes of infants and toddlers. The variety of available services is highly dependent on the children's ages, their degree of hearing loss and communication problems, the extent of their functional hearing, the local and regional educational philosophy, and other factors such as the family's financial resources and commitment to learning a new communication system. Collaborative interventions are the most supportive for families.

Speech-language pathology service models often incorporate a specific type of communication modality, according to the preference of the clinician, center, school, or family. Different language-learning options include oralism, Cued Speech, an English-based sign system, American Sign Language (ASL), total communication, and the bilingual-bicultural approach.

Most hearing children enter public school with the ability to process and integrate spoken information. They have mastered sentence patterns; have a fairly extensive vocabulary; and are ready to read, write, and compute. Children with a hearing loss have the same ability to learn, and they must experience a linguistically rich environment in order to learn (California Department of Education, 2000).

Infants, toddlers, and preschool children with all degrees of hearing loss may have a variety of possible service delivery systems available to them, ranging from home visits by interventionists, to provision of services in a special preschool, to enrollment in a general education preschool with education/therapy services brought to the child in that environment. With the advent of universal newborn hearing screening in birthing hospitals, parents of infants with early identified hearing loss may immediately seek assistance from their school district (Moore-Brown & Montgomery, 2001).

In general, school-age children with mild and moderate to severe hearing losses will be enrolled in general education classrooms in community schools. Consultation and collaboration services from speech-language pathologists, educational audiologists, teachers of children with hearing loss, and other interventionists are brought to the child's classroom. On occasion, the child may leave the general education classroom for individual or small group sessions and may spend part of a day in a special class for intensive small group instruction. Aural/oral language teaching is usually employed as the mode of communication in these learning environments, coupled with the child's use of individually worn hearing aids and/or a classroom FM amplification system.

An infant-toddler program should have the following components: service coordination by a knowledgeable professional, appropriate assessment in all areas of development, design of an individual family service plan (see Chapter 33), assistance with parent–child interactions, modeling and demonstration of speech and language experiences, information to help families decide on communication modes and educational methods, emotional support, direct instruction to the child (if warranted), and transition services to a preschool program beginning at 2½ years of age.

A well-defined preschool program is characterized by a communication-based, developmentally appropriate preschool curriculum and comprehensive services for children 3–5 years of age. Transition planning from preschool to school admission occurs when the child reaches age 5 or 6 (Brannen et al., 2000).

Young school-age children with a severe or profound degree of loss may spend most school days in a special classroom taught by a teacher of children with hearing loss, with other service providers coming into the classroom or taking a child or children out for individualized instruction. This self-contained class may mix with children without hearing losses for some academic subjects or for other school activities. The children grouped in a specific classroom are usually taught exclusively by a specific language method, such as aural/oral, a sign system, or total communication, depending on the method selected by their parents. As children with all degrees of hearing loss (mild to profound) reach middle-school age, they are often included in general education classes with hearing children and receive various types of in-class support, including notetakers and sign interpreters (Montgomery, 1997).

Other school options for children with severe to profound hearing loss include private schools as well as state schools for students who are deaf. Students who are deaf or hard of hearing in elementary and secondary school programs should be provided instruction in the local school district's adopted core curriculum (IDEA 2004; Moore-Brown & Montgomery, 2001). In addition, the students should receive instruction in specialized curriculum areas such as Deaf studies; use of assistive technology, including **teletypewriter (TTY)**/telecommunications devices; ASL; speech and speech reading; auditory training; social skills; and career and vocational education. Content and performance standards in each of these areas must be developed by the education staff. Modifications and accommodations for each curricular area should be addressed at the individualized education program meetings at least yearly. It is important that the students have the full range of activities, including after-class and extracurricular options with appropriate accommodations (e.g., sign language interpreters; closed captioning; C-print, a real-time computer-aided speech-to-text transcription system). Transition from high school to adult life is also a responsibility of the school system (see Chapter 34).

Mandated school services include, but are not limited to, hearing assessment, hearing aid fittings, speech-language therapy, and special education. CIs, however, are not purchased by school districts. IDEA 2004 specifically states that an assistive technology device and related service does not include a medical device that is surgically implanted or the replacement of such a device. In most states, mapping of the CI is not covered either. However, this service may be subject to judicial decision in fair hearing (*Stratham School District v. Beth and David P. IDLER D* 2003).

Language-Learning Options

Various language-learning methods are available to children with severe or profound hearing loss. Aural/oral educational methods emphasize the teaching of listening skills, speech reading, speech articulation and spoken language. Examples of oral approaches include Cued Speech, which utilizes a limited number of hand shapes next to the face to express phonetic sounds with spoken language, and the auditory-verbal method, which emphasizes the training of residual hearing without reliance on visual stimuli (Lim & Simser 2005).

English-oriented sign systems are intended to facilitate the learning of English by combining ASL vocabulary, coined signs, and fingerspelling (letter-for-letter spelling of whole words) in an attempt to represent English sentence structure. Proponents of total communication incorporate aural/oral and manual communication modes, such as listening skills, speech reading, English-oriented signing or ASL, gesture/mime, and anything that facilitates the child's comprehension of what is spoken and/or signed. Advocates of the bilingual-bicultural approach propose that children must first be immersed in ASL so that they have full access to and can acquire the meaningful use of a language before they can attain a less available (spoken) language. ASL has its own unique grammatical patterns and is structurally different from a spoken language, as it is visually received and spatially expressed. Furthermore, ASL is not English in any way; it is a different language within a distinct culture (Seal, 1997).

OUTCOME

A wide range of audiological, familial, linguistic, social, and environmental factors can affect speech development, English literacy, language competence, social development, educational outcomes, and career options in individuals with hearing losses. These factors include age of onset and severity of hearing loss, family response and resources, age of exposure to a language system, psychosocial supports, and the nature of other disabilities or **comorbid** conditions. Formulating a prognosis for the child's ultimate language, educational, and psychosocial development based on any single variable, however, is not possible given the current state of knowledge. Instead, the focus should be on the earliest identification of hearing loss and the prompt access to intervention that is individually tailored, family-centered, and carefully monitored.

SUMMARY

Hearing loss can be temporary or permanent, conductive or SN, congenital or acquired. It can affect one or both ears and may exist alone or with other disabilities. Regardless of the degree or the cause of the hearing loss, it is important for professionals working with children with hearing loss and their families to understand the anatomy and physiology of the hearing mechanism and the impact of the hearing loss on the perception and processing of spoken language. Hearing loss in childhood offers a unique opportunity to witness adaptation to

perceptual impairment and human resilience in the face of a disruption in communication channels. The child's and family's innate strengths, capacities, and vulnerabilities must be viewed within a larger social, linguistic, educational, cultural, and environmental context. Hearing loss does not have to impede typical development, place an individual at a functional disadvantage, or alter ultimate outcomes. Professionals who wish to address the needs of the child with a hearing loss must recognize and make recommendations based on the unique needs of the individual child and family.

REFERENCES

Agency for Healthcare Research and Quality. (2002). *Diagnosis, natural history, and late effects of otitis media with effusion* [Summary, Evidence Report/Technology Assessment: Number 55; AHRQ Publication Number 02-E026]. Retrieved December 5, 2006, from http://www.ahrq.gov/clinic/epcsums/otdiagsum.htm

American National Standards Institute. (1969). *Specifications for audiometers* (ANSI S3.6–1969). New York: Author.

Anderson, I., Weichbold, V., D'Haese, P., et al. (2004). Cochlear implantation in children under the age of two: What do the outcomes show us? *International Journal of Pediatric Otorhinolaryngology, 68*, 425–431.

Anderson, K., & Goldstein, H. (2004). Speech perception benefits of FM and infrared devices to children with hearing aids in a typical classroom. *Language, Speech, and Hearing Services in Schools, 35*, 169–184.

Bagatto, M., Scollie, S., Seewald R., et al. (2002). Real-ear-to-coupler difference predictions as a function of age for two coupling procedures. *Journal of the American Academy of Audiology, 13*, 407–415.

Barbi, M., Binda, S., Caroppo, S., et al. (2003). A wider role for congenital cytomegalovirus infection in SN hearing loss. *Pediatric Infectious Disease Journal, 22*, 39–42.

Bergeron, C., Dubourg, L., Chastagner, P., et al. (2005). Long-term renal and hearing toxicity of carboplatin in infants treated for localized and unresectable neuroblastoma: Results of the SFOP NBL90 study. *Pediatric Blood & Cancer, 45*, 32–36.

Berlin, C., Hood, L., Morlet, T., et al. (2003). Auditory neuropathy/dys-synchrony: Diagnosis and management. *Mental Retardation and Developmental Disabilities Research Reviews, 9*, 225–231.

Berlin, C., Hood, L., Morlet, T., et al. (2005). The battery principle re-visited physiologically, with special attention to auditory neuropathy and Cued Speech. *Perspectives on Hearing and Hearing Disorders in Childhood (ASHA Division 9), 15*, 5–9.

Bess, F., & Humes, L. (2003). *Audiology: The fundamentals* (3rd ed.). Philadelphia: Lippincott, Williams & Wilkins.

Brannen, S.J., Cooper, E.B., Dellegrotto, J.T., et al. (2000). *Developing educationally relevant IEPs: A technical assistance document for speech-language pathologists.* Rockville, MD: American Speech-Language-Hearing Association.

California Department of Education. (2000). *Guidelines for program standards for deaf and hard of hearing.* Sacramento: Author.

Campbell, T., Dollaghan, C., Rockette, H., et al. (2003). Risk factors for speech delay of unknown origin in 3-year-old children. *Child Development, 74,* 346–357.

Casby, M. (2001). Otitis media and language development: A meta-analysis. *American Journal of Speech-Language Pathology, 10,* 65–80.

Christiansen, J., & Leigh, I. (2004). Children with CIs: Changing parent and deaf community perspectives. *Archives of Otolaryngology-Head and Neck Surgery, 130,* 673–677.

Cohen, N. (2004). CI candidacy and surgical considerations. *Audiology & Neuro-otology, 9,* 197–202.

Cohen, N., Roland, J., & Marrinan, M. (2004). Meningitis in cochlear implant recipients: The North American experience. *Otology and Neurotology, 25,* 275–281.

Cohn, L.S., Kelley, P.M., Fowler, T.W., et al. (1999). Clinical studies of families with hearing loss attributable to mutations in the connexin 26 gene (GJB2/DFNB1). *Pediatrics, 103,* 546–550.

Cone-Wesson, B., Dowell, R., Tomlin, D., et al. (2002). The steady-state response: Comparisons with the auditory brainstem response. *Journal of the American Academy of Audiology, 13,* 173–187.

Davis, A. (1999, November). *A report of parental expectations upon being informed their child has a permanent hearing loss.* Paper presented at the annual convention of the American Speech-Language-Hearing Association, San Francisco.

Dawson, P., Decker, J., & Psarros C. (2004). Optimizing dynamic range in children using the nucleus cochlear implant. *Ear and Hearing, 25,* 230–241.

Driscoll, C., Kei, J., Bates, D., et al. (2002). Transient evoked otoacoustic emissions in children studying in special schools. *International Journal of Pediatric Otorhinolaryngology, 64,* 51–60.

Geers, A., Nicholas, J., & Sedey, A. (2003). Language skills of children with early cochlear implantation. *Ear and Hearing, 24*(1, Suppl.), 46S–58S.

Gravel, J.S., & Wallace, I. (2000). Effects of otitis media with effusion on hearing in the first three years of life. *Journal of Speech, Language and Hearing Research, 43,* 631–644.

Hall, J., III, Smith, S., & Popelka, G. (2004). Newborn hearing screening with combined otoacoustic emissions and auditory brainstem responses. *Journal of the American Academy of Audiology, 15,* 414–425.

Haller, A., & Montgomery, J. (2004). Noise-induced hearing loss in children: What educators need to know. *Teaching Exceptional Children, 36,* 22–27.

Herer, G.R. (2004, September). *Universal newborn hearing screening: Successful seven year outcomes for 47,920 newborns.* Unpublished data reported at the meeting of the XXVII International Congress of Audiology, Phoenix.

Individuals with Disabilities Education Improvement Act of 2004, PL 108-446, 20 U.S.C. §§ 1400 *et seq.*

Jahn, A., & Santos-Sacchi, J. (Eds.). (2001). *Physiology of the ear* (2nd ed.). San Diego: Singular Publishing Group.

Janecke, A., Hirst-Stadlmann, A., Gunther, B., et al. (2002). Progressive hearing loss, and recurrent sudden SN hearing loss associated with GJB2 mutations—phenotypic spectrum and frequencies of GJB2 mutations in Austria. *Human Genetics, 111,* 145–153.

Jayarajan, V., Nandi, R., & Caldicott, B. (2005). An innovation in insert visual reinforcement audiometry in children. *Journal of Laryngology and Otology, 119,* 132–133.

Jerger, J., & Musiek, F. (2000). Report of the consensus conference on the diagnosis of auditory processing disorders in school-age children. *Journal of the American Academy of Audiology, 11,* 467–474.

Joint Committee on Infant Hearing. (1990). *Joint Committee on Infant Hearing Position Statement 1990.* Retrieved December 5, 2006, from http://www.jcih.org/JCIH1990.pdf

Joint Committee on Infant Hearing. (2000). Year 2000 position statement: Principles and guidelines for early hearing detection and intervention programs. *Pediatrics, 106,* 798–817.

Kemaloglu, Y., Gunduz, B., Gokmen, S., et al. (2005). Pure tone audiometry in children. *International Journal of Pediatric Otorhinolaryngology, 69,* 209–214.

Kemperman, M., Koch, S., Kumar, S., et al. (2004). Evidence of progression and fluctuation of hearing impairment in branchio-oto-renal syndrome. *International Journal of Audiology, 43,* 523–532.

King, A., Parsons, C., & Moore, D. (2000). Plasticity in neural coding of auditory space in the mammalian brain. *Proceedings of the National Academy of Sciences of the United States of America, 97,* 11821–11828.

Koomen, L., Grobbee, D., Roord, J., et al. (2003). Hearing loss at school age in survivors of bacterial meningitis: Assessment, incidence, and prediction. *Pediatrics, 112,* 1049–1053.

Kuder, S.J. (1997). *Teaching students with language and communication disabilities.* Boston: Allyn & Bacon.

Kuhl, P. (2004). Early language acquisition: Cracking the speech code. *Nature Reviews Neuroscience, 5,* 831–843.

Li, Y., Bain, L., & Steinberg, A. (2003). Parental decision making and the choice of communication modality for the child who is deaf. *Archives of Pediatrics & Adolescent Medicine, 157,* 162–168.

Li, Y., Womer, R., & Silber, J. (2004). Predicting cisplatin ototoxicity in children: The influence of age and the cumulative dose. *European Journal of Cancer, 40,* 2445–2451.

Lilly, D. (2005). The evolution of aural acoustic-immittance measurements. *The ASHA Leader, 6,* 24.

Lim, S., & Simser, J. (2005). Auditory-verbal therapy for children with hearing impairment. *Annals Academy of Medicine Singapore, 34,* 307–312.

Lonsbury-Martin, B. (2005). Otoacoustic emissions: Where are we today. *The ASHA Leader, 19,* 6–7.

Luetke-Stahlman, B., & Nielson, D. (2004). *Deaf students can be great readers.* Los Alamitos: Modern Signs Press.

Manrique, M., Cervera-Paz, F., Huarte, A., et al. (2004). Prospective long-term auditory results of cochlear implantation in prelinguistically deafened children: The importance of early implantation. *Acta Oto-laryngologica. Supplementum, 552,* 55–63.

Mitchell, C., Ellingson, R., Henry, J., et al. (2004). Use of auditory brainstem responses for the early detection of ototoxicity from aminoglycosides or chemotherapeutic drugs. *Journal of Rehabilitation Research and Development, 41,* 373–383.

Montgomery, J., Herer, G., Glattke, T., et al. (2005, April). *Hearing loss, mental retardation or both.* Poster Session presented at the annual meeting of the American Academy of Audiology, Washington, DC.

Montgomery, J.K. (1997). Inclusion in the secondary school. In L. Power-deFur & F.P. Orelove (Eds.), *Inclusive education: Practical implementation of the least restrictive environment* (pp. 181–192). Gaithersburg, MD: Aspen Publications.

Moore-Brown, B.J., & Montgomery, J.K. (2001). *Making a difference for America's children: Speech-language pathologists in public schools.* Eau Claire, WI: Thinking Publications.

Morales-Angulo, C., Gallo-Teran, J., Azuara, N., et al. (2004). Etiology of severe/profound, pre/perilingual bilateral hearing loss in Cantabria (Spain). *Acto Otorrhinolaryngologica Espana, 55,* 351–355.

Mullin, W., Gerace, W., Mestre, J., et al. (2003). *Fundamentals of sound with applications to speech and hearing.* Boston: Allyn & Bacon.

Nance, W. (2003). The genetics of deafness. *Mental Retardation and Developmental Disabilities Research Reviews, 9,* 109–119.

National Center for Hearing Assessment & Management. (2006). *Enacted state newborn hearing screening legislation.* Retrieved December 20, 2006, from http://www .infanthearing.org/legislative/summary/index.html

National Institute on Deafness and Other Communication Disorders. (1997). *Recommendations of NIDCD Working Group on early identification of hearing impairment on acceptable protocols for use in state-wide universal newborn screening programs.* Bethesda, MD: NIDCD Clearinghouse.

Neumann, K., Dettmer, G., Euler, H., et al. (2006). Auditory status of persons with intellectual disability at the German Special Olympic games. *International Journal of Audiology, 45,* 83–90.

Nicholas, J., & Geers, A. (2003). Personal, social, and family adjustment in school-age children with a cochlear implant. *Ear and Hearing, 24*(1, Suppl.), 69S–81S.

Nikolopoulos, T., Gibbin, K., & Dyar, D. (2004). Predicting speech perception outcomes following cochlear implantation using Nottingham children's implant profile (NChIP). *International Journal of Pediatric Otorhinolaryngology, 68,* 137–141.

Northern, J.L., & Downs, M.P. (2002). *Hearing in children* (5th ed.). Philadelphia: Lippincott, Williams & Wilkins.

Ort, S., Beus, K., & Isaacson, J. (2004). Pediatric temporal bone fractures in a rural population. *Otolarygology—Head and Neck Surgery, 131,* 433–437.

Osberger, M., Zimmerman-Phillips, S., & Koch, D. (2002). Cochlear implant candidacy and performance trends in children. *Annals of Otology, Rhinology, & Laryngology, 189* (Suppl.), 62–65.

Paradise, J., Dollaghan, C., Campbell, T., et al. (2003). Otitis media and tympanostomy tube insertion during the first three years of life: Developmental outcomes at age four years. *Pediatrics, 112,* 265–277.

Parisier, S., Chute, P., Popp, A., et al. (2001). Outcome analysis of cochlear implant reimplantation in children. *Laryngoscope, 111,* 26–32.

Parry, G., Hacking, C., Bamford, J., et al. (2003). Minimal response levels for visual reinforcement audiometry in infants. *International Journal of Audiology, 42,* 413–417.

Picton, T., John, M., Dimitrijevic, A., et al. (2003). Human auditory steady-state response. *International Journal of Audiology, 42,* 177–219.

Roberts, J., Hunter, L., Gravel, J., et al. (2004). Otitis media, hearing loss, and language learning: Controversies and current research. *Journal of Developmental and Behavioral Pediatrics, 25,* 110–122.

Robinette, M., & Glattke, T. (Eds.). (2002). *Otoacoustic emissions: Clinical applications* (2nd ed.). New York: Thieme.

Roizen, N. (2003). Nongenetic causes of hearing loss. *Mental Retardation and Developmental Disabilities Research Reviews, 9,* 120–127.

Schauwers, K., Gillis, S., Daemers, K., et al. (2004). Cochlear implantation between 5 and 20 months of age: The onset of babbling and the audiologic outcome. *Otology and Neurotology, 25,* 263–270.

Scollie, S., & Seewald, R. (2001). Hearing aid selection and verification in children. In J. Katz (Ed.), *Handbook of clinical audiology* (pp. 687–706). Philadelphia: Lippincott, Williams & Wilkins.

Seal, B.C. (1997). Educating students who are deaf and hard of hearing. In L. Power-deFur & F.P. Orelove (Eds.), *Inclusive education: Practical implementation of the least restrictive environment* (pp. 259–271). Gaithersburg, MD: Aspen Publishers.

Segal, S., Eviatar, E., Lapinsky, J., et al. (2003). Inner ear damage in children due to noise exposure from cap pistols and firecrackers: A retrospective review of 53 cases. *Noise Health, 5,* 13–18.

Sharma, A., Tobey, E., Dorman, M., et al. (2004). Central auditory maturation and babbling development in infants with cochlear implants. *Archives of Otolaryngology—Head and Neck Surgery, 130,* 511–516.

Sheahan, P., Miller, I., Sheahan, J., et al. (2003). Incidence and outcome of middle ear disease in cleft lip and/or cleft palate. *International Journal of Pediatric Otorhinolaryngology, 67,* 785–793.

Shott, S., Joseph, A., & Heithaus, D. (2001). Hearing loss in children with Down Syndrome. *International Journal of Pediatric Otorhinolaryngology, 61,* 199–205.

Sininger, Y., & Cone-Wesson, B. (2001). Threshold prediction using auditory brainstem response and steady-state evoked potentials with infants and young children. In J. Katz (Ed.), *Handbook of clinical audiology* (pp. 298–322). Philadelphia: Lippincott Williams & Wilkins.

Sininger, Y., & Starr, A. (Eds.). (2001). *Auditory neuropathy: a new perspective on hearing disorders.* San Diego: Singular Publishing Group.

Smith, R., Bale, J.J., & White, K. (2005). SN hearing loss in children. *The Lancet, 365*(9462), 879–890.

Smoski, W.J. (2005). *Speech audiometry.* Retrieved April 30, 2005, from http://www.emedicine.com/ent/topic 371.htm

Stelmachowicz, P., Pittman, A., Hoover, B., et al. (2004). The importance of high-frequency audibility in the speech and language development of children with hearing loss. *Archives of Otolaryngology-Head and Neck Surgery, 130,* 556–562.

Stevens, J., Eames, M., Kent, A., et al. (2003). Long term outcome of neonatal meningitis. *Archives of Disease in Childhood Fetal and Neonatal Edition, 88,* 179–184.

Stratham School District v. Beth and David P. IDLER D, N.H. 2003. U.S. District Court, New Hampshire.

Stueve, M., & O'Rourke, C. (2003). Estimation of hearing loss in children: Comparison of auditory steady-state response, auditory brainstem response, and behavioral test methods. *American Journal of Audiology, 12,* 125–136.

Svirsky, M., Teoh, S., & Neuburger H. (2004). Development of language and speech perception in congenitally, profoundly deaf children as a function of age at cochlear implantation. *Audiology & Neuro-otology, 9,* 224–233.

Thibodeau, L. (2000). Speech audiometry. In R. Roeser, M. Valente, & H. Hosford-Dunn (Eds.), *Audiology: Diagnosis.* New York: Thieme.

Uchanski, R., & Geers, A. (2003). Acoustic characteristics of the speech of young cochlear implant users: A comparison with normal-hearing age-mates. *Ear and Hearing, 24*(1, Suppl.), 90S–105S.

Waltzman, S., Cohen, N., Green, J., et al. (2002). Long-term effects of cochlear implants in children. *Otolaryngology—Head and Neck Surgery, 126*, 505–511.

Waltzman, S., Roland, J., & Cohen, N. (2002). Delayed implantation in congenitally deaf children and adults. *Otology and Neurotology, 23*, 333–340.

White, K., & Maxon, A. (2005). *Early identification of hearing loss: Universal newborn hearing screening (an implementation guide).* Retrieved May 29, 2005, http://www.infanthearing.org/impguide/index.html

Witt, P., & Rapley, J. (2003). *Craniofacial, cleft palate.* Retrieved May 9, 2005, from http://www.emedicine.com/plastic/contents.htm

Wolf, B., Spencer, R., & Gleason, T. (2002). Hearing loss is a common feature of symptomatic children with profound biotinidase deficiency. *The Journal of Pediatrics, 140*, 242–246.

Yoshinaga-Itano, C. (2003). Early intervention after universal neonatal hearing screening: Impact on outcomes. *Mental Retardation and Developmental Disabilities Research Reviews, 8*, 252–266.

Young, N. (2002). Infant cochlear implantation and anesthetic risk. *Annals of Otology, Rhinology, & Laryngology, 189* (Suppl.), 49–51.

Zeng, F., Kong, Y., Michalewski, H., & Starr, A. (2005). Perceptual consequences of disrupted auditory nerve activity. *Journal of Neurophysiology, 93*, 3050–3063.

13 The Brain and Nervous System

Amanda L. Yaun and Robert Keating

Upon completion of this chapter, the reader will

- Understand the anatomy of the brain and the function and interaction of its parts
- Be knowledgeable about the function of the peripheral nervous system and the autonomic nervous system
- Be aware of the structure and function of the neuron, the functional unit of the central nervous system
- Be able to describe the origin and function of cerebrospinal fluid and its associated blockage in hydrocephalus
- Be aware of current and future trends in evaluating the nervous system

Long viewed as an incredibly complex computer, the central nervous system (CNS) is considerably more complicated than any machine made to date (Tanaka & Gleeson, 2000). Each component of the nervous system controls some aspect of behavior and affects our interaction with the world around us. An impairment in any part of this system makes us less able to adapt to the environment and can lead to disorders as diverse as intellectual disability, learning disabilities, autism spectrum disorders (ASDs), cerebral palsy, meningomyelocele, and epilepsy (Lequin & Barkovich, 1999). This chapter provides an overview of the interrelationships between the individual elements of the CNS. It also illustrates examples of CNS dysfunction and its effects on the child.

THE BRAIN AND SPINAL CORD

The brain and the spinal cord comprise the mature CNS and have six main structures: the cerebral hemispheres, basal ganglia, thalamus, brainstem, cerebellum, and spinal cord (Crossman & Neary, 2000; Goldberg, 2000).

The Cerebral Hemispheres

During embryonic development, the primitive precursor to the CNS, the neural tube, develops three bulges that form the main components of the brain (see Chapter 2). The forward-most bulge, called the prosencephalon, gives rise to the left and right cerebral hemispheres. Each hemisphere consists of an outer cerebral cortex (where most neurons, or brain cells, are located), subcortical white matter (where the "wiring" of the brain is located), and deep masses of gray matter (containing specialized groupings of neurons), collectively called the basal ganglia. Within each hemisphere is a fluid-filled cavity called the lateral ventricle. The hemispheres are joined together by a band of fibers called the **corpus callosum** that permits the exchange of information between the two hemispheres (Figure 13.1a–b). Various conditions may lead to partial formation of the corpus callosum or, in more severe cases, complete failure resulting in agenesis (lack of development) of the corpus callosum. The importance of this exchange is emphasized by the results of a surgical procedure called a **corpus**

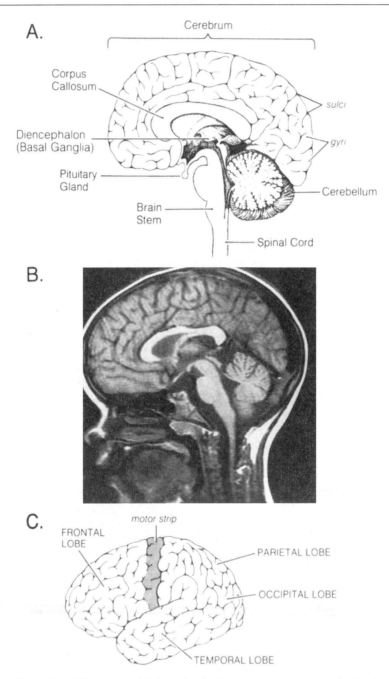

Figure 13.1. A) Lateral view of the brain showing the component elements: cerebral hemispheres, diencephalon, cerebellum, brainstem, and spinal cord. B) Lateral view of brain by magnetic resonance imaging (MRI) scan. Note the excellent reproduction of the structures of the brain. C) Side view of the left hemisphere. The cortex is divided into four lobes: frontal, parietal, temporal, and occipital. The motor strip, lying at the back of the frontal lobe, is highlighted. It initiates voluntary movement and is damaged in **spastic** cerebral palsy.

callosotomy. In this operation, a portion of the corpus callosum is cut in an attempt to control a severe seizure disorder (McInerney et al., 1999; Shimizu 2005; Shimizu & Maehara, 2000). It has proven quite effective in decreasing the spread of seizure activity, but in some adults has resulted in a decline in language and visual-perceptual skills and in manual dexterity (Funnell, Corballis, & Gazzaniga, 1999). This is presumed to occur because the operation interferes with interhemispheric exchange of information (see Chapter 29; Sorenson et al., 1997).

During early fetal life, the surface of the cerebral hemisphere is smooth. As the complexity of the brain increases during the third trimester, involutions called fissures and **sulci** appear. Fissures, which are deeper than sulci, are visible earlier during development and separate each hemisphere into four functional areas or lobes. The frontal lobe occupies the front, or anterior, third of the hemisphere; the parietal lobe sits in the middle-upper part of the hemisphere; the temporal lobe is in the lower-middle region; and the occipital lobe takes up the back, or posterior, quarter of each hemisphere (Figure13.1c). The sulci are smaller involutions within each lobe and the regions between the sulci are called convolutions, or **gyri.** Some gyri show little variation in location and contour from one person to another, whereas others show considerable variability.

The surface of the cerebral hemisphere is called the cortex and is composed principally of nerve cell bodies. Below this gray matter lie the nerve fibers (axons), or white matter. The cerebral cortex initiates motion and thought processes, as well as processes sensory input. Each cortical lobe is responsible for particular activities and functions.

The Frontal Lobe   The frontal lobe controls both voluntary motor activity and important aspects of cognition (Brodal, 1998). Within the frontal lobe the different areas of the body are represented topographically along a strip called the primary motor cortex. The tongue and larynx, or voice box, are controlled from the lowest point, followed in an upward sequence by the face, hand, arm, trunk, thigh, and foot (Figure 13.2). The tongue, larynx, and hand occupy a particularly large area along this strip due to the complexity of speech and fine motor activity.

A nerve impulse initiated in the motor strip passes down the **pyramidal (corticospinal) tract** that connects the cortex with the spinal cord. Reaching the spinal cord, the impulse passes across a synapse to an anterior horn cell. This neuron relays the transmission via its axon to a peripheral nerve that connects to an appropriate muscle. The muscle subsequently contracts in response to the original signal from the motor cortex. In **spinal muscular atrophy** of childhood (Werknig-Hoffmann disease), the motor neurons die, resulting in hypotonia (low muscle tone or "looseness" of the muscle) and weakness (see Chapter 14; Andersson & Rando, 1999; Cole & Siddique, 1999; Talbot, 1999).

Conversely, if there is damage to either the motor cortex or the pyramidal tract, increased tone in the form of spasticity results. In spasticity, the underlying involuntary muscle contractions controlled by the brainstem and spinal cord are no longer inhibited by pyramidal tract activity. As a result, voluntary movement becomes less fluid, as is seen in cerebral palsy and other movement disorders (see Chapter 26). Therapeutic approaches to spasticity include measures that manipulate neurotransmitters to reduce tone. For example, the drug baclofen, which increases the activity of GABA, an inhibitory neurotransmitter, has been adminis-

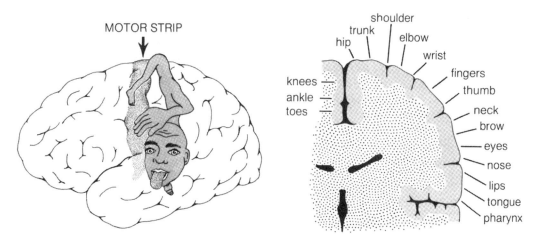

Figure 13.2.   The motor strip. This cartoon shows a representation of body parts at various points on the strip. Note that the areas representing facial and hand muscles are very large. This is because of the intricate control necessary for speech and fine motor coordination. A cross-section of the motor strip is shown to the right.

tered into the spinal fluid using an implantable pump in individuals with cerebral palsy to decrease spasticity (see Chapter 26; Butler & Campbell, 2000).

Damage to the motor cortex can also lead to seizures that begin as focal twitchings and can generalize to involve large muscle groups (Jacksonian epilepsy; see Chapter 29). The frontal lobe subserves abstract thinking. With functional imaging techniques (discussed later), the frontal lobe has been identified as the origin of executive function (Barkley, 2000; Pineda et al., 1998). This high-level abstract thinking involves planning and organizing for future activities and is deficient in children with attention-deficit/hyperactivity disorder (ADHD) and learning disabilities (Lazar & Frank, 1998; see Chapters 24 and 25).

The Parietal Lobe   Touch, pain, vibration, proprioception, and temperature sensation all are processed within the parietal lobe. In addition, the parietal lobe contributes to the integration of other stimuli, promoting a "whole" impression from various sensory inputs. The primary sensory cortex, which receives information from the skin and membranes of the body and face, is located in the somatosensory area. Via the thalamus, this area receives fibers that convey touch and proprioceptive (joint position) sensations from the opposite side of the body. Irritative lesions of this area may produce paresthesias (e.g., numbness with pins-and-needles sensation) on the opposite side of the body. A destructive lesion (e.g., a tumor) in this area produces impairment in sensibility, such as difficulty localizing or measuring the intensity of painful stimuli. Though the primary visual cortex is elsewhere (occipital lobe), some higher levels of visual processing take place in the parietal lobe. There is evidence that the visual-perceptual problems experienced by children with learning disabilities and the difficulties in performing fine motor tasks found in children with ADHD may be related to abnormalities in this region (Vaidya et al., 1998).

The Temporal Lobe   The temporal lobe is primarily involved in communicating and sensation. The dominant hemisphere (the left side in more than 90% of people) is responsible for producing and comprehending speech as well as contributing to the memory of auditory and visual experiences. It receives input from each ear, with point-to-point projection of the cochlea upon the acoustic area of the temporal lobe. Within the base of each temporal lobe rests

two structures, the hippocampus and amygdala, which serve special cognitive functions. The hippocampus plays an important role in memory and allows for the rapid learning of new information. The amygdala is involved in sensory processing and emotions and is part of the general-purpose "fight or flight" defense response control system.

Both the amygdala and hippocampus have been shown to be structurally abnormal in ASDs, with the degree of abnormality linked to the severity of impairment (Schuman et al., 2004). It is unclear if variation in the hippocampus is a cause or an effect of the disorder's symptomatology. Studies in both animals and humans suggest that there can be dynamic changes in the hippocampus related to experience and behavior (Maguire et al., 2000). Dysfunction of the amygdala has strongly been implicated in the social deficits of ASDs. Specifically, lesion studies as well as fMRI studies have shown that the amygdala is involved in the ability to read and relate to the emotions of others (Schultz, 2005; Shaw et al., 2004).

Temporal lobe dysfunction can contribute to a number of disorders; the two most common are receptive aphasia and complex partial seizures (Parry-Fielder et al., 1997). In receptive aphasia, the temporal lobe may have been damaged by a tumor, vascular insufficiency, or trauma (Van Hout, 1997). The individual is unable to understand spoken words but is able to speak, frequently in an unintelligible fashion (see Chapter 22). Complex partial seizures also arise in the temporal lobe (Bourgeois, 1998). Before the seizure begins, the individual may experience a déjà vu, or flashback, phenomenon, caused by stimulation of this area of the brain. The person may also have visual **hallucinations**, hear bizarre sounds, or appreciate olfactory auras, which again emanate from the temporal lobe (see Chapter 29).

Treatment of refractory complex partial seizures may involve surgical removal of the seizure focus (Cross, 1999). This surgery has been shown in adults to be superior to prolonged medical management in terms of seizure control and quality of life (Wiebe et al., 2001). Although adults who undergo this neurosurgical procedure often sustain some language or memory loss, children appear less likely to experience this complication. This suggests that the child's brain is more flexible than the adult brain, such that the nondominant hemisphere can take over some of the language functions of the damaged area. In fact, children as old as 6 years have undergone total dominant hemispherectomies (removal of the left hemisphere for intractable generalized seizures with a left seizure focus) and have been able to recover speech function, presumably by incorporating other cortical locations in a new functional role (Chungani & Muller, 1999; deBode & Curtiss, 2000; Neville & Bavelier, 1998). This is known as **plasticity** (Vicari et al., 2000). With hemispherectomy, the degree of language recovery varies according to the underlying cause of the seizure disorder (Jonas et al., 2004).

In the temporal lobe, the primary auditory cortex receives input from both ears by way of the cochlear nerves and through multiple synapses in the brainstem. Irritation of this cortex may cause a buzzing or roaring sensation. Because of the bilateral representation, unilateral damage does not result in deafness but may result in mild hearing loss. Bilateral lesions can result in complete hearing loss.

The Occipital Lobe The primary visual receptive cortex is located in the occipital lobe. The right occipital lobe receives impulses from the right half of each retina, whereas the left visual cortex receives impulses from the left half of each retina. The upper portion of this cortical area represents the upper half of each retina, whereas the lower portion represents the lower half. Irritation of this visual cortex can produce such visual hallucinations as flashes of light, rainbows, brilliant stars, or bright lines. Destructive lesions can cause defects in the visual fields on the opposite side without loss of macular (central) vision.

Visual stimuli are first interpreted in the visual-receptive area. The image is processed further in an adjacent part of the occipital lobe before being passed on to the temporal and parietal lobes. Here the location in space and the identity of the viewed object are further determined. In both the temporal and parietal lobes, the image is related to what is heard and felt so that an interpretation can be made. Cortical visual impairment (cortical blindness) may result from severe damage to the occipital region (Huo et al., 1999). In this condition, despite a normal visual apparatus and pathway, the occipital lobe does not receive the image and the person appears to be functionally blind (see Chapter 11).

Interconnections The white matter of the adult cerebral hemispheres contains myelinated ("insulated") nerve fibers of many sizes. Some of these fibers serve to connect various regions of the brain. The most important of these interconnections is the corpus callosum, a large arrangement of fibers that connects portions of one hemisphere with corresponding parts of the opposite hemisphere (Figure 13.1a–b).

A second type of interconnection is formed by projection fibers, which connect the cerebral cortex with lower portions of the brain or spinal cord. As an example, the internal capsule is a collection of fibers that project from the cortex to the spinal cord; nerve impulses carried by these fibers control distant muscles. Destructive lesions such as tumors or stroke may compress or destroy the internal capsule and the pyramidal (motor) tract it contains, resulting in hemiplegia (spasticity and weakness) on the opposite side of the body.

Finally, association fibers connect the various portions of a cerebral hemisphere. Short association fibers, or U fibers, connect adjacent gyri. Those fibers located in the deeper portions of the white matter are termed intracortical fibers, and those just beneath the cortex are called subcortical fibers. Long association fibers connect more widely separated areas.

The Basal Ganglia and Thalamus

Deep beneath the cortical surface resides the diencephalon (Figures 13.1a and 13.3) which consists of the thalamus and hypothalamus. Adjacent to the diencephalon are the basal ganglia and related structures. In humans, this primitive part of the brain modulates instructions from the motor cortex in directing voluntary movements (Roberts, 1992). In lower vertebrates it directly controls motor activity. Anatomically, the basal ganglia include the caudate nucleus and the putamen (together called the corpus striatum), the globus pallidus, and the other gray areas at the base of the forebrain. Together, the putamen and the globus pallidus form the lentiform nucleus. The caudate nucleus is separated from the lentiform nucleus and the thalamus by the internal capsule. Functionally, these collections of neurons together with their connections and neurotransmitters form an associated motor system. Damage to the basal ganglia produces various movement disorders. Although voluntary movement is possible, involuntary jerking or twisting, referred to collectively as **choreoathetosis,** may occur. Alternately, there may be dystonic posturing or rigidity. These manifestations can be seen in children with dyskinetic cerebral palsy (see Chapter 26; Cote & Crutcher, 2000).

Immediately adjacent to the basal ganglia is the thalamus. All sensory input to the cortex must first pass through the thalamus. In this way, the thalamus acts as a gate or filter for the cerebral cortex, and has been implicated in a variety of movement disorders as well as in absence seizures (previously called petit mal seizures; see Chapter 29). The thalamus is also thought to be part of a neuronal network concerned with cognitive function, especially language.

The Brainstem

In contrast to the voluntary actions controlled by the cerebral hemispheres, the brainstem controls more reflexive and involuntary activities. It is comprised of three distinct areas (midbrain, pons, and medulla) and connects the cerebral hemispheres to the spinal cord (Figure 13.3). Within it are the cranial nerves that control functions such as vision, hearing, swallowing, and articulation (Klemm & Vertes, 1990). These nerves also affect facial expression, eye and tongue movement, salivation, and even breathing. In addition to the cranial nerve nuclei, the brainstem is composed of a vast array of fiber tracts bringing messages into and out of

the brain. The corticospinal (pyramidal) tracts provide for the passage of neural impulses from the cortex to the spinal cord. Conversely, there are tracts bringing sensory information to the cortex via the thalamus. Therefore, any abnormality in this region affects function in distant locations. Children with cerebral palsy may have damage to the brainstem or to pathways that end in the brainstem; this damage thus offers an explanation for the high incidence of excessive salivation, swallowing problems, strabismus, and speech disorders in these children (see Chapter 26).

The Cerebellum

The cerebellum (Figure 13.1a–b) resides in back of and immediately below the cerebral hemispheres and coordinates voluntary muscle activity. Its principal role is to dampen skeletal muscular activity by providing for the smooth transition between activation of **agonist** muscles (that work together) and inhibiting of their counterpart antagonist muscles. Normal muscle coordination requires that the functions of the cerebellum be integrated with those of the cerebral hemispheres and the basal ganglia. Although voluntary movement can occur without the cere-

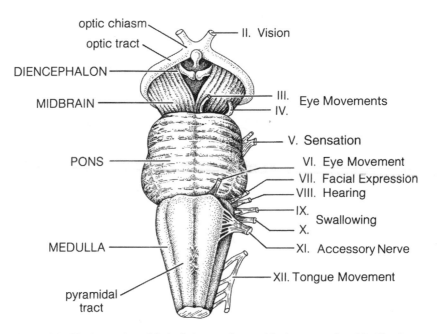

Figure 13.3. The three regions of the brainstem are shown: midbrain, pons, and medulla. The placement and function of 11 of the 12 cranial nerves are illustrated. (The first cranial nerve [smell] is not shown. It lies in front of the second cranial nerve, below the frontal lobe.) Note that the pyramidal tract runs from the cortex (not shown) into the brainstem. The pyramidal fibers cross over in the medulla. Thus, the right hemisphere controls left-side movement, and the left hemisphere controls right-side movement.

bellum, such movements are erratic and uncoordinated. For example, an ataxic gait may be seen with cerebellar tumors, with progressive neurological disorders (e.g., ataxia telangiectasia), as a side effect of medication, or with inebriation (Menkes & Sarnat, 2000). The cerebellum may also have some influence on cognitive function through interconnections with the prefrontal cortex (Diamond, 2000). Cerebellar abnormalities have been found in children with ASDs.

The Spinal Cord

The spinal cord transmits motor and sensory messages between the brain and the rest of the body. In addition to permitting voluntary movement, the spinal cord acts to provide protective reflex arcs in both the upper and lower extrem-

ities, such as the deep tendon reflex elicited when the knee is tapped. The spinal cord is an elongated, cylindrical mass of nerve tissue that is continuous with the brainstem at its upper end and occupies the upper two thirds of the adult spinal canal within the vertebral column (Figure 13.4). It widens laterally in the neck and the lower back regions. These enlargements correspond to the origins of the nerves of the upper and lower extremities. The nerves of the brachial plexus originate at the cervical enlargement; the nerves of the lumbosacral plexus arise from the lumbar enlargement. Injury to the brachial plexus may occur during a difficult vaginal delivery resulting in weakness of the upper extremity (Dodds & Wolfe, 2000).

The spinal cord is divided into approximately 30 segments—8 cervical (neck), 12 tho-

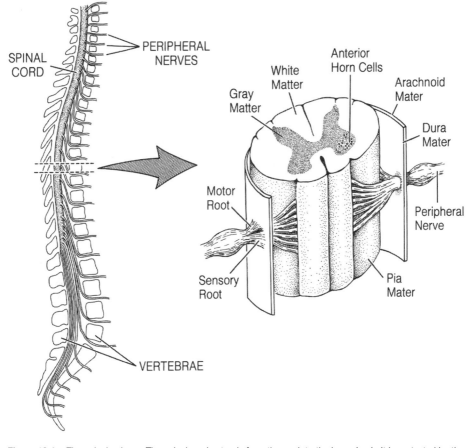

Figure 13.4. The spinal column. The spinal cord extends from the neck to the lower back. It is protected by the bony vertebrae that form the spinal column. The enlargement to the right shows a section of the cord taken from the upper back region. Note the meninges (the dura, arachnoid, and pia mater) surrounding the cord and the peripheral nerve on its way to a muscle. This nerve contains both motor and sensory components. The spinal cord, like the brain, has both gray and white matter. The gray matter consists of various nerve cells, the most important of which are the anterior horn cells. These are destroyed in polio. The white matter contains nerve fibers wrapped in myelin, which gives the cord its glistening appearance.

racic (chest), 5 lumbar (lower back), 5 sacral (pelvic), and a few small coccygeal (tailbone) segments—that correspond to attachments of groups of nerve roots. Individual segments vary in length; they are about twice as long in the mid-thoracic region as in the cervical of upper lumbar area.

There are no sharp boundaries between segments within the cord itself. Each segment contributes to four roots: a ventral (front) and a dorsal (back) root arising from the left half and a similar pair from the right half; each root is made up of many individual **rootlets.** The dorsal nerve roots allow sensory input to ascend to the brainstem, whereas the ventral roots deliver motor input from the brainstem to the appropriate muscle.

If the spinal cord is damaged (e.g., because of trauma or a congenital malformation such as meningomyelocele—see Chapter 28), messages from the brain are short-circuited before they reach the peripheral nerves below the area of abnormality. The result may be a loss of both sensation and movement in the affected limbs. The paralysis, which is initially flaccid but ultimately spastic, may involve the legs (paraplegia) or all four extremities (quadriplegia) depending on the level of the damage.

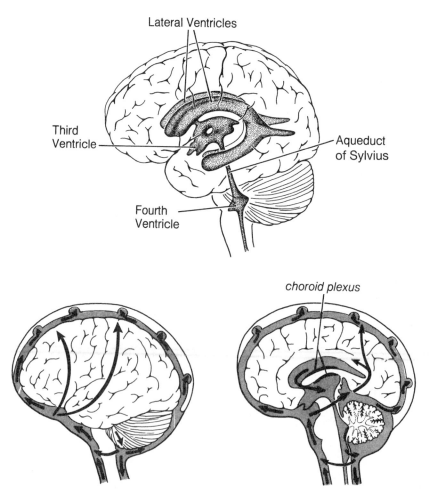

Figure 13.5. The ventricular system of the brain. The major parts of the ventricular system are shown (top). The flow of cerebrospinal fluid (CSF) is shown (bottom). The fluid is produced by the choroid plexus in the roof of the lateral and third ventricles. Its primary route is through the aqueduct of Sylvius, into the fourth ventricle, and then into the spinal column, where it is absorbed. A secondary route is around the surface of the brain. A blockage, most commonly of the aqueduct of Sylvius, leads to hydrocephalus. (From Milhorat, T.H. [1972]. *Hydrocephalus and the cerebrospinal fluid.* Philadelphia: Lippincott Williams & Wilkins. Copyright © 1972, The Williams & Wilkins Co., Baltimore; adapted by permission.)

Cerebral Fluid Dynamics and Hydrodynamics

Long considered simply an aqueous environment for the suspension of the brain, the cerebrospinal fluid (CSF) is now known to perform many other functions. In addition to physically supporting the neural elements and serving to buffer the brain and spinal cord from excessive motion, CSF acts to provide nutritional support as well as to remove excessive hormones and neurotransmitters. CSF may also serve as a "relief valve," adjusting its volume when there are increases in intracranial pressure. Furthermore, its hydrodynamic properties no doubt influence the formation of the brain.

Approximately a pint of CSF is produced each day by the choroid plexus in the brain. This fluid moves throughout the lateral and third ventricles and communicates with the fourth ventricle via the aqueduct of Sylvius (Figure 13.5). At the level of the fourth ventricle, the CSF exits at the foramina of Luschka and Magendie to circulate over the surface of the brain as well as over the spinal cord and its **meningeal** coverings. Removal of CSF occurs at the arachnoid granulations over the superior surface of the brain, which act as one-way valves and allow CSF to move into the blood stream.

Should an imbalance develop between production and absorption of CSF, hydrocephalus may ensue (Figure 13.6). This buildup of CSF within the ventricles may be caused by an obstruction of CSF flow within the ventricles (frequently at the aqueduct of Sylvius) or at the exit foramina (Luschka and Magendie). This is known as a noncommunicating hydrocephalus. In contrast, communicating hydrocephalus is caused by an obstruction at the level of the arachnoid granulations. In addition to inadequate absorption, it is also possible (though rare) to have an oversupply of CSF, as is seen in the setting of a tumor of the choroids plexus. This may overwhelm the ability of the arachnoid granulations to absorb the fluid.

When fluid builds up inside the skull of an infant, the **sutures** (the joints connecting the skull bones) expand and dissipate the increased pressure, at the expense of an increase in head circumference. This may present as a bulging fontanel (or "soft spot"). The same situation in the older child whose sutures have closed, however, may quickly lead to headache, vomiting, lethargy, and **focal neurological changes.** This buildup of fluid can be life threatening at any age and is considered a medical emergency.

When hydrocephalus occurs, it is necessary to restore the balance between production and absorption of CSF. This is often accomplished by performing a shunting procedure that increases the removal of CSF. The shunt's objective is to bypass the obstruction, whether at the level of the arachnoid granulations or within the ventricular system. This usually involves the diversion of CSF from the head to another site, preferably the abdomen. The complication rate from this procedure is low, and the long-term outcome reasonably good. Once

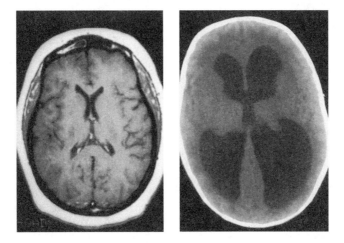

Figure 13.6. Normal computed tomography (CT) scan (left) and CT scan showing hydrocephalus (right). In the image to the right, note the rounded appearance of the frontal horns (top) as well as the differentially enlarged occipital horns (bottom). This is known as culpocephaly and is frequently seen in individuals with spina bifida.

placed, however, numerous obstacles remain in maintaining a working shunt and avoiding infection. Many children require shunt revisions as a result of either obstruction or infection. Despite present-day imperfections, the management of hydrocephalus has been simplified and often allows for a near-typical lifestyle.

In children with noncommunicating hydrocephalus in which there is an obstruction within the ventricular system, either congenital (aquaductal stenosis) or acquired (tumor), there is a surgical alternative to shunting. This procedure (endoscopic third ventriculostomy) involves making a perforation in the floor of the third ventricle to create a new route of outflow for the CSF, thus bypassing the obstruction (Koch & Wagner, 2004; Ruggiero et al., 2004). Endoscopic third ventriculostomy has the benefit of avoiding implants, but it is not feasible in all individuals with hydrocephalus. In addition, there is a small but serious risk of injury to nearby vascular or neural structures.

THE PERIPHERAL NERVOUS SYSTEM

The peripheral nerves allow neural impulses to continue from the CNS (brain and spinal cord) to distant muscles. These nerve tracts have both motor and sensory fibers that run in opposite directions. Motor, or **efferent,** fibers transmit neural impulses from the brain to initiate movement. Sensory, or **afferent,** fibers carry signals from the muscle to the brain that indicate the position of a joint and the tone of the muscle following the movement. Hyperexcitability of sensory neurons in the patient with cerebral palsy contributes to spasticity. There are also a number of hereditary neuropathies that interfere with the **peripheral nervous system** (Ouvrier, 1996).

The regeneration capacity of the peripheral nervous system differs substantially from that of the CNS. Although the CNS is now considered capable of regeneration, the ease of repair in the peripheral nervous system is far greater. This ability to promote the regrowth of peripheral nerves is responsible for the success seen in the neural reconstruction for brachial plexus palsy. At present, the success rate ranges from 60% to 90% for reestablishing meaningful neurological function in children undergoing a neural reconstruction (Xu, Cheng, & Gu, 2000).

Voluntary movement is controlled by the **somatic** component of the **peripheral nervous system.** Complex coordination between the motor and sensory system is necessary to ensure normal muscle tone. An imbalance can lead to increased or decreased muscle tone. Injury to the motor neurons will affect voluntary as well as reflex activities of the involved muscle.

Involuntary activities involving control of the cardiovascular, digestive, endocrine, urinary, respiratory, and reproductive systems are undertaken by the **autonomic** nervous system. Control of these functions begins in the diencephalon and terminates in the end organs. In contrast to the graded response with voluntary movement demonstrated by the somatic nervous system, the autonomic nervous system involves an on/off type of control. The best example of this is the "fight or flight" response (Figure 13.7). When a person feels threatened physically or psychologically, several physiological changes take place simultaneously. The pupils dilate, the hair stands on end, and the functioning of the digestive system is suspended so that blood can be diverted to more important areas, such as the brain. Heart rate and blood pressure increase, and the air passages of the lung expand in size. All of these changes prepare the individual to react to the emergency.

Although the autonomic nervous system works involuntarily in maintaining **homeostasis,** there are nonetheless voluntary adjustments that come from the cerebral cortex to modulate these effects. This is perhaps best illustrated by the development of bowel and bladder control. In an infant, when the bladder or bowel fills, the outlet muscles release automatically, and the infant urinates or defecates. Between the ages of 12 and 18 months, however, the child gradually gains control over these functions. The cerebral cortex begins to send inhibitory signals to reduce the normal autonomic nervous system reflexive activity. As any parent knows only too well, however, this coordination and fine tuning may take months to master. Individuals who have sustained damage to either the corticospinal tracts or the spinal cord are unable to inhibit the autonomic nervous system in this way (Low, 1994). This explains the great difficulty that children with cerebral palsy or meningomyelocele or those who have sustained a traumatic brain injury (see Chapter 30) may have in controlling bladder and bowel function.

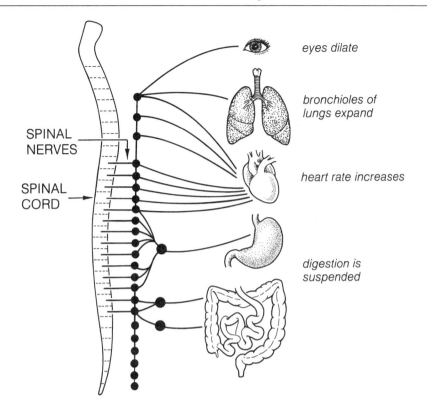

Figure 13.7. Autonomic nervous system. These nerves control such involuntary motor activities as breathing, heart rate, and digestion. This system is involved in "fight or flight" reactions.

THE MICROSCOPIC ARCHITECTURE OF THE BRAIN

The Neuron

Neurons are similar to other cells in that they have a cell body consisting of a nucleus and cytoplasm. Unlike other cells, however, they have a long process called an axon, which extends from the cell body, and many shorter, jutting processes called dendrites (Figure 13.8). The axon carries impulses away from the nerve cell body, sometimes for a distance of greater than a meter. Dendrites receive impulses from other neurons and carry them a short distance toward the cell body. The size and shape of dendrites may change with neuronal activity, suggesting that these changes represent the anatomical basis of memory.

As the brain begins to organize by 5 months' gestation (a process that continues into early childhood) the axons and dendrites grow and differentiate. The major developmental features of this organizational period include 1)

the establishment and differentiation of neurons; 2) the attainment of proper alignment, orientation, and layering of cortical neurons; 3) the elaboration of dendrites and axons; 4) the establishment of synaptic contacts; and 5) cell death and selective elimination of neuronal processes and **synapses.**

As the neuron develops, growing axons are able to recognize various molecules that are on the surface of and that are diffusing away from other axons and cells and use these as cues to navigate the circuitous pathway to their final destination. These axons need to "perceive" this guidance information, distinguishing the correct pathway from the incorrect one. In addition, axons need to move forward, sometimes rapidly, make turns, avoid obstacles, and stop when the target is reached. These guidance functions—sensory, motor, and integrative—are contained within the specialized tip of a growing axon, the growth cone (Sanes, Reh, & Harris, 2000).

During neuronal differentiation, the primitive neurons begin to express their distinctive

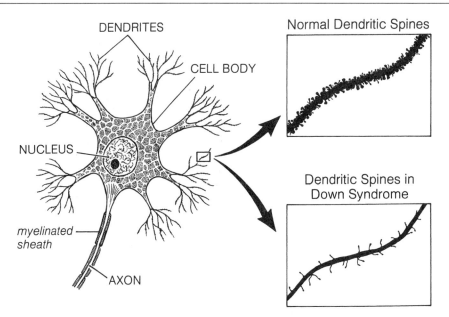

DENDRITES

CELL BODY

NUCLEUS

myelinated sheath

AXON

Normal Dendritic Spines

Dendritic Spines in Down Syndrome

Figure 13.8. Illustration of a nerve cell, showing its component elements. The enlargements show the minute dendritic spines that increase the number of synapses or junctures among nerve cells. Note the diminished size and number of dendritic spines in a child with Down syndrome.

physical and biochemical features. This arborization is much like the growth of a tree from a sapling. It even involves pruning, such that new connections are established while others are abolished. For example, in the visual cortex, the formation of synapses is most rapid between 2 and 4 months after term, a time critical for the development of visual function. Maximum synaptic density is attained at 8 months of age, when elimination of synapses begins; by age 11 months, approximately 40% of synapses have been lost (Volpe, 2001).

As axons grow toward their respective dendritic targets, the dendrites respond by increasing the number of spines, or projections, along their surface (Figure 13.8). The spines increase the surface area of the dendrites, permitting more elaborate and sophisticated communication between neurons. In fact, increased dendritic outgrowth has been associated with enhanced memory. In contrast, deficient development of the dendritic arborization has been observed in individuals with cognitive impairments, most prominently in Down syndrome (Huttenlocher, 1991).

Synapses

Proper function of the nervous system requires not only formation of the needed connection between an axon from one neuron and dendrite from a second neuron, but also of communication between these two neurons once that connection is established. The point of contact between two neurons is called a synapse (Figure 13.9). Synapses can be either chemical or electrical with distinct characteristics for each type. In electrical synapses, there is a short distance between the two neurons and there is a communication between the cytoplasm of the cells. Because of this, there is very little delay as an electric current passes from one neuron to the next and the transmission is usually bidirectional.

In contrast, in chemical synapses there is a larger gap between the two neurons and no direct communication of the cytoplasm. In order to bridge the gap between the two cells, small vesicles of specific chemicals (neurotransmitters) are released from the axon of one neuron. These chemicals travel the distance between the cells to reach the receptors for that particular neurotransmitter on the dendrite of the second neuron. The effect on the postsynaptic cell can be either excitatory or inhibitory. Because of the process involved, there is a delay in transmission and the signal is unidirectional. Within a network, the two types of synapses work together to foster synchrony (Kopell & Ermentrout, 2004).

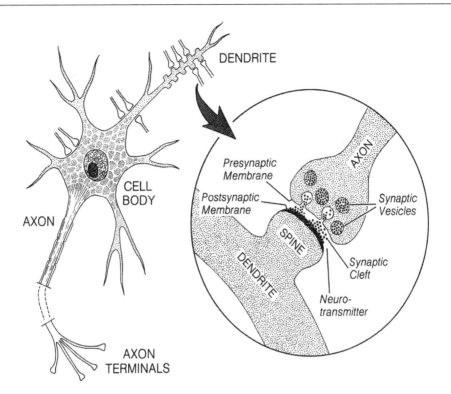

Figure 13.9. Central nervous system (CNS) synapse. The enlargement shows the abutting of an axon against a dendritic spine. The space separating the two is the synaptic cleft. Neurotransmitter bundles are released into the cleft from vesicles in the presynaptic membrane. These permit transmission of an impulse across the juncture.

Neurotransmitters

Neurotransmitters are chemicals that are released by one cell to cause an effect on a second cell. They differ from hormones in the scale of their action. Whereas hormones are released in the bloodstream and can affect cells distant from the originating cell, neurotransmitters are released within the synapse and affect cells that are in very close proximity. For a substance to be considered a neurotransmitter, it has to be synthesized within and released from the presynaptic neuron and exert a defined effect on the postsynaptic neuron.

The steps involved in the chemical transmission at a synapse involve first the synthesis of the neurotransmitter within the presynaptic neuron. Many of the neurotransmitters share common precursor. For example, dopamine and norepinephrine are all synthesized from a common precursor amino acid (tyrosine). After synthesis, the neurotransmitter is packaged and stored in vesicles awaiting release. At the proper signal the vesicles release the neurotransmitter into the synapse and it travels the distance between the two neurons. The postsynaptic neuron has receptors that are specific for the neurotransmitter and when activated have a characteristic affect on that neuron. The excess neurotransmitter within the synapse is then removed either by reuptake or by enzymatic breakdown. The function of the CNS can be altered by manipulating any of the steps in chemical transmission. For example, the most widely used medications for depression and anxiety belong to a group of prescription drugs known as selective serotonin reuptake inhibitors (SSRIs). These medications block the reuptake of serotonin after its release in the synaptic cleft, thereby increasing the availability and the duration of action of the serotonin in specific brain regions.

Within the central, peripheral, and autonomic nervous systems there are a variety of identified neurotransmitters. Table 13.1 provides a simplified summary of the characteristics of some of the major neurotransmitters.

Myelination

The neurons and neuronal processes of the brain and spinal cord form two distinct regions

Table 13.1. Characteristics of some of the major neurotransmitters

Neurotransmitter	Location	Function	Associated disorder
Acetylcholine	Nucleus basalis Neuromuscular junction Autonomic nervous system	Stimulates muscle contraction at the neuromuscular junction	Myasthenia gravis (loss of receptors) Botulism (impaired release)
Dopamine	Substantia nigra	Initiation and control of movement	Parkinson's disease (deficiency) Schizophrenia (excess)
Norepinephrine	Locus ceruleus Sympathetic nervous system	Maintains vigilance and responsiveness	Alzheimer's disease
Serotonin	Raphe nuclei	Involved in the sleep–wake cycle, emotions, food intake, thermoregulation, and sexual behavior	Depression (deficiency)
Histamine	Hypothalamus	Regulation of hormones	
GABA	Inhibitory interneurons throughout the brain and spinal cord	Principal inhibitory neurotransmitter	Epilepsy (deficiency)
Glycine	Inhibitory interneurons in the spinal cord	Inhibits antagonist muscles	Nonketotic hyperglycinemia (excess)
Glutamate	Excitatory neurons throughout the brain and spinal cord	Principal excitatory neurotransmitter	Huntington disease (excess) Acute brain injury (excess)

Source: Kandel, Schwartz, and Jessell. (2000).

of the CNS, the gray matter and the white matter. The gray matter contains the nerve cell bodies, appearing grayish in color. The white matter is made up of axons sheathed with a protective shiny white covering called myelin that promotes the rapid conduction of nerve impulses. During fetal life, most of the axons have no myelin coating. They gradually develop this glistening casing after birth. Effective **myelination** is necessary for the development of voluntary gross and fine motor movement and the suppression of **primitive reflexes.** The majority of myelination is complete by 18 months of age, around the time a child can run (Volpe, 2001); however, this process continues to a lesser degree throughout adolescence and into early adulthood (Sowell et al., 2001). Deficient myelination formation has been found in a number of conditions including prematurity, congenital hypothyroidism, and malnutrition (Porter & Tennekoon, 2000; Rodriguez-Pena et al., 1993).

TECHNIQUES FOR EVALUATING THE NERVOUS SYSTEM

Neuroimaging techniques

In the 1990s, considerable advances in neuro-radiological investigation permitted a better understanding of the living brain (Inder &

Huppe, 2000; Zimmerman, Gibby, & Carmody, 2000). High-speed computed tomography (CT) scans, which are produced from multiple, thin-cut X rays, became a mainstay for the evaluation of the child with hydrocephalus, trauma, craniofacial disorders, new-onset seizures, and tumors of the brain and skull (Maytal et al., 2000). The inherent strength of CT resides in its excellent bone definition. Three-dimensional CT now routinely provides sophisticated reconstruction of complex skull base disorders, whereas CT angiography offers good resolution in characterizing blood vessel or flow abnormalities with additional information from adjacent bony structures. The quick and painless acquisition of images means that CT scans can often be obtained without the need for sedation, as opposed to magnetic resonance imaging (MRI) scans, which take longer to acquire and make sedation necessary in younger children. This also makes CT ideally suited for emergency situations which require rapid acquisition of brain images (e.g., in looking for evidence of intracranial hemorrhage after trauma).

CT can be supplemented with the addition of intravenous contrast. Contrast helps define areas of breakdown of the blood-brain barrier. Addition of contrast is especially helpful in defining infection or tumor. Most infections and many tumors will appear bright with the addition of contrast aiding in visualization the lesion. Conversely, IV contrast does not typically aid in clinical scenarios such as closed head injury or hydrocephalus. Caution should be used with administering contrast in any child with dehydration or abnormal renal function.

Despite the strengths of CT scanning, MRI scanning has surpassed all other modalities for evaluating brain structure (Rivkin, 2000). It is particularly useful in investigating developmental abnormalities of the brain, in assessing the causes of epilepsy (Gaillard, 2000; Goyal et al., 2004) and in identifying chronic hemorrhage (Kidwell et al., 2004). Although technological advances in CT have resulted in improved image quality, MRI scans are superior in defining brain anatomy and soft tissue (as opposed to bony) abnormalities. MRI exploits subtle magnetic differences in water and other molecules of the brain to evaluate regions in great anatomic detail. A variant approach, an MRI technique called diffusion-weighted imaging (DWI), is the only technique that permits a noninvasive assessment of water molecular diffusion, which reflects tissue configuration at a microscopic level. This technique is particularly useful in detecting brain abnormalities caused by ischemia (lack of adequate blood flow resulting in tissue damage). MRI can also be used to perform magnetic resonance spectroscopy (MRS) to detect metabolic abnormalities in the brain as seen in certain inborn errors of metabolism. MRI scanning, which uses no radiation, is safe and usually provides superior resolution to CT scanning. It is, however, more expensive and time consuming than CT scanning and more difficult to perform in emergency situations. It also provides slightly different information, so in some instances CT and MRI are complementary.

Whereas standard CT and MRI primarily provide anatomical and structural information about the CNS, other neuroradiological approaches are now available for assessing the functional state of the CNS. Single photon emission computed tomography (SPECT) and positron emission tomography (PET) are techniques that demonstrate metabolically active regions in the brain. A radioactively labeled compound, most commonly glucose, is injected into the bloodstream and SPECT or PET is then used to assess its selective uptake in various brain regions. This technique has been used to diagnose strokes, tumors, and brain injury following head trauma (Abdel-Dayem et al., 1998) and to predict gross motor development in children

with cerebral palsy (Yim et al., 2000). These modalities have also been employed in the evaluation of seizure disorders prior to surgery (Chugani & Chugani, 1999; So, 2000). In this instance, the studies can differentiate areas that are functionally hyperactive secondary to seizure activity from areas that are hypoactive as a result of structural lesions.

Another approach to functional imaging is functional MRI (fMRI). This combines the excellent resolution of MRI with the capacity to study the effects of attention and activity (e.g., reading, speaking, moving) on brain function (Baving, Laucht, & Schmidt, 1999; Rubia et al., 1999). It does this by detecting minute changes in regional blood flow and metabolism. In epilepsy, fMRI is useful in localizing language and memory function as well as identifying possible seizure foci (Detre, 2004) and may one day replace more invasive testing of these functions. This technique affords significantly superior resolution to PET and will most likely supplant it in the future. Table 13.2 summarizes the advantages and disadvantages of each of these different imaging techniques.

Electroencephalography

Whereas CT and MRI show the structure of the brain, and SPECT, PET, and fMRI show metabolic activity of the brain, there are additional tests that can be useful in assessing the function of the brain. Electroencephalography (EEG) utilizes scalp electrodes to measure the electrical activity of the brain (see Chapter 29). This is a noninvasive test that is able to detect the summation of neuronal discharges in the superficial layers of the cerebral cortex. In epilepsy, EEG can show a pattern that is indicative of epileptiform ("seizure-like") activity. Coupled with continuous video monitoring, EEG becomes a powerful tool to match seizure type with the location of the seizure focus (Pandian et al., 2004). It can also detect seizures that may not be evident clinically and can show the effects of various treatments, both medical and surgical, on seizure activity. EEG is also useful in evaluating cognitive status changes associated with diffuse neurological dysfunction (as might occur in encephalitis or infection of the brain).

Electromyography and Nerve Conduction Studies

To this point, the discussion of techniques for evaluation of the nervous system has focused on

Table 13.2.   Advantages and disadvantages of each neuroimaging technique

Imaging technique	Advantages	Disadvantages
Computed tomography (CT)	High resolution of bony anatomy; quick and readily available; usually does not require sedation	Lower resolution of brain structures compared to MRI
Magnetic resonance imaging (MRI)	Extremely high resolution of brain structures; images obtained in multiple planes; no radiation exposure	Takes longer to acquire images compared with CT; often requires sedation
Positron emission tomography (PET)/single photon emission computed tomography (SPECT)	Shows brain function in addition to structure by tracking the uptake of radioactive glucose	Limited availability at many centers
Functional MRI (fMRI)	Shows function by detecting variation in regional blood flow; lends better structural resolution than PET/SPECT	Requires significant patient cooperation; not feasible for individuals who are very young or who have severe intellectual disability

the evaluation of the CNS. Although there is limited imaging to assess the peripheral nervous system (e.g., MRI to evaluate the brachial plexus, or nerves that arise from the spinal cord to control the arms), functional testing is readily available in the form of electromyography (EMG) and nerve conduction studies (NCS). These studies involve placement of needle electrodes at various points on the body to test both motor and sensory function of the peripheral nerves. EMG and NCS can be used to define traumatic injury or peripheral neuropathy and can demonstrate the aftereffects of toxic exposure (Avaria et al., 2004). In addition, these studies can be a helpful aid in surgical cases that involve dissection near either sensory or motor pathways (Sala et al., 2002).

SUMMARY

The nervous system is composed of central and peripheral elements. The CNS (the brain and spinal cord) is complex in both its structure and function. Various techniques allow better assessment of the brain for diagnosis of a broad range of clinical pathology. As our understanding of both normal and abnormal neurological function improves, better therapeutic avenues will be forthcoming.

REFERENCES

Abdel-Dayem, H.M., Abu-Judeh, H., Kumar, M., et al. (1998). SPECT brain perfusion abnormalities in mild or moderate traumatic brain injury. *Clinical Nuclear Medicine, 23*, 309–317.

Andersson, P.B., & Rando, T.A. (1999). Neuromuscular disorders of childhood. *Current Opinion in Pediatrics, 11*, 497–503.

Avaria, M.A., Mills, J.L., Kleinsteuber, K., et al. (2004). Peripheral nerve conduction abnormalities in children exposed to alcohol in utero. *Journal of Pediatrics, 144* (3), 338–343.

Barkley, R.A. (2000). Genetics of childhood disorders: XVII. ADHD, Part 1: The executive functions and ADHD. *Journal of the American Academy of Child and Adolescent Psychiatry, 39*, 1064–1068.

Baving, L., Laucht, M., & Schmidt, M.H. (1999). Atypical frontal brain activation in ADHD: Preschool and elementary school boys and girls. *Journal of the American Academy of Child and Adolescent Psychiatry, 38*, 1363–1371.

Bourgeois, B.F. (1998). Temporal lobe epilepsy in infants and children. *Brain and Development, 20*, 135–141.

Brodal, P. (1998). *The central nervous system: Structure and function* (2nd ed.). New York: Oxford University Press.

Butler, C., & Campbell, S. (2000). Evidence of the effects of intrathecal baclofen for spastic and dystonic cerebral palsy. AACPDM Treatment Outcomes Committee Review Panel. *Developmental Medicine and Child Neurology, 42*, 643–645.

Chugani, H.T., & Chugani, D.C. (1999). Basic mechanisms of childhood epilepsies: Studies with positron emission tomography. *Advances in Neurology, 79*, 883–891.

Chugani, H.T., & Muller, R.A. (1999). Plasticity associated with cerebral resections. *Advances in Neurology, 81*, 241–250.

Cole, N., & Siddique, T. (1999). Genetic disorders of motor neurons, *Seminars in Neurology, 19*, 407–418.

Cote, L., & Crutcher, M.D. (2000). The basal ganglia. In E.R. Kandel et al. (Eds.), *Principles of neural science* (4th ed., pp. 853–867). New York: McGraw-Hill.

Cross, J.H. (1999). Update on surgery for epilepsy. *Archives of Disease in Childhood, 81*, 356–359.

Crossman, A.R., & Neary, D. (2000). *Neuroanatomy: An illustrated colour text* (2nd ed.). Philadelphia: Churchill Livingstone.

de Bode, S., & Curtiss, S. (2000). Language after hemispherectomy. *Brain and Cognition, 43*(1–3), 135–138.

Detre, J.A. (2004). FMRI: Applications in epilepsy, *Epilepsia, 45*(Suppl. 4), 26–31.

Diamond, A. (2000). Close interrelation of motor development and cognitive development and of the cerebellum and prefrontal cortex. *Child Development, 71,* 44–56.

Dodds, S.D., & Wolfe, S.W. (2000). Perinatal brachial plexus palsy. *Current Opinion in Pediatrics, 12,* 40–47.

Funnell, M.G., Corballis, P.M., & Gazzaniga, M.S. (1999). A deficit in perceptual matching in the left hemisphere of a callosectomy patient. *Neuropsychologia, 37,* 1143–1154.

Gaillard, W.D. (2000). Structural and functional imaging in children with partial epilepsy. *Mental Retardation and Developmental Disabilities Research Reviews, 6,* 220–226.

Goldberg, S. (2000). *Clinical neuroanatomy made ridiculously simple* (2nd ed.). Miami, FL: Medmaster.

Goyal, M., Bangert, B.A., Lewin, J.S., et al. (2004). High-resolution MRI enhances identification of lesions amenable to surgical therapy in children with intractable epilepsy. *Epilepsia, 45*(8), 954–959.

Huo, R., Burden, S.K., Hoyt, C.S., et al. (1999). Chronic cortical visual impairment in children: Aetiology, prognosis, and associated neurological deficits. *British Journal of Ophthalmology, 83,* 670–675.

Huttenlocher, P.R. (1991). Dendritic and synaptic pathology in mental retardation. *Pediatric Neurology, 7,* 79–85.

Inder, T.E., & Huppe, P.S. (2000). In vivo studies of brain development by magnetic resonance techniques. *Mental Retardation and Developmental Disabilities Research Reviews, 6,* 59–67.

Jonas, R., Nguyen, B.S., Hu, B., et al. (2004). Cerebral hemispherectomy: Hospital course, seizure, developmental, language, and motor outcomes. *Neurology, 62,* 1712–1721.

Kandel, E.R., Schwartz, J.H., & Jessell, T.M. (Eds.). (2000). *Principles of neural science* (4th ed.). New York: McGraw-Hill.

Kidwell, C.S., Chalela, J.A., Saver, J.L., et al. (2004). Comparison of MRI and CT for detection of acute intracerebral hemorrhage. *Journal of American Medical Association, 292*(15), 1823–1830.

Klemm, W.R., & Vertes, R.P. (Eds.). (1990). *Brainstem mechanisms of behavior.* Hoboken, NJ: John Wiley & Sons.

Koch, D., & Wagner, W. (2004). Endoscopic third ventriculostomy in infants of less than one year of age: Which factors influence the outcome? *Child's Nervous System, 20,* 405–411.

Kopell, N., & Ermentrout, B. (2004). Chemical and electrical synapses perform complementary roles in the synchronization of interneuronal networks. *Proceedings of the National Academy of Sciences of the United States of America, 101*(43), 15482–15487.

Lazar, J.W., & Frank, Y. (1998). Frontal systems dysfunction in children with attention-deficit/hyperactivity disorder and learning disabilities. *The Journal of Neuropsychiatry and Clinical Neurosciences, 10,* 160–167.

Lequin, M.H., & Barkovich, A.J. (1999). Current concepts of cerebral malformation syndromes. *Current Opinion in Pediatrics, 11,* 492–496.

Low, P.A. (1994). Autonomic neuropathies. *Current Opinion in Neurology, 7,* 402–406.

Maguire, E.A., Gadian, D.G., Johnsrude, I.S., et al. (2000). Navigation-related structural change in the hippocampi of taxi drivers. *Proceedings of the National Academy of Sciences, 97*(8), 4398–4403.

Maytal, J., Krauss, J.M., Novak, G., et al. (2000). The role of brain computed tomography in evaluating children with new onset of seizures in the emergency department. *Epilepsia, 41,* 950–954.

McInerney, J., Siegel, A.M., Nordgren, R.E., et al. (1999). Long-term seizure outcome following corpus callosotomy in children. *Stereotactic and Functional Neurosurgery, 73*(1–4), 79–83.

Menkes, J.H., & Sarnat, H.B. (Eds.). (2000). *Child neurology* (6th ed.). Philadelphia: Lippincott, Williams & Wilkins.

Neville, H.J., & Bavelier, D. (1998). Neural organization and plasticity of language. *Current Opinion in Neurobiology, 8,* 254–258.

Ouvrier, R.A. (1996). Hereditary neuropathies in children: The contribution of the new genetics. *Seminars in Pediatric Neurology, 3,* 140–151.

Pandian, J.D., Cascino, G.D., So, E.L., et al. (2004). Digital video-electroencephalographic monitoring in the neurological-neurosurgical intensive care unit. *Archives of Neurology, 61,* 1090–1094.

Parry-Fielder, B., Nolan, T.M., Collins, K.J., et al. (1997). Developmental language disorders and epilepsy. *Journal of Paediatric Child Health, 33*(4), 277–280.

Pineda, D., Ardila, A., Rosselli, M., et al. (1998). Executive dysfunctions in children with attention deficit hyperactivity disorder. *International Journal of Neuroscience, 96,* 177–196.

Porter, B.E., & Tennekoon, G. (2000). Myelin and disorders that affect the formation and maintenance of this sheath. *Mental Retardation and Developmental Disabilities Research Reviews, 6,* 47–59.

Rivkin, M.J. (2000). Developmental neuroimaging of children using magnetic resonance techniques. *Mental Retardation and Developmental Disabilities Research Reviews, 6,* 68–80.

Roberts, P.A. (1992). *Neuroanatomy* (3rd ed.). New York: Springer-Verlag.

Rodriguez-Pena, A., Ibarrola, N., Iniguez, M.A., et al. (1993). Neonatal hypothyroidism affects the timely expression of myelin-associated glycoprotein in the rat brain. *Journal of Clinical Investigations, 91,* 812–818.

Rubia, K., Overmeyer, S., Taylor, E., et al. (1999). Hypofrontality in attention deficit hyperactivity disorder during higher-order motor control: A study with functional MRI. *American Journal of Psychiatry, 156,* 891–896.

Ruggiero, C., Cinalli, G., Spennato, P., et al. (2004). Endoscopic third ventriculostomy in the treatment of hydrocephalus in posterior fossa tumors in children. *Child's Nervous System, 20,* 828–833.

Sala, F., Krzan, M.J., & Deletis, V. (2002). Intraoperative neurophysiological monitoring in pediatric neurosurgery: Why, when, and how? *Child's Nervous System, 18,* 264–287.

Sanes, D.H., Reh, T.A., & Harris, W.A. (Eds.). (2000). *Development of the central nervous system.* San Diego: Academic Press.

Schultz, R.T. (2005). Developmental deficits in social perception in autism: The role of the amygdala and fusiform face area. *International Journal of Developmental Neuroscience, 23*(2–3), 125–141.

Schumann, C.M., Hamstra, J., Goodlin-Jones, B.L., et al. (2004). The amygdala is enlarged in children but not adolescents with autism; the hippocampus is enlarged at all ages. *The Journal of Neuroscience, 24*(28), 6392–6401.

Shaw, P., Lawrence, E.J., Radbourne, C., et al. (2004). The impact of early and late damage to the human amygdala on 'theory of mind' reasoning. *Brain, 127,* 1535–1548.

Shimizu, H. (2005). Our experience with pediatric epilepsy surgery focusing on corpus callosotomy and hemispherotomy. *Epilepsia, 46*(Suppl. 1), 30–31.

Shimizu, H., & Maehara, T. (2000). Neuronal disconnection for the surgical treatment of pediatric epilepsy. *Epilepsia, 41*(Suppl. 9), S28–S30.

So, E.L. (2000). Integration of EEG, MRI, and SPECT in localizing the seizure focus for epilepsy surgery. *Epilepsia, 41*(Suppl. 3), S48–S54.

Sorenson, J.M., Wheless, J.W., Baumgartner, J.E., et al. (1997). Corpus callosotomy for medically intractable seizures. *Pediatric Neurosurgery, 27,* 260–267.

Sowell, E.R., Thompson, P.M., Tessner, K.D., et al. (2001). Mapping continued brain growth and gray matter density reduction in dorsal frontal cortex: Inverse relationships during postadolescent brain maturation. *The Journal of Neuroscience 21*(22), 8819–8829.

Talbot, K. (1999). Spinal muscular atrophy. *Journal of Inherited Metabolic Diseases, 22,* 545–554.

Tanaka, T., & Gleeson, J.G. (2000). Genetics of brain development and malformation syndromes. *Current Opinion in Pediatrics, 12,* 523–528.

Vaidya, C.J., Austin, G., Kirkorian, G., et al. (1998). Selective effects of methylphenidate in attention deficit hyperactivity disorder: A functional magnetic resonance study. *Proceedings of the National Academy of Sciences of the United States of America, 95,* 14494–14499.

Van Hout, A. (1997). Acquired aphasia in children. *Seminars in Pediatric Neurology, 4,* 102–108.

Vicari, S., Albertoni, A., Chilosi, A.M., et al. (2000). Plasticity and reorganization during language development in children with early brain injury. *Cortex, 36,* 31–46.

Volpe, J.J. (2001). *Neurology of the newborn* (4th ed.). Philadelphia: W.B. Saunders.

Wiebe, S. Blume, W.T., Girvin, J.P., et al. (2001). A randomized, controlled trial of surgery for temporal-lobe epilepsy. *The New England Journal of Medicine, 345*(5), 311–318.

Xu, J., Cheng, X., & Gu, Y. (2000). Different methods and results in the treatment of obstetrical brachial plexus palsy. *Journal of Reconstructive Microsurgery, 16,* 7–20; discussion, 420–422.

Yim, S.Y., Lee, I.Y., Park, C.H., et al. (2000). A qualitative analysis of brain SPECT for prognostication of the gross motor development in children with cerebral palsy. *Clinical Nuclear Medicine, 25*(4), 268–272.

Zimmerman, R.A., Gibby, W.A., & Carmody, R. (2000). *Neuroimaging: Clinical and physical principles.* New York: Springer-Verlag.

14 Muscles, Bones, and Nerves

Diana M. Escolar, Laura L. Tosi,
Ana Carolina Tesi Rocha, and Annie Kennedy

Upon completion of this chapter, the reader will

- Understand how the musculoskeletal and neuromuscular systems function and are integrated

- Recognize the most common signs and symptoms of neuromuscular and musculoskeletal disorders

- Be familiar with some of the most common musculoskeletal and neuromuscular diseases of childhood and their treatments

---

The musculoskeletal (MSK) system consists of bone, muscles, and joints and is connected by **ligaments** and **tendons.** The neuromuscular (NM) system is the "electrical network" that connects the brain to the MSK system; it consists of the spinal motor neurons, the peripheral nerves, and the junction between the nerves and muscles, or neuromuscular junction. The brain initiates the command for movement, but movement can occur only if the NM and MSK systems respond in an organized fashion. Signals from the brain travel down the spinal cord to the spinal motor neuron, which gives rise to peripheral nerves. Signals are then transferred from the peripheral nerves to the neuromuscular junction, where they initiate muscle contraction. As the MSK system begins to move, signals are sent to the brain through the sensory system, providing information about the body's position in space (Figure 14.1).

Together, the NM and MSK systems are responsible for our ability to move; impairments of these systems are a major cause of developmental disability in childhood. This chapter explores how the operation of these systems can be altered, how to recognize the signs and symptoms of NM and MSK disorders, and how an integrated health care and school system can improve the lives of children affected by such disorders.

COMPONENTS OF THE MUSCULOSKELETAL SYSTEM

The bones of the skeleton form the internal scaffolding of the body. They range in size from the ½-inch-long bones of the finger (**phalanges**) to the thigh bone (**femur**), which is roughly 18 inches long in adults. Some bones, such as the skull, are flat; others, such as the femur, are tubular. Even though bones are hard and immobile, they are a dynamic organ system contributing not only to structural support but also to the blood and metabolic systems of the body. And just as the body depends on the skeleton for support, the skeletal system relies on the body for its maintenance and growth.

As growth takes place and the bone is subject to different stresses, the bone responds by changing its shape, a process called remodeling. These changes usually increase the tensile strength and stability of the bone, making it less susceptible to fracture. On average, a section of a child's bone lasts about a year and is then replaced by new bone. In an adult, the reshaping continues even though growth has stopped. The average bone segment of an adult lasts about 7 years. In other words, bone is a living organ that constantly grows and remodels in response to physiological stresses.

The main function of skeletal muscle is to contract by shortening and thus produce move-

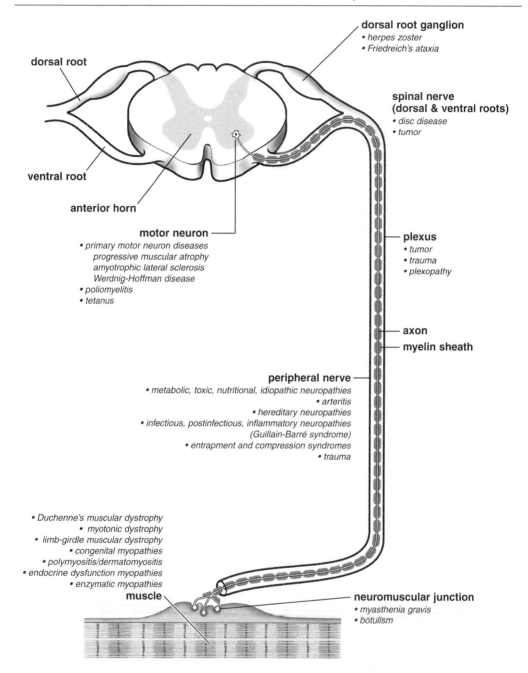

dorsal root ganglion
- *herpes zoster*
- *Friedreich's ataxia*

dorsal root

**spinal nerve
(dorsal & ventral roots)**
- *disc disease*
- *tumor*

ventral root

anterior horn

motor neuron
- *primary motor neuron diseases
  progressive muscular atrophy
  amyotrophic lateral sclerosis
  Werdnig-Hoffman disease*
- *poliomyelitis*
- *tetanus*

plexus
- *tumor*
- *trauma*
- *plexopathy*

axon
myelin sheath

peripheral nerve
- *metabolic, toxic, nutritional, idiopathic neuropathies*
- *arteritis*
- *hereditary neuropathies*
- *infectious, postinfectious, inflammatory neuropathies
  (Guillain-Barré syndrome)*
- *entrapment and compression syndromes*
- *trauma*

- *Duchenne's muscular dystrophy*
- *myotonic dystrophy*
- *limb-girdle muscular dystrophy*
- *congenital myopathies*
- *polymyositis/dermatomyositis*
- *endocrine dysfunction myopathies*
- *enzymatic myopathies*

muscle

neuromuscular junction
- *myasthenia gravis*
- *botulism*

Figure 14.1. The neuromuscular (NM) system. The central components of the nervous system include the brain and spinal cord. Descending corticospinal pathways carry signals from the brain through the spinal cord, which are then transmitted to motor (efferent, or output) nerves, the first segment of the peripheral nervous system. Signals are then transmitted across the neuromuscular junction to muscles, initiating contraction and causing movement through the action of muscles on the musculoskeletal (MSK) system. Sensory (afferent, or input) nerves carry signals back to the spinal cord, which are then transmitted to the brain, which integrates this information to monitor the state of the NM and MSK systems from moment to moment.

ment of the limbs across joints. Cells called muscle fibers comprise muscle. Smooth movement requires the coordination of all of the muscle groups around a joint. Most joints have attached muscles that pull in different direc-

tions. **Antagonist** muscles oppose one another in the movement of a joint, whereas **agonist** muscles pull together to produce movement. For example, when the arm is flexed, the biceps contracts, as does the **brachialis**; the triceps, however, relaxes. If both muscle groups contracted simultaneously, the arm would be held stiffly in an isometric contraction. Thus, when the brain tells the arm to move, it actually sends a number of messages that tell some muscles to contract and others to relax.

SIGNS AND SYMPTOMS OF NEUROMUSCULAR AND MUSCULOSKELETAL DISORDERS

Some children with MSK and NM disorders have signs and symptoms detectable at birth. Others may not manifest symptoms until school age, and teachers are often the first to raise concerns about a child's performance. This section describes general signs and symptoms that should raise suspicion of a NM or MSK disorder and prompt early referral to a physician for further evaluation.

Muscular Symptoms

It is important to differentiate changes in strength of muscle from changes in the tone of the muscle. Muscle tone is the inherent ability of the muscle to respond to stretch, whereas muscle strength is a measure of the force that the muscle exerts. Children can have high tone and an overreactive response to a normal stimulus (hypertonia) or low tone with a response under what would be expected (hypotonia). Many NM or MSK disorders are linked to disturbances in tone. Increased muscle tone (**spasticity**) can be seen in disorders affecting the upper motor neuron or its axons (central nervous system pathology), whereas low muscle tone can be seen in both upper and lower motor neuron involvement.

Muscle weakness is a common sign in all NM disorders and may be **proximal** (involving muscles or body segments closer to the center of the body) or **distal** (involving muscles or body segments farther from the center of the body). Proximal muscle weakness affects the pelvic and shoulder girdle muscles (seen in primary disorders of muscle, called myopathies). Strong pelvic muscles are needed for the child to rise from a seated position and to climb stairs. Children with hip girdle weakness often need to pull on a handrail to walk up steps or to push off with their hands in order to rise from a chair. To get up off the floor, these children often resort to a Gower's maneuver: First they turn to face the floor, then use their hands on the floor to push themselves up, and finally walk their hands up their thighs to regain an erect posture. Children with weak shoulder girdle muscles have difficulty reaching objects on a high shelf, climbing monkey bars, or doing push-ups. Distal muscle weakness (seen in primary disorders of peripheral nerves, which are called neuropathies) affects the hands and feet (i.e., distal extremities). These children may trip and fall frequently because they cannot lift their feet or toes when walking and because they have difficulty standing on their tiptoes when trying to reach an object that is too high. They also may not be able to walk on their heels and may "slap" their feet while walking (a condition called foot drop). Children with distal muscle weakness of the hands often have trouble holding a pen or pencil, finishing long writing activities on time, or using scissors.

Abnormal muscle enlargement (**hypertrophy**), especially of the calves, in combination with weakness can alert one to the presence of **Duchenne muscular dystrophy (DMD)**, whereas fatigability of muscles is a sign of **myasthenia gravis** (see detailed discussion later in the chapter). Excessive muscle cramping during exercise may also signal an underlying NM or MSK disorder. Some of these disorders affect the respiratory muscles, resulting in an abnormal sleep pattern or sleep apnea (brief periods of respiratory arrest). These children typically suffer from severe sleepiness during the day and often appear fatigued or easily distractible; they may also take frequent catnaps.

Sensory Symptoms

Sensory symptoms such as pain or numbness in the hands and feet, changes in skin color, and decreased sensation (e.g., the child might not realize that he has cut his foot until he sees blood) result from disorders of the peripheral sensory nerves (e.g., peripheral neuropathies). Sensory nerve fibers travel through the peripheral nerves to the brain to give feedback on where the body is in space, so these children often have an uncoordinated gait (**ataxia**), slap their feet on the ground too forcefully, and feel very unsteady in the dark, requiring visual input for balance.

Spinal Curvature

Scoliosis is a lateral curvature of the spinal column, whereas kyphosis is an excessive anterior (forward) curvature of the spine. Although in most cases the cause of scoliosis is unknown, both kyphosis and scoliosis can be part of numerous MSK and NM disorders. Idiopathic scoliosis occurs most frequently during the adolescent growth spurt, especially in girls. The appearance of either scoliosis or kyphosis in a younger child should prompt careful evaluation.

Contractures and Gait Abnormalities

If a NM or MSK disorder prevents full range of motion around a joint, a joint **contracture** (shortening of the soft tissue around a joint) can develop, resulting in a fixed loss of joint motion. In an ankle joint contracture, the Achilles tendon becomes very short and the child will toe walk. Toe walking, limping, wide-leg walking, or other gait abnormalities should prompt medical attention to rule out one of these disorders.

PHYSICAL EXAMINATION OF THE MUSCULOSKELETAL SYSTEM

If the child can walk, observing the gait pattern is very valuable. During normal gait, the head and trunk should be level, with minimal sway from side to side. It is helpful to listen to the sound of the feet on the floor. Each footstep should be even, like a metronome, with equal pauses between foot strikes. Watch to see whether the child can maintain balance while standing on one leg and swinging through the opposite leg. The leg that is swinging through should clear the ground, and the foot should not drag; each step should be large enough to allow for forward progression of the body. More complex gait patterns can be better studied using videotape or computerized gait analysis.

If the child crawls, his or her ability to get up on all fours and move in a reciprocal (right then left) pattern should be documented. If the child is unable to crawl, it is still important to document whether he or she can sit independently and how he or she sits. Is the head held independently and the back straight? Are the limbs straight or contracted?

Children with disorders that cause an imbalance of the muscles around the spine can develop a significant spinal curvature. Because spinal curves are best managed when they are still small, the spine of a child who is at particular risk (e.g., a child with spastic cerebral palsy, meningomyelocele, or muscular dystrophy) should be examined regularly. Early clues suggesting scoliosis are unequal heights of the shoulders or a slanting of the waist. The ribs attach to the thoracic (upper) spine and may follow the curve of the vertebrae, causing a rib rise

or "rib hump" when the child bends forward. School screening examinations for scoliosis are designed to look for these physical exam findings to detect scoliosis as early as possible.

The hips, knees, and ankles should be examined for range of motion. Loss of motion in a joint can result from many causes. For example, bone abnormalities in the opposing surfaces of a joint or contractures can limit motion. Often an X ray of the joint is helpful in distinguishing between these two possibilities.

The hip exam, like the spine exam, should be performed often, as early treatment of hip problems is easier than later treatment. The examiner should be able to abduct (spread apart) the hips easily and symmetrically. Loss of hip **abduction** may indicate a hip dislocation or **subluxation.** Another easy way to assess whether the hip is dislocated is to look at the knee heights with the hips and knees flexed and the ankles together. If the knee heights are unequal, the hip may be dislocated or the legs may be of unequal length for some other reason.

The knee joint must be straight for standing but must flex to 90 degrees for comfortable sitting and flex even farther for easy stair climbing. Tightness of the hamstring muscles can limit knee movement. The ankle should be examined for plantarflexion (foot down) and dorsiflexion (foot up). The ability to dorsiflex beyond a neutral position (90 degrees) is important for both walking and sitting and should be tested with the knee both extended and flexed. The goal for every child is to maintain the feet in a plantargrade (flat on the floor) position and to maintain as much flexibility in the feet as possible.

Other important aspects of the musculoskeletal exam involve studying the rotation of the lower extremities. There are three possible areas (thigh, shin, and foot) where an internal twist can occur, causing the child to walk with a toe-in ("pigeon-toed") gait. There can be an internal twist in the femur bone, described as increased femoral anteversion. This can be assessed with the child **prone** by palpating or by looking at the amount of internal rotation compared with external rotation. If there is more internal rotation than external rotation, the femur is anteverted. If the leg appears to turn in when there is no discernible increase in femoral anteversion, then testing for internal tibial torsion (internal rotation in the tibia, or shin bone) can be performed by measuring the thigh-foot angle. Finally, internal rotation of the forefoot can also cause intoeing and can be best demonstrated by loss of the straight lateral (or outside) border of the foot. The foot instead appears *c*-shaped or bean shaped. If this internal foot position is accompanied by loss of ankle dorsiflexion, then the diagnosis of **clubfoot** is likely.

The upper extremities should also be examined for range of motion of the shoulders, elbows, and hands. The arms should be able to be placed above the head. The elbows should straighten fully. All fingers should be able to be straightened and brought out of the palm fully. The hands should be tested for feeling, as occasionally sensation may be diminished. Testing the ability of the child to grasp an object and place it in a desired spot demonstrates selective control, a skill necessary to operate hand controls.

Abnormal physical exam findings are often followed by X rays of the involved areas, which can help detect limits in movement caused by bony deformity. X rays are helpful in detecting the shapes of bone but are a poor gauge of the quality of bone. Almost one third of the bone must be lost before changes are detectable by X ray. Bone quality is best measured by a bone density scan which can detect early loss of bone mass.

DISORDERS OF THE MUSCULOSKELETAL SYSTEM

Musculoskeletal disorders may involve abnormalities of just one limb or joint or the entire skeleton. This section discusses the different types of MSK disorders, providing an example of each.

Skeletal Dysplasias: Achondroplasia

The skeletal dysplasias are a large, genetically diverse group of conditions characterized by abnormalities in the development, growth and maintenance of the skeleton. Many of these disorders result in disproportionate short stature (Savarirayan & Rimoin, 2002). There are approximately 175 different skeletal dysplasias (Orioli, Castilla, & Barbosa-Neto, 1986; Stoll et al., 1989).

Achondroplasia is the most common form of short stature that is associated with disproportionately shortened limbs. It occurs in 1 of every 15,000–25,000 live births. The disorder has been found to result from a point mutation in the gene coding for fibroblast growth factor receptor 3 or FGFR3 (Matsui, Yasui, & Kimura, 1998).

The condition is inherited as an autosomal-dominant trait (see Chapter 1), and most individuals have the same genetic mutation, so the physical manifestations of the condition tend to be similar across individuals (Bellus et al., 1995).

Thoracolumbar kyphosis (curvature of the mid-lower spine in the front to back plane) is present to some degree in most infants with achondroplasia as a result of their enlarged heads, hypotonia, and ligamentous laxity (double jointedness). The kyphosis typically improves spontaneously once the child begins to walk, but 10%–15% of children require bracing or surgical correction of the curvature (Ain & Browne, 2004; Ain & Shirley, 2004). Careful monitoring is essential, and support for the back, particularly in the very young child, may be helpful.

The major impairments of the extremities are short limbs, limited elbow and hip **extension,** and knee and leg deformities that can impede locomotion. Genu verum (bowed legs) occurs in 40% of individuals with achondroplasia, but only 25% will experience a clinically significant deformity that requires surgical correction (Beals, 2005). Significant advances have been made in limb-lengthening procedures, but it still takes about 3 years to achieve the desired lengthening. Growth hormone therapy has achieved only limited success in people with achondoplasia (Hagenas & Hertel, 2003).

Connective Tissue Disorders: Osteogenesis Imperfecta

Connective tissue, disorders are caused by the mechanical failure of collagen, which "connects" tissue. This results in joint hypermobility and, in the case of children with osteogenesis imperfecta (OI), brittle bones. Other examples of connective tissue disorders include Ehlers Danlos syndrome and Marfan syndrome.

Osteogenesis imperfecta (OI) is caused by a failure of formation of type I collagen, the scaffolding on which bone mineral is laid down. Blue sclera (the part of the eye that is normally white) and poor dentition, along with fractures and bone deformity, are the most common characteristics of this disorder. The clinical diagnosis of OI is supported by a skin biopsy to test for the underlying genetic defect (Minch & Kruse, 1998). OI has a prevalence of 1 in 20,000 births. Although hundreds of genetic variants have been identified, most result from a mutation in the COL1A1 (on chromosome 17) and COL1A2 (on chromosome 7) genes.

Orthopedic care has been the mainstay of management and involves measures to prevent fractures, to treat acute fractures, and to correct bony deformities. People with OI are particularly susceptible to disuse osteoporosis (bone weakness); therefore, promoting mobility in daily life and following injury is essential. Placing rods inside the bones for support at the time of a fracture or in conjunction with osteotomies (surgical cuts through the bone to correct deformities) can improve the bone alignment, shorten time to rehabilitation, and help prevent future fractures. Deformity of the spine occurs in 40%–80% of individuals with OI. Because thoracic curves can decrease lung capacity (Widemann et al., 1999), orthopedic consultation is recommended for monitoring curve progression with spine fusion surgery being performed if necessary (Engelbert et al., 1998).

The bone fragility seen in OI is due to disturbed organization of bone tissue, decreased bone mass, and altered bone geometry. While healthy growing children form 7% more bone than they resorb (lose) during growth and remodeling, children with mild OI only form 3% more bone than they resorb. Children with moderate to severe OI form essentially the same amount of bone as they resorb. This imbalance forms the rationale for treating children with OI with bisphosphonates (e.g., Fosamax, typically used to treat osteoporosis in post menopausal women), because this medication reduces osteoblast-mediated bone resorption (Shaw & Bishop, 2005; Zeitlin, Fassier, & Glorieux, 2003). Recent data suggest that these agents are most effective in younger children with severe forms of the disorder. However, older children on bisphosphonate therapy do report a reduction in bone pain and improvement in confidence and general well-being (Pizones et al., 2005).

Joint Disorders: Arthrogryposis

The most common joint disorder is rheumatoid **arthritis.** This section instead profiles arthrogryposis, as it is associated with developmental disabilities and arthritis is not. The term *arthrogryposis* is used to describe the prenatal onset of multiple congenital contractures. Although originally described as a single disorder, it is now clear that it is not a disease entity but a descriptive term for a clinical condition caused by limitation of normal joint motion during fetal growth. Arthrogryposis can result from a wide range of disorders including 1) abnormalities of muscle function, 2) abnormalities of the nerves

that connect the muscles, 3) abnormalities of connective tissue, 4) limitation of space within the uterus, 5) vascular compromise leading to loss of neurons, and 6) maternal illness. Congenital contractures occur in 1 in 3,000–5,000 live births. Although more than 150 different entities resulting in multiple congenital contractures have been recognized, clinicians commonly classify arthrogryposis as involvement of the limbs only, involvement of limbs with other abnormality, or involvement of limbs with major central nervous system dysfunction.

The term *arthrogryposis multiplex congenita*, or *amyloplasia*, is usually reserved for children with the most severe form. The condition occurs in about 1 in every 10,000 births. All four limbs are typically involved. Affected children have a defect primarily in muscle development (Hall, 2002). The primary defect is a loss of anterior horn cells in the spinal column, resulting in the partial paralysis of muscles during intrauterine life (Gordon, 1998). It can be inherited as an X-linked trait (i.e., the mother is a carrier) or an autosomal-recessive disorder, and several candidate genes have been identified (Tanamy et al., 2001; Zori et al., 1998).

Although spinal deformity at birth is uncommon, 30%–67% of children will develop scoliosis during childhood. Most curves are resistant to bracing. Physical therapy (PT) and occupational therapy (OT), however, are helpful in maintaining joint motion and maximizing functional development. In cases of arthrogryposis associated with other congenital anomalies, the child may have other medical problems that must be addressed.

Long-term orthopedic management is directed at maximizing function. Because arthrogryposis can be caused by many disorders, there is no single management plan. The common goals are independent ambulation or wheel chair mobility, self-care, and the ability to be employed and live independently. The initial treatment of any contracture involves gentle stretching and range-of-motion exercises. Once the joint is in a proper position, a lightweight splint may help prevent recurrence. If joint position is not acceptable, casting or soft-tissue release followed by casting may improve joint position.

DISORDERS OF THE NEUROMUSCULAR SYSTEM

In order for a muscle to produce movement across a joint, a signal must begin in the brain (upper motor neuron), pass through the spinal cord to an anterior horn cell (lower motor neuron) and then to a peripheral nerve, ending at a neuromuscular junction. Then, the electrical impulse must jump across the gap (synapse) at this junction, using the neurotransmitter acetylcholine. Finally, the message must pass to the muscle fiber, stimulating it to contract and resulting in movement. These components, from the anterior horn cell to the muscle, form the NM system (Figure 14.1). A defect anywhere in this system leads to weakness and decreased movement. The following sections discuss each level of this system and give examples of associated disorders.

Anterior Horn Cells: Spinal Muscular Atrophy

The nerve cells (neurons) in the spinal column that control movement are called anterior horn cells. The most well know disease associated with damage to the anterior horn cell is **polio.** Fortunately, thanks to the polio vaccine, this viral illness is almost extinct. Now, the most common disorder affecting the anterior horn cell in children is spinal muscular atrophy (SMA). It is caused by a congenital and progressive loss of these neurons and results in muscle weakness and atrophy (Strober & Tennekoon, 1999) with typical intellectual function (Gendron & MacKenzie, 1999; Mailman et al., 2002; Talbot, 1999). The disease, inherited as an autosomal-recessive trait (see Chapter 1), affects about 1 in 20,000 children and is caused by a mutation or change in the gene called SMN (survival motor neuron) that is located at the tip of the chromosome 5 (Jablonka et al., 2000). SMA has been divided into three clinical variants: SMA I (onset before 6 months of age), SMA II (onset between 6 and 18 months), and SMA III (later diagnosis, up to adulthood).

Infants with the SMA I (previously called Werdnig-Hoffmann disease) may appear typical at birth, but they soon develop low muscle tone and weakness, affecting proximal and distal muscles in the child's arms and legs as well as trunk. As a result, these infants cannot hold up their heads and have difficulty breathing, which leads to progressive respiratory failure. Although these infants have typical cognitive functioning, they rarely survive beyond 2 years of age because of the respiratory compromise. Symptoms of SMA II include a characteristic symmetrical weakness that is most severe in the proximal muscles, and respiratory muscles may also be involved. These children generally have low muscle tone, muscle weakness, and absence of deep tendon reflexes. The children can sit, but never walk. Spinal curvature often develops. Symptoms of SMA type III usually appear around 18 months of age. They include weakness, with a similar distribution to that of SMA II. Respiratory muscle weakness and spinal curvature sometimes develop but to a lesser degree than in types I or II. The disease progresses slowly, and children with SMA II can usually walk, at least until adolescence. Wheelchair use is often required later in life, but life span is usually not affected.

Care of children with SMA requires aggressive respiratory therapy to prevent pneumonia as well as ongoing monitoring of respiratory capacity (Barois & Estournet-Mathiaud, 1997). Occupational and speech-language therapy may be helpful with feeding and speech issues. As the disease progresses, oxygen or home ventilation may be required (Bach, Niranjan, & Weaver, 2000). Because scoliosis can reduce respiratory capacity, the spine should be fused while the child has good forced vital capacity. Once scoliosis begins to progress, surgery becomes increasingly difficult and eventually impossible in the face of respiratory deterioration (Phillips et al., 1990).

Disorders of the Peripheral Nerves: Charcot-Marie-Tooth Disease

Disorders of the peripheral nerves lead to paralysis of the muscles that are supplied by these nerves. Localized or generalized weakness occurs, depending on which nerves are involved. The term *neuropathy* is nonspecific and implies that one or several nerves are affected. *Peripheral neuropathy* refers to a neuropathy in which the more distal parts of the nerves (i.e., those of the fingers and toes) are affected first. It progresses toward the mid-line of the body as the disease worsens.

Charcot-Marie tooth (CMT) disease is the most common type of hereditary peripheral neuropathy, affecting 1 in 2, 500 individuals in the United States. CMT, also known as hereditary motor and sensory neuropathy (HMSN), involves a group of disorders caused by mutations in genes that affect the function and development of the peripheral nerves. In practical terms, it is useful to know whether the neuropathy affects one or both sensory and motor nerves, as the manifestation and rehabilitation depends on this. The most common form of

HSMN is type Ia, which is a sensory-motor neuropathy caused by a defective protein that forms myelin, the outer sheath over of the nerve (Bertorini et al., 2004; Sevilla & Vilchez, 2004; Shy, 2004).

Onset of symptoms of CMT depends on the specific type and may occur at birth or not until adulthood. Most cases present in adolescence or early adulthood. People with CMT typically present with weakness and wasting of the foot and lower leg muscles, which may result in foot drop and a high-stepped gait with frequent tripping or falls. Foot deformities, such as high arches (which is also called **pes cavus**) and hammertoes (a condition in which the ends of the toes curl downward), are characteristic as a result of weakness of the small muscles in the feet. Initially, though, the children can present with pes planus (flat feet) and need arch supports. The degeneration of motor nerves results in muscle weakness and atrophy in the arms, legs, hands, or feet, and the degeneration of sensory nerves results in a reduced ability to feel heat, cold, and pain. Because of the muscle weakness, contractures develop with time and sometimes curvature of the spine may occur (Shy, 2004).

In general, CMT is slowly progressive, and people with most forms of CMT have a normal life span. There is no cure for CMT, but PT, OT, braces and other orthopedic devices, and orthopedic surgery can help individuals with CMT live fairly functional lives despite the disabling symptoms of the disease (Bertortini et al., 2004; McDonald, 2001; Shy, 2004).

Diseases of the Neuromuscular Junction: Myasthenia Gravis

The peripheral nerves end at the neuromuscular junction. For a nerve impulse to cross the synapse separating the nerve and muscle, the chemical neurotransmitter acetylcholine must be released from the nerve terminal, travel through the space between the nerve and muscle, bind to its receptor on the muscle membrane (much like a key fitting into a keyhole), and generate the muscle membrane impulse that will transmit the signal to the contractile structures within the muscle cell. Impairment of any of these mechanisms prevents the impulse from generating muscle movement and results in disorders called myasthenic syndromes (from *myo* meaning muscle and *asthenia* meaning fatigability). Although in rare instances myasthenic syndromes are genetic in

origin, they are most often acquired as autoimmune disorders. The most common symptoms are fatigability after repetitive movements and fluctuation of the symptoms throughout the day. Myasthenia often affects the muscles of the face first, with droopy eyelids or indistinct speech. It may then progress to other muscle groups, interfering with eating, walking, or even breathing.

Treatment of acquired myasthenia is generally targeted to improve neuromuscular transmission and increase muscle strength while suppressing the production of abnormal antibodies. Immunosuppression with steroids is usually used as a first line of therapy and, if there is a lack of response, then other immunosuppressants, such as azathioprine or cyclosporine (Sandimmune) are used (Harvard & Fonseca, 1990). Thymectomy (Kogut et al., 2000), the surgical removal of the thymus, (small gland resting under the breast plate which plays key role in autoimmune response) can result in permanent remission in about 30% of cases. Although most individuals continue to require immunosuppressant therapy, such therapy can improve the symptoms or cure some individuals, possibly by rebalancing the immune system. Mestinon (pyridostigmine) is a common symptomatic treatment that slows the removal of acetylcholine at the synapse, thus giving temporary increase of muscle strength.

Disorders of Muscle

Disorders of muscle can involve voluntary and/or involuntary muscle function. Voluntary (skeletal) muscles are essential for movement and respiration, whereas involuntary muscles control cardiac and gastrointestinal function. The most common muscle disorders of childhood are inherited and include the muscular dystrophies and congenital myopathies.

Duchenne Muscular Dystrophy
DMD is the most common form of muscular dystrophy in childhood. It is a progressive skeletal muscle disorder caused by a genetic mutation in the X-linked dystrophin gene, resulting in absence of a critical protein, dystrophin (Hoffman et al., 1987). The incidence of DMD is approximately 1 in 3,300 male births (Jeppesen et al., 2003). This disorder is associated with a high spontaneous mutation rate (van Essen et al., 1992), so almost one third of boys with DMD have no family history of muscular dystrophy.

Lower-than-average IQ scores have been described in individuals with DMD, although results have not been consistent and many children have typical cognition (Felisari et al., 2000). Certain cognitive areas (i.e., verbal memory, digit span, and auditory comprehension) are more affected than others (Hinton et al., 2000). Deletions localized in specific part of the dystrophin gene are preferentially associated with cognitive impairment (Giliberto et al., 2004).

The disease manifests clinically in early childhood, although abnormal muscle **creatine kinase (CPK)** levels and pathological muscle changes can be seen in an affected newborn. Delay in walking and frequent falls are characteristic initial symptoms. Children with DMD usually walk on their tiptoes, and manifestations of proximal hip girdle muscle weakness become apparent by 3–4 years of age, when the child starts having difficulties climbing in the playground, getting up from the floor, and running. Muscle weakness is present initially in the neck **flexor** muscles, and the child needs to turn on his side when getting up from a **supine** position on the floor, showing the initial sign of the Gower's maneuver. Hypertrophy (abnormal enlargement) of the calf muscles is typical, often becoming very prominent by age 3–4 years (Figure 14.2). Hypertrophy of other muscles may also develop. Muscle mass, however, is usually decreased in later stages of the disease. Hip girdle muscles are affected before shoulder girdle muscles. Because of weakness of the hip **extensor** muscle, these individuals tend to rock from side to side when walking, producing a waddling gait.

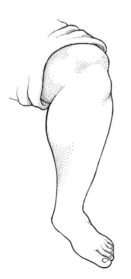

Figure 14.2. Abnormal enlargement of calf muscles associated with Duchenne muscular dystrophy (DMD).

As muscle deterioration proceeds, climbing stairs becomes difficult, requiring the use of both hands on a railing or crawling on all fours. In addition, shoulder girdle weakness begins to appear and affects daily activities. Contractures of heel cords, requiring vigorous daily stretching, may be a significant concern as early as 4–5 years of age. Leg and hip flexors (skeletal muscles that bend the leg over the hip) are other areas that may become contracted because of the alteration in gait resulting from the muscle weakness. If contractures are allowed to advance to a fixed equinovarus (foot flexed down and turned inward) position, the individual walks on the toes and often falls.

Accelerated deterioration in strength and balance often results from intercurrent disease or surgically induced immobilization. If tendon releases are performed, immediate mobilization in a walking splint or cast is necessary to prevent deterioration in muscle strength from disuse. When ambulation is no longer possible, typically by adolescence, contractures in the lower extremities become more pronounced and soon involve the shoulders. The need for daily PT and OT services at school and daily stretching exercises at home are imperative.

Kyphoscoliosis may develop after ambulation is lost. Maintaining an erect posture with long-leg braces or a stander may help prevent scoliosis and contractures and improve pulmonary function. It is useful to have a stander at school for the child to use for at least half an hour each day, plus another stander at home to use for an additional hour per day. Proper wheelchair sizing and solid seating and back support are important. Both manual and power wheelchairs are useful.

Cardiac and respiratory involvement often occurs in the later stages of disease. OT evaluation at school is essential at this stage to assess self-feeding, self-care, torso positioning within the classroom, and writing. A keyboard should be provided to complete school tasks, and an assistive technology evaluation should be completed. A voice recorder is useful for taking notes or a note taker can be appointed. Some students may require a classroom aide in order to participate fully in the academic environment and safely navigate the school building.

Baseline back X-ray films should be obtained for comparison with future films to monitor the development of scoliosis. The use of solid seat and back inserts in properly fitted wheelchairs is helpful in preventing scoliosis by keeping truncal posture erect. For some boys, long-leg braces can be fitted to allow braced upright standing to prevent curvature. Surgery is usually scheduled once the scoliosis films show 30–50 degree curvature (Brook et al., 1996). The optimal time for surgical intervention is while lung and cardiac function are satisfactory (Finder et al., 2004). Failure to repair scoliosis at this point can result in increased hospitalization rates, worsening of pulmonary function, and poor quality of life (Finder et al., 2004).

There is accumulating evidence that medical treatment of DMD should start as soon as the diagnosis is made (Dubowitz et al., 2002; Kinali et al., 2002). Daily prednisone (a steroid medication) stabilizes or improves strength; it is the only proven treatment for this disease (Griggs et al., 1993). The synthetic steroid deflazacort, which is presently available only in Europe and South America, appears to delay clinical progression of the disease and has fewer side effects than prednisone, although it shows an increase risk for asymptomatic cataract formation (Biggar et al., 2001; Campbell & Jacob, 2003; Moxley et al., 2005). There is some evidence that herbal supplements such as creatine and glutamine may improve strength and energy (Escolar et al., 2005). As with so many other incurable diseases, much hope resides in molecular genetic advancements. Different approaches to "fix" the gene or remedy the effects of the genetic abnormality have been proposed but are not yet ready for clinical application.

Congenital Myopathies Congenital myopathies are caused by mutations on genes that code for the structural proteins of muscle, such as actinin (causing nemaline myopathy), or functional proteins, such as the ryanodine receptor (in central core disease) or myotubularine (in centronuclear myopathy). These disorders usually manifest in infancy with marked hypotonia and weakness, feeding difficulties, and respiratory insufficiency. Within each disorder, there is a spectrum of severity (Dubowitz & Fardeau, 1995). Children with congenital myopathies are distinguished from those with muscular dystrophies because their level of CPK in blood is normal or only mildly elevated. They also have a different pattern of abnormalities seen on muscle biopsy. They usually have thin limbs rather than the hypertrophy seen in DMD. Extraocular muscles can be affected, and feeding difficulties are seen early. Finally, the disease course is static rather than progressive, so in contrast to DMD, the child's function tends to improve rather than worsen over time.

Care of the child with a congenital myopathy will depend on the severity of the disorder. No pharmacological treatment exists for any form of the disorders. These children have typical cognitive development, so education should be provided at the appropriate age and grade level. However, some children may be nonverbal because of facial and tongue weakness, so an **augmentative and alternative communication** evaluation is essential. Rehabilitation therapy centers on improving daily living skills.

General Principles for the Management of Musculoskeletal and Neuromuscular Disorders

Educational Services Children with acute NM disorders such as myasthenia gravis or inflammatory myopathies often require prolonged admissions to the hospital and are therefore absent from school for extended periods. Some require homebound instruction during convalescence. Once the child returns to school, supportive measures such as PT and OT need to be in place (Table 14.1). Children with fluctuating disorders such as myasthenia gravis may require rest periods throughout the day or a shortened school day. Children with chronic

Table 14.1. School accommodations for children with neuromuscular and musculoskeletal disorders

Physical and occupational therapy

   Stretching

   Range-of-motion exercises

   Muscle cramp massage

   Safety training (on stairs and playground)

   Hallway safety

   Accommodating activities of daily living to changing physical needs (e.g., toileting, lunchtime/cafeteria safety)

   Adapted or modified physical education and sports for individuals with disabilities

   Consultation for body positioning, seating, and gross- and fine-motor function

   Assistive technology

Other school accommodations

   Provision of an additional set of textbooks to avoid having to transport books from one classroom to another

   Access to an elevator

   Consideration of students' physical needs when designing class schedule

   Preferential seating in the classroom

   Consideration of students' physical needs when developing a school emergency evacuation plan

   Consideration of students' needs when planning field trips and school events

disorders such as congenital and hereditary progressive myopathies, as well as chronic polyneuropathies, require specialized rehabilitation care as noted previously. In terms of chronic treatment, steroids are the most common medication used. Two adverse events, behavior problems and weight gain, may have implications in daily living. Changes in behavior related to the chronic treatment could have implications in school performance and patient relationships. Steroids can cause depression, hyperactivity, and psychosis. Caregivers and teachers need to be aware of the possibility of these side effects and immediately communicate personality changes to the child's primary care doctor. Sometimes a simple adjustment of the dose or suspension of the medication can improve these symptoms. Because attention-deficit/hyperactivity disorder (ADHD; see Chapter 24) can occur with DMD, it is essential to distinguish between an adverse effect of the medication and a symptom of ADHD.

A child receiving steroids also tends to have increased appetite and weight gain. Unwanted weight gain, while never a happy occurrence, can be very detrimental in children with NM disease, especially those with muscular dystrophies. The increased body weight becomes a burden on the already weak muscles, and this can obscure all the benefits that can be gained by steroid treatment. This problem can be avoided if the child follows a healthy nutritional plan. Children on steroids should bring lunch to school in order to follow their diet.

Medical Care In addition to disease-specific medical care, children with NM disease should have routine immunizations as recommended for all children by the American Academy of Pediatrics (American Academy of Pediatrics, Committee on Infectious Diseases, 2007). They should also receive the pneumococcal and annual influenza (flu) vaccine.

Children with myopathies and muscular dystrophy are at increased risk for sleep apnea. Symptoms may be noticeable during daytime and often involve fatigue, falling asleep during class, or morning headaches. A polysomnographic (sleep) study with continuous CO_2 monitoring is the best way to assess the need for ventilatory support. Provision of noninvasive nocturnal ventilation can significantly increase quality of life (Baydur et al., 2000). The decisions regarding long-term ventilation, be it invasive or noninvasive, should involve the child, his or her caregivers, and his or her medical team.

Rehabilitation Management No large prospective studies have been performed to evaluate the effectiveness of PT, stretching exercises, and braces in patients with neuromuscular disorders, so scientific evidence for solid recommendations is absent. However, the current thought is that PT and rehabilitation is likely to play an important role in maximizing functional status and tone, as well as in delaying the need to use a wheelchair.

In muscular dystrophies there is a general consensus that high-resistance exercises, especially those involving eccentric contractions (i.e., weight lifting, abdominal crunches), are damaging to the muscle cell membrane and should be avoided (Ansved, 2003). However, the impact of a sedentary life is equally negative (McDonald, 2002). Therefore, active, nonresistive exercises are encouraged; swimming is a good example. Keeping an active lifestyle will also prevent excessive weight gain, especially if the child is receiving steroids. Daily extended walks will help maintain strength and retard contracture formation. Swivel walkers may be used to provide low-energy ambulation (Sibert et al., 1987). Both the nature and quantity of activity should be modified so that fatigue does not remain after a night's sleep. Wheelchair games can be played when ambulation is lost. Children with NM disorders who are confined to bed because of the disease, injury, or surgery require PT, including range-of-motion exercises, with return to more active exercise, including walking, as soon as possible. In the event of leg fractures, walking casts should be used as soon as possible (Siegel, 1977). Similarly, every effort should be made to limit the amount of time the child spends in a cast to the minimum needed to achieve fracture healing.

Avoid Contractures Nighttime stretching orthoses or splinting should be recommended as soon as tightness of the heel cords is noticed (Hyde et al., 2000). A standing board tilted at 20 degrees may be used for 20 minutes twice per day to provide constant stretching of the Achilles tendon in children who do not ambulate. If strenuous stretching is not effective, surgical release of tight heel cords may be beneficial (Goertzen et al., 1995). Temporary bracing after tendon surgery is necessary for optimal results.

Avoid Disuse that Leads to Low Bone Mass and Pathologic Fractures In children with neuromuscular and musculoskeletal disorders, a fracture can occur with little or no trauma (e.g., from gentle range of motion exercises during PT). Such fractures are called pathologic fractures and may result from bone fragility (especially OI), as a secondary effect of a medication (e.g., steroids, antiepileptic drugs), or as weakness from disuse (Sambrook & Jones, 1995). Children with pathological fractures may have swelling and increased warmth of the fractured extremity. Weight-bearing activities are important for the maintenance of bone density, which in turn helps decrease the risk of fractures. Thus, having the child stand is extremely important, as bones have internal receptors that recognize weight-bearing activity and send signals to make bones stronger in response. Children who cannot stand independently can use standing frames to build up their bones. Similarly, it is essential that these children be given diets rich in calcium and vitamin D.

SUMMARY

The MSK and NM systems support the physical structure of the body and help carry out movement. Diseases affecting these systems can have a significant impact on a child's functional capacity and independence. The first challenge to treatment is to determine the highest level of function that a child can realistically attain. The child's care team should include family members, primary care physicians, therapists, surgeons, and rehabilitative specialists, as each member of the team brings insights from a different perspective. The goals are to gain or retain function, conserve energy, and improve quality of life. Attempts to reach these goals may involve a combination of medical and nonmedical therapies, including medications, bracing, PT and OT, seating systems, adaptive equipment, and, when necessary, surgery. The treatment efforts may need to be short or long term. Many of the disorders are under active investigation, with the goal of developing new treatment approaches, including the repair of genetic material, more effective medications, and improved surgical techniques.

REFERENCES

Ain, M.C., & Browne, J.A. (2004). Spinal arthrodesis with instrumentaiton for thoracolumbar kyphosis in pediatric achonrdoplasia. *Spine, 29*(18), 2075–2080.

Ain, M.C., & Shirley, E.D. (2004). Spinal fusion for kyphosis in achondroplasia. *Journal of Pediatric Orthopedics, 24*(5), 541–545.

American Academy of Pediatrics, Committee on Genetics. (1995). Health Supervision for children with achondroplasia. *Pediatrics, 95*, 443–451.

American Academy of Pediatrics, Committee on Infectious Diseases. (2007). Recommended Immunization Schedules for Children and Adolescents–United States, 2007. *Pediatrics, 119*, 207–214.

Ansved, T. (2003). Muscular dystrophies: Influence of physical conditioning on the disease evolution. *Current Opinion in Clinical Nutrition and Metabolic Care, 6*(4), 435–439.

Bach, J.R., Niranjan, V., & Weaver, B. (2000). Spinal muscular atrophy type 1: A noninvasive respiratory management approach. *Chest, 117*(4), 1100–1105.

Barois, A., & Estournet-Mathiaud, B. (1997). Respiratory problems in spinal muscular atrophies. *Pediatric Pulmonology, 16*(Suppl.), 140–141.

Baydur, A., Layne, E., Aral, H., et al. (2000). Long term non-invasive ventilation in the community for patients with musculoskeletal disorders: 46 year experience and review. *Thorax, 55*(1), 4–11.

Beals, R.K. (2005). Surgical correction of bowlegs in achondroplasia. *Journal of Pediatric Orthopedics, 14*(4), 245–249.

Bellus, G.A., Hefferon, T.W., Rosa, I., et al. (1995). Achondroplasia is defined by recurrent G380R mutations of FGFR3. *American Journal of Human Genetics, 56*, 368–373.

Bertorini, T., Narayanaswami, P., & Rashed, H. (2004). Charcot-Marie-Tooth disease (hereditary motor sensory neuropathies) and hereditary sensory and autonomic neuropathies. *Neurologist, 10*(6), 327–337.

Biggar, W.D., Gingras, M., Fehlings, D.L., et al. (2001). Deflazacort treatment of Duchenne muscular dystrophy. *The Journal of Pediatrics, 138*(1), 45–50.

Brook, P.D., Kennedy, J.D., Stern, L.M., et al. (1996). Spinal fusion in Duchenne's muscular dystrophy. *Journal of Pediatric Orthopedics, 16*(3), 324–331.

Campbell, C., & Jacob, P. (2003). Deflazacort for the treatment of Duchenne Dystrophy: A systematic review. *BMC Neurology, 3*, 7.

Dubowitz, V., & Fardeau, M. (1995). Proceedings of the 27th ENMC sponsored workshop on congenital muscular dystrophy. 22–24 April 1994, The Netherlands. *Neuromuscular Disorders, 5*(3), 253–258.

Dubowitz, V., Kinali, M., Main, M., (2002). Remission of clinical signs in early Duchenne muscular dystrophy on intermittent low-dosage prednisolone therapy. *European Journal of Paediatric Neurology, 6*(3), 153–159.

Engelbert, R.H., Pruijs, H.E., Beemer, F.A., et al. (1998). Osteogenesis imperfecta in childhood: Treatment strategies. *Archives in Physical Medicine and Rehabilitation, 79*, 1590–1594.

Escolar, D.M., Buyse, G., Henricson, E., et al. (2005). CINRG randomized controlled trial of creatine and glutamine in Duchenne muscular dystrophy. *Annals of Neurology, 58*(1), 151–155.

Felisari, G., Martinelli Boneschi, F., Bardoni, A., et al. (2000). Loss of Dp140 dystrophin isoform and intellectual impairment in Duchenne dystrophy. *Neurology, 55*(4), 559–564.

Finder, J.D., Birnkrant, D., Carl, J., et al. (2004). Respiratory care of the patient with Duchenne muscular dystrophy: ATS consensus statement. *American Journal of Respiratory and Critical Care Medicine, 170*(4), 456–465.

Gendron, N.H., & MacKenzie, A.E. (1999). Spinal muscular atrophy: Molecular pathophysiology. *Current Opinions in Neurology, 12*(2), 137–42.

Giliberto, F., Ferreiro, V., Dalamon, V., et al. (2004). Dystrophin deletions and cognitive impairment in Duchenne/Becker muscular dystrophy. *Neurological Research, 26*(1), 83–87.

Goertzen, M., Baltzer, A., & Voit, T. (1995). Clinical results of early orthopaedic management in Duchenne muscular dystrophy. *Neuropediatrics, 26*(5), 257–259.

Gordon, N. (1998). Arthrogryposis multiplex congenita. *Brain Development, 20,* 507–511.

Griggs, R.C., Moxley, R.T., III, Mendell, J.R., et al. (1993). Duchenne dystrophy: Randomized, controlled trial of prednisone (18 months) and azathioprine (12 months). *Neurology, 43*(3, Pt. 1), 520–527.

Hagenas, L., & Hertel, T., (2003). Skeletal dysplasia, growth hormone treatment and body proportion: Comparison with other syndromic and non-syndromic short children. *Hormone Research, 60*(Suppl. 3), 65–70.

Hall, J.G. (2002). Don't use the term "amyoplasia" loosely. *American Journal of Medical Genetics, 111*(3), 344.

Harvard, C.W., & Fonseca, V. (1990). New treatment approaches to myasthenia gravis. *Drugs, 39*(1), 66–73

Hinton, V.J., De Vivo, D.C., Nereo, N.E., et al. (2000). Poor verbal working memory across intellectual level in boys with Duchenne dystrophy. *Neurology, 54*(11), 2127–2132.

Hoffman, E.P., Brown, R.H., Jr., & Kunkel, L.M. (1987). Dystrophin: The protein product of the Duchenne muscular dystrophy locus. *Cell, 51*(6), 919–928.

Hyde, S.A., Fløytrup, I., Glent, S., et al. (2000). A randomized comparative study of two methods for controlling Tendo Achilles contracture in Duchenne muscular dystrophy. *Neuromuscular Disorders, 10*(4–5), 257–263.

Jablonka, S., Rossoll, W., Schrank, B., et al. (2000). The role of SMN in spinal muscular atrophy. *Journal of Neurology, 247* (Suppl. 1), 137–142.

Jeppesen, J., Green, A., Steffensen, B.F., et al. (2003). The Duchenne muscular dystrophy population in Denmark, 1977–2001: Prevalence, incidence and survival in relation to the introduction of ventilator use. *Neuromuscular Disorders, 13*(10), 804–812.

Kinali, M., Mercuri, E., Main, M., et al. (2002). An effective, low-dosage, intermittent schedule of prednisolone in the long-term treatment of early cases of Duchenne dystrophy. *Neuromuscular Disorders, 12* (Suppl. 1), S169–S174.

Kogut, K.A., Bufo, A.J., Rothenberg, S.S., et al. (2000). Thoracoscopic thymectomy for myasthenia gravis in children. *Journal of Pediatric Surgery, 35*(11), 1576–1577.

Lahoti, O., & Bell, M.J. (2005). Transfer of pectoralis major in arthrogryposis to restore elbow flexion: Deteriorating results in the long term. *The Journal of Bone and Joint Surgery: British Volume, 87*(6), 858–860.

Mailman, M.D., Heinz, J.W., Papp, A.C., et al. (2002). Molecular analysis of spinal muscular atrophy and modification of the phenotype by SMN2. *Genetics in Medicine, 4*(1), 20–26.

Matsui, Y., Yasui, N., Kimura, T., et al. (1998). Genotype phenotype correlation in achondroplasia and hypochondroplasia. *The Journal of Bone and Joint Surgery: British Volume, 80,* 1052–1056.

McDonald, C.M. (2001). Peripheral neuropathies of childhood. *Physical Medicine and Rehabilitation Clinics of North America, 12*(2), 473–490.

McDonald, C.M. (2002). Physical activity, health impairments, and disability in neuromuscular disease. *American Journal of Physical Medicine & Rehabilitation, 81*(11, Suppl.), S108–S120.

Minch, C.M., & Kruse, R.W. (1998). Osteogenesis imperfecta: A review of basic science and diagnosis. *Orthopedics, 21,* 558–567, 568–569.

Moxley, R.T., III, Ashwal, S., Pandya, S., et al. (2005). Practice parameter: Corticosteroid treatment of Duchenne dystrophy: Report of the Quality Standards Subcommittee of the American Academy of Neurology and the Practice Committee of the Child Neurology Society. *Neurology, 64*(1), 13–20.

Orioli, I.M., Catilla, E.E., & Barbosa-Neto, J.G. (1986). The birth prevalence rates for the skeletal dysplasias. *Journal of Medical Genetics, 23*(4), 328–332.

Phillips, D.P., Roye, D.P., Jr., Farcy, J.P., et al. (1990). Surgical treatment of scoliosis in a spinal muscular atrophy population. *Spine, 15*(9), 942–945.

Pizones, J., Plotkin, H., Parra-Garcia, J.I., et al. (2005). Bone healing in children with osteogenesis imperfecta treated with bisphosphonates. *Journal of Pediatric Orthopedics,25*(3), 332–335.

Sambrook, P.N., & Jones, G. (1995). Corticosteroid osteoporosis. *British Journal of Rheumatology, 34,* 8–12.

Savarirayan, R., & Rimoin, D.L. (2002). The skeletal dysplasias. *Best Practice and Research in Clinical Endocrinology and Metabolism, 16*(3), 547–560.

Sevilla, T., & Vilchez, J.J. (2004). Different phenotypes of Charcot-Marie-Tooth disease caused by mutations in the same gene. Are classical criteria for classification still valid? *Neurologia, 19*(5), 264–271.

Shaw, N.J., & Bishop, N.J. (2005). Bisphosphonate treatment of bone disease. *Archives of Disease in Childhood, 90*(5), 494–499.

Shaw, N.J., White, C.P., Fraser, W.D., et al. (1994). Osteopenia in cerebral palsy. *Archives of Disease in Childhood, 71,* 235–238.

Shy, M.E. (2004). Charcot-Marie-Tooth disease: An update. *Current Opinion in Neurology, 17*(5), 579–585.

Sibert, J.R., Williams, V., Burkinshaw, R., (1987). Swivel walkers in Duchenne muscular dystrophy. *Archives of Disease Childhood, 62*(7), 741–742.

Siegel, I.M. (1977). Fractures of long bones in Duchenne muscular dystrophy. *The Journal of Trauma, 17*(3), 219–222.

Stoll, C., Dott, B., Roth, M.P., et al. (1989). Birth prevalence rates of skeletal dysplasias. *Clinical Genetics, 35* (2), 88–92.

Strober, J.B., & Tennekoon, G.I. (1999). Progressive spinal muscular atrophies. *Journal of Child Neurology, 14*(11), 691–695.

Talbot, K. (1999). Spinal muscular atrophy. *Journal of Inherited Metabolic Disease, 22*(4), 545–554.

Tanamy, M.G., Magal, N., Halpern, G.J., et al. (2001). Fine mapping places the gene for arthrogryposis multiplex congenita neuropathic type between D5S394 and D5S2069 on chromosome 5qter. *American Journal of Medical Genetics, 104*(2), 152–156.

van Essen, A.J., Busch, H.F., te Meerman, G.J., (1992). Birth and population prevalence of Duchenne muscular dystrophy in The Netherlands. *Human Genetics, 88* (3), 258–266.

Widemann, R.F., Bitan, F.D., Laplaza, F.J., et al. (1999). Spinal deformity, pulmonary compromise, and quality of life in osteogenesis imperfecta. *Spine, 24,* 1673.

Zeitlin, L., Fassier, F., & Glorieux, F.H. (2003). Modern approach to children with osteogenesis imperfecta. *Journal of Pediatric Orthopedics, Part B, 12*(2), 77–87.

Zori, R.T., Gardner, J.L., Zhang, J., et al. (1998). Newly described form of X-linked arthrogryposis maps to the long arm of the human X chromosome. *American Journal of Medical Genetics, 78,* 450–454.

15 Patterns in Development and Disability

Louis Pellegrino

Upon completion of this chapter, the reader will

- Understand the basic definitions of development and disability
- Understand constitutional and contextual contributions to development
- Understand how typical and atypical patterns of development are assessed
- Understand how disturbances in expected patterns of development lead to the diagnosis of specific developmental disabilities
- Understand how the diagnosis and etiology of disability differ

---

BJ

BJ is a 3-year-old boy who demonstrates skills that are significantly below his age level. He sat independently at 12 months of age and walked for the first time at 22 months of age. He began using single words at 24 months of age and just recently started putting words together. BJ responds inconsistently to single-step commands and is beginning to point out body parts following verbal direction. He is mainly interested in exploratory play and is starting to show an interest in simple pretend play. He is able to remove his socks and shoes, but he is otherwise dependent on his parents for dressing and undressing. Although BJ is not yet toilet trained, he is beginning to show an interest and inconsistently indicates a need for a diaper change. His parents say that his skills are most like those of a 1½-year-old.

BJ and other children who have significant developmental delays raise concerns about the possibility that they may have a developmental disability. The terms *development* and *disability* are frequently used together to describe a range of problems that are usually recognized in childhood but that may have lifelong functional implications. Both terms have become so much a part of common usage that it is easy to lose sight of their precise meaning, either when used separately or together. This book is devoted to describing how disability arises from disturbances in typical patterns of development. What follows is an attempt to describe in general terms what constitutes typical and atypical development.

WHAT IS DEVELOPMENT?

Development can refer to anything that changes over time (e.g., a photographic negative develops), but it is most often used to describe an organic process of change. For the purposes of this discussion, the term *development* is used with reference to changes in human thought, behavior, and function. Development is distinguished from growth, which refers more specifically to physical increases in height, weight, head size, and sexual maturation. Although the concepts *growth* and *development* are obviously connected, the techniques used to measure and describe them tend to be separate.

As applied to the individual human being, the term *development* can take on different meanings. On the one hand, each person changes in response to a specific set of life circumstances and experiences. In this sense every human being has a unique developmental history that can never be replicated. On the other hand, it is well known that individuals experience changes in cognition, emotion, and in specific abilities that seem to relate to a common "blueprint" that transcends particular life histories or cultures. For example, most children learn to walk at about the same time and seem to follow a fairly consistent protocol leading to the acquisition of this particular skill. Similarly, children universally and spontaneously learn to speak their native language and do so in a predictable sequence of steps without any explicit instruction in vocabulary or grammar. More general changes in behavior and social-emotional responses also occur in predictable ways. Infants begin to exhibit "stranger anxiety" at about 8 or 9 months of age. Toddlers demonstrate limit-testing behavior in the service of increased autonomy. School-age children become enamored of rules and enjoy a sense of industrious accomplishment. Preteens and teens experience a renewed sense of independence and identity in the context of intensified peer relations.

Human development is wonderfully varied but reasonably predictable, and for the purposes of this discussion, may be defined as follows: *Development* refers to the characteristic, predictable ways that behavior changes during the human life cycle. At its most basic level, *behavior* refers to any action that one person can perform and that another person can observe. Moving a leg, sneezing, saying a word, or composing a symphony are all forms of human behavior. Behavior can be characterized as simple (moving an arm) or complex (playing a concerto). Some forms of behavior are inherently more meaningful than others (e.g., talking versus coughing). With regard to the definition of development, behavior that is most directly relevant to real-life situations tends to be of greatest interest. Behavior is also used as a proxy for aspects of cognition and emotion that are critically important to development but that cannot be observed directly. Observation and interpretation of behavior is the bread and butter of developmental assessment.

Development and the Nervous System

Development is dependent on the brain, and the predictable behavioral changes that characterize development occur in parallel with the maturation of the central nervous system (Figure 15.1). Functional and structural changes in the human nervous system are most dramatically evident during fetal life and early childhood but continue into adulthood (see Chapters 2 and 13). Early brain development is dominated by a genetically predetermined series of events resulting in the establishment of basic brain structures. By the end of the second trimester of pregnancy, the maximum number of neurons (brain cells) that an individual will ever possess are already present in the fetal brain. Subsequent brain development is dominated by processes that increase the connectivity and functionality of existing neuronal elements. Myelination is a process that involves elaboration of supportive structures that improve transmission of electrical impulses from one part of the nervous system to another. Myelination is most exuberant during early childhood (especially during the first 3 years) but continues into adulthood. Synaptogenesis is the elaboration of connections, or synapses, between individual neurons. This process peaks between 7 and 8 years of age; thereafter, there is a drop off in the total number of synapses related to a "pruning back" of underutilized connections (Volpe, 2001).

These processes promote and are intimately connected with developmental change. For example, myelination of key corticospinal pathways (pathways from the cortex of the brain to the spinal cord that orchestrate movement) during the first year of life is one of the main determinants of early gross motor development (Volpe, 2001). There also seem to be critical changes in the functional organization of the brain toward the end of the second year of life that create an opportunity for explosive language development that typically occurs between 18 and 24 months of age (Neville & Mills, 1997). Changing nervous system plasticity (the ability of the nervous system to change or adapt) over the course of the human life cycle also creates opportunities and constraints on development. The well-known observation that young children are much more easily able to become fluent in a foreign language than adults or older children (beyond 8 or 9 years of age) is an example of this. Indeed, there appears to be a sensitive period for language acquisition during these early years; children who miss this opportunity will most likely never develop fluency in any language (Grimshaw et al., 1998; Ross & Bever, 2004). The good news for adults is that although there is decreased brain plasticity with age, learning continues unabated through the entire life cycle. The brain works by creating a rich network of functional connections within and across many cortical and subcortical domains, and these networks are continually enhanced and elaborated throughout the life span.

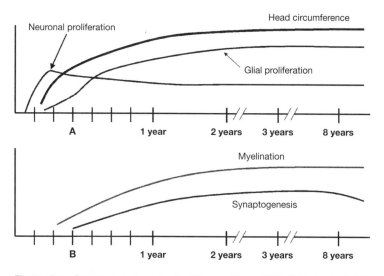

Figure 15.1. Patterns in brain maturation (*Source:* Volpe, 1995). A) During the 1st trimester of pregnancy, central nervous system development is dominated by formation of basic brain structures in association with proliferation of brain cells (neurons). The peak number of neurons is achieved at the end of this period. Proliferation of supporting elements (glial cells) begins by the end of the second trimester and continues through early childhood. B) Myelination (formation of the "insulation" of neuronal connections) proceeds in parallel with the development of glial cells and continues into adult life. Synaptogenesis (formation of the network of connections between neurons) is most exuberant during early childhood and begins to level off in late childhood.

Development in Context

Developmental change is driven from both within and without. Neurological maturation is the internal driving force; external influences derive from the environment. The "environment" is actually not a single entity: it consists of the physical environment and the social context. The physical environment is the Newtonian universe of light and heat, cause and effect, friction and gravity to which all organisms must be adapted. The social context consists of the people, activities, and social settings that embrace the developing individual and that are defined by history and culture. Various developmental theories have tended to emphasize these different influences to a greater or lesser extent. Gesell (Knobloch & Pasamanick, 1974) emphasized the maturational aspects of development; Piaget (1990) emphasized the development of cognitive and problem solving abilities relative to the physical environment; Vgotsky (1986) emphasized the importance of the sociocultural system in providing the basis for the development of higher cognitive processes. Bronfenbrenner (1979) took this a step further by describing the embedded structures of the social environment (Figure 15.2). He defined a variety of developmental settings within which the individual is immersed and which serve as the engine for developmental change. Bronfenbrenner's formulation is appealing because it provides a way to think about developmental change as it occurs in real-life settings. For example, the development of language would be viewed as arising within the context of the home and the parent–child relationship and not simply as something that "happens" to the child. Bronfenbrenner also recognized that the process of development involves *everyone* embedded within a particular developmental setting (the child is not the only person who develops). Development is seen to be a property of the social landscape as much as a property of individuals, and recognition is given to cultural differences that influence both the nature and interpretation of developmental change. The individual is seen as a nexus of potential action that is only actuated when placed in this larger social and cultural context.

Dynamic Systems Theory

Contemporary theories of development attempt to transcend older distinctions by conceptualizing the human organism as an amalgam of func-

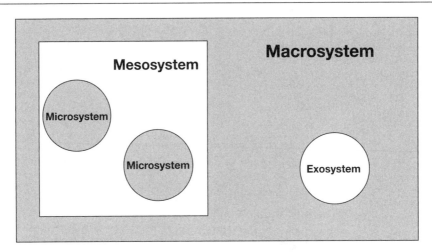

Figure 15.2. Development in context (*Source:* Bronfenbrenner, 1979). Bronfenbrenner's framework describes a series of embedded settings within which development occurs. The microsystem is a setting, such as home or school, in which a child actually participates. *Mesosystem* refers to the collection of microsystems for a particular child. *Exosystem* refers to settings that a child does not directly participate in but that still affect the child's development (e.g., a parent's place of work). *Macrosystem* refers to the cultural milieu that defines the unique characteristics of the various subsystems. (From Pellegrino, L., & Meyer, G. [1995]. Interdisciplinary care of the child with cerebral palsy. In J.P. Dormans & L. Pellegrino [Eds.], *Caring for children with cerebral palsy: A team approach* [p. 66]. Baltimore: Paul H. Brookes Publishing Co.; reprinted by permission.)

tional components or systems that cooperate in an ongoing process of adaptation to changing environmental circumstances. Dynamic systems theory, in particular, emphasizes that behavior is task specific and focuses on process rather than product when describing the determinants of developmental change (Thelen & Smith, 1996). For example, motor development is traditionally described as a direct consequence of neurological maturation. In this sense, milestones such as rolling, sitting, and walking are considered to be genetically and neurologically "pre-programmed" events. Dynamic systems theory places neurologic maturation on par with several other cooperating systems, including musculoskeletal components, sensory integrative mechanisms, and individual-specific characteristics such as body and head size (Campbell, 1995). Developmental sequences, rather than being rigidly predetermined, are in a sense, discovered through a dynamic process of adaptation. Skills are self-assembled as a child engages in a series of trial and error processes, drawing upon relevant functional systems and organized around a specific task. In this connection, dynamic systems theory provides a more satisfying explanation for variations in development that are difficult to explain otherwise. For example, many infants who are otherwise typical in their motor development may show unexpected departures from the expected

sequence of motor milestones. Healthy preterm infants are especially known for this. Many of these children exhibit transient differences in muscle tone in early infancy that result in relatively low muscle tone (looseness) in the trunk or torso and relatively high muscle tone (stiffness) in the legs. This pattern makes it relatively difficult for them to maintain a sitting posture but tends to affect other activities to a lesser degree. Infants who are unable to sit may be able to crawl or even pull to stand in apparent defiance of the expected sequence of milestones. Maturational theories cannot easily explain this phenomenon. Dynamic systems theory would suggest that muscle tone differences make certain tasks more difficult (in this example, sitting), but have less of an effect other tasks (crawling, pulling to stand).

Another example relates to the well-researched recommendation that infants should sleep on their backs to reduce the risk of sudden infant death syndrome (SIDS) (American Academy of Pediatrics, 1992). Implementation of the recommendation has had the desired effect of reducing SIDS, but it has also resulted in changes in the expected pattern of motor development during the first year of life (Davis et al., 1998). Infants who sleep on their backs (supine position) tend to learn to roll, sit, crawl, and pull to stand later than infants who sleep on their bellies (prone position). Infants in both groups walk independently at about the same time. A purely maturationalist perspective cannot explain this difference. Dynamic systems theory would suggest that the prone position offers mechanical advantages over the supine position relative to the emergence of these motor activities. Infants who spend more time on their backs are therefore at a temporary disadvantage with regard to early motor development (the dramatic advantages of the supine position—reducing the rate of SIDS—clearly outweigh any short term disadvantages, however).

Dynamic systems theory offers a conceptual framework for explaining both expected patterns of development and normal variations in these patterns. It allows for the possibility that similar functional outcomes can be arrived at by different pathways and that each individual pursues a unique developmental trajectory that will never be replicated in quite the same way again.

PATTERNS IN DEVELOPMENT

In order to make reproducible observations of development, it is necessary to break it down into component parts. The component parts have been variously described as developmental strands, streams, and domains (Table 15.1). Most developmental screening and psychometric instruments rely on this fragmentation of development into domains. There is some variability in how these domains are defined, however. Development may be defined in terms of broad functional domains; this type of scheme tends to emphasize adaptation to real-life situations (e.g., whether a child can get dressed, walk to school, give a report, or play with friends at recess). Development may also be defined in terms of specific skill sets. These skill sets tend to refer to specific abilities that are easily observed and tested in children, such as speech (putting words together to form a phrase), gross motor skills (jumping in place), symbolic play (engaging in pretend play with dolls), and academic skills (reading at grade level). These two schemes are not mutually exclusive; in fact, skill sets make specific contributions to larger functional domains, and functional domains provide a frame of reference for specific skill sets. For example, the ability to manipulate small objects (a specific type of fine motor skill) contributes to the ability to work with buttons and zippers when getting dressed (a broad functional category). In practice, both types of schemes are drawn upon in different contexts to help characterize a particular child's developmental pattern.

Table 15.1. Defining developmental domains

By functional domains	Communication/socialization
	Conversation skills
	Literacy (reading and writing)
	Social engagement
	Activities of daily living
	Dressing skills
	Toileting skills
	Feeding skills
	Electronic/computer literacy
	Mobility
	Ambulatory skills
By skill sets	Language
	Expressive Language
	Receptive Language
	Problem solving
	Visual-spatial skills
	Visual-motor skills
	Social and play
	Sensory
	Vision
	Hearing
	Motor
	Fine motor
	Gross motor
	Oral motor
	Attention and impulse control
	Academic

Developmental Milestones

Reproducibility in the observation of developmental change also requires the definition of specific markers, or milestones, that can be generally agreed upon and reliably reproduced. Much of the early work in defining a variety of milestones was done by Arnold Gesell and his colleagues at Yale University in early to mid-20th century (Knobloch & Pasamanick, 1974). Gesell amassed an enormous amount of information regarding a wide range of skills and abilities in various domains at different ages. He was able to gather from this a finite list of specific behaviors that were easily observed and which emerged during a relatively narrow range of ages. These items have become familiar components of many development screening and assessment instruments (Capute & Accardo, 2005; Frankenburg et al., 1992).

Milestones can be very useful in a variety of ways. Referencing particular milestones allows us to describe a child's pattern of skills, and milestones provide a means for tracking developmental progress. Milestones can become problematic, however, if they are misapplied or misinterpreted. Although many milestones reflect intrinsically important functional accomplishments, others are not critically important in and of themselves. For example, walking independently and speaking in sentences are intrinsically important milestones, whereas stacking blocks or placing a peg in a pegboard are useful proxies for other, more important skills (e.g., using utensils, writing with a pencil). Therapeutic interventions should not be directed toward achieving milestones per se, but rather toward achieving meaningful functional goals that are represented by milestones.

Another pitfall in interpreting milestones is the mistaken notion that a particular milestone is associated with an exact age. When we say that children walk at a year of age, we are actually providing an estimate of the age of onset of that skill. Based on a more precise, standardized assessment of this milestone, a more exact statement can be articulated (Figure 15.3). According to one assessment tool (Piper et al., 1994) a small minority of children take their first step between 8 and 9 months of age, 50% have taken their first step by 11 months of age, 75% by about 12.5 months of age, and 90% by 13.5 months of age. So a more precise statement would be "a majority of children start walking

by 12 months of age" or "almost all typically developing children can walk by 14 months of age." Standardized measures of development tend to use 75% of children achieving a milestone as the typical age for that skill and use the 90% mark as the age beyond which a child is said to be late or delayed in achieving that skill (Piper et al., 1992).

Development as a Rate Phenomenon

Developmental delay is often described in terms of how many months or years a child is behind in the attainment of a particular milestone or set of skills. For example, a child who begins walking at 18 months of age is said to be "6 months delayed" for developing that skill. In this sense the developmental "gap" can be defined as the chronological age minus the developmental age (in this case, 18 months − 12 months = 6 months). It is often more useful, however, to conceptualize development as a percentage of expected attainment. In the previous example, the child would be said to be developing at about 67% of expected for walking (12 months / 18 months × 100 = 67). Defining development in this way puts the spotlight on the rate of de-

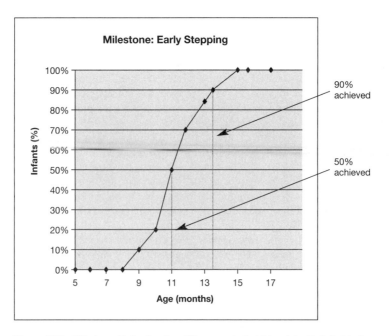

Figure 15.3. Milestone: Early stepping. Fifty percent of children take their first independent steps by 11 months; 90% have achieved this milestone by 13.5 months. (From Piper, M.C., & Darrah, J. [1994]. *Motor assessment of the developing infant* [p. 165]. Philadelphia: W.B. Saunders; Copyright © 1994 Elsevier; adapted by permission.)

velopment. Focusing on rate gives a clearer picture of developmental change over time. A child who is "6 months delayed" at 18 months (developing at 67% of the expected rate) has a more serious delay than a child who is 6 months delayed at 4 years of age (developing at 88% of the expected rate). Using rates of development allows us to track and compare degrees of delay across a range of ages. At any given moment in time, the rate of development can be estimated by calculating the developmental quotient, which is defined as follows:

$$\text{Developmental quotient} =$$
$$\text{Developmental age / Chronological age} \times 100$$

In practice, the developmental age usually represents an average level of attainment across a variety of skills and domains, rather than an estimate of the level of attainment for a single skill, and chronological age may be adjusted for prematurity (e.g., an adjusted chronological age of 15 months for the previous example may be used for a child born at 28 weeks' gestation, or 3 months early). Conceptualizing development as a rate phenomenon provides the basis for analyzing developmental trajectories and contributes to diagnostic and prognostic statements. Developmental rates are used to assess differential patterns of function and behavior; this in turn yields data useful to the diagnostic process. For example, recognizing that a child's speech is developing at 50% of the expected rate, with age-appropriate development in all other areas, suggests that the child may have a specific language impairment. Rates also provide a key element in determining prognosis and outcome

(Figure 15.4). If a child is developing at a slower rate, over time that child will tend to fall further and further behind other children who are developing at a more typical rate. In order to "catch up," a child with developmental delays must show a significant acceleration in the attainment of new skills. In general, the slower a child's rate of development (especially if the developmental quotient falls well below 50), the more difficult, and thus less likely, it is for that child to catch up developmentally.

In order to get a true picture of a child's development, it is necessary to describe the evolution of skills over a sufficient interval of time. This can be done by direct assessment of a child on multiple occasions or by eliciting historical information about a child's development from an involved and observant caregiver, teacher, or therapist. Making diagnoses or prognostic judgments based on direct observations of a child's skills on a single occasion is often problematic. Following a child over time leads to a clearer picture of that child's developmental trajectory. For example, if a child who has delays gains 6 months of new skills at the 6-month reexamination, he or she is tracking at a typical rate and, although still delayed, may well catch up over time. If that child gains 3 months, it would suggest that the delay may evolve into a disability.

DEFINING DISABILITY

The term *disability*, like the term *development*, is widely used and widely misunderstood. At its most basic level, the term refers to a decrement in the ability to perform some action, engage in

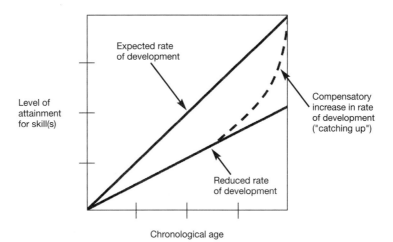

Figure 15.4. Developmental rates. If a child is developing at a slower than expected rate, there must be a compensatory acceleration in the acquisition of skills in order for the child to "catch up."

some activity, or participate in some real-life situation or setting. Like development, disability can be thought of with respect to person-specific factors (e.g., the inability to walk as a result of a neuromuscular disorder) or to environment-contingent factors (barriers or obstacles that lead to functional limitations for individuals). Historically, the tendency has been to define disability mainly with respect to an individual's physical, cognitive, or psychological impairment. The trend more recently has been to define disability in relation to the ecological/environmental context.

Various classification schemes have been put forward over several decades in an attempt to better define disability and place it into a meaningful conceptual framework. Two frequently referenced models, the World Health Organization (WHO) International Classification of Impairments, Disability and Handicaps (ICIDH; WHO, 1980) and the National Center for Medical Rehabilitation Research (NCMRR; National Institutes of Health, 1993) Model of Disability, are presented in Table 15.2. WHO has presented an updated multidimensional model in which disability is defined with respect to several functional and contextual factors (Rosenbaum & Stewart, 2004; Ustun et al., 2003; WHO, 2001). Key to this model is the notion that ability and functional capacities occur on a continuum (i.e., *disability* is a relative term) and that both person-specific and context-specific factors are determinants with respect to the expression of disability. For example, mobility may be limited both by a person's inability to walk and by lack of wheelchair access in the community.

PATTERNS OF DISABILITY

Disability is also defined in terms of specific developmental or functional diagnoses. Developmental disabilities, in particular, are conditions that are first recognized during early childhood as departures from expected patterns of development. There are three ways that these departures occur (Capute & Accardo, 1996). First, a child may have delays. *Delay* refers simply to a slower than expected rate in the acquisition of skills, usually defined with reference to widely accepted developmental milestones. A child with delays demonstrates skills that are typical of a younger child. Second, a child may deviate or diverge from an expected developmental path. In this case, a child demonstrates functional or behavioral characteristics that are not typical for any child at any age. Third, a child may demonstrate an uneven pattern of skills, such that in some areas (developmental domains) progress is fairly typical, whereas in other areas the child demonstrates a significant departure (delay or deviation) from the expected course. This phenomenon is referred to as *dissociation*. The following examples serve to illustrate these concepts.

BJ: THE CHILD WITH DELAYED DEVELOPMENT

BJ, the 3-year-old described at the beginning of this chapter, provides an example of global development delay, or delay that involves multiple developmental domains. BJ exhibits a significantly

Table 15.2.   Models of disability

World Health Organization International Classification of Impairments, Disability and Handicaps (ICIDH; 1980)	National Center for Medical Rehabilitation Research (NCMRR) Model of Disability (NIH; 1993)
Disease: Deviation from normal structure or function	*Pathophysiology:* Interruption or interference with normal physiology or development
Impairment: Loss or abnormality of psychological, physiological, or anatomical structure or function at the organ level	*Impairment:* Losses or abnormalities of cognitive, emotional, physiological, or anatomical structure or function
	Functional Limitation: Restriction or lack of ability to perform an action within expected parameters for a particular organ or organ system
Disability: Restriction of ability to perform an activity resulting from an impairment	*Disability:* An inability or limitation in performing tasks, activities, and roles to levels expected within the physical and social context
Handicap: A disadvantage experienced as the result of an impairment or disability	*Societal Limitation:* Restrictions attributable to societal or physical barriers which prevent access to opportunities for full participation in society

delayed rate of development, and as his parents suggest, his current skills are most consistent with those usually observed in children between 18 and 20 months of age (this is consistent with an estimated developmental quotient of 53%). If he continues to develop at a persistently delayed rate, there would be concern that this child's global delays represent an early manifestation of a long-term intellectual disability (i.e., mental retardation; see Chapter 17).

JAKE: THE CHILD WITH DIVERGENT DEVELOPMENT

Jake is a 4-year-old with a history of difficulties with language, communication, and socialization skills. He was slightly late in beginning to speak but was using complete sentences by 3 years of age. Despite a large vocabulary and well-developed grammatical skills, Jake has trouble with social communication. He rarely uses speech to communicate wants and needs and instead prefers to drag people by the hand to get their attention or to help him obtain a desired object. Jake's spontaneous speech consists mainly of repeated phrases from television shows. He seems oblivious to the feelings of others and tends to treat people as though they were objects. Jake is obsessively interested in letters and numbers and has poor imitative and pretend play skills. He can dress himself, he was toilet trained by 3 years of age, and he recently taught himself to ride a bicycle without training wheels.

This child, although demonstrating age appropriate skills in many areas, has a significant disturbance in communication, socialization, and play skills consistent with an autism spectrum disorder (ASD; see Chapter 23). Although some delays are evident, the most prominent features in Jake's profile of skills are those social and behavioral characteristics that deviate from expected patterns and would not be typical for any child at any age.

SARAH: THE CHILD WITH DISSOCIATED DEVELOPMENT

Sarah is a 7-year-old who attends second grade in a public school. She had some mild difficulties with early speech development (mainly problems with pronouncing certain words) but this has since

resolved. She was on time or early in the attainment of all other skills and milestones. She was very successful in preschool and was consistently described by her teachers as being exceptionally mature and intelligent. She began to experience difficulties with reading decoding skills in first grade and was diagnosed with dyslexia by the beginning of second grade. She now receives resource room support for reading and is doing better. She continues to excel in other academic areas.

For this child, problems with reading stand out against a background of well-developed social, cognitive, and academic skills. Other children may have specific weakness in other academic or functional domains (e.g., children with specific difficulties learning math, children with specific difficulties in attention and impulse control). The unevenness in Sarah's profile of skills is an example of developmental dissociation. More complex patterns of dissociation are frequently seen with children who have a variety of academic and functional difficulties; these are referred to collectively as *learning disabilities* (see Chapter 25).

These cases illustrate relatively pure examples of delayed, divergent, and dissociated development. Most children with developmental problems are more complex and frequently exhibit elements of all three types of developmental disturbance. Given this complexity, it can be challenging to accurately analyze and describe the pattern of skills a particular child exhibits and more challenging still to encapsulate this in the form of a diagnosis. In the process of assessing children with developmental difficulties, certain fairly consistent themes, constellations of behavioral characteristics, and patterns of skills emerge that make specific diagnoses possible. A particular developmental diagnosis, or developmental disability, is defined by these recognizable patterns (see Table 15.3). The concept of *developmental disability* integrates what is known about typical and atypical development into a cogent diagnostic framework and may be defined as follows: A *developmental disability* is a specific diagnostic entity characterized by a disturbance in or departure from expected patterns of development that results in predictable patterns of impairment, functional limitation, and disadvantage with regard to participation in real-life situations and settings. Section III of this book is devoted to describing specific forms of developmental disability in detail.

Table 15.3. Patterns of development associated with specific developmental disabilities[a]

Developmental diagnosis	Delays	Divergence	Dissociation
Intellectual disability	*Significant early delays across developmental domains associated with long-term dysfunction*	Atypical behavior patterns (e.g., self-injurious behavior), especially in severe or profound intellectual disability	Language skills tend to be more severely affected than other areas
Cerebral palsy	*Significant delays in motor skills and mobility*	*Significantly pathological motor control, muscle tone, and involuntary motor responses in some*	Motor and mobility dysfunction most prominent
Autism spectrum disorders	Delays in language, play and basic social skills common.	*Prominent disturbances in social communication and socialization skills; atypical play interests and behavioral patterns*	Relatively few difficulties with problem-solving, self-care and motor skills, in many
Communication disorders	*Delays in language skills most prominent*	Atypical communication skills in some (pragmatic language dysfunction)	*Relatively few difficulties with nonlanguage skills*
Learning disability	*Delays and dysfunction of specific aspects of learning (e.g., reading, math, writing)*	Mildly atypical social and behavioral characteristics occasionally observed	*Prominent discrepancy between areas of weakness and areas of strength*
Attention-deficit/ hyperactivity disorder (ADHD)	*Delayed/weak attention, response inhibition and executive function*	Mildly atypical social and behavioral characteristics occasionally observed	*Prominent discrepancy between areas of weakness and areas of strength*
Hearing impairment	*Delays in language and communication skills of variable degree, related to severity and timing of hearing loss and type of interventions*	*Prominent, pathological disturbance in the hearing apparatus*	Relatively few difficulties with nonlanguage domains

[a]Italicized descriptors represent the most prominent features of the specific diagnosis.

DISABILITY DIAGNOSES VERSUS ETIOLOGIC DIAGNOSES

As described previously, developmental disabilities are defined and diagnosed strictly on the basis of a child's functional and behavioral characteristics. A disability diagnosis (also called a developmental or functional diagnosis) is therefore made without reference to a specific medical cause. An etiological diagnosis, on the other hand, defines the exact cause of an illness or disorder (*etiology* refers to the cause of a medical condition). In contrast to a disability diagnosis, pursuit of an etiological diagnosis often involves specialized medical testing (e.g., genetic tests, brain imaging studies; see Chapters 1, 13, and 17). For children with developmental issues, both developmental disability and etiological diagnoses must be considered. When a child is diagnosed with a developmental disability, such

as cerebral palsy or an ASD, it is natural to wonder what caused the disability in the first place. It is important to recognize that although the processes involved in diagnosing disability differ qualitatively from those involved in diagnosing etiology, they do occur in parallel, and the results of one diagnostic process tend to shed light on the other. For example, specific brain imaging findings are often associated with spastic cerebral palsy in preterm infants (see Chapter 26).

The relationship between etiological diagnoses and disability diagnoses is complex. For example, Down syndrome (see Chapter 18) is a specific etiological diagnosis that is known to be a cause of intellectual disability. Many other specific genetic and neurological conditions have also been associated with intellectual disability, so it may be said that intellectual disability can be a consequence of certain medical conditions. Conversely, intellectual ability is also known to vary in the general population, and individuals at the lower end of this expected range of ability may meet the functional criteria for an intellectual disability. For these individuals, there is often no discrete, medically defined pathological cause for their disability. In these cases, learning and cognitive disabilities tend to "run in the family" and may not be associated with a definable neurological or genetic abnormality. Intellectual disability is therefore an example of a development disability that has multiple etiologies, some of which are related to discrete pathological conditions and some of which are related to the continuum of intellectual ability present in the general population.

Cerebral palsy and some forms of learning disability provide an important counterpoint to this. Cerebral palsy can result from a number of causes, but in all cases, it is thought to be the consequence of a discrete pathological process that disrupts normal brain function (see Chapter 26). In other words, one would not expect to find cerebral palsy as a variant of motor function in the general population. By contrast, some forms of learning disability are thought to represent variations in information processing that exist in the general population. In other words, certain types of learning disability may not be the consequence of a discrete pathological process at all. For example, studies of children with reading disabilities suggest the reading decoding skills vary on a continuum and that reading disability or dyslexia represents a difference of degree (typically developing children with very weak reading skills) rather than of kind (atypically developing children whose reading skills differ in a fundamental way from those of other children) (Shaywitz et al., 1990).

A specific etiological diagnosis may be made based on the medical and physical examination findings alone, but in many instances, additional laboratory testing is required to identify or confirm a diagnosis. Genetic and neurological tests are most relevant to the diagnosis of etiology in the evaluation of developmental disabilities. In general, the tests that will be used must be determined on a case-by-case basis (see Chapter 17).

SUMMARY

Human development is a complex phenomenon that may be operationally defined with respect to the characteristic patterns of behavioral change and functional adaptation that occur during the course of the human life cycle. The precise determinants of these behavioral changes have been the subject of intense scientific and philosophical debate. Developmental disabilities are conceptualized as unexpected departures from typical patterns of development. Specific diagnoses are based on the recognition of patterns of disturbance within and among specific developmental domains and the predictable functional consequences that arise from these disturbances. Developmental disabilities may be the consequence of a specific pathological process or may be the functional manifestation of the extremes of ability present in the general population. Our understanding of both developmental disabilities and their varied causes continues to improve, but it is still far from complete. The chapters that follow in Section III describe in much greater detail what is known, and what is still to be learned, about the major types of developmental disability.

REFERENCES

American Academy of Pediatrics Task Force on Infant Positioning and SIDS. (1992). Positioning and SIDS. *Pediatrics, 89,* 1120–1126.

Bronfenbrenner, U. (1979). *The ecology of human development.* Cambridge, MA: Harvard University Press.

Campbell, S. (1995). The child's development of functional movement. In S. Campbell (Ed.), *Physical therapy for children* (pp. 3–37). Philadelphia: W.B. Saunders.

Capute, A.J., & Accardo, P.J. (Eds.). (1996). *Developmental disabilities in infancy and childhood* (2nd ed.). Baltimore: Paul H. Brookes Publishing Co.

Capute, A.J., & Accardo, P.J. (2005). *The Capute Scales: Cognitive Adaptive Test/Clinical Linguistic and Auditory Milestone Scale (CAT/CLAMS).* Baltimore: Paul H. Brookes Publishing Co.

Davis, B.E., Moon, R.Y., Sachs, H.C. et al. (1998). Effects of sleep position on infant motor development. *Pediatrics, 102,* 1135–1140.

Frankenburg, W., Dodds, J., Archer, P., et al. (1992). The Denver II: A major revision and restandardization of the Denver Developmental Screening Test. *Pediatrics, 89,* 91–97.

Grimshaw, G.M., Adelstein, A., Bryden, M.P., et al. (1998). First-language acquisition in adolescence: Evidence for a critical period for verbal language development. *Brain and Language, 63*(2), 237–255.

Knobloch, H., & Pasamanick, B. (Eds.). (1974). *Gesell and Amatruda's developmental diagnosis* (3rd ed.). New York: Harper & Row.

National Institutes of Health. (1993). *Research plan for the National Center for Medical Rehabilitation Research.* (NIH Publication No. 93-3509). Bethesda, MD: Author.

Neville, H., & Mills, D. (1997). Epigenesis of language. *Mental Retardation and Developmental Disabilities Research Reviews, 3,* 282–292.

Piaget, J. (1990). *The child's conception of the world.* New York: Littlefield Adams Quality Paperbacks.

Piper, M.C., & Darrah, J. (1994). *Motor Assessment of the Developing Infant*. Philadelphia: W.B. Saunders.

Piper, M.C., Pinnell, L.E., Darrah, J., et al. (1992). Construction and validation of the Alberta Infant Motor Scale (AIMS). *Canadian Journal of Public Health 83* (Suppl. 2), S46–S50.

Rosenbaum, P., & Stewart, D. (2004). The World Health Organization International Classification of Functioning, Disability, and Health: A model to guide clinical thinking, practice and research in the field of cerebral palsy. *Seminars in Pediatric Neurology, 11*(1), 5–10.

Ross, D.S., & Bever, T.G. (2004). The time course for language acquisition in biologically distinct populations: evidence from deaf individuals. *Brain and Language, 89*(1), 115–121.

Shaywitz, S.E., Shaywitz, B.A., Fletcher, J.M., et al. (1990). Prevalence of reading disability in boys and girls: results of the Connecticut Longitudinal Study. *Journal of the American Medical Association, 264*, 998–1002.

Thelen, E., & Smith, L. (1996). *A dynamic systems approach to development of cognition and action*. Cambridge, MA: The MIT Press.

Ustun, T.B., Chatterji, S., Bickenbach, J., (2003). The International Classification of Functioning, Disability and Health: A new tool for understanding disability and health. *Disability and Rehabilitation, 25*(11–12), 565–571.

Volpe, J. (Ed.). (1995). *Neurology of the newborn* (3rd ed.). Philadelphia: W.B. Saunders.

Volpe, J. (Ed.). (2001). *Neurology of the newborn* (4th ed.). Philadelphia: W.B. Saunders.

Vygotsky, L. (1986). *Thought and language* (A. Kozulin, Trans.). Cambridge, MA: The MIT Press.

World Health Organization. (1980). *International Classification of Impairments, Disabilities and Handicaps (ICIDH)*. Geneva: Author.

World Health Organization. (2001). *ICF: Introduction*. Retrieved March 23, 2005, Health Web site: http://www3.who.int/icf/intros/ICF-Eng-Intro.pdf

III Developmental Disabilities

16 Epidemiology of Developmental Disabilities

Marshalyn Yeargin-Allsopp,
Carolyn Drews-Botsch, and Kim Van Naarden Braun

Upon completion of this chapter, the reader will

- Appreciate the principles of epidemiology
- Understand how common various developmental disabilities are
- Recognize common social and demographic characteristics of children with the specified developmental disabilities

---

Developmental disabilities are an important clinical and public health issue and are much more common than many people realize. For example, about 17% of children in the United States have some type of a disability, and about 2% of all children will require lifelong care for their disability (Boyle & Cordero, 2005). Developmental disabilities are also very costly; Boyle and Cordero (2005) estimated that the economic costs of four disabilities—intellectual disability, cerebral palsy, hearing loss, and vision impairment—exceeded $50 billion annually, based on 2003 dollars. The epidemiology of developmental disabilities and disorders is a rapidly changing field that is an important complement to clinical research studies and clinical practice. Results from epidemiologic studies can inform the development of prevention programs and the identification of the clinical and educational needs of children with developmental disabilities (Paneth, 2005). This chapter discusses basic epidemiologic concepts and their application to foster better understanding of the occurrence of **autism spectrum disorders (ASDs),** intellectual disability, cerebral palsy, **attention-deficit/hyperactivity disorder (ADHD),** communication and speech disorders, hearing loss, and vision impairment.

The findings and conclusions in this chapter are those of the authors and do not necessarily represent the views of the Centers for Disease Control and Prevention.

WHAT IS EPIDEMIOLOGY?

Epidemiology is the study of the distribution of diseases in populations. The goals of epidemiologic investigations are to determine the extent of disease in specific subgroups of the population, to understand the natural history of the disease, and to identify risk factors and causes (Paneth, 2005). The underlying assumption is that diseases are not randomly distributed but are concentrated within specific subgroups of the population. By understanding the characteristics of individuals with disease at the population level, the factors that cause the disease can be identified. Epidemiologic studies can be divided into two types: descriptive and analytic. Descriptive studies evaluate the distribution of disease in a population; analytic studies compare the distribution of disease in more than one population with the purpose of identifying factors that are associated with differential chances of having the disease or disorder.

Measures of Disease Occurrence

The occurrence of disease in a population is generally measured as some type of ratio to account for differences in population size. The numerator is a count of the number of cases of disease within society in general, and the denominator is a count of the underlying population. Counting the number of cases requires operationally defining the condition and then counting all the individuals who meet that definition. The two basic measures of disease occurrence are 1) incidence, which measures the number of newly developing cases, and 2) prevalence, which measures the number of cases of disease present in a population at a given point in time. Incidence and prevalence are numerically related through the average length of time those individuals remain affected. Thus, factors that influence the incidence, the cure rate, and the case fatality rate all affect the prevalence of disease in a population.

Two types of incidence can be described. The first is the risk or cumulative incidence. This risk is defined as the proportion of individuals in a closed population (i.e., one in which individuals can neither enter nor exit) who will develop disease in a predefined period of time. Incidence can also be described as a rate or as incidence density. The numerator for the incidence rate is defined as the number of new cases of the disease developing in the population divided by the amount of person-time spent at risk.

However, use of incidence measures is rare in developmental disability research for two reasons. First, theoretically, the population at risk includes all pregnancies because most developmental disabilities are believed to originate before birth. Therefore, all pregnancies, even those lost or terminated prior to birth, should be included in the denominator, and all of those which would have developed the disability should be included in the numerator. Clearly, this is a nearly impossible task. Consequently, there is no way to precisely measure incidence of most developmental disabilities. A second characteristic of developmental disabilities that limits the ability to estimate incidence is that the manifestation of disease is often insidious, making it difficult to identify the timing of incident events. For example, although many children exhibit recognized abnormalities in development in the first and second years of life, the average age of diagnosis is considerably later for both cerebral palsy and autism (Stanley, Blair, & Alberman, 2000). As a result of these challenges, most epidemiologic studies of developmental disabilities use disease prevalence as a measure of occurrence.

Measures of Disease Association

One of the primary objectives of epidemiology is to study the causes of disease. However, an exposure cannot be presumed causal just because an individual develops disease following an exposure. To determine whether such a risk factor is potentially causal, one must compare the disease experience of those with such a factor to that in those without the factor. In comparing the experience in the two groups, there are standard measures of association to describe and quantify the strength of the association between a risk (or protective) factor and disease outcome (Rothman & Ray, 2002). The risk ratio or rate ratio is used to describe the risk (or rate) of disease in the exposed group relative to those in the unexposed group; it is calculated as the incidence risk (or rate) of disease in the exposed group divided by the incidence risk (or rate) of disease in the unexposed group. One can also calculate analogous difference measures—the risk difference and the rate difference—by subtracting the incidence among unexposed individuals from the incidence among exposed individuals.

The measure of association often differs according to the type of study design. For cohort studies, the choice between difference and ratio measures is often up to the discretion of the investigator. Case-control studies (starting with a sample of individuals with a particular disease and a sample of similar individuals who did not develop disease) commonly estimate odds ratios, which are calculated as follows: [(probability of exposure among diseased individuals)/(probability that diseased individuals are not exposed)]/[(probability of exposure among nondiseased individuals)/(probability that nondiseased individuals are not exposed)]. The **prevalence odds ratio (POR)** is usually the measure of choice for studies of developmental disabilities because most such studies rely on the prevalence of disease rather than incident cases; it is calculated as [prevalence in subgroup 1/(1-prevalence in subgroup1)]/ [prevalence in subgroup 2/(1-prevalence in subgroup2)].

Bias

When evaluating an association, the epidemiologist must consider whether or not the observed association is valid. In other words, on average, does the observed association represent the true relationship between exposure and outcome, or are the data skewed—or biased—in some way? There are three main types of bias that arise in epidemiologic studies: information bias, selection bias, and confounding.

Information bias occurs because the variables in the study are not measured accurately. The errors may be in assessing the outcome, the exposure, and/or covariates that are included in the study and are extremely common in epidemiologic studies. One source of information bias results from combining individuals with etiologically distinct conditions. For example, intellectual disability caused by Down syndrome and that resulting from fetal alcohol syndrome have different risk factors (the former maternal age and the latter alcohol intake) and therefore should be studied separately. In general, errors in measurement of the exposure and/or outcome bias the observed association towards the null (i.e., suggesting no effect), creating a conservative bias in studies in which an association has been observed (Hofler, 2005). However, if the measurement of exposure (e.g., parental report, clinical diagnosis) differs by the outcome, the direction of bias is unpredictable. This is of particular concern for associations that are highly visible to the community, such as the alleged association between autism and childhood vaccinations (Andrews et al., 2002).

Selection bias occurs because of differences in who is selected for evaluation. In a **cohort study,** such bias would occur if there were differences in loss to follow-up by exposure status and/or the risk of outcome. For example, if individuals with high socioeconomic status (SES) who have children with a disability migrate from an area in search of more ideal services, this could create a selection bias.

Confounding occurs when a covariate is an independent risk factor for the disease; that is, it is correlated, positively or negatively, with the exposure of interest and is not in the causal pathway between the exposure and disease. For example, because social class is associated with cognitive development (Drews et al., 1995) and prematurity (Foster et al., 2000), social class will be a confounder in studies assessing the impact of prematurity on cognitive development. However, unlike the bias resulting from misclassification and selection bias, the investigator can limit the bias resulting from confounding by controlling for the covariate in the analysis.

HOW COMMON ARE VARIOUS DISABILITIES?

The following sections discuss the occurrence of ASDs, intellectual disability, cerebral palsy, ADHD, speech and communication disorders, hearing loss, and vision impairment.

Autism Spectrum Disorders

There is current debate about the prevalence of ASDs and whether they have increased over time. (See Figure 16.1 for a comparison of

rates.) Recent studies have concluded that the current prevalence of ASDs is approximately 1 in 150 children (Autism and Developmental Disabilities Monitoring [ADDM] Network, 2007a, 2007b; Bertrand et al., 2001; Kadesjö, Gillberg, & Hagberg, 1999). However, the observed prevalence has varied considerably over time, in part due to differences in the definition of *autism* in use at the time and changes in awareness of the disorder (see Chapter 23).

Autism affects more boys than girls, with sex ratios generally ranging from 2:1 to 4:1 (Fombonne, 2003; Gillberg & Wing 1999). The observed male-to-female ratio increases as IQ scores increases, ranging from close to 1:1 for children with IQ scores lower than 50 (Fombonne, 1999; Yeargin-Allsopp et al., 2003) to about 6:1 for children with high-functioning autism (Fombonne, 2003).

Older studies report that as many as 75%–80% of children with autism also have intellectual disability (Bryson et al., 1988; Gillberg, 1984). More recent studies have reported lower proportions (Baird et al., 2006; Icasiano et al., 2004). For example, in one study, only 26% of the 97 children with one of the ASD subtypes had intellectual disability (ADDM Network, 2007a, 2007b; Chakrabarti & Fombonne, 2001).

Few data are available concerning variations in the prevalence of autism by racial or ethnic group because most studies have been conducted in northern European countries or Japan (Dyches et al., 2004), where the populations are relatively homogeneous. However, some studies report a lower prevalence in racial/ethnic minorities (Dyches et al., 2004; Sanua, 1984), whereas other studies have not found a significant difference in rates among white and black children (Yeargin-Allsopp et al., 2003).

Kanner (1943, p. 248) observed that children with autism were from "highly intelligent families," and other early reports also concluded that there was an association between autism and higher social class (Cox et al., 1975). In recent studies, associations have been found between the prevalence of autism and social class and maternal education (Bhasin & Schendel, 2006; Croen et al., 2002). However, this association may result from selection bias.

Some studies (Glasson et al., 2004), but not all studies (Steinhausen et al., 1986), have shown maternal age to be associated with autism. Croen et al. (2002) found that the prevalence of autism in children born to mothers 35 years of age was four times higher than in children whose mothers were 20 years of age (Croen et

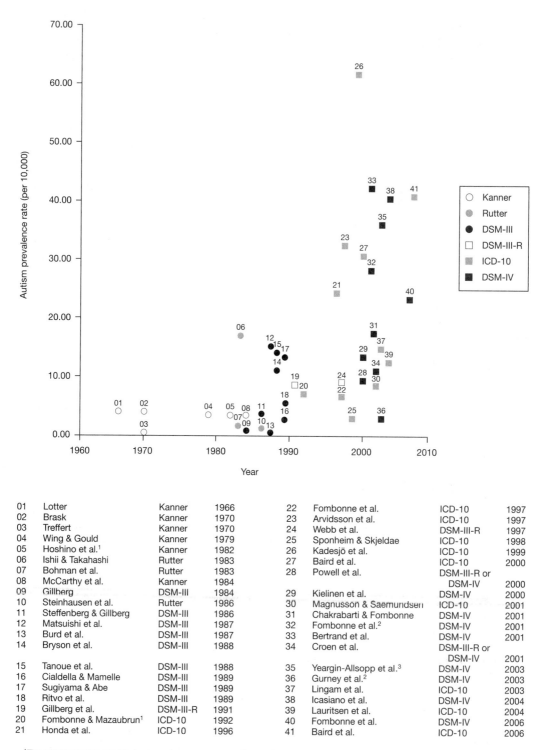

01	Lotter	Kanner	1966
02	Brask	Kanner	1970
03	Treffert	Kanner	1970
04	Wing & Gould	Kanner	1979
05	Hoshino et al.[1]	Kanner	1982
06	Ishii & Takahashi	Rutter	1983
07	Bohman et al.	Rutter	1983
08	McCarthy et al.	Kanner	1984
09	Gillberg	DSM-III	1984
10	Steinhausen et al.	Rutter	1986
11	Steffenberg & Gillberg	DSM-III	1986
12	Matsuishi et al.	DSM-III	1987
13	Burd et al.	DSM-III	1987
14	Bryson et al.	DSM-III	1988
15	Tanoue et al.	DSM-III	1988
16	Cialdella & Mamelle	DSM-III	1989
17	Sugiyama & Abe	DSM-III	1989
18	Ritvo et al.	DSM-III	1989
19	Gillberg et al.	DSM-III-R	1991
20	Fombonne & Mazaubrun[1]	ICD-10	1992
21	Honda et al.	ICD-10	1996

22	Fombonne et al.	ICD-10	1997
23	Arvidsson et al.	ICD-10	1997
24	Webb et al.	DSM-III-R	1997
25	Sponheim & Skjeldae	ICD-10	1998
26	Kadesjö et al.	ICD-10	1999
27	Baird et al.	ICD-10	2000
28	Powell et al.	DSM-III-R or DSM-IV	2000
29	Kielinen et al.	DSM-IV	2000
30	Magnusson & Saemundsen	ICD-10	2001
31	Chakrabarti & Fombonne	DSM-IV	2001
32	Fombonne et al.[2]	DSM-IV	2001
33	Bertrand et al.	DSM-IV	2001
34	Croen et al.	DSM-III-R or DSM-IV	2001
35	Yeargin-Allsopp et al.[3]	DSM-IV	2003
36	Gurney et al.[2]	DSM-IV	2003
37	Lingam et al.	ICD-10	2003
38	Icasiano et al.	DSM-IV	2004
39	Lauritsen et al.	ICD-10	2004
40	Fombonne et al.	DSM-IV	2006
41	Baird et al.	ICD-10	2006

[1]The prevalence rate provided represents an average prevalence rate.
[2]The prevalence study provided overall rate only.
[3]64% had "mental retardation" based on IQ data, and 68% had cognitive impairment based on IQ and developmental tests.

Figure 16.1. Comparison of autism prevalence rates. (*Key:* DSM-III, *Diagnostic and Statistical Manual of Mental Disorders, Third Edition;* DSM-III-R, *Diagnostic and Statistical Manual of Mental Disorders, Third Edition, Revised;* ICD-10, *International Classification of Diseases, Tenth Edition;* DSM-IV, *Diagnostic and Statistical Manual of Mental Disorders, Fourth Edition.*)

al., 2002). Data from metropolitan Atlanta for 1996 also showed a 70% higher prevalence of autism associated with other disabilities in children born to older mothers (Bhasin & Schendel, 2006).

Genetics is believed to play a strong role in the etiology of autism (Lamb et al., 2000). The recurrence risk in siblings of affected children is 2% to 6% (Rutter et al., 1999). In addition, the concordance rate among same-sex dizygotic twins is much lower than among monozygotic twins (Bailey et al., 1995). Even though autism is believed to have a strong genetic component, the recent increase in prevalence has prompted both parents and investigators to search for environmental factors that have resulted in more cases of autism (see Chapter 5).

Intellectual Disability

Three quarters of individuals with intellectual disability are usually reported to have mild intellectual disability (Murphy et al., 1998). Many reviews of international epidemiological studies have suggested that the prevalence of severe intellectual disability is approximately 3–4 per 1,000 in children and adults (Leonard & Wen, 2002). The reported prevalence of mild intellectual disability has been much more variable than for severe intellectual disability. It is not known whether these variations represent true differences in the prevalence of mild intellectual disability in the population or methodological differences in the studies. Roeleveld, Zielhuis, and Gabreels (1997) concluded that 30 per 1,000 is a reasonable estimate of the prevalence of mild intellectual disability.

The observed prevalence of intellectual disability varies by a number of population characteristics including age, sex, and SES. The observed prevalence of intellectual disability usually peaks at 10 to 14 years of age. Murphy reported a prevalence of intellectual disability of 1 per 1,000 in children younger than the age of 5 versus 97 per 1,000 in children 10 through 14 years of age (Murphy, Yeargin-Allsopp, et al., 1995). The higher prevalence in later childhood probably results from the diagnosis of children, particularly those with mild intellectual disability, occurring within educational settings, rather than from incident cases occurring during the school years (Murphy et al., 1998).

Intellectual disability is found more commonly in males than in females, with an observed male-to-female ratio of approximately 1.5:1 (Leonard & Wen, 2002). In several stud-

ies, the excess of males was higher for mild intellectual disability, with ratios ranging from 1.4:1 in the Netherlands to 1.8:1 in Sweden (Murphy, Yeargin-Allsopp, et al., 1995, Roeleveld et al., 1997). The male-to-female ratio for severe intellectual disability has been reported to be 1.2:1 (Roeleveld et al., 1997). Biologic factors, such as fragile X syndrome and other X-linked conditions (Chelley & Mandel; Tariverdian & Vogel, 2000), could result in a greater occurrence of intellectual disability among boys than among girls (Partington et al., 2000). Social factors, such as behaviors that might cause boys to receive greater attention and thus get tested, are believed to be responsible for at least some of the male preponderance in mild intellectual disability.

The inverse relationship between socioeconomic status and prevalence of intellectual disability has been well documented (Yeargin-Allsopp et al., 1995). Studies have consistently shown that mild intellectual disability is largely of unknown etiology and is highly correlated with lower SES (Drews et al., 1995; Yeargin-Allsopp et al., 1995). Drews and colleagues (1995) examined intellectual disability associated with neurological conditions (nonisolated intellectual disability) and without neurological conditions (isolated intellectual disability). Their findings support the idea that there are two distinct types of intellectual disability: a milder, isolated form, which is mainly influenced by social and demographic factors, and a nonisolated form, which is more likely to be severe and affected by biological or pathological factors (Drews et al., 1995).

Racial and ethnic differences in the prevalence of intellectual disability have also been reported. In the United States, black children and children born to Hispanic and Asian mothers have higher rates of intellectual disability than do white children (Murphy, Yeargin-Allsopp, et al., 1995; Croen, Grether, & Selvin, 2001; Yeargin-Allsopp et al., 1995). Confounding by socioeconomic factors is assumed to contribute to these observed differences. However, an excess of intellectual disability among black children compared with white children in metropolitan Atlanta remained after controlling for the sociodemographic factors (Yeargin-Allsopp et al., 1995).

Maternal age at delivery is another risk factor (Drews et al., 1995). This association varies with the level of intellectual disability. Children whose mothers were teenagers (ages 15–19) at the time of delivery had a slightly increased risk for mild intellectual disability than did children of older mothers. On the other hand, children whose mothers were older (ages 40–44) had a greater risk for moderate to severe intellectual disability than did children whose mothers were in their twenties at the time of delivery (Chapman, Scott, & Mason, 2002). The latter finding may be related to the increased risk of various chromosomal disorders with increased maternal age.

A review by Leonard and Wen (2002) found that the proportion of intellectual disability cases with a known etiology varied from 22% in metropolitan Atlanta to 77% in Sweden. The proportion with a known etiology varies with the intensity of the diagnostic workup, the definition of a known cause, and the source of data used to identify an etiology. The causes of intellectual disability also differ by level of severity of intellectual disability. Approximately three quarters of children with severe intellectual disability have an identified cause of their disability (Leonard & Wen, 2002; Yeargin-Allsopp et al., 1997). In contrast, most studies have reported a recognized etiology for fewer than half (25%–40%) of children with mild intellectual disability. However, the low proportion of children with mild intellectual disability with a recognized etiology has been challenged as a result of improved diagnostic capabilities (Shevell et al., 2003) and examination of the contribution of environmental factors, such as lead and mercury exposure (Mendola et al., 2002).

More than 500 genetic diseases are known to cause intellectual disability; however, most are rare and do not contribute substantially to the overall prevalence (Murphy et al., 1998). Chromosomal disorders are the most common known cause of intellectual disability, accounting for 5%–19% of all cases (Schaefer & Bodensteiner, 1992; Yeargin-Allsopp et al., 1997) and a higher proportion of cases of severe intellectual disability. Down syndrome (1 per 800 live births; National Center on Birth Defects and Developmental Disabilities, 2004) accounts for 10%–15% of all intellectual disability cases among live-born children (Leonard & Wen, 2002) and at least two thirds of all genetic causes of intellectual disability (Stromme & Hagberg, 2000; Yeargin-Allsopp et al., 1997). Other prominent causes of intellectual disability include fragile X syndrome (1 per 4,000 males and 1 per 8,000 females; Turner et al., 1996); and Prader-Willi syndrome (1 per 12,000 to 15,000) (Leonard & Wen, 2002).

Prenatal events are believed to contribute to the majority of causes of intellectual disability (Yeargin-Allsopp et al., 1997). These include maternal drinking (Leonard & Wen, 2002), smoking (Drews et al., 1996), medications (Holmes et al., 2005), medical conditions (e.g., thyroid disease; Qian, Wang, & Chen, 2000), urinary tract infections (McDermott et al., 2001), maternal phenylketonuria (Waisbren et al., 1997), and intrauterine infections (Murphy et al., 1998). Birth defects are more common in children with intellectual disability; however, this association may result from a shared etiology. Low birth weight (LBW; less than 2,500 grams), preterm delivery (prior to 37 weeks' gestation), and intrauterine growth restriction all have been associated with intellectual disability (Leonard & Wen, 2002). Twins and other multiples are at increased risk for intellectual disability (Boyle, Keddie, & Holmgreen, 1997), probably because of the effect of multiple gestations on fetal growth and gestational age.

Perinatal asphyxia was once thought to be a major contributor to intellectual disability and other developmental disabilities; however, a strong association has not been supported (Yeargin-Allsopp et al., 1997). In addition, relatively few cases of intellectual disability are now due to perinatal infections, including Group B *streptococcus* (CDC, 1997) and herpes simplex virus (American Academy of Pediatrics, 2003). Neonatal screening has been shown to be effective in preventing intellectual disability resulting from a number of metabolic and endocrine disorders (CDC, 1999).

Postnatal causes account for 3%–15% of the cases of intellectual disability with a known etiology (Murphy et al., 1998; Yeargin-Allsopp et al., 1997). Many of these causes are preventable, including lead exposure (Mendola et al., 2002), injuries (CDC, 1996; Yeargin-Allsopp et al., 1997), traumatic brain damage, and postnatally acquired infections (CDC, 1996; Yeargin-Allsopp et al., 1997).

Cerebral Palsy

Most cerebral palsy is considered to be prenatal in origin, with the resulting motor disability manifesting itself as the child fails to reach developmental motor milestones. Despite methodological differences, the prevalence of cerebral palsy from population-based studies has been remarkably similar—ranging from 1.2 to 2.8 per 1,000 live births, with the majority of rates at about 2.0 per 1,000 live births (Clark & Hankins, 2003).

Blair and Stanley (1997) did not find consistent trends in the overall birth prevalence of cerebral palsy in the period from 1958 to1989 in five different registry systems. The lack of a reduction in prevalence is surprising given the remarkable improvements in obstetric and neonatal care and in neonatal survival during that time period. However, among neonatal survivors with birth weights less than 1,500 grams, the prevalence of cerebral palsy appeared to increase between the mid-1960s and the late 1980s (Winter et al., 2002). In contrast, several studies of children born in the mid-1990s suggest a possible downward trend in the rate of cerebral palsy in very low birth weight (VLBW) neonatal survivors (Grether & Nelson 2000; O'Shea et al., 1998; Surman, Newdick, & Johnson, 2003).

There is a higher prevalence of cerebral palsy among males than females, with sex ratios ranging from 1.1 to 1.5:1 (Jarvis et al., 2005). Prematurity is the most prominent risk factor for cerebral palsy (O'Shea, 2002). In terms of the effect of race, a study in metropolitan Atlanta showed that among children born with LBW, black children had lower rates of cerebral palsy than did white children; however, among children with birth weights greater than 2,500 grams, black children had higher rates than whites (Winter et al., 2002).

Twins and higher-order multiples also have a greater risk of cerebral palsy than singletons. For the most part, this increased risk seems to be attributable to premature delivery. However, death of a co-twin in utero is a risk factor for cerebral palsy in the surviving twin. At least some cases of cerebral palsy in singletons are believed to be attributable to the early in utero death of an unrecognized co-twin (Scher et al., 2002).

Preeclampsia is associated with a reduced occurrence of cerebral palsy among infants with VLBW. However, there is a modest increase in risk of cerebral palsy associated with preeclampsia in normal birth weight infants (Collins & Paneth, 1998). It is unclear why preeclampsia would be protective in preterm infants, given that preeclampsia often occurs in infants who have lower birth weight for gestational age, a risk factor for cerebral palsy. One suggestion is that this is an artifact of selection due to higher mortality in infants born very preterm to mothers with preeclampsia (Murphy et al., 1996).

Congenital infections, primarily rubella and cytomegalovirus (CMV), cause various neurological impairments, including cerebral palsy, primarily in term infants (Gilbert, 1996). A number of markers of maternal infection in pregnancy, such as clinical chorioamnionitis, maternal fever and antibiotic use, uterine tenderness, and neonatal sepsis, have been linked to cerebral palsy in preterm infants in some studies (O'Shea, 2002) but not all studies (Grether et al., 2003). Although it is unclear whether the link between maternal infection and cerebral palsy is independent of factors associated with preterm birth, these same markers of maternal infection, including biomarkers of neonatal inflammatory response, have been associated with cerebral palsy in term infants (Schendel, 2001). A variety of coagulation abnormalities, both hereditary and acquired (e.g., antiphospholipid antibodies, the factor V Leiden), have been linked to neonatal stroke and cerebral palsy in term infants (Nelson, 2002). Obstetric complications and birth asphyxia, long thought to be the main causes of cerebral palsy, in fact account for only a small proportion of cerebral palsy (Nelson, 2002).

Between 10% and 16% of cases of cerebral palsy result from postnatal causes (Cans et al., 2004; CDC, 1996; Stanley et al., 2000); however, some of the reported variability may relate to differences in the age limits applied in the definition of cerebral palsy. This low occurrence of cerebral palsy resulting from postnatal events such as infection, cerebrovascular events, and head injuries does not account for the observed increases in the prevalence of cerebral palsy with age (Cans et al., 2004; CDC, 1996).

Attention-Deficit/ Hyperactivity Disorder

The reported prevalence of ADHD has been quite variable (2%–18%), particularly when clinical studies are included (Brown et al., 2001). Much of this variability can be attributed to evolving diagnostic criteria, the use of the different diagnostic tools, differences in the source of the information about a child's behavior, and differences in how the information is combined (Rowland, Lesesne, & Abramowitz, 2002). The *Diagnostic and Statistic Manual of Mental Disorders, Fourth Edition* (DSM-IV; American Psychiatric Association, 1994) reports a prevalence of 3%–7%, but it is unclear how this estimate was derived. When limiting studies to those from school-based settings using *DSM-IV* criteria, the prevalence rates were considerably higher and showed less variation (11%–16%) (Cantwell, 1996).

With the exception of a higher ratio of boys to girls (about 4:1), other demographic characteristics of ADHD have not been well described (Cantwell, 1996). A number of explanations have been advanced for the excess of boys with ADHD, including referral bias because of greater disruptive behaviors in boys and potentially an underdiagnosis of inattentive subtypes in girls. It is unclear if differences exist by socioeconomic status or race. However, a school-based epidemiologic study suggested little racial difference in the rate of ADHD (Rowland, Umbach, et al., 2002). The study's findings did suggest racial/ethnic variations in the prevalence of medication use for ADHD, with the highest use among whites and the lowest among Hispanics.

Many conditions, including emotional and behavioral disorders, oppositional defiant disorder and/or conduct disorder, obsessive-compulsive disorder, **anxiety disorders,** and depression, are found more often in children with ADHD than in unaffected children (Cantwell, 1996). Some of these conditions have symptoms similar to ADHD, making it difficult to distinguish between a diagnosis of ADHD and a co-occurring disorder in epidemiologic studies. The challenges in accurate assessment of co-morbidities might result in spurious high ADHD prevalence estimates (Rowland, Lesesne, & Abramowitz, 2002). Furthermore, it is unclear if these conditions have a similar etiologic mechanism or if one of the conditions produces the other.

ADHD has been described as a complex genetic condition. The prevalence of ADHD is higher in families with a family history of ADHD, and concordance among monozygotic twins is higher than among dizygotic twins (Acosta, Arcos-Burgos, & Muenke, 2004). Few nongenetic risk factors have been identified. The most convincing of these are LBW, which could be a proxy measure for preterm delivery (Botting, Powls, & Cook, 1997), and environmental lead exposure (Bellinger et al., 1994).

Speech and Communication Disorders

Chronic speech disorders are defined as difficulty producing speech sounds or problems with voice quality. The prevalence of such disorders is 16 per 1,000 children younger than the age of 18 years (American Speech-Language-Hearing Association, 2004). In the 2000–2001 school year, 19% of school-age children received services for speech or language disorders under IDEA Part B; this figure does not include children who had speech or language problems that were secondary to another condition (U.S. Department of Education, 2002).

Specific language impairment refers to a significant deficit in linguistic functioning that does not result from deficits in hearing, intelligence, or motor functioning (Shamas, Wiig, & Secord, 1998). Estimates of the prevalence of specific language impairment during preschool and early school years range from 2% to 8%, with an overall median prevalence of 6% (8% for boys and 6% for girls) (Tomblin, Smith, & Zhang, 1997). Over the 10-year period from the 1991–1992 to the 2000–2001 school years, there was a 10% increase in the number of children receiving services for a speech or language impairment (U.S. Department of Education, 2002). In 2003, 1,129,260 children received services for speech or language impairments under IDEA Part B. After specific learning disabilities, it is the second most common disability classification (U.S. Department of Education, 2004).

Hearing Loss

The reported prevalence of permanent bilateral childhood hearing loss is 0.6–2.6 per 1,000 children (Yeargin-Allsopp & Drews-Botsch, in press). Data from the Metropolitan Atlanta Developmental Disabilities Surveillance Program showed that the rate of hearing loss in that population was 1.1 per 1,000 children ages 3–10 years and that the rate increased steadily with age—a trend that was seen for all levels of severity. Differences in methods of clinical assessment, as well as ascertainment for studies, may be responsible for much of the observed difference in reported prevalence. Hearing loss was found to be more common among boys than girls and more common among black children than white children in metropolitan Atlanta in 2000 (Karapurkar Bhasin et al., 2006). The majority of hearing losses in children was sensorineural (79%). Approximately 30% of children in metropolitan Atlanta with a hearing loss were found to have another developmental disability, most often intellectual disability (Van Naarden Braun & Decouflé, 1999).

Of note, universal newborn hearing screening programs are identifying children with congenital hearing loss in the United States at an earlier age than in the past. However, it is also important to screen children for hearing loss at later ages. Fortnum and colleagues (2001) reported that late-onset and progressive hearing impairments—for example, those due to disorders such as CMV, postnatally acquired loss, and genetic disorders that present after the newborn period—are more prevalent than previously thought. They found that the prevalence of permanent childhood hearing loss of 40 decibels or greater in children in the United Kingdom born from 1980 through 1995 rises with age and that as many as 2 per 1,000 children age 9 years or older may have hearing losses of this level. This increase in prevalence has implications for service needs for children with hearing loss.

More than 400 syndromes are associated with hearing loss and account for up to 50% of cases (Kenneson, Van Naarden Braun, & Boyle, 2002). A specific syndrome can be identified in about 30% of these cases. The remaining 70% of genetic cases are nonsyndromic, either familial or sporadic. Of the familial nonsyndromic cases, 75%–80% are autosomal recessive, 20%–25% are autosomal dominant, and 1%–1.5% are X-linked. Variants in one locus, Gap Junction Beta 2 or GJB2 (connexin 26), account for up to half of cases of nonsyndromic sensorineural hearing loss in some populations, most notably among the Ashkenazi Jewish population, whites of northern European descent, the Japanese population, and individuals from Ghana (Kenneson et al., 2002).

Vision Impairment

Recent estimates of the prevalence of vision impairment among children in the United States range from 0.2 to 0.9 per 1,000 children (Yeargin-Allsopp & Drews-Botsch, in press). This observed range probably relates to different ascertainment methods, different survival rates of VLBW infants, and different case definitions (low vision versus legal blindness). In 1991, the prevalence of low vision (defined as a best corrected visual acuity of 20/70 in the better eye) among children 3–10 years of age in metropolitan Atlanta was 0.8 per 1,000 children. This prevalence was similar to that of legal blindness (defined as a best corrected visual acuity of 20/200 or worse, or a visual field of 20 degrees or less in the better eye) in 10-year-old children in the same population ascertained during the period of 1985 through 1987 (Drews et al., 1992).

As was observed for hearing loss, the prevalence of vision impairment in 1991 increased with age (up to 7 years). The prevalence of vision impairment was higher in boys than girls and higher in black children than white children (Karapurkar Bhasin et al., 2006).

Prenatal causes accounted for 43% of low vision, whereas 27% of the etiologies were perinatal in origin. Postnatal etiologies were relatively uncommon, as most causes of traumatic and postnatal vision loss causes unilateral vision loss (Rahi & Dezateux, 1998). Of the prenatal etiologies, 38% were genetic, with the largest percentage being caused by ocular or oculocutaneous albinism. The distribution of timing of insult associated with the vision impairment differed significantly by birth weight categories, with children of normal birth weight having a larger percentage of prenatal etiologies and children with LBW having a larger percentage of perinatal etiologies, including retinopathy or prematurity.

SUMMARY

The epidemiology of developmental disabilities and disorders is a rapidly evolving field that is an important complement to clinical investigation and practice. Epidemiologic data can assist in developing prevention programs and in identifying the clinical and educational burden of providing services to children with developmental disabilities. However, the nature of developmental disabilities makes such investigations difficult. Therefore, in developing and using this knowledge, clinicians, educators, and investigators need to clearly define these conditions, understand their developmental timing, subdivide the conditions into etiologically homogeneous subgroups, identify the population to which the measure of occurrence applies, and recognize the possible sources of error and bias that may result from the methods used. As the field of developmental disabilities epidemiology evolves, the information available to clinicians and parents will improve, allowing for better decisions for the families, children, and communities affected by these prevalent conditions.

REFERENCES

Acosta, M.T., Arcos-Burgos, M., & Muenke, M. (2004). Attention deficit/hyperactivity disorder (ADHD): Complex phenotype, simple genotype? *Genetics in Medicine, 6*, 1–15.

American Academy of Pediatrics. (2003). Group B streptococcal infections. In L.K. Pickering (Ed.), *Redbook:*

2006 report of the Committee on Infectious Diseases (27th ed., pp. 620–627). Elk Grove Village, IL: Author.

American Psychiatric Association. (1980). *Diagnostic and statistical manual of mental disorders* (3rd ed.). Washington, DC: Author.

American Psychiatric Association. (1987). *Diagnostic and statistical manual of mental disorders* (3rd ed., rev.). Washington, DC: Author.

American Psychiatric Association. (1994). *Diagnostic and statistical manual of mental disorders* (4th ed.). Washington, DC: Author.

American Speech-Language-Hearing Association. (2004). *Communication facts: Incidence and prevalence of communication disorders and hearing loss in children.* Retrieved November 11, 2005, from http://www.asha.org/members/research/reports/children.htm

Andrews, N., Miller, E., Taylor, B., et al. (2002). Recall bias, MMR, and autism. *Archives of Disease in Childhood, 87*(6), 493–494.

Arvidsson, T., Danielsson, B., Forsberg, P., et al. (1997). Autism in 3- to 6-year-old children in a suburb of Goteborg, Sweden. *Autism, 1*, 163–171.

Autism and Developmental Disabilities Monitoring Network Surveillance Year 2000 Principal Investigators; Centers for Disease Control and Prevention. (2007a). Prevalence of autism spectrum disorders—Autism and Developmental Disabilities Monitoring Network, six sites, United States, 2002. *Morbidity and Mortality Weekly Report Surveillance Summaries, 56*(1), 1–11.

Autism and Developmental Disabilities Monitoring Network Surveillance Year 2002 Principal Investigators; Centers for Disease Control and Prevention. (2007b). Prevalence of autism spectrum disorders—Autism and Developmental Disabilities Monitoring Network, 14 sites, United States, 2002. *Morbidity and Mortality Weekly Report Surveillance Summaries, 56*(1), 12–28.

Bailey, A., Le Couteur, A., Gottesman, I., et al. (1995). Autism as a strongly genetic disorder: Evidence from a British twin study. *Psychological Medicine, 25*, 63–77.

Baird, G., Charman, T., Baron-Cohen, S., et al. (2000). A screening instrument for autism at 18 months of age: A 6-year follow-up study. *Journal of the American Academy of Child & Adolescent Psychiatry, 39*, 694–702.

Baird, G., Simonoff, E., Pickles, A., et al. (2006). Prevalence of disorders of the autism spectrum in a population cohort of children in South Thames: The Special Needs and Autism Project (SNAP). *The Lancet, 368*, 210–215.

Baker, H.C. (2002) A comparison study of autism spectrum disorder referrals 1997 and 1989. *Journal of Autism and Developmental Disorders, 32*(2), 121–125.

Barbaresi, W.J., Katusic, S.K., Colligan, R.C., et al. (2005). The incidence of autism in Olmsted County, Minnesota, 1976–1997: Results from a population-based study. *Archives of Pediatrics and Adolescent Medicine, 159*, 37–44.

Bhasin, T.K., & Schendel, D. (2006). Sociodemographic risk factors for autism in a US metropolitan area. *Journal of Autism and Developmental Disorders* [Epub ahead of print] PMID: 16951989.

Bellinger, D., Leviton, A., Allred, E., et al. (1994). Pre- and postnatal lead exposure and behavior problems in school-aged children. *Environmental Research, 66*(1), 12–30.

Bertrand, J., Mars, A., Boyle, C., et al. (2001). Prevalence of autism in a United States population: The Brick Township, New Jersey, investigation. *Pediatrics, 108,* 1155–1161.

Blair, C., & Stanley, F.J. (1997). Issues in the classification and epidemiology of cerebral palsy. *Mental Retardation and Developmental Disabilities Research Reviews, 3,* 184–193.

Bohman, M., Bohman, I.L., Bjorck, P.O., et al. (1983). Childhood psychosis in a northern Swedish country: Some preliminary findings from an epidemiological survey. In M.H. Schmidt & H. Remschmidt (Eds.), *Epidemiological Approaches in Child Psychiatry, 29,* 433–445.

Botting, N., Powls, A., & Cooke, R.W.I. (1997). Attention deficit hyperactivity disorder and other psychiatric outcomes in very low birthweight children at 12 years. *Journal of Child Psychology and Psychiatry, and Allied Disciplines, 38,* 931–941.

Boyle, C.A., & Cordero, J.F. (2005). Birth defects and disabilities: A public health issue for the 21st century. *American Journal of Public Health, 95*(11), 1884–1886.

Boyle, C.A., Keddie, A., & Holmgreen, P. (1997). The risk of mental retardation in twins. *Society for Pediatric Epidemiology Research, 11,* A10.

Brask, B.H. (1970). A prevalence investigation of childhood psychosis. *Nordic Symposium Care of Psychotic Children,* 145–153.

Brown, R.T., Freeman, W.S., Perrin, J.M., et al. (2001). Prevalence and assessment of attention-deficit/hyperactivity disorder in primary care settings. *Pediatrics, 114*(2), 511–512.

Bryson, S., Clark, B., & Smith, I.M. (1988). First report of a Canadian epidemiological study of autistic syndromes. *Journal of Child Psychology and Psychiatry, and Allied Disciplines, 29,* 433–446.

Burd, L., Fisher, W., & Kerbeshian, J. (1987). A prevalence study of pervasive developmental disorders in North Dakota. *Journal of the American Academy of Child & Adolescent Psychiatry 26*(5), 700–703.

California Department of Developmental Services. (1999). *Changes in the population of persons with autism and pervasive developmental disorders in California's developmental services system: 1987–1998. A report of the legislature.* Sacramento: Author.

California Department of Developmental Services. (2003, April). *Autistic spectrum disorders: Changes in the California caseload; An update: 1999 through 2002.* Sacramento: Author.

Cans, C., McManus, V., Crowley, M., et al. (2004). Surveillance of cerebral palsy in Europe Collaborative Group. Cerebral palsy of post-neonatal origin: Characteristics and risk factors. *Paediatric and Perinatal Epidemiology, 18,* 214–220.

Cantwell, D.P. (1996). Attention deficit disorder: A review of the past 10 years. *Journal of the American Academy of Child and Adolescent Psychiatry, 35,* 978–987.

Centers for Disease Control and Prevention. (1996). Postnatal causes of developmental disabilities in children aged 3–10 years—Atlanta, Georgia, 1991. *Morbidity and Mortality Weekly Report, 45,* 130–134.

Centers for Disease Control and Prevention. (1997). Decreasing incidence of perinatal Group B streptococcal disease. United States, 1993–1995. *Morbidity and Mortality Weekly Report, 46,* 473–477.

Centers for Disease Control and Prevention. (1999). Mental retardation following diagnosis of a metabolic disorder in children aged 3–10 years—metropolitan Atlanta, Georgia, 1991–1994. *Morbidity and Mortality Weekly Report, 48,* 353–356.

Centers for Disease Control and Prevention. (2005). *Metropolitan Atlanta Developmental Disabilities Surveillance Program unpublished data.*

Chakrabarti, S., & Fombonne, E. (2001) Pervasive developmental disorders in preschool children. *Journal of the American Medical Association, 285*(24), 3093–3099.

Chapman, D.A., Scott, K., & Mason, C. (2002). Early risk factors for mental retardation: Role of maternal age and maternal education. *American Journal of Mental Retardation, 1,* 46–59.

Chelly, J., & Mandel, J.L. (2001). Monogenic causes of X-linked mental retardation. *Nature Review Genetics, 2,* 669–680.

Cialdella, P., & Mamelle, N. (1989), An epidemiological study of infantile autism in a French department (Rhone): A research note. *The Journal of Child Psychology and Psychiatry, 30,* 165–175.

Clark, S.L., & Hankins, G.D. (2003). Temporal and demographic trends in cerebral palsy—fact and fiction. *American Journal of Obstetrics and Gynecology, 188,* 628–633.

Collins, M., & Paneth, N. (1998). Pre-eclampsia and cerebral palsy: Are they related? *Developmental Medicine and Child Neurology, 40,* 207–211.

Cox, A., Rutter, M., Newman, S., et al. (1975). A comparative study of infantile autism and specific developmental receptive language disorder II. Parental characteristics. *The British Journal of Psychiatry, 126,* 146–159.

Croen, L.A., Grether, J., Hoogstrate, J., et al. (2002). The changing prevalence of autism in California. *Journal of Autism and Developmental Disorders, 32*(3), 207–215.

Croen, L.A., Grether, J.K., & Selvin, S. (2001). The epidemiology of mental retardation of unknown cause. *Pediatrics, 107*(6), E86. Retrieved January 23, 2006, from http://pediatrics.aappublications.org/cgi/content/full/107/6/e86

Davidson, P.W., Myers, J., & Weiss, B. (2004). Mercury exposure and child development outcomes. *Pediatrics, 113*(4), 1023–1027.

Drews, C.D., Murphy, C.C., Yeargin-Allsopp, M., et al. (1996). The relationship between idiopathic mental retardation and maternal smoking during pregnancy. *Pediatrics, 97,* 547–553.

Drews, C.D., Yeargin-Allsopp, M., Decouflé, P., et al. (1995). Variation in the influence of selected sociodemographic risk factors for mental retardation. *American Journal of Public Health, 85,* 329–334.

Drews, C.D., Yeargin-Allsopp, M., Murphy, C.C., et al. (1992). The prevalence of legal blindness among 10-year-old children in Metropolitan Atlanta, 1985–1987. *American Journal of Public Health, 82,* 1377–1379.

Dyches, T.T., Wilder, L.K., Sudweeks, R.R., et al. (2004). Multicultural issues in autism. *Journal of Autism and Developmental Disorders, 34*(2), 211–222.

Fombonne, E. (1999). The epidemiology of autism: A review. *Psychological Medicine, 29,* 769–786.

Fombonne, E. (2003). Epidemiological surveys of autism and other pervasive developmental disorders: An update. *Journal of Autism and Developmental Disorders, 33*(4), 365–382.

Fombonne, E., & du Mazaubrun, C. (1992). Prevalence of infantile autism in four French regions. *Social Psychiatry and Psychiatric Epidemiology, 27*(4), 203–210.

Fombonne, E., du Mazaubrun, C., Cans, C., et al. (1997). Autism and associated medical disorders in a French epidemiological survey. *Journal of the American Academy of Child & Adolescent Psychiatry, 36*(11), 1561–1569.

Fombonne, E., Simmons, H., Ford, T., et al. (2001). Prevalence of pervasive developmental disorders in the British nationwide survey of child mental health. *Journal of the American Academy of Child & Adolescent Psychiatry, 40*(7), 820–827.

Fombonne, E., Zakarian, R., Bennett, A., et al. (2006). Pervasive developmental disorders in Montreal, Quebec, Canada: Prevalence and links with immunizations. *Pediatrics, 118,* 139–150.

Fortnum, H.M., Summerfield, A.Q., Marshall, D.H., et al. (2001). Prevalence of permanent childhood hearing impairment in the United Kingdom and implications for universal neonatal hearing screening: Questionnaire based ascertainment study. *British Medical Journal, 323,* 536–540.

Foster, H.W., Wu, L., Bracken, M.B., et al. (2000). Intergenerational effects of high socioeconomic status on low birthweight and preterm birth in African Americans. *Journal of the National Medical Association, 92*(5), 213–221.

Gilbert, G.L. (1996). Congenital fetal infections. *Seminars in Neonatology, 1,* 91–105.

Gillberg, C. (1984). Infantile autism and other childhood psychoses in a Swedish urban region: Epidemiological aspects. *Journal of Child Psychology and Psychiatry, and Allied Disciplines, 25*(1), 35–43.

Gillberg, C., Steffenburg, S., & Schaumann, H. (1991). Is autism more common now than ten years ago? *The British Journal of Psychiatry, 158,* 403–439.

Gillberg, C., & Wing, L. (1999). Autism: Not an extremely rare disorder. *Acta Psychiatrica Scandinavica, 99,* 399–406.

Glasson, E.J., Bower, C., Petterson, B., et al. (2004). Perinatal factors and the development of autism: A population-based study. *Archives of General Psychiatry, 61*(6), 618–627.

Grether, J.K., & Nelson, K.B. (2000). Possible decrease in prevalence of cerebral palsy in premature infants [letter]. *The Journal of Pediatrics, 136,* 133.

Grether, J.K., Nelson, K.B., Walsh, E., et al. (2003). Intrauterine exposure to infection and risk of cerebral palsy in very preterm infants. *Archives of Pediatrics & Adolescent Medicine, 157,* 26–32.

Gurney, J.G., Fritz, M.S., Ness, K.K., et al. (2003). Analysis of prevalence trends of autism spectrum disorder in Minnesota. *Archives of Pediatrics and Adolescent Medicine, 157*(7), 622–627.

Hjördís Ósk Atladóttir, M.B., Parner, E.T., Schendel, D., et al. (2007). Time trends in reported diagnoses of childhood neuropsychiatric disorders: A Danish cohort study. *Archives of Pediatrics and Adolescent Medicine,* 193–198.

Hofler, M. (2005). The effect of misclassification on the estimation of association: A review. *International Journal of Methods in Psychiatric Research, 14*(2), 92–101.

Holmes, L.B., Coull, B.A., Dorfman, J., et al. (2005). The correlation of deficits in IQ with midface and digit hypoplasia in children exposed in utero to anticonvulsant drugs. *The Journal of Pediatrics, 146*(1), 118–122.

Honda, H., Shimizu, Y., Misumi, K., et al. (1996). Cumulative incidence and prevalence of childhood autism in children in Japan. *The British Journal of Psychiatry, 169*(2), 228–235.

Hoshino, Y., Kumashiro, H., Yashima, Y., et al. (1982). The epidemiological study of autism in Fukushima-ken. *Folia Psychiatric Neurology, Japan, 36*(2), 115–124.

Icasiano, F., Hewson, P., Machet, P., et al. (2004). Childhood autism spectrum disorder in the Barwon region. A community based study. *Journal of Pediatrics and Child Health, 40,* 696–701.

Ishii, T., & Takahashi, O. (1983). The epidemiology of autistic children in Toyota, Japan. *Japanese Journal of Child & Adolescent Psychiatry, 24,* 311–321.

Jarvis, S., Glinianaia, S.V., Arnaud, C., et al. (2005). Case gender and severity in cerebral palsy varies with intrauterine growth. *Archives of Disease in Childhood, 90*(5), 474–479.

Kadesjö, B., Gillberg, C., & Hagberg, B. (1999). Brief report: Autism and Asperger syndrome in seven-year-old children: A total population study. *Journal of Autism and Developmental Disorders, 29*(4), 327–332.

Kanner, L. (1943). Autistic disturbances of affective contact. *Nervous Child, 2,* 217–250.

Karapurkar Bhashin, T., Brocksen, S., Avchen, R., et al. (2006). Prevalence of 4 DDS in 8 year old children; Metropolitan Atlanta Developmental Disabilities Surveillance Program, 1996 and 2000. *Morbidity and Mortality Weekly Report, 55,* 1–9.

Kenneson, A., Van Naarden Braun, K., & Boyle, C. (2002). GJB2 (connexin 26) variants and nonsyndromic sensorineural hearing loss. *Genetics in Medicine, 4*(4), 258–274.

Kielinen, M., Linna, S.L., & Moilanen, I. (2000). Autism in Northern Finland. *European Child and Adolescent Psychiatry, 9,* 162–167.

Lamb, J.A., Moore, J., Bailey, A., et al. (2000). Autism: Recent molecular genetic advances. *Human Molecular Genetics, 9*(6), 861–868.

Lauritsen, M.B., Pedersen, C.B., & Mortensen, P.B. (2004) The incidence and prevalence of pervasive developmental disorders: A Danish population-based study. *Psychological Medicine, 34,* 1–8.

Leonard, H., & Wen, X. (2002) The epidemiology of mental retardation: Challenges and opportunities in the new millennium. *Mental Retardation and Developmental Disabilities Research Reviews, 8*(3), 117–134.

Lingam, R., Simmons, A., Andrews, N., et al. (2003). Prevalence of autism and parentally reported triggers in a north east London population. *Archives of Disease in Childhood, 88*(8), 666–670.

Lotter, V. (1966) Epidemiology of autistic conditions in young children: Some characteristics of the parent and children prevalence. *Social Psychiatry, 1,* 124–137.

Magnusson, P., & Saemundsen, E. (2001). Prevalence of autism in Iceland. *Journal of Autism and Developmental Disorders, 31,* 153–163.

Matsuishi, T., Shiotsuki, Y., Yoshimura, K., et al. (1987). High prevalence of infantile autism in Kurume City, Japan. *Journal of Child Neurology, 2*(4), 268–271.

McCarthy, P., Fitzgerald, M., & Smith, M.A. (1984). Prevalence of childhood autism in Ireland. *Irish Medical Journal, 77,* 129–130.

McDermott, S., Daguise, V., Mann, H., et al. (2001). Perinatal risk for mortality and mental retardation associated with maternal urinary tract infections. *The Journal of Family Practice, 50,* 433–437.

Mendola, P., Selevan, S., Gutter, S., et al. (2002). Environmental factors associated with a spectrum of neurodevelopmental deficits. *Mental Retardation and Developmental Disabilities Research Reviews, 8*(3), 188–197.

Murphy, C.C., Boyle, C., Schendel, D., et al. (1998). Epidemiology of mental retardation in children. *Mental Retardation and Developmental Disabilities Research Reviews, 4,* 6–13.

Murphy, C.C., Yeargin-Allsopp, M., Decouflé, P., et al. (1995). The administrative prevalence of mental retardation in 10-year-old children in metropolitan Atlanta, 1985 through 1987. *American Journal of Public Health, 85*(3), 319–323.

Murphy, D.J., Squier, M.V., Hope, P.L., et al. (1996). Clinical associations and term of onset of cerebral white matter damage in very preterm babies. *Archives of Disease in Childhood, 75,* F27–F32.

National Center on Birth Defects and Developmental Disabilities. (2004). *Risk factors for Down syndrome.* Atlanta, GA: Centers for Disease Control and Prevention. Retrieved December 28, 2005, from http://www.cdc.gov/ncbddd/bd/ds.htm

Nelson, K.B. (2002). The epidemiology of cerebral palsy in term infants. *Mental Retardation and Developmental Disabilities Research Reviews, 8,* 146–150.

Newschaffer, C., Falb, D., & Gurney, J.G. (2005). National autism prevalence trends from United States special education data. *Pediatrics, 115,* 277–282.

O'Shea, T.M. (2002). Cerebral palsy in very preterm infants: New epidemiologic insights. *Mental Retardation and Developmental Disabilities Research Reviews, 8,* 135–145.

O'Shea, T.M., Preisser, J.S., Klinepeter, K.L., et al. (1998). Trends in mortality and cerebral palsy in a geographically based cohort of very low birth weight neonates born between 1982 to 1994. *Pediatrics, 101*(4), 642–647.

Paneth, N. (2005). *Nature and uses of epidemiology.* Retrieved January 23, 2006, from http://www.pitt.edu/~super1/courses/epi.htm

Partington, M., Mowat, D., Einfeld, S., et al. (2000). Genes on the X chromosome are important in undiagnosed mental retardation. *American Journal of Medical Genetics, 92,* 57–61.

Powell, J.E., Edwards, A., Edwards, M., et al. (2000). Changes in the incidence of childhood autism and other autistic spectrum disorders in preschool children from two areas of the West Midlands, UK. *Developmental Medicine and Child Neurology, 42*(9), 624–628.

Qian, M., Wang, D., & Chen, Z. (2000). A preliminary meta-analysis of 36 studies on impairment of intelligence development induced by iodine deficiency. *American Journal of Preventive Medicine, 24*(2), 75–77.

Rahi, J.S., & Dezateux, C. (1998). Epidemiology of visual impairment in Britain. *Archives of Disease in Childhood, 78*(4), 381–386.

Ritvo, E.R., Freeman, B.J., Pingree, C., et al. (1989). The UCLA–University of Utah Epidemiologic Survey of Autism: Prevalence. *American Journal of Psychiatry, 146*(2), 194–245.

Roeleveld, N., Zielhuis, G.A., & Gabreels, F. (1997). The prevalence of mental retardation: A critical review of recent literature. *Developmental Medicine and Child Neurology, 39,* 125–32.

Rothman, K.J., & Ray, W. (2002). Should cases with a known cause of their disease be excluded form study? *Pharmacoepidemiology and Drug Safety, 11*(1), 11–14.

Rowland, A.S., Lesesne, C.A., & Abramowitz, A.J. (2002). The epidemiology of attention-deficit/hyperactivity disorder (ADHD): A public health view. *Mental Retardation and Developmental Disabilities Research Reviews, 8,* 162–170.

Rowland, A.S., Umbach, D.M., Stallone, L., et al. (2002). Prevalence of medication treatment for attention deficit hyperactivity disorder among elementary school children: Johnston County, NC. *American Journal of Public Health, 92,* 231–234.

Rutter, M., Silberg, J., O'Connor, T., et al. (1999). Genetics and child psychiatry: II. Empirical research findings. *Journal of Child Psychology and Psychiatry, and Allied Disciplines, 40,* 19–55.

Sanua, V.D. (1984). Is infantile autism a universal phenomenon? An open question. *International Journal of Social Psychiatry, 30,* 163–177.

Schaefer, G.B., & Bodensteiner, J.B. (1992). Evaluation of the child with idiopathic mental retardation. *Pediatric Clinics of North America, 39,* 929–943.

Schendel, D.E. (2001). Infection in pregnancy and cerebral palsy. *Journal of the American Medical Women's Association, 56,* 105–108.

Scher, A.L., Petterson, B., Blair, E., et al. (2002). The risk of mortality or cerebral palsy in twins: A collaborative population-based study. *Pediatric Research, 52,* 671–681.

Shamas, G.H., Wiig, E.H., & Secord, W.A. (1998). *Human communication disorders: An introduction* (5th ed.). Boston: Allyn & Bacon.

Shevell, M., Ashwal, S., Donley, D., et al. (2003). Practice parameter: Evaluation of the child with global developmental delay. *Neurology, 60,* 367–380.

Sponheim, E., & Skjeldal, O. (1998). Autism and related disorders: Epidemiological findings in a Norwegian study using IDC-10 diagnostic criteria. *Journal of Autism and Developmental Disorders, 28,* 217–227.

Stanley, F., Blair, E., & Alberman, E. (2000). *Cerebral palsies: Epidemiology and causal pathways.* London: Mac Keith Press.

Steffenberg, S., & Gillberg, C. (1986). Autism and autistic-like conditions in Swedish rural and urban areas: A population study. *The British Journal of Psychiatry, 149,* 81–87.

Steinhausen, H.C., Gobel, D., Breinlinger, M., et al. (1986). A community survey of infantile autism. *Journal of the American Academy of Child and Adolescent Psychiatry, 25,* 189–190.

Stromme, P., & Hagberg, G. (2000). Aetiology in severe and mild mental retardation: A population-based study of Norwegian children. *Developmental Medicine and Child Neurology, 42,* 76–86.

Sugiyama, T., & Abe, T. (1989). The prevalence of autism in Nahoya, Japan: A total population study. *Journal of Autism and Developmental Disorders, 19*(1), 87–96.

Surman, G., Newdick, H., & Johnson, A. (2003). Cerebral palsy rates among low-birthweight infants in the 1990s. *Developmental Medicine and Child Neurology, 45,* 456–462.

Tanoue, Y., Oda, S., Asano, F., et al. (1988). Epidemiology of infantile autism in southern Ibaraki, Japan: Differences in prevalence in birth cohorts. *Journal of Autism and Developmental Disorders, 18*(2), 155–166.

Tariverdian, G., & Vogel, F. (2000). Some problems in the genetics of X-linked mental retardation. *Cytogenetics and Cell Genetics, 91,* 278–284.

Tidmarsh, L., & Volkmar, F.R. (2003). Diagnosis and epidemiology of autism spectrum disorders. *Canadian Journal of Psychiatry, 48*(8), 517–525.

Tomblin, J.B., Smith, E., & Zhang, X. (1997). Epidemiology of specific language impairment: Prenatal and perinatal risk factors. *Journal of Communication Disorders, 30,* 325–344.

Treffert, D.A. (1970) Epidemiology of infantile autism. *Archives of General Psychiatry, 22*(5), 431–438.

Turner, G., Webb, T., Wake, S., et al. (1996). Prevalence of fragile X syndrome. *American Journal of Medical Genetics, 64,* 196–197.

U.S. Department of Education. (2002). *Twenty-fourth Annual Report to Congress on the Implementation of the Individuals with Disabilities Education Act, Section 618.* Jessup, MD: ED Pubs, Education Publication Center, U.S. Department of Education.

U.S. Department of Education. (2004). *Individual with Disabilities Education Act (IDEA) Data. Number of Children Served Under IDEA by Disability and Age Group, 1994–2003.* Retrieved January 21, 2005, from http://www.ideadata.org/tables27th/ar_aa9.xls

Van Naarden Braun, K., & Decouflé, P. (1999). Relative and attributable risks for moderate to profound bilateral sensorineural hearing impairment associated with lower birth weight in children 3 to 10 years old. *Pediatrics, 104*(4), 905–910.

Waisbren, S.E., Rokni, H., Bailey, I., et al. (1997). Social factors and the meaning of food in adherence to medical diets: Results of a maternal phenylketonuria summer camp. *Journal of Inherited Metabolic Disease, 20*(1), 21–27.

Webb, E.V., Lobo, S., Hervas, A., et al. (1997). The changing prevalence of autistic disorder in a Welsh health district. *Developmental Medicine and Child Neurology, 39*(3), 150–152.

Wing, L., & Gould, J. (1979). Severe impairments of social interaction and associated abnormalities in children: Epidemiology and classification. *Journal of Autism and Developmental Disorders, 9,* 11–29.

Winter, S., Autry, A., Boyle, C., et al. (2002). Trends in the prevalence of congenital cerebral palsy in Atlanta, Georgia. *Pediatrics, 10,* 1220–1225.

World Health Organization. (1990). *International Classification of Diseases (ICD-10).* Geneva: Author.

Yeargin-Allsopp, M., Drews, C.D., Decouflé, P., et al. (1995). Mild mental retardation in black and white children in metropolitan Atlanta: A case-control study. *American Journal of Public Health, 85,* 324–328.

Yeargin-Allsopp, M., & Drews-Botsch, C. (in press). Epidemiology of neurodevelopmental disabilities. In M. Shevell (Ed.), *Clinical and scientific aspects of neurodevelopmental disabilities: International review of child neurology.* London: Mac Keith Press.

Yeargin-Allsopp, M., Murphy, C.C., Cordero, J.F., et al. (1997). Reported biomedical causes and associated medical conditions for mental retardation among 10-year-old children, metropolitan Atlanta, 1985 to 1987. *Developmental Medicine and Child Neurology, 39,* 142–149.

Yeargin-Allsopp, M., Rice, C., Karpurkar, T., et al. (2003). Prevalence of autism in a US metropolitan area. *Journal of the American Medical Association, 289,* 49–55.

17 Developmental Delay and Intellectual Disability

Mark L. Batshaw, Bruce Shapiro, and Michaela L.Z. Farber

Upon completion of this chapter, the reader will

- Understand the definition of *developmental delay* and implications of the terms *mental retardation* and *intellectual disability*
- Be aware of the various causes of intellectual disability
- Recognize the various interventions in intellectual disability
- Be aware of the different levels of functioning and independence that individuals with intellectual disability can achieve

The term *global developmental delay* is most commonly used as a temporary diagnosis in young children at risk for developmental disabilities, especially intellectual disabilities. In this context, it indicates a failure to achieve age-appropriate neurodevelopmental milestones in the areas of language, motor, and social-adaptive development (Beirne-Smith, Ittenbach, & Patton, 2001).

DANIEL

Daniel's mother, Marina, noticed many signs in his early development that indicated atypical development. (In the following paragraphs, the typical ages for these developmental milestones are indicated in parentheses after the age at which Daniel achieved them.)

As an infant, Daniel showed little interest in his environment and was not very alert. Although Marina tried to breast-feed him, his suck was weak, and he frequently regurgitated his formula. He was floppy and had poor head control. His cry was high pitched, and he was difficult to comfort. He would sit in an infant seat for hours without complaint.

In social and motor development, Daniel lagged behind the norm. In language skills, he did not start babbling until 13 months (6 months). He smiled at 5 months (2 months) and was not very responsive to his parents' attention. In terms of gross motor development, Daniel could hold his head up at 4 months (1 month), roll over at 8 months (5 months), and sit up at 14 months (6 months). He transferred objects from one hand to the other at 14 months (5 months).

When evaluated with the Bayley Scales of Infant Development–Third Edition (BSID-III; Bayley, 2006) at 16 months of age, Daniel's mental age was found to be 7 months, and he received a Mental Developmental Index (MDI; similar to an IQ score) of less than 50. He progressed from an early intervention program to a special preschool program, and prior to school entry at age 6, Daniel was retested on the Stanford-Binet Intelligence Scales, Fifth Edition (SB5; Roid, 2003). His score indicated a mental age of 2 years, 8 months, and an IQ score of 40. Concomitant impairments in adaptive behavior were demonstrated by the Vineland Adaptive Behavior Scales, Second Edition (Vineland-II; Sparrow et al., 2005), which revealed communicative, self-care, and social skill challenges.

EARLY IDENTIFICATION OF DEVELOPMENTAL DELAY

Global developmental delay is recognized by the failure to meet age-appropriate expectations based on the typical sequence of development. In the first months of life, delayed development can be indicated by a lack of visual or auditory response, an inadequate suck, and/or floppy or spastic muscle tone. Later in the first year, lack of language and motor delays in sitting and walking may suggest developmental delay. When a child continues to show significant delays in all developmental spheres, intellectual disability is the most likely diagnosis. Unfortunately, some medical practitioners continue to use the term *global developmental delay* long after a more specific diagnosis can be made. Although developmental delay is the most common presenting concern in children who turn out to have an intellectual disability, sensory impairment, an autism spectrum disorder (ASD), or cerebral palsy, it does not always indicate a developmental disability. Isolated mild delays in expressive language (particularly in boys) or in gross motor abilities usually resolve over time. These mild early delays, however, often signal an increased risk of the child having academic or behavioral difficulties that will become evident by school age.

Early identification of atypical development is more likely to occur with more severe impairments. In order to facilitate early identification, all children should receive developmental surveillance as part of their routine pediatric care (Rydz et al., 2005). This includes obtaining a history of developmental concerns from the parents, recording developmental milestones and performing a screening test (e.g., the Denver Developmental Screening Test II [Frankenburg et al., 1992], the Ages & Stages Questionnaires® [ASQ; Bricker et al., 1999], or the Parent Evaluations of Developmental Status [PEDS; Glascoe, 1997; see also http://www .pedstest.com]). Unfortunately, many children come from underserved populations and do not have a "medical home" with systematic screening, assessment, and family supports. Even when followed in a clinic, there may be little time for the staff to take a developmental history or to perform a developmental screening test. Furthermore, the available developmental screening tests themselves are not sufficiently sensitive to detect many developmental disabilities.

It is important to emphasize that screening tests are not designed to supplant a formal neurodevelopmental and psychological assessment. They are designed to be used in asymptomatic populations in order to identify individuals at risk. The usefulness of a screening instrument is determined by its ability to appropriately classify children who do or do not have significant developmental delays—that is, its sensitivity

and specificity, respectively. Sensitivity is the ability to detect affected children (measured by the true positive rate). Specificity is the ability to classify typical children as typical (measured by the true negative rate). The ideal screening instrument would detect all of the children who require further assessment (no false negatives) and none of those who do not (no false positives). Unfortunately, many screening instruments misclassify too many children to be clinically useful.

Given these difficulties, the best approach to early identification is multifaceted. Infants at high risk should be closely monitored and entered into early intervention programs if appropriate (Guralnick, 2005). High-risk conditions include the following:

- Prematurity

- Low birth weight (Wilson-Costello et al., 2005)

- Perinatal complications

- Chronic physical health conditions (Akinbami, LaFleur, & Schoendorf, 2002)

- Exposure to environmental hazardous substances (O'Dowd, 2002)

- Maternal functioning compromised by depression (Petterson & Albers, 2001), substance abuse (Hoyme et al., 2005), lack of education (Neiss & Rowe, 2000), involvement in maltreatment (Carrey et al., 1995), or domestic violence (Koenen et al., 2003)

- Low socioeconomic family background (Turkheimer et al., 2003).

In addition, all parents should be educated to look for and report delays in developmental achievements. Clinic staff and physicians should routinely note developmental milestones, much like they note height and weight. In addition, children should receive neonatal hearing screening and a developmental screening battery and tests of vision and hearing every 6–12 months during early childhood (Committee on Children with Disabilities, 2001; Hayes, 2003; Jacobson & Jacobson, 2004).

Parents usually seek an evaluation for developmental delay once their child fails to meet specific developmental milestones (Table 17.1). In early infancy, these include a lack of responsiveness, unusual muscle tone or posture, and feeding difficulties (Bear, 2004). Between 6 and 15 months of age, motor delay is the most com-

Table 17.1. Presentations of intellectual disability by age

Age	Area of concern
Newborn	Dysmorphisms (structural abnormalities)
	Major physiologic dysfunction (e.g., eating, breathing)
2–4 months	Failure to interact with the environment (e.g., parent suspects child is deaf or has a visual impairment)
6–18 months	Gross motor (e.g., sitting, crawling, walking)
18 months–3 years	Language
3–5 years	Language
	Behavior (including play)
	Fine motor (e.g., cutting, coloring)
5+ years	Academic Achievement
	Behavior (e.g., attention, anxiety, mood, conduct)

Source: Shapiro and Batshaw (2002).

mon complaint. Language and behavior problems are the common concerns after 18 months. If there is evidence of a significant developmental lag over time, the child should then be sent for a comprehensive evaluation. Ideally, this evaluation should include an examination by at least a physician (pediatrician, neurodevelopmental pediatrician, developmental-behavioral pediatrician, child psychiatrist, or pediatric neurologist) experienced in early childhood development and/or developmental disabilities, preferably in tandem with a clinical/educational psychologist or a social worker with similar experience. Depending on the child's age and impairments, he or she also may need to be seen for early intervention assessment by an early childhood educator, speech-language pathologist, and/or audiologist. If the child displays motor impairments, physical and occupational therapists should also be involved. Following the assessment, an individual family service plan (IFSP) is developed in the context of an early intervention program (see Chapter 33).

DEFINING INTELLECTUAL DISABILITY

The most commonly used definition of intellectual disability (mental retardation) comes from the Individuals with Disabilities Education Act (IDEA) of 1997 (PL 105-17). It defines mental retardation as ". . . significantly subaverage general intellectual functioning, existing concurrently with deficits in adaptive behavior and manifested during the developmental period, that adversely affects a child's educational performance" (34 C.F.R. §300.7[c][6]). The most commonly used medical diagnostic criteria for intellectual disability are those contained in the American Psychiatric Association (APA)'s *Diagnostic and Statistical Manual of Mental Disorders, Fourth Edition, Text Revision* (*DSM-IV-TR*; 2000) (see Table 17.2). The use of the term *mental retardation* is controversial because it has a pejorative context. Rather than being used as a designation to assist people, mental retardation has been used as a means of limiting them. Despite this, mental retardation, as a diagnosis, is not likely to disappear any time soon because this term is written into laws that provide protection and support for individuals with this diagnosis. We feel more comfortable, however, using the term *intellectual disability* and will do so throughout this book. In terms of defining mental retardation, as noted previously, there is general agreement that a person must have significantly subaverage intellectual functioning and impairment in adaptive abilities, but, as will be described, disagreements over the details of this definition have arisen for both biological and philosophical reasons.

Intellectual Functioning

The first controversial issue in the definition involves the assessment of intellectual functioning. The average level of intellectual functioning in a population corresponds to the apex of a bell-shaped curve. Two standard deviations on either side of the mean encompass 95% of a population sample and approximately define the range of typical intellectual functioning (Figure 17.1). By definition, the average intelligence quotient, or IQ score, is 100, and the standard deviation (a statistical measure of dispersion from the mean) of most IQ tests is 15 points. Historically, a person scoring more than 2 standard deviations below the mean, or below 70, has been considered to have an intellectual disability (mental retardation).

Statisticians, however, point out that there is a measurement variance of approximately 5 points in assessing IQ by most psychometric tests. In other words, repeated testing of the same individual will produce scores that vary by as much as 5 points (APA, 2000). Thus, it has been proposed that the demarcation of intellectual disability be changed from an IQ score of 70 to a range of 65–75, using the presence or absence of significant impairments in adaptive skills

Table 17.2. Diagnostic criteria for Mental Retardation

A. Significantly subaverage intellectual functioning: an IQ of approximately 70 or below on an individually administered IQ test (for infants, a clinical judgment of significantly subaverage intellectual functioning).

B. Concurrent deficits or impairments in present adaptive functioning (i.e., the person's effectiveness in meeting the standards expected for his or her age by his or her cultural group) in at least two of the following areas: communication, self-care, home living, social/interpersonal skills, use of community resources, self-direction, functional academic skills, work, leisure, health, and safety.

C. The onset is before age 18 years.

Code based on degree of severity reflecting level of intellectual impairment:

317	**Mild Mental Retardation:**	IQ level 50–55 to approximately 70
318.0	**Moderate Mental Retardation:**	IQ level 35–40 to 50–55
318.1	**Severe Mental Retardation:**	IQ level 20–25 to 35–40
318.2	**Profound Mental Retardation:**	IQ level below 20–25
319	**Mental Retardation, Severity Unspecified:**	when there is a strong presumption of Mental Retardation but the person's intelligence is untestable by standard tests

Reprinted with permission from the *Diagnostic and Statistical Manual of Mental Disorders, Fourth Edition, Text Revision* (p. 49). Copyright © 2000 American Psychiatric Association.

to establish the diagnosis. Using this schema, intellectual disability would be diagnosed in an individual with an IQ score between 70 and 75 who exhibits significant impairments in adaptive behavior, whereas it would not be diagnosed in an individual with an IQ of 65–70 who does not have impairments in adaptive skills.

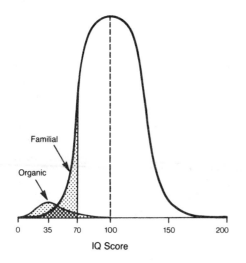

Figure 17.1. Bimodal distribution of intelligence. The mean IQ score is 100. An IQ score of less than 70, or 2 standard deviations below the mean, can indicate intellectual disability. The second, smaller curve takes into account individuals who have intellectual disability because of birth trauma, infection, inborn errors, or other organic causes. This explains why more individuals have severe to profound intellectual disability than are predicted by the familial curve alone. (From Zigler, E. [1967]. Familial retardation: A continuing dilemma. *Science, 155,* 292, Figure 1. Copyright © 1967 by the American Association for the Advancement of Science. Reprinted with permission from the American Association for the Advancement of Science.)

Beyond any measurement variability, a more fundamental concern of some theorists is the underlying value of an IQ score. Gardner (1983) challenged the dichotomous (verbal versus performance) structure of intelligence assessed by most IQ tests. He proposed that intelligence comprises a wider range of abilities, not only the traditional linguistic and logical-mathematical skills, but also musical, spatial, bodily-kinesthetic, and interpersonal characteristics as well. This approach has not gained wide acceptance, as it does not have a clear neuropsychological or neuroanatomical basis. And, although it is acknowledged that a single IQ score averages a person's cognitive abilities and may not capture all forms of intelligence, there is evidence that a significantly subnormal IQ score is a meaningful predictor of future cognitive functioning.

Yet, it must be emphasized that cognitive functioning is not always uniform across all neurodevelopmental domains. An example is found in the study by Wang and Bellugi (1993) comparing neuropsychological testing results in children with Down syndrome and Williams syndrome. Although the Full-Scale IQ scores on the Wechsler Intelligence Scale for Children–Revised (Wechsler, 1974) in both groups were similar, the pattern of cognitive strengths and weaknesses was very different. The individuals with Williams syndrome had much stronger skills in language but much poorer visual-perceptual abilities than did the children with Down syndrome. When volumetric analysis of magnetic resonance imaging (MRI) scans was performed, the cortical areas involved in language acquisition were much more developed in individuals with Williams syndrome; conversely the basal ganglia area that is involved in visual-perception was more developed in individuals with Down syndrome.

Finally, there are the concerns over predictive validity and cultural bias. Infant psychological tests are notoriously poor predictors of adult IQ scores, although they clearly differentiate severe impairments from typical functioning. In addition, cultural bias has been suggested as one explanation for differences in IQ scores found among individuals from various racial, ethnic, and socioeconomic groups.

Adaptive Impairments

Individuals fulfilling the diagnosis of intellectual disability not only must have limitations in their intellectual abilities but also must be impaired in their ability to adapt or function in daily life. Earlier definitions did not elaborate on the specifics of these adaptive impairments. The American Association on Mental Retardation (AAMR; 2002) and the APA (2000), however, have defined mental retardation as including at least two of the following impairments in adaptive behavior: communication, self-care, home living, social/interpersonal skills, use of community resources, self-direction, functional academic skills, work, leisure, health, and safety (Table 17.2).

CLASSIFICATION OF INTELLECTUAL DISABILITY

Intellectual disability is a heterogeneous group of conditions that arise from many different causes and has many different expressions. Although the diagnosis of intellectual disability is important, the classification of intellectual disability is as important. Etiologic evaluation, neurobiological mechanisms, management, planning, and prognosis are all predicated on the ability to classify the disorder. There are many methods for classification, but this chapter focuses on four: degree of intellectual impairment, required supports, domains of disability, and etiology.

Degree of Intellectual Impairment

There is controversy about classifying the levels of intellectual disability. The *DSM-IV-TR* (APA, 2000) subdivides intellectual disability into four degrees of severity. As noted in Table 17.2, per the APA, an individual is classified as having mild intellectual disability if his or her IQ level is 50 to approximately 70; moderate, IQ level 35 to approximately 50; severe, IQ level 20 to approximately 35; and profound, IQ level below 20–25. This classification has met with widespread acceptance in the medical community; although it has also been suggested that intellectual disability should be simply dichotomized into mild (IQ score of 50 to approximately 70) and severe (IQ score below 50). This is based on the discrete biological division between mild retardation and the more severe forms of intellectual disability, with different etiologies and outcomes. This dichotomy has not been widely accepted for clinical purposes because the medical, educational, and habilitative needs are quite different between individuals with moderate and profound impairments.

Required Supports

The AAMR takes a different approach in defining the degree of severity of intellectual disability, relying not on IQ scores but rather on the patterns and intensity of support needed (i.e., requiring intermittent, limited, extensive, or pervasive support; AAMR, 2002). This definition marks a philosophical shift from an emphasis on degree of impairment to a focus on the abilities of individuals to function in an inclusive environment. This shift is controversial, as it assumes that adaptive behaviors can be independent of cognition and does not provide clear guidelines for establishing diagnostic eligibility of children with IQ scores in the upper limits of the range connoting intellectual disability (MacMillan, Gresham, & Siperstein, 1995). This chapter (as well as the others in the book) uses the APA's categories in discussing medical issues and the AAMR's categories in discussing educational and other interventions, emphasizing the capabilities rather than the impairments of individuals with intellectual disability.

Domains of Disability

Another way of classifying intellectual disability is to use the terminology in disability classification developed by the National Center for Medical Rehabilitation Research (NCMRR; Msall et al., 2003). This model defines five domains: pathophysiology, impairment, functional limitation, disability, and societal limitation (Table 17.3). Pathophysiology focuses on the

Table 17.3. Relationship between disabilities domain and treatment in Down syndrome, fetal alcohol syndrome, and Prader-Willi syndrome

Pathophysiology	Impairment	Functional limitation	Disability	Societal limitation	Treatment
Deletion of chromosome 15	Prader-Willi syndrome	Intellectual disability Feeding disorder	Learning and adaptive skills below age level Obesity	Noninclusive school settings Stereotyping because of obesity and intellectual disability Underestimating abilities	Education Activities to promote weight loss
In utero alcohol exposure	Fetal alcohol syndrome	Intellectual disability Behavioral disturbances	Learning and adaptive skills below age level but variable Severe hyperactivity common	Noninclusive school settings Stigma because of etiology Overestimating abilities because of variable cognitive profile	Education Mental health interventions as required
Trisomy 21	Down syndrome	Intellectual disability	Learning and adaptive skills below age level	Noninclusive school settings Stereotyping because of intellectual disability Underestimating abilities	Education Programs to raise societal awareness

From Michael E. Msall, Roger C. Avery, Michelle R. Tremont, Julie C. Lima, Michelle L. Rogers, and Dennis P. Hogan. Functional Disability and School Activity Limitations in 41,300 School-Age Children: Relationship to Medical Impairments. *Pediatrics,* March 2003: *111*(3), 549; adapted by permission.

Note: Even though each child may have similar degrees of intellectual disability, the pattern of disability and type of treatments may vary widely.

cellular, structural, or functional events resulting from injury, disease, or genetic abnormality that underlie the developmental disability. Impairment refers to the losses that result from the pathophysiological event. Functional limitation describes the restriction or lack of ability to perform a normal function. Disability is the inability to perform or limitation in the performance of activities. Societal limitations focus on barriers to full participation in society. Table 17.3 illustrates how this system could be applied to children with Down syndrome, Prader-Willi syndrome, or fetal alcohol syndrome (FAS). The advantage of this approach is that it leads directly from diagnosis to treatment and focuses on how to overcome limitations. It also acknowledges the change in emphasis in the diagnosis of intellectual disability from impairment and functional limitations to disability and societal limitations. This is consistent with the move from focusing on the intensity of the disability (e.g., severe) to the support needed to function in society (e.g., requiring extensive support). This approach is also in keeping with the process for developing an individualized education program (IEP) for a school-age child (see Chapter 34).

Etiology

The epidemiology of intellectual disability suggests that there are two overlapping populations: Mild intellectual disability is more likely to be associated with environmental factors such as lower socioeconomic status and neglectful or abusive parenting (Durkin, 2002; Noble, Tottenham, & Casey, 2005; Leonard & Wen, 2002), whereas severe intellectual disability is more typically linked to a biological origin (Hou, Wang, & Chuang, 1998; Strømme &

Hagberg, 2000). There is often, however, an interaction between nature and nurture. Postnatal environmental influences mediate biological processes through mechanisms that may be indirect and not fully understood at present. In addition, postnatal environmental factors may affect the expression of the neurodevelopmental dysfunction. For example, a child may have an initial biological insult (e.g., intrauterine growth restriction [IUGR]) that can be compounded by postnatal environmental variables (e.g., poor nutrition, parental neglect). Mothers who never finished high school are four times more likely to have children with mild intellectual disability than are women who completed high school (Mendola et al., 2002). The explanation for this is unclear but may involve a genetic component (i.e., inheritance of a cognitive impairment) and socioeconomic factors (e.g., poverty, undernutrition) as well as inattentive or harsh parenting practices. Although African American children appear to be more than twice as likely to have IQ scores in the range of mild intellectual disability than Caucasian children, this increase is probably attributable to poverty and other adverse social conditions and is likely to be remediable (Yeargin-Allsopp et al., 1995). For example, application of early intervention services to high-risk infants who are also at socioeconomic risk has resulted in improved cognitive outcomes (Campbell et al., 2001).

The specific origins of mild intellectual disability are identifiable in less than 50% of individuals (Aicardi, 1998). Cultural, social, and familial factors play an important role here. Conversely, the most common biological causes are genetic syndromes with multiple minor congenital anomalies (e.g., velocardiofacial syndrome [VCFS]), fetal deprivation (e.g., IUGR), perinatal impairment (e.g., encephalopathy, infection), intrauterine exposure to drugs of abuse (especially fetal alcohol spectrum disorders [FASDs]; Burd et al., 2003; O'Leary, 2004), and X-chromosome abnormalities (e.g., Klinefelter syndrome; Lanfranco et al., 2004). Although definite genetic causes are less common (5% versus 47% in severe intellectual disability), familial clustering is frequent (Gillberg, 1998).

In children with severe intellectual disability, a biological origin of the condition can be identified in about three quarters of cases (Aicardi, 1998). The most common diagnoses are Down syndrome, fragile X syndrome, and FASDs, which together account for almost one third of all identifiable cases of severe intellectual disability (Macmillan, 1998; Moser, 1995).

One way of dividing the biological origins of intellectual disability is by their timing in the developmental sequence. In general, the earlier the problem, the more severe its consequences. This is consistent with finding a prenatal cause in about three quarters of individuals with an identifiable cause of severe intellectual disability (Acosta et al., 2002). Chromosomal disorders (e.g., Down syndrome, Prader-Willi syndrome, VCFS), nonchromosomal dysmorphic syndromes (e.g., Rubinstein-Taybi syndrome), and abnormalities of brain development (e.g., microcephaly) that affect early embryogenesis are the most common and severe. In addition, 10% are attributable to single-gene defects (e.g., inborn errors of metabolism; see Chapter 20). Together, these groups of genetically based causes of intellectual disability account for more than two thirds of identifiable causes and encompass more than 500 disorders (see http://www.ncbi.nlm.nih.gov/omim for more information). Insults occurring in the first and second trimesters as a result of substance abuse (e.g., FASD), infections (e.g., cytomegalovirus), and other pregnancy problems (e.g., IUGR) occur in 10% of cases (see Chapter 2). Fetal deprivation in the third trimester due to placental damage, preeclampsia, or hemorrhage (see Chapter 3) and problems in the perinatal period (see Chapter 4) now account for less than 10% of cases of severe intellectual disability. Five percent are the result of postnatal brain damage, most commonly brain infections and traumatic brain injury (see Chapter 30).

PREVALENCE OF INTELLECTUAL DISABILITY

Based on the previous discussion, the prevalence of intellectual disability depends on the definition used, the method of ascertainment, and the population studied (see Chapter 16; Fernell, 1996; Roeleveld, Zielhuis, & Gabreels, 1997; Strømme & Valvatne, 1998). Approximately 1.5 million people between the ages of 5 and 65 years in the United States were receiving services for intellectual disability in 1993 (Centers for Disease Control and Prevention, 1996). According to statistics and based on the *DSM-IV-TR* (APA, 2000) definition, 2.5% of the population could be predicted to have intellectual disability, and another 2.5% to have superior intelligence (Figure 17.1). Of individuals with intellectual disability, the IQ scores of 85% should fall 2–3 standard deviations below the mean, in the range of mild intellectual disability. If individuals who score low on IQ tests because of cultural or societal disadvantage are excluded from the count of those with mild intellectual disability, however, the prevalence is only about half these predictions, somewhere between 0.8% and 1.2% (McLaren & Bryson, 1987). Whatever the prevalence, intellectual disability appears to peak at 10–14 years of age, acknowledging that children with mild impairments are identified significantly later than those with more severe impairments. This issue is discussed further in Chapter 16.

Overall, the recurrence risk in families with one child who has severe intellectual disability of unknown origin is 3%–9% (Van Naarden Braun et al., 2005). Recurrence risk for intellectual disability of known origin, however, varies according to the cause. A family whose child has intellectual disability following neonatal meningitis does not have a significantly increased risk of having future affected children, whereas a woman who has had one child with a FASD has a 30%–50% risk of having other affected children if she continues to abuse alcohol during pregnancy. The risk of recurrent Down syndrome ranges from less than 1% for trisomy 21 to more than 10% for a balanced translocation (see Chapter 1; Mikkelsen, Poulsen, & Tommerup, 1989; Wolff et al., 1989). If the cause of intellectual disability is a Mendelian disorder (see Chapter 1) such as neurofibromatosis (an autosomal dominant trait), Hurler syndrome (an autosomal recessive trait), or fragile X syndrome (an X-linked trait), the recurrence risk ranges from 0% to 50%, depending on the inheritance pattern of the specific disorder (Ropers & Hamel, 2005).

ASSOCIATED IMPAIRMENTS

An intellectual disability is often accompanied by other impairments. Although a mild intellectual disability is frequently an isolated disorder, it may be paired with motor or communication impairments that affect the child's developmental outcome. The prevalence of these associated impairments correlates with the severity of the disability (Ferrell et al., 2004; Jansen et al., 2004; McBrien, 2003; Seager & O'Brien, 2003). These associated impairments include cerebral palsy, seizure disorders, sensory impairments, and psychological/behavioral disorders (Table 17.4), as well as communication disorders, feeding difficulties, and attention-deficit/hyperactivity disorder (ADHD). More than half of children with severe intellectual disability and one

quarter of children with mild intellectual disability have sensory impairments, of which vision impairments, especially strabismus and refractive errors, are the most common. Speech-language impairments, beyond those related to the cognitive impairment, also are frequent. Approximately 20% of children with severe intellectual disability have cerebral palsy, which may also be associated with feeding problems and failure to thrive (see Chapter 26). Seizure disorders also occur in about 20% of children with intellectual disability (see Chapter 29; Caplan & Austin, 2000). Finally, psychiatric and behavior disorders such as mood disorders (see Chapter 21), ASDs (see Chapter 23), and self-injurious behavior occur in up to half of children with intellectual disability (Bouras, 1999; Dekker & Koot, 2003). In considering intervention strategies, identifying these additional impairments and working toward their treatment is essential.

Associated impairments may make distinguishing intellectual disability from other developmental disabilities difficult. Certain distinguishing features, however, usually exist (Table 17.5). In isolated intellectual disability, language and nonverbal reasoning skills are significantly delayed, whereas gross motor skills tend to be less affected. Conversely, in cerebral palsy, motor impairments are more prominent than cognitive impairments. In communication disorders, expressive and/or receptive language skills are more delayed than motor and nonverbal reasoning skills. In ASDs, social skills impairments and atypical behaviors are superimposed on cognitive (especially communication) impairments. In some instances, repeated assessments may be necessary to determine the primary developmental disability.

Table 17.4. Percentages of children with intellectual disability (ID) who have associated developmental disabilities

Associated disability	Severe ID (%)	Mild ID (%)
None	17	63
Cerebral palsy	19	6
Seizure disorders	21	11
Sensory impairments	55	24
Psychological/behavioral disorders	50	25

From Kiely, M. (1987). The prevalence of mental retardation. *Epidemiologic Reviews, 9,* 194; adapted by permission of Oxford University Press.

Table 17.5. Developmental delays in various developmental disabilities during preschool years

Disorder	Motor	Language	Problem solving (nonverbal reasoning)	Social-adaptive
Intellectual disability	Variable	2	2	2
Autism spectrum disorder	N/A	3	Variable	3
Cerebral palsy	3	Variable	Variable	2
Language disorder/ deafness	N/A	2	N/A	Variable
Blindness	1	N/A	Variable	1

Key: 3, severe impairment; 2, moderate impairment; 1, mild impairment; N/A, not affected.

MEDICAL DIAGNOSTIC TESTING

No single method exists for detecting all causes of intellectual disability (Shevell et al., 2000; van Karnebeek et al., 2005). As a result, diagnostic testing should be based on the medical history and a physical examination (Battaglia & Carey, 2003; Moeschler et al., 2006). For example, a child with an unusual facial appearance or multiple congenital anomalies should be referred to a geneticist. Even minor anomalies may be worth pursuing with high-resolution chromosomal banding, fluorescent *in situ* hybridization (FISH), array comparative genomic hybridization (array CGH), and chromosome painting for subtelometric rearrangements (Devriendt & Vermeesch, 2004; Irons, 2003; Poplawski, 2003). A male with unusual physical features and/or a family history of intellectual disability should probably have molecular studies for fragile X syndrome. A child with a progressive neurological disorder will need extensive metabolic investigation, and a child with seizure-like episodes should have an electroencephalogram. Finally, children with abnormal head growth or asymmetrical neurological findings warrant a neuroimaging procedure such as MRI. These tests, however, should not be seen as screening tools to be used in all children with intellectual disability, as their yield of useful results is low unless there is a specific reason for performing the test. Table 17.6 lists tests that may be used to investigate intellectual disability and how commonly they reveal a cause.

Although these are the most common reasons for performing diagnostic tests, it now seems clear that some children with subtle physical or neurological findings also may have determinable biological origins of their intellectual disability. It has been shown that about 6% of unexplained intellectual disability can be accounted for by microdeletions (very minute chromosomal abnormalities) that require extensive testing to identify (McFadden & Friedman, 1997; Xu & Chen, 2003). In addition, MRI scans have been found to document a significant number of subtle markers of cerebral dysgenesis in about 10% of children with intellectual disability (Barkovich & Raybaud, 2004).

How intensively one should investigate the cause of a child's intellectual disability is based on a number of factors. First, what is the degree of intellectual disability? One is less likely to find a biological cause in a child with mild intellectual disability than in a child with a severe disability. Second, is there a specific diagnostic path to follow? If there is a medical history, a family history, or physical findings pointing to a specific cause, a diagnosis is more likely to be made. Conversely, in the absence of these indicators, it is difficult to choose specific tests to perform. Third, are the parents planning on having additional children? If so, one would be more likely to intensively seek disorders for which prenatal diagnosis or a specific early treatment option is available. Finally, and most important, what are the parents' wishes? Different parents have different levels of investment in searching for the cause; some focus exclusively on treatment. Others are so directed on obtaining a diagnosis that they have difficulty accepting intervention until a specific cause has been determined. Both extremes and everything in between must be respected, and sup-

Table 17.6. Tests that may be used in the evaluation of the child with intellectual disability

Test	Yield	Comment
In-depth history		Includes pre-, peri-, and postnatal events (including seizures), developmental attainments, and three-generation pedigree in family history
Physical examination		Particular attention to minor/subtle abnormalities
		Neurological examination for focality and skull abnormalities
		Behavioral phenotype
Vision/hearing evaluation		
Karyotype	3.7%	
Fragile X screen	2.6%	Preselection on clinical grounds may increase yield to 7.6%
Neuroimaging	40%–55%	Magnetic resonance imaging (MRI) preferred
		Positives increased by abnormalities of skull contour or size or focal neurological examination
		Identification of specific etiologies is rare
		Most conditions that are found do not alter treatment plan
		Need to weigh risk of sedation against possible yield
Thyroid (thyroid hormone, thyroid stimulating hormone)	~4%	Near 0% in settings with universal newborn screening program
Serum lead	?	Necessary if there are identifiable risk factors for excessive environmental lead exposure
Metabolic testing	~1%	Testing for urine organic acids, plasma, amino acids, ammonia, lactate, and a capillary blood gas
		Focused testing based on clinical findings warranted
Subtelomeric deletion	6.6%	Obtain in the presence of dysmorphisms with a normal karyotype and fragile X DNA study; higher in severe intellectual disability
MECP2 for Rett syndrome	?	For females with severe intellectual disability
Electroencephalogram (EEG)	~1%	May be deferred in absence of history of seizures

Sources: Curry, Stevenson, Aughton, et al. (1997); Shevell, Ashwal, Donley, et al. (2003).

portive anticipatory guidance should be provided in the context of parent education for the "here and now" as well as for the future.

PSYCHOLOGICAL TESTING

The routine evaluation for intellectual disability should include an individual intelligence test. The most commonly used test in children are the Bayley Scales of Infant Development–Third Edition (BSID-III; Bayley, 2006) and the Wechsler scales: the Wechsler Preschool and Primary Scale of Intelligence–Third Edition (WPPSI-III; Wechsler, 2002) and the Wechsler Intelligence Scale for Children–Fourth Edition (WISC-IV; Wechsler, 2003). These and a few other tests are briefly described next and further outlined in Appendix E.

Infant Developmental Tests

The BSID-III is used to assess language, visual problem-solving skills, behavior, fine motor skills, and gross motor skills of children between 1 month and 42 months of age. A Mental Developmental Index (MDI) and a Psychomotor Development Index (PDI; a measure of motor competence) score are derived from the results. Less commonly used infant tests include the Battelle Developmental Inventory-2 (Newborg et al., 2004) and the Mullen Scales of Early Learning (Mullen, 1989).

Intelligence Tests in Children

The most commonly used psychological tests for children older than 3 years of age are the Wechsler scales. The WPPSI-III (Wechsler,

2002) is used for children with mental ages of 3–7 years. The WISC-IV (Wechsler, 2003) is used for children who function between a 6-16 year mental age. The Wechsler Adult Scale of Intelligence–Third Edition (WAIS-III; Wechsler, 1997) is used for individuals with cognitive abilities above 16 years. The Wechsler Abbreviated Scale of Intelligence (WASI; Wechsler, 1999) is also being used more commonly. The Stanford-Binet Intelligence Scales, Fifth Edition (SB5; Roid, 2003) and the Kaufman Assessment Battery for Children, Second Edition (KABC-II; Kaufman & Kaufman, 2004) are used as well but much less frequently.

Tests of Adaptive Functioning

As noted in the *DSM-IV-TR* (APA, 2000) definition of mental retardation, in addition to testing intelligence, adaptive skills also should be measured, including social functioning (Bielecki & Swender, 2004). The most commonly used test of adaptive behavior is the Vineland-II (Sparrow et al., 2005). These tests involve semistructured interviews with parents and/or caregivers and teachers that assess adaptive behavior in four domains: communication, daily living skills, socialization, and motor skills. The test has three forms, with 244–577 items. Other tests of adaptive behavior (Wodrich, 1997) include the Woodcock-Johnson Scales of Independent Behavior (Bruininks et al., 1996) and the Adaptive Behavior Assessment System, Second Edition (ABAS-II; Harrison & Oakland, 2003).

Interpretation of Test Results

In infants and young children with typical development, there is substantial variability in IQ scores on repeated cognitive testing and consequently poor predictive validity until around 10 years of age. Accuracy is enhanced if repeated testing confirms a stable rate of cognitive development. The predictive value of infant tests is further limited because such tests are primarily dependent on nonlanguage items, whereas language skills remain the best predictors of future IQ scores (Bayley, 1958). These tests do permit the differentiation of infants with severe intellectual disability from typically developing infants but are less helpful in distinguishing between a typically developing child and one with a mild intellectual disability (Maisto & German, 1986). In general, however, there is less variability seen with cognitive growth in children with intellectual disability, so predictive validity is enhanced compared with children with typical development.

Although children with intellectual disability usually score below average on all subscale scores, they occasionally score in the typical range in one or more performance areas in the Wechsler Scales. Overall, these scales are quite accurate in predicting adult IQ scores when administered to school-age children. The evaluator, however, must ensure that situations that may lead to falsely low IQ scores do not confound the test performance. Conditions such as motor impairments, communication disorders, sensory impairments, speaking a language other than English, extremely low birth weight, or severe sociocultural deprivation may invalidate certain intelligence tests and require modification of others, and they always involve caution in interpretation.

There is usually (but not always) a good correlation between scores on the intelligence and adaptive scales (Bloom & Zelko, 1994). Adaptive abilities, however, are more responsive to intervention efforts than is the IQ score. They are also more variable, which may relate to the underlying condition and to environmental expectations. For example, although individuals with Prader-Willi syndrome have stability of adaptive skills through adulthood, individuals with fragile X syndrome may have increasing impairments over time (Jacquemont et al., 2004).

TREATMENT APPROACHES

The most useful treatment approach for children with intellectual disability consists of multimodal efforts directed at many aspects of the child's life—education, social, and recreational activities; behavior problems; and associated impairments. Support for parents, siblings, and other caregivers (both family members and unrelated caregivers) is also important (see Chapter 40).

Educational Services

Education is the single most important discipline involved in intervention for children with intellectual disability and their families (see Chapters 33 and 34). The achievement of good outcomes in an educational program is dependent on the interaction between the student and teacher. Educational programs must be relevant to the child's needs and address the child's individual strengths and challenges. The child's developmental level and his or her requirements for support and goals for independence provide a basis for establishing an IFSP or an IEP.

It also needs to be remembered that children's learning always begins in a familial context that later is shared with the educational system. Education for infants and toddlers (birth to 3 years) is more likely to take place in their families' homes than in out-of-home formalized education centers. Starting at age 3, although some children may still reside with their parents (as primary teachers) other children begin attending some form of group socializing, out-of-home or center-based care, or preschool environment. Their teaching begins to be shared or relegated to multiple teaching providers. At age 5, many children enter kindergarten for half- or full-day sessions and are introduced to a more formal learning school environment.

Leisure and Recreational Needs

In addition to education, the child's social and recreational needs should be addressed (Bielecki & Swender, 2004). Children's peer socialization in play and recreational activities constitutes an important part of their social-emotional development and builds resilience. As such, children's socialization competencies and experiences (e.g., dealing with social conflict, managing anger, making needs known, expressing affection or unhappiness) can exert a significant influence upon their developmental outcomes and school readiness and participation, and it eventually also can influence children's future success in adult life. In the ideal world, children with intellectual disability would participate as equals in all recreation and leisure activities. Although young children with intellectual disability are not usually excluded from play activities, parents still may have a difficult time finding age appropriate adaptive play equipment (cost can be a significant factor) or socially oriented play groups (transportation costs and availability of inclusive programs are additional compromising factors). Furthermore, adolescents with an intellectual disability are often excluded by their typically developing peers from participating in extracurricular sports and social activities. Yet, participation in sports or related fun exercise regimens must be encouraged with all children (as functionally appropriate) because it offers many benefits, including weight management, development of physical coordination, maintenance of cardiovascular fitness, and improvement of self-image (see Chapter 38).

Adolescent social activities are equally important to the social and emotional development of youth with intellectual disabilities. Such opportunities should include a variety of social activities, including those with youth of the opposite gender and with youth who do not have disabilities. Such activities, however, need to be based on the youth's functionally adaptive age appropriate behaviors. Examples of normalizing activities include participation in summer camps; school dances; school or family trips; dating or socialization in youth groups or school clubs; visits to movies, restaurants, and other socializing establishments; and other typical recreational events. Such activities should also include opportunities for increasing social-emotional independence away from direct parental oversight and exposure to novel experiences, in which the individual has the opportunity to test, grapple with, and practice his or her overall developmental competencies (see Chapter 41).

Behavior Therapy

Although most children with intellectual disability do not have behavior disorders, these problems do occur with a greater frequency in this population than among children with typical development (Bouras, 1999). To facilitate the child's socialization, significant behavior problems must be addressed (Chapter 35). Behavior problems may result from organic problems, primary or associated secondary psychiatric disorders, unrealistic parental expectations, and/or other family difficulties and school-related adjustment difficulties. Typically, behavior problems represent attempts by the child to communicate, gain attention, or avoid frustration. In assessing the behavior, one must first consider whether the behavior is appropriate for the child's "cognitive" age rather than for his or her chronological age. The child's chronological age, however, needs to be considered in order to address the manifested behavior in the environmental context of the child's functioning. When intervention is needed, an environmental change, such as a more appropriate classroom environment, may improve behavior problems for some children. For other children, behavior management techniques (see Chapter 35) and/or the use of psychotropic medication may be appropriate.

Use of Medication

Medication is not useful in treating the core symptoms of intellectual disability; no drug has been found to improve cognitive function. Medication may be helpful, however, in treating associated behavioral and emotional disorders. These drugs are generally directed at specific symptom complexes, including ADHD (e.g., stimulants [Ritalin, Concerta, Focalin, Metadate CD, Daytrana, Methylin, Adderall]), self-injurious behavior (e.g., risperidone [Risperdal]), aggression (e.g., carbamazepine [Tegretol], valproate [Depakote], aripiprazole [Abilify]), and depression and/or obsessive-compulsive disorder (e.g., fluoxetine [Prozac], sertraline [Zoloft]; Holinger et al., 2003; Shedlack et al., 2005; Singh et al., 2005). The properties of these psychopharmaceutical drugs are outlined in Appendix C. Before long-term therapy with any drug is initiated, a short trial should be conducted. Even if a medication proves successful, its use should be reevaluated at least yearly to assess the need for continued treatment.

Treating Associated Impairments

Any associated impairment—cerebral palsy; sensory impairments; seizure disorders; speech disorders; ASDs; and other disorders of language, behavior or perception—must also be treated to achieve an optimal outcome for the child. This may require ongoing physical therapy, occupational therapy, speech-language therapy, behavioral therapy, adaptive equipment, eyeglasses, hearing aids, medication, and so forth. Failure to adequately identify and treat these problems may hinder successful **habilitation** and result in difficulties in the home, school, or neighborhood environment.

Family Counseling

All families benefit from anticipatory guidance regarding their child's health and development, but this is especially true for those families with children suspected of or identified with intellectual disability. Many families adapt well to having a child with intellectual disability, but some have difficulty (Scorgie & Sobsey, 2000). Among the significant factors that have been associated with family coping skills are the severity of the child's disability, number of siblings, stability of the parents' relationship, parental age, mental and physical health of the family, financial stability, expectations and acceptance of the child's diagnosis, supportiveness of the extended family, and availability of community programs and respite care services. In families in which the emotional demands of having a child with intellectual disability are great, family counseling should be an integral part of the treatment plan (see Chapter 40).

Periodic Reevaluation

The needs of children and their families change over time and more information must be provided. Children's health, learning, adaptive, and behavioral goals must be reassessed, and developmentally based and school related programming needs to be adjusted. A periodic review should include information about the child's health status as well as his or her functioning at home, at school, and in other social contexts. Other information, such as formal **psychoeducational** testing, may be needed. Reevaluation should be undertaken at routine intervals, at any time the child is not meeting expectations, and when he or she is moving from one service provision system to another. Reevaluations are needed during early childhood and preschool years to ensure that the program remains appropriate as the child matures. They are especially necessary during adolescence to prepare for the transition to adulthood (Bates et al., 2003; see Chapter 41).

OUTCOME

Save in the extremes, IQ scores alone are not good predictors of outcome (Braddock et al., 2001). Outcome for an individual with intellectual disability depends on the interplay of many factors including the underlying cause; the degree of disability; the presence of associated medical and developmental deficits; the capabilities of the family; and the supports, community services, and training provided to the child and family (Seltzer & Krauss, 2001). As adults, many people with intellectual disability requiring intermittent support are able to gain functional literacy and some economic and social independence. Such adults may, however, need periodic assistance, especially when under social or economic stress. Some marry and live successfully in the community, either independently or in supervised settings (APA, 2000; Aylward, 2002). Life expectancy usually is not adversely affected.

For individuals with intellectual disability requiring limited support, the goals of education are to enhance adaptive abilities, functional academics, and vocational skills so that these individuals are better able to live in the adult world (Cummins, 2001). Contemporary gains including supported employment have benefited these individuals the most. Supported employment challenges the view that prerequisite skills must be taught before there can be successful vocational adaptation. Instead, individuals are trained by a coach to do a specific job in the setting in which the person is to work. This approach bypasses the need for extended time mastering "prerequisite skills" and has resulted in successful work adaptation in the community for many people with intellectual disability. Outcome studies have documented the benefits and effectiveness of this approach (Stephens et al., 2005). People with intellectual disability requiring limited support (e.g., individuals with Down syndrome) can generally live at home or in a supervised setting in the community.

As adults, people with intellectual disability requiring extensive to pervasive support may perform simple tasks in supervised settings. These individuals, however, may have associated impairments such as cerebral palsy and sensory impairments that further limit their adaptive functioning. Yet, most people with this level of intellectual disability are able to live in the community with supportive adaptations in their environment and with supervisory oversight (see Chapter 41). Family-based, community-supported care is preferable to institutional care for these individuals, but it is often difficult to achieve for a variety of reasons (e.g., parents' advanced ages, lack of economic support, familial or community reluctance). As a result, some of these individuals with severe medical problems, behavioral disturbances, or disrupted families require out-of-home living in such settings as foster homes, alternative living units, group homes, nursing homes, or residential schools. People who require extensive or pervasive supports have increased utilization health care, mentoring, and behavioral health and may have a shortened life span (Hollins et al., 1998; Katz, 2003).

SUMMARY

Development is an ordered process that is linked to the maturation of the central nervous system. With intellectual disability, development is altered so that intellectual and adaptive skills are impaired. In most cases of mild intellectual disability the underlying cause is unclear

and may be tied to environmental effects. In three quarters of individuals with severe intellectual disability, however, there is a definable biologic cause. The vast majority of people with intellectual disability require only intermittent support and are often able to achieve some economic and social independence. The early identification of a global developmental delay is important to ensure appropriate treatment and to enable the child to develop and use all of his or her capabilities. Treatment should be multimodal, supporting the educational, mental and physical health, adaptive behavior, and communication skills of individuals with intellectual disability.

REFERENCES

Acosta, M., Gallo, V., & Batshaw, M.L. (2002). Brain development and the ontogeny of developmental disabilities. *Advances in Pediatrics, 49,* 1–57.

Aicardi, J. (1998). The etiology of developmental delay. *Seminars in Pediatric Neurology, 5,* 15–20.

Akinbami, L.J., LaFleur, B.J., & Schoendorf, K.C. (2002). Racial and income disparities in childhood asthma in the United States. *Ambulatory Pediatrics 2*(5), 382–387.

American Association on Mental Retardation. (2002). *Mental retardation: Definition, classification, and systems of supports* (10th ed.). Washington, DC: Author.

American Psychiatric Association. (2000). *Diagnostic and statistical manual of mental disorders* (4th ed., text rev.). Washington, DC: Author.

Aylward, G.P. (2002). Cognitive and neuropsychological outcomes: More than IQ scores. *Mental Retardation and Developmental Disability Research Reviews, 8*(4), 234–340.

Barkovich, A.J., & Raybaud, C.A. (2004). Malformations of cortical development. *Neuroimaging Clinics of North America, 14*(3), 401–423.

Bates, K., Bartoshesky, L., & Friedland, A. (2003). As the child with chronic disease grows up: Transitioning adolescents with special health care needs to adult-centered health care. *Delaware Medical Journal, 75*(6), 217–220.

Battaglia, A., & Carey, J.C. (2003). Diagnostic evaluation of developmental delay/mental retardation: An overview. *American Journal of Medical Genetics Part C: Seminars in Medical Genetics, 117*(1), 3–14.

Bayley, N. (1958). Value and limitations of infant testing. *Children, 5,* 129–133.

Bayley, N. (2006). *Bayley Scales of Infant Development: Third edition manual.* San Antonio, TX: Harcourt Assessment.

Bear, L.M. (2004). Early identification of infants at risk for developmental disabilities. *Pediatric Clinics of North America, 51*(3), 685–701.

Beirne-Smith, M., Ittenbach, R.F., & Patton, J.R. (2001). *Mental retardation* (6th ed). Upper Saddle River, NJ: Prentice Hall.

Bielecki, J., & Swender, S.L. (2004). The assessment of social functioning in individuals with mental retardation: A review. *Behavior Modification, 28*(5), 694–708.

Bouras, N. (Ed.). (1999). *Psychiatric and behavioural disor-*

ders in developmental disabilities and mental retardation. New York: Cambridge University Press.

Bloom, A.S., & Zelko, F.A. (1994). Variability in adaptive behavior in children with developmental delay. *Journal of Clinical Psychology, 50,* 261–265.

Braddock, D., Emerson, E., Felce, D., et al. (2001). Living circumstances of children and adults with mental retardation or developmental disabilities in the United States, Canada, England and Wales, and Australia. *Mental Retardation and Developmental Disabilities Research Reviews, 7*(2)., 115–121.

Bricker, D., & Squires, J., with Mounts, L., Potter, L., Nickel, R., et al. (1999). *Ages & Stages Questionnaires© (ASQ): A parent-completed, child-monitoring system* (2nd ed.). Baltimore Paul H. Brookes Publishing Co.

Bruininks, R.H., Woodcock, R.W., Weatherman, R.F., et al. (1996). *Scales of Independent Behavior–Revised (SIB-R).* Chicago: Riverside.

Burd, L., Cotsonas-Hassler, T.M., Martsolf, J.T., et al. (2003). Recognition and management of fetal alcohol syndrome. *Neurotoxicology and Teratology, 25*(6), 681–688.

Campbell, F.A., Pungello, E.P., Miller-Johnson, S., et al. (2001). The development of cognitive and academic abilities: growth curves from an early childhood educational experiment. *Developmental Psychology, 37*(2), 231–342.

Caplan, R., & Austin, J.K. (2000). Behavioral aspects of epilepsy in children with mental retardation. *Mental Retardation and Developmental Disabilities Research Reviews, 6*(4), 293–299.

Carrey, N.J., Butter, H.J., Persinger, M.A., et al. (1995). Physiological and cognitive correlates of child abuse. *Journal of the American Academy of Child and Adolescent Psychiatry, 34*(8), 1067–1075.

Centers for Disease Control and Prevention. (1996). State-specific rates of mental retardation—United States, 1993. *Morbidity and Mortality Weekly Report, 45*(3), 61–65.

Committee on Children with Disabilities. (2001). Role of the pediatrician in family-centered early intervention services. *Pediatrics, 107*(5), 1155–1157.

Cummins, R.A. (2001). Living with support in the community: predictors of satisfaction with life. *Mental Retardation and Developmental Disabilities Research Reviews, 7*(2), 99–104.

Council on Children with Disabilities, Section on Developmental Behavioral Pediatrics; Bright Futures Steering Committee; and Medical Home Initiatives for Children with Special Needs Project Advisory Committee. (2006). Identifying infants and young children with developmental disorders in the medical home: An algorithm for developmental surveillance and screening. *Pediatrics, 118*(1), 405–420. Erratum in *Pediatrics, 118*(4),1808–1809.

Curry, C.J., Stevenson, R.E., Aughton, D., et al. (1997). Evaluation of mental retardation: Recommendations of a consensus conference. American College of Medical Genetics. *American Journal of Medical Genetics, 72,* 468–477.

Dekker, M.C., & Koot, H.M. (2003). DSM-IV disorders in children with borderline to moderate intellectual disability. I: Prevalence and impact. *Journal of the American Academy of Child and Adolescent Psychiatry, 42* (8), 915–922.

Devriendt, K., & Vermeesch, J.R. (2004). Chromosomal phenotypes and submicroscopic abnormalities. *Human Genomics, 1*(2), 126–133.

Durkin, M. (2002). The epidemiology of developmental disabilities in low-income countries. *Mental Retardation and Developmental Disabilities Research Reviews, 8*(3), 206–211.

Fernell, E. (1996). Mild mental retardation in schoolchildren in a Swedish suburban municipality: Prevalence and diagnostic aspects. *Acta Paediatrica, 85*(5), 584–588.

Ferrell, R.B., Wolinsky, E.J., Kauffman, C.I, et al. (2004). Neuropsychiatric syndromes in adults with intellectual disability: issues in assessment and treatment. *Current Psychiatry Reports, 6*(5), 380–390.

Frankenburg, W.K., Dodds, J.B., Archer, P., et al. (1992). *Denver II* (2nd ed.). Denver, CO: Denver Developmental Materials.

Gardner, H. (1983). *Frames of mind: The theory of multiple intelligences.* New York: Basic Books.

Gillberg, C. (1998). Mental retardation. In J. Aicardi (Ed.), *Clinics in developmental medicine: Nos. 115–118. Diseases of the nervous system in childhood* (2nd ed., pp. 822–826). New York: Cambridge University Press.

Glascoe, F. (1997). Parents' concerns about children's development: Prescreening technique or screening test. *Pediatrics, 99,* 522–528.

Guralnick, M.J. (Ed.). (2005). *The developmental systems approach to early intervention.* Baltimore: Paul H. Brookes Publishing Co.

Harrison, P.L., & Oakland, T. (2003). *Adaptive Behavior Assessment System–Second Edition (ABAS-II).* San Antonio, TX: Harcourt Assessment.

Hayes D. (2003). Screening methods: Current status. *Mental Retardation and Developmental Disabilities Research Reviews, 9*(2):65–72.

Holinger, D.P., Bellugi, U., & Mills, D.L., et al. (2003). Patients with and without intellectual disability seeking outpatient psychiatric services: Diagnoses and prescribing pattern. *Journal of Intellectual Disability Research, 47*(Pt. 1), 39–50.

Hollins, S., Attard, M.T., von Fraunhofer, N., et al. (1998). Mortality in people with learning disability: Risks, causes, and death certification findings in London. *Developmental Medicine and Child Neurology, 40,* 50–56.

Hou, J.W., Wang, T.R., & Chuang, S.M. (1998). An epidemiological and aetiological study of children with intellectual disability in Taiwan. *Journal of Intellectual Disability Research, 42*(Pt. 2), 137–143.

Hoyme, H.E., May, P.A., Kalberg, W.O., et al. (2005). A practical clinical approach to diagnosis of fetal alcohol spectrum disorders: Clarification of the 1996 institute of medicine criteria. *Pediatrics, 115*(1), 39–47.

Individuals with Disabilities Education Act Amendments of 1997, PL 105-17, 20 U.S.C. §§ 1400 *et seq.*

Irons, M. (2003). Use of subtelomeric fluorescence in situ hybridization in cytogenetic diagnosis. *Current Opinion in Pediatrics, 15*(6), 594–597.

Jacobson, J., & Jacobson, C. (2004). Evaluation of hearing loss in infants and young children. *Pediatric Annals, 33*(12), 811–821.

Jacquemont, S., Farzin, F., Hall, D., et al. (2004). Aging in individuals with the FMR1 mutation. *American Journal on Mental Retardation, 109*(2), 154–164.

Jansen, D.E., Krol, B., Groothoff, J.W., et al. (2004). People with intellectual disability and their health problems: A review of comparative studies. *Journal of Intellectual Disability Research, 48*(Pt. 2), 93–102.

Katz, R.T. (2003). Life expectancy for children with cerebral palsy and mental retardation: Implications for life care planning. *NeuroRehabilitation, 18*(3), 261–270.

Kaufman, A.S., & Kaufman, N.L. (2004). *Kaufman Assessment Battery for Children, Second Edition (KABC-II)*. Circle Pines, MN: AGS Publishing.

Kiely, M. (1987). The prevalence of mental retardation. *Epidemiologic Reviews, 9*, 194–218.

Koenen, K.C., Moffitt, T.E., Caspi, A., et al. (2003). Domestic violence is associated with environmental suppression of IQ in young children. *Development and Psychopathology, 15*(2), 297–311.

Lanfranco, F., Kamischke, A., Zitzmann, M., et al. (2004). Klinefelter's syndrome. *The Lancet, 364*(9430), 273–283.

Leonard, H., & Wen, X. (2002). The epidemiology of mental retardation: Challenges and opportunities in the new millennium. *Mental Retardation and Developmental Disabilities Research Reviews,8*(3), 117–134.

Macmillan, C. (1998). Genetics and developmental delay. *Seminars in Pediatric Neurology, 5*, 39–44.

MacMillan, D.L., Gresham, F.M., & Siperstein, G.N. (1995). Heightened concerns over the 1992 AAMR definition: Advocacy versus precision. *American Journal on Mental Retardation, 100*, 87–97.

Maisto, A.A., & German, M.L. (1986). Reliability, predictive validity, and interrelationships of early assessment indices used with developmentally delayed infants and children. *Journal of Clinical Child Psychiatry, 15*, 547–554.

McBrien, J.A. (2003). Assessment and diagnosis of depression in people with intellectual disability. *Journal of Intellectual Disability Research, 47*(Pt. 1), 1–13.

McFadden, D.E., & Friedman, J.M. (1997). Chromosome abnormalities in human beings. *Mutation Research, 396*(1–2), 129–140.

McLaren, J., & Bryson, S.E. (1987). Review of recent epidemiological studies of mental retardation: Prevalence, associated disorders, and etiology. *American Journal of Mental Retardation., 92*(3), 243–354.

Mendola, P., Selevan, S.G., Gutter, S., et al. (2002). Environmental factors associated with a spectrum of neurodevelopmental deficits. *Mental Retardation and Developmental Disabilities Research Reviews, 8*(3), 188–197.

Mikkelsen, M., Poulsen, H., & Tommerup, N. (1989). Genetic risk factors in human trisomy 21. *Progress in Clinical Biological Research, 311*, 183–197.

Moeschler, J.B., Shevell, M., & the Committee on Genetics. (2006). Clinical genetic evaluation of the child with mental retardation or developmental delays. *Pediatrics, 117*, 2304–2316.

Moser, H.W. (1995). A role for gene therapy in mental retardation. *Mental Retardation and Developmental Disabilities Research Reviews, 1*, 4–6.

Msall, M.E., Avery, R.C., Tremont, M.R., et al. (2003). Functional disability and school activity limitations in 41,300 school-age children: Relationship to medical impairments. *Pediatrics, 111*(3), 548–553.

Mullen, E. (1989). *Mullen Scales of Early Learning*. Cranston, RI: T.O.T.A.L. Child.

Neiss, M., & Rowe, D.C. (2000). Parental education and child's verbal IQ in adoptive and biological families in the National Longitudinal Study of Adolescent Health. *Behavior Genetics, 30*(6), 487–495.

Newborg, J. (2004). *Battelle Developmental Inventory–Second edition (BDI-2)*. Chicago: Riverside.

Noble, K.G., Tottenham, N., & Casey, B.J. (2005). Neuroscience perspectives on disparities in school readiness and cognitive achievement. In C. Rouse, J. Books-Gunn, & S. McLanahan, *The future of the children: School readiness, 15*(1), 71–89.

O'Dowd P. (2002). Controversies regarding low blood lead level harm. *Medicine and Health, Rhode Island, 85* (11), 345–348.

O'Leary, C.M. (2004). Fetal alcohol syndrome: Diagnosis, epidemiology, and developmental outcomes. *Journal of Paediatrics and Child Health, 40*(1–2), 2–7.

Petterson, S.M., & Albers, A.B. (2001). Effects of poverty and maternal depression on early child development. *Child Development, 72*(6), 1794–1813.

Poplawski, N.K. (2003). Investigating intellectual disability: A genetic perspective. *Journal of Paediatrics and Child Health, 39*(7), 492–506.

Roeleveld, N., Zielhuis, G.A., & Gabreels, F. (1997). The prevalence of mental retardation: A critical review of recent literature. *Developmental Medicine and Child Neurology, 39*, 125–132.

Roid, G. (2003). *Stanford-Binet Intelligence Scales, Fifth Edition (SB5)*. Chicago: Riverside.

Ropers, H.H., & Hamel, B.C. (2005). X-linked mental retardation. *Nature Review Genetics, 6*(1), 46–57.

Rydz, D., Shevell ,M.I., Majnemer, A., et al. (2005). Developmental screening. *Journal of Child Neurology, 20* (1), 4–21.

Scorgie, K., & Sobsey D. (2000). Transformational outcomes associated with parenting children who have disabilities. *Mental Retardation, 38*, 195–206.

Seager, M.C., & O'Brien, G. (2003). Attention deficit hyperactivity disorder: Review of ADHD in learning disability: The Diagnostic Criteria for Psychiatric Disorders for Use with Adults with Learning Disabilities/Mental Retardation[DC-LD] criteria for diagnosis. *Journal of Intellectual Disability Research, 47*(Suppl. 1), 26–31.

Seltzer, M.M., & Krauss, M.W. (2001). Quality of life of adults with mental retardation/developmental disabilities who live with family. *Mental Retardation and Developmental Disability Research Reviews, 7*(2), 105–114.

Shapiro, B.K., & Batshaw, M.L. (2002). Mental retardation. In F.D. Burg, J.A. Ingelfinger, R.A. Polin, et al. (Eds.), *Gellis and Kagan's current pediatric therapy* (17th ed., pp. 399–402). Philadelphia: W.B. Saunders.

Shedlack, K.J., Hennen, J., Magee, C., et al. (2005). Assessing the utility of atypical antipsychotic medication in adults with mild mental retardation and comorbid psychiatric disorders. *The Journal of Clinical Psychiatry, 66*(1), 52–62.

Shevell, M., Ashwal, S., Donley, D., et al. (2003). Practice parameter: Evaluation of the child with global developmental delay: Report of the Quality Standards Subcommittee of the American Academy of Neurology and the Practice Committee of the Child Neurology Society. *Neurology, 60*(3), 367–380.

Shevell, M.I., Majnemer, A., Rosenbaum, P., et al. (2000). Etiologic yield of subspecialists' evaluation of young children with global developmental delay. *Journal of Pediatrics, 136*, 593–598.

Singh, A.N., Matson, J.L., Cooper, C.L., et al. (2005). The use of risperidone among individuals with mental retardation: Clinically supported or not? *Research in Developmental Disabilities, 26*(3), 203–318.

Stephens, D.L., Collins, M.D., & Dodder, R.A. (2005). A longitudinal study of employment and skill acquisition among individuals with developmental disabilities. *Research in Developmental Disabilities, 26*(5), 469–486.

Sparrow, S.S., Bella, D.A., & Crichetti, D.V. (2005). *Vineland Adaptive Behavior Scales, Second Edition (Vineland-II)*. Circle Pines, MN: AGS Publishing.

Strømme, P., & Hagberg, G. (2000). Aetiology in severe

and mild mental retardation: A population-based study of Norwegian children. *Developmental Medicine and Child Neurology, 42,* 76–86.

Strømme, P., & Valvatne, K. (1998). Mental retardation in Norway: Prevalence and sub-classification in a cohort of 30,037 children born between 1980 and 1985. *Acta Paediatrica, 7,* 291–296.

Turkheimer, E., Haley, A., Waldron, M., et al. (2003). Socioeconomic status modifies heritability of IQ in young children. *Psychological Science, 14*(6), 623–628.

van Karnebeek, C.D., Jansweijer, M.C., Leenders, A.G., et al. (2005). Diagnostic investigations in individuals with mental retardation: A systematic literature review of their usefulness. *European Journal of Human Genetics, 13*(1), 6–25.

Van Naarden Braun, K., Autry, A., & Boyle, C. (2005). A population-based study of the recurrence of developmental disabilities—Metropolitan Atlanta Developmental Disabilities Surveillance Program, 1991–1994. *Paediatric and Perinatal Epidemiology, 19*(1), 69–79.

Wang, P.P., & Bellugi, U. (1993). Williams syndrome, Down syndrome, and cognitive neuroscience. *American Journal of Diseases of Childhood, 147,* 1246–1251.

Wechsler, D. (1974). *Wechsler Intelligence Scale for Children–Revised.* San Antonio, TX: Harcourt Assessment.

Wechsler, D. (1997). *Wechsler Adult Intelligence Scale–Third Edition (WAIS-III).* San Antonio TX: Harcourt Assessment.

Wechsler, D. (1999). *Wechsler Abbreviated Screening Inventory (WASI).* San Antonio, TX: Harcourt Assessment.

Wechsler, D. (2002). *Wechsler Preschool and Primary Scale of Intelligence–Third Edition (WPPSI-III).* San Antonio, TX: Harcourt Assessment.

Wechsler, D. (2003). *Wechsler Intelligence Scale for Children–Fourth Edition (WISC-IV).* San Antonio, TX: Harcourt Assessment.

Wilson-Costello, D., Friedman, H., Minich, N., et al. (2005). Improved survival rates with increased neurodevelopmental disability for extremely low birth weight infants in the 1990s. *Pediatrics, 115,* 997–1003.

Wodrich, D.L. (1997). *Children's psychological testing: A guide for nonpsychologists* (3rd ed.). Baltimore: Paul H. Brookes Publishing Co.

Wolff, G., Back, E., Arleth, S., et al. (1989). Genetic counseling in families with inherited balanced translocations: Experience with 36 families. *Clinical Genetics, 35*(6), 404–416.

Xu, J., & Chen, Z. (2003). Advances in molecular cytogenetics for the evaluation of mental retardation. *American Journal of Medical Genetics Part C: Seminars in Medical Genetics, 117*(1), 15–24.

Yeargin-Allsopp, M., Drews, C.D., Decoufle, P., et al. (1995). Mild mental retardation in black and white children in metropolitan Atlanta: A case-control study. *American Journal of Public Health, 85,* 324–328.

18 Down Syndrome

Nancy J. Roizen

Upon completion of this chapter, the reader will

- Recognize the physical characteristics of Down syndrome
- Understand the medical complications of this disorder
- Know the typical cognitive, developmental, and behavioral characteristics of a child with Down syndrome
- Learn about educational and other interventions

Down syndrome was one of the first symptom complexes associated with intellectual disability to be identified as a syndrome. In fact, evidence of the syndrome dates back to ancient times. Archaeological excavations have revealed a skull from the 7th century A.D. that displays the physical features of an individual with Down syndrome. Portrait paintings from the 1500s depict children with a Down syndrome–like facial appearance. In 1866, Dr. John Langdon Down, for whom the syndrome is named, published the first complete physical description of Down syndrome, including the similarity of facial features among affected individuals. In 1959, researchers identified the underlying chromosomal abnormality (an additional chromosome 21) that causes Down syndrome (Lejeune, Gautier, & Turpin, 1959).

JASON AND ANN

In most ways, Jason is like all of the other 8-year-olds in the neighborhood. He plays soccer, skates, swims, is a Boy Scout, and is in the second grade. Jason has a great sense of humor and is a bit mischievous. His mother makes every effort to provide him with a balance of social and academic opportunities. But Jason has had experiences that most of the other children have not. He has a unilateral hearing loss and attention-deficit/hyperactivity disorder (ADHD), which has improved since he started taking methylphenidate (Concerta). In his school, Jason was the first child with Down syndrome to be included in the general education kindergarten. His reading skills are at a preprimer level. At the local Down syndrome family support group, Jason's mother is inspired by Ann, who also has Down syndrome and has done exceptionally well. Ann has recently graduated from high school, drives a car, and has a job doing office work.

CHROMOSOMAL FINDINGS

Three types of chromosomal abnormalities can lead to Down syndrome: trisomy 21 (which accounts for about 95% of individuals with the disorder), translocation (4%), and mosaicism (1%). Trisomy 21 results from nondisjunction, most commonly during meiosis I of the egg (see Figure 1.3 in Chapter 1). Translocation Down syndrome involves the attachment of the long arm of an extra chromosome 21 to chromosome 14, 21, or 22 (see Figure 1.5). Mosaic trisomy implies that some, but not all cells, have the defect. This results from nondisjunction during mitosis of the fertilized egg.

Studies indicate that children with translocation Down syndrome do not differ cognitively or medically from those with trisomy 21. Children with mosaic Down syndrome, perhaps because their trisomic cells are interspersed with normal cells, typically score higher on IQ tests than those with trisomy 21 or translocation Down syndrome (Fishler & Koch, 1991). Medical complications tend to be similar among the three groups, however (McClain et al., 1996).

PREVALENCE

The prevalence of Down syndrome births is presently 13.7 per 10,000 or 1/732. In definitions of prevalence, maternal age has been consistently linked to Down syndrome. At 20 years of age, women have about a 1 in 2,000 chance of having a child with trisomy 21; at 45 years of age, the likelihood increases to 1 in 20 (Figure 7.1; Trimble & Baird, 1978). There is no increased risk of translocation Down syndrome with increased maternal age, but one third of individuals with translocation Down syndrome inherit the translocation from a parent who is a carrier (Jones, 2006). Chromosome analysis can identify parents who are at risk of producing other children with translocation Down syndrome. Although trisomic Down syndrome occurs in more males (59%) than females (41%), translocation Down syndrome more often occurs in females (74%; Staples et al., 1991). The reason for these phenomena is unclear.

CAUSE

The sequencing of chromosome 21 (Hattori et al., 2000) revealed that it has many more genes than predicted, greater than 400 identified as of 2005 (University of Colorado at Denver and Health Sciences Center & Eleanor Roosevelt Institute at the University of Denver, n.d.). There are sets of genes involved in specific metabolic pathways or biological systems (Roizen & Patterson, 2003); for example, there are at least 10 genes that exert influence on the structure and function of the central nervous system. The overexpression of one of these genes (amyloid precursor protein, or APP) might account for the early age of onset of Alzheimer's disease in individuals with Down syndrome (Capone, 2004). The cause of the clinical findings in Down syndrome, however, appears to be more complicated. Nonspecific small effects of many genes on chromosome 21 may more fully explain the clinical findings (Olson et al., 2004).

Although the underlying mechanism remains unclear, much has been learned about the embryology and neuropathology of Down syndrome. It is likely that the trisomy causes malformations as a result of incomplete rather than deviant development of the embryo. For example, although the heart may be normally formed, the wall separating the two sides of the heart may not close completely creating an endothelial cushion defect, an **atrial septic defect,** or a **ventricular septal defect.** Similarly,

the separation of the **trachea** and esophagus may be incomplete, resulting in a **tracheoesophageal fistula** (an area of connection between the two). Examination of the brain tissue of individuals with Down syndrome reveals multiple developmental abnormalities, including delayed myelination, fewer neurons, decreased synaptic density, and decreased acetylcholine neurotransmitter receptors (Zigman, Silverman, & Wisniewski, 1996).

EARLY IDENTIFICATION

Routinely, women 35 years of age and older are offered prenatal diagnostic testing for Down syndrome with amniocentesis. In women of any age, a variety of prenatal screening options are available in the first and second trimesters that utilize a blood screening test and sometimes a fetal ultrasound (see Chapter 7; Malone et al., 2005). Identification of Down syndrome prior to birth enables the physician to provide genetic counseling to the family and, if the pregnancy is continued, cardiac planning, parental accommodation, and appropriate medical evaluation of the newborn infant.

Because of the distinctive pattern of physical features, infants with Down syndrome can be identified fairly easily at birth. An index developed by Rex and Preus (1982) based on eight physical features predicts Down syndrome with an accuracy rate of 75%. These characteristics include three palm print (dermatoglyphic) patterns, Brushfield spots (colored speckles in the iris of the eye), ear length, internipple distance, neck skinfold, and widely spaced first toes. Individuals with XXXY, XXXXY, and XXXX syndromes (see Chapter 1), however, bear a physical resemblance to individuals with Down syndrome in the newborn period (Jones, 2006). Therefore, all children suspected of having Down syndrome should have a chromosomal analysis performed to ensure correct diagnosis and to provide accurate genetic counseling about future pregnancies.

MEDICAL COMPLICATIONS IN DOWN SYNDROME

Children with Down syndrome have an increased risk of abnormalities in almost every organ system (Roizen & Patterson, 2003; van Trotsenburg et al., 2006). Knowledge of the possible complications enables the caregiver to evaluate the child for the more common disorders, and to monitor, prevent and be vigilant for other medical problems (Table 18.1).

Congenital Heart Defects

In a population based study of infants with Down syndrome, 44% had congenital heart defects, the most common being **endocardial cushion defect** (resulting in a connection between the **atria,** or upper chambers, and **ventricles,** or lower chambers), **ventricular septal defect** (a connection between the two lower chambers), and **atrial septal defect** (a connec-

Table 18.1. Medical complications in Down syndrome

Disorder	% affected
Congenital heart defect	44
Endocardial cushion defect	20
Ventricular septal defect	15
Atrial septal defect	4
Other	5
Ophthalmic disorders (often more than one)	60
Refractive errors	35
Strabismus	27
Nystagmus	20
Blepharitis	9
Tear duct obstruction	6
Cataracts	5
Ptosis	5
Hearing loss	66
Endocrine abnormalities	50–90
Subclinical hypothyroidism	25–40
Overt hypothyroidism	4–30
Diabetes	0.5–1
Growth problems	50–90
Obesity	60
Short stature	50–90
Orthopedic abnormalities	16
Subclinical atlantoaxial subluxation	15
Symptomatic atlantoaxial subluxation	1
Dental problems, periodontal disease, and malocclusion	60–100
Gastrointestinal malformations	5
Celiac disease	1–7
Epilepsy	6
Leukemia	0.6–1
Skin conditions	50
Alzheimer's disease after 40 years	21

Sources: American Academy of Pediatrics, Committee on Genetics (2001); Cohen, for the Down Syndrome Medical Interest Group (1999).

tion between the two upper chambers; (Freeman et al., 1998). A major complication of congenital heart disease is pulmonary vascular obstructive disease. This leads to increased back pressure in the arteries that connect the heart to the lungs and results in congestive heart failure. Progression of this potentially fatal complication is more rapid in children with Down syndrome than in children with the same heart defects and normal chromosomes (Suzuki et al., 2000).

Sensory Impairments

Vision and hearing problems occur with increased frequency in children with Down syndrome. A survey of 77 randomly selected children with Down syndrome found that more than 60% had ophthalmic disorders requiring treatment or monitoring. The most common of these disorders were refractive errors, strabismus (crossed eyes), nystagmus (jiggling of the eyes), blepharitis (inflammation of the eyelids), tear duct obstruction, cataracts, and **ptosis** (droopy eyelids) (Roizen, Mets, & Blondis, 1994). In children with no ophthalmic abnormalities observed during general pediatric checkups, 35% actually had an identifiable disorder when examined by an ophthalmologist. Thus, in the first few weeks of life, and subsequently at periodic intervals, all children with Down syndrome should receive an ophthalmological examination.

Hearing loss occurs in approximately two thirds of children with Down syndrome. It can be conductive (bone conduction of sound), sensorineural (involving the cochlea or auditory nerve), or combined, and it can be unilateral or bilateral (see Chapter 12; Shott, 2000). Conductive hearing problems result from narrow throat structures and immune variation (Roizen & Patterson, 2003) that predispose these children to recurrent ear infections. Chapman et al. (1998) estimated that 10% of the language impairment in children with Down syndrome is accounted for by the hearing impairments. These children also may develop **sleep apnea** (brief periods of arrested breathing during sleep) as a consequence of upper airway obstruction from enlarged tonsils and adenoids (Shott, 2000; Donnelly et al., 2004).

Endocrine Abnormalities

Congenital hypothyroidism due to poor development of the thyroid gland is found in 0.8%–

1.8% of newborns with Down syndrome, a rate about 28–54 times that seen in the general population (Fort et al., 1984; Tuysuz & Beker, 2001). In addition, 25%–40% of children with Down syndrome beyond the neonatal period manifest an elevated level of thyroid stimulating hormone (TSH) in the presence of normal thyroid hormone. Only 7% of these children ultimately developed overt hypothyroidism (Rubello et al., 1995). So most individuals with Down syndrome do not require thyroxine (thyroid hormone) replacement therapy.

Children with Down syndrome are at great risk for becoming overweight. A major factor in the development of obesity is the presence of a lower resting metabolic rate; children with Down syndrome require fewer calories to gain weight (Bauer et al., 2003). In general, newborns with Down syndrome have proportional weight for height, but in the first year of life they become light for their height. During the next few years, however, the children gain relatively more weight than height, and by early childhood, half are overweight, with some developing metabolic syndrome, a precursor for diabetes.

Diabetes occurs in 1% of children with Down syndrome compared to 4 per 10,000 in the general population (Anwar, Walker, & Frier, 1998).

In addition to being overweight, individuals with Down syndrome have short stature. The average adult height is 5 feet in males and 4½ feet in females with the syndrome (Toledo et al., 1999).

Orthopedic Problems

Children with Down syndrome have an increased prevalence of orthopedic problems that are probably related to abnormally loose ligaments. These include atlantoaxial subluxation, or partial dislocation of the upper spine (Figure 18.1); patellar (knee cap) instability; and flat feet. These children also can develop juvenile rheumatoid arthritis.

Atlantoaxial subluxation is the most controversial and perplexing of these problems, occurring in approximately 15% of children with Down syndrome (American Academy of Pediatrics [AAP], Committee on Sports Medicine and Fitness, 1995). This involves the partial dis-

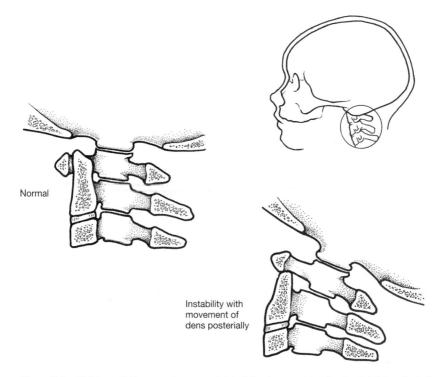

Normal

Instability with
movement of
dens posteriorly

Figure 18.1.   Children with Down syndrome are at risk of developing subluxation (partial dislocation) of the atlantoaxial or atlanto-occipital joint, as shown in this illustration (right side). A typical neck region is shown for comparison (left side). This subluxation predisposes these children to spinal injury with trauma. This abnormality can be detected by X ray or magnetic resonance imaging scan of the neck.

placement of the upper vertebra, potentially leading to spinal nerve entrapment. Only 1% of children with Down syndrome become symptomatic, however, and the subluxation rarely leads to paralysis. Symptoms of subluxation include easy fatigability, difficulties in walking, abnormal gait, neck pain, limited neck mobility, **torticollis** (painful head tilt), a change in hand function, the new onset of urinary retention or incontinence, incoordination and clumsiness, sensory impairments, and spasticity (AAP Committee on Sports Medicine and Fitness, 1995).

Dental Problems

The most serious dental problem is early-onset **periodontal disease** that can rapidly progress (Hennequin et al., 1999). This involves both gingivitis (gum inflammation) and regression of the jaw bone that anchors the teeth (see Chapter 32). The periodontal disease is a manifestation of the immune variations in children with Down syndrome. In addition to having periodontal disease, almost all children with Down syndrome have **malocclusions** (abnormal contact of opposing teeth), and many have dental anomalies (e.g., fused teeth, microdontia [small teeth], missing teeth). **Primary** and permanent teeth erupt later than usual. Interestingly, dental caries occurs less often in children with Down syndrome than in the general population; the reason for this is unclear but is probably related to differences in immunity and tooth shape.

Gastrointestinal Problems

Gastrointestinal malformations are found in approximately 5% of children with Down syndrome. Most of these abnormalities present with symptoms in the newborn period such as poor feeding, vomiting, or aspiration pneumonia. The malformations include stenosis (narrowing) or atresia (blockage) of the duodenum, the first section of the small intestine (3%), **imperforate** (closed) anus (0.9%), Hirschsprung disease (congenitally enlarged colon; 0.5%), tracheoesophageal fistula (an abnormal connection between the trachea and esophagus) or **esophageal atresia** (0.4%), and pyloric stenosis (narrowing of the stomach outlet; 0.3%) (Roizen & Patterson, 2003). Gastroesophageal reflux is known to be common in children with Down syndrome. Celiac disease (sensitivity to wheat and other grains) has been found in 1%–7% of children with Down syndrome (Celiac Guidelines Committee, 2005).

Epilepsy

Epilepsy occurs in 6% of individuals with Down syndrome (Johannsen et al., 1996). This is more common than in the general population but about average for children with moderate intellectual disability. Seizure types include generalized tonic-clonic (55% of all seizures in children with Down syndrome), infantile spasms (13%), myoclonic (6%), atonic plus tonic-clonic (6%), and simple partial (6%) (see Chapter 29). Seizures occur most commonly in individuals younger than 3 years and older than 13 years of age. Sixty-two percent of the seizures have an identifiable cause, the most common being infections and hypoxia resulting from congenital heart disease. Children with Down syndrome who have infantile spasms have a better outcome than children with infantile spasms who do not have Down syndrome.

Hematologic Disorders

Although there is little information about the specific mechanisms of the abnormalities, almost every cellular element of the **hematopoietic** (blood) system has been found to be at risk for an abnormality in Down syndrome. For example, erythrocytosis (too many red blood cells) and elevated numbers of white blood cells (transient leukemia) can be found in the newborn. Therefore, a complete blood count is indicated at birth for infants with Down syndrome. Platelets may be either increased or decreased (Pueschel & Pueschel, 1992). Few of these abnormalities lead to serious problems, but 10%–20% of the children with transient leukemia in the newborn period later develop acute myelogenous leukemia (Ahmed et al., 2004). This is thought to be due to a mutation in the gene that encodes for GATA-1 that is required for development of young platelets (Ahmed et al., 2004). One in 150 children with Down syndrome will develop either acute myelogenous leukemia or acute lymphoblastic leukemia during their lifetime (Lange, 2000).

Skin Conditions

Several skin conditions, mostly of immune origin, are observed more frequently in individuals with Down syndrome than in the general population. Some of these conditions noticeably affect the appearance, and therefore the quality of life, of the child and thus require treatment. By puberty, half or more of these individuals will experience atopic dermatitis (**eczema**), **cheilitis** (inflammation of the lips), ichthyosis (dry and scaly skin), **onychomycosis** (fungal infection of the nails), **seborrheic dermatitis** (dandruff), **vitiligo** (patches of depigmentation), and/or **xerosis** (dryness of eyes) (Ercis, Balci, & Atakan, 1996). Less common skin diseases are syringomas (sweat gland cysts) and **alopecia** (hair loss).

NEURODEVELOPMENT AND BEHAVIOR

Infants with Down syndrome typically have central hypotonia (floppiness without weakness) and associated delayed gross motor development. Most children with Down syndrome do not sit up until 11 months of age or walk until 19 months (Winders, 1997). Developmental milestones in boys with Down syndrome are generally reached slightly later than in girls with the disorder. Although continued progress in the gross motor area is slow, significant physical disabilities are rare. Children with Down syndrome learn to run, ride bicycles, and participate in sports (see Chapter 38).

In the first 2 years of life, children with Down syndrome, primarily because of their social responsiveness, appear to have less cognitive impairment than is apparent later in childhood (Brown et al., 1990). By 2 years of age significant language delays become evident; children with Down syndrome often do not speak their first word until 18 months of age (Kumin, 2001). Their receptive language is generally better than their expressive language. Even after children with Down syndrome speak in sentences, problems with intelligibility interfere with effective communication. Therefore, speech therapy that addresses the development of expressive speech and intelligibility is needed for many years (Chapman et al., 1991; Chapman et al., 1998; Kumin, 2001; Miller, Leddy, & Leavitt, 1999). Formal psychological testing at school age shows that 85% of children with Down syndrome have IQ scores that range from 40 to 60, which label them as having mild to moderate intellectual disability. Although these children generally have poor verbal short-term memory skills, their visual-motor skills are relatively strong (Wang, 1996). This cognitive pattern is consistent with functional neuroimaging studies that reveal impairments within and between the frontal and parietal lobes of the brain, including the inferior frontal gyrus, that contains Broca's speech area.

Children with Down syndrome are stereotyped as being amiable and happy. Tempera-

ment studies, however, have shown them to have profiles comparable to typically developing children (Chapman & Hesketh, 2000). In a survey of 261 children with Down syndrome 29% were found to have behavior and psychiatric disorders with the following percentages of specific problems: aggressive behavior (7%), ADHD (6%), oppositional disorder (5%), stereotypic behavior (3%), elimination difficulties (2%), phobias (2%), autism spectrum disorders, or ASDs (1%); eating disorders (1%); self-injurious behavior (1%); and Tourette syndrome (0.4%) (Myers & Pueschel, 1991). A second study found an even higher frequency of ASDs (7%) in children with Down syndrome (Kent et al., 1999), and other studies have reported a delay in the diagnosis of ASDs among children who have Down syndrome when compared with children who have ASDs but not Down syndrome (Rasmussen et al., 2001).

Some individuals with Down syndrome may experience a deterioration of cognitive or psychological functioning in adolescence, often manifested as worsening of behavior or academic performance. Many times, this deterioration can be attributed to unrecognized hypothyroidism or depression. If such diagnoses are confirmed, medical and psychiatric treatment can reverse these problems. It appears, however, that virtually all individuals with Down syndrome older than 50 have pathological plaques and tangles in their brain, which are the hallmarks of Alzheimer's disease. Yet, even in adults with Down syndrome who have a decline in function, a mental health disorder such as anxiety, depression, or **obsessive-compulsive disorder** accounts for more than half (55%) of the cases; about one fifth (21%) have Alzheimer's disease (Pearlson et al., 1998).

EVALUATION AND TREATMENT

Several of the comorbid medical conditions occur with sufficient frequency that an organized approach to medical management is indicated. Some conditions require routine monitoring: congenital heart disease, hearing loss, vision deficits, thyroid disorders, and celiac disease. Gum disease and obesity are to be prevented. And, vigilance must be maintained for disorders that occur more frequently in children with Down syndrome than in the general population, such as diabetes and leukemia. The AAP (2001) and the Down Syndrome Medical Interest Group (Cohen, 1999) have developed guidelines for medical management of individ-

	Infancy						Early childhood					Late childhood					Adolescence			
Age	1	2	4	6	9	12	15	18	24	3	4	5	6	8	10	12	14	16	18	21
	(in months)									(in years)										
Procedures																				
Karyotype	•																			
Thyroid screen	•		•		•			•	•	•		•	•	•	•	•	•	•	•	•
Complete blood count	•[1]																			
Echocardiogram	•[2]																			
Neck X rays										•[3]										
Celiac panel								•												
Sensory																				
Vision	O[4]	S	S	S	S	S	S	S	O	O	O	O	O	O	O	O	O	O	O	O
Hearing	O[5]	S	S	O	S	S	O	S	O	O	O	O	O	O	O	O	O	O	O	O
Consultation																				
Cardiology	•																			
Ophthalmology			•		•			•		•		•		•	•	•	•	•	•	•
Ear, nose, and throat			•[6]					•		•		•		•	•	•	•	•	•	•
Genetic	•																			
Dental								•	•	•		•	•	•	•	•	•	•	•	•
Referrals																				
Early intervention	•———————————————→																			

• = to be performed   S = subjective, by history   O = objective, by a standard testing method

[1]Special attention to increased red and white blood cells

[2]Even in absence of murmur

[3]Earlier, if having surgery

[4]Must see red reflex to rule out cataracts

[5]Neonatal screening, auditory brainstem response (ABR)

[6]Depending on view of tympanic membrane

Figure 18.2. Recommendations for preventive health care for children and adolescents with Down syndrome. (*Sources:* American Academy of Pediatrics, Committee on Genetics, 2001; Cohen for the Down Syndrome Medical Interest Group, 1999.)

uals with Down syndrome (Figure 18.2). Several others have focused on children in specific age groups including infants and young children (Saenz, 1999), adolescents (Roizen, 2002), and adults (Smith, 2001).

Congenital heart disease in children with Down syndrome may be difficult to identify based on physical findings alone, as it is not always accompanied by a cardiac murmur, nor does it commonly produce a "blue baby." Yet, because children with Down syndrome tend to develop pulmonary vascular disease sooner than other children with the same defect do, early identification and treatment are essential. Although children with Down syndrome were

once considered poor risks for cardiac surgery, data now indicate that they have a similar outcome as other children with the same heart defect (Malec et al., 1999). The one exception is complete atrioventricular septal defect, which has a higher overall surgical mortality in children with Down syndrome. A cardiac evaluation, including an echocardiogram, is the standard of care for the newborn with Down syndrome.

Within the first 6 months of life, all children with Down syndrome need an ophthalmologic evaluation to identify cataracts and strabismus (see Chapter 11). Subsequently, these children should be evaluated annually or semiannually to detect refractive errors and other ophthalmic disorders (e.g., cataracts) that may develop after the first decade of life (Roizen et al., 1994).

Infants with Down syndrome who fail their newborn hearing screen will need a hearing evaluation by 3 months of age. If they have a hearing loss, by 6 months of age, they will need hearing aids and additional early intervention services that address the hearing loss. Not all losses are present at birth, and children with Down syndrome are at increased risk for recurrent middle-ear infections leading to conductive hearing losses and possibly even sensorineural hearing losses (Shott, 2000). Therefore, the child with Down syndrome should have an ear cleaning, a check for middle ear fluid, and a hearing evaluation every 6 months from birth to 3 years of age and then annually (Cohen, 1999; Shott, Joseph, & Heithaus, 2001).

If there is the suspicion of sleep apnea (marked by snoring and sleep disturbance), a **polysomnogram** (sleep study) should be performed (Shott, 2000). If the diagnosis is confirmed and found to be associated with enlarged adenoids, antibiotic treatment is used and the adenoids are subsequently removed surgically. If the adenoidectomy does not correct the mechanical obstruction, sleeping with continuous positive airway pressure (CPAP) or, in infrequent cases, a **tracheostomy** may be necessary to keep the airway open (Shott, 2000).

As with all newborns, children with Down syndrome are routinely screened for congenital hypothyroidism (see Chapter 8). In addition, they should have thyroid function tests performed at 4–6 months of age, at 1 year, and then annually (AAP Committee on Genetics, 2001). More frequent thyroid function tests are indicated if the child displays accelerated weight gain, behavior problems, plateauing of height, or an unexpected lack of cognitive progress. If there is clinical and laboratory evidence of hypothyroidism, treatment with thyroxine is indicated. It is now recommended that children with Down syndrome also be screened for celiac disease at 30 months using a IgG tissue transglutaminase (Celiac Guidelines Committee, 2005). Growth should be monitored using growth charts for typical children and those for children with Down syndrome (Cronk et al., 1988).

Because of the high prevalence of periodontal disease, daily cleaning of teeth should begin as soon as they erupt. As with all children, regular dental visits should also begin at this time. Orthodontic intervention is needed by

most children with Down syndrome and becomes possible when the child is able to cooperate with and tolerate the therapy.

The evaluation of children for atlantoaxial subluxation by X-ray studies is customarily done on entrance to preschool and sometimes prior to elective surgery. If the child participates in Special Olympics activities (see Chapter 38), an additional radiograph is usually obtained at that time to make sure that subluxation has not developed, which would place the child at increased risk for sports injuries. Signs and symptoms of spinal cord compression, such as the onset of weakness in gait, torticollis, neck pain, or bowel and bladder incontinence indicate the need for further testing (AAP Committee on Sports Medicine and Fitness, 1995). Children with radiologic findings indicating neck instability of an unacceptable degree and children with symptomatic subluxation are treated surgically with a neck fusion.

Several other medical problems, such as diabetes and leukemia, occur more frequently in children with Down syndrome than in the general population. Although screening for these disorders is not routinely done, it is appropriate to lower the threshold for evaluation for individuals with Down syndrome. The clinician also should be alert to symptoms of psychiatric illness (e.g., depression) and refer the individual for appropriate evaluation and treatment when indicated (see Chapter 21).

INTERVENTION

The parents of a newborn with Down syndrome should be provided with a balanced view of the condition (Skotko, 2005). They should be given up-to-date print materials on infants with Down syndrome, the telephone number of the point-of-entry to the early intervention system, local and national parent support/advocacy programs such as the National Down Syndrome Society and the National Down Syndrome Congress (see Appendix D), respite care options, and Supplemental Security Income (SSI) (see Chapter 42). Children with Down syndrome have a long history of involvement in early intervention programs. Studies of early intervention in Down syndrome indicate improved development especially in fine motor, social, and self-help skills (Guralnick, 1997).

The educational program of the child with Down syndrome needs to provide the optimal environment for learning. Thus, a balance of inclusion and learning environments with typical children and therapeutic interventions need to be planned for each child (Chapter 34). The plan needs to consider the child's opportunities for socialization in the home and community and his or her developmental and educational strengths and needs. Most frequently, children with Down syndrome have strengths in visual motor skills and weakness in verbal short-term memory (Wang, 1996) A visual approach that uses aids such as written instructions, visual organizers, and schedules employs this strength. Such plans need to be reviewed and altered at regular intervals.

In their role as advocates for their child with Down syndrome, most parents consider using alternative and complementary therapies for improvement of cognitive function and appearance (Prussing et al., 2005). Eighty-seven percent of parents do at some time treat their child with an alternative therapy, most commonly combination nutritional therapy (e.g., Nutri-vene) (Prussing et al., 2004). Although there are many studies of alternative therapies in individuals with Down syndrome, few meet even the minimal methodology criteria of scientific studies (Roizen, 2005). Alternative therapies include mixtures and individual vitamins (e.g., vitamins A, C, and E), minerals (e.g., selenium, zinc), and hormones (e.g., growth, thyroid); cell therapy or injections of fetal lamb brains; facial plastic surgery; and drugs (e.g. piracetam). None of these has been shown to be effective (Roizen, 2005). Some studies in adults with Down syndrome treated with donepezil (a drug that increases the level of acetylcholine, which is thought to be decreased in Alzheimer's disease) show improvement in language and dementia scores (Prasher, 2004; Roizen, 2005).

OUTCOME

Since the 1970s, the prognosis for a productive and positive life experience for individuals with Down syndrome has increased substantially, largely due to the efforts of parent advocacy groups. Children with Down syndrome were among the first children with disabilities to be "mainstreamed" in public schools, and they have been the pioneers in the trend toward inclusion. In a 25-year follow-up study, however, parents reported that access to inclusive educational placements and services lessened as their children neared and attained adulthood at age 21. The most difficult challenges included medical complications, teasing or ostracism, disappointments in their child's ability to achieve certain adult milestones (e.g., obtaining a driver's license), and a lack of adequate services and supports in adulthood (Hanson, 2003).

Life expectancy for individuals with Down syndrome has improved greatly since the 1980s (Friedman, 2001; Yang, Rasmussen, & Friedman, 2002). Between 1983 and 1997, the median life span increased from 25 to 49 years, with congenital heart defects, dementia, hypothyroidism, and leukemia being the causes of death that were out of proportion to the general population (Yang, Rasmussen, & Friedman, 2002). Life expectancy tables indicate that more than half of individuals with Down syndrome will survive into their fifties and that 13.5% will be alive at age 68 years (Baird, 1989).

With the introduction in the 1980s of supported employment (in which individuals with disabilities have a job coach), adults with Down syndrome often hold jobs with improved pay and benefits and better working conditions. To succeed in supported employment, a person needs a healthy sense of self-esteem that is nurtured from early childhood, the ability to complete tasks without assistance, a willingness to separate emotionally from his or her parents and family members, and access to personal recreational activities. All of these should be goals of educational programs for individuals with Down syndrome.

SUMMARY

Down syndrome is characterized by a recognizable pattern of physical features, an increased risk for specific medical problems, and intellectual disability requiring intermittent to limited support. As children with Down syndrome are usually identified at birth, the early intervention system frequently has them as their youngest enrollees. Although much remains to be learned and accomplished, the educational and medical systems are probably more knowledgeable and comfortable with the special needs of children with Down syndrome than with any other single diagnostic disability group.

The AAP Committee on Genetics (2001) and the Down Syndrome Medical Interest Group (Cohen, 1999) have proposed standards of medical care that include periodic monitoring for medical problems that occur frequently in children with Down syndrome. With optimal audiologic, cardiac, endocrinologic, ophthalmologic, and orthopedic functioning, children with Down syndrome have the opportunity for good health and developmental functioning.

REFERENCES

Ahmed, M., Sternberg, A., Hall, G., et al. (2004). Natural history of GATA1 mutations in Down syndrome. *Blood, 103,* 2480–2489.

American Academy of Pediatrics, Committee on Genetics. (2001). Health supervision for children with Down syndrome. *Pediatrics, 107,* 442–449.

American Academy of Pediatrics, Committee on Sports Medicine and Fitness. (1995). Atlantoaxial instability in Down syndrome: Subject review. *Pediatrics, 96,* 151–154.

Anwar, A.J., Walker, J.D., & Frier, B.M. (1998). Type I diabetes mellitus and Down's syndrome: Prevalence, management and diabetic complications. *Diabetes Medicine, 15,* 160–163.

Baird, P.A., & Sadovnick, A.D. (1989). Life tables for Down syndrome. *Human Genetics, 82,* 291–292.

Bauer, J., Teufel, U., Doege, C., et al. (2003). Energy expenditure in neonates with Down syndrome. *Journal of Pediatrics, 143,* 264–266.

Brown, F.R., Greer, M.K., Aylward, E.H., et al. (1990). Intellectual and adaptive functioning in individuals with Down syndrome in relation to age and environmental placement. *Pediatrics, 85,* 450–452.

Capone, G. (2004). Down syndrome genetic insights and thoughts on early intervention. *Infants and Young Children, 17,* 45–58.

Celiac Guidelines Committee of the North American Society for Pediatric Gastroenterology, Hepatology and Nutrition. (2005). Guideline for the diagnosis and treatment of celiac disease in children: Recommendations of the North American Society for Pediatric Gastroenterology, Hepatology and Nutrition. *Journal of Pediatric Gastroenterology and Nutrition, 40,* 1–19.

Chapman, R.E., Schwartz, S.E., & Kay-Raining Bird, E. (1991). Language skills of children and adolescents with Down syndrome, I: Comprehension. *Journal of Speech, Language, and Hearing Research, 34,* 1106–1120.

Chapman, R.E., Seung, H.-K., Schwartz, S.E., et al. (1998). Language skills of children and adolescents with Down syndrome, II: Production deficits. *Journal of Speech, Language, and Hearing Research, 41,* 861–873.

Chapman, R.S., & Hesketh, L.J. (2000). Behavioral phenotype of individuals with Down syndrome. *Mental Retardation and Developmental Disabilities Research Reviews, 6,* 84–95.

Cohen, W.I., for the Down Syndrome Medical Interest Group. (1999). Health care guidelines for individuals with Down syndrome: 1999 revision (Down syndrome preventive medical checklist). *Down Syndrome Quarterly, 4,* 1–15.

Connolly, J.A. (1978). Intelligence levels on Down's syndrome children. *American Journal of Mental Deficiency, 83,* 193–196.

Cronk, C., Crocker, A.C., Pueschel, S.M., et al. (1988). Growth charts for children with Down syndrome: 1 month to 18 years of age. *Pediatrics, 81,* 102–110.

Donnelly, L.F., Shott, S.R., LaRoze, C.R., et al. (2004). Causes of persistent obstructive sleep apnea despite previous tonsillectomy and adenoidectomy in children with Down syndrome as depicted on static and dynamic cine MRI. *American Journal of Radiology, 183,* 175–181.

Ercis, M., Balci, S., & Atakan, N. (1996). Dermatological manifestations of 71 Down syndrome children admitted to a clinical genetics unit. *Clinical Genetics, 50,* 317–320.

Fishler, K., & Koch, R. (1991). Mental development in Down syndrome mosaicism. *American Journal on Mental Retardation, 96,* 345–351.

Fort, P., Lifshitz, F., Bellisario, R., et al. (1984). Abnormalities of thyroid functioning in infants with Down syndrome. *Journal of Pediatrics, 104,* 545–549.

Freeman S.B., Taft L.F., Dooley K.J., et al. (1998). Population-based study of congenital heart defects in Down syndrome. *American Journal of Medical Genetics, 80,* 213–217.

Friedman, J.M. (2001). Racial disparities in median age at death of persons with Down syndrome: United States, 1968–1997. *Morbidity and Mortality Weekly Report, 50,* 463–465.

Guralnick, M.J. (Ed.). (1997). *The effectiveness of early intervention.* Baltimore: Paul H. Brookes Publishing Co.

Hanson, M. (2003). Twenty-five years after early intervention a follow-up of children with Down syndrome and their families. *Infants and Young Children, 16,* 354–365.

Hattori, M., Fujiyama, A., Taylor, T.D., et al. (2000). The DNA sequence of human chromosome 21. *Nature, 405,* 311–319.

Hennequin, M., Faulks, D., Veyrune, J.-L., et al. (1999). Significance of oral health in persons with Down syndrome: A literature review. *Developmental Medicine and Child Neurology, 41,* 275–283.

Johannsen, P., Christensen, J.E., Goldstein, H., et al. (1996). Epilepsy in Down syndrome: Prevalence in three age groups. *Seizure, 5,* 121–125.

Jones, K.L. (2006). *Smith's recognizable patterns of human malformation* (6th ed.). Philadelphia: Elsevier Saunders.

Kent, L., Evans, J., Paul, M., et al. (1999). Comorbidity of autistic spectrum disorders in children with Down syndrome. *Developmental Medicine and Child Neurology, 41,* 153–158.

Kumin, L. (2001). Speech intelligibility in individuals with Down syndrome: A framework for targeting specific factors for assessment and treatment. *Down Syndrome Quarterly, 6,* 1–8.

Lange, B. (2000). The management of neoplastic disorders of haematopoiesis in children with Down's syndrome. *British Journal of Haematology, 110,* 512–524.

Lejeune, J., Gautier, M., & Turpin, R. (1959). Etude des chromosomes somatiques de neuf enfants mongoliens. [Study of somatic chromosomes of new children with mongolism] *Compte Rendu d'Academy Science, 248,* 1721–1722.

Malec, E., Mroczek, T., Pajak, J., et al. (1999). Results of surgical treatment of congenital heart defects in children with Down's syndrome. *Pediatric Cardiology, 20,* 351–354.

Malone, F.D., Canick, J.A., Ball, R.H., et al. (2005). First-trimester or second-trimester screening, or both, for Down's syndrome. *The New England Journal of Medicine, 353,* 2001–2011.

McClain, A., Bodertha, J., Meyer, J., et al. (Eds.). (1996). *Mosaic Down syndrome.* Richmond: Richmond Medical College of Virginia/Virginia Commonwealth University.

Miller, J.F., Leddy, M., & Leavitt, L.A. (Eds.). (1999). *Improving the communication of people with Down syndrome.* Baltimore: Paul H. Brookes Publishing Co.

Myers, B.A., & Pueschel, S.M. (1991). Psychiatric disorders in persons with Down syndrome. *Journal of Nervous and Mental Diseases, 179,* 609–613.

Olson, L.E., Richtsmeier, J.T., Leszl, J., et al. (2004). A chromosome 21 critical region does not cause specific Down syndrome phenotypes. *Science, 306,* 687–690.

Pearlson, G.D., Breiter, S.N., Aylward, E.H., et al. (1998). MRI brain changes in subjects with Down syndrome with and without dementia. *Developmental Medicine and Child Neurology, 40,* 326–334.

Prasher, V.P. (2004). Review of donepezil, revastigmine, galantamine, and menantine for the treatment of dementia in Alzheimer's disease in adults with Down syndrome: Implications for the intellectual disability population. *International Journal of Geriatric Psychiatry, 19,* 509–515.

Prussing, E., Sobo, E.J., Walker, E., et al. (2004). Communication with pediatricians about complementary/alternative medicine: Perspectives from parents of children with Down syndrome. *Ambulatory Pediatrics, 4,* 488–494.

Prussing, E., Sobo, E.J., Walker, E., et al. (2005). Between "desperation" and disability rights: A narrative analysis of complementary/alternative medicine use by parents for children with Down syndrome. *Society of Scientific Medicine, 60,* 587–598.

Pueschel, S.M., & Pueschel, J.K. (Eds.). (1992). *Biomedical concerns in persons with Down syndrome.* Baltimore: Paul H. Brookes Publishing Co.

Rasmussen, P., Borjesson, O., Wentz, E., et al. (2001). Autistic disorders in Down syndrome: Background factors and clinical correlates. *Developmental Medicine and Child Neurology, 43,* 750–754.

Rex, A.P., & Preus, M. (1982). A diagnostic index for Down syndrome. *The Journal of Pediatrics, 100,* 903–906.

Roizen, N.J. (2002). Medical care and monitoring for the adolescent with Down syndrome. *Adolescent Medicine: State of the Art Reviews, 13,* 345–357.

Roizen, N.J. (2005). Complimentary and alternative medicine in Down syndrome. *Mental Retardation and Developmental Disabilities Research Reviews, 11,* 149–155.

Roizen, N.J., Mets, M.B., & Blondis, T.A. (1994). Ophthalmic disorders in children with Down syndrome. *Developmental Medicine and Child Neurology, 36,* 594–600.

Roizen, N.J., & Patterson, D. (2003). Down's Syndrome. *The Lancet, 361,* 1281–1289.

Rubello, D., Pozzan, G.B., Casara, D., et al. (1995). Natural course of subclinical hypothyroidism in Down's syndrome: Prospective study results and therapeutic considerations. *Journal of Endocrinologic Investigation, 17,* 35–40.

Saenz, R.B. (1999). Primary care of infants and young children with Down syndrome. *American Family Physician, 59,* 381–390, 392, 395–396.

Shott, S.R. (2000). Down syndrome: Common pediatric ear, nose and throat problems. *Down Syndrome Quarterly, 5,* 1–6.

Shott, S.R., Joseph, A., & Heithaus, D. (2001). Hearing loss in children with Down syndrome. *International Journal of Pediatric Otorhinolaryngology, 61,* 199–205.

Skotko, B. (2005). Mothers of children with Down syndrome reflect on their postnatal support. *Pediatrics, 115,* 64–77.

Smith, D.S. (2001). Health care management of adults with Down syndrome. *American Family Physician, 64,* 1031–1038.

Staples, A.J., Sutherland, G.R., Haan, E.A., et al. (1991). Epidemiology of Down syndrome in South Australia, 1960–89. *American Journal of Human Genetics, 49,* 1014–1024.

Suzuki, K., Yamaki, S., Mimori, S., et al. (2000). Pulmonary vascular disease in Down's syndrome with complete atrioventricular septal defect. *American Journal of Cardiology, 86,* 434–437.

Toledo, C., Alembik, Y., Aguirre Jaime, A., et al. (1999). Growth curves of children with Down syndrome. *Annals of Genetics, 42,* 81–90.

Trimble, B.K., & Baird, P.A. (1978). Maternal age and Down syndrome: Age-specific incidence rates by single-year intervals. *American Journal of Medical Genetics, 2,* 1–5.

Tuysuz, B., & Beker, D.B. (2001). Thyroid dysfunction in children with Down's syndrome. *Acta Paediatrics, 90,* 1389–1393.

University of Colorado at Denver and Health Sciences Center & Eleanor Roosevelt Institute at the University of Denver. (n.d.). *Chromosome 21 gene function and pathway database.* Retrieved December 8, 2006, from http://chr21db.cudenver.edu

Van Trotsenburg, A.S., Heymans, H.S., Tijssen, J.G., et al. (2006). Comorbidity, hospitalization, and medication use and their influence on mental and motor development of young infants with Down syndrome. *Pediatrics, 118,* 1633–1639.

Wang, P. (1996). A neuropsychological profile of Down syndrome: Cognitive skills and brain morphology. *Mental Retardation and Developmental Disabilities Research Reviews, 2,* 102–108.

Winders, P.C. (Ed.). (1997). *Gross motor skills in children with Down syndrome: A guide for parents and professional.* Bethesda, MD: Woodbine House.

Yang, Q., Rasmussen, S.A., & Friedman, J.M. (2002). Mortality associated with Down's syndrome in the USA from 1983 to 1997: A population-based study. *The Lancet, 359,* 1019–1025.

Zigman, W., Silverman, W., & Wisniewski, H.M. (1996). Aging and Alzheimer's disease in Down syndrome: Clinical and pathological changes. *Mental Retardation and Developmental Disabilities Research Reviews, 2,* 73–79.

19

X-Linked Syndromes Causing Intellectual Disability

Gretchen A. Meyer

Upon completion of this chapter the reader will

- Understand the clinical implications of a CGG triplicate repeat
- Recognize the family characteristics of a person with fragile X syndrome
- Know the clinical features of full mutation and permutation alleles in males and females
- Be aware of the association between autism spectrum disorders and fragile X syndrome
- Know the medical complications that are associated with fragile X syndrome

---

Fragile X syndrome (FXS) is the most common inherited genetic cause of intellectual disabilities worldwide. The causative genetic mutation in FXS was discovered in 1991 (Verkerk, Pieretti, & Sutcliffe, 1991). However, the fact that X-linked genes may be involved in the inheritance of intellectual disability was suspected over 70 years ago based on the fact that the prevalence of intellectual disability, among all ethnically diverse populations worldwide, was as much as two to three times higher in males than in females (Crawford, Acuna, & Sherman, 2001; Crawford et al., 2002; Leonard & Wen, 2002; Tzeng et al., 2005). As part of the research involving the human genome, the genetic sequencing of the entire X chromosome was recently completed (Ross, Grafham, & Coffey, 2005), confirming that an unusually large number of genes reside on the X chromosome that are critically important for brain development, nerve cell function, learning, and memory. In fact, up to 10% of all currently known genetic errors causing intellectual disability reside on the X chromosome, despite the fact that the X chromosome contains only 4% of the total genome (Inlow & Restifo, 2004). Collectively, X-linked disorders characterized primarily by intellectual disability are referred to as

X-linked mental retardation (XLMR) disorders. The most common of these disorders is FXS, causing 30–40% of all XLMR disorders (Stevenson & Schwartz, 2002). Other XLMR disorders include Rett syndrome, Coffin-Lowry syndrome, Aarskog syndrome, and Börjeson-Forsson-Lehmann syndrome (see Appendix B).

The prevalence of X-linked intellectual disability is estimated to be 2–6 per 1,000 births (Stevenson & Schwartz, 2002). As of October 2004, a total of 142 syndromic and 63 "nonspecific," or nonsyndromic, XLMR disorders had been identified (Chiurazzi et al., 2004). Research has shown that certain of these genes can cause a syndromic type of intellectual disability in one family member and intellectual disability alone in another. Therefore, the distinction between syndrome and nonsyndromic XLMR disorders is becoming less clear (Kleefstra & Hamel, 2005). Nonsyndromic XLMR syndromes tend to be named numerically, by the order in which the genetic defect was discovered.

The X-linked pattern of inheritance has been described in depth in Chapter 1. Males who inherit an X-chromosome containing a mutation generally exhibit more severe symptoms than females because they only possess one copy of the gene (the one with the genetic mutation). Females, in contrast, may inherit an X chromosome from one parent with a genetic mutation but usually have an X chromosome from the other parent without an identical mutation. Due to varying degrees of X chromosome inactivation, the severity of the female's symptoms can vary from none to very severe. Rarely, a female could inherit an X chromosome from each parent with identical mutations (homozygote). In this circumstance, the child would likely demonstrate severe symptoms.

The first reported cases of FXS were described by Martin and Bell (1943). They described 11 males and 2 females in two generations of a family who had a number of similar clinical symptoms. The affected men had severe intellectual disability, language impairments, and behavior problems, whereas the women had mild intellectual disability and a "highly nervous temperament." Over subsequent decades, researchers have learned that this disorder is a form of X-linked intellectual disability. Furthermore, scientists now know that individuals with FXS have an abnormality of the X chromosome that causes the bottom tip of the long arm to become threadlike. This is known as a "fragile" site. In 1991, the underlying gene defect, an abnormality in the fragile X mental retardation gene (named FMR1), associated with expansion of repetitive triplets of specific nucleotide bases (CGG), was discovered (Verkerk, Pieretti, & Sutcliffe, 1991).

TONY, CARLOS, JEAN, AND SYLVIA

Tony was 4 years old when his parents first learned that he had FXS. He had been referred to a specialist because of speech and language delay, marked hyperactivity, and self-stimulatory behavior (including repetitive hand flapping when excited or anxious, and spinning the wheels of his toy cars while holding them at eye level). Extensive testing revealed that he also had mild intellectual disability. A family history revealed that Tony's maternal uncle, 16-year-old Vincent, attends a school for teenagers with special needs and is reading at the first-grade level. Tony's mother, Sylvia, reports that she was excessively shy as a young girl, and although she is only 36 years old, she is already having symptoms of menopause. Tony's maternal grandfather (Sylvia's father), 59-year-old Carlos, is currently undergoing a neurological evaluation because of recent concerns for memory loss, trouble walking, and hand tremors. Tony has a 9-year-old

sister, Jean, who is in the fourth grade; although she is very shy, she is doing well at school.

A DNA test for FXS was done on all five members of this family; Sylvia was found to have 120 CGG repeats; Vincent, 1,500; Jean, 100; Tony, 1,000, and Carlos, 150. Tony was enrolled in a small, structured preschool program that focuses on language development and uses behavior management techniques. Tony recently began taking a stimulant medication, which has significantly decreased his hyperactivity. The behavioral strategies are helping to decrease his overfocus on the wheels of his toy cars. Jean is also coping better; in addition to receiving services at school, she is seeing a counselor who is helping her overcome her shyness and social anxiety. Sylvia's father, Carlos, was found to have white matter abnormalities on an MRI scan of his brain. He was diagnosed with fragile X-associated tremor/ataxia syndrome (FXTAS), is receiving therapy and medication, and was glad to finally have an answer for his neurological problems.

THE GENETICS OF FRAGILE X SYNDROME

The discovery of the genetic basis of FXS provided an understanding of some unique aspects of the FXS's inheritance pattern that had previously been difficult to explain using a simple, X-linked model. FXS is caused by an expanded section of DNA on the X chromosome at the distal end of the long arm (Xq27.3). The sequence of DNA that is repeated in excess consists of a series of three nucleotide bases, cytosine-guanine-guanine (CGG_n), also known as a triplet repeat. Most individuals have between 5 and 40 copies of this CGG triplet repeat. A repeat number in this range would, thus, be referred to as a normal allele (CGG_{5-40}). When the CGG triplet is repeated between 41 and 58 times, this is called an intermediate allele, or gray zone (CGG_{41-58}). Triplet repeats of between 59 and 200 are premutation alleles (CGG_{59-200}), and those greater than 200 are full mutations ($CGG_{>200}$) (Cronister et al., 2005; Nolin et al., 2003).

Genes contain the blueprint for the encoding of proteins necessary for the body to function. The protein product of the FMR1 gene has been dubbed the fragile X mental retardation protein (FMRP). The expansion of the CGG_n repeats to greater than 200 essentially acts like a switch and "turns off" production of

FMRP by causing methylation at the upstream promoter region of the gene and shutting down messenger RNA (mRNA) translation. The result is a severe decrease or absence of FMRP (Stevenson & Schwartz, 2002; Kenneson et al., 2001).

Normal alleles (CGG_{5-40}) are passed from parent to offspring in a stable fashion. Thus, while the repeat sequence may expand or contract slightly, the change in number is generally minimal. Premutation alleles (CGG_{59-200}), however, are unstable and tend to expand when transmitted. The greater the number of repeats in the maternal premutation allele, the greater is the chance that the child will inherit a full mutation allele ($CGG_{>200}$). Interestingly, if an FMR1 premutation is passed from an unaffected father to his daughter, the allele nearly always undergoes contraction rather than expansion. In this way, a daughter can never inherit a full mutation allele from her father, even if he possesses a full mutation himself. Fathers who pass this mutation on to their daughters are known as transmitting males.

Counseling should be offered to individuals with FXS and to their families by a knowledgeable genetics specialist (geneticist/genetic counselor) because of the extremely complex nature of this inherited disorder. In addition to counseling from the genetics specialist, the child's primary physician should take time to discuss the basics of this disorder with the parents in a supportive way. Many parents will experience guilt, particularly the parent through whom the genetic abnormality was transmitted. All professionals who interact with the family must be cognizant of this reaction and offer reassurance that no one is to blame for errors that exist within one's genes.

CLINICAL FEATURES IN MALES

Full Mutation

Males that possess a FMR1 full mutation allele ($CGG_{>200}$) are considered to be fully affected and have FXS. Common physical features shared by affected males include a long, narrow face; prominent jaw and forehead; large, protruding ears; a high, arched palate; and loose connective tissues (causing hyperextensible joints, flat feet, and mitral valve prolapse). After puberty, the majority of affected men have markedly enlarged testicles (**macroorchidism**). Some of these physical characteristics are subtle during childhood and become more pronounced with

age, making early identification difficult based on physical features alone. Boys with FXS tend to be hypotonic (have low muscle tone) and often lack coordination. It is not uncommon for them to be larger than their peers as young children and to have large heads (macrocephaly) (Hagerman, 2002; Terracciano, Chiurazzi, & Neri, 2004).

In addition to physical features, males with FXS manifest impairments in cognitive abilities, communication, and behavioral patterns that follow characteristic patterns of strengths and weaknesses. Developmental delays are evident in infancy, with nearly 100% of males with a full mutation scoring in the "delayed" range for both language and non-language skills when evaluated at 12 months of age with a standardized developmental screening tools. Thus, with a high index of suspicion and careful developmental screening, the diagnosis can be made in children as young as 12–18 months of age (Mirrett et al., 2004). Ultimately, more than 80% of males with FXS have IQ scores in the range of mild to moderate intellectual disability (Loesch et al, 2002).

A relative cognitive strength among males with FXS is the ability to process multiple parts of information as a whole (simultaneous processing). Other strengths demonstrated by boys with FXS include the ability to verbally label objects; a large single-word vocabulary; visual matching; memory for situations; memory for favorite songs, videos, and movies; and adaptive functioning. Finally, individuals with FXS often have a delightful sense of humor, which may help them tremendously in social interactions. Cognitive weaknesses include sequential tasks, visual-spatial skills, auditory memory, and higher level thinking and reasoning. In addition, children with FXS have impairments in executive functioning (planning, sustaining attention and effort, self-monitoring, making use of feedback, and generating problem-solving strategies) (Cornish, Sudhalter, & Turk, 2004; Loesch et al., 2002; The National Fragile X Foundation, 2004).

Speech and language delays are usually present from the preschool period (Kau, Meyer, & Kaufman, 2002). When speech does develop, it tends to be **echolalic** (parrot-like), cluttered (rushed and poorly articulated), and perseverative. The conversations of boys with FXS are frequently interrupted by tangential statements, poor topic maintenance, or perseveration on one idea. These pragmatic language difficulties tend to worsen with anxiety. Although both expressive and receptive language are significantly delayed in early childhood, receptive language appears to develop at a faster rate than expressive language, creating a notable discrepancy between the two language abilities (Cornish, Sudhalter, & Turk, 2004).

Over the years, it has become apparent that individuals with FXS demonstrate a unique behavioral style characterized by **stereotypies** (e.g., hand flapping), lack of eye contact or gaze avoidance, hyperactivity, inattention, aggression, and anxiety (Cornish, Sudhalter, & Turk, 2004; Hatton et al., 2002; Kau et al., 2004; Reiss & Dant, 2003). Sixty to ninety percent of males with FXS demonstrate aspects of this behavioral phenotype to some degree. Sensory integration difficulties are common, particularly tactile defensiveness. For example, children with FXS often become easily overwhelmed by sensory stimuli such as noises in large crowds, noise and odors in cafeterias, or even the light touch of a teacher's hand. When present, these sensory integration dysfunctions can have a marked impact on an individual's behavioral response to the environment and can be the root of tantrums, rage, or even aggression.

Premutation

Males who have FMR1 premutation alleles (CGG_{50-200}) were once thought to be completely unaffected and were referred to only as transmitting males. Research has now shown that males with premutations can manifest symptoms in one of two possible ways. Hagerman et al. (1996) described a subset of males who demonstrated typical intellectual functioning but had learning disabilities with specific weaknesses in visual-spatial processing, auditory memory, quantitative concepts, and executive functioning. There have been at least two separate reports of males with FMR1 premutation alleles who have also been found to have an autism spectrum disorder (ASD) (Aziz et al., 2003; Goodlin-Jones et al., 2004).

A second possible manifestation of a FXS premutation in men occurs in 40% of male premutation carriers over the age of 50 years. Since 2000, researchers have described a neurological syndrome involving intention tremor, ataxia, dementia, parkinsonism, and autonomic dysfunction. This condition, FXTAS, is the focus of much active research (Hagerman et al., 2004; Loesch et al., 2005). Neuroimaging of the brains of these men reveals white matter changes in the middle cerebellar peduncles. Upon post-

mortem examination, characteristic eosinophilic intranuclear inclusions have been found throughout the brain in both neurons and astrocytes (Jacquemont et al., 2003). In a recent study of newly diagnosed men with late-onset ataxia, 4% were found to have CGG repeat expansions in the premutation range (Brussino et al., 2005).

CLINICAL FEATURES IN FEMALES

Full Mutation

In general, women with the full FMR1 mutation ($CGG_{>200}$) may look typical or may have only a slightly altered physical appearance, with a narrow face and large ears (Riddle et al., 1998). The cognitive profile of women with the full mutation is also much more variable and less severe than that seen in males with FXS. In infancy, delays in development are evident by 12 month of age in 50%–75% of girls screened with a standardized developmental screening tool (Mirrett et al., 2004). Typically, about half of the women have normal intellectual functioning but may exhibit non–language-based learning disabilities. The other half has intellectual disability, usually in the mild range. The degree of variance among women is due to individual differences in the ratio of X chromosome inactivation.

The cognitive profile of strengths and weaknesses seen in females with FXS appears similar to that described in males, but females may demonstrate overall higher levels of functioning. Specific areas of strength, like those in boys, may include vocabulary, short-term visual memory, reading, and spelling. Weaknesses may include abstract thinking, visual-spatial and visual motor skills, quantitative processing and number concepts, pragmatic language, topic maintenance, auditory memory, and attention span. Speech and language development, language pragmatics, and the spectrum of behavioral difficulties also parallel those seen in males, although they may vary in degree or severity in any individual child (Cornish, Sudhalter, & Turk, 2004; Reiss & Dant, 2003; Rogers, Wehner, & Hagerman, 2001).

Premutation

Among females with a premutation of FMR1 (CGG_{50-200}), most do not manifest significant physical, cognitive, or behavioral abnormalities. A subgroup of female carriers does, however, demonstrate one or more phenotypic features similar to those described in males or females with a full mutation. When physical features are present, they are generally limited to an elongated face, prominent ears, and/or hyperflexible finger joints. Frequently, females with a premutation, despite being clinically unaffected in other areas, manifest significant levels of shyness and anxiety. They also have an increased reported incidence of depression and obsessive-compulsive behavior (Hagerman & Hagerman, 2004). Moreover, it has been shown that the likelihood of a female carrier exhibiting the described behavioral characteristics rises when the number of CGG repeats is greater than 100 (Johnston et al., 2001) and, thus, is inversely related to the amount of FRMP ultimately encoded by the FMR1 gene (Tassone et al., 2000a).

There are two other distinct ways in which women with a FMR1 premutation allele can be affected clinically. Up to 20% experience premature ovarian failure (prior to the age of 40) (Hagerman & Hagerman, 2004; Welt, Smith, & Taylor, 2004). When this occurs, there is early aging of the ovaries, a consequence of which is an increased rate of spontaneous twinning. Secondly, although FXTAS was initially thought to be a phenomenon seen only in older adult men with a premutation allele, it has recently also been described in females with premutations. The incidence is not yet known, but it is estimated that it is less than the 40% seen in men (Hagerman et al., 2004).

FRAGILE X SYNDROME AND AUTISM SPECTRUM DISORDERS

Many of the behaviors that are commonly seen in individuals with FXS, such as perseverative speech, tendency toward social anxiety, poor eye contact, motor stereotypies, and sensory integration dysfunctions, are reminiscent of similar behaviors seen in children with ASDs. An association between ASDs and FXS has been discussed and researched for over 20 years, since it was first postulated by Brown et al. in 1982. When using standard diagnostic assessment tools, it now appears that as many as 33% of children with an FMR1 full mutation meet *DSM-IV* diagnostic criteria for an ASD (Rogers et al., 2001). More recent reports have documented cohorts of both males and females with premutation alleles being diagnosed with ASDs at a higher rate than in the population without FMR1 mutations (Aziz et al., 2003; Goodlin-Jones et al., 2004). The consensus amongst those

who work with individuals with FXS and those who conduct research regarding FXS is that up to 25% of individuals with FXS may display enough behaviors and characteristics that overlap with ASDs to meet the criteria for a secondary diagnosis of an ASD (Demark, Feldman, & Holden, 2003; Kaufmann et al., 2004; Philofsky et al., 2004; & Sabaratnam et al., 2003). Because the behaviors are quite similar, it may be difficult to discern whether a particular child has an ASD or simple FXS-like behaviors (Bailey et al., 2001). In any one individual child, it is more important that the specific behavioral strengths and weaknesses be noted, described accurately, and addressed through treatment than it is for this distinction to be made. More generally, however, the link between ASDs and FXS is providing a crucial avenue through which researchers may ultimately learn about the neurological basis for the behaviors and developmental challenges of both FXS and ASDs.

DIAGNOSIS OF FRAGILE X SYNDROME

Until 1991, when the fragile X gene defect was identified, the diagnosis could only be confirmed when the well-known fragile site was detected on the long arm of the X chromosome (Xq27.3). A special culture medium deficient in folic acid was necessary in order to detect the fragile site. This technique was quite effective at identifying affected males, but it was expensive and could be done only in specialized laboratories. Furthermore, carrier women and transmitting males were not accurately identified in this way Despite these limitations, chromosome analysis can still be useful in identifying other chromosomal anomalies when a child is being evaluated for developmental delay and thus may be a useful adjunct to DNA testing in some individuals.

The current gold standard for diagnosing FXS is a DNA test for FMR1. There are two methods that labs utilize to examine the DNA for the FMR1 mutation. Southern blot analysis has the advantage of being able to detect mosaic patterns (where not all cells are affected) as well as carrier females. Its disadvantages are that it cannot detect the precise number of CGG copies present, and it is a much slower process. The polymerase chain reaction (PCR) method, however, can be completed much more rapidly than Southern blot analysis (24–48 hours versus 1–2 weeks) and can identify the precise number of CGG copies present. The use of one or both of these DNA tests allows detection of 99% of patients with a premutation or full mutation of FMR1 (Maddalena et al., 2001). In 1% or less of individuals with FXS, mechanisms other than CGG expansion, such as deletion or point mutation, are responsible for the syndrome (Hammond et al., 1997. In these cases, linkage studies and/or studies for rare mutations may be needed and are available on a research basis. Newborn screening for FXS is not currently available on a widespread basis. However, research is underway to study its feasibility, cost-effectiveness, and accuracy (Bailey, 2004).

FXS testing should be considered in the following conditions: 1) individuals of either sex with intellectual disability, developmental delay, or an ASD, particularly if they have a family history of FXS or any relatives with intellectual disability; 2) individuals with a family history of either FXS or undiagnosed intellectual disability who are seeking reproductive counseling; and 3) fetuses of mothers with a FMR1 premutation allele (American College of Medical Genetics, 1994).

Despite recent advances in laboratory techniques for the diagnosis of FXS, the fact remains that the physical features of FXS in affected infants and toddlers can be subtle and often may go unrecognized (Stoll, 2001). Longitudinal studies are now underway investigating the patterns of behavior and trajectories of development in affected youngsters. What families and experts alike have noted is that the temperament and behavior of the children may change significantly over time. Infants, for example, have been found to be more hyposensitive to sensory stimuli. By the preschool age, however, most are reported to be oversensitive and are described as having high activity, low adaptability and attention, and impulsivity (Kau, Meyer, & Kaufmann, 2002).

It is critical that pediatricians maintain a strong index of suspicion and that a careful family history be obtained at all times. Sadly, a recent study indicated that despite the fact that parents had already recognized a delay in the first child's development and brought it to the attention of their child's medical provider, half of the families had already had a second child before their first child was diagnosed with FXS. Forty-three percent of these second children were also affected with FXS (Bailey, Skinner, & Sparkman, 2003; Centers for Disease Control and Prevention, 2002). In addition, there have been many advances into strategies for intervention for youngsters affected with FXS. An earlier diagnosis can afford a child earlier access to needed therapeutic and educational services (Mirrett, Roberts, & Price, 2003).

MEDICAL MANAGEMENT

Children with FXS should receive all routine pediatric care, including immunizations (American Academy of Pediatrics, Committee on Genetics, 1996). In addition, periodic physical examinations should be done to identify the presence of medical complications related to FXS. These complications include ophthalmic disorders, orthopedic abnormalities, serous otitis media, mitral valve prolapse, seizure disorders, and macroorchidism.

Ophthalmic disorders in FXS include strabismus, myopia, ptosis, and nystagmus (Hagerman, 2002). The most common of these is strabismus; if present, refraction or patching may help prevent the development of amblyopia. Orthopedic abnormalities relate to the underlying connective tissue abnormality and include flat feet, scoliosis, and loose joints; orthotics may occasionally be useful, but surgery is rarely needed. Recurrent middle-ear infections are common in FXS and may require antibiotic prophylaxis or, if persistent, surgical aspiration and placement of pressure-equalization tubes. In cases of recurrent ear infections or serous otitis media, it is critical that the child's hearing status be monitored closely. Serous fluid in the middle ear can cause a fluctuating hearing loss that may further impair the child's language skills and attention span. If there is a heart murmur, an echocardiogram should be obtained; and if mitral valve prolapse is detected, antibiotic prophylaxis should be considered prior to surgical or dental procedures. Seizures occur in about 20% of affected individuals and are most commonly complex partial or generalized tonic-clonic types. If properly treated, the seizures need not dramatically alter the life of the child or family (Incorpora et al., 2002). Macroorchidism may become evident before adolescence in some boys with FXS; parents should be reassured that this does not require treatment, result in precocious puberty, or affect sexual functioning (Slegtenhorst-Eegdeman et al., 1998).

Medications prescribed to address specific behavioral and psychiatric characteristics have proven helpful and should be considered on an individual basis. Stimulants have been effective in treating hyperactivity and inattention. Serotonin reuptake inhibitors (SSRIs; e.g., fluoxetine [Prozac]) are being used successfully for obsessive-compulsive behaviors, anxiety, social inhibition; the atypical neuroleptics (e.g., risperidone [Risperdal]) have been used to treat aggression (Tsiouris & Brown, 2004).

EDUCATIONAL AND THERAPEUTIC INTERVENTION STRATEGIES

Educational and therapeutic interventions for individuals with FXS should be based on each person's unique profile of strengths and weaknesses, with strategies directed at the various cognitive, communicative, and behavior impairments that person exhibits. Most often, a child with FXS will be eligible for specialized educational and therapeutic services. Children younger than 3 years old may qualify for state-funded early intervention services, which may vary from individual therapy provided in the child' home to a center-based, classroom-type program. An early intervention program is designed to meet the individual needs of the infant and is written into a plan known as an individualized family service plan (IFSP; see Chapter 34). Once children are 3 years old, they then become eligible for educational and therapeutic services through the local public school system. An individualized educational plan (IEP)program, which is similar to the IFSP but designed to be implemented in a classroom environment, is developed for the child (see Chapter 34).

Because those with FXS syndrome have difficulties with organization skills, auditory memory, and inattention, a highly structured learning environment is helpful as well as a consistent daily schedule. It is important to prepare the individual for any changes in routine ahead of time. Verbal instructions should be concrete and clear, with visual cues given whenever possible. As a result of these children's strength in visual memory, a multisensory approach to learning new skills is more effective than a purely auditory approach (The National Fragile X Syndrome, 2004). Computer learning also may be helpful in promoting visual learning and attention. A sight word approach to reading rather than an emphasis on phonics is recommended. Children with FXS learn arithmetic best when manipulatives and visual associations are utilized. For the development of daily living skills, a behavior-based (shaping) technique seems to work well (see Chapter 35). Speech-language therapy is essential to helping children with FXS improve listening skills, auditory memory, ability to follow directions, and the so-cial rules of language (pragmatics). In addition, many of these children benefit from formal social skills training. Occupational therapy may be indicated to assist a child whose joint laxity is interfering with self-help or handwriting skills. In severe cases, assistive technology should be included. Occupational therapy is also extremely useful when a child has sensory integration dysfunction. The establishment of a daily "sensory diet" can help to alleviate many behavioral problems and prevent others before they occur.

OUTCOME

Outcome in FXS primarily depends on the degree of impairment experienced by the individual. Males with a full mutation tend to have intellectual disability requiring limited to extensive support throughout life. Furthermore, because of their associated communicative, behavior, and social skills impairments, they tend to be less independent than would be predicted based on their cognitive abilities alone. Females with a full mutation may succeed in society without support or may require supervision, depending on the degree of clinical involvement. The most prominent long-term problem facing females with the full mutation is the development of psychiatric disorders (Einfeld et al., 1999). Shyness and social anxiety superimposed on mild cognitive impairments can significantly interfere with independence. Fertility is normal in males and females with a full mutation and in males with a premutation. Females with a premutation often experience fertility problems and/or premature ovarian failure. Longevity in both males and females is likely to be normal.

SUMMARY

FXS is the most common inherited cause of intellectual disabilities. It is an X-linked disorder but has a unique inheritance pattern and variable presentation of clinical symptoms. The majority of fully affected boys and more than half of fully affected girls have a characteristic pattern of physical, cognitive, and behavior impairments. A fraction of carrier girls and boys may manifest less severe but similar symptoms. Older men who are carriers of the gene defect and females with the premutation may develop a unique tremor/ataxia syndrome. Because of an expansion of a triplet base pair repeat, CGG, the X chromosome becomes fragile and the FMR1 gene is inactivated. This results in decreased or absent production of FMRP, a protein important in early brain development. Although there is currently no specific treatment for this disorder, special education, behavior management techniques, social skills training, and pharmacotherapy can improve outcome for affected individuals.

REFERENCES

American Academy of Pediatrics, Committee on Genetics. (1996). Health supervision for children with fragile X syndrome. *Pediatrics, 98,* 297–300.

American College of Medical Genetics. (1994). Fragile X syndrome, policy statement on diagnostic and carrier testing. *American Journal of Medical Genetics, 53,* 380–381.

Aziz, M., Stathopulu, E., Callias, M., et al. (2003). Clinical features of boys with fragile X premutations and intermediate alleles. *American Journal of Medical Genetics, 121B,* 119–127.

Bailey, D.B., Skinner, D., & Sparkman, K.C. (2003). Discovering fragile X syndrome: Family experiences and perceptions. *Pediatrics, 111,* 407–416.

Bailey, D.B., Jr. (2004). Newborn screening for fragile X syndrome. *Mental Retardation and Developmental Disabilities Research Reviews, 10,* 3–10.

Bailey, D.B., Jr., Hatton, D.D., Skinner, M., et al. (2001). Autistic behavior, FMR1 protein, and developmental trajectories in young males with fragile X syndrome. *Journal of Autism and Developmental Disorders, 31,* 165–74.

Brown, W.T., Jenkins, E.C., Friedman, E., et al. (1982). Autism is associated with the fragile X syndrome. *Journal of Autism and Developmental Disorders, 12*(3), 303–308.

Brussino, A., Gellera, C., Saluto, A., et al. (2005). FMR1 gene premutation is a frequent genetic cause of late-onset sporadic cerebellar ataxia. *Neurology, 64,* 145–147.

Centers for Disease Control and Prevention (CDC). (2002). Delayed diagnosis of fragile X syndrome: United States, 1990–1999. *Morbidity and Mortality Weekly Report, 51*(33), 740–742.

Chiurazzi, P., & Oostra, B.A. (2000). Genetics of mental retardation. *Current Opinion in Pediatrics, 12,* 529–535.

Chiurazzi, P., Tabolacci, E., & Neri, G. (2004). X-linked mental retardation (XLMR): From clinical conditions to cloned genes. *Critical Reviews in Clinical Laboratory Sciences, 41*(2), 117–158.

Cornish, K., Sudhalter, V., & Turk, J., (2004). Attention and language in fragile X. *Mental Retardation and Developmental Disabilities Research Reviews, 10*(1), 11–16.

Crawford, D.C., Acuna, J.M., & Sherman, S.L. (2001). FMR1 and the fragile X syndrome: Human genome epidemiology review. *Genetics in Medicine, 3*(5), 359–371.

Crawford, D.C., Meadows, K.L., Newman, J.L., et al. (2002). Prevalence of the fragile X syndrome in African-Americans. *American Journal of Medical Genetics, 110*(3), 226–233.

Cronister, A., DiMaio, M., Mahoney, M.J., et al. (2005). Fragile X syndrome carrier screening in the prenatal genetic counseling setting. *Genetics in Medicine, 7*(4), 246–250.

Demark, J.L., Feldman, M.A., & Holden, J.J.A. (2003). Behavioral relationship between autism and fragile X syndrome. *American Journal on Mental Retardation, 108* (6), 314–326.

Einfeld, S., Tonge, B., & Turner, G. (1999). Longitudinal course of behavioral and emotional problems in fragile X syndrome. *American Journal of Medical Genetics, 87,* 436–439.

Goodlin-Jones, B.L., Tassone, F., Gane, L.W., et al. (2004). Autism and the fragile X premutation. *Journal of Developmental & Behavioral Pediatrics, 25,* 392–398.

Hagerman, P.J., & Hagerman, R.J. (2004). The fragile-X mutation: A maturing perspective. *American Journal of Human Genetics, 74,* 805–816.

Hagerman, R.J. (2002). The physical and behavioral phenotype. In R.J. Hagerman & P.J. Hagerman (Eds.), *Fragile X syndrome: Diagnosis, treatment, and research* (pp. 3–109). Baltimore: The Johns Hopkins University Press.

Hagerman, R.J., Leavitt, B.R., Farzin, F., et al. (2004). Fragile-X-associated tremor/ataxia syndrome (FXTAS) in females with the FMR1 premutation. *American Journal of Human Genetics, 74,* 1051–1056.

Hagerman, R.J., Stanley, L.W., O'Conner, R., et al. (1996). Learning-disabled males with a fragile X CGG expansion in the upper premutation size range. *Pediatrics, 97,* 122–126.

Hammond, L.S., Macias, M.M., Tarleton, J.C., et al. (1997). Fragile X syndrome and deletions in FMR1: New case and review of the literature. *American Journal of Medical Genetics, 72,* 430–434.

Hatton, D.D., Hooper, S.R., Bailey, D.B., et al. (2002). Problem behavior in boys with fragile X syndrome. *American Journal of Medical Genetics, 108*(2), 105–116.

Incorpora, G., Sorge, G., Sorge, A., et al. (2002). Epilepsy in fragile X syndrome. *Brain & Development, 24*(8), 766–769.

Inlow, J.K., & Restifo, L.L. (2004). Molecular and comparative genetics of mental retardation. *Genetics, 166,* 835–881.

Jacquemont, S., Hagerman, R.J., Leehey, M., et al. (2003). Fragile X premutation tremor/ataxia syndrome: Molecular, clinical, and neuroimaging correlates. *American Journal of Human Genetics, 72,* 869–878.

Johnston, C., Eliez, S., Dyer-Friedman, J., et al. (2001). Neurobehavioral phenotype in carriers of the fragile X premutation. *American Journal of Medical Genetics, 103*(4), 314–319.

Kau, A.S., Meyer, W.A., & Kaufmann, W.E. (2002). Early development in males with fragile X syndrome: A review of the literature. *Microscopy Research Technology, 57*(3), 174–178.

Kau, A.S., Tierney, E., Bukelis, I., et al. (2004). Social behavior profile in young males with fragile X syndrome: Characteristics and specificity. *American Journal of Medical Genetics, A, 126*(1), 9–17.

Kaufmann, W.E., Cortell, R., Kau, A.S., et al. (2004). Autism spectrum disorder in fragile X syndrome: Communication, social interaction, and specific behaviors. *American Journal of Medical Genetics A, 129,* 225–34.

Kenneson, A., Zhang, F., Hagedorn, C.H., et al. (2001). Reduced FMRP and increased FMR1 transcription is proportionally associated with CGG repeat number in intermediate-length and premutation carriers. *Human Molecular Genetics, 10,* 1449–1454.

Kleefstra, T., & Hamel, B.C.J. (2005). X-linked mental retardation: Further lumping, splitting, and emerging phenotypes. *Clinical Genetics, 67,* 451–467.

Leonard, H., & Wen, X. (2002). The epidemiology of mental retardation: Challenges and opportunities in the new millennium. *Mental Retardation and Developmental Disabilities Research Reviews, 8,* 117–134.

Loesch, D.Z., Churchyard, A., Brotchie, P., et al. (2005). Evidence for, and a spectrum of, neurological involvement in carriers of the fragile X pre-mutation: FXTAS and beyond. *Clinical Genetics, 67,* 412–417.

Loesch, D.Z., Huggins, R.M. Bui, Q.M., et al. (2002). Effect of the deficits of fragile X mental retardation protein on cognitive status of fragile X males and females assessed by robust pedigree analysis. *Journal of Developmental & Behavioral Pediatrics, 23*(6), 416–424.

Maddalena, A., Richards, C.S., McGinniss, M.J., et al. (2001). Technical standards and guidelines for fragile X: The first of a series of disease-specific supplements to the Standards and Guidelines for Clinical Genetics Laboratories of the American College of Medical Genetics, Quality Assurance Subcommittee of the Laboratory Practice Committee. *Genetics in Medicine, 3,* 200–205.

Martin, J.P., & Bell, J. (1943). A pedigree of mental defect showing sex-linkage. *Journal of Neurology and Psychiatry, 6,* 154–157.

Mirrett, P., Roberts, J.E., & Price, J. (2003). Early intervention practices and communication intervention strategies for young males with fragile X syndrome. *Language, Speech, and Hearing Services in Schools, 34,* 331.

Mirrett, P.L., Bailey, D.B., Roberts, J.E., et al. (2004). Developmental screening and detection of developmental delays in infants and toddlers with fragile X syndrome. *Journal of Developmental & Behavioral Pediatrics, 25,* 21–27.

The National Fragile X Foundation. (2004). *Lesson planning guide for students with fragile X syndrome: A practical approach for the classroom.* San Francisco: Author.

Nolin, S.L., Brown, W.T., Glicksman, A., et al. (2003). Expansion of the fragile X CGG repeat in females with premutation or intermediate alleles. *American Journal of Human Genetics, 72,* 454–464.

Philofsky, A., Hepburn, S.L., Hayes, A., et al. (2004). Linguistic and cognitive functioning and autism symptoms in young children with fragile X syndrome. *American Journal on Mental Retardation, 109,* 208–218.

Reiss, A.L., & Dant, C.C. (2003). The behavioral neurogenetics of fragile X syndrome: Analyzing gene–brain–behavior relationships in child developmental psychopathologies. *Developmental Psychopathology, 15,* 927–968.

Riddle, J.E., Cheema, A., Sobesky, W.E., et al. (1998). Phenotypic involvement in females with the FMR1 gene mutation. *American Journal on Mental Retardation, 102,* 590–601.

Rogers, S.J., Wehner, D.E., & Hagerman, R. (2001). The behavioral phenotype in fragile X: Symptoms of autism in very young children with fragile X syndrome, idiopathic autism, and other developmental disorders. *Journal of Autism and Developmental Disorders, 22,* 409–417.

Ross, M.T., Grafham, D.V., & Coffey, A.J. (2005). The DNA sequence of the human genome. *Nature, 434,* 325–327.

Sabaratnam, M., Murthy, N.V., Wijeratne, A., et al. (2003). Autistic-like behaviour profile and psychiatric morbidity in Fragile X Syndrome: A prospective ten-year follow-up study. *European Child and Adolescent Psychiatry, 12,* 172–177.

Slegtenhorst-Eegdeman, K.E., de Rooij, D.G., Verhoef-Post, M., et al. (1998). Macroorchidism in FMR1 knockout mice is caused by increased sertoli cell proliferation during testicular development. *Endocrinology, 139,* 156–162.

Stevenson, R.E., & Schwartz, C.E. (2002). Clinical and molecular contributions to the understanding of X-linked mental retardation. *Cytogenetic Genome Research, 99*(1–4), 265–275.

Stevenson, R.E., Schwartz, C.E., & Schroer, R.E., (2000). X-linked mental retardation. *Oxford Monographs on Medical Genetics No. 39.* New York: Oxford University Press.

Stoll, C. (2001). Problems in the diagnosis of fragile X syndrome in young children are still present. *American Journal of Medical Genetics, 100,* 110–115.

Tassone, F., Hagerman, R.J., Taylor, A.K., et al. (2000a). Clinical involvement and protein expression in individuals with the FMR1 premutation. *American Journal of Medical Genetics, 91,* 144–152.

Terracciano, A., Chiurazzi, P., & Neri, G. (2004). Fragile X syndrome. *Journal of Developmental and Behavioral Pediatrics, 25,* 392–398.

Tsiouris, J.A., & Brown, W.T., (2004). Neuropsychiatric symptoms of fragile X syndrome: Pathophysiology and pharmacotherapy. *CNS Drugs, 18,* 687–703.

Tzeng, C.C., Tsai, L.P., Hwu, W.L., et al. (2005). Prevalence of the FMR1 mutation in Taiwan assessed by large-scale screening of newborn boys and analysis of DXS548-FRAXAC1 haplotype. *American Journal of Medical Genetics A, 133*(1), 37–43.

Verkerk, A.J.M.H., Pieretti, M., Sutcliffe, J.S., et al. (1991). Identification of a gene (FMR1) containing a CGG repeat coincident with a breakpoint cluster region exhibiting length variation in fragile X syndrome. *Cell, 65,* 905–914.

Welt, C.K., Smith, P.C., & Taylor, A.E., (2004). Evidence of early ovarian aging in fragile X premutation carriers. *Journal of Clinical Endocrinology and Metabolism, 89*(9), 4569–4574.

20 Inborn Errors of Metabolism

Mark L. Batshaw and Mendel Tuchman

Upon completion of this chapter, the reader will

- Understand the term *inborn error of metabolism*
- Know the differences among a number of these inborn errors, including amino acid disorders, organic acidemias, fatty acid oxidation defects, mitochondrial disorders, peroxisomal disorders, and lysosomal storage diseases
- Identify the characteristic clinical symptoms and diagnostic tests for these disorders
- Know which of these disorders have newborn screening tests available
- Recognize different approaches to treatment
- Understand the outcome and range of developmental disabilities associated with inborn errors of metabolism

The food we eat contains fats, proteins, and carbohydrates that must be broken down into smaller components and then metabolized by hundreds of enzymes that maintain body functions. Approximately 1 in 2,500 children are born with a deficiency in one of the enzymes that normally **catalyzes** an important biochemical reaction in the cells (McKusick et al., 2005). These children are said to have an inborn error of metabolism. Such an enzyme deficiency can result in the accumulation of a toxic chemical compound behind the enzyme block or lead to a deficiency of a product normally produced by the deficient enzyme (Figure 20.1). The result may be organ damage/dysfunction (often the brain), various degrees of disability, or even death. For example, children with phenylketonuria (PKU) have a deficiency in the enzyme that normally converts one amino acid (phenylalanine) to another (tyrosine). An inherited deficiency of this enzyme (phenylalanine hydroxylase) leads to the accumulation of phenylalanine, which at high levels is toxic to the brain. If untreated soon after birth, PKU leads to severe mental retardation (Figure 20.1). In contrast, in children with congenital adrenal

hypoplasia, an inherited enzyme deficiency leads to decreased production of certain hormones (e.g., cortisol) that are essential for normal body function. Females with this deficiency may be born with ambiguous genitalia because they produce abnormal amounts of male steroid sex hormone (testosterone) in utero (van der Kamp & Wit, 2004). Fortunately, for both of these disorders, newborn screening tests and early treatment have permitted affected children to grow up with typical intelligence and normal physiological functioning. Not all inborn errors of metabolism can be as effectively treated, however, because of delays in diagnosis or lack of an effective intervention. This chapter provides examples from a range of inborn errors of metabolism to explain diagnostic and therapeutic advances that are improving the outcome of patients with these disorders.

LISA

Lisa was discharged from the hospital at 3 days of age. Her parents were surprised and upset when they were called back a week later, after doctors reported that she had a positive PKU screening test. Amino acid studies confirmed the diagnosis of PKU, and Lisa was placed on a formula that was low in phenylalanine. As Lisa grew, her parents could hardly believe there was a problem because Lisa looked and acted normally and achieved her developmental milestones on time. The visits to the metabolism clinic were difficult reminders of her "silent disorder." Once Lisa entered elementary school, she began resisting her dietary restrictions, and her parents had difficulty maintaining good metabolic control. Lisa was born in 1970, when the importance of strict metabolic control for life in PKU was not widely appreciated. Her parents stopped her low-phenylalanine diet at age 7. Psychometric testing at 10 years of age showed that Lisa had an IQ score of 85. Despite some learning and behavioral difficulties, she graduated from high school and began working. When she became pregnant, however, she refused to go back on a phenylalanine restricted diet, despite her parents' and health care providers' explanation of the serious risks to her baby. Her child was born with a small head, and at age 5, has intellectual disability requiring limited supports.

DARNEL

Darnel babbled at 6 months and sat without support shortly thereafter. His parents became concerned by 1 year of age, however, when he had made no further progress. If anything, he seemed less steady in sitting and was uninvolved with his surroundings. His pediatrician worried that Darnel might have an autism spectrum disorder. By 18 months, there were graver concerns. Darnel was no longer able to roll over; he was very floppy and did not appear to respond to light or sound. His pediatrician referred Darnel to a genetics clinic, where an extensive workup eventually diagnosed him as having Tay-Sachs disease, a genetic disorder affecting lipid metabolism in the brain. Over the next 3 years, Darnel slipped into an unresponsive condition and required tube feeding. He finally succumbed to aspiration pneumonia. As a result of the diagnosis, his mother decided to undergo prenatal diagnosis in subsequent pregnancies. She now has two healthy children and underwent one termination of an affected fetus.

TYPES OF INBORN ERRORS OF METABOLISM

Inborn errors of metabolism are a relatively recently discovered group of diseases. PKU, one of the first disorders identified, was described by Fölling in 1934. About 300 additional disorders have been identified since the 1950s, and a number of new ones are described each year (McKusick et al., 2005). The majority of these enzyme deficiencies are inherited as autosomal recessive traits, in which both parents carry a defective gene but are both healthy. A few are transmitted as X-linked disorders or through mitochondrial inheritance (see Chapter 1). Prenatal diagnosis is available for most of these disorders (see Chapter 7).

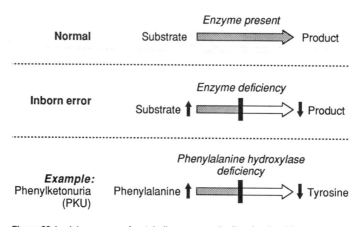

Figure 20.1.   Inborn errors of metabolism are genetic disorders involving an enzyme deficiency. This enzyme block leads to the accumulation of a toxic substrate and/or the deficient synthesis of a product needed for normal body function. In phenylketonuria (PKU) there is a toxic accumulation of phenylalanine behind the deficient enzyme, phenylalanine hydroxylase.

Although there are many different ways of categorizing these disorders, inborn errors of metabolism are often divided into those that are clinically "silent" for a relatively long period before being recognized, those that produce acute metabolic crises, and those that cause progressive organ damage or dysfunction (Table 20.1). Among the silent disorders are certain abnormalities involving amino acids (e.g., PKU) or hormones (e.g., congenital hypothyroidism). Disorders producing acute toxicity include certain inborn errors in the metabolism of small molecules, including ammonia, amino acids, organic acids, fatty acids, lactic acid, and carbohydrates (Burlina, Bonafe, & Zacchello, 1999). Inborn errors of metabolism causing progressive disorders include most **glycogen** storage and peroxisomal and lysosomal storage disorders. The specific names of the disorders are often derived from their deficient enzyme (e.g., **ornithine transcarbamylase [OTC] deficiency,** an ammonia metabolism disorder). Silent disorders such as PKU do not manifest life-threatening crises, but if untreated, lead to brain damage and developmental disabilities over time. These disorders contrast with inborn errors that cause acute symptoms, such as OTC deficiency, that may be life threatening in infancy. In both cases, an affected baby is generally protected in the womb because the maternal circulation can remove the toxic chemical or provide the missing product. After birth, however, the infant must rely on his or her own metabolic pathways, and if they are abnormal, toxicity occurs rapidly or over time depending on the severity of the defect. In progressive disorders, there is the gradual accumulation, beginning in the womb, of large molecules that cannot cross the cell membrane or the placenta. These molecules are stored in the cells of various body organs, including the brain, where they ultimately cause damage, leading to physical and/or neurological deterioration.

CLINICAL MANIFESTATIONS

The clinical manifestations of the various inborn errors of metabolism fall along a spectrum, from lack of overt symptoms to life-threatening episodes. The group of silent disorders, such as PKU, does not manifest symptoms such as lethargy, coma, or regression of skills. Instead, untreated children develop very slowly and are typically not identified as having intellectual disability until later in childhood.

Life-threatening crises characterize the second group of inborn errors of metabolism. Infants with these disorders appear to be unaffected at birth, but by a few days of age they develop vomiting, respiratory distress, and lethargy before slipping into coma. These symptoms, however, mimic those observed in other severe newborn illnesses (see Chapter 4) such as sepsis (blood-borne infection), brain hemorrhage, heart and lung abnormalities, and gastrointestinal obstruction, which can make the correct diagnosis difficult. If specific metabolic testing of the blood and urine is not performed, the disease will go undetected. Undiagnosed and untreated, virtually all affected children will die quickly. One study reported that 60% of children with newborn onset inborn errors of the **urea** cycle (causing elevated ammonia level) had at least one sibling who died before the disorder was correctly diagnosed in a subsequent affected child (Batshaw et al., 1982). Even with "heroic" treatment, which may include **dialysis** to "wash out" the toxin (ammonia), many infants do not survive, and severe developmental disabilities are common in those who do (Msall et al., 1984).

In children with neonatal-onset disease, DNA analysis typically shows mutations that cause the absence of the enzyme or the formation of a nonfunctional enzyme. Enzyme activity levels are generally undetectable (see Chapter 1). Some children with the same inborn error of metabolism, however, have less severe mutations that result in reduced amount of enzymes or enzymes that are only partially dysfunctional. These children have later onset of clinical signs and more variable symptoms. Here, symptoms of behavioral changes and cyclical vomiting and lethargy are often provoked by excessive protein intake or intercurrent infections (Gropman & Batshaw, 2004). Al-

Table 20.1.   Examples of inborn errors of metabolism

Type I: Silent disorders
   Phenylketonuria (PKU)
   Congenital hypothyroidism

Type II: Disorders presenting in acute metabolic crisis
   Urea cycle disorders (ornithine transcarbamylase [OTC] deficiency)
   Organic acidemias (multiple carboxylase deficiency)

Type III: Disorders with progressive neurological deterioration
   Tay-Sachs disease
   Gaucher disease
   Metachromatic leukodystrophy

though these children have a better outcome than those with neonatal-onset disease, they remain at risk for life-threatening metabolic crises throughout life. In addition, although their developmental disabilities may be less severe than those in children with neonatal-onset disease, children with later onset disease rarely escape without some residual impairment, ranging from attention-deficit/hyperactivity disorder (ADHD) and learning disabilities to intellectual disability.

The third clinical presentation of inborn errors of metabolism is in the form of a slowly progressive disorder (Haltia, 2003). Examples include the following:

- Glycogen storage diseases, such as Pompe disease

- Lysosomal storage disorders, such as Tay-Sachs disease (Cooper, 2003; Fernandes Filho & Shapiro, 2004)

- Ceroid lipofuscinosis such as Batten disease (Goebel & Wisniewski, 2004)

- Mucopolysaccharide disorders (Muenzer & Fisher, 2004)

- Metachromatic leukodystrophy (Gieselmann, 2003; Gieselmann et al., 2003)

- Mitochondrial disorders, such as Leigh encephalopathy (Scaglia et al., 2004; Thorburn, 2004)

- Peroxisomal disorders, including adreno-leukodystrophy (Moser et al., 2004) and Zellweger syndrome (Wanders, 2004)

In the more severe of these disorders, there is a gradual and progressive loss of motor and/or cognitive skills beginning in infancy or early childhood that if left untreated commonly leads to death in childhood. In the case of Tay-Sachs disease (Darnel's disorder) the affected child appears to develop typically until 3–6 months of age, at which point skill development halts. For the next 1–2 years, the child gradually loses all skills; begins having seizures; and exhibits decreased muscle tone, vision, hearing, and cognition. Death usually results from malnutrition or from aspiration pneumonia. Unfortunately, no effective treatment currently exists for this disorder. Enzyme replacement therapy, however, has been recently found to be successful in treating several other lysosomal disorders (notably Gaucher disease, Fabry disease, and Hurler syndrome) in which target organs, other than the brain, are accessible to the recombinant enzyme (Brady & Schiffmann 2004). Bone marrow transplantation, stem cell transplantation, and gene therapy also offer hope for the future (Muenzer & Fisher 2004).

MECHANISM OF BRAIN DAMAGE

The causes of brain damage in the various inborn errors of metabolism are not completely understood. Research is starting to provide some clues that may eventually lead to improved treatment. For example, thyroid hormone has been found to be necessary for the normal growth of neurons, their processes, and surrounding myelin in the brain. Untreated, a congenital thyroid hormone deficiency is thought to lead to poor postnatal brain growth and result in microcephaly (Oerbeck et al., 2003; Rovet, 2005).

Neurotoxins appear to play a role in certain other metabolic disorders. For example, in nonketotic hyperglycinemia, an inborn error of amino acid metabolism, there is an accumulation of **glycine,** leading to uncontrolled seizures (Chien et al., 2004). Glycine appears to produce excito-toxicity at a neurotransmitter receptor, leading to the influx of calcium ions and water into the neuron. This causes swelling and, eventually, cell death. Experimental drugs are being tested to block this receptor from being overstimulated (Hoover-Fong et al., 2004). In Lesch-Nyhan syndrome, which is caused by a defect in **purine** metabolism, deficits in the **dopamine** neurotransmitter system are associated with self-injurious behavior (McCarthy, 2004; Nyhan 1997).

In some disorders, more than one neurotoxin may be involved. Scientists believe that in inborn errors of the urea cycle the accumulating toxins, ammonia, and/or glutamine directly cause the nerve cells to swell and also indirectly cause excito-toxic damage to the brain (Batshaw, 1994; Cooper, 2001). If children are rescued from the ammonia-induced coma within a day or two, the neurotoxic effect can subside and outcome can be fairly good (Gropman & Batshaw, 2004). If the coma is prolonged, however, irreversible brain damage occurs.

ASSOCIATED DISABILITIES

The toxic accumulation of metabolic compounds or deficient synthesis of essential products results in a range of developmental disabilities in children with inborn errors of metabolism. The most common are intellectual disability and cerebral palsy. However, there are also rather specific impairments in certain inborn errors. These are sometimes associated with distinctive pathological features in the brain, which may eventually permit a better understanding of brain development and function. For example, boys with the X-linked Lesch-Nyhan syndrome exhibit choreoathetosis (a form of abnormal movements, dyskinetic cerebral palsy; see Chapter 26) and compulsive, self-injurious behavior (McCarthy, 2004). Children with glutaric acidemia type I and other organic acidemia and mitochondrial disorders can have dyskinetic cerebral palsy associated with calcifications of basal ganglia (Desai et al., 2003; Mordekar & Baxter, 2004). In Zellweger syndrome, a disorder of the **peroxisome** formation, children exhibit multiple malformations that are more commonly associated with chromosomal disorders, including an abnormal facial appearance, kidney cysts, and congenital heart defects (Grayer, 2005).

DIAGNOSTIC TESTING

A child with developmental disabilities of unknown origin should be referred for a genetic/metabolic evaluation if he or she has any of the following signs or symptoms: cyclical behavioral changes, vomiting and lethargy, enlargement of the liver or spleen, evidence of neurological deterioration, and/or a family history suggestive of an inherited disorder. The increasing number of clinically available biochemical and molecular tests can lead to a specific diagnosis and possibly effective therapy and a better outcome. Even in currently untreatable disorders, a specific diagnosis may permit effective genetic counseling. A metabolic evaluation is not required, however, for all children with intellectual disability. It is expensive and the diagnostic yield is quite low. Thus, meticulous clinical evaluation should determine if a metabolic work up is warranted.

Diagnoses of inborn errors of amino acid and organic acid metabolism rely primarily on blood and urine tests to detect toxins and/or biochemical markers. The most common tests include blood ammonia, lactic acid, acylcarnitines, and amino acids and urine for organic acids analysis. The metabolic evaluations are individualized based on the specific biochemical pathway that is suspected to be involved. OTC deficiency, the most common inborn error of the urea cycle, illustrates one such defective pathway (Figure 20.2). When pro-

teins are broken down into their amino acids components, the amino acids that are not reused for making new proteins are degraded to produce energy, and during this process ammonia waste is normally released. The ammonia is then converted into the nontoxic product urea through six enzymatic steps in the urea cycle (OTC is the second enzyme). Urea is then excreted in the urine, thus eliminating nitrogen from ammonia. If any one of the six enzymes is deficient, ammonia will accumulate and can cause severe neurological symptoms (Batshaw, 1994). In those individuals with some residual enzyme activity, the disorder may only manifest under certain environmental stresses (e.g., infectious illness), and the disorders may only be correctly diagnosed during those acute episodes. To diagnose this disorder, levels of ammonia and amino acids are measured in blood, and orotic acid is measured in the urine. Many other inborn errors of amino acid and organic acid metabolism can be identified using similar blood and urine tests.

Brain degenerative conditions such as lysosomal storage disorders can be suspected by microscopic analysis of various tissues and some biochemical testing (e.g., **mucopolysaccharides** in urine) but are typically diagnosed by measuring the suspected deficient enzyme activity in the blood or cultured skin cells (Meikle et al., 2004; Wilcox, 2004). Imaging studies (e.g., magnetic resonance imaging [MRI] with magnetic resonance spectroscopy [MRS], computed tomography [CT] scan), electroencephalogram (EEG), and other neurological measures (e.g., nerve conduction velocity, electromyography) may also prove helpful in diagnosing these disorders.

NEWBORN SCREENING

Because individual inborn error of metabolisms are rare (typically occurring in fewer than 1 in 10,000 births) and the diagnosis is easily missed, efforts have been directed at developing newborn mass screening methods for the detection of the more common and treatable disorders (Carreiro-Lewandowski, 2002). As explained previously, rapid diagnosis and treatment is important for achieving a favorable outcome. As a result, screening efforts have focused on newborn infants. The first newborn screening test was developed for PKU in 1959 (Guthrie & Susi, 1963), and it was successful in detecting more than 90% of affected infants. Subsequently, methods have been established for screening other disorders, including congenital

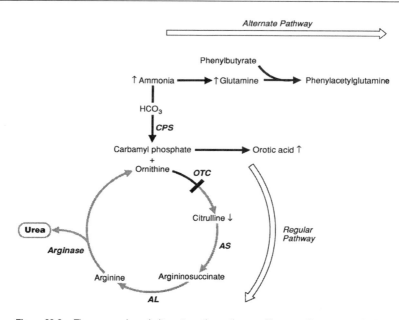

Figure 20.2. The urea cycle and alternate pathway therapy. There are five enzymes in this cycle that convert toxic ammonia, a breakdown product of protein, to nontoxic urea, which is excreted in the urine. The enzymes, shown in boldface italic type, are CPS (carbamyl phosphate synthetase), OTC (ornithine transcarbamylase), AS (argininosuccinate synthetase), AL (argininosuccinate lyase), and arginase. Inborn errors at each step of the urea cycle have been described, with the most common being OTC deficiency. In OTC deficiency, behind the block there is accumulation of ammonia, glutamine, and orotic acid and deficient production of citrulline. Treatment has been directed at providing an alternate pathway for waste nitrogen excretion by giving the drug sodium phenylbutyrate, which combines with glutamine to form phenylacetylglutamine, a nontoxic product that can be excreted in the urine. This results in a decrease in the accumulation of ammonia.

hypothyroidism, galactosemia, homocystinuria, biotinidase deficiency, maple syrup urine disease, and fatty acid oxidation defects, as well as certain other genetic disorders that are not associated with developmental disabilities, including cystic fibrosis, adrenal insufficiency, sickle cell anemia, and alpha$_1$-antitrypsin deficiency (a disorder affecting the liver and lungs). This expanded testing, now employing tandem mass spectrometry in state-run screening laboratories, can measure more than 30 inborn errors of metabolism and is offered to families in the newborn nurseries (Banta-Wright & Steiner, 2004; Carlson, 2004). The specific inborn errors of metabolism tested for vary among states based on local legislation (Rinoldo et al., 2004). State specific information is provided on the National Newborn Screening and Genetics Resource Center web site (http://genes-r-us.uthscsa.edu).

To perform the newborn screening test, a few drops of blood are drawn from the infant's heel and placed on a filter paper. The dried blood sample is mailed to the screening laboratory, where results are obtained within a few days. Although these tests have proved to be remarkably effective, parents should be reminded that a positive test only indicates a higher than normal likelihood of a genetic disorder that needs to be confirmed or ruled out by additional confirmatory testing in the specialized clinic. In addition, the tests detect only a fraction of disorders that cause developmental disabilities, whereas parents might incorrectly assume that these tests are diagnostic for all disorders.

THERAPEUTIC APPROACHES

Figure 20.3 illustrates the varying approaches to treating inborn errors of metabolism. These methods include 1) **substrate** deprivation (dietary restriction), 2) externally supplying the deficient product, 3) stimulating an alternative pathway, 4) providing a vitamin co-factor, 5) replacing an enzyme, 6) transplanting an organ, and 7) using gene therapy. With the exception of gene therapy, which is not yet a practical option, each of these approaches is illustrated by specific disorders in Table 20.2.

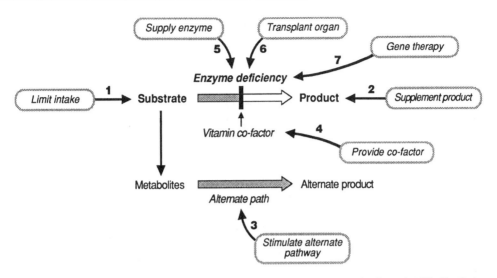

Figure 20.3.   Approaches to treatment of inborn errors of metabolism. Treatment can be directed at 1) limiting the intake of a potentially toxic compound, 2) supplementing the deficient product, 3) stimulating an alternate metabolic pathway, 4) providing a vitamin co-factor to activate residual enzyme activity, 5) supplying the enzyme itself, 6) transplanting a body organ containing the deficient enzyme, and 7) gene therapy.

Substrate Deprivation (Dietary Restriction)

A relatively straightforward method of treating an inborn error of metabolism is to establish dietary restrictions that limit the child's intake of a potentially toxic amino acid. For example, children with PKU are placed on a phenylalanine-restricted diet in order to prevent the phenylalanine accumulation that causes brain damage (Huijbregts et al., 2002). This involves using a special phenylalanine-restricted formula and low-protein foods. One study showed that the IQ scores of children who began this treatment within the first month of life were around 100, whereas the scores of those initially treated later in childhood were 20–50 points lower (Table 20.3; Hanley, Linsao, & Netley, 1971).

Scientists initially thought that only those children with PKU who were younger than 6 years needed to follow a phenylalanine-restricted diet, as was done with Lisa. For older children, it was thought that phenylalanine would be much less toxic. In addition, the high cost and rejection of this rather unpleasant and restrictive diet made continuation difficult. Initial studies to determine whether children with PKU experienced a loss in intellectual functioning following dietary treatment discontinuation suggested that IQ scores did not decline over time (Waisbren et al., 1987). In a subsequent study, however, researchers found that children with PKU

who maintained the diet through age 10 actually experienced a modest gain in IQ scores compared with children who stopped the diet at age 6. The differences in IQ scores between the two groups were statistically significant (Michals et al., 1988). Thus, metabolic specialists now suggest that the phenylalanine-restricted diet be continued indefinitely.

An elevated phenylalanine level poses a serious threat for the fetus of a woman with PKU who is without dietary control, as described with Lisa (Lee et al., 2005). Before newborn screening and effective treatment were available, men and women with PKU had severe intellectual disability and did not often bear children. Since effective treatment became available, most women with PKU became mothers. These women, however, had typically stopped following the phenylalanine-restricted diet during childhood. Unexpectedly, almost all of the children born to these women were found to have small heads, intellectual disability, and other congenital abnormalities, including congenital heart disease, cleft lip and palate, and gastrointestinal and urinary abnormalities. These children, however, do not have PKU; they are only carriers. Instead, the intellectual disability and other abnormalities are caused by the teratogenic effect of the mother's high phenylalanine levels on the developing fetus. Studies have shown that lowering the phenylalanine levels in the pregnant mother with PKU significantly

Table 20.2.   Examples of treatment approaches for inborn errors of metabolism

Approaches	Disorder	Specific treatment
Substrate deprivation	Phenylketonuria (PKU)	Phenylalanine restriction
	Maple syrup urine disease	Branch chain amino acid restriction
	Galactosemia	Galactose restriction
Externally supplementing the deficient product	Congenital hypothyroidism	Thyroid hormone (Synthroid)
	Glycogen storage disease	Cornstarch
	Urea cycle disorders (except argininemia)	Arginine
Stimulating an alternative pathway	Urea cycle disorders	Phenylbutyrate (Buphenyl)
	Organic acidemias	Carnitine
	Isovaleric acidemia	Glycine
	Tyrosinemia	NTBC
Providing a vitamin co-factor	Multiple carboxylase deficiency	Biotin
	Homocystinuria	Pyridoxine
	Methylmalonic acidemia	Vitamin B_{12}
Replacing an enzyme	Fabry disease	Agalsidase beta (Fabrazyme)
	Gaucher disease	Alglucerase (Ceredase)
	Hurler disease	Alpha-L-iduronidase (laronidase [Aldurazyme])
Transplanting an organ	Metachromatic leukodystrophy	Bone marrow
	Ornithine transcarbamylase (OTC) deficiency	Liver

improves the chances for typical development of offspring. As a result, it is now advised that women with PKU resume a phenylalanine-restricted diet prior to conception (Rohr et al., 2004; Rouse & Azen, 2004).

Another example of substrate deprivation therapy has shown promise in animal models of PKU (Gamez et al., 2004). Here, the use of a recombinant enzyme to degrade phenylalanine in the intestine before its absorption could reduce the phenylalanine load and allow less severe dietary restriction (Gamez et al., 2004). In certain lysosomal storage disorders, inhibition of glycosphingolipid synthesis would have the analogous effect of reducing lysosomal products that are toxic to the brain (Cox, 2005).

Externally Supplementing the Deficient Product

Some children with inborn errors of metabolism are given replacements for the enzyme product they are missing. For example, children with congenital hypothyroidism receive a thyroid supplement to compensate for the thyroid hormone they lack. Similarly, children with congenital adrenal hyperplasia receive steroid hormone replacement. This treatment, if administered early, effectively corrects the metabolic disor-

der. Children with hypothyroidism who are treated in the first months of life develop typical intelligence (Palma Sisto, 2004) although, as with children who have PKU, these children have some residual impairment in attention and learning (Rovet, 2005).

Stimulating an Alternative Pathway

Physicians are now able to treat some metabolic disorders by stimulating an alternative pathway that detours around the enzymatic block. For example, children with inborn errors of the urea cycle cannot convert toxic ammonia to nontoxic urea. Treatment by dietary protein restriction alone has proved unsuccessful, because the degree of restriction required to prevent an accumulation of ammonia does not allow a sufficient diet for sustained growth or prolonged survival (Shih, 1976). A novel approach is to use the drug sodium phenylbutyrate (Buphenyl) to stimulate an alternate pathway for ammonia excretion. By providing a detour around the enzymatic block and converting the ammonia to an alternate nontoxic product, phenylacetylglutamine, instead of urea (Figure 20.2), this drug allows the majority of children with urea cycle disorders to survive, although many have developmental disabilities (Batshaw et al., 2001).

Table 20.3. Results of treating phenylketonuria (PKU) diagnosed at various stages

	Number of children by age at diagnosis (months)				
	Birth–2	2–6	6–12	12–24	24+
Number of cases	38	6	11	19	20
IQ score					
90+	27	0	0	1	2
0–89	6	3	0	2	1
70–79	4	1	3	2	0
Less than 70	1	2	8	14	17
Mean IQ score	93.5	71.6	54.5	55.5	40.8

From Hanley, W.B., Linsao, L.S., & Netley, C. (1971). The efficiency of dietary therapy for phenyketonuria. Reprinted from *CMAJ* 1971:104 Page 1089 by permission of the publisher. © 1971 Canadian Medical Association.

Another example of using a detour is the inhibition of a pathway upstream to prevent the formation of toxic products behind the enzymatic block. In hereditary tyrosinemia type I, the drug 2-(2-nitro-4-trifluoromethylbenzoyl)-1,3-cyclohexanedione (NTBC), an herbicide derivative, was found to inhibit tyrosine degradation in affected children, preventing the formation of a toxic compound that is suspected to cause liver and renal tubular disease and liver cancer in affected children (Crone et al., 2003; Grompe, 2001). Similarly, a recently approved medication miglustat (Zavesca) for the treatment of Gaucher disease, inhibits the formation of glucosylcermide, reducing the accumulated substrate load (Jeyakumar et al., 2001; Platt et al., 2001). It is being tested for other lysosomal storage disorders as well (Niemann-Pick Type C, Late Onset Tay-Sachs, and Type 3 Gaucher disease).

Providing a Vitamin Co-factor

For a few inborn errors of metabolism, providing a large dose of a vitamin co-factor results in amplification of residual enzyme activity or enhanced enzyme stability and clinical improvement. This approach has been used most effectively in treating children with an organic acidemia called multiple carboxylase deficiency (Morrone et al., 2002). These children, who develop symptoms of acidosis and coma because of a defect in their enzyme (holocarboxylase synthetase), show remarkable improvement if biotin is provided at a very high (but nontoxic) dosage. Similar vitamin therapy can help children with certain forms of another organic

acidemia called methylmalonic aciduria (using vitamin B_{12}) and an amino acid disorder called homocystinuria (using vitamin B_6; Morrone et al., 2002). Vitamin therapy has unfortunately spawned a "quick-fix" approach to treating everything from cancer, to Down syndrome, to schizophrenia, although there is no evidence that megavitamin therapy is effective in treating these disorders (Nutrition Committee of the Canadian Paediatric Society, 1990).

Replacing an Enzyme

The previously discussed methods of therapy use indirect approaches to improve the child's condition. Supplying the missing enzyme is a more direct approach to actually correct the inborn error. Injections of a synthetic enzyme first proved successful in treating the lysosomal storage disorder Gaucher disease, which is associated with the accumulation of glucocerebroside in cells of the liver, spleen, and bone marrow. With severe infantile Gaucher disease, the enzyme accumulates in the brain as well. Individuals who receive biweekly injections of the deficient enzyme showed marked improvements, including significant shrinkage of the liver and spleen (Desnick, 2004). This enzyme, however, cannot cross the blood–brain barrier, making replacement therapy ineffective for those children with severe infantile Gaucher disease. As of 2006, specific enzyme replacement therapy has been approved for Fabry disease, mucopolysaccharidosis type I (Hurler disease), and mucopolysaccharidosis type VI (Maroteaux-Lamy syndrome) and is being tested for other lysosomal storage diseases (Wraith et al., 2005).

Although replacement therapy seems ideal, it is not without shortcomings. These synthetic enzymes are some of the most expensive drugs in the world. In addition, the enzyme must be injected at frequent intervals throughout the individual's life, and antibodies can develop against the foreign protein, just as antibodies against insulin develop in some individuals with diabetes.

Transplanting an Organ

Some deficient enzymes can be replaced by transplanting a body organ that contains the enzyme. For example, bone marrow transplantation has been attempted in individuals with certain lysosomal and peroxisomal storage disorders, including juvenile metachromatic leukodystrophy, adrenoleukodystrophy, and Hurler syndrome. These disorders, marked by neurological and physical deterioration, and early death, are caused by the deficiency of enzymes found in many body organs, including bone marrow cells. In a number of studies, bone marrow transplantation has resulted in the arrest of or improvement in symptoms (Krivit, 2004; Muenzer & Fisher, 2004).

In addition to bone marrow transplants, liver transplantation has been used to treat certain inborn errors of amino acid metabolism, most notably newborn onset OTC deficiency and hereditary tyrosinemia type I. It has been associated with biochemical correction and improvement in symptoms (McBride et al., 2004). Organ transplantation, however, carries significant mortality and morbidity, and transplant recipients require immunosuppression therapy for life.

Using Gene Therapy

In theory, the ideal treatment for an inborn error of metabolism would involve the insertion of a normal gene to compensate for a defective one. This insertion would allow for the production of a normal enzyme, thereby permanently correcting or curing the disorder. In clinical research studies, however, gene therapy trials have not yet been successful or have been associated with severe adverse events (Bosch & Heard, 2003; Cavazzana-Calvo et al., 2005; Raper et al., 2003).

OUTCOME

The range of outcomes in inborn errors of metabolism varies enormously. In disorders that can be detected by newborn screening, such as

PKU, affected children have generally done well. Their intellectual functioning generally falls within the average range, if somewhat lower than that of their parents. They are, however, at increased risk for having learning disabilities and ADHD (Huijbregts et al., 2002). Less favorable outcomes occur in other inborn errors of amino acid and organic acid metabolism. Although these children are surviving longer now, many manifest developmental disabilities. Among children with metabolic disorders associated with progressive neurological disorders, such as certain lysosomal storage diseases, there has been only limited improvement in mortality and morbidity (Wraith, 2002).

SUMMARY

Although inborn errors of metabolism are rare, their consequences are often devastating. Fortunately, therapy is effective for a number of these disorders. Affected children, however, often must continue treatment for the rest of their lives, which may prove difficult to accomplish. For therapy to succeed, it must be started early. Researchers continue to look for new therapeutic strategies for these diseases. It is hoped that these new therapeutic approaches will continue to improve the outcome for children with inborn errors of metabolism. The expansion in the number of disorders that are tested by newborn screening also bodes well for early treatment and improved outcome.

REFERENCES

Banta-Wright S.A., & Steiner R.D. (2004). Tandem mass spectrometry in newborn screening: A primer for neonatal and perinatal nurses. *Journal of Perinatal and Neonatal Nursing, 18*, 41–58.

Batshaw, M.L. (1994). Inborn errors of urea synthesis: A review. *Annals of Neurology, 35*, 133–141.

Batshaw, M.L., Brusilow, S., Waber, L., et al. (1982). Treatment of inborn errors of urea synthesis: Activation of alternative pathways of waste nitrogen synthesis and excretion. *The New England Journal of Medicine, 306*, 1387–1392.

Batshaw, M.L., MacArthur, R.B., & Tuchman M. (2001). Alternative pathway therapy for urea cycle disorders: Twenty years later. *The Journal of Pediatrics, 138*(1, Suppl.), S46–S54; discussion S54–55.

Bosch A., & Heard J.M. (2003). Gene therapy for mucopolysaccharidosis. *International Review of Neurobiology, 55*, 271–296.

Brady, R.O., & Schiffmann, R. (2004). Enzyme-replacement therapy for metabolic storage disorders. *The Lancet Neurology, 3*, 752–756

Burlina, A.B., Bonafe, L., & Zacchello, F. (1999). Clinical and biochemical approach to the neonate with a suspected inborn error of amino acid and organic acid metabolism. *Seminars in Perinatology, 23*, 162–173.

Carlson M.D. (2004). Recent advances in newborn screening for neurometabolic disorders. *Current Opinion in Neurology, 17,* 133–138.

Carreiro-Lewandowski, E. (2002). Newborn screening: An overview. *Clinical Laboratory Science, 15,* 229–238.

Cavazzana-Calvo, M., Lagresle, C., Hacein-Bey-Abina, S., et al. (2005). Gene therapy for severe combined immunodeficiency. *Annual Review of Medicine, 56,* 585–602.

Chien, Y.H., Hsu, C.C., Huang, A., et al. (2004). Poor outcome for neonatal-type nonketotic hyperglycinemia treated with high-dose sodium benzoate and dextromethorphan. *Journal of Child Neurology, 19,* 39–42.

Copper, A.J. (2001). Role of glutamine in cerebral nitrogen metabolism and ammonia neurotoxicity. *Mental Retardation and Developmental Disabilities Research Reviews, 7,* 280–286

Cooper, J.D. (2003). Progress towards understanding the neurobiology of Batten disease or neuronal ceroid lipofuscinosis. *Current Opinion in Neurology, 16,* 121–128.

Cox, T.M. (2005). Substrate reduction therapy for lysosomal storage diseases. *Acta Paediatrica Supplement, 94,* 69–75.

Crone, J., Moslinger, D., Bodamer, O.A., et al. (2003). Reversibility of cirrhotic regenerative liver nodules upon NTBC treatment in a child with tyrosinaemia type I. *Acta Paediatrica, 92,* 625–628.

Desai, N.K., Runge, V.M., Crisp, D.E., et al. (2003). Magnetic resonance imaging of the brain in glutaric acidemia type I: A review of the literature and a report of four new cases with attention to the basal ganglia and imaging technique. *Investigative Radiology, 38,* 489–496.

Desnick, R.J. (2004). Enzyme replacement and enhancement therapies for lysosomal diseases. *Journal of Inherited Metabolic Disease, 27,* 385–410.

Fernandes Filho, J.A., & Shapiro B.E. (2004). Tay-Sachs disease. *Archives of Neurology, 61,* 1466–1468.

Fölling, A. (1934). Excretion of phenylalanine in urine: An inborn error of metabolism associated with intellectual disability. *Hoppe-Seyler's Zeitschrift für Physiologische Chemie, 227,* 169–176.

Gamez, A., Wang, L., Straub, M., et al. (2004). Toward PKU enzyme replacement therapy: PEGylation with activity retention for three forms of recombinant phenylalanine hydroxylase. *Molecular Therapy, 9,* 124–129.

Gieselmann V. (2003). Metachromatic leukodystrophy: recent research developments. *Journal of Child Neurology, 18,* 591–594.

Gieselmann, V., Franken, S., Klein D., et al. (2003). Metachromatic leukodystrophy: Consequences of sulphatide accumulation. *Acta Paediatrica Supplement, 92,* 74–79; discussion, 45.

Goebel, H.H., & Wisniewski, K.E. (2004). Current state of clinical and morphological features in human NCL. *Brain Pathology, 14,* 61–69.

Grayer J. (2005). Recognition of Zellweger syndrome in infancy. *Advances in Neonatal Care, 5,* 5–13.

Grompe, M. (2001). The pathophysiology and treatment of hereditary tyrosinemia type I. *Seminars in Liver Disease, 21,* 563–571

Gropman, A.L., & Batshaw M.L. (2004). Cognitive outcome in urea cycle disorders. *Molecular Genetics and Metabolism, 81,* S58–S62.

Guthrie, R., & Susi, A. (1963). A simple method for detecting phenylketonuria in large populations of newborn infants. *Pediatrics, 32,* 338–343.

Haltia, M. (2003). The neuronal ceroid-lipofuscinoses. *Journal of Neuropathology and Experimental Neurology, 62,* 1–13.

Hanley, W.B., Linsao, L.S., & Netley, C. (1971). The efficiency of dietary therapy for phenylketonuria. *Canadian Medical Association Journal, 104,* 1089.

Hoover-Fong, J.E., Shah S., Van Hove J.L., et al. (2004). Natural history of nonketotic hyperglycinemia in 65 patients. *Neurology, 63,* 1847–1853.

Huijbregts, S.C., de Sonneville, L.M., van Spronsen, F.J., et al. (2002). The neuropsychological profile of early and continuously treated phenylketonuria: orienting, vigilance, and maintenance versus manipulation-functions of working memory. *Neuroscience and Biobehavioral Reviews, 26,* 697–712.

Jeyakumar, M., Norflus, F., Tifft, C.J., et al. (2001). Enhanced survival in Sandhoff disease mice receiving a combination of substrate deprivation therapy and bone marrow transplantation. *Blood, 97,* 327–329.

Krivit, W. (2004). Allogeneic stem cell transplantation for the treatment of lysosomal and peroxisomal metabolic diseases. *Springer Seminars in Immunopathology, 26,* 119–132.

Lee, P.J., Ridout, D., Walter J.H., et al. (2005). Maternal phenylketonuria: report from the United Kingdom Registry 1978–1997. *Archives of Disease in Childhood, 90,* 143–146.

McBride, K.L., Miller, G., Carter S., et al. (2004). Developmental outcomes with early orthotopic liver transplantation for infants with neonatal-onset urea cycle defects and a female patient with late-onset ornithine transcarbamylase deficiency. *Pediatrics, 114,* e523–e526.

McCarthy, G. (2004). Medical diagnosis, management and treatment of Lesch Nyhan disease. *Nucleosides Nucleotides Nucleic Acids, 23,* 1147–1152.

McKusick, V.A., et al. (2005). *Online Mendelian Inheritance in Man.* Retrieved October 10, 2006, from http://www.ncbi.nlm.nih.gov/omim

Meikle, P.J., Fietz, M.J., & Hopwood J.J. (2004). Diagnosis of lysosomal storage disorders: Current techniques and future directions. *Expert Review of Molecular Diagnostics, 5,* 677–691.

Michals, K., Azen, C., Acosta, P., et al. (1988). Blood phenylalanine levels and intelligence of 10-year-old children with PKU in the National Collaborative Study. *Journal of the American Dietetic Association 88,* 1226–1129.

Msall, M., Batshaw, M.L., Suss, R., et al. (1984). Neurologic outcome in children with inborn errors of urea synthesis: Outcome of urea-cycle enzymopathies. *The New England Journal of Medicine, 310,* 1500–1505.

Mordekar, S.R., & Baxter, P.S. (2004). 'Cerebral palsy' due to mitochondrial cytopathy. *Journal of Paediatrics and Child Health, 40,* 714–5.

Morrone, A., Malvagia, S., Donati, M.A., et al. (2002). Clinical findings and biochemical and molecular analysis of four patients with holocarboxylase synthetase deficiency. *American Journal of Medical Genetics, 111,* 10–18.

Moser, H., Dubey, P., & Fatemi, A. (2004). Progress in X-linked adrenoleukodystrophy. *Current Opinion in Neurology, 17,* 263–269.

Muenzer, J., & Fisher, A. (2004). Advances in the treatment of mucopolysaccharidosis type I. *The New England Journal of Medicine, 350,* 1932–1934.

Nutrition Committee of the Canadian Paediatric Society. (1990). Megavitamin and megamineral therapy in childhood. *Canadian Medical Association Journal, 143,* 1009–1013.

Nyhan, W.L. (1997). The recognition of Lesch-Nyhan syndrome as an inborn error of purine metabolism. *Journal of Inherited Metabolic Disease, 20,* 171–178.

Oerbeck B., Sundet K., Kase B.F., et al. (2003). Congenital hypothyroidism: Influence of disease severity and L-thyroxine treatment on intellectual, motor, and school-associated outcomes in young adults. *Pediatrics, 112,* 923–930.

Palma Sisto, P.A. (2004). Endocrine disorders in the neonate. *Pediatric Clinics of North America, 51,* 1141–1168.

Platt, F.M., Jeyakumar, M., Andersson, U., et al. (2001). Inhibition of substrate synthesis as a strategy for glycolipid lysosomal storage disease therapy. *Journal of Inherited Metabolic Disease, 24,* 275–290.

Raper, S.E., Chirmule, N., Lee, F.S., et al. (2003). Fatal systemic inflammatory response syndrome in a ornithine transcarbamylase deficient patient following adenoviral gene transfer. *Molecular Genetics and Metabolism, 80*(1–2), 148–158.

Rinaldo, P., Tortorelli, S., & Matern, D. (2004). Recent developments and new applications of tandem mass spectrometry in newborn screening. *Current Opinion in Pediatrics, 16,* 427–433.

Rohr, F., Munier, A., Sullivan, D., et al. (2004). The Resource Mothers Study of Maternal Phenylketonuria: Preliminary findings. *Journal of Inherited Metabolic Disease, 27,* 145–155.

Rouse, B., & Azen, C. (2004). Effect of high maternal blood phenylalanine on offspring congenital anomalies and developmental outcome at ages 4 and 6 years: The importance of strict dietary control preconception and throughout pregnancy. *The Journal of Pediatrics, 144,* 235–239.

Rovet, J.F. (2005). Children with congenital hypothyroidism and their siblings: Do they really differ? *Pediatrics, 115,* e52–e57.

Scaglia, F., Towbin, J.A., Craigen, W.J., et al. (2004). Clinical spectrum, morbidity, and mortality in 113 pediatric patients with mitochondrial disease. *Pediatrics, 114,* 925–931.

Shih, V.E. (1976). Hereditary urea-cycle disorders. In S. Grisolia, R. Baguena, & F. Mayor (Eds.), *The urea cycle* (pp. 367–414). Hoboken, NJ: John Wiley & Sons.

Thorburn, D.R. (2004). Mitochondrial disorders: Prevalence, myths and advances. *Journal of Inherited Metabolic Disease, 27,* 349–362.

van der Kamp, H.J., & Wit, J.M. (2004). Neonatal screening for congenital adrenal hyperplasia. *European Journal of Endocrinology, 151*(Suppl. 3), U71–U75.

Waisbren, S.E., Mahon, B.E., Schnell, R.R., et al. (1987). Predictors of intelligence quotient and intelligence quotient change in persons treated for phenylketonuria early in life. *Pediatrics, 79,* 351–355.

Wanders, R.J. (2004). Metabolic and molecular basis of peroxisomal disorders: A review. *American Journal of Medical Genetics Part A, 126,* 355–375.

Wilcox, W.R. (2004). Lysosomal storage disorders: The need for better pediatric recognition and comprehensive care. *The Journal of Pediatrics, 144*(5, Suppl.), S3–S14.

Wraith, E.J., Hopwood, J.J., Fuller, M., et al. (2005). Laronidase treatment of mucopolysaccharidosis I. *BioDrugs, 19,* 1–7.

Wraith, J.E. (2002). Lysosomal disorders. *Seminars in Neonatology, 7,* 75–83.

21 Behavioral and Psychiatric Disorders in Children with Disabilities

Adelaide Robb and Mark Reber

> Upon completion of this chapter, the reader will
>
> - Understand that individuals with developmental disabilities have a relatively high prevalence of psychiatric disorders
> - Be able to describe the types and symptoms of psychiatric disorders among people with developmental disabilities
> - Be able to discuss interventions in children who have a dual diagnosis of a developmental disability and a psychiatric disorder

Children with developmental disabilities face all of the challenges faced by children with typical development and manifest the range of psychiatric illnesses that typically developing children do, but they may also face psychiatric illnesses specific to their disorder. The presence of a developmental disability, especially intellectual disability, often alters the symptomatic presentation of psychiatric disorders and makes accurate diagnosis more difficult. Recognition of these problems with developmental transitions and psychiatric disorders is crucial for caregivers of these children. When these disorders go unrecognized or untreated, children can fail in educational and social settings, be unmanageable at home, and show aggression and self-injury. These comorbid conditions may ultimately determine children's outcome and placement. If the conditions are identified early, however, treatment can be started and long-term adverse effects minimized. It is a distinct challenge for parents and individuals who work with children with disabilities to be alert to the possible presence of a psychiatric disorder and obtain early diagnosis and treatment. This chapter addresses developmental transitions, as well as identification and treatment of behavioral and psychiatric disorders in children with disabilities.

WILLIAM

William, age 14, has Asperger syndrome, attention-deficit/hyperactivity disorder (ADHD), and obsessive-compulsive disorder (OCD). He was in a special educational setting for high school students with Asperger syndrome and was being treated with two **antipsychotic medications,** a mood stabilizer, a **stimulant,** and the selective **serotonin reuptake inhibitor** (SSRI) fluoxetine (Prozac). He had been stable for a long period with resolution of his previous psychiatric symptoms, so the family asked that his medication regimen be simplified. In consultation with his family, the child psychiatrist began slowly tapering off the mood stabilizers, antipsychotic medications, and the SSRI. Eight months into this process, the school and parents noted that William had become withdrawn and sad over 4 weeks. He was crying at school, not eating lunch or dinner, no longer playing or reading favorite books, not sleeping at night, and saying that he was a bad person who should be dead. The psychiatrist restarted William on a higher dose of Prozac (which had originally been prescribed to treat OCD symptoms). Over the next 2 weeks, William started smiling and eating again. His sleep improved, and he was back to being himself by the end of 4 weeks.

PREVALENCE AND CAUSES OF PSYCHIATRIC DISORDERS AMONG CHILDREN WITH DEVELOPMENTAL DISABILITIES

In their landmark study of the epidemiology of childhood psychiatric disorders on the Isle of Wight, Rutter, Graham, and Yule (1970) found emotional disturbances in 7%–10% of typically developing children. Yet, 30%–42% of children with intellectual disability demonstrated psychiatric disorders (Rutter et al., 1970). In a Swedish study, Gillberg et al. (1986) found that 57% of children and adolescents with mild intellectual disability and 64% with severe intellectual disability met diagnostic criteria for a psychiatric disorder (Gillberg et al. 1986). Additional studies have confirmed these results, indicating a four- or five-fold increase in the prevalence of psychiatric disorder in children with intellectual disability and the absence of any decline in frequency with age (Borthwick-Duffy, 1994; Bregman, 1991; Koller et al., 1983).

Children both with and without developmental disabilities are at risk for the same types of psychiatric disorders. However, certain maladaptive behavior disorders—stereotypic movement disorder (i.e., repetitive, self-stimulating, nonfunctional motor behavior, which may include self-injurious behavior [SIB]) and pica (i.e., the persistent ingesting of nonfood items)—are found principally among individuals with severe to profound levels of intellectual disability.

In some cases, the cause of psychiatric disorders in individuals with developmental disabilities is the direct result of a biochemical abnormality. For example, in the inborn error of metabolism Lesch-Nyhan syndrome (see Appendix B), abnormalities in the dopamine neurotransmitter system cause affected individuals to exhibit a compulsive form of SIB (Zimmerman, Jinnah, & Lockhart, 1998). In other cases, conditions that affect the developing brain are risk factors for psychiatric disorder. Among such conditions are prenatal exposure to alcohol sufficient to cause alcohol-related neurodevelopmental disorder (see Chapter 5), congenital infections, Chapter 6, such as rubella (which is associated with autism spectrum disorders [ASDs]), and perinatal or neonatal hypoxic-ischemic encephalopathy (brain disorders due to lack of oxygen or blood flow) (see Chapter 4). The increased risk of psychiatric disturbance in neurobiological disorders may be attributable to factors such as irritability, affective instabil-ity, distractibility, and communication impairments (Feinstein & Reiss, 1996). Risk may also increase in the presence of conditions such as epilepsy, developmental language disorders, and sensory impairments, which are independently associated with an increased incidence of psychiatric disorders.

The cause of most psychiatric disorders among children with developmental disabilities is likely, however, to be a complex interaction among biological (including genetic), environmental, and psychosocial factors. For example, a young man who has sustained a significant traumatic brain injury (see Chapter 30) with resulting cognitive impairment may become depressed because of a combination of neurotransmitter changes due to brain injury, a familial predisposition to depression, his parents' grief, and his own despair over loss of previous abilities.

PSYCHIATRIC DISORDERS OF CHILDHOOD AND ADOLESCENCE

The following sections cover a number of psychiatric disorders described in the *Diagnostic and Statistical Manual of Mental Disorders, Fourth Edition, Text Revision* (*DSM-IV-TR*; American Psychiatric Association, 2000). Two important disorders, ASDs and ADHD, are not discussed here because separate chapters are devoted to these conditions (see Chapters 23 and 24).

Oppositional Defiant and Conduct Disorders

In order for a child to be diagnosed with oppositional defiant disorder (ODD), there must be a pattern of negative, hostile, and defiant behaviors lasting for at least 6 months. Children must have at least four of the following eight symptoms: 1) often loses temper, 2) often argues with adults, 3) often breaks rules or fails to comply with adult requests, 4) deliberately annoys people, 5) blames others for one's mistakes, 6) is touchy or easily annoyed, 7) is angry and resentful, and 8) is spiteful and vindictive. These behaviors must occur outside of a psychotic or mood disorder, and they must cause impaired function at home and/or school. This diagnosis is usually given to preadolescent children.

To be diagnosed with a conduct disorder (CD), an individual must demonstrate a pattern of behavior in which other people's rights are violated, norms are ignored, or rules are broken. This behavior must have occurred for at least 12 months. The four main problem areas are 1) aggression to people and animals, 2) destruction of property, 3) deceitfulness or theft, and 4) serious violation of rules. Aggression includes bullying and threatening, starting physical fights, using a weapon in fights, being physically cruel to people or animals, stealing while confronting a victim, and forcing someone into sexual activity. Destruction includes deliberate fire setting or destruction of property. Deceitfulness or theft includes breaking into a house or car, lying to obtain goods or services, and stealing or shoplifting. Serious violation of rules includes staying out at night (but not overnight) before age 13, running away from home overnight at least twice, and frequent truancy from school before age 13. Conduct disorders are rarely diagnosed in preadolescent children. If someone meets criteria for conduct disorder, he or she does not receive a concurrent diagnosis of ODD.

Both of these disorders are often associated with ADHD, and the treatment for one may improve the co-morbid condition as well (Kutcher et al., 2004). Treatment of both CD and ODD includes the use of the same behavior management techniques that are useful in ADHD. Similarly, both disorders may benefit from stimulant and other ADHD medication (Connor, Barkley, & Davis, 2000). The difference is that although stimulant medication is the treatment of choice for ADHD, behavioral therapy is the preferred treatment for ODD and CD. Behavioral therapy involves setting consistent limits, behavioral expectations, and consequences for violating the limits. This intervention must be similar at home and school so that the child knows that the rules are in force for all settings. For young children, a positive reinforcement system employing stickers and/or a behavior chart targeting two principal areas, being respectful and following directions, can cover most rules and activities during the day (see Chapter 35). Achieving a certain number of stickers or "yeses" on the behavior chart leads to praise and a small reward, such as participation in an activity with the parent after school. Some special education programs also give children a chance to go to a "prize closet" at the end of a week following five "good days." Prizes might include a fun pencil or eraser. For older children and adolescents, tokens are used to reinforce following rules. These can be traded for desired activities, such as an extra 30 minutes of television or free computer time. In this way, adolescents earn and pay for

their privileges in the same way that adults use wages to buy what they need or want.

Impulse Control Disorders

These disorders include intermittent explosive disorder and trichotillomania. Intermittent explosive disorder is diagnosed after there are several discrete episodes of failure to resist aggressive impulses, with resultant assaults or destruction of property. The severity of the assault must be out of proportion to the precipitating psychosocial stressor. An example might be a child who is told that he cannot have cake until he has finished his lunch. The child then throws his plate across the room, breaks his chair, and start kicking his little sister over the incident. In the literature, treatment of intermittent explosive disorder in adults includes the use of **beta-blockers** such as propranolol, certain antiepileptic/mood stabilizing drugs (e.g., valproic acid [Depakote]), and novel antipsychotics (e.g., risperidone [Risperdal]) (Jenkins, & Maruta, 1987). Children with mild to moderate intellectual disability are more likely to have this disorder than their typically developing peers.

Trichotillomania involves the recurrent pulling out of hair (anywhere on body) that is noticeable. It is not associated with an underlying skin or physical condition causing hair loss. Consultation with a dermatologist to rule out skin problems such as tinea capitis (ringworm), which can cause hair loss, may be appropriate. There is a sense of tension that makes the child pull out the hair and a sense of relief after this is done. Children who have trichotillomania may eat the hair, which can cause bezoars (hair balls) in the stomach or gastrointestinal track that need to be surgically or endoscopically removed. In children with hair loss, it is important to ask the parent and child if the child is pulling out and eating hair. Treatment of this disorder is similar to that for OCD, with the use of SSRIs (e.g., fluoxetine) and cognitive-behavioral therapy. There are numerous manuals for the use of cognitive behavioral therapy in pediatric psychiatry disorders such as the manuals used for two National Institute of Mental Health (NIMH) studies: 1) the Treatment of Adolescent Depression Study (TADS) for adolescent depression (TADS Team, 2004), and 2) the Pediatric OCD Treatment Study (POTS) (POTS Team, 2004). In treating patients who are young or have more cognitive impairment, the manuals can be simplified to suit the person's developmental level.

Anxiety Disorders

Anxiety disorders include the *DSM-IV-TR* classifications Generalized Anxiety Disorder, **Panic Disorder**, Social Phobia, OCD, and **Posttraumatic Stress Disorder (PTSD)**.

Generalized Anxiety Disorder

The diagnosis of generalized anxiety disorder, including overanxious disorder of childhood, requires at least 6 months of excessive anxiety and worry about many events or situations such as school, play, sports, friends, and family. It is hard to control the worry, and the child has symptoms that accompany the worry including restlessness or feeling keyed up, being easily fatigued, having problems concentrating, and experiencing irritability, muscle tension, and disturbed sleep. There are problems at home or school because of the anxiety, and it is unrelated to another psychiatric or medical illness. Treatment includes cognitive-behavioral therapy to reduce worry and at times medication such as SSRIs. One paper in the literature reported on the use of sertraline (Zoloft) in the treatment of generalized anxiety disorder in children (Rynn, Siqueland, & Rickels, 2001), and a second paper reported on the use of fluvoxamine (Luvox) for several anxiety disorders in children (Walkup et al., 2001). Both papers showed that these medications were safe and effective in treating this disorder.

Panic Disorder

Panic attacks do not usually begin until puberty. They consist of recurrent and unexpected episodes combined with worry about having more panic attacks, worry about the consequence of an attack (e.g., that the child might die or go crazy), or a significant change in behavior due to the attacks (e.g., stopping exercising because of a fast heartbeat, rapid breathing, and sweating—feeling like a heart attack). Panic attacks include at least four of the symptoms listed in Table 21.1. Because these symptoms can mimic other disorders such as heart problems, stomach disorders, seizures, and asthma, appropriate treatment is often delayed while the child is sent to specialists to rule out medical causes. In patients with panic disorder, there is often a history of anxiety disorder or panic attacks in other family members. Adolescents with panic disorder may begin to avoid certain places or situations such as crowds, public transportation, and other places where a

Table 21.1. Symptoms of Panic Disorder

1. Rapid or racing heartbeat
2. Sweating, trembling, or shaking
3. Feeling short of breath or as if smothering
4. Feeling as if choking
5. Chest pain or discomfort
6. Nausea or abdominal distress
7. Feeling dizzy, lightheaded, or faint
8. Feeling of unreality or detachment (like floating or in a dream)
9. Fear of losing control or going crazy
10. Fear of dying
11. Numbness and tingling
12. Hot flashes or chills

Note: At least four symptoms need to be present during an attack for a diagnosis of panic disorder.

panic attack could occur. This avoidance can lead to comorbid agoraphobia (fear of leaving the house). Patients with panic disorder can be treated with high-potency benzodiazepines such as alprazolam (Xanax) and clonazepam (Klonopin) alone or in combination with SSRIs. Patients with panic disorder can also be helped through cognitive-behavioral therapy to develop a list of things that are least to most likely to cause a panic attack. Patients then work their way through the list, facing the different issues that cause the attacks. The therapist helps the adolescent ride out the attacks and observes how the anxiety decreases over time.

Social Phobia

A **phobia** particularly relevant to children is social phobia, which includes school phobia. Social phobia involves a marked and persistent fear of one or more social or performance situations in which a person is exposed to strangers or to scrutiny by others and worries that he or she will do something embarrassing. To be diagnosed with this disorder, a child must have appropriate relationships with family members and friends but be afraid of other peers and adults. Exposure to the social situation (e.g., a birthday party) provokes anxiety and the child may cry, have a tantrum, freeze, or shrink from situations with unfamiliar people. The child may not be aware that the fear is unreasonable, and the fear must cause an impairment in social functioning. Social phobia is classified as generalized if it takes place in multiple settings. The symptoms must last for more than 6 months. Treatment includes cognitive-behavioral therapy to reduce anxiety in social situations, speech making and acting classes for people with performance anxieties, and the use of SSRIs. Extreme cases of social phobia in childhood may include children who are too frightened to speak in the classroom, eat in the cafeteria, or use the restroom at school. This can lead to a marked impairment in school performance and should not be dismissed as simple shyness. Some children with a variant of social phobia may have selective mutism, in which they refuse to speak to unfamiliar people or children; SSRIs may be helpful in this case (Black & Udhe, 1994). Girls with fragile X syndrome have been found to have severe shyness that may be a manifestation of social phobia (Hagerman et al., 1992).

Obsessive-Compulsive Disorder A child with OCD has obsessions, compulsions, or both. Obsessions are recurrent thoughts, images, or impulses that are experienced as intrusive and inappropriate and cause anxiety or distress. The obsessions are not excessive worries about real-life problems (as in generalized anxiety), and the individual attempts to ignore, suppress, or neutralize the obsessions. Children may not be aware that the obsessions and compulsions are unreasonable; furthermore, children with a developmental disability may not realize that the obsessions are a product of the mind. Compulsions are repetitive behaviors (e.g., hand washing) or mental acts (e.g., praying, counting) that are done to neutralize an obsession or as part of following rigid rules. A child with obsessions about germs would have washing compulsions to neutralize the germs. The compulsions are designed to reduce distress or to prevent some dreaded act. For example, a child might refuse to step on green tiles in the school corridor because his or her mother might die if the child stepped on green tiles. Children, especially younger ones, are more likely to have compulsions without the accompanying obsessions; thus, a child might have an elaborate 2-hour bedtime ritual without knowing why it must be done in a certain way. Some children develop the rapid onset of OCD after a streptococcal skin or throat infection. Common compulsions in children include ordering and arranging, counting, tapping, touching, and collecting/hoarding. In order to meet the *DSM-IV-TR* criteria for the diagnosis, the obsessions and compulsions must occupy more than 1 hour per day and interfere with functioning.

Treatment of OCD in children and adolescents includes cognitive-behavioral therapy, which is aimed at experiencing the obsessive thought without carrying out the compulsion designed to reduce the anxiety. This form of cognitive-behavioral therapy is called exposure and response prevention. A child with fear of germs would be asked to touch a doorknob and then be prevented from washing her hands. Children have weekly assignments in this therapy. Several medications are also approved for the treatment of OCD including clomipramine (Anafranil), sertraline (Zoloft), fluoxetine (Prozac) and fluvoxamine (Luvox) (DeVaugh-Geiss et al., 1992; Geller et al., 2001; March, Biederman, et al., 1998; Riddle et al., 2001). One paper in the literature described the difference in outcome among children with OCD who were treated with sertraline, placebo, cognitive-behavioral therapy, and a combination of medication and therapy (POTS Team, 2004). Combination therapy helped the most children, followed by cognitive-behavioral therapy alone, then sertraline, and placebo. OCD can be comorbid with other developmental disabilities, especially ADHD and ASDs.

Posttraumatic Stress Disorder PTSD is an anxiety disorder that occurs after exposure to a traumatic event in which the person experiences or witnesses an actual or threatened death, serious injury, or threat. In children with developmental disabilities, this may occur after physical abuse or after the injury that caused the disability. Children with intellectual disability are particularly at risk for PTSD, as they have more limited coping skills. The person's response to the inciting event involves intense fear, helplessness, or horror, and the child may have disorganized or agitated behavior. For a diagnosis of PTSD, one must have symptoms for at least 1 month and have impairment of functioning as a result of the symptoms. The symptoms are broken down into three categories: 1) reexperiencing the trauma, 2) avoidance and numbing, and 3) increased arousal. Reexperiencing behavior includes recurrent recollections of the event (in children, this may manifest as a repetitive theme in play), dreams of the event (children may have distressing dreams that are not trauma specific), flashbacks of the event (children may reenact the trauma), intense mental distress at physical or mental cues that remind one of the event, and physiological reactivity on exposure to cues that remind one of the event. Avoidance behavior includes efforts to avoid thoughts or feelings associated with the trauma, efforts to avoid people and places associated with the trauma, inability to recall important aspects of the trauma, decreased interest or participation in activities, feelings of detachment or estrangement, restricted range of feelings, and a sense of a shortened future. Symptoms of increased arousal include difficulty sleeping, irritability or angry outbursts, difficulty concentrating, hypervigilance, and an exaggerated startle response. PTSD is characterized by duration, either acute (3 months or less) or chronic (more than 3 months), and by delayed onset (starts 6 months after the stressor).

Treatment of PTSD includes both **psychotherapy** and SSRIs (March, Amaya-Jackson, et al., 1998). Patients must practice talking through the thoughts and events that remind them of the incident that elicited the PTSD. Play therapy, in which a child has a chance to relive and triumph over the trauma, may also help the child work through the loss. Therapy must be modified based on the cognitive level of the child.

Mood Disorders

Major Depression   Children carrying a diagnosis of **major depression** must have a 2-week period with at least five of the following symptoms that represent a change from previous functioning: 1) depressed mood by subjective report or as observed by others (children and adolescents may have an irritable mood), 2) decreased interest or pleasure in most activities, 3) significant change in weight or appetite (children may fail to make expected weight gains), 4) insomnia or hypersomnia (excessive sleep), 5) psychomotor agitation or retardation, 6) fatigue or loss of energy, 7) feelings of worthlessness or guilt, 8) decreased concentration or indecisiveness, and 9) recurrent thoughts of death and dying. Symptoms must not be due to bereavement and must cause impairment in the child's daily function. Children with major depression can be treated with medication or psychotherapy or a combination of both. Studies have shown that several SSRIs are superior to a placebo in the treatment of depression (Emslie et al., 2002; Wagner et al., 2003; Wagner et al., 2004). A NIMH study found that for adolescents with major depression, a placebo and cognitive-behavioral therapy alone were similar in improvement, whereas fluoxetine was better, and fluoxetine plus cognitive-behavioral therapy had the best outcome (TADS Team, 2004).

Bipolar Disorder   Bipolar disorder consists of swings between depression and **mania** or both together (mixed bipolar disorder). A manic episode consists of a distinct period of abnormally and persistently elevated, expansive, or irritable mood lasting at least 1 week. The mood disturbance must have three of the following symptoms if happy and four if irritable: 1) inflated self-esteem or grandiosity, 2) decreased need for sleep, 3) more talkative or pressured speech or vocalizations (in nonverbal children), 4) flight of ideas or racing thoughts, 5) distractibility, 6) increased goal directed activity or psychomotor agitation, and 7) excessive involvement in pleasurable activities that have a high potential for painful consequences (e.g., sexual touching of self and others). A mixed episode is diagnosed when criteria are met for both manic and major depressive episodes nearly every day for 1 week. Hypomania consists of symptoms of mania without impairment or hospitalization, fewer symptoms, or duration of symptoms for less than 1 week.

Individuals with bipolar disorder are treated with mood stabilizers such as lithium or valproic acid (Depakote, which is also used as an antiepileptic drug). They may also benefit from antipsychotic medication such as risperidone (Risperdal), aripiprazole (Abilify), olanzapine (Zyprexa), quetiapine (Seroquel), and ziprasidone (Geodon) in conjunction with mood stabilizers or as monotherapy (use of antipsychotics alone rather than in combination with a primary mood stabilizer such as lithium or valproic acid). Children with bipolar disorder must have consistent bedtimes and routines so that lack of sleep does not precipitate either a manic or mixed episode.

Psychotic Disorders

Psychotic disorders consist of alterations in thinking or perceptions that are not connected with reality. The primary psychotic disorder is **schizophrenia.** It consists of two or more of the following symptoms that are present for at least a 1-month period, less if treated: 1) **delusions** (fixed idiosyncratic false belief; e.g., that someone is following the person), 2) hallucinations (sensory perception without stimulus; e.g., hearing a voice when no one else is present), 3) disorganized speech and grossly disorganized or catatonic (statue-like) behavior, and 4) negative symptoms (apathy, lack of emotions, poor or nonexistent social functioning). Only one criterion needs to be met if the delusions are bizarre, the voice keeps a running commentary on the person's behavior, or two or more voices are conversing with each other. Patients with a mood disorder or an ASD may have symptoms that are confused with schizophrenia. Other medical conditions that can mimic schizophrenia include epilepsy, effects of an illegal drug, and brain tumors. Once the diagnosis has been confirmed, treatment with antipsychotics will reduce the delusions and hallucinations, thereby improving psychosocial functioning.

Eating Disorders

Two important types of eating disorders occur in children with developmental disabilities, rumination and binge eating. In rumination disorder, infants or young children repeatedly regurgitate without nausea or gastrointestinal illness for at least 1 month. It is a common form of self-stimulatory behavior in children with moderate to severe intellectual disability. Treatment includes behavioral interventions and the use of gastrointestinal motility agents (e.g., laxatives). The second common eating disorder is binge eating, whereby the child eats large amounts of food during short periods of time. Individuals with binge eating disorder do not engage in the accompanying purging behaviors seen in bulimia and do not have a distortion of body image. Children who do binge are at risk for choking and death from this eating pattern. In Prader-Willi syndrome, binge eating is a frequent complication and contributes to the morbid obesity seen among people with this disorder. Children with binge eating disorder need nutritional guidance and counseling, parental and school oversight of meals, limited access to food outside of meals, and an exercise routine. For some children with a severe binge eating disorder, admission to a long-stay residential setting with strict oversight of meals and activity levels can dramatically change the child's weight and improve the underlying medical condition.

Adjustment Disorders

These disorders involve the development of emotional or behavioral symptoms in response to an identifiable stressor and occur within 3 months of the onset of that stressor. The symptoms or behaviors are clinically significant and cause marked distress, in excess of what would be expected from exposure to the stressor, or

significant impairment in social or occupational (academic) functioning. With the exception of an ASD, individuals do not have another major psychiatric disorder and do not have bereavement. Once the stressor ends, the symptoms do not persist for more than 6 months. Adjustment Disorder with Anxiety has symptoms such as nervousness, worry, or jitteriness or, in children, fears of separation from parents. Adjustment Disorder with Depressed Mood includes depressed mood, tearfulness, or hopelessness as the predominant symptoms. Adjustment Disorder with Mixed Emotions and Conduct manifests as altered emotions, such as depression or anxiety, plus problematic behavior such as truancy, vandalism, reckless driving, or fighting.

Children with developmental disabilities may be at higher risk for adjustment disorders because they have limited coping skills and frequently have medical illnesses or require procedures that produce stress. When children with developmental disabilities enter the hospital for a medical procedure or illness, parents, caregivers, and health care providers must be prepared for exaggerated emotional and behavioral responses to being in the hospital and to being kept away from their normal routine. Children may cry, have tantrums, or act out. They may alternatively become quiet and withdrawn, refusing to eat or cooperate with the staff. Patience and reassurance will generally help the child navigate the stressful situation and return to his or her baseline emotional and behavioral functioning.

Maladaptive Behavior Disorders

Some individuals with severe to profound levels of intellectual disability develop behavioral symptoms that are qualitatively different from those seen in people without developmental disabilities. These symptoms, which include repetitive self-stimulating behavior, SIB, and pica, rarely occur in typically developing children.

Individuals who engage in SIB generally display a specific pattern for producing injury. They may bang their heads, bite their hands, pick at their skin, hit themselves with their fists, or poke their eyes. They may do this once or twice a day, in association with tantrums, or as often as several hundred times an hour. Tissue destruction, infection, internal injury, loss of vision, and even death may result. These behaviors may be accompanied by additional repetitive, stereotyped behaviors, such as hand waving and body rocking. When these repetitive behaviors interfere with activities of daily living or result in significant injury to the individual, a diagnosis of stereotypic movement disorder with SIB is made.

Although serious SIB occurs in fewer than 5% of people with intellectual disability, these behaviors cause enormous distress to the individuals and their caregivers, can result in severe body injury, and may lead to residential placement with the separation of the individual from the family and from other community contacts. Some children with SIB also demonstrate severe aggressive behavior toward their caregivers or peers.

SIB is a puzzling and disturbing phenomenon that prompts one to ask why these individuals hurt themselves. Although no simple answer exists, there is evidence for both environmental and biological causes, in a context of enormous individual variation (Buitelaar, 1993; Mace & Mauk, 1995; Schroeder et al., 1999). Some children exhibit SIB as a result of environmental events (i.e., **operant control;** Loschen & Osman, 1992). For example, a girl who is nonverbal may demonstrate head banging that is reinforced once she learns that this action captures the attention she craves. Other environmental factors that can reinforce this behavior include access to desired items (e.g., food), avoidance of task demands (e.g., chores), and certain sensory effects (e.g., bright lights from eye pressing; Mace & Mauk, 1995). The inference that the sensations produced through self-induced painful stimulation may somehow be gratifying has led to the notion that SIB plays a role in regulating physiologic states, such as arousal. Guess and Carr (1991) proposed a biobehavioral model in which the regulation of normal sleep, wake, and arousal patterns is delayed or disturbed in some individuals (Guess & Carr, 1991). These individuals then develop stereotypic movements and SIB as a way to self-regulate arousal in under- or overstimulating environments; they ultimately also get environmental reinforcement for the behavior. There is also a relationship between SIB and pain in nonverbal children with severe cognitive impairment. These children have been found to increase their SIB during an ear infection, constipation, or other conditions associated with pain (Breau et al., 2003). Other biological factors are suggested by the increased prevalence of SIB in certain genetic syndromes, including de Lange syndrome, Lesch-Nyhan syndrome, Prader-Willi syndrome, and Rett syndrome

(see Appendix B). Psychiatric disorders such as ASDs, depression, mania, and schizophrenia are also risk factors for SIB. General medical conditions and medication side effects can be acute precipitants of SIB. For example, a painful middle-ear infection may lead to head banging. Evaluating any individual for the cause of SIB demands the systematic testing of a broad range of behavioral and biomedical hypotheses (Sternberg, Taylor, & Babkie, 1994).

Although the brain mechanisms underlying most forms of SIB remain unknown, several neurotransmitters are thought to be involved. These include dopamine, which mediates certain reinforcement systems in the brain; serotonin, the depletion of which is sometimes associated with violent behavior; gamma-aminobutyric acid (GABA), an inhibitory neurotransmitter; and opioids, the brain's natural painkillers (Verhoeven et al., 1999). The atypical antipsychotic risperidone has been found to be useful in treating this disorder (Zarcone et al., 2001) together with applied behavior analysis (Chapter 35). As of 2006, risperidone was FDA approved for the treatment of violent and aggressive behavior, including SIB in individuals with ASDs.

Pica, the persistent craving and ingesting of nonfood items, is a typical behavior of toddlers. When children older than 2 years display pica, however, professionals should explore the possibility that the child has a psychiatric disorder or a nutritional deficiency. It should be noted that pica in older children can also be a typical behavior of people with severe to profound levels of intellectual disability. Irrespective of the cause, pica can seriously affect a child's well-being. It can result in toxicity from ingested materials such as medications or lead-containing plaster or paint chips. It also can cause physical damage to the individual's gastrointestinal tract. Behavior management techniques (see Chapter 35) have been found to be the most effective intervention for pica (Johnson, Hunt, & Siebert, 1994).

EVALUATION

Psychiatric needs can be met only if parents, teachers, and other staff who work with children with disabilities are aware of the possible existence of emotional disturbances. Ideally, the referral for evaluation should be made to mental health professionals (e.g., psychiatrists, psychologists, social workers) with specific training, experience, and expertise in the psychiatric disorders of children with developmental disabilities. Often this requires referral to a specialized tertiary care center with a multidisciplinary team, such as a university hospital. Less experienced mental health professionals who undertake such evaluations should have access to consultation from a specialized center.

The mental health professional first takes a detailed history of the current symptoms and problematic behaviors from parents or other caregivers. For example, identification of recent changes in sleep pattern, appetite, or mood provides important evidence of depression. In addition, an individual and family medical history should be obtained. The family history may reveal, for example, other members with depression. A review of the individual's past medical and psychological assessments may indicate prior behavior or psychiatric problems. Following the history taking, an interview is conducted posing both structured and open-ended questions to the child and parents. If impairments in communication and cognitive skills are significant, the professional can still gain important information from the direct observation of the child both alone and in the presence of the parents (King et al., 1994).

The evaluation should also focus on the social system and setting in which the psychiatric disorder occurs. Thus, the professional should evaluate the current level of family functioning by assessing 1) family members' ability to cope with the child's psychiatric disorder and therapy; 2) their current morale, problem-solving abilities, external social supports, and practical resources (e.g., finances, insurance); 3) the system of beliefs that sustains their efforts; and 4) the stability of the parents' relationship. It is important to understand how individual family members are reacting and adjusting to the child's underlying developmental disability as well as any current mental health problems (see Chapter 40).

Following the comprehensive interview, the child may be referred for psychological testing or behavioral assessment. Although standardized behavior rating scales are available, they are insufficient by themselves as diagnostic tools. A single, structured psychological testing instrument may not be able to cover the range of developmental levels and behavioral baselines exhibited by individuals with developmental disabilities. These instruments are important, however, for confirming or adding to information obtained from the history and interview. They can also be extremely helpful in measuring changes that occur during the course

of intervention (Aman, Burrow, & Wolford, 1995; Demb et al., 1994; Linaker & Helle, 1994; Reiss & Valenti-Hein, 1994).

Standardized rating scales may be combined with a functional behavior analysis. This type of assessment is most useful for children with severe behavioral abnormalities for which specific family or behavior therapies are being considered. Behavior analysis provides direct observation of the child in a natural setting, yielding a clear description of the abnormal behavior itself and its antecedents and consequences (see Chapter 35).

It is important to note that many of the symptoms of a psychiatric disorder can actually be caused by a variety of medical disorders and treatments. For example, hypothyroidism, common in individuals with Down syndrome, can cause emotional disturbances that present as anxiety or depression. In excessive (and sometimes therapeutic) dosages, drugs used to treat associated impairments such as epilepsy can cause symptoms of hyperactivity or depression (Alvarez, 1998). Careful evaluation for medical conditions or drug reactions should be a part of any assessment of new-onset behavioral or psychiatric symptoms.

After the evaluations have been completed, the professional can begin to work to formulate an intervention plan based not only on the psychiatric diagnosis but also on the developmental level of the child, accompanying medical conditions, the family's strengths and challenges, and the needs and limitations of the settings where the child spends his or her time.

TREATMENT

Treatment of psychiatric illness in children and adolescents with developmental disabilities involves some or all of the modalities described in the following sections. Intervention must be tailored to each child's needs at home, at school, and with peers. The treatment modalities utilized may need to be adjusted as the child matures and as his or her needs change.

Educational Interventions

Educational interventions can include a variety of supports to help a child succeed in the classroom (see Chapter 34). Children may be placed in smaller self-contained classes or included in the general education class but with extra aides or a one-to-one helper. When the child becomes upset, the aide can help the child become calm, avoiding the need to leave the classroom. The child may also benefit from therapy sessions with the school counselor and a behavioral psychologist. There should be close collaboration between the school personnel and the child's medical team.

Rehabilitation Therapy

There is evidence that language impairments significantly contribute to the development of certain behavior problems. Some aggressive behaviors and SIBs have been linked to the inability to communicate needs, and teaching functional communication skills has been shown to decrease SIB. Thus, speech-language therapy and training in augmentative and alternative communication systems (see Chapter 22) may be an important part of the intervention program. Similarly, if the child has a physical disability, the pain from contractures, an inability to ambulate, or difficulty reaching for desired objects may lead to behavior and mood alterations. Physical and occupational therapy may result in an improvement in motor function, with associated improvement in behavior and mood.

Psychotherapy

There is ample evidence that various forms of psychological/behavioral therapy (individual, group, and family) can benefit a child or adolescent with developmental disabilities and psychiatric disorders, if it is adapted to the child's mental age and communication abilities (Hollins, Sinason, & Thompson, 1994; Nezu & Nezu, 1994; Sigman, 1985). Table 21.2 shows

different types of psychotherapy and the *DSM-IV-TR* disorders that they are most useful in treating. Goals of therapy are to relieve symptoms and help the child to understand the nature of his or her disability and associated feelings and to gain a recognition of and appreciation for his or her strengths. Psychotherapy, particularly group work, can also enhance social skills and help the child deal with stigmatization, rejection, peer pressure, and attempts at exploitation (American Academy of Child and Adolescent Psychiatry, 1999). Regrettably, individuals with developmental disabilities are seriously underserved regarding psychotherapy, despite the fact that psychotherapy can provide a supportive relationship, help restore self-esteem, and enhance the capacity to recognize and master emotional conflicts and solve problems. Psychotherapy also can be added to behavior therapy and pharmacotherapy when these approaches have not adequately resolved symptoms or improved quality of life. Ideally, the therapist should have expertise in working with individuals with developmental disabilities.

Behavior therapy is perhaps the most widely researched psychotherapeutic intervention for children and adolescents with intellectual disabilities (see Chapter 35). There is extensive literature supporting the effectiveness of behavioral approaches in psychiatric disorders (National Institutes of Health, 1989). When used in conjunction with comprehensive assessment, accurate medical and psychiatric diagnoses, and programmatic intervention, behavior therapy is among the most powerful available interventions. As with other forms of psychotherapy and pharmacotherapy, however,

Table 21.2.   Types of psychotherapy and uses in different disorders

Therapy	Behavior	CBT	Social skills	Group	Individual	Supportive/ educational	Parent training
ADHD	X		X	X			X
ODD and Conduct Disorder	X		X	X			X
Generalized Anxiety Disorder		X			X	X	
Social Phobia		X	X	X	X	X	X
Panic Disorder		X			X	X	
PTSD		X			X	X	
OCD		X			X		
Major Depression		X			X	X	
Bipolar Disorder					X	X	X
ASDs	X		X	X		X	X
Schizophrenia		X			X	X	X

Key: CBT, cognitive-behavioral therapy; ADHD, attention-deficit/hyperactivity disorder; ODD, oppositional defiant disorder; PTSD, posttraumatic stress disorder; OCD, obsessive-compulsive disorder; ASDs, autism spectrum disorders.

it should be implemented only under the supervision of licensed professionals who have been specifically trained in this methodology.

Pharmacotherapy

Medication can play an important role in treating the psychiatric disorders that occur in children with developmental disabilities (Efron et al., 2003). Table 21.3 lists the various medications in each of the groups that are described next. Additional information on uses and side effects of these medications can be found in Appendix C.

Antidepressants Anitdepressants are used to treat major depression and anxiety disorders including OCD, generalized anxiety disorder, and **separation anxiety** disorder (DeVaugh-Geiss et al., 1992; Emslie et al., 2002; Geller et al., 2001; March, Biederman, et al., 1998; Riddle et al., 2001; Wagner et al., 2003; Wagner et al., 2004). The class of antidepressants most commonly used in children and adolescents is the SSRIs. In 2006, the Food and Drug Administration (FDA) required drug companies to start putting "black box" warnings on the packaging of all categories of antidepressants, as well as atomoxetine (Strattera) and quetiapine (Seroquel), which is approved for bipolar depression. The warning states that these medications have been associated, in short-term studies, with a two-fold increase in suicidal ideation and attempts compared to placebo. No suicides have actually been reported. Per the FDA, all children under the age of 18 started on any antidepressant for any indication must be monitored weekly for the first 4 weeks, then biweekly for the second 4 weeks, then monthly. Patients are to be monitored for any change in mental state and for the emergence of suicidal ideation or plans. With these controls in place, antidepressants can continue to be useful in the treatment of pediatric mood and anxiety disorders and remain an important part of treatment for these illnesses (Hammad, Laughren, & Racoosin, 2006).

Antihypertensives Beta-blockers, such as propranolol, are used to treat explosive and aggressive behavior, whereas alpha-2 adrenergic receptor agonists (e.g., clonidine [Catapres], guanfacine [Tenex]) are used to treat tic disorder, Tourette syndrome, and ADHD. These medications are sedating and can also lower blood pressure; thus, they should be used cautiously (Ahmed & Takeshita, 1996).

Antipsychotic Medications Antipsychotic medications have been used primarily to treat aggression and SIB in children with intellectual disability or ASDs. There is, in fact, more safety data on risperidone in children with intellectual disability and ASDs than in their typically developing peers. In 2006 risperidone became the first antipsychotic approved for the treatment of aggressive behavior in individuals with ASD. Many of the other novel neuroleptics have also been studied in individuals with ASDs. Although these medications are much more likely to cause weight gain, they are less likely to cause a movement disorder (Martin et al., 2004; Stigler et al., 2004).

Benzodiazepines Benzodiazepines are helpful in reducing anxiety in the short term. Children with developmental disabilities, however, may have paradoxical reactions to these medications and may become agitated rather than calm and sleepy. Because chronic use of these agents can cause chemical and behavioral dependency, they should not be used for long-term control of anxiety symptoms.

Mood Stabilizers Mood stabilizers include lithium and antiepileptic medication (Findling et al., 2005). They are most commonly used to treat bipolar disorder and aggressive behaviors. Lithium is effective in treating current episodes and in preventing future bipolar episodes. It is a salt that is excreted through the kidneys and causes increased thirst and urination. It must be used with caution in combination with certain other drugs that can lead to toxic lithium levels, including nonsteroidal anti-inflammatory drugs (e.g., ibuprofen) and certain anticonvulsants (e.g., topiramate [Topamax]) that are excreted by the kidneys. Lithium toxicity can occur with rapid onset if normal fluid intake is decreased, for example with vomiting, diarrhea, or acute illness; this in turn can result in coma, kidney failure, or the need for dialysis.

Stimulants and Atomoxetine Stimulants of both the amphetamine and methylphenidate classes are first-line treatments for ADHD. Both families of drugs now have long-acting preparations available that can improve control of ADHD symptoms throughout the day. Side effects include loss of appetite, insomnia, tics, headache, and gastrointestinal side effects (Pearson et al., 2003). The use of atomoxetine has been studied in children with ADHD (Newcorn et al., 2005) and ASDs and has been

Table 21.3. Medications used to treat psychiatric disorders

	Generic name	Trade name	Type	Uses	Other formulations
Antidepressants	Fluoxetine	Prozac, Sarefem	SSRI	Depression, anxiety, OCD	Liquid and weekly
	Fluvoxamine	Luvox	SSRI	OCD	None
	Sertraline	Zoloft	SSRI	Depression, anxiety, OCD	Liquid
	Paroxetine	Paxil, Paxil CR	SSRI	Depression, anxiety, OCD	Liquid (not in CR)
	Citalopram	Celexa	SSRI	Depression	Liquid
	Escitalopram	Lexapro	SSRI	Depression, anxiety	Liquid
	Venlafaxine	Effexor, Effexor XR	SNRI	Depression, anxiety	None
	Duloxetine	Cymbalta	SNRI	Depression	None
	Buproprion	Wellbutrin, Wellbutrin SR, Wellbutrin XL	Dopamin-ergic	Depression, ADHD	None
Antihypertensives	Propranolol	Inderal, Inderal LA	Beta blocker	Aggressive be-havior	None
	Clonidine	Catapres, Cat-apres-TTS patch	Alpha-2-adrenergic agonist	ADHD, tics, sleeping agent	Weekly skin patch
	Guanfacine	Tenex	Alpha-2-adrenergic agonist	ADHD, tics	None
Antipsychotics	Clozapine	Clozaril	Atypical	Treatment-resistant schizophrenia, bipolar disor-der (not FDA approved for acute bipolar mania)	None
	Risperidone	Risperdal, Risperdal M-Tab, Risperdal Consta	Atypical	Schizophrenia, bipolar disor-der, aggres-sive behavior in children with autism spectrum dis-orders	Liquid, oral dis-solving tab-lets (M-Tab), 2-week injec-tion (Consta)
	Olanzapine	Zyprexa, Zyprexa Zydis	Atypical	Schizophrenia, bipolar dis-order, acute agitation	Oral dissolving tablets, daily injection
	Ziprasidone	Geodon	Atypical	Schizophrenia, bipolar disor-der, acute ag-itation	Daily injection
	Quetiapine	Seroquel	Atypical	Schizophrenia, bipolar disor-der (acute mania and bi-polar depres-sion)	None
	Aripiprazole	Abilify Abilify Discmelt	Atypical (plus serotonin agonist)	Schizophrenia, bipolar disor-der	Liquid, oral dissolving tablets

	Generic name	Trade name	Type	Uses	Other formulations
	Haloperidol	Haldol, Haldol Decanoate	Typical	Schizophrenia, Tourette syndrome, agitation, severe behavior disorders	Liquid, daily injection, monthly injection
	Pimozide	Orap	Typical	Tourette syndrome	None
Benzodiazepines	Lorazepam	Ativan	Typical	Anxiety	Liquid, daily injection
	Alprazolam	Xanax, Xanax XR	High potency	Panic, anxiety	None
	Clonazepam	Klonopin, Klonopin Wafers	High potency	Panic, anxiety	Oral dissolving tablets
Mood stabilizers	Lithium carbonate	Lithobid, Eskalith Eskalith-CR	Mood stabilizer	Bipolar disorder (acute mania and maintenance)	Liquid
	Valproic acid	Depakote, Depakote ER, Depacon, Depakene	Antiepileptic drug	Bipolar disorder	Liquid, intravenous, sprinkles
	Carbamazepine	Tegretol, Tegretol XR, Carbatrol, Equetro	Antiepileptic drug	Bipolar disorder	Chewable tablet, liquid
	Oxcarbazepine	Trileptal	Antiepileptic drug	Not FDA approved yet for bipolar disorder, but used	Liquid
	Lamotrigine	Lamictal	Antiepileptic drug	Bipolar maintenance	Chewable tablets
Stimulants and atomoxetine	Methylphenidate -racemic mixture	Ritalin, Ritalin LA, Metadate CD, Concerta	Synthetic stimulant	ADHD	Sprinkles for Ritalin LA and Metadate CD
	Dexmethylphenidate	Focalin, Focalin XR	Synthetic stimulant	ADHD	Sprinkles for XR
	Dextroamphetamine	Dexedrine, Dexedrine ER spansules	Stimulant	ADHD	Chewable generic tablet, ER spansule
	Mixed amphetamine salts	Adderall, Adderall XR	Stimulant	ADHD	Sprinkles for XR
	Modafanil	Provigil, Sparlon	Unknown	ADHD (not FDA approved for ADHD due to concern about Stevens-Johnson syndrome)	None
	Atomoxetine	Strattera	NRI	ADHD	None

Key: SSRI, selective serotonin reuptake inhibitor; OCD, obsessive-compulsive disorder; CR, controlled release; SNRI, serotonin norepinephrine reuptake inhibitor; XR, extended release; SR, slow release; XL, extra long; ADHD, attention-deficit/hyperactivity disorder; LA, long acting; TTS, transdermal system; ER, extended release; FDA, Food and Drug Administration; CD, controlled delivery; NRI, norepinephrine reuptake inhibitor. For further information see Appendix C.

found to control hyperactive/impulsive symptoms with an effect size similar to methylphenidate.

SUMMARY

Children with developmental disabilities are at higher risk of having psychiatric and behavioral disorders at some time during the course of their childhood or adolescence. By being aware of the possibility of psychiatric disorders that can affect a child's behavior, parents, educators, and clinicians can identify the problem early and intervene. Early intervention leads to more rapid resolution of the difficulties and allows the child to function more effectively and happily at home, at school, and in the community.

REFERENCES

Ahmed, I., & Takeshita, J. (1996). Clonidine: A critical review of its role in the treatment of psychiatric disorders. *CNS Drugs, 6*, 53.

Alvarez, N. (1998). Barbiturates in the treatment of epilepsy inpeople with intellectual disability. *Journal of Intellectual Disabilities, 42*(Suppl. 1), 16–23.

Aman, M.G., Burrow, W.H., & Wolford, P.L. (1995). The Aberrant Behavior Checklist Community: Factor validity and effect of subject variables for adults in group homes. *American Journal on Mental Retardation, 100*, 293–294.

American Academy of Child and Adolescent Psychiatry. (1999). Practice parameters for the assessment and treatment of children, adolescents and adults with mental retardation and comorbid mental disorders. *Journal of the American Academy of Child and Adolescent Psychiatry, 38*(Suppl. 12), 5S–31S.

American Psychiatric Association. (2000). *Diagnostic and statistical manual of mental disorders* (4th ed., text rev.). Washington, DC: Author.

Black, B., & Udhe, T. (1994). Treatment of elective mutism with fluoxetine: A double-blind, placebo-controlled study. *Journal of the American Academy of Child and Adolescent Psychiatry, 33*, 1000–1006.

Borthwick-Duffy, S.A. (1994). Epidemiology and prevalence of psychopathology in people with mental retardation. *Journal of Consulting and Clinical Psychology, 62*, 17–27.

Breau, L.M., Camfield, C.S., Symons, F.J., et al. (2003). Relation between pain and self-injurious behavior in nonverbal children with severe cognitive impairments. *The Journal of Pediatrics, 142*(5), 498–503.

Bregman, J.D. (1991). Current developments in the understanding of mental retardation, Part II: Psychopathology. *Journal of the American Academy of Child and Adolescent Psychiatry, 30*, 861–872.

Buitelaar, J.K. (1993). Self-Injurious behavior in retarded children: Clinical phenomena and biological mechanisms. *Acta Paedopsychiatrica, 56*, 105–111.

Connor, D.F., Barkley, R.A., & Davis, H.T. (2000). A pilot study of methylphenidate, clonidine, or the combination in ADHD comorbid with aggressive oppositional defiant or conduct disorder. *Clinical Pediatrics, 39*(1), 15–25.

Demb, H.B., Brier, N., Huron, R., et al. (1994). The adolescent behavior checklist: Normative data and sensitivity and specificity of a screening tool for diagnosable psychiatric disorders in adolescents with mental retardation and other development disabilities. *Research in Developmental Disabilities, 15*, 151–165.

DeVaugh-Geiss, J., Moroz, G., Biederman, J., et al. (1992). Clomipramine hydrochloride in childhood and adolescent obsessive-compulsive disorder: A multicenter trial. *Journal of the American Academy of Child and Adolescent Psychiatry, 31*, 45–49.

Efron, D., Hiscock, H., Sewell, J.R., et al. (2003). Prescribing of psychotropic medications for children by Australian pediatricians and child psychiatrists. *Pediatrics, 111*(2), 372–375.

Emslie, G.J., Heiligenstein, J.H., Wagner, K.D., et al. (2002). Fluoxetine for acute treatment of depression in children and adolescents: A placebo-controlled, randomized clinical trial. *Journal of the American Academy of Child and Adolescent Psychiatry, 41*(10), 1205–1215.

Feinstein, C., & Reiss, A.L. (1996). Psychiatric disorder in mentally retarded children and adolescents: The challenges of meaningful diagnosis. *Child and Adolescents Psychiatric Clinics of North America, 5*, 1031–1037.

Findling, R.L., McNamara, N.K., Youngstrom, E.A., et al. (2005). Double-blind 18-month trial of lithium versus divalproex maintenance treatment in pediatric bipolar disorder. *Journal of the American Academy of Child and Adolescent Psychiatry, 44*(5), 461–469.

Geller, D.A., Hoog, S.L., Heiligenstein, J.H., et al. (2001). Fluoxetine treatment for obsessive-compulsive disorder in children and adolescents: A placebo-controlled clinical trial. *Journal of the American Academy of Child and Adolescent Psychiatry, 40*(7), 773–779.

Gillberg, C., Persson, E., Grufman, M., et al. (1986). Psychiatric disorders in mildly and severely mentally retarded urban children and adolescents: Epidemiological aspects. *British Journal of Psychiatry, 149*, 68–74.

Guess, D., & Carr, E. (1991). Emergence and maintenance of stereotypy and self-injury. *American Journal on Mental Retardation, 96*, 299–320.

Hagerman, R.J., Jackson, C., Amiri, K., et al. (1992). Girls with fragile X syndrome: Physical and neurocognitive status and outcome. *Pediatrics, 89*(3), 395–400.

Hammad, T.A., Laughren, T., & Racoosin, J. (2006). Suicidality in pediatric patients treated with antidepressant drugs. *Archives of General Psychiatry, 63*(3), 332–339.

Hollins, S., Sinason, V., & Thompson, S. (1994). Individual, group and family psychotherapy. In N. Bouras (Ed.), *Mental health in mental retardation*. New York: Cambridge University Press.

Jenkins, S.C., & Maruta, T. (1987). Therapeutic use of propranolol for intermittent explosive disorder. *Mayo Clinic Proceedings, 62*, 204.

Johnson, C.R., Hunt, F.M., & Siebert, M.J. (1994). Discrimination training in the treatment of pica and food scavenging. *Behavior Modification, 18*, 214–229.

King, B.H., DeAntonio, C., McCracken, J.T., et al. (1994). Psychiatric consultation in severe and profound mental retardation. *American Journal of Psychiatry, 151*, 1802–1808.

Koller, H., Richardson, S.W., Katz, M., et al. (1983). Behavioral disturbance since childhood in a 5-year birth cohort of all mentally retarded young adults in a city. *American Journal of Mental Deficiency, 87*, 386–395.

Kutcher, S., Aman, M., Brooks, S.J., et al. (2004). International consensus statement on attention-deficit/

hyperactivity disorder (ADHD) and disruptive behaviour disorders (DBDs): Clinical implications and treatment practice suggestions. *European Neuropsychopharmacology, 14*(1), 11–28.

Linaker, O.M., & Helle, J. (1994). Validity of the schizophrenia diagnosis of the Psychopathology Instrument For Mentally Retarded Adults (PIRMA): A comparison of schizophrenic patients with and without mental retardation. *Research in Developmental Disabilities, 15*, 473–486.

Loschen, E.L., & Osman, O.T. (1992). Self-injurious behavior in the developmentally disabled: Assessment techniques. *Psychopharmacology Bulletin, 28*, 433–438.

Mace, F.C., & Mauk, J.E. (1995). Bio-behavioral diagnosis and treatment of self-injury. *Mental Retardation and Developmental Disabilities Research Reviews, 1*, 104–110.

March, J.S., Amaya-Jackson, L., Murray, M.C., et al. (1998). Cognitive-behavioral psychotherapy for children and adolescents with posttraumatic stress disorder after a single-incident stressor. *Journal of the American Academy of Child and Adolescent Psychiatry, 37*(6), 585–593.

March, J.S., Biederman, J., Wolkow, R., et al. (1998). Sertraline in children and adolescents with obsessive-compulsive disorder: A multicenter randomized controlled trial. *Journal of the American Medical Association, 280*(20), 1752–1756.

Martin, A., Scahill, L., Anderson G.M., et al. (2004). Weight and leptin changes among risperidone-treated youths with autism: 6-month prospective data. *The American Journal of Psychiatry, 161*(6), 1125–1127.

National Institutes of Health. (1989). Treatment of destructive behaviors in persons with developmental disabilities. *NIH Consensus Development Conference Statement, 7*(9), 1–14.

Newcorn, J.H., Spencer, T.J., Biederman, J., et al. (2005). Atomoxetine treatment in children and adolescents with attention-deficit/hyperactivity disorder and comorbid oppositional defiant disorder. *Journal of the American Academy of Child & Adolescent Psychiatry, 44*(3), 240–248.

Nezu, C.M., & Nezu, A.M. (1994). Outpatient psychotherapy for adults with mental retardation and concomitant psychopathology: Research and clinical imperatives. *Journal of Consulting and Clinical Psychology, 62*, 34–42.

Pearson, D.A., Santos, C.W., Roache, J.D., et al. (2003). Treatment effects of methylphenidate on behavioral adjustment in children with intellectual disability and ADHD. *Journal of the American Academy of Child and Adolescent Psychiatry, 42*(2), 209–216.

The Pediatric OCD Treatment Study (POTS) Team. (2004). Cognitive-behavior therapy, sertraline and their combination for children and adolescents with obsessive-compulsive disorder: The pediatric OCD treatment study (POTS) randomized controlled trial. *Journal of the American Medical Association, 292*(16), 1969–1976.

Reiss, S., & Valenti-Hein, D. (1994). Development of a psychopathology rating scale for children with mental retardation. *Journal of Consulting and Clinical Psychology, 62*, 28–33.

Riddle, M.A., Reeve, E.A., Yaryura-Tobias, J.A., et al. (2001). Fluvoxamine for the treatment of anxiety disorders in children and adolescents. *Journal of the American Academy of Child and Adolescent Psychiatry, 40*(2), 222–229.

Rutter, M., Graham, P., & Yule, W. (1970). *A neuropsychiatric study in childhood.* London: Spastics International.

Rynn, M.A., Siqueland, L., & Rickels, K. (2001). Placebo-controlled trial of sertraline in the treatment of children with generalized anxiety disorder. *American Journal of Psychiatry, 158*(12), 2008–2014.

Schroeder, S.R., Reese, R.M., Hellings, J., et al. (1999). The causes of self-injurious behavior and their clinical implications. In N.A. Wieseler & R.H. Hanson (Eds.), *Challenging behavior of persons with mental health disorder and severe developmental disabilities* (pp. 65–87). Washington, DC: American Association on Mental Retardation.

Sigman, M. (1985). Individual and group psychotherapy with mentally retarded adolescents. In M. Sigman (Ed.), *Children with emotional disorder and developmental disabilities* (pp. 259–276). New York: Grune & Stratton.

Sternberg, L., Taylor, R.L., & Babkie, A. (1994). Correlates of interventions with self-injurious behavior. *Journal of Intellectual Disability Research, 38*, 475–485.

Stigler, K.A., Potenza, M.N., Posey D.J., et al. (2004). Weight gain associated with atypical antipsychotic use in children and adolescents: Prevalence, clinical relevance, and management. *Pediatric Drugs, 6*(1), 33–44.

Treatment for Adolescents with Depression Study (TADS) Team. (2004). Fluoxetine, cognitive-behavioral therapy, and their combination for adolescents with depression: Treatment for Adolescents with Depression Study (TADS) randomized controlled trial. *Journal of the American Medical Association, 292*(7), 807–820.

Verhoeven, W.M., Tuinier, S., van den Berg, Y.W., et al. (1999). Stress and self-injurious behavior: Hormonal and serotonergic parameters in mentally retarded subjects. *Pharmacopsychiatry, 32*, 13–20.

Wagner, K.D., Ambrosini, P., Rynn, M., et al. (2003). Efficacy of sertraline in the treatment of children and adolescents with major depressive disorder: Two randomized controlled trials. *Journal of the American Medical Association, 290*(8), 1033–1041.

Wagner, K.D., Robb, A.S., Findling, R.L., et al. (2004). A randomized, placebo-controlled trial of citalopram for the treatment of major depression in children and adolescents. *American Journal of Psychiatry, 161*(6), 1079–1083.

Walkup, J.T., Labellarte, M.J., Riddle, M.A., et al. (2001). Fluvoxamine for the treatment of anxiety disorders in children and adolescents. *Journal of the American Medical Association, 344*(17), 1279–1285.

Zarcone, J.R., Lindauer, S.E., Morse, P.S., et al. (2001). Effects of risperidone on destructive behavior of persons with developmental disabilities: III. Functional analysis. *American Journal on Mental Retardation, 109* 310–321.

Zimmerman, A.W., Jinnah, H.A., & Lockhardt, P.J. (1998). Behavioral neuropharmacology. *Mental Retardation and Developmental Disabilities Research Reviews, 4*, 26–35.

22 Communication Disorders

Sheela Stuart

Upon completion of this chapter, the reader will

- Be able to describe the different elements of speech and of language
- Understand the typical course of language development
- Be familiar with the biological processes that underlie speech and language
- Know the major types of speech and language disorders and their causes
- Be aware of the methods of speech and language assessment
- Recognize the treatment alternatives for these communication disorders

As humans, one of the major means of participating in our lives is through communication. We complain, calm, greet, request, inform, question, praise, compliment, argue, demand, order, correct, beg, invite, cajole (and so the list continues). Although there are many different elaborate, sophisticated, versatile, and creative ways of communicating, the means most frequently used is talking. Therefore, families herald a child's first words with joy, and when there is a problem in the development of his or her ability to talk, anxiety abounds. The following letter is an example of this type of situation.

LETTER FROM A WORRIED GRANDMOTHER

Dear Children's Hospital Professionals: My grandson, David, is 2½ years old. Although as a baby he cooed and babbled and began walking at 12 months, he has never talked. He often grunts and points to things he wants and recently has begun to consistently make a few sounds for "mama," "daddy," "up," "bow wow," and "cup." He has never been seriously ill. He has had some colds and we were afraid these had caused problems with his hearing. However, he recently received a complete audiological evaluation and he hears perfectly.

His pediatrician also recommended that David be evaluated by a speech-language pathologist.

During this evaluation, the therapist played with David while she made a videotape recording of this part of the session. She also tried to get him to say words and imitate animal sounds that she made, and they spent some time looking in the mirror while she tried to get him to imitate facial expressions. She also asked him to look at some pictures in a book and do some things she requested (point to the picture of the baby, put the block in the box, behind the bear, and so forth). In addition, she used a long interview sheet and asked David's mother about many things such as how he plays, what he does to interact with his parents and with other children, whether he follows directives, and so forth. In her report, the speech-language pathologist indicated she had used these instruments: the Rossetti Infant-Toddler Language Scale, the Preschool Language Scale–4, and the MacArthur-Bates Communicative Development Inventories. Her reported conclusion was that David's receptive language was at approximately the 18- to 20-month level and his expressive language was at approximately the 9- to 12-month level.

Although we know what we were told, we do not understand it. Our family handles things much better if we know what's going on. What causes this type of problem? Will David eventually talk? My daughter is considering having a second child.

Is this type of problem likely to occur a second time? Is there anything in addition to the therapy we can do? Thank you in advance for your help.

Sincerely,

A Worried Grandmother

This chapter provides information that addresses these questions. The various aspects that compose talking (speech and language) and their development are described. There also is a discussion of the underlying causes that result in disorders of speech and language. Finally, the focus of therapy and compensatory approaches for overcoming communication disorders are described.

COMPONENTS OF COMMUNICATION

Communication has been studied by many different professionals, including linguists, psychologists, anthropologists, literature scholars, speech-language pathologists, neuropsychologists, and even engineers and biologists. Because each profession's interest in communication comes from a different perspective, the resulting information includes a variety of terminology and at times contrasting viewpoints.

Regardless of the perspective, however, it is agreed that the human brain is the underlying mechanism that supports and coordinates the separate processes of communication. The brain also is a dynamic organ that functions in a varying manner depending upon the age, personal experiences, and even the gender of the individual.

The brain includes interconnected pathways between areas that regulate, integrate, and formulate communicative messages. Many of the specific functions related to hearing, speech, and language are found in the cerebrum (cerebral cortex). The frontal lobe of the cerebrum has the primary motor area and Broca's speech production area. The temporal lobe contains the primary auditory area and Wernicke's speech comprehension area. The occipital lobe is concerned with vision, and the parietal lobe is concerned with somatesthetic (bodily) sensations.

The **neural network** that interconnects the many brain regions makes it possible for auditory, visual, and conceptual brain regions that serve speech and language functions to differ, at least slightly, from one person to the next (Ojemann, 1991). It is useful to understand some general information about the complex activities of understanding language (receptive) and producing language (expressive).

An example of **receptive language** functioning would be when a person hears the word *cup*, the sound signal is transmitted along the auditory pathways, which then sends the signal to Wernicke's area, where neurons that correspond to that particular combination of sounds are activated. Neurons are then activated to store a visual picture of a cup, and other neurons store concepts about how cups are used.

If a person wishes to name the object *cup*, he or she would first activate the internal visual picture of a cup (e.g., shape, uses, materials used for cups). These ideas would be channeled through the speech area of the brain (Broca's area) located in the frontal lobe. Here, these thoughts are converted into patterns of motor movement, then transmitted to the motor strip located in the frontal lobe, where impulses for muscle movement needed to produce the sound /kup/ are transmitted.

To answer David's grandmother's questions, it will be helpful to summarize the basic components that, directed by the brain, provide the basis for listening and talking. Figure 22.1 outlines the components of human communication: hearing, speech (voice and **articulation**), language (including form, which consists of **phonology,** and **grammar,** and function, which consists of **semantics** and **pragmatics**), and **fluency** (rhythm and emphasis).

Hearing

To develop typical speech, children must perceive speech sounds. Normal hearing (see Chapter 12) is also vital so that children have an active model and can monitor and modify what they say. Hearing related to speech and language includes being able to perceive the sounds (auditory perception) and being able to decode the different sounds for meaning (auditory processing). At birth infants are able to listen and discriminate between different speech sounds. A child immediately begins to listen to the stream of speech sounds within his or her environment and begins attaching meaning to these sounds. During his or her first year, the baby will learn to recognize sequences of sounds and word boundaries; among the first recognized words is the child's name (Mandel, Jusczyk, & Pisoni, 1994).

Speech

Speech is the production of articulated sounds and syllables. The areas composing speech are

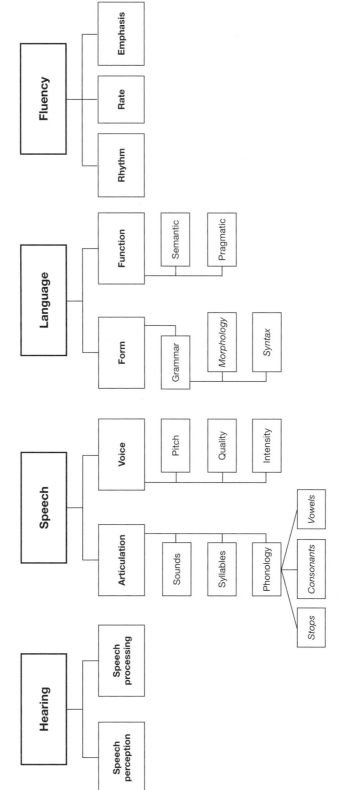

Figure 22.1. Components of human communication.

voice (used to produce the sounds) and articulation (used to shape the sounds). A brief description of voice and articulation follows.

Voice is the sound source for producing words (talking). Breath from the lungs is channeled through the larynx and provides the power source to set the vocal folds vibrating, producing sound. Once voice is produced, the voice sounds must be shaped into specific speech sounds. This process is called articulation. Articulation is the shaping of voice sounds into specific sound patterns by a series of rapid movements of various structures in the mouth including the tongue and lips (forming shapes and coming together or moving apart).

Language

Language is a set of rules regarding form (comprising phonology and grammar) and function (comprising semantics and pragmatics). Form consists of the rules that govern the way in which sounds and words are combined to transmit meaning. Within the area of language form, there are rules for phonology and for grammar. Phonology is part of speech and incorporates the rules for combining types of **phonemes** (i.e., consonants and vowels), pauses, and stress to form words. Grammar incorporates rules for using the smallest meaningful units of language (**morphemes**) and word order (**syntax**) to convey specific information. Syntax consists of the rules governing the order of words used to accomplish different communication functions (e.g., questions, statements, commands).

Function comprises rules governing the use of specific words to convey meaning (semantics) and use of specific words to accomplish communicative functions within personal interactions (pragmatics). Semantics is the system of meaning conveyed by various words, phrases, and sentences. Pragmatics is the rule system for using of language in personal interactions and social situations. Simply put, these rules are guidelines for what to say and when to say it.

Fluency

Achieving the goal of communication through talking also requires that a child produce words in a particular easy, fluid manner. This process is called fluency. Fluency is the joining of sounds, syllables, words, and phrases within oral language without hesitations or repetitions. It involves rate, rhythm, and emphasis.

TYPICAL DEVELOPMENT OF SPEECH AND LANGUAGE

Infants start as preintentional communicators (relying on crying and movement to express needs and wants), become intentional communicators (relying on vocalization, gestures, and facial expression), and finally communicative intent becomes encoded into words and language.

Infants begin listening to speech and language in utero (Querleu & Renard, 1981) and at birth demonstrate a pattern of **phonetic** perception that is universal. By 6 months of age, linguistic experience alters the infant's phonetic perception, equipping him or her with language specific phonetic prototypes and assisting in organizing speech sounds into categories. These phonetic prototypes are now considered to be the building blocks for acquiring word meanings. All of these milestones occur before the end of the first year (Kuhl, 2000).

First words are produced at around 12 months of age and are related to child's world of objects and events. Research (Strauss & Ziv, 2001; Tomasello, 2000) has revealed that the process of acquiring words and expanding language is highly correlated with joint attention, social cognition, and cultural influences. A child's own preferences and tendencies, as well as the caregivers' use of language and the course of communication/interactions throughout each day, contribute to the language acquisition process (Goldfield & Snow, 2005). Implications of individual differences include the recognition that there are many ways to learn a language but that typically developing children arrive at predictable levels of communicative competence by specific ages. These provide the basis for formal testing norms used in assessing language skills. For more information regarding speech and language development and actual examples of typical development at specific ages, see American Speech-Language Hearing Association (ASHA; 2007).

Cultural Diversity and Bilingualism

The United States continues to be an increasingly diverse society. Although English is the dominant language of the United States, many children grow up in homes in which English is neither the first language nor the only language they experience. For children acquiring language in a bilingual/multilingual environment, the acquisition process is more complex, so it is possible that the overall language acquisition could be slower than if the child is exposed to only one language. During the learning process, a child from a bilingual environment may include language forms from the other language. The previously described and other learning behaviors can be misinterpreted, therefore putting a bilingual child at risk for being falsely identified as having a language disorder.

COMMUNICATION DISORDERS AND INTERVENTION APPROACHES

The grandmother's brief description of David's levels of communicative functioning indicates that he has delays in both speech and language development. The grandmother also mentioned some standardized instruments and techniques that were used by the speech-language pathologist in the evaluation session. In addition to conducting the testing described by David's grandmother in the letter, the speech-language pathologist also obtained parental report (including medical history, language environment, and specific concerns) and engaged in direct observation of spontaneous communication and communicative interaction. In addition, the speech-language pathologist obtained reports from other professionals (e.g., developmental pediatrician, occupational therapist, physical ther-

apist) and from preschool and/or child care providers. All of these data were gathered, discussed in depth with the family, and analyzed using systematic methods. The final measurement of David's communication skills was the summary of this information, which provided an approximate level of communicative functioning that was then compared with norms of development for his chronological age. In David's case, receptive language skills were 10–12 months behind and **expressive language** skills were 18 months behind those normed for his chronological age of 30 months. This information provided the basis for the diagnosis of a communication disorder and the need for an intervention plan. Table 22.1 lists some indications that there is a need for referral for speech-language assessment, and Table 22.2 lists commonly used measures of speech and language skills.

Statistically, 5%–10% of all children have a type of speech and language disorder. In some instances, this disorder is a symptom related to another etiology (e.g., hearing loss, cognitive disabilities, and/or syndromes). In addition, recent studies (Fisher, 2005; Fisher, Lai, & Monaco, 2003) have found that a specific type of communication disorder is related to genetic abnormality. Half of the members of a London family, scientifically referred to as KE, have a

Table 22.1. Indications for speech-language evaluation

Age for referral	Indications for referral
Birth to 6 months	Does not respond to environmental sounds or voices
3–4 months	Does not gesture or make sounds to indicate he or she wants you to do something
	Has no interactive eye gaze
1 year	Does not follow simple commands or understand simple questions (e.g., "Roll the ball," "Kiss the doll," "Where's your shoe?")
	Does not say 8–10 words spontaneously
	Does not identify three body parts on self or doll
2 years	Does not use some one- or two-word questions (e.g., "Where kitty?" "Go bye-bye?" "What's that?")
	Does not use at least 50 understandable, different words
	Does not refer to self by name or pronoun (e.g., "me," "mine")
3 years	Does not understand differences in meaning (e.g., *go/stop, in/on, big/little, up/down*)
	Does not respond to *wh-* questions (e.g., *who, what, where*)
	Does not tell you about something in two- or three-word "sentences"
4 years	Has difficulty learning new concepts and words
	Still echoes speech
	Has unclear speech
	Does not explain events

Table 22.2.   Frequently used measures of speech and language skills

Test	Ages	Description
Bankson-Bernthal Test of Phonology (BBTOP; Bankson & Bernthal, 1990)	2–16 years	Identifies error patterns according to distinctive features and phonological processes
Peabody Picture Vocabulary Test–Third Edition (PPVT-III; Dunn & Dunn, 1997)	2½–adult	Tests receptive vocabulary
MacArthur-Bates Communicative Development Inventories (CDIs), Second Edition (Fenson et al., 2007)	8–37 months	Develops a profile of communicative behaviors in words and gestures (CDI: Words and Gestures, 8–18 months); Spanish version available
		Develops a profile of communicative behaviors in words and sentences (CDI: Words and Sentences, 16–30 months); Spanish version available
		Measures expressive vocabulary and grammar (CDI-III, 30–37 months)
Expressive One-Word Picture Vocabulary Test–2000 Edition (EOWPVT-2000; Brownell, 2000)	2–15 years	Tests expressive vocabulary
Goldman-Fristoe Test of Articulation–2 (GFTA-2; Goldman & Fristoe, 2000)	2–16 years	Assesses articulation of consonant sounds
The Rossetti Infant-Toddler Language Scale (Rossetti, 1990)	Birth to 36 months	Develops a profile of communicative behaviors in six areas: interaction-attachment, pragmatics, gesture, play, language comprehension, and language expression
Clinical Evaluation of Language Fundamentals–Third Edition (CELF-3; Semel, Wiig, & Secord, 1995)	6–21 years	Has multiple subtests of expressive and receptive language, tapping grammar semantics, phonology, sentence recall, and paragraph comprehension; Spanish version available
Clinical Evaluation of Language Fundamentals–Preschool (CELF-Preschool; Wiig, Secord, & Semel, 1992)	3–6 years	Contains multiple subtests of receptive language, tapping semantics, morphology, syntax, and expressive language and assesses phonology, sentence recall, and auditory memory
Preschool Language Scale–4 (PLS-4; Zimmerman, Steiner, & Pond, 2002)	Birth to 6 years	Has subscales on auditory comprehension and expressive communication; Spanish version available

communication disorder described as "verbal **dyspraxia**." The family's communication disorder has been found to be directly linked to a point of mutation on chromosome 7q31 that affects the transcription of ribonucleic acid (RNA) produced by a regulator gene FOXP2. Shriberg and colleagues (2005, 2006) provided in detail the types of speech **prosody** and voice metrics of a mother and daughter (affected members of the KE family, having cognitive, language, and speech challenges) who were identified with a breakpoint in a balance 7;13 chromosomal translocation that disrupted the transcription gene, FOXP2. In yet other instances, the cause of the problem is still unknown.

Regardless of the possible source of challenges in developing speech and language, if caregivers have questions about their child's communicative development and functioning, they should first review typical development information such as that provided by the ASHA through its written materials and/or web site. If concerns continue, caregivers should consult a certified speech-language pathologist, and, if the diagnosis confirms a speech-language disorder, as in David's case, early identification and intervention can make a significant, positive impact.

It is beyond the scope of this chapter to provide detailed descriptions of the speech-language disorders associated with specific developmental disabilities, but the chapter includes general information about areas of difficulty (e.g., producing accurate speech sounds, learning the rules of speech sounds, learning to decode and produce language). It is important for caregivers to gain a general understanding of such problems as they further their knowledge through Internet resources and work closely with the speech-language pathologists in carrying out intervention techniques. The chapter also describes some key principles for building an intervention program in which all members of the child's environment(s) are involved in facilitating the growth and development of speech-language skills.

SPEECH DISORDERS

Speech disorders are caused by problems making sounds correctly and most frequently are due to articulation difficulties, phonological processing disorders, or **resonance** disorders. Articulation difficulties entail not making the sound in the proper area of the oral mechanism and/or not having proper movements of the oral mechanism (tongue, lips, teeth, jaw) to produce the sound properly. Phonological processing relates to learning the rules about sounds in specific positions within words and about how sounds go together. A phonological processing disorder involves not learning these rules and thus producing the wrong sounds in the wrong places. Resonance disorders result from abnormal amounts of nasality. Hypernasality (too much nasality) is often caused by structural malformations such as cleft palate. Hyponasality (too little nasality) is often caused by structural malformations such as enlarged **adenoids** and tonsils or structural anomalies such as a deviated septum.

There is a developmental progression in the ability to accurately articulate phonemes. In English, the sounds /p/ and /b/ may be correctly produced by 12–24 months of age, but sounds such as /r/ and /l/ may take a child up to age 6 years to correctly produce (Goldman-Fristoe, 2000). Sound patterns such as vowel-consonant and consonant-vowel-consonant require practice to produce correctly, especially in different positions within words. The child's abilities depend on the interaction of hearing/attending (i.e., listening to others produce the sounds and self-monitoring his or her productions) and the control and coordination of the movement and placement of tongue, lips, and jaw.

LANGUAGE DISORDERS

Many children with developmental disabilities struggle with language development. Sometimes language development problems are the result of hearing impairments; other times, the cause of the language disorder is unknown.

Language Disorders Resulting from Hearing Impairments

As noted previously, there are many causes, with hearing being one of the first considerations. There are different types of hearing loss. In conductive hearing loss, there is difficulty with the sound reaching the inner ear. Sensorineural hearing loss involves a problem either with the inner ear itself or with transfer of messages from the inner ear to the brain. (For specifics, see Chapter 12.) The degree of hearing loss is directly correlated with the delay in language development. Even a mild hearing loss, when combined with a home environment that does not offer intensive language learning, can result in a delay in language acquisition.

Research (Roberts et al., 2004) has investigated the possible link between otitis media with effusion (a common problem for infants and toddlers) and hearing loss with resulting disruption of language development. The results were very specific to typically developing children and indicated that on average, otitis media with effusion often results in only a temporary hearing loss, which in these studies was found to not be a substantial risk factor for later speech and language development problems. These results, however, do not change the overall need for awareness that a hearing loss has potential to negatively affect language development.

Designing appropriate therapy for a child with a hearing loss requires understanding of the type and severity of loss, the age at which the hearing loss occurred, and the utility of assistive devices in restoring some hearing ability. Over the years, various approaches have gained popularity, but three primary communication methods have been used in intervention and education for children with hearing impairments: the oral/aural approach, total communication, and a bilingual/bicultural (bi-bi) approach. The oral/aural approach emphasizes maximal use of residual hearing, instruction in lipreading, and articulation therapy to improve speech output. Total communication employs aspects of the oral/aural approach but includes a manual sign system as a supplement. The bi-bi approach is yet another adaptation of total communication and is modeled after English as a second language programs. This approach emphasizes initially teaching the child sign language, assisting him or her in gaining communicative proficiency, and emphasizing the positive aspects of the Deaf culture. Then, efforts are introduced to acquire English as a second language (in terms of verbal, reading, and writing abilities). In the bi-bi approach, there is less emphasis on maximizing residual hearing through the use of assistive listening devices. Therefore, people who favor this approach frequently resist the advent of progressive technologies such as cochlear implants (Ratner, 2005).

Cochlear implants are prostheses that work by placing electrodes within or near the cochlea and applying an electrical current to the electrode site. This stimulates the auditory nerve and bypasses nonfunctional parts of the inner ear (i.e., the hair cells of the cochlea). Cochlear implants do not result in restoration of unimpaired hearing. In addition, it is agreed that for a child to receive benefits from this technology, he or she must also receive intensive speech-language therapy and appropriate educational support.

Parents make the final decision about which approaches to use after they receive in-depth education and information about the options, as provided through consultation with audiologists, speech-language pathologists, and educators. Teamwork that incorporates interactive, detailed planning and collaborative implementation results in the greatest success (Ratner, 2005).

Language Disorders of Unknown Etiology

Research into language disorders with heretofore unknown etiology is being pursued by several professionals in several fields, including neuropsychology, speech-language pathology, and genetics. Through the use of imaging techniques and electroencephalogram (EEG), there have been recent efforts to link language disorders with genetic transmission. Fisher (2005) and Fisher et al. (2003) reported on a family in which approximately half of the members were affected with a severe speech and language disorder that appeared to be transmitted as an autosomal dominant trait. Future investigation may offer insight into the molecular genetics of the developmental process that culminates in speech and language.

Individual Variation

Regardless of the etiology, the manner and extent to which language development is affected varies from child to child. Ultimately there is an effect on how the child is able to listen to talking within the environment, analyze it, associate it with a multitude of experiences, and use his or her communication system to respond and or imitate. For example, the child may be slow to remember the specific names of objects; may not understand or use functional words such as *the*, *am*, and *to*; may not understand the implication of word endings (*-ing*, *-ed*, *-s*); and often are late in being able to produce multiword sentences. Children with a disorder on the autism spectrum may be able to imitate the production of these items through echolalia but cannot generate this language to get their needs met. Children with Asperger syndrome may have accurately developed linguistic elements of language but make pragmatic errors in areas such as turn taking and topic sharing. Some children experience problems in more than one area.

INTERVENTION

Therefore, the plan and intervention techniques must be designed to meet the individual needs. The brief description of David's levels of functioning indicates that he has delays in learning both speech and language. It is most important to answer his grandmother's questions regarding outcome (e.g., "Will David eventually talk?"), but doing so requires a great deal more information than the letter supplies. It will require family history, observation of interactive and play skills, and a phonetic inventory. A best practice scenario would also require the speech-language pathologist to spend considerable time discussing general impressions from the evaluation and delineating factors involved in potential recovery from a communication disorder. For example, research has identified important contributors to recovery: early identification, specific causes, and severity of the communication impairment (Bashir & Scavuzzo, 1992).

In addition, it is now accepted that the "who, how, and where" of intervention is very important. Building an intervention program that is carried out collaboratively with people who regularly interact with the child—that is, caregivers such as parents, extended family members, and preschool staff—and consideration of places and activities in which the child is regularly involved is essential to success. Therapy in natural environments in collaboration with caregivers achieves at least three major benefits for children: 1) enhanced relationships among family members, therapists, educational staff, and parents; 2) modeling and support to facilitate caregivers in their work addressing the child's problems; and 3) better ability to assess a child's functioning and set appropriate, meaningful outcome goals (Bowen & Cupples, 2004; Hanft & Pikington, 2000).

Therefore, the ideal approach for designing therapy for David would be accomplished through a family-centered, team approach in the child's natural environments. Ideally, the initial meeting would be held in David's home or child care center, allowing an opportunity to observe him and his activities. The focus of initial discussions in planning would need to address issues such as those suggested by Hanft and Pikington (2000): 1) What does the David need to learn or do next? 2) Which intervention strategies and natural environments will facilitate David's specific developmental outcome? 3) Whose expertise is needed to help David achieve the identified, agreed-on desired outcomes? 4) How and where should services be provided?

In this case, observing and recognizing key opportunities for David to use communication to participate within the activities and routines that occur within all of his environments will be vital to the intervention plan. The therapist's challenge will be to find creative ways to translate expertise and knowledge into meaningful interventions to support David's learning while participating. This will mean that in addition to the speech-language intervention activities, such as targeting words for model and imitation within joint attention activities and reinforcing all types of vocalization and word approximations, some compensatory therapy approaches will also be developed. In a compensatory approach, strategies and supports are designed for children to bypass their communicative limitations. Because the consistent goal for every child is functional communication that supports participation in all of the activities of his or her life, the compensatory approach may include signing, using low-tech symbols, and using speech-generating devices with various levels of complexity.

Augmentative and Alternative Communication

Parents often fear that the introduction of a compensatory approach will foster dependence on an artificial means of communication and further delay verbal development. The opposite is true. Even when it seems likely that oral speech may eventually develop, augmentative and alternative communication (AAC) is still often used to prevent delayed communication development and to support communicative participation in daily activities.

AAC includes sign language, picture communication boards, object symbols, adapted books, and low-tech or high-tech speech-generating devices. Parents, preschool teachers, siblings, and friends learn various ways to use the specific customized items when interacting with the child whose verbal speech abilities do not adequately meet his or her communicative needs. Each of these items should be used within the naturally occurring routines of a child's daily activities to support interactions. The specific signs, pictures on a board, object symbols, and messages in a speech-generating device are chosen on the basis of the child's needs within activities.

Sign language provides a visual and tactile representation of spoken words and can be "ready" vocabulary for very important communications for the child with limited verbal output. The signs often include the names for favorite toys, activities, and people, as well as phrases to control some actions. For example, the signs WANT MORE PLEASE, and THANK YOU have many applications over the course of a day. Most parents and teachers are encouraged to choose 20 or 30 signs relevant to their child and the situations he or she regularly encounters. If the child is unable to make the signs perfectly, approximations are accepted. The goal is for the child to have an easy, consistent means of transferring information.

Picture boards and object symbols can be used in a number of ways, such as highlighting vocabulary choices for home routines (e.g., *cereal, yogurt*) or as complex as a sequence of actual photos organized to tell the story of a visit to the zoo. The pictures or symbols may be organized to offer special tactile cues for children with visual impairments or may include unique objects to request individual interests (e.g., string for a child with an autism spectrum disorder).

Speech-generating devices contain prerecorded messages in a single form or in combination. As they can be very simple or very complex, the style is selected depending on the child's abilities and needs. Through the power of touching a button or pressing a switch, the device will speak a message that supports the child's participation in activities such as partaking in circle time in educational settings, asking a question, and introducing him- or herself.

It is imperative that the child's caregivers, educators, professionals, friends, and other relevant individuals collaborate to design the AAC system. However, there is a need for an AAC system designer to take the lead. This person should have special insight into customizing systems to compensate for various disorders and ensuring that the system supports many communication functions (e.g., questions, jokes, commentary, requests) (Batorowicz, McDougall, & Shepherd, 2006).

It is imperative that the AAC system designer does not fall prey to some common misconceptions that have denied many individuals the right to communication. The following are some of the more common fallacies:

- There are established prerequisites (e.g., cognitive milestones, receptive language strengths, demonstrable communicative intent, yes/no consistency) that must be satisfied before the individual becomes a candidate for an AAC system.

- AAC should be taught through a series of isolated sequential skills that will then be generalized into a communication process.

- Children's young age or motor or cognitive impairments prevent them from using AAC (National Joint Committee for the Communication Needs of Persons with Severe Disabilities, 2003).

SUMMARY

The ability to communicate provides a primary means of participating in our lives and the lives of others. Therefore, disorders of communication have a profound impact on the very essence of our being. Returning to David's story, it is clear that he has already received an evaluation that has identified specific areas of need. Following the best case scenario, it can be projected that he will receive therapy that will stimulate his verbal productions and that he will have the advantage of an AAC system. With these ongoing supports, David will immediately be able to use his symbols to participate in activities such as choosing between swimming and going to the library and using his speech-generating device to "talk" to his Grandmother on the telephone and "read" his bedtime story.

REFERENCES

American Speech-Language-Hearing Association. (2007). *How does your child hear and talk?* Retrieved February 7, 2007, from http://www.asha.org/public/speech/development/child_hear_talk.htm

Bankson, N.B., & Bernthal, J.E. (1990). *Bankson-Bernthal Test of Phonology (BBTOP).* Chicago: Riverside.

Bashir, A.S., & Scavuzzo, A. (1992). Children with language disorders: Natural history and academic success. *Journal of Learning Disabilities, 25,* 53–65.

Batorowicz, B., McDougall, S., & Shepherd, T. (2006). AAC and community partnerships: The participation path to community inclusion. *AAC: Augmentative and Alternative Communication, 22*(3), 178–195.

Bowen, C., & Cupples, L. (2004). The role of families in optimizing phonological therapy outcomes. *Child Language Teaching and Therapy, 20*(3), 245–260.

Brownell, R. (2000). *Expressive One-Word Picture Vocabulary Test–2000 Edition (EOWPVT-2000).* Novato, CA: Academic Therapy Publications.

Dunn, L.M., & Dunn, L.M. (1997). *Peabody Picture Vocabulary Test–Third Edition (PPVT-III).* Circle Pines, MN: AGS Publishing.

Fenson, L., Marchman, V.A., Thal, D.J., et al. (2007). *MacArthur-Bates Communicative Development Inventories: Users guide and technical manual.* Baltimore: Paul H. Brookes Publishing Co.

Fisher, S. (2005). Dissection of molecular mechanisms underlying speech and language disorders. *Applied Psycholinguistics, 26,* 111–128

Fisher, S., Lai, C., & Monaco, A. (2003). Deciphering the genetic basis of speech and language disorders. *Annual Review of Neuroscience, 26,* 57–80

Goldfield, B., & Snow, C. (2005). Individual differences: Implications for the study of language acquisition. In J.B. Gleason (Ed.), *The development of language* (6th ed., pp. 292–323). Upper Saddle River, NJ: Pearson Education.

Goldman, R., & Fristoe, M. (2000). *Goldman-Fristoe Test of Articulation–2 (GFTA-2).* Circle Pines, MN: AGS Publishing.

Hanft, B., & Pilkington, K. (2000). Therapy in natural environments: The means or end goal for early intervention. *Infants and Young Children, 12,*(4), 1–13.

Kuhl, P. (2000). A new view of language acquisition. *Proceedings of the National Academy of Sciences, 97*(22), 11850–11857.

Mandel, D.R., Jusczyk, P.W., & Pisoni, D.B. (1994). *Do 4½ month olds know their own names?* Paper presented at the 127th meeting of the Acoustical Society of America, Cambridge, MA.

National Joint Committee for the Communication Needs of Persons with Severe Disabilities. (2003). Position statement on access to communication services and supports: Concerns regarding the application of restrictive "eligibility" policies. *ASHA Supplement, 23,* 19–20

Ojemann, G.A. (1991). Cortical organization of language. *Journal of Neuroscience, 11,* 2281–2287.

Querleu, D., & Renard, K. (1981). Les perceptions auditives du fœtus humain [Auditory perception of the human fetus]. *Médecine et hygiene, 39,* 2101–2110.

Ratner, N. (2005). Atypical language development. In J.B. Gleason (Ed.), *The development of language* (6th ed. pp. 324–394). Upper Saddle River, NJ: Pearson Education.

Roberts, J., Burchinal, M., & Zeisel, S. (2002). Otitis media in early childhood in relation to children's school-age language and academic skills. *Pediatrics, 110*(4), 696–706

Roberts, J., Hunter, L., Gravel, J., et al. (2004). Otitis media, hearing loss, and language learning: Controversies and current research. *Developmental and Behavioral Pediatrics, 25*(2), 110–122.

Rossetti, L. (1990). *The Rossetti Infant-Toddler Language Scale.* East Moline, IL: LinguiSystems.

Semel, E., Wiig, E.H., & Secord, W.A. (1995). *Clinical Evaluation of Language Fundamentals–Third Edition (CELF-3).* San Antonio, TX: Harcourt Assessment.

Shriberg, L., Ballard, K., Tomblin, J.B., et al. (2006). Speech, prosody, and voice characteristics of a mother and daughter with a 7;13 translocation affecting FOXP2. *Journal of Speech, Language, and Hearing Research, 49,* 500–525.

Shriberg, L., Lewis, B., Tomblin, J.B., et al. (2005). Toward diagnostic and phenotype markers for genetically transmitted speech delay. *Journal of Speech, Language, and Hearing Research, 48,* 834–852.

Strauss, S., & Ziv, M. (2001). Children request teaching when asking for names of objects. *Behavioral and Brain Sciences, 246,* 1118–1119.

Tomasello, M. (2000). First steps toward a usage-based theory of language acquisition. *Cognitive Linguistics, 11,* 61–82.

Wiig, E.H., Secord, W., & Semel, E. (1992). *Clinical Evaluation of Language Fundamentals–Preschool (CELF–Preschool).* San Antonio, TX: Harcourt Assessment.

Zimmerman, I.L., Steiner, V.G., & Pond, R.E. (2002). *Preschool Language Scale–4 (PLS-4).* San Antonio, TX: Harcourt Assessment.

23 Autism Spectrum Disorders

Susan L. Hyman and Kenneth E. Towbin

Upon completion of this chapter, the reader will

- Be familiar with the core features of autism and related disorders
- Distinguish among the diagnostic criteria for Autistic Disorder, Asperger's Disorder, Pervasive Developmental Disorder-Not Otherwise Specified, Childhood Disintegrative Disorder, and Rett's Disorder
- Understand the issues related to prevalence of autism spectrum disorders
- Be familiar with interventions and outcomes

Autism spectrum disorders (ASDs) are a class of neurodevelopmental disorders characterized by an impairment in social reciprocity, atypical communication, and repetitive behaviors. The term *autism spectrum* indicates that the disorders in this category occur along a continuum and is commonly used as a synonym for the category **pervasive developmental disorders**. The *Diagnostic and Statistical Manual of Mental Disorders, Fourth Edition, Text Revision (DSM-IV-TR*, American Psychiatric Association [APA], 2000) uses the equivalent term *Pervasive Developmental Disorders (PDDs)*, because symptoms pervade all areas of development. Included in this group of disorders are the specific diagnoses of Autistic Disorder, Asperger's Disorder, Rett's Disorder, and Childhood Disintegrative Disorder (CDD). Pervasive Developmental Disorder-Not Otherwise Specified (PDD-NOS) is a classification used when symptoms are present but specific criteria for one of the other diagnoses in this category are not met. Because the continuum of disorders is popularly referred to as the autism spectrum disorders (ASDs) rather than the *DSM-IV-TR* terminology of Pervasive Developmental Disorders, this chapter uses the term *ASDs*. Some research studies cited have been done with people with Autistic Disorder. This will be specifically noted in the text because the findings might be different for people with other ASDs.

The symptoms of ASDs are neurologically based. Scientific evidence indicates a genetic predisposition for ASDs, although there is likely to be gene–environment interaction (Muhle, Trentacoste, & Rapin, 2004). ASDs may occur in conjunction with other functionally defined diagnoses such as intellectual disability and learning disabilities, biologically based behaviors such as tics, and medical conditions including epilepsy. Advances in understanding the core symptoms and early implementation of educational, communication, and behavioral treatment approaches have positively affected the outcome of children with ASDs (National Research Council, 2001).

CHRISTOPHER

Christopher and Katie are fraternal twins who were born after an uncomplicated pregnancy. The children's parents, both trained as engineers, recall that Katie was somewhat colicky and that Christopher seemed content in comparison. He seemed advanced in the first year of life compared with his sister. Christopher smiled and babbled on time, and his parents remember that from a very early age, he was quite interested in toys with letters or numbers. By the time he was 1 year old, Christopher could identify some letters, and his parents thought he was rather precocious. They noticed that by 15 months of age, however, Katie was using words and beginning to play appropriately with toys. Christopher, conversely, had many words used as labels but never said "momma" or "dadda" and seemed to be consumed with naming and ordering letters and numbers. He could repeat phrases from his movies but did not make novel phrases at 2 years of age. At times, Christopher's parents worried that he was deaf because he seemed to ignore them.

The parents took Christopher to the doctor, and the pediatrician referred Christopher to an early intervention program. His hearing was normal, but he had significant delays in receptive and social language. Christopher was diagnosed as having an ASD and began an intense, disorder-specific program.

DIAGNOSTIC CATEGORIES WITHIN THE AUTISM SPECTRUM

ASDs are defined by the presence or absence of behaviors in three areas: social reciprocity, communication, and repetitive behaviors (APA, 2000). The number and distribution of symptoms, the pattern of early language development, the cognitive ability, and the timing of regression all are used to make a specific diagnosis within this category of disorders.

Autistic Disorder

Autism (or Autistic Disorder, per the *DSM-IV-TR*) is a discrete diagnosis within the ASDs. It is defined by a pattern of six symptoms distributed across three areas (Table 23.1). At least two symptoms must be in the area of social reciprocity. Dr. Leo Kanner first described the syndrome of autism (derived from the Greek word for self-absorption) in 1943 (Kanner, 1943). He observed a series of patients in his practice of child psychiatry with social aloofness and a desire for "preservation of sameness." Although Kanner believed autism was an organic condition, through the 1950s most psychiatrists considered autism to be caused by poor parenting. Some thought it was a form of childhood schizophrenia. With better behavioral description, it became clear that the ASDs were discrete from schizophrenia and occurred along a gradient. Progressive modification of the *DSM* (APA, 2000) has altered diagnostic criteria so both younger children or children with lower functioning and children with typical cognitive abilities can be identified as having ASDs.

Asperger's Disorder

Dr. Hans Asperger was a contemporary of Dr. Kanner (Asperger, 1944/1991). Asperger observed children with apparently typical lan-

guage who had difficulties with socialization, could not conform to social demands, and had repetitive behaviors. The *DSM-IV-TR* indicates that Asperger's Disorder (also called Asperger syndrome) can be diagnosed if three symptoms—two related to social reciprocity and one to habitual behaviors—are present. Language development must be grossly within normal limits (two-word phrases by 2 years of age; longer phrases by 3 years of age). Pragmatic language impairments are common, and adaptive behaviors may be delayed. There is considerable overlap between the diagnosis of high-functioning autism (Autistic Disorder in someone with typical intelligence) and Asperger's Disorder (Szatmari, 2000). Children with Asperger's Disorder may not be diagnosed until school age, when the social demands of the classroom make the symptoms functionally apparent.

Pervasive Developmental Disorder-Not Otherwise Specified

The diagnosis PDD-NOS is used to describe children who do not have the number or distribution of symptoms for another diagnosis within the ASDs or have atypical presentation but have functional impairments in the relevant areas. There is no minimum number of symptoms necessary to diagnose PDD-NOS. This results in significant heterogeneity among individuals given this clinical diagnosis. The comorbidity of cognitive, language, and behavioral symptoms with PDD-NOS may result in significant functional impairment, although fewer symptoms of autism are present.

Childhood Disintegrative Disorder

CDD is a very rare condition in which all aspects of development proceed typically until 3–5 years of age, when skills in all domains regress (Hendry, 2000). Language, cognitive ability, social reciprocity, play, motor skills, and basic adaptive functions such as bowel and bladder skills deteriorate. Behaviors subsequently stabilize at a lower level of functioning. CDD probably represents a common final pathway for a number of neurologic insults. Work up for a neurodegenerative disorder is indicated if late regression is documented. Epileptic aphasia (Landau-Kleffner Syndrome) is not the same as CDD, as children with LKS may lose only language. Characteristic electroencephalogram (EEG) findings are present during sleep (Trevithan, 2004) in LKS.

Table 23.1. Diagnostic criteria for Autistic Disorder

A. A total of six (or more) items from the following groups:

Group 1[a]	Group 2[b]	Group 3[c]
1. Marked impairment in the use of multiple nonverbal behaviors such as eye-to-eye gaze, facial expression, body postures, and gestures to regulate social interaction	1. Delay in, or total lack of, the development of spoken language (not accompanied by an attempt to compensate through alternative modes of communication such as gesture or mime)	1. Encompassing preoccupation with one or more stereotyped and restricted patterns of interest that is abnormal either in intensity or focus
2. Failure to develop peer relationships appropriate to developmental level	2. In individuals with adequate speech, marked impairment in the ability to initiate or sustain a conversation with others	2. Apparently inflexible adherence to specific, nonfunctional routines or rituals
3. A lack of spontaneous seeking to share enjoyment, interests, or achievements with other people (e.g., by a lack of showing, bringing, or pointing out objects of interest)	3. Stereotyped and repetitive use of language or idiosyncratic language	3. Stereotyped and repetitive motor mannerisms (e.g., hand or finger flapping or twisting, complex whole-body movements)
4. Lack of social or emotional reciprocity	4. Lack of varied, spontaneous make-believe play or social imitative play appropriate to developmental level	4. Persistent preoccupation with parts of objects

B. Delays or abnormal functioning in at least one of the following areas with onset prior to age 3 years:
   1. Social interaction
   2. Language as used in social communication
   3. Symbolic or imaginative play

C. The disturbance is not better accounted for by Rett's Disorder or Childhood Disintegrative Disorder.

Reprinted with permission from the *Diagnostic and Statistical Manual of Mental Disorders, Fourth Edition, Text Revision* (p. 75). Copyright © 2000 American Psychiatric Association.

[a]Qualitative impairments in social interaction, as manifested by at least two criteria from Group 1.

[b]Qualitative impairments in communication as manifested by at least one criterion from Group 2.

[c]Restricted, repetitive, and stereotyped patterns of behavior, interests, and activities, as manifested by at least one criterion from Group 3.

Rett's Disorder

Rett's Disorder (also called Rett syndrome) is a specific neurogenetic syndrome that is classified as an ASD because it involves the loss of previously obtained language and social milestones Rett's Disorder is predominantly seen in girls. The deterioration in function is accompanied by the development of a set of mid-line stereotyped hand movements. Rett's Disorder is associated with a mutation in the methyl-CpG-binding protein 2 (MeCP2) gene on the X chromosome (Huppke & Gartner, 2005). Affected children have a history of a normal birth and infancy, with slowing of head growth and a loss or plateauing of cognitive, language, and motor skills in the second year of life (Nomura & Sagawa, 2005). Spasticity in the lower extremities, seizures, constipation, and hyperventilation/breathholding are also common findings. Although affected children lose language and social interest with their initial deteriora-

tion, social approach and interest often returns. Understanding the relationship between the genetic mutation and developmental regression may help direct future research examining brain development in children with ASDs and Rett's Disorder.

Broader Autism Phenotype

The term *broader autism phenotype (BAP)* reflects the current conceptualization that each symptom of the autism phenotype exists along a continuum with typical behavior (Dawson et al., 2002). Subtle differences in pragmatic language organization and psychiatric symptoms such as anxiety (Piven et al., 1997) or mood disorders (deLong & Nohria, 1994) may occur with greater frequency in family members of people with ASDs. Understanding that there is a gradient of symptoms is an important step in understanding how multiple genes must interact to result in an ASD.

DIAGNOSTIC FEATURES OF AUTISM SPECTRUM DISORDERS

There is significant heterogeneity among people diagnosed with ASDs given the number of symptoms and possible patterns. Core symptoms are divided into the three areas, which are discussed next.

Qualitative Impairments in Social Reciprocity

The deficits in social reciprocity that are critical to the diagnosis of an ASD reflect an intrinsic inability to read and comprehend the feelings, experiences, and motives of others. These basic social understanding skills allow interpretation of the verbal and nonverbal messages of others, including nuanced facial expression, vocal inflection, gesture, social intention, and emotional tone. Because of these symptoms, children with ASDs have social difficulties with peers (Travis & Sigman, 1998). Infants with typical development learn that eye contact with adults and vocalizations are associated with attention. They learn to look at their parents when their name is called, as well as to distinguish their parents' facial expressions and the inflection in their voices (Bruinsma, Koegel, & Koegel, 2004). Some infants with ASD are quiet and content babies with decreased gaze.

Understanding that other people have a different point of view is referred to as theory of mind. This basic difference interferes with the capacity of people with ASDs to understand social language and intent of others (Rogers, 1998). Although individuals with ASDs have varying degrees of difficulty in initiating, responding to, and maintaining social interactions, they may be highly responsive to specific individuals or situations. Patterns of relating to other people may be atypical. They may have diminished eye contact, decreased use of facial expression, and exaggerated or absent gestures. People without ASDs generally look at the eyes of a person to whom they are speaking, whereas most people with ASDs tend to look at the person's mouth (Klin et al., 2002). Some people with ASD have intense eye gaze without the social awareness of when to look away. People with ASDs may have difficulty in integrating verbal and nonverbal components of communication. Although some are aloof, many children with ASDs respond to affection and are affectionate with their families (Travis & Sigman, 1998).

There is a broad range of social skills in individuals with ASDs. Symptoms related to atypical social reciprocity are closely tied to the presence or absence of symptoms in the area of language.

Atypical Communication Development

Difficulty with social communication is present in varying degrees in all people with ASDs (Rapin & Dunn, 2003). Language delays may relate to intellectual disability or exist in isolation. Delays in language are the first area of concern identified by most families whose children are later diagnosed with ASDs. Typical early language is often reported, including the emergence of single words; however, when early milestones are scrutinized, it becomes apparent many children with ASDs have had atypical development in receptive and expressive language (Mars, Mauk, & Dowrick, 1998). Language milestones are lost between 18 and 24 months by at least half of children with autistic disorder (Rogers, 2004). Loss of social milestones is less often reported but occurs with some frequency (Richler et al., 2006).

Early language of children with ASDs is often characterized by imperative labeling (using words for naming instead of communicating); echolalia (echoing speech); abnormal prosody, or inflection; and improper use of pronouns. Echoing adult words is common in typical development, as toddlers gain vocabulary and learn to process what is said to them. In children with ASDs, however, echolalic speech may persist in a perseverative fashion. Perseverative language may occur to provide structure and a known outcome in a social situation that the child with an ASD does not understand. Once functional language is established, prosody may be sing-song, robotic, or imitative of the inflection used by the original speaker. Young children with ASDs also may have difficulty assigning pronouns because they may not see how words need to be rearranged to have meaning to another person (Rapin & Dunn, 2003).

Communication requires a synthesis of many behaviors that are nonverbal. Children with ASDs may have a basic inability to both perceive and imitate facial expression (Dawson, Webb, & McPartland, 2005). Studies have shown that the brains of people with Autistic Disorder process faces as if they were objects. As a result, every time the facial expression of the communication partner is changed, the person with an ASD must reidentify the face (Schultz et al., 2000). This neurobiologic finding may be one factor that influences social processing and pragmatic language in people with ASDs.

Receptive language problems may also affect communication. Learning may be more efficient with visual, rather than auditory, cues. Unusual eye contact, body posture, gestures, and other nonverbal aspects of communication may have an impact on communication. Without specific intervention, nonverbal communication impairments may be problematic even with the development of conversational language.

Atypical Behavior

Although the differences in social "give and take" may be central to the diagnosis of ASDs, repetitive, perseverative, and stereotyped behaviors are often the most visible symptoms. Strict adherence to routines is common among people with ASDs. This can extend to food aversions, rituals related to daily routines, or obsessions. Young children with ASDs may have attachments to unusual items, such as string, rather than to soft or cuddly toys. Children with ASDs may not use toys in their intended manner but may focus instead on a part of a toy—for example, the wheels on a toy truck, which they may spin repetitively. They may line things up, stare out of the corners of their eyes, or visually inspect aspects of objects. Pretend play may not develop spontaneously, and once taught, it may take on a rote quality.

Interruption of a ritual or preoccupation may upset a child with an ASD and lead to distress or a temper tantrum. Stereotyped movements such as pacing, spinning, running in circles, drumming, flipping light switches, rocking, hand waving, arm flapping, and toe walking are common. Self-injurious behavior, including biting and head banging, may also occur. Unusual responses to sensory input are commonly reported. These include insensitivity to pain or heat and overreaction to environmental noises, touch, or odors. For example, although the child may appear "deaf" to the language of others but hear the television, or they may cover their ears and scream because of hyperacusis (unusual sensitivity to certain sounds).

The core symptoms of ASD vary with age and ability. For example, some people may have a total absence of language and communicative intent, whereas others engage in "professorial" speech with no conversational regard for the interest of the listener. Current challenges include development of more precise ways to elicit and quantify the core symptoms for early and accurate diagnosis.

CAUSES OF AUTISM SPECTRUM DISORDERS

ASDs do not form a single disorder and are without a single etiology. The weight of evidence now points to a genetic predisposition with environmental interactions (see Chapter 16).

The Genetics of Autism

The evidence for a genetic etiology for ASDs comes from both family studies and twin studies. The recurrence risk for an ASD in subsequent siblings of a child with ASD is 3%–5% (Chakrabarti & Fombonne, 2001). This is tenfold higher than what would be expected in the general population. An identical twin of a child with autism, however, has a 65% chance of having an ASD. Almost all identical twins of individuals with ASDs have some symptoms, although fraternal twins have been reported to have no greater rate of autism than other siblings (Folstein & Rutter, 1977). This strongly supports a genetic component of ASDs. It should be emphasized that these rates suggest an interaction of multiple genes (see Chapter 1). It is also likely that as yet unknown environmental factors influence gene expression and brain development in these disorders. Genetic research has followed three strategies, which are discussed next.

Family Studies   In family studies, also called linkage analysis, patterns of genes or specific DNA markers in family members with and without Autistic Disorder or an ASD are investigated. This strategy has identified genes that may be related to ASDs on multiple chromosomes, including 2, 7, and 15 (Muhle et al., 2004).

Candidate Genes Studies   Identification of a trait of interest allows specific investigation of associated genes in families with individuals with ASDs. A number of genes of interest relate to early brain development (Muhle et al., 2004). The interaction of genes and environmental events in early pregnancy is an area of active study. Candidate genes related to neurotransmitter generation and receptor function are of great interest because of potential for medical treatment of symptoms (Scott & Deneris, 2005).

***Association with Genetic Disorders
of Known Etiology*** ASDs tend to be associated with other genetic disorders that have
known etiologies. It is understood that brain
functioning in certain genetic disorders, such
as tuberous sclerosis and fragile X syndrome,
places individuals at a greater risk for having
ASDs (see Chapter 19 and Appendix B). This
knowledge allows for investigation of the relationship between known biologic abnormalities
and behaviors symptomatic of autism.

Brain Structure and Function in Autism Spectrum Disorders

Neuroimaging techniques are used to study
brain development and function. Although head
circumference is normal at birth, children with
ASDs (other than Rett's Disorder) have large
heads in early childhood. The reason for this is
not yet known. Magnetic resonance imaging
(MRI) studies of children with ASDs note a
greater volume of white matter in cortex and
cerebellum in early childhood, but by middle
childhood, the head size is in the normal range
(Redcay & Courchesne, 2005). There may be abnormal genetic regulation of early brain growth
and/or synaptic development. Anatomic findings
on MRI, however, do not consistently identify
the same structural asymmetries or size differences. Improvements in imaging, such as diffusion tensor imaging (which images specific neural tracts) will advance understanding of brain
structure and function.

It is possible to indirectly examine how
neurons in different parts of the brain behave in
terms of neurotransmitter activity and energy
utilization by using functional MRI and spectroscopy. Most studies have been done with
higher functioning adolescents and adults. One
finding was that theory of mind tasks require
the networking of the medial prefrontal cortex,
temporoparietal junction, and temporal poles
with other brain regions (Vollm et al., 2005).
High-functioning adolescents with ASDs demonstrate impairments in processing faces in the
fusiform gyrus (Schultz et al., 2000) and in processing the eye gaze of others in the superior temporal sulcus (Pelphrey, Morris, & McCarthy,
2005). In addition, imitation may be impaired
because mirror neurons do not communicate
properly (Williams, Waiter, et al., 2005).

Few brains of individuals with ASDs have
been examined histologically. The findings to
date suggest that prenatal events alter cell number and density in the cerebellum and limbic
system. Abnormal development of the brain

stem nuclei and the inferior olive, as well as het-
erotopias (abnormally placed neurons) have
been reported in isolated cases (Bailey et al.,
1998). Modern techniques have identified additional pathological changes in some individuals'
brains, including atypical inflammation and disordered cellular organization in the cortex
(Casanova, Buxhoeveden, & Gomez, 2004; Vargas et al., 2005). To further basic understanding
of the neurobiology of these disorders, post-
mortem study of the brains of individuals with
ASDs must occur. Autism Speaks and the National Institutes of Health have sponsored a
brain bank to make pathologic material available to researchers (see http://www.Memoriesof
Hope.org).

Obstetric Complications

Epidemiologic studies have not strongly associated any specific prenatal or birth complications with the development of ASDs. Obstetric
optimality scores that reflect the overall health
of the pregnancy, delivery, and newborn period
are lower in children with ASDs (Zwaigenbaum
et al., 2002). The prenatal events that predispose a child to develop an ASD may compromise fetal well-being in subtle and inconsistent
ways.

Environmental Exposures

It is likely that environmental factors interact
with genes to cause the symptoms of ASDs. To
date, the only established environmental risk
factors for ASDs are a few medications (discussed in the next section) that a mother might
have been prescribed early in pregnancy (Hyman,
Arndt, & Rodier, 2005).

Teratogens Substances that result in
an increased risk of birth defects in the developing fetus are termed *teratogens*. These include
maternal medications, drugs of abuse, chemicals, and radiation. Thalidomide is a drug that
was used to treat nausea in pregnant women in
the 1960s. It was associated with limb deformities in exposed fetuses (see Chapter 2). Many
years later, ophthalmologists studying the abnormalities of eye movement in adults who
were exposed to thalidomide in utero found
that these adults also had a very high prevalence
of ASDs. In addition, increased rates of ASDs
have been reported in children who were exposed during early pregnancy to valproic acid
(used to treat seizures and bipolar disorder) and
mesoprostol (which may fail when used to in-

duce early termination of pregnancy) (Hyman et al., 2005).

No known environmental or chemical exposures have been associated with an increased risk for ASDs to date. The epidemiologic study that compared the rates of ASD in Brick Township, New Jersey, to other communities in New Jersey did not identify increased risk in that locale (Bertrand et al., 2001). Recent reports of increased airborne mercury in locations with higher rates of children with ASDs require further study with more rigorous methodology that includes actual air sampling (Palmer et al., 2006). Although existing data do not implicate specific chemical agents, it is certainly plausible that substances to which mothers and newborns are exposed may affect brain development in a way that leads to ASDs in susceptible individuals.

Vaccinations There has been significant controversy about the alleged association of the measles, mumps, and rubella (MMR) vaccine, developmental regression, and ASDs (Wakefield et al., 1998). Population-based studies do not demonstrate an increase in the rate of diagnosis of ASDs with the introduction of MMR (Demicheli et al., 2005). Madsen et al. (2002) compared the rate of ASDs in more than 400,000 children in Denmark who received the MMR vaccine with about 100,000 children who did not get the vaccine. There was no difference in the rate of ASDs. Epidemiologic data does not support an association of the MMR vaccination with autism.

A second hypothesis relates the ethylmercury-based preservative, thimerosal (used as a preservative in pediatric vaccines prior to 2001) to symptoms of ASD in genetically susceptible children (Bernard et al., 2001). The rate of diagnosis of ASDs actually increased after removal of thimerosal from vaccines in Denmark (Madsen et al., 2003), although this was attributed to the broadened diagnostic criteria and increased awareness of ASDs in families and providers. The neurologic symptoms that are known to be associated with specific types of mercury toxicity depend on the type of mercury and age at and length of exposure. Neurologic symptoms of ASDs and acute, chronic and prenatal mercury toxicity affect sensory functions, motor abilities, and learning, but the specific symptoms are not the same (Nelson & Bauman, 2003). Methylmercury, the type of mercury ingested in fish and marine mammals, has not yet been associated with autism in populations with high pre- and postnatal exposure (Davidson, Myers, & Weiss, 2004).

In sum, no studies provide scientific documentation of a causal association of thimerosal containing vaccines and ASDs. In addition, current vaccines administered to children in the U.S. other than some influenza vaccines are typically thimerosal free (see http://www.fda.gov/cber/vaccine/thimerosal.htm#t1). Despite these factors, chelation therapy to bind and excrete heavy metals is pursued as a clinical intervention by families of children with ASDs. No clinical trials have been published to date that examine the safety and efficacy of this practice (Levy & Hyman, 2005).

Infections Prenatal infection with rubella increases the risk for cerebral palsy, intellectual disability, visual impairments, and ASDs, depending on the timing of infection (Chess, 1971). Vaccination-based immunity in women has all but eliminated this cause of ASDs in the United States. Other virus and bacterium that commonly infects pregnant women are not routinely associated with ASDs in the offspring, although rare cases of ASD have been reported in children with congenital CMV. A mother's own immunologic response to infections such as influenza might cause subtle differences in brain development, which might predispose a susceptible fetus to an ASD (Shi et al., 2003).

Another issue that has been raised is the possibility of infections in early childhood being associated with ASDs. Children who have severe neurologic injury after meningitis or encephalitis may have symptoms of ASDs. There is no evidence to indicate overgrowth of intestinal yeasts or bacteria (Levy & Hyman, 2005) cause ASDs.

Gender and Autism Spectrum Disorders

There is a 4:1 male to female predominance of ASDs. The gender ratio is closer to 1:1 for children with ASDs who have IQ scores of less than 50 (Yeargin-Allsopp et al., 2003). The excess of identified males may be the result of differential genetic or hormonal susceptibility, teratogenic effects, or application of the diagnostic criteria.

EARLY IDENTIFICATION OF AUTISM SPECTRUM DISORDERS

By *DSM-IV-TR* definition, the symptoms of ASDs must be present by 3 years of age. Even when parents are concerned about a child's early development, the diagnosis of an ASD may not be made for 2–3 years (Mars et al., 1998). As with many other disorders, the more severe the symptoms, the earlier the child is referred for evaluation. The age of diagnosis has decreased with increased awareness by pediatricians, parents, and preschool teachers. Children with Asperger syndrome and high-functioning autism, however, tend to be diagnosed at school age.

Delayed language development, repetitive behaviors, and atypical social responsivity are common early parental concerns. Systematic review of videotapes from the first of year life demonstrates differences in infants with ASDs by 1 year of age. They may not respond to their name and are less interested in faces and voices than other infants. Infants later diagnosed with ASDs may have had poor eye contact, absence of a social smile, irritability, and a dislike of being held. As toddlers, they may have had sleep difficulties, limited diets, tantrums, and inattention to language. Because of limited response to the language of others, initial concerns may have been around hearing impairment. Overall, ASDs cannot be thought of in terms of age of onset of symptoms but rather in terms of age of recognition (Volkmar, Stier, & Cohen, 1985).

Early diagnosis is based on the recognition of the core features of ASDs as they appear in early childhood. Atypical development of pretend play, pointing to share interest, use of eye gaze to engage another person in communication, and social interest can distinguish toddlers at high risk for ASD as young as 18 months of age. These observations are the basis for the Checklist for Autism in Toddlers (CHAT; Baron-Cohen et al., 2000) and the Modified Checklist for Autism in Toddlers (M-CHAT; Robins et al., 2001). The M-CHAT is a brief parent questionnaire suitable for screening toddlers prior to 3 years of age. Other tests that can be used to screen for ASDs in toddlers include the Screening Tool for Autism (STAT; Stone et al., 2004) and the Pervasive Developmental Disorder Screening Test-II (PDDST-II; Siegel, 2004). The routine use of general developmental and behavioral screening tests by primary care providers, however, is likely to be the best screening mechanism to identify children with ASD. This approach identifies general delays and results in earlier referral for diagnostic and treatment services. Because of the importance of early diagnosis in leading to early intervention, there has been much interest in the accurate screening and diagnosis at younger and younger ages. (See Table 23.2 for more information about screening tools.)

Evaluation of the Child with an Autism Spectrum Disorder

Assessment for ASDs requires time, collaboration among health care and educational professionals, and knowledge of the disorders. The evaluation follows directly from the diagnostic criteria that focus on impairments in social reciprocity, language, and restricted patterns of behavior (Filipek et al., 2000).

Multidisciplinary Assessment Most children are initially referred to school-based assessment teams or early intervention services by their primary care providers or by parents because of language delays (see Chapter 33). Initial multidisciplinary evaluation of developmental concerns should involve formal assessments of 1) receptive and expressive language, 2) cognitive function, 3) hearing, 4) fine and gross motor function, 5) social and emotional skills, and 6) adaptive skills.

If an ASD is suspected, referral should be made to a professional experienced in making diagnoses, such as a neurodevelopmental or developmental-behavioral pediatrician, child neurologist, child psychiatrist, child psychologist, or speech-language pathologist. The assessment should include a detailed medical history, with particular attention paid to 1) social development; 2) developmental milestones, especially in language; 3) other medical conditions; 3) family history, including behavioral, medical, neurologic, developmental, and psychiatric illnesses; and 4) current family functioning and circumstances. As noted previously, more than one quarter of children with Autistic Disorder have a reported loss of language and/or social milestones in the second year of life. An underlying medical condition needs to be considered in these cases. Ten percent of children with ASDs are reported to have medical conditions that might be etiologic (Chakrabarti & Fombonne, 2001). A general physical and neurological examination for intercurrent medical conditions that might exacerbate behavior and for underlying causes of the ASD should take place. The physical examination should include an examination of the skin, as children with neurocutaneous syndromes (e.g., tuberous sclerosis) are at higher risk for ASDs. Head circumference should be monitored and with conventional neurologic assessment of macro and microcephaly.

Diagnostic Measures Diagnosis of an ASD is based on the application of the *DSM-IV-*

TR criteria (APA, 2000). The history and clinical observation requires input from parents, therapists, and teachers who are familiar with the child in multiple settings. Because many children with ASDs are anxious in new settings, it may take multiple visits to obtain a reliable assessment. Structured history through the Autism Diagnostic Inventory (Lord, Rutter, &Le Couter, 1994) and observation of symptoms through the Autism Diagnostic Observation Schedule (Lord et al., 2000) are used primarily in research settings to standardize application of the *DSM-IV-TR* criteria.

Laboratory Testing and Neuroimaging

There is no standard medical workup for children with ASDs. Etiologic workup is determined by history and physical examination (American Academy of Pediatrics [AAP], 2001). DNA analysis for fragile X syndrome is often recommended in children with cognitive limitations and symptoms of ASDs. Karyotyping should also be considered. A chromosomal abnormality is identified in up to 5% of children with ASDs and cognitive limitations. Advances in chromosome analysis such as subtelomeric analysis (see Chapter 1) has not increased diagnostic yield to date. As the genes for ASD are identified, it is likely that testing for specific gene alterations will be routinely recommended.

Although abnormalities may be seen on MRI in children with ASDs, the yield for diagnostic or treatable conditions identified by routine neuroimaging studies is low. Similarly, in the absence of a history of seizures, routine screening with EEGs is not indicated (Filipek et al., 2000). General metabolic screening rarely has positive results if the history and physical examination is negative. Although additional medical and biological evaluations are often pursued, there is no scientific evidence to support measurement of heavy metal levels in hair, blood, or urine; immunologic parameters in blood; stool flora; urine peptides; or yeast metabolites in urine in children with ASDs (Levy & Hyman, 2005).

ASSOCIATED CONDITIONS

ASDs may be associated with intellectual disability, as well as many other conditions. These are discussed next.

Intellectual Disability

Most studies report that up to three quarters of individuals with Autistic Disorder also have in-

Table 23.2. Screening and diagnostic tests for autism spectrum disorders (ASDs)

Screening tests for ASDs in toddlers

Modified Checklist for Autism in Toddlers (M-CHAT; Dumont-Mathew & Fein, 2005): ages 18–36 months

Screening Tool for Autism in Two-Year-Olds (STAT; Stone et al., 2004)

Pervasive Developmental Disorder Screening Test (PDDST; Seigel, 2004)

Screening tests for older children

Social Communication Questionnaire (SCQ; Berument et al., 2002): older than 3 years of age

Social Reciprocity Scale (Constantino, 2004): school age

Standardized tests that support a clinical diagnosis of autism

Childhood Autism Rating Scale (CARS; Schopler, Reichler, & Renner, 1993): older than 2 years of age

Gilliam Autism Rating Scale, Second Edition (GARS-2; Gilliam, 2005): older than age 3

"Gold standard" companion measures designed to elicit symptoms of ASDs for diagnostic purposes

Autism Diagnostic Interview (ADI; Lord et al., 1994): semistructured interview with the caregiver that allows for scoring whether autism is present

Autism Diagnostic Observation Schedule (ADOS; Lord et al., 2000): structured interactions for children of different language abilities to allow for observation of symptoms of ASDs per the *Diagnostic and Statistical Manual of Mental Disorders, Fourth Edition, Text Revision (DSM-IV-TR;* American Psychiatric Association, 2000) criteria for both Autistic Disorder and Pervasive Developmental Disorder

The above two measures are often used together to characterize cases for research related to autism.

Note: Clinical application of the diagnostic criteria from *DSM-IV-TR* by an experienced clinician is the mainstay of diagnosis.

tellectual disability. Yeargain-Alsop et al. (2003) reported that 68% of the children between 3 and 10 years of age identified with ASDs in the Atlanta area also had intellectual disability. Only 40% of preschool children diagnosed with ASDs were found to have comorbid intellectual disability at the time of the first evaluation (Chakrabarti & Fombonne, 2001). With more inclusive diagnostic criteria for ASD, it is likely that increasing numbers of individuals with typical cognitive abilities and with significant intellectual disability will be identified as having ASDs. Brain insults responsible for causing ASDs can disrupt other neurologic functions and result in intellectual disability.

Overlap of symptoms between intellectual disability and the ASDs also complicates the diagnostic process. Careful clinical assessment is necessary to determine if social development is atypical for the child's mental age. Symptoms of ASD such as a lack of interest in peer play, lack of pretend play, and repetitive behaviors may also be seen in people with severe intellectual disability without ASDs (de Bildt et al., 2004).

Learning Disabilities

Learning disabilities are common among individuals who have ASDs. Specific impairments in **executive function**—the cognitive tasks related to taking in, organizing, processing and acting on information—also may be present in people with ASDs (Ozonoff et al., 2004).

Epilepsy

Overall, epilepsy is reported in about one quarter of individuals with ASDs and most commonly presents in infancy and adolescence (Tuchman & Rapin, 2002). There is also an increased likelihood of having an abnormal EEG without seizures in people with ASDs. The implications of this finding are unclear, and the role of anticonvulsant treatment in the absence of seizures has not been evaluated.

Tic Disorders

Up to 9% of children with ASDs also have tics or brief involuntary motor movements. Tourette syndrome can be diagnosed when both vocal and motor tics last 6 months. Tourette syndrome may be associated with inattention and hyperactivity, obsessions, and learning disabilities. Individuals who have Tourette syndrome but not an ASD have appropriate social reciprocity (Ringman & Jankovic, 2000).

Sleep Disorders

Sleep disturbances are reported in 50%–70% of children with ASDs. Although often considered most problematic in the preschool years, symptoms persist in many children. Night waking, delayed sleep onset, and early morning waking are all reported (Wiggs & Stores, 2004). Poor sleep may be associated with daytime inattention and irritability. Underlying biologic causes may relate to abnormal melatonin synthesis and release or disordered sleep cycles. Until the etiology is better understood, the mainstay of treatment is behavioral intervention. Medical treatment with melatonin, antihistamines, and other sedating agents may be used to augment behavioral treatment.

Gastrointestinal Symptoms

Increased prevalence of abdominal pain, gastroesophageal reflux, diarrhea, constipation, and bloating among children with ASDs has been suggested (Erickson et al., 2005). Although high rates of gastrointestinal symptoms are reported among children with ASDs attending subspecialty clinics, no increased rate of complaint was identified in studies examining primary care records in the United Kingdom for children prior to diagnosis. In a clinical series of children with ASDs who were referred for evaluation of accompanying gastrointestinal (GI) concerns, the children were reported to have a greater than anticipated rate of lymphonodular hyperplasia on intestinal biopsy (Wakefield, Anthony, & Murch, 2000). Additional study is necessary to determine if this evidence of inflammatory response represents a specific disease state. Abdominal discomfort may be responsible for acute behavioral changes. Children with ASDs often have specific food aversions and rituals and are at risk for nutritional compromise. Symptoms of GI disease need to be assessed and treated in children with ASDs as with any other children.

Psychiatric Conditions

Children with ASDs are at greater risk for depression, mood disorders, symptoms of attention-deficit/hyperactivity disorder, and anxiety. Comorbid diagnosis may be most evident in adolescents with adequate language and insight to allow standard application of diagnostic criteria.

Genetic Disorders Associated with Autism Spectrum Disorders

ASDs occurs with greater frequency among children with specific genetic disorders. Children with these disorders need to be monitored for symptoms of ASDs.

Tuberous Sclerosis Tuberous sclerosis is an autosomal dominant disorder caused by a defect in the TSC2 gene that codes for the protein tuberin. This neurocutaneous condition results in characteristic skin lesions (depigmented oblong patches called ash leaf spots), acne-like adenoma sebaceum, and benign growths (**tubers**) in the brain (Smalley, 1998). Common features are intellectual disability and seizures. Although, only 1%–4% of people with ASDs are likely to have tuberous sclerosis, a substantial number of children with tuberous sclerosis have symptoms of autism. All children being evaluated for an ASD should be examined to rule out neurocutaneous conditions.

Fragile X Syndrome At one time fragile X syndrome, the most prevalent cause of inherited intellectual disability, was believed to be a common genetic cause of ASDs. With careful clinical diagnosis, it has become clear that a large number of individuals with fragile X syndrome have many symptoms of ASDs but do not meet full criteria for the diagnosis. Up to 2% of boys with an ASD also have fragile X (Wassink, Piven, & Pitel, 2001).

Chromosome 15 Deletion Prader-Willi syndrome and Angelman syndrome share a common region for chromosomal deletion on chromosome 15 (15q11-q13). People with Prader-Willi syndrome have profound obesity, short stature, skin picking behaviors, and mild cognitive limitations. Angelman syndrome is characterized by intellectual disability, a happy affect, ataxic movements, hand clapping, and a characteristic facial appearance. A subgroup of children within ASD has been identified who also have a deletion or duplication in this region on chromosome 15 (Muhle et al., 2004).

Other Syndromes Associated with Autism Spectrum Disorders An increased rate of ASDs has been reported in Moebius syndrome (facial diplegia) and Joubert syndrome (cerebellar hypoplasia). Both of these syndromes may involve disruption of early embryologic brain development. Other genetic syndromes that have been associated with ASDs include Down syndrome, CHARGE syndrome, and Smith-Lemli-Opitz syndrome. The co-occurrence of these syndromes and the behaviors of autism may help researchers learn more about the neurobiology of ASDs (Muhle et al., 2004).

TREATMENT APPROACHES

It is important to diagnose children with ASDs early and accurately. Early educational programs focus on teaching social language and enhancing appropriate behaviors to children with ASDs. It is believed that treatment is most ef-

fective if started early. The National Research Council (2001) recommended intervention that is intensive, multidisciplinary, and continuous. Goals of autism treatment include 1) fostering development, 2) promoting learning, 3) reducing rigidity and stereotypy, 4) eliminating maladaptive behaviors, and 5) alleviating family distress (Rutter, 1985). A comprehensive approach usually requires a combination of an **individualized educational program,** behavioral supports, social and pragmatic language skills development, and family support.

Educational Approaches

The mainstay of treatment is education (National Research Council, 2001). Disorder-specific programs should be instituted as soon as a diagnosis is made. There are many different approaches to preschool education for children with ASDs. Successful programs share the characteristics of early entry, active participation in an intensive program offered daily throughout the year, planned teaching opportunities organized with the attention span of the child in mind, and sufficient adult staffing to meet the needs of the individual child and his or her program. An increase in tested IQ scores has been documented in young children with autism who participate in disorder-specific interventions (Harris et al., 1991). This finding may be in part the result of maturation, and increased motivation to participate in testing. In the absence of well-designed studies, one must be careful in ascribing treatment effects to either educational or complementary interventions that are instituted during early childhood.

Although there are philosophical differences between some of the teaching strategies, most preschool programs utilize the following: 1) structured teaching periods, 2) reinforcement of spontaneous communication, 3) instruction of specific skills using principles of reinforcement, and 4) incidental learning (i.e., use of spontaneously occurring "teachable moments"). Some of the more common approaches are described next.

TEACCH The TEACCH (Treatment and Education of Autistic and related Communication handicapped Children) was one of the initial disorder-specific educational programs that recognized the need for an intensive and coordinated approach to skill building and developing communication abilities (Mesibov, Shea, & Schopler, 2005). It was designed to address the needs of the child and family across the school experience and includes classroom teaching, parent training, and other support services. The approach is eclectic and involves the use of behavioral strategies to enhance communication and social interaction, as well as visual organization and cuing; in addition, it emphasizes the parents' roles as co-therapists.

Applied Behavior Analysis

The behavioral principles of operant learning (see Chapter 35) were used in a program for preschool children with ASDs developed by Dr. Ivor Lovaas (1987). His initial studies demonstrated that intensive and early intervention that specifically teaches the component skills necessary for development was associated with typical classroom performance in almost half of the 20 children with autism studied from 7–11 years of age (McEachin, Smith, & Lovaas, 1993). This model initially tested a 40-hour-per-week program that was based on individual therapy using discrete trial teaching, prompting, and reinforcement. Goals of the first year of treatment were to develop language skills, increase social use of language, increase social approach, promote play skills, and decrease behaviors that competed with the desired goals of therapy. In the second year of treatment, the goal was to extend intervention to a preschool environment in order to encourage interaction with peers and generalize the acquired skills. Later studies reported qualitative improvement even in children who do not have the dramatic response to behavioral treatment because of comorbid intellectual disability (Smith et al., 1997). Modifications in the delivery of applied behavior analysis (ABA) services have addressed teaching language skills and using a variety of behaviorally based strategies for skill development (Koegel, Koegel, & McNerney, 2001). Generalization of skills to the home and classroom are an important component of the treatment plan.

Developmental-Individual Difference-Relationship Based Model

The Developmental-Individual Difference-Relationship Based model (DIR model) is a treatment strategy described by Weider and Greenspan (2003) that builds on social communication learned in relationships with consistent and responsive adults. "Opening and closing circles of communication" in the context of child directed play is the focus of this intervention. It depends on participation by the family and educational team. This type of therapy has been demonstrated to contribute to developmental gains when used as part of an early intervention program (Mahoney & Perales, 2005). It seeks to build shared attention leading to engagement. Communication and problem solving are also practiced, and the adults shape the development of appropriate play and interaction.

Relationship Development Intervention

Relationship Development Intervention (RDI; Connections Center, 2004) is another relationship development approach that addresses social learning as an apprenticeship model. The adults lead the child through learning how to interact and respond in naturalistic settings. Parents are educated to understand the core deficits of ASDs so they can respond and shape their child's responses to language and social situations.

Classroom-Based Programs

For children 3–21 years of age, Autistic Disorder is included as a special category of educational disability under the Individuals with Disabilities Education Improvement Act of 2004 (PL 108-446). This law mandates that specific academic goals should relate to the child's cognitive *and* functional level, and the program should be provided in the least restrictive environment. The Handicapping Condition under federal law is Autism, although under the diagnostic criteria in the *DSM-IV-TR*, Autistic Disorder is only one of the ASDs (or Pervasive Developmental Disorders per the *DSM-IV-TR*).

Children with ASDs should have their individualized needs addressed whether they are educated in small structured classrooms or in inclusive environments. Inclusive education allows for the child to model appropriate behaviors and learn how to participate in the community. Modifying educational materials may require consultant teacher support or team-taught classrooms. Some children with ASDs may benefit from a more structured environment with fewer sensory distractions. A specialized class setting could potentially be *less* restrictive for some children with ASDs because the predictability may result in less personal distress. Many educational strategies can be used to enhance the success of children with ASDs in the classroom (Harrower & Dunlap, 2001; Myles & Southwick, 1999). Future studies need to determine which programs are most effective and for which students.

Behavioral Intervention

An important goal of educating children with ASDs is to teach skills that extend their ability to communicate and socialize with others. Behavior carries meaning and should not be presumed to be a random act. Painful medical conditions and comorbid psychiatric conditions should be considered in cases of acute behavioral deterioration. If the origin of the behavior is considered, it may be possible to teach more effective ways to achieve a similar result (e.g., comfort, communication) and to expand behaviors that increase social adaptability. Behavioral support can be helpful in establishing daily routines, in extinguishing destructive behaviors, and in responding to tantrums. A functional behavioral analysis is indicated if behaviors interfere with classroom functioning (Dalton, 2002). This formal assessment determines why the behaviors are occurring. A functional behavioral plan can then be developed to alter the environmental factors that precipitate the challenging behaviors or teach the child and staff other means of responding (see Chapter 33).

Pragmatic Language and Social Skills Training

Communication attempts by children with ASDs should be rewarded socially or in other ways to foster language development. Bondy and Frost (1998) demonstrated that organizing visual cues helps children with ASDs associate the spoken word with events. This helps them learn the role of communication in obtaining tangible items and can be built into a Picture Exchange Communication System (PECS). There may be comorbid verbal motor dyspraxia or apraxia. This is when the motor coordination of speech is discordant with language understanding. Therapy may include a visual language system (picture or sign) which, in some cases, scaffolds the development of spoken communication. The use of augmentative and alternative communication (AAC) is different from facilitated communication. In AAC, children who do not have efficient oral speech are taught to independently gain access to written, graphic, or computer-assisted technologies for independent communication. Facilitated communication is a technique whereby a facilitator guides the individual with an ASD to type responses. Subconscious guidance by the facilitator has been demonstrated under experimental conditions, and facilitated communication is not endorsed for clinical use (Mostert, 2001).

For children with spoken language, an important objective is the promotion of language skills used in conversation (Quill, 2000). *Pragmatic language* refers to the integration of gesture, expression, proximity, and inflection of language to enhance interpersonal understanding of communication. It involves both production and understanding of these functions in the conversational partner. These skills can make the difference in independent living, employment, and higher education. Encouraging social and pragmatic language development can be accomplished through a variety of approaches, including modeling by peers in inclusive settings, Social Stories (Gray, 2000), formal social skills curricula, supervised social skills group experiences, and tutoring by typically developing peers (Rogers, 2000). Children with ASDs may not generalize rehearsal in a group to other settings unless specifically taught to do so. Moreover, these techniques may not bridge the gap between social interactions and social relationships (Bauminger & Kasari, 2000). Therefore, educational objectives should address mastery of social skills in different settings and with different people.

Medication

Medication should only be considered as a component of a therapeutic program that includes behaviorally based therapy to teach appropriate behaviors and understanding of the reasons why behaviors might occur. Treatment with medication should be for specific target behaviors or a comorbid psychiatric or medical disorder.

Stimulant Medications Hyperactivity and inattention are common symptoms in children with ASDs. If appropriate language and educational interventions are in place and inattention persists, treatment with conventional stimulant medications such as methylphenidate and mixed dextroamphetamine salts can have beneficial effects (Handen, Johnson, & Lubetsky, 2000; see Appendix C). Side effects may include insomnia, decreased appetite, increased moodiness, and repetitive behaviors. Guanfacine and clonidine have been used for treatment of motor hyperactivity with some success (Jaselskis et al., 1992). Potential side effects of these two medications include hypotension and sedation.

Selective Serotonin Reuptake Inhibitors Because of some similarities between perseverative interests and obsessions, selective serotonin reuptake inhibitors (SSRIs) have been used to treat repetitive behaviors, irritability, and self-injury in people with ASDs (Moore et al., 2004). Decreasing anxiety may have additional benefits in enhancing language and social interactions. Side effects may include paradoxical hyperactivity or mood instability. Suicidal behaviors have very rarely been reported with drugs in this class when used to treat adolescent depression, so close monitoring is suggested.

Atypical Neuroleptics Well-designed trials have demonstrated that the atypical neuroleptic risperdone significantly improves irritability, aggression, and self-stimulatory/self-injurious behaviors in children with ASDs and intellectual disability (McCracken et al., 2002; McDougle et al., 2005). Medications in this class, such as olanzapine and aripiprazole, have been used on the basis of small open trials. The major side effect seen is weight gain. Less common side effects from this class of medications include metabolic syndrome (a prediabetic state with elevation of blood lipids), tardive dyskinesia, sedation, and hormonal imbalances. Routine monitoring for side effects is important.

Mood Stabilizers Anticonvulsant drugs used to treat bipolar disorder, such valproic acid and carbamazepine, are also used in the management of explosive behaviors in people with ASDs (Hollander et al., 2001). Both medications need to be monitored with blood levels. By extension, newer anticonvulsants are sometimes used.

Other Medications Other types of medications are being investigated for symptoms of ASDs. Advances in technology are likely to bring to market other medications designed to affect specific neural systems.

Complementary and Alternative Therapies

Almost two thirds of Americans employ treatments that could fall into the category of complementary or alternative medicine (CAM). Up to one third of families are already using CAM therapies at the time that their child receives the formal diagnosis of an ASD (Levy et al., 2003). The AAP Committee on Children with Disabilities (2001) recognized that CAM treatments are commonly used for chronic conditions. The committee encouraged traditional health care providers to understand the issues that families are dealing with, to help educate families in the interpretation of claims made by CAM providers and literature, and to monitor children for side effects if CAM therapies are utilized. The health care professional should advocate for the child to pursue educational and other therapeutic interventions known to enhance outcome and help the families evaluate data regarding the cost, side effects, plausibility of the claims, and the claimed benefits for the treatment they wish to try.

There are increasing numbers of scientific studies examining CAM therapies for safety and efficacy. The most informative study design is the double-blind placebo-controlled trial with an adequate number of subjects with well-defined ASDs whose treatment response is measured using valid tests. In most behavioral studies, up to one third of participants report benefit from placebo. That is why it is so important that placebo controlled trials be reported for treatment.

Dietary treatment is popular. Elimination of gluten and casein (wheat and milk proteins) has been hypothesized to result in decreased symptoms of autism and in decreased intestinal distress in some children. Although there are many anecdotal reports of improvement, two small studies have not demonstrated marked improvement (Elder et al., 2006; Millward et al., 2005). Despite this, the gluten- and casein-restricted diet remains popular, and families who decide to pursue it need to carefully monitor their child's nutritional needs. For example, when milk is removed, alternative sources of calcium, vitamin D, and protein need to be provided.

Vitamins are often used in doses greater than the recommended daily intake in an attempt to effect behavioral change. Vitamin B_6 taken with magnesium is one such treatment used to enhance attention and language. Although several studies suggested benefit, two double-blind placebo-controlled studies could not demonstrate it (Nye & Brice, 2005). Other nutritional treatments that enjoy popularity at the writing of this chapter include supplementation with essential fatty acids, B_{12}, dimethylglycine, and carnosine (Levy & Hyman, 2005). Children should have target behaviors identified and a monitoring system in place to determine if the intervention has a positive effect. Knowledge of potential side effects is also crucial. Other types of CAM are used to treat hypothesized infectious or immune imbalances such as yeast overgrowth in the colon and intestinal dysbiosis (Finegold et al., 2002). The current scientific literature does not support these treatments.

Sometimes the nontraditional use of a prescription medication becomes a CAM therapy. Secretin is one example. Secretin is a hormone that increases pancreatic secretion into the intestine and is usually employed to evaluate pancreatic function during endoscopy. Anecdotal observation of behavioral improvement in three children after secretin with endoscopy resulted in its widespread use. Subsequently, more than 700 children with ASDs have been studied in double-blind placebo-controlled trials of secretin without confirmation of the original improvement (Williams, Wray, & Wheeler, 2005).

Not all CAM therapies are biologic. Facilitated communication, auditory integration training, and optometric training are nonbiologic examples of CAM. The conventional medical literature does not support the use of these interventions. Sensory integration techniques are often used by occupational therapists to stimulate or calm children who demonstrate altered sensory and motor reactivity (Baranek, 2002). Although popular, there is little data to support general implementation of these strategies. Until appropriately designed scientific studies are completed, each child must be evaluated by the family and therapy team for both positive and negative responses to CAM therapies that families chose to employ.

Family Supports

Families should be connected with appropriate parent support organizations at the time of diagnosis (Chapter 40). The stressors of receiving the diagnosis, making decisions, and addressing the child's needs may require referral for additional counseling services for other family members. The needs of siblings must also be addressed. Most studies indicate that the siblings of children with disabilities are resilient (Kaminsky & Dewey, 2002).

OUTCOME

Measured IQ scores and the presence of language that can be used for conversation remains the best predictor of outcome for children with ASDs (Bilstedt, Gillberg, & Gillberg, 2005). More than half of children diagnosed with au-

tism acquire language that can be used for communication (Howlin, 2003). With the expansion of diagnostic criteria to include a large number of individuals with typical cognitive abilities among those with ASDs (e.g., people with Asperger syndrome), the outcome for successful completion of education and community employment may be more optimistic.

It is as yet unknown how function is altered by educational programs. Diagnosis of an ASD at age 2 seems to be accurate (Lord et al., 2006). It is impossible to predict at the time of diagnosis which children will respond positively to intervention and which children will later also be diagnosed with intellectual disability. Therefore the need to provide an intense and disorder-specific intervention program to all children with ASDs is imperative.

SUMMARY

ASDs are neurodevelopmental disorders with a genetic basis, the presentation of which might be modified by environmental factors. These disorders are characterized by abnormalities in communication, social interaction, and repetitive interests and behaviors. Children with ASDs may have associated intellectual disability and severe communication impairments. Individuals with typical cognitive abilities and high-functioning autism or Asperger syndrome have symptoms related to social reciprocity and repetitive behaviors. Advances in early recognition and intervention have had a positive impact on outcome and quality of life for people with ASDs and their families. Individualized, multidimensional treatment is the standard of care and is associated with notable improvements in symptoms.

REFERENCES

American Academy of Pediatrics, Committee on Children with Disabilities. (2001). Technical Report: The pediatrician's role in the diagnosis and management of Autistic Spectrum Disorder in children. *Pediatrics, 107*, E85.

American Psychiatric Association. (2000). *Diagnostic and statistical manual of mental disorders* (4th ed., text rev.). Washington, DC: Author.

Asperger, H. (1991). 'Autistic psychopathy' in childhood (U. Frith, Trans.). In U. Frith (Ed.), *Autism and Asperger syndrome* (pp. 37–92). New York: Cambridge University Press. (Original work published 1944)

Bailey, A., Luthert, P., Dean, A., et al. (1998). A clinico-pathological study of autism. *Brain, 121*, 889–905.

Baranek, G.T. (2002). Efficacy of sensory and motor interventions for children with autism. *Journal of Autism and Developmental Disorders, 32*(5), 397–422.

Barbaresi, W.J., Katusic, S.K., Colligan, R.C., et al. (2005). The incidence of autism in Olmsted County, Minnesota, 1976–1997: Results from a population based study. *Archives of Pediatrics and Adolescent Medicine, 159,* 37–44.

Baron-Cohen, S., Wheelwright, S., Cox, A., et al. (2000). Early identification of autism by the Checklist for Autism in Toddlers (CHAT). *Journal of the Royal Society of Medicine, 93*(10), 521–525.

Bauminger, N., & Kasari, C. (2000). Loneliness and friendship in high functioning children with autism. *Child Development, 71,* 447–456.

Bernard, S., Enayati, A., Redwood, L., et al. (2001). Autism: A novel form of mercury poisoning. *Medical Hypotheses, 56,* 462–471.

Bertrand, J., Mars, A., Boyle, C., et al. (2001). Prevalence of autism in a United States population: The Brick Township, New Jersey, investigation. *Pediatrics, 175,* 444–451.

Berument, S., Rutter, M., Lord, C., et al. (2002). Screening young people for autism with the Developmental Behavior Checklist. *Journal of the American Academy of Child and Adolescent Psychiatry, 41,* 1369–1375.

Billstedt, E,. Gillberg, C., & Gillberg, C. (2005). Autism after adolescence: Population based 13–22 year follow up study of 120 individuals with autism diagnosed in childhood. *Journal of Autism and Developmental Disorders, 35*(3), 351–360.

Bondy, A.S., & Frost, L.A. (1998). The Picture Exchange Communication System. *Seminars in Speech and Language, 19*(4), 373–388.

Bruinsma, Y., Koegel, R.L., & Koegel L.K. (2004). Joint attention and children with autism: A review of the literature. *Mental Retardardation and Developmental Disabilities Research Reviews, 10*(3), 169–175.

Casanova, M.F., Buxhoeveden, D.P., & Gomez, J. (2004). Disruption in the inhibitory architecture of the cell minicolumn: Implications for autism. *Neuroscientist, 9*(6), 496–507.

Centers for Disease Control and Prevention (CDC). (2006). Mental health in the United States: Parental report of diagnosed autism in children aged 4–17 years: United States, 2003–2004. *Morbidity and Mortality Weekly Report, 55*(17), 481–486.

Chakrabarti, S., & Fombonne, E. (2001). Pervasive developmental disorders in preschool children. *Journal of the American Medical Association, 285*(24), 3093–3099.

Chess, S. (1971). Autism in children with congenital rubella. *Journal of Autism and Childhood Schizophrenia, 1*(1), 33–47.

Committee on Children with Disabilities. (2001). American Academy of Pediatrics: Counseling families who choose complementary and alternative medicine for their child with chronic illness or disability. *Pediatrics, 107,* 598–601. (Erratum in *Pediatrics, 108,* 507.)

Connections Center. (2004). *Relationship Development Intervention (RDI).* Retrieved October 11, 2006, from http://www.rdiconnect.com

Constantino, J. (2004). *Social Responsiveness Scale (SRS).* Los Angeles: Western Publishing Services.

Dalton, M.A. (2002). Education rights and the special needs child. *Child and Adolescent Psychiatric Clinics in North America, 11,* 859–868

Davidson, P.W., Myers, G.J., & Weiss, B. (2004). Mercury exposure and child development outcomes. *Pediatrics, 113*(4, Suppl.), 1023–1099.

Dawson, G., Webb, S.J., & McPartland, J. (2005). Understanding the nature of face processing impairment in autism: Insights from behavioral and electro-physiological studies. *Developmental Neuropsychology, 27,* 403–424.

Dawson, G., Webb, S., Schellenberg, G.D., et al. (2002). Defining the broader phenotype of autism: Genetic, brain, and behavioral perspectives. *Developmental Psychopathology, 14*(3), 581–611.

de Bildt, A., Sytema, S., Ketelaars, C., et al. (2004). Interrelationship between Autism Diagnostic Observation Schedule–Generic (ADOS-G), Autism Diagnostic Interview–Revised (ADI-R), and the Diagnostic and Statistical Manual of Mental Disorders (DSM-IV-TR) classification in children and adolescents with intellectual disability. *Journal of Autism and Developmental Disorders, 34*(2), 129–137.

deLong, R., & Nohria, C. (1994). Psychiatric family history and neurological disease in autistic spectrum disorders. *Developmental Medicine and Child Neurology, 36*(5), 441–448.

Demicheli, V., Jefferson, T., Rivetti, A, et al. (2005). Vaccines for measles, mumps and rubella in children. *Cochrane Database of Systematic Reviews,* CD004407.

Dumont-Mathew, T., & Fein, D. (2005). Screening for autism in young children: The Modified Checklist for Autism in Toddlers (M-CHAT) and other measures. *Mental Retardation and Developmental Disabilities Research Reviews, 11,* 253–262.

Elder, J.H., Shankar, M., Shuster, J., et al. (2006). The gluten-free, casein-free diet in autism: Results of a preliminary double blind clinical trial. *Journal of Autism and Developmental Disorders, 36*(3), 413–420.

Erickson, C.A., Stigler, K.A., Corkins, M.R., et al. (2005). Gastrointestinal factors in autistic disorder: A critical review. *Journal of Autism and Developmental Disorders, 35*(6), 713–727.

Filipek, P., Accardo, P., Ashwal, S., et al. (2000). Practice parameter: Screening and diagnosis of autism. *Neurology, 55,* 468–479.

Finegold, S.M., Molitoris, D., Song, Y., et al. (2002). Gastrointestinal microflora studies in late-onset autism. *Clinical Infectious Disease, 35*(Suppl. 1), S6–S16.

Folstein, S., & Rutter, M. (1977). Infantile autism: A genetic study of 21 twin pairs. *Journal of Child Psychology, Psychiatry, and Allied Disciplines, 18,* 297–321.

Fombonne, E. (2001). Is there an epidemic of autism? *American Academy of Pediatrics, 107,* 411–412.

Fombonne, E. (2002). Epidemiological trends in rates of autism. *Molecular Psychiatry, 7,* S4–S6.

Fombonne, E. (2003). Epidemiological surveys of autism and other pervasive developmental disorders: An update. *Journal of Autism and Developmental Disorders, 33,* 365–382.

Gilliam, J.E. (2005). *Gilliam Autism Rating Scale, Second Edition (GARS-2).* Circle Pines, MN: AGS Publishing.

Gray, C. (2000). *The new Social Stories book.* Arlington, TX: Future Horizons.

Greenspan, S.I., & Wieder, S. (1998). *The child with special needs.* Philadelphia: Perseus Books.

Gutstein, S. (2003). *Administration manual for the Relationship Development Assessment (RDA) Part 1 (Version 3.0).* Houston, TX: Connections Center.

Handen, B.L., Johnson, C.R., & Lubetsky, M. (2000). Efficacy of methylphenidate among children with autism and symptoms of attention-deficit hyperactivity disorder. *Journal of Autism and Developmental Disorders, 30*(3), 245–255.

Harris, S.L., Handleman J.S., Gordon R., et al. (1991). Changes in cognitive and language functioning of preschool children with autism. *Journal of Autism and Developmental Disorders, 21*(3), 281–290.

Harrower, J.K., & Dunlap, G. (2001). Including children with autism in general education classrooms: A review of effective strategies. *Behavior Modification, 25*, 762–784.

Hendry, C.N. (2000). Childhood disintegrative disorder: Should it be considered a distinct diagnosis? *Clinical Psychology Review, 20*, 77–90.

Hollander, E., Dolgoff-Kaspar, R., Cartwright, C., et al. (2001). An open trial of divalproex sodium in autism spectrum disorders. *The Journal of Clinical Psychiatry, 62*(7), 530–534.

Howlin, P. (2003). Outcome in high-functioning adults with autism with and without early language delays: implications for the differentiation between autism and Asperger syndrome. *Journal of Autism and Developmental Disorders, 33*, 3–13.

Huppke, P., & Gartner, J. (2005). Molecular diagnosis of Rett syndrome. *Journal of Child Neurology, 20*, 732–736.

Hyman, S.L., Arndt, T.L., & Rodier, P.M. (2005). Environmental agents in autism: Once and future associations. *International Journal Intellectual Disability Reviews.*

Individuals with Disabilities Education Improvement Act of 2004, PL 108-446, 20 U.S.C. §§ 1400 *et seq.*

Jaselskis, C.A., Cook, E.H., Fletcher, K.E., et al. (1992). Clonidine treatment of hyperactive and impulsive children with autistic disorder. *Journal of Clinical Psychopharmacology, 12*, 322–327.

Kadesjö, B., Gillberg, C., & Hagberg, B. (1999). Brief report: Autism and Asperger syndrome in seven-year-old children: A total population study. *Journal of Autism and Developmental Disorders, 29*, 327–31.

Kaminsky, L., & Dewey, D. (2002). Psychosocial adjustment in siblings of children with autism. *Journal of Child Psychology and Psychiatry, 43*, 225–232.

Kanner, L. (1943). Autistic disturbances of affective contact. *Nervous Child, 2*, 217.

Kemper, T.L., & Bauman, M. (1998). Neuropathology of infantile autism. *Journal of Neuropathology and Experimental Neurology, 57*, 645–652.

Klin, A., Jones W., Schultz, R. et al. (2002). Visual fixation patterns during viewing of naturalistic social situations as predictors of social competence in individuals with autism. *Archives of General Psychiatry, 59*, 809–816.

Koegel, R.L., Koegel, L.K., & McNerney, E.K. (2001). Pivotal areas in intervention for autism. *Journal of Clinical Child Psychology, 30*(1), 19–32.

Krause, I., Xiao-Song, H., Gershwin, E., et al. (2002). Brief report: Immune factors in autism: A critical review. *Journal of Autism and Developmental Disabilities, 32*, 337–345.

Levy, S.E., & Hyman, S.L. (2005). Novel treatments for autistic spectrum disorders. *Mental Retardation and Developmental Disabilities Research Reviews, 11*(2), 131–142.

Levy, S.E., Mandell, D.S., Merhar, S., et al. (2003). Use of complementary and alternative medicine among children recently diagnosed with autistic spectrum disorder. *Journal of Developmental and Behavioral Pediatrics, 24*, 418–423.

Lord, C., Risi, S., DiLavore, P.S., et al. (2006). Autism from 2 to 9 years of age. *Archives of General Psychiatry, 63*(6), 694–701.

Lord, C., Risi, S., Lambrecht, L., et al. (2000). The autism diagnostic observation schedule-generic: A standard measure of social and communication deficits associated with the spectrum of autism. *Journal of Autism and Developmental Disorders, 30*, 205–223.

Lord, C., Rutter, M., Goode, S., et al. (1989). Autism diagnostic observation schedule: A standardized observation of communicative and social behavior. *Journal of Autism and Developmental Disorders, 19*, 185–212.

Lord, C., Rutter, M., & Le Couteur, A. (1994). Autism Diagnostic Interview–Revised: A revised version of a diagnostic interview for caregivers of individuals with possible pervasive developmental disorders. *Journal of Autism and Developmental Disorders, 24*, 659–685.

Lovaas, O.I. (1987). Behavioral treatment and normal educational and intellectual functioning in young autistic children. *Journal of Consulting and Clinical Psychology, 55*, 3–9.

Madsen, K.M., Hvliid, A., Vestergaard, M., et al. (2002). A population-based study of measles, mumps, and rubella vaccination and autism. *The New England Journal of Medicine, 347*(19), 1477–1482.

Madsen, K.M., Lauritsen, M.B., Pedersen, C.B., et al. (2003). Thimerosal and the occurrence of autism: Negative ecological evidence from Danish population-based data. *Pediatrics, 112*, 604–606.

Mahoney, G., & Perales, F. (2005). Relationship-focused early intervention with children with pervasive developmental disorders and other disabilities: A comparative study. *Journal of Developmental and Behavioral Pediatrics, 26*(2), 77–85.

Mars, A.E., Mauk, J.E., & Dowrick, P.W. (1998). Symptoms of pervasive developmental disorders as observed in prediagnositc home videos of infants and toddlers. *The Journal of Pediatrics, 132*, 500–504.

McCracken, J.T., McGough, J., Shah, B., et al. (2002). Risperidone in children with autism and serious behavioral problems. *The New England Journal of Medicine, 347*, 314–321.

McDougle, C.J., Scahill, L., Aman, M.G., et al. (2005). Risperidone for the core symptom domains of autism: Results from the study by the autism network of the research units on pediatric psychopharmacology. *American Journal of Psychiatry, 162*(6), 1142–1148.

McEachin, J.J., Smith, T., & Lovaas, O.I. (1993). Long-term outcome for children with autism who received early intensive behavioral treatment. *American Journal on Mental Retardation, 97*, 359–372.

Mesibov, G.B., Shea, V., & Schopler, E. (2005). *The TEACCH approach to autism spectrum disorders.* New York: Kluwer Academic/Plenum Publishers.

Millward, C., Ferriter, M., Calver, S., et al. (2005). Gluten- and casein-free diets for autistic spectrum disorder. *Cochrane Database of Systematic Reviews, 2*, CD003498.

Moore, M.L., Eichner, S.F., & Jones, J.R. (2004). Treating functional impairment of autism with selective serotonin-reuptake inhibitors. *Annals of Pharmacotherapy, 38*, 1515–1519. (Epub 2004 Aug 3.)

Mostert, M.P. (2001). Facilitated communication since 1995: A review of published studies. *Journal of Autism and Developmental Disorders, 31*, 287–313.

Muhle, R., Trentatcoste, S.V., & Rapin, I. (2004). The genetics of autism. *Pediatrics, 113*(5), e472–86.

Myles B.S., & Southwick J. (1999). *Asperger syndrome and difficult moments.* Shawnee Mission, KS: Autism Asperger Publishing Co.

National Research Council. (2001). *Educating children with autism: Committee on Educational Interventions for Children with Autism, Division of Behavioral and Social Sciences and Education.* Washington, DC: National Academies Press.

Nelson, K.B., & Bauman, M.L. (2003). Thimerosal and autism? *Pediatrics, 111*(3), 674–679.

Nomura, Y., & Sagawa, M. (2005). Natural history of Rett syndrome. *Journal of Child Neurology, 20,* 764–768.

Nye, C., & Brice, A. (2005). Combined vitamin B6-magnesium treatment in autism spectrum disorder. *Cochrane Database of Systematic Reviews, 4,* CD003497.

Ozonoff, S., Cook, I., Coon, H., et al. (2004). Performance on Cambridge Neuropsychological test automated battery subtests sensitive to frontal lobe function in people with autistic disorder: Evidence from the Collaborative Programs of Excellence in Autism network. *Journal of Autism and Developmental Disorders, 34,* 139–150.

Palmer, R.F., Blanchard, S., Stein, Z., et al. (2006). Environmental mercury release, special education rates, and autism disorder: An ecological study of Texas. *Health Place, 12*(2), 203–209

Pelphrey, K.A., Morris, J.P., & McCarthy, G. (2005). Neural basis of eye gaze processing deficits in autism. *Brain, 128,* 1038–1048.

Piven, J., Palmer, P., Landa, R., et al. (1997). Personality and language characteristics in parents from multiple-incidence autism families. *American Journal of Medical Genetics, 74,* 398–411.

Quill, K.A. (2000). *DO-WATCH-LISTEN-SAY: Social and communication intervention for children with autism.* Baltimore: Paul H. Brookes Publishing Co.

Rapin, I., & Dunn, M. (2003). Update on the language disorders of individuals on the autistic spectrum. *Brain & Development, 25*(3), 166–172.

Redcay, E., & Courchesne, E. (2005). When is the brain enlarged in autism? A meta-analysis of all brain size reports. *Biological Psychiatry, 58,* 1–9.

Richler, J., Luyster, R., Risi, S., et al. (2006). Is there a 'regressive phenotype' of autism spectrum disorder associated with the measles-mumps-rubella vaccine? A CPEA study. *Journal of Autism and Developmental Disorders, 36*(3), 299–316.

Ringman, J.M., & Jankovic, J. (2000). Occurrence of tics in Asperger's syndrome and autistic disorder. *Journal of Child Neurology, 15*(6), 394–400.

Robins, D., Fein, D., Barton, M., et al. (2001). The Modified Checklist for Autism in Toddlers: An initial study investigating the early detection of autism and pervasive developmental disorders. *Journal of Autism and Developmental Disorders, 32*(2), 131–144.

Rogers, S. (2000). Interventions that facilitate socialization in children with autism. *Journal of Autism and Developmental Disorders, 30,* 399–410.

Rogers, S.J. (1998). Neuropsychology of autism in young children and its implications for early intervention. *Mental Retardation and Developmental Disabilities Research Reviews, 4,* 104–112.

Rogers, S.J. (2004). Developmental regression in autistic spectrum disorders. *Mental Retardation and Developmental Disorders Research Reviews, 10*(2), 139–143.

Rutter, M. (1985). The treatment of autistic children. *Journal of Child Psychology and Psychiatry and Allied Disciplines, 28,* 3–14.

Schopler, E., Reichler, R.J., & Renner, B.R. (1993). *Childhood Autism Rating Scale (CARS).* Circle Pines, MN: AGS Publishing.

Schultz R.T., Grelotti D.J., Klin A., et al. (2000). The role of the fusiform face area in social cognition: Implications for the pathobiology of autism. *Philosophical Transactions of the Royal Society of London. Series B: Biological Sciences, 358,* 415–427.

Scott, M.M., & Deneris, E.S. (2005). Making and break-ing serotonin neurons and autism. *International Journal of Developmental Neuroscience, 23,* 277–285.

Shattuck, P.T. (2006). The contribution of diagnostic substitution to the growing administrative prevalence of autism in US special education. *Pediatrics, 117*(4), 1028–1037.

Shi, L., Fatemi, S.H., Sidwell, R.W., et al. (2003). Maternal influenza infection causes marked behavioral and pharmacological changes in the offspring. *Journal of Neuroscience, 23,* 297–302.

Siegel, B. (2004). *Pervasive Developmental Disorders Screening Test–II (PDDST-II).* San Antonio, TX: Harcourt Assessment.

Smalley, S.L. (1998). Autism and tuberous sclerosis. *Journal of Autism and Developmental Disorders, 28,* 407–414.

Smith, T., Eikeseth, S., Klevstrand, M., et al. (1997). Intensive behavioral treatment for preschoolers with severe intellectual disability and pervasive developmental disorder. *American Journal on Intellectual Disability, 105,* 269–285.

Sponheim, E., & Skjeldal, O. (1998) Autism and related disorders: epidemiological findings in a Norwegian study using ICD-10 diagnostic criteria. *Journal of Autism and Developmental Disorders, 28,* 217–227.

Stone, W.L., Coonrod, E.E., Turner, L.M., et al. (2004). Psychometric properties of the STAT for early autism screening. *Journal of Autism and Developmental Disorders, 34,* 691–701.

Szatmari, P. (2000). The classification of Autism, Asperger's syndrome and pervasive developmental disorder. *Canadian Journal of Psychiatry, 45,* 731–738.

Travis, L.L., & Sigman, M. (1998). Social deficits and interpersonal relationships in autism. *Mental Retardation and Developmental Disabilities Research Reviews, 4,* 65–72.

Trevathan, E. (2004). Seizures and epilepsy among children with regression and autistic spectrum disorder. *Journal of Child Neurology,* S49–S57.

Tuchman, R, Rapin, I. (2002). Epilepsy in autism. *The Lancet Neurology, 1*(6), 352–358.

Vargas, D.L., Nascimbene, C., Krishnan, C., et al. (2005). Neuroglial activation and neuroinflammation in the brain of patients with autism. *Annals of Neurology, 57*(1), 67–81. (Erratum in *Annals of Neurology, 57*(2), 304.)

Volkmar, F.R., Stier, D.M., & Cohen, D.J. (1985). Age of recognition of pervasive developmental disorder. *The American Journal of Psychiatry, 142,* 1450–1452.

Vollm, B.A., Taylor, A.N., Richardson, P. et al. (2005). Neuronal correlates of theory of mind and empathy: A functional magnetic resonance imaging study in a nonverbal task. *Neuroimage, 29,* 90–98.

Wakefield, A.J., Anthony, A., Murch, S.H., (2000). Enterocolitis in children with developmental disorders. *The American Journal of Gastroenterology, 95*(9), 2285–2295.

Wakefield, A.J., Murch, S.H., Anthony, A., et al. (1998). Ileal-lymphoid-nodular hyperplasia, non-specific colitis, and pervasive developmental disorder in children. *The Lancet, 351,* 637–641.

Wassink, T.H., Piven, J., & Pitel, S.R. (2001). Chromosomal abnormalities in a clinic sample of individuals with autistic disorder. *Psychiatric Genetics, 11,* 57–63.

Webb, E.B., Lobo, S., Hervas, A., et al. (1997). The changing prevalence of autistic disorder in a Welsh health district. *Developmental Medicine and Child Neurology, 39,* 150–152.

Weider, S., & Greenspan, S. (2003). Climbing the symbolic ladder in the DIR model through floor time/interactive play. *Autism, 7,* 425–435.

Wiggs, L., & Stores, G. (2004). Sleep patterns and sleep disorders in children with autistic spectrum disorders: Insights using parent report and actigraphy. *Developmental Medicine and Child Neurology, 46,* 372–380.

Williams, J.H., Waiter, G.D., Gilchrist, A., et al. (2005). Neural mechanisms of imitation and 'mirror neuron' functioning in autistic spectrum disorder. *Neuropsychologia* (Epub ahead of print).

Williams, K.W., Wray, J.J., & Wheeler, D.M. (2005). Intravenous secretin for autism spectrum disorder. *Cochrane Database of Systematic Reviews,* CD003495.

Yeargin-Allsopp, M., Rice, C., Karapurkar, T., et al. (2003). Prevalence of autism in a US metropolitan area. *Journal of the American Medical Association, 289*(1), 49–55.

Zwaigenbaum, L., Szatmari, P., Jones, M.B., et al. (2002). Pregnancy and birth complications in autism and liability to the broader autism phenotype. *Journal of the American Academy of Child and Adolescent Psychiatry, 41,* 572–579.

24 Attention Deficits and Hyperactivity

Marianne M. Glanzman and Nathan J. Blum

Upon completion of this chapter, the reader will

- Be familiar with the characteristics of attention-deficit/hyperactivity disorder
- Be aware of some of the causes of inattention and hyperactivity
- Understand the components of the diagnostic process
- Know the different approaches to management
- Be aware of the natural history and outcomes for this disorder

---

Attention-deficit/hyperactivity disorder (ADHD) is one of the most prevalent neurodevelopmental/mental health conditions in childhood. It is characterized by developmentally inappropriate levels of inattention and distractibility and/or hyperactivity and impulsivity that cause impairment in adaptive functioning at home, at school, or in social situations. Treatment improves short-term academic, social, and adaptive functioning (MTA Cooperative Group, 2004a). It is anticipated, though not proven, that comprehensive management can lead to improved long-term outcomes for children with ADHD; however, it is now understood that the condition and its impact tends to persist into adolescence and adulthood in a substantial percentage of individuals (Mick, Faraone, & Biederman, 2004; Wolraich et al., 2005). ADHD has important implications for the individual, as well as his or her family and community (Harpin, 2005; Klassen, Miller, & Fine, 2004).

JASON

Jason, now 7, is in second grade. His teacher reports that he is having great difficulty learning to read. He also is quite disruptive in class, frequently not listening to directions, getting out of his seat, making silly comments, and talking out of turn. Similar problems were reported by his first grade

teacher, but these difficulties were attributed to his adjusting to the new school, as he attended a Montessori kindergarten previously. His parents and soccer coach have also noticed problems with his following directions and paying attention. Jason was adopted shortly after birth so there is no family history available. He has, however, always had a "difficult" temperament. He was a colicky baby with poor sleep patterns. As a preschooler, he was demanding and would exhaust all those around him. His parents and teachers feel that he is still quite immature and demanding, as he requires much more attention than other children his age do.

A comprehensive evaluation revealed that Jason has ADHD, combined type, and a specific reading disability, although he is intellectually gifted. Jason is at significant risk for both academic and behavioral difficulties, so a multimodal treatment plan has been put into place. Medication has been dramatically helpful at school and is used on weekends and during school vacations as well for improved functioning in social situations and activities of daily living. His counselor focuses on the development of a consistent behavior management plan at home and school, as well as social skill instruction. At school, he receives resource room teaching for reading and language arts, enrichment programming in math, and weekly meetings with the school counselor for a social skills group.

DIAGNOSIS AND ATTENTION-DEFICIT/ HYPERACTIVITY DISORDER SUBTYPES

ADHD is a neurobehavioral syndrome; there are no currently available medical or psychological tests to make the diagnosis. Instead, the diagnosis depends on ruling in symptoms of ADHD and ruling out other causes of the symptoms. Through the use of interviews and rating scales to systematically collect information from parents, teachers, and (older) children, the clinician must evaluate whether 1) significant ADHD symptoms are present in more than one setting; 2) the symptoms result in functional impairment; and 3) these symptoms are the result of another psychiatric, medical, or social condition (Pelham, Fabbiano, & Mas-

setti, 2005). The current diagnostic criteria consist of two major clusters of symptoms: inattention and hyperactivity/impulsivity (American Psychiatric Association [APA], 2000). These criteria, outlined in the APA's *Diagnostic and Statistical Manual of Mental Disorders, Fourth Edition, Text Revision (DSM-IV-TR)* are shown in Table 24.1.

Children who display a significant number (at least six) from both symptom clusters are diagnosed with ADHD combined type (ADHD-C), provided the symptoms were evident before age 7, have persisted for at least 6 months, occur across settings, cause impairment, and cannot be better accounted for by another disorder. The selection of 7 years as the age at which symptoms must have been present is controversial because some children who meet all the

---

Table 24.1. Diagnostic Criteria for Attention-Deficit/Hyperactivity Disorder

A. Inattention/distractibility
   1. Often fails to give close attention to details or makes careless mistakes in schoolwork, work, or other activities
   2. Often has difficulty sustaining attention in tasks or play activities
   3. Often does not seem to listen when spoken to directly
   4. Often does not follow through on instructions and fails to finish schoolwork, chores, or duties in the workplace (not due to oppositional behavior or failure to understand instructions)
   5. Often has difficulty organizing tasks and activates
   6. Often avoids, dislikes, or is reluctant to engage in tasks that require sustained mental effort (such as schoolwork or homework)
   7. Often loses things necessary for tasks or activities (e.g., toys, school assignments, pencils, books, or tools)
   8. Is often easily distracted by extraneous stimuli
   9. Is often forgetful in daily activates

B. Hyperactivity
   1. Often fidgets with hands or feet or squirms in seat
   2. Often leaves seat in classroom or in other situations in which remaining seated is expected
   3. Often runs about or climbs excessively in situations in which it is inappropriate (in adolescents or adults, may be limited to subjective feelings of restlessness)
   4. Often has difficulty playing or engaging in leisure activities quietly
   5. Is often "on the go" or acts as if "driven by a motor"
   6. Often talks excessively

Impulsivity
   1. Often blurts out answers before the questions have been completed
   2. Often has difficulty awaiting turn
   3. Often interrupts or intrudes on others (e.g., butts into conversations or games)

To make a diagnosis

A. At least 6 symptoms from just Category A (ADHD, Inattentive Subtype), or just Category B (ADHD, Hyperactive-Impulsive Subtype), or at least 6 symptoms from both categories (ADHD, Combined Subtype)

B. Symptoms are chronic (some symptoms were functionally impairing from before the age of 7), are clearly significantly impairing (in social, academic, or occupational functioning), are present across settings

C. Symptoms do not occur exclusively during the course of a Pervasive Developmental Disorder, Schizophrenia or other Psychotic Disorder, and are not better accounted for by another mental disorder (e.g., Mood, Anxiety, Dissociative, or Personality Disorder).

From the *Diagnostic and Statistical Manual of Mental Disorders, Fourth Edition, Text Revision* (pp. 92–93). Copyright © 2000 American Psychiatric Association.

other criteria for ADHD do not demonstrate functionally impairing symptoms before later elementary or middle school (Voeller, 2004; Weiss, Murray, & Weiss, 2002). ADHD-C is the most commonly diagnosed and studied form of ADHD (Barkley, 1998; Voeller, 2004).

The second most common subtype in children, ADHD predominately inattentive type (ADHD-I), refers to individuals who do not display significant levels of hyperactivity but have significant problems in maintaining attention. There is some evidence to suggest that the specific nature of inattention in this subtype may differ from the inattention shown by those with the combined subtype. A "slow" cognitive tempo is characteristic in ADHD-I. The ratio of girls to boys with this subtype is slightly higher than for the other subtypes, and it is usually identified at a later age. The pattern of psychiatric comorbidity also differs from that of ADHD-C, with fewer disruptive behavior disorders among these individuals and their relatives. Educational impairments are the most prominent difficulty experienced by this group (reviewed in Barkley, 1998; Voeller, 2004).

The third subtype, ADHD-predominantly impulsive/hyperactive type (ADHD-HI), was first identified in *Diagnostic and Statistical Manual of Mental Disorders, Fourth Edition* (*DSM-IV*; APA, 1994) and refers to children who do not display significant levels of attention problems in the presence of hyperactivity and impulsivity. This subtype is most often diagnosed in young children who have not yet reached an age at which attention problems are impairing. Less is known about the developmental course of this subtype or its response to treatment.

Finally, ADHD-not otherwise specified (ADHD-NOS) can be used for individuals who have significant functional impairment from the symptoms of ADHD, but may not meet strict criteria for the diagnosis based on the number of symptoms present or the age of onset criteria. Any of the subtypes can be used with the phrase "in partial remission" when symptoms are present but have improved such that the individual no longer meets strict criteria.

CLINICAL PRESENTATION

The presenting symptoms of ADHD differ with age. During the preschool years, excessive activity level and impulsivity are typically the most prominent symptoms. This is often accompanied by "intense" temperament and cognitive inflexibility. In combination, these symptoms may lead to impulsive aggression toward peers. Given the high activity level and short attention span of the typical preschooler, only children severely affected with ADHD will differ sufficiently from the developmental norm to fully meet the criteria for the disorder. Children who present in the preschool period should be carefully assessed for language, cognitive, sensory, and autism spectrum disorders, all of which have some similarities in presentation to ADHD (DuPaul et al., 2001).

Upon entering elementary school, problems with listening and compliance, task completion, work accuracy, and socializing are common concerns of parents and teachers (Barkley, 1998). In adolescence, observable hyperactivity may decline significantly (Faraone, Biederman, & Mick, 2006). Concerns often focus around work completion, organization, and following rules. Approximately 65% of children with ADHD diagnosed early in childhood continue to meet the criteria for the disorder in adolescence, whereas an additional group will meet criteria for ADHD-NOS because of a reduced number of symptoms. Occasionally, individuals are not diagnosed with ADHD until adolescence, although they must have had symptoms by history that were impairing in childhood in order to meet current diagnostic criteria. Children who were able to cope during the early grades, typically because of low levels of hyperactivity/impulsivity; strong intellectual skills; social, athletic, or other strengths; and supportive families and school personnel, may present in adolescence. Their attentional/executive systems may finally be overwhelmed by the demands for processing increased volumes of reading and writing, as well as the complex social, time management, organizational, and higher-order thinking and language processing skills required of them (Stein & Baren, 2003).

COMMON COEXISTING CONDITIONS

There are several conditions that commonly coexist with ADHD, typically referred to as coexisting or comorbid conditions. Less frequently, another condition mimics ADHD and is the primary cause of inattentive or hyperactive symptoms rather than a condition that coexists with ADHD (see The Evaluation Process section). Coexisting conditions are important to identify during an evaluation because 1) they will often require additional or different treatment and 2) unless treated, they may prevent adequate treatment of ADHD.

Approximately 30%–50% of individuals with ADHD have an externalizing behavior disorder, such as oppositional defiant disorder (characterized by noncompliance and defiance of authority) or conduct disorder (characterized by more serious antisocial behaviors) (Burke, Loeber, & Birmaher, 2002; Waxmonsky, 2003). Estimates of mood disorders (depression, anxiety, bipolar disorder) in ADHD vary considerably from study to study, ranging from 14%–83%. Childhood bipolar disorder is estimated to occur in as many as 10% of individuals with ADHD (Waxmonsky, 2003). Children with bipolar disorder are likely to be chronically highly irritable, with intermittent explosiveness and signs of disordered thinking (e.g., grandiosity). They tend to have significant aggression and are at risk for additional problems including anxiety and conduct disorders (Waxmonsky, 2003). Anxiety disorders occur in approximately 25% of children with ADHD, and may include separation anxiety, generalized anxiety, phobias, or obsessive-compulsive disorder (OCD) (Varley & Smith, 2003). The prevalence of learning disorders in children with ADHD ranges from 10%–40% depending on which test and criteria are utilized (Kronenberger & Dunn, 2003).

Tic disorders, including transient, chronic, or Tourette syndrome are seen in at least 6% of children with ADHD in a community sample over the course of a year, with transient tics being the most common (approximately 5%) and Tourette syndrome being the least common (less than 1%) (Khalifa & von Knorring, 2005). Similar rates of tic disorders are seen in children with ADHD receiving placebos (Palumbo et al., 2004). Persistent tics are often associated with ADHD and other neuropsychiatric conditions, most notably OCD (Scahill et al., 2005). Tics can occur on a spectrum from mild, which may not even be reported by parents to more severe, in which tics have important physical, emotional, and social impact (Power & Glanzman, 2006). In children with both ADHD and Tourette syndrome, ADHD typically causes greater functional impairment than does the tic disorder itself (Denkla, 2006).

ASSOCIATED IMPAIRMENTS

Individuals with ADHD often have associated impairments that are neither directly described by the core features of ADHD nor indicative of one of the common coexisting diagnoses.

Nonetheless, they can be significantly impairing and may require additional interventions. These include deficits in executive, language, social, academic, and adaptive functions as well as problems with sleep patterns and motor coordination.

Although ADHD is defined and diagnosed based on the presence of observed behaviors, neuropsychological investigations suggest that deficits in executive functioning based in the frontal/prefrontal cortex may underlie the characteristic observed behaviors in many children (Weyandt, 2005; Willcutt Doyle, et al., 2005). Executive functions include sustaining and shifting attention, being able to hold information in ultra–short-term memory in order to complete a task (working memory), organizing and prioritizing incoming information, planning ahead, self-monitoring, and inhibiting responses (Martinussen et al., 2005).

Even when criteria for a learning disability are not met, academic underachievement is a concern of many parents of school-age children with ADHD. Difficulty with verbal memory, listening comprehension, and organization of verbal and written output occur in children with ADHD, even in the absence of specific language impairments (McInnes et al., 2003). Although the topic has not been well studied, there appears to be a high rate of pragmatic language difficulties in children with ADHD (Armstrong & Nettleton, 2004). This results in difficulty reading, most often in the form of problems with fluency, comprehension, or engagement and retention of written material (Ghelani et al., 2004; Willicut et al., 2005).

Many children with ADHD have problems with social interactions with peers (Barkley, 2004; Frankel & Feinberg, 2002). They have difficulty "reading" the nuances of social behavior or inhibiting impulsive responses. They may react excessively or overly negatively to the behavior of others, leading some children to enjoy "pushing their buttons" to get a reaction. Some children with ADHD have difficulty initiating or sustaining the verbal turn taking or other reciprocal aspects of peer relations and may find themselves passively or actively ignored and without the deeper friendships that older children begin to develop at school. They may be inflexible or perfectionistic, leading to "bossiness" with peers. Research into the characterization and treatment of social impairment is in its early stages, although it is known that social deficits tend to persist to adulthood (Mannuzza & Klein, 2000).

Research has supported a link between ADHD and sleep disturbances (reviewed in Owens, 2005). The underlying cause of this association is presently unknown. Although stimulant medication can contribute to insomnia, sleep disturbance occurs in children with ADHD prior to medication use as well. They have a greater frequency of problems with sleep initiation, sleep maintenance, decreased rapid eye movement (REM) sleep, increased periodic limb movements, awakening, and decreased daytime alertness (Brown & McMullen, 2001). Although there is not an increased frequency of obstructive sleep apnea in individuals with ADHD, when present, its treatment may improve problems with daytime somnolence, concentration, and behavioral regulation (Bass et al., 2004; Cohen-Zion & Ancoli-Israel, 2004).

Children with ADHD also have an increased incidence of problems with motor coordination that may impair written work in school and participation in athletic activities (Martin et al., 2006; Visser, 2003).

CAUSES OF ATTENTION-DEFICIT/ HYPERACTIVITY DISORDER

Heredity

The most common etiological factor in the development of ADHD is heredity. Siblings of children with ADHD are between five and seven times more likely to be diagnosed with ADHD than children in unaffected families. Each child of a parent with ADHD has a 25% chance of having ADHD (Wilens, Hahsey, et al., 2005). Between 55% and 92% of identical twins will be concordant for ADHD (reviewed in Faraone, Perlis, et al., 2005).

Several genes have been found in preliminary studies to relate to susceptibility to ADHD including those related to the dopamine, norepinephrine, serotonin, acetylcholine, GABA, and glutamate neurotransmitter systems as well as genes associated with neurotransmitter release and neuroimmunology. We all have these genes and there are a few, slightly different forms of each of these genes, called alleles. In molecular genetic studies of families, a specific allele of each of these genes has been found to occur at an unexpectedly high frequency in individuals in the family who have ADHD, whereas different alleles tend to be present in individuals within the family who do not have ADHD. This suggests that specific alleles confer susceptibility to ADHD. The genes thus far identified

do not account for the majority of the variation in ADHD symptoms, however, suggesting that other as yet unidentified genes also confer susceptibility (or protection). Those genes that have been found to be associated with ADHD in more than one study sample include the dopamine transporter and the dopamine type 4 and 5 receptors, dopamine beta hydroxylase (an enzyme that is involved in the conversion of **dopamine** to **norepinephrine**), the serotonin transporter, the serotonin 1B receptor subtype, and SNAP-25 [synaptosomal-associated protein, a membrane protein involved in synaptic release of neurotransmitters] (reviewed in Faraone, Perlis, et al., 2005; Glanzman, in press; Kent, 2004).

Dopamine-related genes are candidate genes for investigating the basis for ADHD because a variety of evidence indicates that dopamine is involved in the modulation of attention and behavioral regulation in the frontal cortex and its connections, particularly the striatum. Norepinephrine is another neurotransmitter that plays an important role in orienting attention and regulating alertness in the frontal cortex and in other areas of the cortex and lower brain. Medications that are effective in ameliorating ADHD symptoms have consistently been shown to affect one or both of these neurotransmitters (Glanzman, in press; Solanto, 2002).

Other Etiologic Factors

Other conditions known to affect brain development may result in ADHD symptoms or increase the risk of those genetically at risk for the disorder. These include prenatal exposures to cigarette smoking, lead, alcohol, and possibly cocaine; prematurity; intrauterine growth restriction; brain infections; and inborn errors of metabolism. Sex chromosome abnormalities (e.g., Klinefelter syndrome, Turner syndrome, fragile X syndrome) and other genetic syndromes (e.g., neurofibromatosis type 1, Williams syndrome, Tourette syndrome) are associated with attention problems or overactivity/ impulsivity (reviewed in Accardo, 1999). In children who do not have a family history of ADHD, there is an increased incidence of complications during labor, delivery, and infancy (Sprich-Buckminster et al., 1993). Premature infants with evidence of low cerebral blood flow were found at 12–14 years of age to have an increased risk for ADHD and motor reaction time abnormalities that were associated with alterations in dopamine type 2/3 receptor binding. This suggests that cerebral ischemia may contribute to long-term changes in dopamine neurotransmission that are related to ADHD motor and behavioral symptoms (Lou et al., 2004).

Structural and Functional Differences in the Brain

Multiple lines of evidence suggest that structural and functional differences exist in the brains of individuals with ADHD (reviewed in Durston, 2003; Glanzman, in press). Magnetic resonance imaging (MRI) scans have shown important differences when the volume of specific areas is compared. Five regions have shown consistent differences—the frontal lobes (particularly the right), caudate nucleus and globus pallidus (nuclei in the basal ganglia), corpus callosum (particularly anteriorly), and the posterior inferior cerebellar vermis (lobules 8–10). The frontal lobes of the brain serve as the "executive center," processing incoming stimuli and coordinating appropriate cognitive, emotional, and motor responses. It is thought that the cerebellum and basal ganglia may also be involved because these areas are critical to motor planning, behavioral inhibition, and motivation. These regions are 5%–9% smaller in individuals with ADHD (reviewed in Durston, 2003; Glanzman, in press). The volume reductions appear to affect both gray and white matter (Glanzman, in press; Sowell et al., 2003) and are present from the youngest ages studied (5 years of age) (Castellanos et al., 2002).

Functional MRI (fMRI) is a noninvasive technique that is used to evaluate variations in regional oxygen uptake in the brain, which correlates with cellular activity. FMRI studies support the role of the prefrontal cortex in executive functions, but to date there are only a few small studies in children with ADHD (reviewed in Glanzman, in press). These studies indicate that subjects with ADHD underactivate the prefrontal cortex and caudate nucleus compared with controls during motor inhibition tasks (Rubia et al.,1999; Vaidya et al.,1998), that stimulant medication can increase activation in these areas (Lou et al., 1989), and that the pattern of response to the stimulant may differ between controls and subjects (Vaidya et al., 1998).

Positron emission tomography (PET) and single photon emission tomography (SPECT) scans also provide information about brain function, but these techniques require injection of a radioactive tracer molecule, which has limited its use in children. Multiple studies in children and adults document underperfusion of frontal-striatal regions, although the specific findings within these areas differ between studies (Durston, 2003, Glanzman & Elia, 2006). Several studies document abnormalities in the frontal-striatal dopamine system including alterations in dopamine uptake in the prefrontal cortex and right midbrain in adults and children, respectively (Ernst et al., 1998; Ernst et al., 1999), and a higher level of binding to the dopamine transporter in both adults (Krause et al., 2003) and children (Cheon et al., 2003). Structural and functional imaging scans are presently important research tools, but they have not been shown to be sufficiently sensitive or specific be used diagnostically (American Academy of Pediatrics [AAP], 2000; Glanzman & Elia, 2006).

THE EVALUATION PROCESS

Evaluating a child for ADHD requires focusing on four areas: 1) the symptoms of ADHD, 2) different conditions that might cause the same symptoms, 3) coexisting conditions, and 4) associated medical, psychosocial, or learning issues that may not reach the threshold for a specific diagnosis but may nonetheless influence the treatment plan. A comprehensive history, physical/neurological examination, and academic assessment should be completed. Findings in these examinations may prompt additional investigations.

The history, generally taken from the parents, with the child's participation depending on age, includes current status and concerns, previous treatments and their effects, prenatal and perinatal events, medical history, developmental, psychiatric and behavioral history, educational course, social and family circumstances, and biological family history for ADHD symptoms and associated disorders. Information from teachers, typically in the form of standardized rating scales, should be included to document impairment in the school setting (AAP, 2000).

The medical examination should focus on growth parameters and physical signs of sensory, genetic, chronic medical, and neurologic disorders. In addition, alertness, social interaction, informal communicative ability and insight, and motor skills should be assessed.

Educational testing (including intellectual and achievement measures) will be necessary for many children and should focus on careful assessment for learning disabilities, memory and processing capabilities, and deficits and areas of academic weakness that may not meet criteria for a learning disability but for which additional support may allow the child to make better academic progress. This should include assessments of reading mechanics and comprehension, spelling, mathematical concepts and computation, and writing skills. Some evaluators will include tests of verbal and visual memory and processing efficiency, which can be useful in identifying reasons for intellectual–achievement discrepancies and can inform choices about educational remediation strategies.

Obtaining information about symptoms of ADHD and related conditions, comparing the level of symptoms with age- and gender-matched peers, and assessing the level of functional impairment is frequently facilitated by the use of standardized interview formats and rating scales for parents and teachers. In addition, rating scales designed for teachers allow the required collection of information from more than one setting. Commonly used scales to specifically assess ADHD symptoms include the ADHD-IV Rating Scale (DuPaul, Power, Anastopoulos, et al., 1998), the Conners' Rating Scales–Revised (CSR-R; Conners, 1997), the SNAP-IV Rating Scale (SNAP-IV; Swanson, n.d.), and the Vanderbilt ADHD Diagnostic Rating Scales (Vanderbilt Children's Hospital, n.d.). (For a review of these measures, see AAP, 2000; Pelham et al., 2005.)

Structured diagnostic interviews are most often used in psychiatric and research settings, as they are quite time consuming and require specialized training for their standardized administration. Commonly used structured diagnostic interviews include the DICA-R (Diagnostic Interview for Children and Adolescents, Revised) (Reich, 2000), and the Kiddie Schedule for Affective Disorders and Schizophrenia (K-SADS; Kaufman, J., Birmaher, B., Brent, D., et al., 1996). (For a review of these measures, see American Academy of Child and Adolescent Psychiatry, 1997; Pelham et al., 2005.)

Because comprehensive information is required, several professionals are typically involved (e.g., physician, psychologist, teacher). The primary person responsible for formulating the diagnosis and communicating the findings and recommendations to the family must be experienced with the range of coexisting conditions. This person is typically a physician (e.g., pediatrician, neurodevelopmental or behavioral pediatrician, neurologist, psychiatrist) or a psychologist. Additional professionals may

be asked to provide input such as speech-language pathologists and occupational therapists. Although such a complex evaluation can be coordinated through a primary care setting, there are also a number of barriers related to knowledge, time, resources, and medical/mental health insurance coverage that limit access to a thorough evaluation for many children (Rushton, Fant, & Clark, 2004).

TREATMENT OF ATTENTION-DEFICIT/ HYPERACTIVITY DISORDER

Most treatment plans for ADHD include education about the disorder, as well as one or more of the following: behavioral and family counseling, educational interventions, and medication. Often a combination of treatments is used because of the multiple aspects of the child's life that are affected by ADHD.

Education About the Disorder and Emotional Support

Parents and older children need to learn as much as possible about ADHD so that they can be effective decision makers and advocates. The clinician can provide some information directly but should also guide the family toward other sources of information such as national support and advocacy organizations, books, videos, Internet sites, and parent support groups. Growing up with ADHD and parenting a child with ADHD are significant challenges. Although providing emotional support alone is not likely to result in significant improvements, without emotional support parents and children may not be able to perform the difficult work needed to address the problems.

Behavioral Counseling and Social Skill Intervention

Behavior therapy is the type of counseling intervention with the best documented efficacy (AAP, 2001). The premise of behavioral therapy is that the likelihood of a specific behavior occurring is determined by what takes place prior to the behavior (the antecedents) and immediately after the behavior (the consequences). (See Chapter 35). Changing the antecedents often involves altering the environment. Seating a child away from distracting stimuli, breaking long tasks into smaller components, and making eye contact when giving instructions are examples of ways in which antecedents can be altered to increase the chances of success for an inattentive child.

Behavior therapy can be done in individual or group sessions and forms the basis for most parent training and classroom management programs. Studies have consistently found that these interventions result in at least short-term improvements in the behavior of children with ADHD (Chronis et al., 2004). A study of a very intensive behavioral intervention that also included social skill building and emotional support found some persistent benefit 15 months after the intervention ended (MTA Cooperative Group, 2004b). Factors that may interfere with effective parent training include parental depression, parental ADHD, and high levels of marital discord (Chronis et al., 2004).

Behavior therapy should be differentiated from other forms of therapy that have little documented efficacy in the treatment of children with ADHD. Individual psychotherapy or play therapy may be helpful for children with coexisting mood, anxiety, or self-esteem problems, but it is not effective in treating the core symptoms of ADHD (Barkley, 2004). Similarly, cognitive or cognitive-behavioral therapy (CBT) that attempts to change behavior by helping individuals change self-defeating thought and behavior patterns has been found to have little, if any, effect in children with ADHD (Barkley, 2004). However, there are some small studies of CBT in adults with ADHD (some of whom also took medication) that suggest that CBT may have some benefit in this group (Safren et al., 2004; Stevenson et al., 2002). Family therapy may be necessary when parents cannot agree on an intervention plan or other family stressors interfere with implementation of a treatment plan.

Interpersonal difficulties such as peer victimization and/or social isolation are common in individuals with ADHD (Frankel & Feinberg, 2002). As a result, social skill interventions may be recommended as part of a comprehensive treatment plan. Social skill groups are often conducted in school or other group settings and teach by modeling, practicing, and reinforcing prosocial behaviors. When social skills interventions for children with ADHD are evaluated as a single intervention, the results have generally been disappointing (Abikoff et al., 2004; Barkley, 2004). The social skills interventions that seem to be the most effective are conducted in naturalistic settings (i.e., at a camp or school rather than in a clinic) and are combined with behavioral parent training (Chronis et al., 2004).

Educational Intervention

Appropriate school programs are extremely important for children with ADHD, many of whom have coexisting learning difficulties. Even those children without a specific learning disability may require substantial repetition of an educational task, yet are easily bored and resist it. A well-trained teacher who is interested in providing special help and an educational program suited to the needs of the child are invaluable. The teacher may need to use environmental modifications and behavior management techniques to maintain the child's attention to tasks and decrease unwanted behavior. The child may need the teacher's assistance to develop organizational skills. Classwork or homework assignments may need to be modified to emphasize the child's strengths and help manage the child's learning weaknesses or disabilities. Tutoring outside of school will be helpful in some cases, especially to ensure that basic concepts that serve as building blocks for more advanced work have been learned thoroughly.

When children with ADHD are in need of more assistance than is typically provided in the classroom, they may qualify for **accommodations** within their general classes or in special education settings under either Section 504 of the Rehabilitation Act of 1973 (PL 93-112) or the Individuals with Disabilities Education Improvement Act of 2004 (IDEA 2004; PL 108-446) (see Chapter 34). Accommodations allow the child with ADHD to gain access to the general education environment and may include 1) regular home–school communication; 2) a behavior program to manage mildly disruptive behaviors; 3) a plan to ensure that the student understands and is following through on instructions; 4) modifications of testing time, format, or environment; 5) an extra set of materials at home; and/or 6) technological assistance such as the use of tape recorders and word processors.

Pharmacological Treatment

Stimulant medications are the most effective and most commonly prescribed medications for ADHD. Atomoxetine (Strattera) is the only nonstimulant medication approved by the Food and Drug Administration (FDA) for the treatment of ADHD. Antidepressants, alpha-2-adrenergic agonists, and neuroleptics are sometimes used (although not FDA-approved for the treatment of ADHD) in children who do not respond to stimulants or atomxetine, who experience side effects from these medications, or who have a condition in addition to ADHD that is better treated by one of these medications. Although combinations of these medications are sometimes used, there is little research available concerning the efficacy and safety of combined pharmacological treatment in ADHD.

Stimulant Medications Stimulant medications, including methylphenidate and amphetamines (See Table 24.2) have been used for the treatment of children with disruptive behaviors since 1937 and have been more frequently used and more thoroughly studied than any other psychopharmacologic treatment in children. In the 1990s, 1%–3% of children in the United States received a stimulant medication for treatment of ADHD (Safer & Malever, 2000; Safer & Zito, 1999), and more than 11 million stimulant prescriptions were written per year. Research into the epidemiology of stimulant use suggests that stimulants may be both overprescribed and underprescribed, depending on the community practitioner. For example, one study found that only 12% of children meeting diagnostic criteria for ADHD were prescribed stimulants (Jensen et al., 1999), whereas another found that more than 70% were prescribed stimulants but that more than half of children prescribed stimulants had few parent-reported ADHD symptoms (Angold et al., 2000). During the 1990s, there was a rapid increase in the prevalence of stimulants prescribed to females (Zito et al., 2003), to preschoolers (Zito et al., 2000), and to children receiving more than one psychotropic medication (Safer, Zito, & dosReis, 2003).

Table 24.2. Stimulant medications commonly used to treat attention-deficit/hyperactivity disorder

Brand name	Generic name of active medicine	Usual duration of action (hours)	Dosages available (milligrams)	Comments
Ritalin	D, L-methylphenidate	3–4	Tablets: 5, 10, 20	
Focalin	D-methylphenidate	3–4	Tablets: 2.5, 5, 10	Contains only the active isomer of methylphenidate; usual dose would be the D, L-methylphenidate dose
Focalin XR	D-methylphenidate	12 (20 mg dose)	Capsules: 5, 10, 20	Capsule can be opened and sprinkled
Methylin	D, L-methylphenidate	3–4	Tablets: 2.5, 5, 10	Tablets are grape flavored and chewable
			Liquid: 5 mg/5milliter and 10mg/5milliliter	
Metadate CD	D, L-methylphenidate	6–8	Capsules: 10, 20, 30, 40, 50, 60	Capsule can be opened and sprinkled
				30% of dose immediately released
Ritalin LA	D, L-methylphenidate	6–8	Capsules: 20, 30, 40	Capsule can be opened and sprinkled
				50% of dose immediately released
Concerta	D, L-methylphenidate	10–12	Tablet: 18, 27, 36, 54	Must be swallowed whole
				22% of dose immediately released
Daytrana	D, L-methylphenidate	Up to 12	Patch: 10, 15, 20, 30	Allows variable duration based on timing of patch removal
Dexedrine	Dextroamphetamine	3–6	Tablet: 5	
Dexedrine Spansules	Dextroamphetamine	6–8	Capsule: 5, 10, 15	
Adderall	Mixed salts of amphetamines	3–6	Tablets: 5, 7.5, 10, 12.5, 15, 20, 30	
Adderall XR	Mixed salts of amphetamines	10–12	Capsule: 5, 10, 15, 20, 25, 30	Capsule can be opened and sprinkled
				50% of dose immediately released

Key: XR, extended release; CD, controlled delivery; LA, long acting.

Beneficial Effects Stimulant medications significantly reduce symptoms of ADHD in 70%–90% of those treated (Wigal et al., 1999). They result in a rapid and often dramatic improvement in attention to task and a decrease in impulsivity and hyperactivity. In addition, they improve academic productivity and accuracy, improve parent–child interactions, and decrease aggression (Connor et al.2002; Wigal et al., 1999). The effect of stimulants on academic performance is less strong than that on behavior, with only about half of the children showing significant improvement (Rapport et al., 1994). Although beneficial effects are very clearly demonstrated in short- to intermediate-term studies (up to 5 years of treatment; Charach, Ickowicz, & Schachar, 2004), the long-term efficacy of stimulants is not nearly as well studied. It should also be noted that response to stimulant treatment is not diagnostic of ADHD, as individuals with other psychiatric or developmental disorders, as well as controls, display similar effects when given stimulant medication (Rapaport et al., 1978).

Formulations Methylphenidate and amphetamines come in a variety of formulations, as shown in Table 24.2. The beneficial effects and side effects of these two types of stimulants are nearly identical, although individual children may respond better to one medication than the other (Elia, 2005). Amphetamine-based stimulants are given at approximately half the dose of the methylphenidate-based stimulants to account for differences in the potency of the two medications (Manos, Short, & Findling, 1999). Pemoline (Cylert), which is in a third category of stimulants, is not listed in Table 24.2 because it is rarely used since reports linked it to severe liver failure (Safer, Zito, & Gardner, 2001).

The onset of action of methylphenidate and amphetamine is usually within 30 minutes of taking the dose. Different formulations vary principally in their duration of action, how much of the medication is released immediately, and how the remainder is released (in a later bolus versus continuously). Although Table 24.2 gives the typical duration of action for the various formulations, there is significant variation among individuals. In addition, methylphenidate patch (Daytrana) gives individuals the capacity to vary the duration of action on a daily basis (up to 12 hours) based on the timing of patch removal (see http://www.daytrana.com).

Side Effects The most common adverse effects of stimulants are decreased appetite, headaches, stomachaches, and sleep problems (Elia, 2005). These symptoms are common in children with ADHD off medication as well, so it is important to determine their nature and frequency prior to starting the stimulant. Decreased appetite is reported in 50%–60% of treated children, but it is often mild and limited to school hours (Efron, Jarman, & Barker, 1997). About 10%–15% of children have substantial weight loss. These children may benefit from caloric, vitamin, and mineral supplementation to prevent weight loss and maintain adequate nutrition, but some will simply not tolerate an effective dose in spite of supplementation.

Less common but potentially more problematic side effects include "**rebound**" effects, tics, and social withdrawal. *Rebound* refers to a temporary worsening of symptoms, including irritability, increased activity, and/or mood swings, when the medication wears off. Although it is estimated that 30% of school-age children experience some rebound effects, the effects are significant enough to require altering the medication regimen only in about 10% of cases (Carlson & Kelly, 2003). Some children do become withdrawn on the medication. This may improve with dose adjustment or switching to another medication.

Tics have been reported to occur in approximately 10% of children treated with stimulants (Lipkin, Goldstein, & Adesman, 1994). However, in a community sample of 3,600 children, tics occurred in 22% of preschoolers, 8% of elementary school children, and 3.4% of adolescents (Gadow & Sverd, 2006). Although early reports suggested that stimulants induced or exacerbated tics, more recent research indicates that this is an uncommon occurrence (Gadow & Sverd, 2006; Palumbo et al., 2004). In addition, tics that appear to be stimulant induced or exacerbated usually subside with time, after the dose is reduced, or when treatment is discontinued. In rare cases, tics that appear to have been induced by stimulants do not resolve or may even worsen over time. Given that Tourette syndrome, chronic motor tics, and OCD appear to have an underlying genetic origin, it is possible that those individuals whose tics appear to be induced by stimulants have a genetic predisposition (reviewed in Power & Glanzman, 2006; Saccomani et al., 2005). Although the presence of tics and a personal or family history of Tourette syndrome are listed as contraindications to stimulant use by the pharmaceutical companies that manufacture these medications, given the previously cited research, this seems unnecessarily restrictive. ADHD symptoms may cause much more functional impairment and thus be the priority for treatment (American Academy of Child and Adolescent Psychiatry, 2002; Denkla, 2006).

Growth velocity slows by approximately 1.2 centimeters per year on average in prepubertal children during at least the first 2 years of continuous treatment with stimulants (MTA Cooperative Group, 2004b). Whether this results in any decrease in ultimate height is less clear. A study of children treated with methylphenidate for at least 6 months during the 1970s found that although these children had decreases in height velocity on the medication, the children treated with stimulants did not have deficits in adult height (Klein & Mannuzza, 1988). However, the average length of treatment in this study was only slightly more that 2 years, which is less than the total duration of stimulant treatment many children with ADHD currently receive. Other recent studies of up to 2 years in duration suggest continued, although minimal, effects on height (Faraone, Biederman, et al., 2005; Wilens, McBurnett, et al., 2005). Thus, stimulants can cause a lag in growth, but short- to intermediate-term treatment does not seem to have a significant effect on adult height. Whether long-term treatment could affect adult height has not been adequately studied.

Other side effects include elevations of pulse or blood pressure and, rarely, activation of mania or psychosis. Typically the elevations of pulse or blood pressure are small and not clinically significant. Significant elevations should prompt an investigation for a potential underlying medical problem that may be exacerbated by the stimulants. Reports of sudden death in children on stimulants raised concerns that stimulants might be at fault, but careful review showed that approximately two thirds of those children had previously undetected cardiac abnormalities. The FDA has recommended that stimulants should generally not be used in individuals with known serious heart disease. This recommendation is on file with the FDA and is listed in the package insert for each stimulant product. The American Heart Association Panel on Psychotropic Medications in Children and Adolescents recommends a careful history for risk factors for sudden death and monitoring of pulse and blood pressure during treatment. In the absence of risk factors, the value of additional cardiac assessment or monitoring is unclear at this time (Wilens et al., 2006).

Potential for Substance Abuse Stimulants are classified as controlled substances by the Drug Enforcement Agency (DEA). They have been used by individuals who want to stay up for long hours, and when injected or taken intranasally stimulants will produce a high. However, children and adolescents taking the medication orally for ADHD do not report euphoria or dependence. Recent research suggests that the relatively slow uptake of methylphenidate into the brain with an oral (as opposed to intravenous) dose prevents oral doses from causing a high (Volkow & Swanson, 2003). The use of slow-release forms, in which the medication is mixed with other substances, makes abuse even less likely to occur. The possibility of diversion (giving or selling medication to others), however, still needs to considered when prescribing these medications. Coaching adolescents about how they will manage questions from peers about their medication or requests to provide it is a wise part of clinical practice for clinicians who prescribe stimulants.

ADHD has been shown to be a risk factor for later substance use disorders, most clearly in the presence of conduct disorder (reviewed in Biederman, 2003). However, multiple studies indicate that the use of stimulant medication does not increase this risk (Wilens et al., 2003) and may, in fact, be protective (Fischer & Barkley, 2003).

Initiating and Monitoring Therapy There is not a direct relationship between an individual's weight and the optimal dose of stimulant medication, so clinicians should have a standard way of assessing medication effectiveness and side effects during a medication trial with a planned titration from lower to higher doses (American Academy of Child and Adolescent Psychiatry, 2002; AAP, 2001). A large, multisite, clinical trial found that children treated with stimulants in the study did better than children treated with these same medications by community physicians (Jensen et al., 2001). Although several factors may have contributed to this finding, a likely factor was the titration protocol used to determine optimal medication dose. Instead of trying a low dose and then increasing until an adequate response was obtained, children in the study were evaluated on at least three different doses, and then the dose that had the best combination of efficacy and side effects was chosen (MTA Cooperative Group, 1999a). Thus, current recommendations are that the initial drug trial assess the child's response to at least two different doses of the medication until the child's behavior is not distinguishable from peers without ADHD, further increases in doses do not result in further behavioral improvement, or the child begins experiencing significant side effects (American Academy of Child and Adolescent Psychiatry, 2002; AAP, 2001). This may be done by obtaining an ADHD teacher rating scale at baseline and increasing the dose on a weekly basis with repeat weekly or twice-weekly rating scales, with the teacher blinded to the child's medication dose. If a child does not respond or has significant side effects on one stimulant, it is reasonable to try a stimulant from the other class (i.e., methylphenidate versus amphetamine) because some children will respond better to one stimulant that to the other (Elia, 2005).

School achievement, behavior, relationships, mood, vital signs, and growth velocity should be monitored at baseline and at regular intervals (every 3–6 months, depending on the frequency of medication or dose changes and the stability of these outcome measures in the past) to ensure continued beneficial responses and the absence of significant adverse effects. No specific blood tests are indicated as part of the monitoring. During childhood, it is important to periodically assess if medication is still required. These evaluations may occur every 1–2 years with the specific timing (e.g., during the summer versus during the school year) dependant on individual circumstances. For children with primarily attention problems, a longer trial may be needed with an evaluation of the medication effect on schoolwork and homework.

As children become adolescents and young adults, additional targets become important that make a longer duration of medication coverage relevant. These include more hours spent doing homework and extracurricular activities, afterschool jobs, the requirement for social decision making with increasingly serious implications, and the need for consistent concentration while driving. Driving performance (but not knowledge) has been shown to be impaired in individuals with ADHD, and effective medication treatment has been shown to improve simulated performance (Cox et al., 2004).

Stimulants in Preschoolers Despite relatively few controlled studies of stimulants in preschool-age children, the use of these medications among preschoolers is increasing (Zito et al., 2000). The few controlled, short-term studies of methylphenidate suggested that it does have beneficial effects in preschool-age children with ADHD (Kratochvil et al., 2004). The percentage of preschool children having a beneficial response may be slightly lower than in elementary school–age children, and side effects may be more common (Ghuman et al., 2001; Kratochvil et al., 2004). Although methylphenidate has been studied more frequently than dextroamphetamine (Dexadrine) or mixed salts of amphetamines (Adderall) in preschool children with ADHD, methylphenidate is not FDA approved for children younger than 6 years of age, whereas the amphetamine products are approved for children older than 3 years of age. Nonetheless, methylphenidate was chosen as the medication for a national multisite clinical trial of treatment in preschool-age children with ADHD that is currently under way. Methylphenidate is also available in liquid and chewable tablet preparations and as a patch which will facilitate its use in preschoolers who may be unable to swallow capsules (see Table 24.2).

Nonstimulant Medications Between 10% and 30% of children with ADHD will not benefit from stimulants or will have adverse side effects that preclude their use. Nonstimulant medications may be helpful for these individuals. Such medications fall into three categories: norepinephrine reuptake inhibitors, antidepressants, and alpha-2-adrenergic agonists.

Norepinephrine Reuptake Inhibitors Currently the only nonstimulant that is FDA approved for the treatment of ADHD in children (6 years of age and older) is the norepinephrine reuptake inhibitor atomoxetine (Strattera). At least six randomized clinical trials in children and adults have demonstrated atomoxetine's efficacy in reducing symptoms of inattention and hyperactivity/impulsivity (Michelson et al., 2002). Atomoxetine may take a few days before one begins to see effects and several weeks to reach the maximum effect. The principle advantage over stimulants is that atomoxetine may improve symptoms 24 hours per day. In addition, it is theoretically less likely to exacerbate tics (Allen et al., 2005). Some children will experience fatigue when the medication is first started. Nausea, vomiting, and stomachaches are more likely to occur if the medication is taken on an empty stomach. Taking the medication with high-fat foods minimizes this side effect. Some children experience weight loss during the first few months of treatment. Other side effects include dizziness, irritability, somnolence, and allergic reactions. Small increases in pulse and blood pressure do occur (Michelson et al., 2001). Although there were not reports of hepatotoxicity in the 4,000 individuals who were studied prior to FDA approval, postmarketing surveillance has identified at least two individuals who had increases in liver enzymes on this medication. Both improved after the medication was stopped. There is insufficient evidence at this time to make recommendations about the monitoring of liver function tests on atomoxetine, but parents should be made aware of the need for a physician to review any persistent gastrointestinal complaints or general malaise.

Antidepressants Several types of antidepressants have been found to be effective in children with ADHD. More than 20 placebo-controlled studies of tricyclic antidepressants (TCAs)—including desipramine (Norpramin), imipramine (Tofranil), and nortriptyline (Pamelor)—have demonstrated that they improve ADHD symptoms, although TCAs appear to have a greater impact on parent and teacher ratings of behavior than on neuropsychological measures of cognitive functioning (Banaschewski et al., 2004; Biederman, Spencer, & Wilens, 2004). About two thirds of children with ADHD who do not respond to a stimulant will improve with a TCA (Biederman et al., 1989).

Compared with stimulants, TCAs have advantages that are similar to those of atomoxetine. They have a longer duration of action, low abuse potential, and tend not to exacerbate tics (Singer et al., 1995). However they have many more potentially problematic cardiovascular, neurologic (tingling, incoordination, tremors), and anticholinergic (blurred vision, dry mouth) side effects that limit their use. Drug levels should be checked, as there can be large interindividual differences in metabolism of these medications (Banaschewski et al., 2004). Electrocardiograms (EKGs) must be obtained at baseline and monitored for cardiovascular changes. Overdoses can be lethal, and a few cases of sudden death, presumably from cardiac arrhythmias, have occurred in children taking appropriate doses of desipramine, although causality could not be clearly established (Popper, 2000).

Bupropion (Wellbutrin) is a chemically distinct antidepressant whose precise mechanism of action in ADHD treatment remains unknown, although it is a weak dopamine reuptake inhibitor. It has been shown to improve ADHD symptoms in both children and adults with ADHD (Pliszka, 2003a). Beneficial effects may be detected as early as 3 days after initiation of treatment, but maximum effects may not be seen until 4 weeks of treatment (Conners et al., 1996). On average, the magnitude of the effects is similar to or slightly less than those of stimulants (Conners et al., 1996). Gastrointestinal complaints, drowsiness, and rashes are the most common side effects. Wellbutrin is associated with a slightly increased risk of drug-induced seizures (about 4 per 1,000 patients). Use of high doses, a previous history of seizures, and the presence of an eating disorder seem to increase the risk for seizures. Bupropion may exacerbate tic disorders.

Alpha-2-Adrenergic Agonists Despite relatively limited studies, the alpha-2-adrenergic agents, clonidine (Catapres) and guanfacine (Tenex), are used for the treatment of ADHD. These medications can reduce hyperactivity and impulsivity, but they may not improve attention span (Tourette Syndrome Study Group, 2002). Studies investigating the combination of clonidine with a stimulant suggest that some children may benefit more from the combination than from a stimulant alone (Hazell & Stuart, 2003; Tourette Syndrome Study Group, 2002). In addition, clonidine has been used for stimulant-related sleep difficulties (Banaschewski et al., 2004).

Sedation is the most common side effect of clonidine and has led clinicians to use the less sedating medication, guanfacine, although there are even fewer studies of this medication. Dizziness and hypotension can occur with these medications, and some children become irritable or depressed while taking them. Alpha-2 adrenergic agonists should not be stopped abruptly, as this can result in rebound hypertension.

TREATMENT WITH COEXISTING CONDITIONS

Intellectual Disability

Individuals with intellectual disability can be diagnosed with ADHD if their inattention or hyperactivity and impulsivity are inconsistent with their developmental level and cause additional functional impairments. Studies suggest that stimulants have similar effects in children with ADHD and intellectual disabilities requiring intermittent to limited supports as in children with ADHD and typical intelligence (Handen et al., 1992). Children with intellectual disabilities, however, have a lower response rate (around 50%) and an increased risk for side effects, such as tics and social withdrawal (Handen et al., 1991). Alpha-2-adrenergic agents and atypical antipsychotics such as risperidone (Risperdal) have also been used to treat hyperactivity and disruptive behaviors in individuals with intellectual disabilities (Turgay et al., 2002).

Internalizing Disorders

Children with ADHD may also experience depression or anxiety disorders. The Multimodal Treatment Study of ADHD found that children with anxiety disorders were one of the few groups that responded as well to psychosocial intervention as to medication (MTA Cooperative Group, 1999b). However, stimulants are effective in the treatment of ADHD in combination with anxiety and mood disorders and remain the first-line medication. Thus the Texas Children's Medication Algorithm recommends that if depression symptoms persist after treatment with stimulants, an SSRI should be added to the stimulant (Emslie et al., 2004). However, the finding that SSRIs can increase suicidal ideation in individuals with depression underscores the need for close monitoring of children being treated for depression (March et al., 2004). In addition, there are no studies comparing this approach to the use of a single medication, such as bupropion or the TCAs, which may improve both depression and ADHD symptoms.

Conduct Disorders

The behavior exhibited by children with a conduct disorder consists of a pattern of persistent and repetitive violation of the rights of others or of age-appropriate social norms or rules. Individuals with ADHD and conduct disorder are at a much higher risk of developing substance abuse, of developing antisocial personality disorder, and of being involved in criminal activity than individuals with ADHD alone (Pliszka, 2003b). Individuals with ADHD and conduct disorder respond to stimulants for their ADHD (Pliszka, 2003b); however, they require intensive multimodal intervention that includes medication, behavior therapy, family therapy, and school-based interventions (Frick, 2001). Treatment must be tailored to the individual

child's symptoms and may include the use of antidepressants, mood stabilizers, or atypical antipsychotics.

MULTIMODAL TREATMENT

The Multimodal Treatment Study of ADHD is the largest clinical trial of ADHD treatments to date (MTA Cooperative Group, 1999a). This multisite study of 576 children between the ages of 7 and 9 years randomized participants into one of four treatment groups: 1) medication management, 2) intensive behavioral treatment, 3) medication and intensive behavioral treatment, and 4) standard community care. The medication management group received primarily methylphenidate titrated to the best of three doses. The behavioral treatment involved 35 group and individual sessions for parents, a summer program for children, teacher consultation, and 60 days of a part-time behaviorally trained paraprofessional working with the child in school. The combined treatment group received both of these interventions; those in the standard community care group were evaluated and referred back to providers in their own community for treatment.

Outcome was assessed 14 months after the initiation of treatment. For improving the core ADHD symptoms, medication alone was nearly as effective as the combined treatment. Those receiving the combined treatment, however, achieved these outcomes on lower doses of medication than the medication only group. Both the combined and medication only treatments were more effective in improving core ADHD symptoms than behavioral treatment or community care. In terms of academic achievement, anxiety/depressive symptoms, and oppositional/aggressive symptoms, there were small benefits of combined treatment compared with medication alone on some but not all outcome measures (Jensen et al., 2001). Thus, this study and other studies of intensive psychosocial interventions (Abikoff et al., 2004) suggest that behavioral interventions have only small additional benefits for children who respond to stimulant medication. Nonetheless, the study revealed some important points about matching psychosocial interventions to individual patients. For example, children with anxiety disorders at the beginning of treatment responded as well to the psychosocial treatment as they did to medication alone. Moreover, in this group, the combined treatment offered greater advantages over medication alone than were found for the rest of the sample. Families who were on public assistance also had greater benefit from the psychosocial intervention than medication alone. Moreover, despite the greater efficacy of medication treatment, the behavioral intervention was rated as more acceptable to parents (MTA Cooperative Group, 2004a).

COMPLEMENTARY AND ALTERNATIVE THERAPIES

There are numerous nonconventional treatments for ADHD (Arnold, 2001a, 2000b; Baumgaertel, 1999). Among these, the only controlled studies involve dietary interventions. Dietary treatments have taken two general approaches, either elimination of foods thought to cause symptoms or addition of dietary supplements, vitamins, or minerals. Controlled studies comparing diets eliminating certain additives, commonly allergenic foods, or both with disguised diets containing these substances have found that approximately 10%–20% of subjects have significant improvements in rating scale measures of some symptoms. Hyperactivity and irritability are more likely to improve than inattention, and younger children may be more likely to respond than older children (Arnold, 2001a; Bateman et al., 2004). In contrast to elimination of allergens and additives, elimination of sugar has not been found to have an observable effect (Wolraich, Wilson, & White, 1995).

Studies of minerals have documented that children with ADHD may be relatively deficit in iron, zinc, and magnesium (Arnold, 2001a; Konofal et al., 2004). Small open label studies of supplementation with these minerals have demonstrated some improvement in ADHD symptoms (Arnold, 2001a, 2001b). A large, double-blind placebo-controlled study of zinc found improvements in hyperactive and impulsive behaviors but not inattentive behaviors. Approximately 29% of the zinc-treated group versus 20% of the placebo group were judged to be responders, and those with lower zinc levels at baseline were more likely to respond (Bilici et al., 2004). Further study of the role of zinc deficiency in ADHD and the effects of supplementation is warranted, as most of the studies have been done in non-Western cultures in which zinc deficiency is more prevalent (Arnold & DiSilvestro, 2005). Megadoses of vitamins or minerals can have negative health effects and are not indicated or expected.

Essential fatty acids (EFAs) are lower in children with ADHD than in controls, and sup-

plementation has shown positive effects in a number of mental health disorders, (reviewed in Richardson & Puri, 2000). Positive (Richardson & Montgomery, 2005) and negative (Voigt et al., 2001) results have been found in ADHD. Positive studies used eicosapentaenoic (EPA, omega-3), docosahexaenoic (DHA, omega-3), and linoleic acid (LA, omega-6) or gama-linoleic acid (GLA, omega 6) together, whereas negative studies used either DHA or LA/GLA alone, suggesting that a combination may be necessary. Because children may be deficient at certain points in the metabolism of certain EFAs, initial measures followed by individualized treatment may be a more appropriate way to assess the effects of supplementation.

Several techniques that "train the brain" are being investigated as alternative treatments (Hirshberg, Chiu, & Frazier, 2005). Electroencephalogram (EEG) biofeedback is the technique that has been studied most extensively. Studies of the quantity of different types of brain waves produced by groups with ADHD versus controls have shown that subjects with ADHD tend to have a lower level of those waves (alpha and beta) associated with alert, thinking states and a higher level of those waves (theta) associated with drowsiness. EEG biofeedback uses computer technology to train the individual to produce more of the brain wave patterns associated with concentration and to suppress those associated with drowsiness (Gruzelier & Egner, 2005; Hirshberg et al., 2005; Monstra, 2005). There is some evidence for its effectiveness (Monstra, 2005; Rossiter, 2004). EEG biofeedback is safe but time consuming and expensive, and it is not clear which symptoms or children can be predicted to respond. Specific training programs to improve working memory and motor control show promising initial results, and further study is indicated (Klingberg et al., 2005).

OUTCOME

Although overt hyperactivity and impulsivity tend to decline as a clinical problem when youth reach adolescence and young adulthood, inattention often persists. It is estimated that ADHD persists into adulthood in 30% to more than 60% of individuals diagnosed with this disorder as children. In many individuals whose symptoms no longer meet the criteria for ADHD, subclinical difficulty with sustained attention and/or impulsivity may persist (Faraone et al., 2006). In general, adults with ADHD complete less formal schooling, have lower-status jobs and work performance ratings, are more likely to have their driver's licenses suspended and to get into car accidents, have higher rates of antisocial behavior (Barkley, 2002; Mannuzza & Klein, 2000), and have higher rates of additional neuropsychiatric disorders (Biederman et al., 2006).

The presence of conduct disorder is the strongest predictor for adverse outcome, placing children and teens at risk for antisocial personality disorder and substance abuse (Barkley et al., 2004). However, underachievement in educational and occupational level in those with ADHD compared with controls persists even when the adults with antisocial personality disorder are excluded from the sample (Mannuzza et al., 1993). Those whose ADHD symptoms improve during adolescence tend to have a much better outcome than those with persistent symptoms (Biederman, Mick, & Farone, 1998; Greenfield, Hechtman, & Weiss, 1988).

SUMMARY

ADHD is a prevalent neurodevelopmental condition that has a significant impact on the lives of affected children, their families, and the educational and medical/mental health systems. The core features of difficulty sustaining mental effort, hyperactivity, and impulsivity lead to impairment in academic, occupational, social, and adaptive functioning without effective intervention. Coping with ADHD is made more complicated by commonly coexisting conditions, including learning disorders, oppositional defiant disorder, and anxiety disorders. ADHD is highly genetic, but adverse conditions in the pre- and perinatal period can contribute to symptoms. Multiple lines of evidence suggest a biological basis involving frontal cortical-basal ganglia-cerebellar pathways and biogenic amine neurotransmitters, particularly dopamine and norepinephrine. Treatments include counseling, particularly that focusing on behavior management; accommodations in the classroom; addressing coexisting conditions; and medication. Fortunately, the knowledge and resources presently available, and the increases in these areas that are sure to occur over the next generation, offer children growing up with ADHD the opportunity to experience success.

REFERENCES

Abikoff, H., Hechtman, L., Klein, R.G., et al. (2004). Social functioning in children with ADHD treated with long-term methylphenidate and multimodal psychosocial treatment. *Journal of the American Academy of Child and Adolescent Psychiatry, 43,* 820–829.

Accardo, P. (1999). A rational approach to the medical assessment of the child with attention-deficit/hyperactivity disorder. *Pediatric Clinics of North America, 46,* 845–856.

Allen, A.J., Kurlan, R.M., Gilbert, D.L., et al. (2005). Atomoxetine treatment in children and adolescents with ADHD and comorbid tic disorders. *Neurology, 65,* 1941–1949.

American Academy of Child and Adolescent Psychiatry. (1997). Practice parameter for the use of stimulant medications in the treatment of children, adolescents, and adults. *Journal of the American Academy of Child and Adolescent Psychiatry, 36*(Suppl. 10), 85S–121S.

American Academy of Child and Adolescent Psychiatry. (2002). Practice parameter for the use of stimulant medications in the treatment of children, adolescents, and adults. *Journal of the American Academy of Child and Adolescent Psychiatry, 41*(Suppl. 2), 26S–49S.

American Academy of Pediatrics. (2000). Clinical practice guideline: Diagnosis and evaluation of the child with attention-deficit/hyperactivity disorder. *Pediatrics, 105,* 1158–1170.

American Academy of Pediatrics. (2001). Clinical practice guideline: Treatment of the school-aged child with attention-deficit/hyperactivity disorder. *Pediatrics, 108,* 1033–1044.

American Psychiatric Association. (1994). *Diagnostic and statistical manual of mental disorders* (4th ed.). Washington, DC: Author.

American Psychiatric Association. (2000). *Diagnostic and statistical manual of mental disorders* (4th ed., text rev.). Washington, DC: Author.

Angold, A., Erkanli, A., Egger, H.L., et al. (2000). Stimulant treatment for children: A community perspective. *Journal of the American Academy of Child and Adolescent Psychiatry, 39,* 975–984.

Armstrong M.B., & Nettleton, S.K. (2004). Attention deficit hyperactivity disorder and preschool children. *Seminars in Speech and Language, 25,* 225–232.

Arnold, L.E. (2001a, Summer). Ingestive treatments for learning disorders. *Perspectives (The International Dyslexia Association),* 21–22.

Arnold, L.E. (2001b). Alternative treatments for adults with attention-deficit hyperactivity disorder (ADHD). *Annals New York Academy of Sciences, 931,* 310–341.

Arnold, L.E., & DiSilvestro, R.A. (2005). Zinc in attention-deficit/hyperactivity disorder. *Journal of Child and Adolescent Psychopharmacology, 15,* 619–627.

Banaschewski, T., Roessner, V., Dittman, R.W., et al. (2004). Non-stimulant medications in the treatment of ADHD. *European Child and Adolescent Psychiatry, 13*(Suppl. 1), 102–116.

Barkley, R.A. (1998). Primary symptoms, diagnostics criteria, prevalence, and gender differences. In R.A. Barkley (Ed.), *Attention-deficit hyperactivity disorder: A handbook for diagnosis and treatment* (pp. 56–96). New York: The Guilford Press.

Barkley, R.A. (2002). Major life activity and health outcomes associated with attention-deficit/hyperactivity disorder. *Journal of Clinical Psychiatry, 63*(Suppl. 12), 10–15.

Barkely, R.A. (2004). Adolescents with attention-deficit/hyperactivity disorder: An overview of empirically-based treatments. *Journal of Psychiatric Practice, 10,* 39–56.

Barkley, R.A., Fischer M, Smallish L, et al. (2004). Young adult follow-up of hyperactive children: Antisocial activities and drug use. *Journal of Child Psychology and Psychiatry, 45*, 195–211.

Bass, J.L., Corwin, M., Gozal, D., et al. (2004). The effect of chronic or intermittent hypoxia on cognition in childhood: A review of the evidence. *Pediatrics, 114*, 805–816.

Bateman, B., Warner, J.O., Hutchinson, E., et al. (2004). The effects of a double-blind, placebo controlled, artificial food colorings and benzoate preservative challenge on hyperactivity in a general population sample of preschool children. *Archives of Diseases in Children, 89*, 506–511.

Baumgaertel, A. (1999). Alternative and controversial treatments for attention-deficit/hyperactivity disorder. *Pediatric Clinics of North America, 46*, 977–992.

Biederman, J. (2003). Pharmacotherapy for attention-deficit/hyperactivity disorder (ADHD) decreased the risk for substance abuse: Findings from a longitudinal follow-up of youths with and without ADHD. *Journal of Clinical Psychiatry, 64*, S11, 3–8.

Biederman, J., Baldessarini, R.J., Wright, V., et al. (1989). A double-blind placebo controlled study of desipramine in the treatment of ADD: I. Efficacy. *Journal of the American Academy of Child and Adolescent Psychiatry, 28*, 777–784.

Biederman, J., Mick, E., & Faraone, S.V. (1998). Normalized functioning in youths with persistent attention-deficit/hyperactivity disorder. *Journal of Pediatrics, 133*, 544–551.

Biederman, J., Monuteaux, M.C., Mick, E., et al. (2006). Young adult outcome of attention deficit hyperactivity disorder: A controlled 10-year follow-up study. *Psychological Medicine, 36*, 167–179.

Biederman, J., Spencer, T., & Wilens, T. (2004). Evidence-based pharmacotherapy for attention-deficit hyperactivity disorder. *International Journal of Neuropsychopharmacology, 7*, 77–97.

Bilici, M., Yildirim F, Kandil, S., et al. (2004). Double-blind, placebo-controlled study of zinc sulfate in the treatment of attention deficit hyperactivity disorder. *Progress in Neuro-Psychopharmacology & Biological Psychiatry, 28*, 181–190.

Brown, T.E., & McMullen, W.J., Jr. (2001). Attention deficit disorders and sleep/arousal disturbance. *Annals of the New York Academy of Sciences, 931*, 271–286.

Burke, J.D., Loeber, R., & Birmaher, B. (2002). Oppositional defiant and conduct disorder: A review of the past 10 years, part 2. *Journal of the American Academy of Child and Adolescent Psychiatry, 41*, 1275–1293.

Carlson, G.A., & Kelly, K.L. (2003). Stimulant rebound: How common is it and what does it mean? *Journal of Child and Adolescent Psychopharmacology, 13*, 137–142.

Castellanos, F.X., Lee, P.P., Sharp, W., et al. (2002). Developmental trajectories of brain volume abnormalities in children and adolescents with attention-deficit/hyperactivity disorder. *The Journal of the American Medical Association, 288*, 1740–1748.

Charach, A., Ickowicz, A., & Schachar, R. (2004). Stimulant treatment over five years: Adherence, effectiveness, and adverse events. *Journal of the American Academy of Child and Adolescent Psychiatry, 43*, 559–567.

Cheon, K.-A., Ryu, Y.H., Kim, Y.-K., et al. (2003). Dopamine transporter density in the basal ganglia assessed with [123I]IPT SPET in children with attention deficit hyperactivity disorder. *European Journal of Nuclear Medicine, 30*, 306–311.

Chronis, A.M., Chacko, A., Fabiano, G.A., et al. (2004). Enhancements to the behavioral parent training paradigm for families of children with ADHD: Review and future directions. *Clinical Child and Family Psychology Review, 7*, 1–27.

Cohen-Zion, M., & Ancoli-Israel, S. (2004). Sleep in children with attention-deficit hyperactivity disorder (ADHD): A review of naturalistic and stimulant intervention studies. *Sleep Medicine Reviews, 8*, 379–402.

Conners, C.K. (1997). *Conners' Rating Scales–Revised (CSR-R)*. North Tonawanda, NY: Multi-Health Systems.

Conners, C.K., Casat, C.D., Gualtieri, C.T., et al. (1996). Bupropion hydrochloride in attention deficit disorder with hyperactivity. *Journal of the American Academy of Child and Adolescent Psychiatry, 34*, 1314–1321.

Connor, D.F., Glatt, S.J., Lopez, I.D., et al. (2002). Psychopharmacology and aggression. I: A meta-analysis of stimulant effects on overt/covert aggression-related behaviors in ADHD. *Journal of the American Academy of Child and Adolescent Psychiatry, 41*, 253–261.

Cox, D.J., Merkel, R.L., Penberthy J.K., et al. (2004). Impact of methylphenidate delivery profiles on driving performance of adolescents with attention-deficit/hyperactivity disorder: A pilot study. *Journal of the American Academy of Child and Adolescent Psychiatry, 43*, 269–275.

Denkla, M.B. (2006). Attention deficit hyperactivity disorder: The childhood comorbidity that most influences the burden of disability in Tourette syndrome. *Advances in Neurology, 99*, 17–21.

DuPaul, G.J., McGoey, K.E., Eckert, T.L. et al. (2001). Preschool children with attention-deficit/hyperactivity disorder: Impairments in behavioral, social, and school functioning. *Journal of the American Academy of Child and Adolescent Psychiatry, 40*, 508–515.

DuPaul, G.J., Power, T.J., Anastopoulos, A.D., et al. (1998). *ADHD Rating Scale-IV: Checklists, norms, and clinical interpretations*. New York: The Guilford Press.

Durston, S. (2003). A review of the biological basis of ADHD: What have we learned from imaging studies? *Mental Retardation and Developmental Disabilities Research Reviews, 9*, 184–195.

Efron D., Jarman, F., & Barker, M. (1997). Side effects of methylphenidate and dexamphetamine in children with attention-deficit hyperactivity disorder: A double-blind crossover trial. *Pediatrics, 100*, 662–666.

Elia, J. (2005, January). Attention deficit/hyperactivity disorder: Pharmacotherapy. *Psychiatry*, 27–35.

Emslie, G.J., Hughes, C.W., Crimson, M.L., et al. (2004). A feasibility study of the childhood depression medication algorithm: The Texas children's medication algorithm project (CMAP). *Journal of the American Academy of Child and Adolescent Psychiatry, 43*, 519–527.

Ernst, M., Zametkin, A.J., Matochik, J.A., et al. (1998). DOPA decarboxylase activity in ADHD adults. An [F18] fluorodopa PET study. *Journal of Neuroscience, 18*, 5901–5907.

Ernst, M., Zametkin, A.J., Matochik, J.A., et al. (1999). High midbrain [F18] DOPA accumulation in children with ADHD. *American Journal of Psychiatry, 156*, 1209–1215.

Faraone, S.V., Biederman, J., & Mick, E. (2006). The age-dependent decline of attention deficit hyperactivity disorder: A meta-analysis of follow-up studies. *Psychological Medicine, 36*, 159–165.

Faraone, S.V., Biederman, J., Monuteaux, M., et al. (2005). Long-term effects of extended-release mixed amphetamine salts treatment of attention-deficit/hyperactivity disorder on growth. *Journal of Child & Adolescent Psychopharmacology, 15,* 191–202.

Faraone, S.V., Perlis, R.H., Doyle, A.E., et al. (2005). Molecular genetics of attention-deficit/hyperactivity disorder. *Biological Psychiatry, 57,* 1313–1323.

Fischer, M., & Barkley, R.A. (2003). Childhood stimulant treatment and risk for later substance abuse. *Journal of Clinical Psychiatry, 64*(Suppl. 11), 19–23.

Frankel, F., & Feinberg, D. (2002). Social problems associated with ADHD vs. ODD in children referred for friendship problems. *Child Psychiatry and Human Development, 33,* 125–146.

Frick, P.J. (2001). Effective interventions for children and adolescents with conduct disorder. *Canadian Journal of Psychiatry, 46,* 597–608.

Gadow, K.D., & Sverd, J. (2006). Attention deficit hyperactivity disorder, chronic tic disorder, and methylphenidate. *Advances in Neurology, 99,* 197–207.

Ghelani, K., Sidhu, R., Jain, U., et al. (2004). Reading comprehension and reading related abilities in adolescents with reading disabilities and attention-deficit/hyperactivity disorder. *Dyslexia: The Journal of the British Dyslexia Association, 10,* 364–384.

Ghuman, J.K., Ginsburg, G.S., Subramaniam, G., et al. (2001). Psychostimulants in preschool children with attention-deficit/hyperactivity disorder: Clinical evidence from a developmental disorders institution. *Journal of the American Academy of Child and Adolescent Psychiatry, 40,* 516–524.

Glanzman, M. (in press). Genetics, imaging, and neurochemistry in attention deficit hyperactivity disorder (ADHD). In P.J. Accardo (Ed.), *Capute and Accardo's neurodevelopmental disabilities in infancy and childhood, third edition, volume II: The spectrum of developmental disabilities.* Baltimore: Paul H. Brookes Publishing Co.

Glanzman, M., & Elia, J. (2006). Neurodevelopmental and neuropsychiatric disorders. In M. Charron (Ed.), *Practical pediatric PET imaging* (pp. 334—360). New York: Springer.

Greenfield, B. Hechtman, L., & Weiss, G. (1988). Two subgroups of hyperactives as adults: Correlations of outcome. *Canadian Journal of Psychiatry, 33,* 505–508.

Gruzelier, J., & Egner, T. (2005). Critical validation studies of neurofeedback. *Child and Adolescent Psychiatric Clinics of North America, 14,* 83–104.

Handen, B.L., Breaux, A.M., Janosky, J., et al. (1992). Effects and noneffects of methylphenidate in children with mental retardation and ADHD. *Journal of the American Academy of Child and Adolescent Psychiatry, 31,* 455–461.

Handen, B.L., Feldman, H., Gosling, A., et al. (1991). Adverse side effects of methylphenidate among mentally retarded children with ADHD. *Journal of the American Academy of Child and Adolescent Psychiatry, 30,* 241–245.

Harpin, V.A. (2005). The effect of ADHD on the life of an individual, their family, and community from preschool to adult life. *Archives of Diseases in Childhood, 90*(Suppl. 1), i2–i7.

Hazell, P.L., & Stuart, J.E. (2003). A randomized controlled trial of clonidine added to psychostimulant medication for hyperactive and aggressive children. *Journal of the American Academy of Child and Adolescent Psychiatry, 42,* 886–894.

Hirshberg, L.M., Chiu, S., & Frazier, J.A. (2005). Emerging brain-based interventions for children and adolescents: overview and clinical perspective. *Child and Adolescent Psychiatric Clinics of North America, 14,* 1–19.

Individuals with Disabilities Education Improvement Act of 2004, PL 108-446, 20 U.S.C. §§ 1400 *et seq.*

Jensen, P.S. (2000). Current concepts and controversies in the diagnosis and treatment of attention deficit hyperactivity disorder. *Current Psychiatry Reports, 2,* 102–109.

Jensen, P.S., Hinshaw, S.P., Swanson, J.M., et al. (2001). Findings from the NIMH Multimodal Treatment Study of ADHD (MTA): Implications and applications for primary care providers. *Journal of Developmental and Behavioral Pediatrics, 22,* 60–73.

Jensen, P.S., Kettle, L., Roper, M.T., et al. (1999). Are stimulants overprescribed? Treatment of ADHD in four U.S. communities. *Journal of the American Academy of Child and Adolescent Psychiatry, 38,* 797–804.

Kaufman, J., Birmaher, B., Brent, D., et al. (1996). *Kiddie Schedule for Affective Disorders and Schizophrenia (K-SADS).* Retrieved December 18, 2006, from http://www.wpic.pitt.edu/ksads/default.htm

Kent, L. (2004). Recent advances in the genetics of attention deficit hyperactivity disorder. *Current Psychiatry Reports, 6,* 143–148.

Khalifa, N., & von Knorring, A-L. (2005). Tourette syndrome and other tic disorders in a total population in children: Clinical assessment and background. *Acta Paediatrica, 94,* 1608–1614.

Klassen, A.F., Miller, A., & Fine, S. (2004). Health-related quality of life in children and adolescents who have a diagnosis of attention-deficit/hyperactivity disorder. *Pediatrics, 114,* 541–547.

Klein, R.G., & Mannuzza, S. (1988). Hyperactive boys almost grown up III. Methylphenidate effects on ultimate height. *Archives of General Psychiatry, 45,* 1131–1134.

Klingberg, T., Fernell, E., Olesen, P.J., et al. (2005). Computerized training of working memory in children with ADHD: A randomized, controlled trial. *Journal of the American Academy of Child and Adolescent Psychiatry, 44,* 177–186.

Konofal, E., Lecendreux, M., Arnulf, I., et al. (2004). Iron deficiency in children with attention-deficit/hyperactivity disorder. *Archives of Pediatrics & Adolescent Medicine, 158,* 1113–1115.

Kratochvil, C.J., Greenhill, L.L., March, J.S., et al. (2004). The role of stimulants in the treatment of preschool children with attention-deficit hyperactivity disorder. *CNS Drugs, 18,* 957–966.

Krause, K.H., Dresel, S.H., Krause, J., et al. (2003). The dopamine transporter and neuroimaging in attention deficit hyperactivity disorder. *Neuroscience & Biobehavioral Reviews, 27,* 605–613.

Kronenberger, W.G., & Dunn, D.W. (2003). Learning disorders. *Neurologic Clinics, 21,* 941-952.

Lipkin, P.H., Goldstein, I.J., & Adesman, A.R. (1994). Tics and dyskinesias associated with stimulant treatment in attention-deficit hyperactivity disorder. *Archives of Pediatrics & Adolescent Medicine, 148,* 859–861.

Lou, H.C., Henriksen, L., Bruhn, P., et al. (1989). Striatal dysfunction in attention deficit and hyperkinetic disorder. *Archives of Neurology, 46,* 48–57.

Lou, H.C., Rosa, P., Pryds, O., et al. (2004). ADHD: Increased dopamine receptor availability linked to attention deficit and low neonatal blood flow. *Developmental Medicine and Child Neurology, 46,* 179–183.

Mannuzza, S., & Klein, R.G. (2000). Long-term prognosis in attention-deficit/hyperactivity disorder. *Child and Adolescent Psychiatric Clinics of North America, 9,* 711–726.

Mannuzza, S., Klein, R.G., Bessler, A., et al. (1993). Adult outcome of hyperactive boys: Educational achievement, occupational rank, and psychiatric status. *Archives of General Psychiatry, 50,* 565–576.

Manos, M.J., Short, E.J., & Findling, R.L. (1999). Differential effectiveness of methylphenidate and Adderall in school-aged youths with attention-deficit/hyperactivity disorder. *Journal of the American Academy of Child and Adolescent Psychiatry, 38,* 813–819.

March, J,. Silva, S., Petrycki, S., et al. (2004). Fluoxetine, cognitive-behavioral therapy, and their combination for adolescents with depression: Treatment for Adolescents with Depression Study (TADS) randomized controlled trial. *The Journal of the American Medical Association, 292,* 807–820.

Martin, N.C., Piek, J.P., & Hay, D. (2006). DCD and ADHD: A genetic study of their shared etiology. *Human Movement Science, 25,* 110–124.

Martinussen, R., Haysen, J., Hogg-Johnson, S., et al. (2005). A meta-analysis of working memory in children with attention-deficit/hyperactivity disorder. *Journal of the American Academy of Child and Adolescent Psychiatry, 44,* 377–384.

McInnes, A., Humphries, T., Hogg-Johnson, S., et al. (2003). Listening comprehension and working memory are impaired in attention-deficit hyperactivity disorder irrespective of language impairment. *Journal of Abnormal Child Psychology, 31,* 427–443.

Michelson, D., Allen, A.J., Busner, J., et al. (2002). Once-daily atomexetine treatment for children and adolescents with attention deficit hyperactivity disorder: A randomized, placebo-controlled study. *American Journal of Psychiatry, 159,* 1896–1901.

Michelson, D., Faries, D., Wernicke, J., et al. (2001). Atomoxetine in the treatment of children and adolescents with attention-deficit/hyperactivity disorder: A randomized placebo-controlled, dose-response study. *Pediatrics, 108(5),* e83.

Mick, E., Faraone, S.V., & Biederman, J. (2004). Age-dependent expression of attention-deficit/hyperactivity disorder symptoms. *Psychiatric Clinics of North America, 27,* 215–224.

Monstra, V.J. (2005). Electroencephalographic biofeedback (neurotherapy) as a treatment for attention deficit hyperactivity disorder: Rationale and empirical foundation. *Child and Adolescent Psychiatric Clinics of North America, 14,* 55–82.

MTA Cooperative Group. (1999a). A 14-month randomized clinical trial of treatment strategies for attention-deficit/hyperactivity disorder. *Archives of General Psychiatry, 56,* 1073–1086.

MTA Cooperative Group. (1999b). Moderators and mediators of treatment response for children with attention-deficit/hyperactivity disorder: The Multimodal Treatment Study of children with attention-deficit/hyperactivity disorder. *Archives of General Psychiatry, 56,* 1088–1096.

MTA Cooperative Group. (2004a). National Institute of Mental Health Multimodal Treatment Study of ADHD follow-up: 24-Month outcomes of treatment strategies for attention-deficit/hyperactivity disorder. *Pediatrics, 113,* 754–761.

MTA Cooperative Group. (2004b). National Institute of Mental Health Multimodal Treatment Study of ADHD follow-up: Changes in effectiveness and growth after the end of treatment. *Pediatrics, 113,* 762–769.

Owens, J.A. (2005). The ADHD and sleep conundrum: A review. *Journal of Developmental and Behavioral Pediatrics, 26,* 312–322.

Palumbo, D., Spencer, T., Lynch, J., et al. (2004). Emergence of tics in children with ADHD: Impact of once-daily OROS methylphenidate therapy. *Journal of Child & Adolescent Psychopharmacology, 14,* 185–194.

Pelham, W.E., Fabbiano, G.A., & Massetti, G.M. (2005). Evidence-based assessment of attention deficit hyperactivity disorder in children and adolescents. *Journal of Clinical Child and Adolescent Psychology, 34,* 449–476.

Pliszka, S.R. (2003a). Non-stimulant treatment of attention-deficit/hyperactivity disorder. *CNS Spectrums, 8,* 253–258.

Pliszka, S.R. (2003b). Psychiatric comorbidities in children with attention deficit hyperactivity disorder: Implications for management. *Pediatric Drugs, 5,* 741–750.

Popper, C.W. (2000). Pharmacologic alternatives to psychostimulants for the treatment of attention-deficit/hyperactivity disorder. *Child and Adolescent Psychiatric Clinics of North America, 9,* 605–646.

Power, T.J., & Glanzman, M.M. (2006). Tic disorders. In G.G. Bear & K.M. Minke (Eds.), *Children's needs III: Development, prevention, and intervention* (pp. 1055–1068). Bethesda, MD: National Association of School Psychologists.

Rapaport, J., Buchsbaum, M., Zahn, T.P., et al. (1978). Dextroamphetamine: Cognitive and behavioral effects in normal prepubertal boys. *Science, 199,* 560–563.

Rapport, M.D., Denney, C., DuPaul, G.J., et al. (1994). Attention deficit disorder and methylphenidate: Normalization rates, clinical effectiveness, and response prediction in 76 children. *Journal of the American Academy of Child and Adolescent Psychiatry, 33,* 882–893.

Rehabilitation Act of 1973, PL 93-112, 29 U.S.C. §§ 701 et seq.

Reich, W. (2000). Diagnostic Interview for Children and Adolescents (DICA). *Journal of the American Academy of Child & Adolescent Psychiatry, 39,* 59–66.

Richardson, A.J., & Montgomery, P. (2005). The Oxford-Durham study: A randomized, controlled trial of dietary supplementation with fatty acids in children with developmental coordination disorder. *Pediatrics, 115,* 1360–1366.

Richardson, A.J., & Puri, B.K. (2000). The potential role of fatty acids in attention-deficit/hyperactivity disorder. *Prostaglandins, Leukotrienes, and Essential Fatty Acids, 63,* 79–87.

Rossiter, T. (2004). The effectiveness of neurofeedback and stimulant drugs in treating AD/HD: part II. Replication. *Applied Psychophysiology and Biofeedback, 29,* 233–243.

Rubia, K., Overmeyer, S., Taylor, E., et al. (1999). Hypofrontality in attention deficit hyperactivity disorder during higher order motor control: A study with functional MRI. *American Journal of Psychiatry, 156,* 891–896.

Rushton, J.L., Fant, K.E., & Clark, S.J. (2004). Use of

practice guidelines in the primary care of children with attention-deficit/hyperactivity disorder. *Pediatrics, 114*, e23–e28.

Saccomani, L., Fabiana, V., Manuela, B., et al. (2005). Tourette syndrome and chronic tics in a sample of children and adolescents. *Brain & Development, 27*, 349–352.

Safer, D.J., & Malever, M. (2000). Stimulant treatment in Maryland public schools. *Pediatrics, 106*, 533–539.

Safer, D.J., & Zito, J.M. (1999). Psychotropic medications for ADHD. *Mental Retardation and Developmental Disabilities Research Reviews, 5*, 237–242.

Safer, D.J., Zito, J.M., & dosReis, S. (2003). Concomitant psychotropic medication for youths. *American Journal of Psychiatry, 160*, 438–449.

Safer, D.J., Zito, J.M., & Gardner, J.E. (2001). Pemoline hepatotoxicity and postmarketing surveillance. *Journal of the American Academy of Child and Adolescent Psychiatry, 40*, 622–629.

Safren, S.A., Sprich, S., Chulvick, S., et al. (2004). Psychosocial treatments for adults with attention-deficit/hyperactivity disorder. *Psychiatric Clinics of North America, 27*, 349–360.

Scahill, L., Sukhodolsky, D.G., Williams, S.K., et al. (2005). Public health significance of tic disorders in children and adolescents. *Advances in Neurology, 96*, 240–248.

Singer, H.S. (2005). Tourette syndrome: From behavior to biology. *The Lancet Neurology, 4*, 149–159.

Singer, H.S., Brown, J.E., Quaskey, S., et al. (1995). The treatment of attention-deficit hyperactivity disorder in Tourette's syndrome: A double-blind, placebo-controlled study with clonidine and desipramine. *Pediatrics, 95*, 74–81.

Solanto, M.V. (2002). Dopamine dysfunction in AD/HD. *Behavioral Brain Research, 130*, 65–71.

Sowell, E.R., Thompson, P.M., Welcome, S.E., et al. (2003). Cortical abnormalities in children and adolescents with attention-deficit/hyperactivity disorder. *The Lancet, 362*, 1699–1707.

Sprich-Buckminster, S., Biederman, J., Milberger, S., et al. (1993). Are perinatal complications relevant to the manifestations of ADD? Issues of comorbidity and familiarity. *Journal of the American Academy of Child and Adolescent Psychiatry, 32*, 1032–1037.

Stein, M.A., & Baren, M. (2003). Welcome progress in the diagnosis and treatment of ADHD in adolescence. *Contemporary Pediatrics, 20*, 83–108.

Stevenson, C.S., Whitmont, S., Bornholt, L., et al. (2002). A cognitive remediation program for adults with attention deficit hyperactivity disorder. *Australian and New Zealand Journal of Psychiatry, 36*, 610–616.

Tourette Syndrome Study Group. (2002). Treatment of ADHD in children with tics: A randomized controlled trial. *Neurology, 58*, 527–536.

Swanson, J.M. (n.d.). *SNAP-IV Rating Scale.* Retrieved December 18, 2006, from http://www.adhd.net

Turgay, A., Binder, C., Snyder, R., et al. (2002). Long-term safety and efficacy of risperidone for the treatment of disruptive behavior disorders in children with subaverage IQs. *Pediatrics, 110*(3), e34.

Vaidya, C.J., Austin, G., Kirkorian, G., et al. (1998). Selective effects of methylphenidate in attention deficit hyperactivity disorder: A functional magnetic imaging study. *Proceedings of the National Academy of Science of the United States of America, 95*, 14494–14499.

Vanderbilt Children's Hospital. (n.d.). *Vanderbilt ADHD Diagnostic Parent Rating Scale.* Retrieved December 18, 2006, from http://www.vanderbiltchildrens.com/uploads/documents/ccdr_adhd_scale.pdf

Vanderbilt Children's Hospital. (n.d.). *Vanderbilt ADHD Diagnostic Teacher Rating Scale.* Retrieved December 18, 2006, from http://www.brightfutures.org/mental health/pdf/professionals/bridges/adhd.pdf

Varley, C.K., & Smith, C.J. (2003). Anxiety disorders in the child and teen. *Pediatric Clinics of North America, 50*, 1107–1138.

Visser, J. (2003). Developmental coordination disorder: A review of research on subtypes and comorbidities. *Human Movement Science, 22*, 479–493.

Voeller, K.K. (2004). Attention-deficit hyperactivity disorder (ADHD). *Journal of Child Neurology, 19*, 798–814.

Voigt, R.G., Llorente, A.M., Jensen, C.L., et al. (2001). A randomized, double-blind, placebo-controlled trial of docosahexanoic acid supplementation in children with attention-deficit/hyperactivity disorder. *Pediatrics, 139*, 189–196.

Volkow, N.D., & Swanson, J.M. (2003). Variables that affect the clinical use and abuse of methylphenidate in the treatment of ADHD. *American Journal of Psychiatry, 160*, 1909–1918.

Waxmonsky, J. (2003). Assessment and treatment of attention deficit hyperactivity disorder in children with comorbid psychiatric illness. *Current Opinion in Pediatrics, 15*, 476–482.

Weiss, M., Murray, C., & Weiss, G. (2002). Adults with attention deficit/hyperactivity disorder: Current concepts. *Journal of Psychiatric Practice, 8*, 99–111.

Weyandt, L.L. (2005). Executive function in children, adolescents, and adults with attention-deficit/hyperactivity disorder: An introduction to the special issue. *Developmental Neuropsychology, 27*, 1–10.

Wigal, T., Swanson, J.M., Regino, R., et al. (1999). Stimulant medications for the treatment of ADHD: Efficacy and limitations. *Mental Retardation and Developmental Disabilities Research Reviews, 5*, 215–224.

Wilens, T.E., Faraone, S.V., Biederman, J., et al. (2003). Does stimulant therapy of attention-deficit/hyperactivity disorder beget later substance abuse? A meta-analytic review of the literature. *Pediatrics, 111*, 179–185.

Wilens, T.E., Hahsey, A.L., Biederman, J., et al. (2005). Influence of parental SUD and ADHD on ADD in their offspring: Preliminary results from a pilot-controlled family study. *American Journal on Addictions, 14*, 179–187.

Wilens, T.E., McBurnett, K., Stein, M., et al. (2005). ADHD treatment with once-daily OROS methylphenidate: Final results from a long-term open-label study. *Journal of the American Academy of Child and Adolescent Psychiatry, 44*, 1015–1023.

Wilens, T.E., Prince, J.B., Spencer, T.J., et al. (2006). Stimulants and sudden death: What is a physician to do? *Pediatrics, 118*, 1215–1219.

Willcutt, E.G., Doyle, A.E., Nigg, J.T., et al. (2005). Validity of the executive function theory of attention-deficit/hyperactivity disorder: A meta-analytic review. *Biological Psychiatry, 57*, 1336–1346.

Willcutt, E.G., Pennington, B.F., Olson, R.K., et al. (2005). Neuropsychological analysis of comorbidity between reading disability and attention deficit hyperactivity disorder: In search of the common deficit. *Developmental Neuropsychology, 27*, 35–78.

Wolraich, M.L., Wibbelsman, C.J., Brown, T.E., et al.

(2005). Attention-deficit/hyperactivity disorder among adolescents: A review of the diagnosis, treatment, and clinical implications. *Pediatrics, 115,* 1734–1746.

Wolraich, M.L., Wilson, D.B., & White, J.W. (1995). The effect of sugar on behavior or cognition in children. *The Journal of the American Medical Association, 274,* 1617–1621.

Zito, J.M. Safer, D.J., dosReis, S., et al. (2000). Trends in the prescribing of psychotropic medications to preschoolers. *The Journal of the American Medical Association, 23,* 1025–1030.

Zito, J.M., Safer, D.J., dosReis, S., et al. (2003). Psychotropic practice patterns for youth: A 10 year perspective. *Archives of Pediatrics & Adolescent Medicine, 157,* 17–25.

25 Specific Learning Disabilities

Bruce Shapiro, Robin P. Church, and M.E.B. Lewis

Upon completion of this chapter, the reader will

- Know the definitions of the term *specific learning disability*
- Be aware of impairments associated with specific learning disabilities
- Recognize some of the methods of early identification
- Be aware of some intervention strategies
- Know the mandates of current federal law in both special and general education that have an impact on the education of students with learning disabilities
- Know the range of outcomes for children and adolescents with specific learning disabilities

A child may have difficulty learning for many reasons. Intellectual disability, cerebral palsy, seizure disorders, receptive and expressive language disorders, and hearing and vision impairments all can interfere with learning. This chapter focuses on children whose difficulty with learning is not primarily the result of any of these disorders. These children instead appear to have an impairment in some aspect of language and/or visual-perceptual development that interferes with learning. Specific reading disability, or dyslexia, is the principal focus of discussion, as it is both the most common specific learning disability (SLD) and the one about which the most is known.

DONALD

Donald developed typically as a young child and seemed as bright and alert as his sisters, although he began to talk somewhat later than they had. In kindergarten, however, he was found to have learning difficulties. On a test of early reading skills, he scored well below average in knowledge of the alphabet, phonemic awareness, and early word recognition skills, although his math skills fell within the average range. In first grade, Donald entered a general education class and soon began to fail. He could not learn phonics, and his spelling errors seemed bizarre. Yet, he learned to add and subtract easily. Donald went through a battery of tests that identified specific reading disability in the presence of above-average intellectual functioning—his Full-Scale IQ score on the Wechsler Intelligence Scale for Children–Fourth Edition (WISC-IV) was 110.

The school decided to keep Donald in a general education class with an itinerant special education teacher providing extra help. This approach was not effective, however, and Donald fell further behind the other children in language arts. He started misbehaving in school and avoiding going to school, using headaches as an excuse. At the end of first grade, his reading was more than 1 year delayed, whereas his arithmetic skills were well above an age-appropriate level.

When he entered second grade, Donald was anxious and unhappy. During that year, he attended a general education class but received pull-out services in reading daily for 45 minutes. Donald and three other students worked with a reading specialist who used a structured phonics approach to learning to read. Donald also worked with a speech-language specialist who focused on phonological skills. His parents also worked with him at night. He remained a poor reader, but he could feel the excitement of gaining new knowledge. He developed friendships with the other children, although his less sensitive schoolmates continued to tease him.

At the end of second grade, Donald was retested and found to have made substantial progress during the previous school year. His decoding skills had accelerated to a low-average range, but his fluency remained slow and methodical. He remained a little more than a year behind in reading, but his rate of learning had accelerated. He continued to receive extra reading services daily for another year. By this time, he excelled in mathematics, which helped to offset his difficulty with reading and spelling. He still found school difficult, but he stopped avoiding it. His behavior problems also faded. With the continued support of his teachers and parents, Donald is likely to have a good outcome.

DEFINING SPECIFIC LEARNING DISABILITIES

The Individuals with Disabilities Education Improvement Act of 2004 (IDEA 2004; PL 108-446) maintains the same definition of specific learning disability as in the Individuals with Disabilities Education Act (IDEA) Amendments of 1997 (PL 105-17): "A disorder in one or more of the basic psychological processes involved in understanding or in using language, spoken or written, which disorder may manifest in imperfect ability to listen, think, speak, read, write, spell, or do mathematical calculations" (§ 602[26][a]). The term *specific learning disability* replaces such older terms as *perceptual disabilities, brain injury, minimal brain dysfunction, dyslexia,* and *developmental aphasia.* The term, however, excludes learning problems that are the result of visual, hearing, or motor disabilities; of intellectual disability; of emotional disturbance; or of environmental, cultural, or economic disadvantage.

Unfortunately, there are several problems with this definition. First, it fails to define the core features of SLD. The definition does not provide guidelines regarding what the "basic psychological processes" of learning are or how marked an "imperfect ability" to learn must be to constitute a disability. It is a definition of ex-

clusion; all other causes for the learning problems must be eliminated. This is problematic because SLDs can coexist with other conditions, most notably attention-deficit/hyperactivity disorder (ADHD; see Chapter 24). Visual, hearing, or motor disabilities; intellectual disability; emotional disturbance; and environmental, cultural, or economic disadvantage were excluded from the definition to prevent "double dipping" from existing federal programs that deal with those issues. It is clear, however, that a child with SLD may also have one of these other conditions. Finally, this definition does not address origin or the response to treatment (Shapiro & Gallico, 1993).

The way this definition has been operationalized is also problematic. The common approach for diagnosing SLD has been to document a severe discrepancy between ability and achievement. This has been done by demonstrating a significant difference between the child's potential to learn, or IQ score, and his or her actual educational achievement (Gregg & Scott, 2000). Evidence now suggests, however, that this discrepancy approach has poor sensitivity and specificity in discriminating students with specific reading disability from those with low IQ scores and poor reading (Francis et al., 2005). In one study, this approach correctly identified less than half of children who were receiving special education services, particularly underidentifying young and African American students (Shapiro, 1996). In fact, children with high IQ scores who have specific reading disability do not differ from those with lower IQ scores in reading skills (Siegel, 1998). Discrepancy formulas also have shown poor validity in projecting the child's later school performance in reading. Only 17% of children classified as having specific reading disability in first grade on the basis of ability; achievement discrepancy remained in this classification by sixth grade (Shaywitz et al., 1992). In addition, the discrepancy model incorrectly assumes that IQ scores measure the basic skills involved in the various SLDs. In many studies, the discrepancy formula was no better in identifying SLD than simply applying a criterion of low achievement (Fletcher et al., 1994). Lastly, a discrepancy approach relies on tests that invariably have measurement error. Decisions based on such scores would argue for a more robust approach to assessment and identification processes (Francis et al., 2005). For all of these reasons, there is now serious doubt about the utility and validity of the discrepancy concept for specific reading disability. It is less clear whether the discrepancy model has better classification abilities for other SLDs (Berninger & Abbott, 1994).

IDEA 2004 builds on the base of knowledge that questions the appropriateness of relying entirely on the discrepancy model (Council for Exceptional Children, 2004). Although the discrepancy model is not abandoned under this legislation, a variety of tools and assessment strategies may be used to determine eligibility. The new bill adds language stating that "a local education agency shall not be required to take into consideration whether a child has a severe discrepancy between achievement and intellectual ability . . . "; it further states that "in determining whether a child has a specific learning disability, a local educational agency may use a process that determines if the child responds to scientific, research-based intervention" (sec 614, (b), 6, B page 60). This approach is often called a response to intervention (RTI) model. A brief description of such a model follows. To ensure homogeneity of the process of eligibility determination, each state will develop regulations to be applied by local schools. Most states have not yet formalized the regulations.

RESPONSE TO INTERVENTION

Vaughn and Fuchs (2003) advocated redefining learning disability as an inadequate response to instruction. This approach is a promising alternative to traditional testing methods for identifying students with learning disabilities. They identify several important benefits of such an approach: 1) identification of students using an at-risk rather than a deficit model, 2) earlier identification, 3) reduction of identification bias, and 4) a strong focus on student outcome. Such a model involves the provision of intensive, systematic instruction to very small groups of students who are at risk of academic failure for a defined period of time. The simplest form of RTI involves students receiving instruction in their general education classroom with their progress carefully and regularly monitored. Those who do not progress receive additional services from a learning or reading specialist. Again, their progress is carefully and regularly monitored. Those who still fail to progress are referred for special education evaluation (Fuchs et al., 2003; Olitsky & Nelson, 2003). A more costly approach to RTI involves intensive instruction provided daily in a very small group setting. Those who make progress at the end of the prescribed time (usually 12–16 weeks) are

then returned to the general education program. Those who do not made adequate gains receive a second round of intensive intervention. Students who remain unresponsive to such intensive intervention are then referred for comprehensive evaluation. Despite widespread support for RTI, potential issues remain. These include relying on the instructional environment, insuring instructional validity, defining intensive instruction, personnel preparation, and availability of trained teachers.

PREVALENCE

The U.S. Department of Education, National Center for Education Statistics (2003), reported that of the more than 6.4 million students receiving special education services during the 2001–2002 school year, slightly less than half (2.8 million) were classified as having SLD. This represents approximately 5% of the total school-age population. The size of this category has more than tripled since its original creation in 1977, with a particular acceleration in the 1990s. Although this expansion may represent early or improved diagnosis, it also may be a consequence of a certain amount of overdiagnosis or of the inclusion of children with more subtle learning problems in a category previously reserved for students with more obvious disabilities. It should be emphasized, too, that prevalence figures depend on the definition of disability. Because the definition of SLD is problematic, it follows that prevalence figures may be unreliable and vary from author to author or study to study (Francis et al., 1996).

In addition, reporting differences among schools affect the prevalence of SLD. Individual school districts exercise considerable autonomy in defining, describing, and coding disabilities at the time services are determined. Districts in the same state may not code or assign services for learning disabilities in the same way. In districts where families are persistent and involved, the correct and discrete identification of a child's disability is more certain. In districts where disabilities are not specified correctly or include other aspects that contribute to learning difficulties, such as attention or behavior issues, overembracing terms such as *multiple disorder* may be used. This camouflages the exact nature of a child's problems with learning and distorts the design of an effective and useful education program in the form of a well-derived individual education program (IEP). Needless to say, the accuracy of exact numbers of students identified as having specific learning disabilities can be affected by these factors.

SPECIFIC READING DISABILITY

Mechanisms

Specific reading disability (also called developmental dyslexia) is by far the most common form of SLD, accounting for approximately 80% of affected children (Flynn & Rabar, 1994). Theoretically, any defect in the processing or interpretation of written words can lead to specific reading disability. Efficient reading depends on rapidly, accurately, and fluently decoding and recognizing the phonemes (speech sounds) of single words (Talcott et al., 2000; Wolf, Bowers, & Biddle, 2000). Phonological awareness includes phoneme awareness (the understanding that speech is made up of discrete sounds) as well as a metacognitive understanding of word boundaries within spoken sentences, of syllable boundaries within spoken words, and of how to isolate these phonemes to establish their location within syllables and words (Clark & Uhry, 1995). Phonological awareness manifests in the ability to analyze and manipulate sounds within syllables (e.g., to count, delete, and reorder them). If a child does not realize that syllables and words are composed of phonemes and that these segments can be divided according to their acoustic boundaries, reading will be slow, labored, and inaccurate, and comprehension will be poor (Fletcher et al., 1994). A second possible mechanism may be a defect in phonetic representation in working memory, wherein the child can understand the syntactic structure of a sentence but is unable to maintain it in working memory long enough to comprehend the meaning (Mann, 1994).

Poor reading has been linked to phonological processing deficits, but these deficits alone are not sufficient to explain specific reading disabilities. Several mechanisms have been proposed to explain the relationship between poor reading and phonological processing deficits.

Wolf and Bowers (1999) proposed three subtypes of specific reading disability. In addition to the phonological deficit model, the authors posited a second type of reading disability characterized by poor fluency that results from disrupted orthographic processing, which in turn results from slow naming speed. The third type is caused by a combination of both types of deficit. Children who manifest the double deficit, phonological deficits and naming speed deficit, are the poorest readers. This hypothesis has not been universally accepted. One group failed to find a phonological deficit in the absence of a naming speed deficit and noted that the double-deficit groupings identified children with different neuropsychological profiles (Waber et al., 2004). Others have reviewed the topic and found little support for the theory that underlies the double-deficit hypothesis, namely that rapid serial processing and temporal integration of letter identities are the primary means by which orthographic codes are formed (Vellutino et al., 2004; Vukovic & Siegel, 2006). They also question the independence of phonological and rapid naming skills and the specificity of deficits in rapid naming for reading.

Taking these findings into account, a biologically based definition of specific reading disability has been proposed by Lyon, Shaywitz, and Shaywitz:

> Dyslexia is a specific learning disability that is neurobiological in origin. It is characterized by difficulties with accurate and/or fluent word recognition and by poor spelling and decoding abilities. These difficulties typically result from a deficit in the phonological component of language that is often unexpected in relation to other cognitive abilities and the provision of effective classroom instruction. Secondary consequences may include problems in reading comprehension and reduced reading experience that can impede growth of vocabulary and background knowledge. (2003, p. 2)

Genetics

Since the turn of the 20th century, it has been hypothesized that reading disabilities are heritable. Often several members of a family have a specific reading disability, and the underlying phonological processing impairments in this disorder appear to be highly heritable (Pennington & Gilger, 1996). Genetic studies using linkage and association techniques have shown a relationship between specific reading disability and loci on chromosomes 1, 2, 3, 6, 15, and 18 (Demonet et al., 2004; Fisher & DeFries, 2002).

Children with certain genetic syndromes also may have an increased risk of manifesting a particular type of learning disability, although less commonly specific reading disability. For example, girls with Turner syndrome and fragile X syndrome (see Appendix B and Chapter 19, respectively) and boys with Klinefelter syndrome (Appendix B) tend to have visual-perceptual learning disabilities (Mazzocco, 2001; Reiss & Freund, 1990). Casey et al. (2000) studied parents of children with Tourette syndrome and found that these parents showed language-based learning problems. Children with neuro-fibromatosis, type I (see Appendix B), have both visual-perceptual and language-based learning disabilities (Cutting, Koth, & Denckla, 2000).

Neural Substrates

Reading is a dynamic process that develops with age and experience. It encompasses a wide variety of skills that develop at varying times. Early instruction focuses on learning to read and targets decoding. Later instruction uses reading to learn and the focus shifts to comprehension. Beginning, inexperienced readers employ a "bottom-up" approach that uses analytic and synthetic processes. Experienced readers use a "top-down" approach that results in faster, more efficient reading. Top-down, or conceptual, approaches assume that the path from text to meaning extends from prior knowledge that is applied to the process of acquiring the sound–symbol connection of reading. Compensated poor readers recruit additional brain areas to read.

Neuroimaging studies include a series of techniques that give important information about brain structure and function. They show associations, but causality should not be inferred. The brain works as an entity, and abnormalities that occur earlier or later in the process may show differences in a region of interest. Care should be noted when findings are observed, because some of the findings may be the result of poor reading rather than the cause. With these caveats noted, a new model of brain function during reading is emerging based on neuroimaging studies.

Functional brain imaging studies have shed insights into the developmental sequence underlying reading acquisition. This model involves three major brain areas in reading (see Table 25.1). Posterior systems predominate during early reading acquisition (Turkeltaub et al., 2003; Simos et al., 2002). As children become older and are more skilled at reading, they begin to engage parietal and superior temporal areas, with anterior regions coming on line last.

Children who are identified as having dyslexia do not increase activation of the word form area, even after repeated trials of word exposure. As they grow older, they show the opposite—activation of the anterior system. Anterior activation is not the sole processing difference, however, as those with dyslexia also activate their right anterior inferior frontal gyrus as well as the right posterior occipital-temporal region (Sandak et al., 2004).

Shaywitz and colleagues (2004) underscored the importance of dysfunction of the left hemisphere brain systems in specific reading disability. They provided a year of intensive reading remediation to a group of children with specific reading disability. After the intervention, the children made gains in reading fluency. Neuroimaging studies showed increased activation of the anterior and dorsal systems. A study in adults with a lifetime history of developmental dyslexia demonstrated that reading remediation in older individuals might be different. This study showed both left and right hemisphere increases following successful reading intervention (Eden et al., 2004).

The findings of functional magnetic resonance imaging (fMRI) and positron emission tomography (PET) help delineate the reading process but do not tell the complete story. It is possible to have deficits that are associated not only with where the activation occurs, but also when it occurs. Techniques such as magnetoencephalography (MEG) are likely to increase our understanding of how neural systems function together (Figure 25.1).

Table 25.1. Brain systems involved with reading

System	Brain areas	Function
Dorsal	Temporo-parietal areas (including angular gyrus supramarginal gyrus in the inferior parietal lobe, and posterior superior temporal gyrus [Wernicke's area])	Analyze the written word, transform orthography (word configuration) into the linguistic structures
Ventral	Occipito-temporal area, (includes inferior occipital-temporal/fusiform area and middle and inferior temporal gyri)	Skilled reading and automatic instant word recognition (word form area)
Anterior	Inferior frontal gyrus and insular cortex (Broca's area)	Articulation, silent reading, and naming

Sources: Sandak et al. (2004); Shaywitz and Shaywitz (2005).

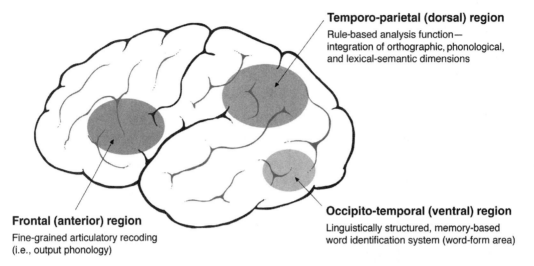

Temporo-parietal (dorsal) region
Rule-based analysis function—
integration of orthographic, phonological,
and lexical-semantic dimensions

Frontal (anterior) region
Fine-grained articulatory recoding
(i.e., output phonology)

Occipito-temporal (ventral) region
Linguistically structured, memory-based
word identification system (word-form area)

Figure 25.1. An overview of the major reading circuits defined by functional neuroimaging studies. (From Pugh, K.R., Mencl, W.E., Jenner, A.R., et al. [2000]. Functional neuroimaging studies of reading and reading disability [developmental dyslexia]. *Mental Retardation and Developmental Disabilities Research Reviews, 6*(3), 209. Copyright © 2000 Wiley-Liss, Inc. Adapted by permission of Wiley-Liss, Inc., a subsidiary of John Wiley & Sons, Inc.)

SPECIFIC MATHEMATICS DISABILITY

Three to six percent of children have performance on tests of mathematical ability that is discrepant from their IQ scores (Shalev & Gross-Tsur, 2001). This percentage may be higher than the true frequency of SLD in mathematics (SLD math). One reason for this is that there is much more variation in the teaching of mathematics. Consequently, poor performance may be due to a lack of adequate instruction in areas that are covered by the assessment measures. Another reason for discrepant performance on math tests may relate to impairments in reading or executive function rather than mathematics. SLD math commonly is seen in the presence of other specific learning disabilities and cognitive disorders. Of children with SLD math, approximately 17% had coexisting specific reading disability and 26% had ADHD (Gersten, Jordan, & Flojo, 2005; Shalev & Gross-Tsur, 2001). Of kindergarten children with developmental language disorders, 26% had significantly impaired arithmetic skills (Manor et al., 2001). Marshall and colleagues (1999) found that inattention exerts a specific and deleterious effect on the acquisition of arithmetic computation skills. This has led some to defer the diagnosis of SLD math in the presence of ADHD until the ADHD is properly managed (Shalev & Gross-Tsur, 2001). Finally, assessment of mathematics encompasses a variety of skills and neuropsychological processes, some of which may be impaired whereas others are relatively spared.

Difficulty with mathematics may manifest in different ways. Counting, basic calculation, problem solving, place values (base-10 concepts), equivalence, measurement, time, relations (as in algebra), and geometry are but some of the ways that mathematics is expressed. Despite the wide range of expression, SLD math is defined by deficiencies in fact mastery and calculation fluency (Jordan et al., 2003).

SLD math evolves over time. Early presentations exhibit difficulty with retrieval of basic arithmetic facts and in computing arithmetic exercises. These have been related to immature counting skills. Older children have difficulty in learning arithmetic tables and comprehending algorithms of adding, subtracting, multiplying and dividing. These manifest as misuse of signs, forgetting to carry, misplacing digits, or approaching problems from left to right (Shalev, 2004). Ten- to 11-year-olds with SLD math showed persistent poor math performance on reexamination 6 years later (Shalev et al., 2005).

Neuobiological evidence of SLD math is still evolving, and the exact mechanism of SLD math remains to be delineated. Evidence derived from clinical syndromes, neuroimaging, and genetics suggest a number of brain-based disorders.

Although the clinical syndromes point to a major role of the parietal lobe in dyscalculia, the relationship is not simple. Different types of mathematic skills require coordination of different brain functions and, by extension, activation of different brain areas on fMRI. Complicating this is the finding that people who have difficulty with math will recruit other brain areas and use other psychological mechanisms to compensate for the impairment in brain function.

There is a paucity of studies that focus on the genetics of SLD math. Yet, familial occurrences of SLD math have been described. Shalev and colleagues (2001) found that approximately half of siblings of children with developmental dyscalculia also had dyscalculia (Shalev et al., 2001). In a study of twins, one of whom had SLD math, Alarcon et al. (1997) found significantly higher rates of SLD math in identical (monozygotic) twins than fraternal (dizygotic) twins.

Several psychological mechanisms have been proposed for SLD math. Rourke and Finlayson (1978) found that children with SLD math showed poor nonverbal skills (visual-spatial and tactile-perceptual), whereas children with SLD math and specific reading disability showed poorer verbal skills (verbal and auditory-perceptual). Geary (2004) posits three subtypes of SLD math based on memory and cognitive deficits: 1) procedural subtype, 2) semantic memory subtype, and 3) visuospatial subtype. Others have associated SLD math with executive function and working memory (McLean & Hitch, 1999). Dehaene and Cohen (1995) advocated a "triple-code model" wherein simple arithmetic operations are processed by the verbal system within the left hemisphere and more complex arithmetic procedures that require magnitude estimations and visual representations are bilaterally localized.

IMPAIRMENTS ASSOCIATED WITH SPECIFIC LEARNING DISABILITIES

Donald's case is unusual in that he has an isolated specific reading disability. One quarter to one half of children with SLDs have additional impairments that interfere with school functioning. These may include executive function impairments, ADHD, social skills impairments, and emotional and behavior disorders. These behavior and emotional problems may be externalizing (e.g., aggression, oppositional-defiant behavior) or internalizing (e.g., shyness, depression). Failure to detect and treat these additional impairments is a common reason for failed intervention programs (Kube & Shapiro, 1996).

As comorbid conditions may adversely affect outcome, it may be most appropriate to categorize children not only on the basis of their learning impairments but also according to comorbid conditions (Rock, Fessler, & Church, 1996).

Memory Impairments

Impairments in the ability to listen, remember, and repeat auditory stimuli have been associated with reading disability. The holding of information in immediate and working memory is essential in learning to read. A number of studies comparing children with equivalent IQ scores but low or high reading abilities have reported impairments in the poor readers on the Digit Span subtest of the Wechsler Intelligence Scale for Children–Third Edition (WISC-III; Wechsler, 1991) (see D'Angiulli & Siegel, 2003). Executive dysfunction coupled with memory deficits may adversely affect the student's ability to choose the appropriate strategy for solving a problem. As a result, the student's ability to use cognitive behavioral techniques may be limited because he or she cannot remember a sequence of problem-solving steps.

Impairments in Executive Functions

According to Pennington (1991), executive functions involve the ability to maintain an appropriate problem-solving set of procedures for attaining a future goal. This includes the ability to 1) inhibit or defer a response; 2) formulate a sequential, strategic plan of action; and 3) encode relevant information in memory for future use (Welsh & Pennington, 1988). These metacognitive abilities are necessary for organizational skills, planning, future-oriented behavior, maintaining an appropriate problem-solving set of procedures, impulse control, selective attention, vigilance, inhibition, and creativity in thinking. These abilities involve an awareness of what skills, strategies, and resources are needed to perform a task effectively. They also require the ability to use self-regulatory mechanisms to ensure the successful completion of a task. Yet students with SLDs are often impulsive rather than reflective when presented with a problem-solving task. This failure to consider alternative solutions often results in errors or poor quality in the solution. Executive functions become essential in middle school to complete homework and long-term projects, to sustain attention during lectures, and to set future goals. Disruption in this organization and control of behavior often manifests itself as disruption in the classroom.

Attention-Deficit/ Hyperactivity Disorder

Approximately one third of children with SLDs also have ADHD, making this the most common comorbid condition (Shaywitz, Fletcher, & Shaywitz, 1995). Studies have found that the prevalence of ADHD in children with SLDs is higher than the prevalence of SLDs in children with ADHD (see Schulte, Conners, & Osborne, 1999). The symptoms typically include inattention, impulsivity, and hyperactivity (see Chapter 24).

Social Skills Impairments

Some children with SLDs may have impairments in social skills. Such children tend to be socially isolated, may have few close friends, and infrequently participate in social activities. In turn, they are often overlooked or rejected by their peers because of their odd behavior and poor school and/or athletic performance. Teachers tend to rate these children as having social adjustment difficulties and being easily led. There may be many reasons for these problems, including poor social comprehension, inability to take the perspective of others, poor pragmatic language skills, and misinterpretation of body language (Shapiro & Gallico, 1993).

Emotional and Behavior Disorders

Although associated impairments may represent endogenous biological conditions, they also may result from the child's experiences of school failure. Children with SLDs can exhibit a range of emotional and behavior disturbances, including conduct disorders, withdrawal, poor self-esteem, and depression. These individuals are less likely to take pride in their successes and more likely to be overcome by their failures. More than one third of students with SLDs receive a failing grade in one or more courses each school year. These children often exhibit chronic frustration and anxiety as they attempt to meet the demands of skill-based tasks such as phonological decoding, comprehension, spelling, and math. This school failure, combined with social skills impairments, may lead to peer rejection, poor self-image, and withdrawal from participation in school activities (McKinlay, Ferguson, & Jolly, 1996). Eventually, these children may avoid going to school all together or

act out in class to obtain the attention they do not receive through good grades. The overall dropout rate of children with SLDs is twice that found in the general population (U.S. Department of Education, Office of Special Education Programs, 1991).

HEALTH PROBLEMS SIMULATING SPECIFIC LEARNING DISABILITIES

Some children who do not have SLDs may demonstrate learning differences in school as a consequence of another developmental disability, a chronic illness, or psychosocial problems. If these children are misdiagnosed as having SLDs, efforts directed solely at treating the learning problem will have limited success. Instead, the underlying problem must be identified and addressed. Once this problem has been treated, the learning problem may well improve or disappear.

For example, if a child has an unidentified sensory impairment, learning is likely to be impaired. The provision of hearing aids to a child with hearing loss or of glasses to the child with a refractive error may lead to a significant improvement in school performance. Children with epilepsy (see Chapter 29) also may have problems in school resulting either from poorly controlled seizures or from side effects of antiepileptic drugs. Modifying the drug regimen may significantly improve both attention and learning. Children with psychiatric disorders also may fail in school. The use of psychotropic drugs and psychotherapy often leads to significantly improved school performance, although some of these drugs can have an adverse effect on attention. (For specific information on medication side effects, see Appendix C.)

An increased incidence of learning problems also has been described in children with such chronic illnesses as diabetes, human immunodeficiency virus infection (see Chapter 6), cancer, and chronic kidney and liver disease. In these situations, SLD may exist, but learning difficulties also may result from other causes such as physiological derangement, excessive school absences, attention impairments, or depression. A secondary learning problem rather than a primary SLD is suggested if learning improves once the medical condition is brought under control (Sexson & Madan-Swain, 1993).

Children who were born prematurely have an increased incidence of learning disabilities (Litt et al., 2005). Acute disorders such as meningitis, encephalitis, and traumatic brain injury (TBI) also can result in the subsequent development of learning problems. TBI is the most common of these and is an increasingly recognized cause of behavior and learning problems in children (see Chapter 30). The injury may result in either temporary or permanent neurological impairments. Affected children present special challenges in the classroom as a result of the evolving nature of their recovery (Savage & Wolcott, 1994). During the acute phase of recovery, disorders of attention and other executive functions, higher language skills, and behavior are common. Because of this, TBI has been identified as a separate category of disability under IDEA 2004 (see Chapter 34), to distinguish it from SLDs and other related disorders. When recovery is completed, some children with TBI may have residual SLDs.

Finally, psychosocial influences may affect the child's ability to learn. A child who is hungry cannot pay attention or learn well (Durkin, 1989). A child who comes from a home that does not value learning rarely achieves well in school. And a home beset with family problems or abuse is a poor setting in which to encourage the child's school performance (Coles, 1987). Improvement in these psychosocial areas would likely result in improved school performance but has proven very difficult to achieve. Until a complete picture of why students in a particular school are identified as having profiles of underachievement—and until the role of factors such as poverty, prematurity, nutrition, and environmental threats (i.e., lead poisoning, other environmental toxins) are fully understood and accommodated—educators will continue to struggle to reconcile cognitive disabilities and effective instructional practices.

What is vital to the improvement of this state of affairs is greater attention to how school teams obtain and use information that identifies SLDs and the resources available to treat the disorder in the school, school district, and community. All existing information should be used in the educational process. Medical or educational assessments by qualified examiners, combined with the assessment data developed by the school, serve as the foundation for developing an effective educational program and optimizes the use of related services (see Chapter 34).

ASSESSMENT PROCEDURES

Assessment is undertaken to explain the reasons for a student's difficulty in the classroom and to propose a method of therapy. It should delineate a student's areas of strength and challenges

and permit the development of a comprehensive plan that would optimize his or her academic function. Often, assessment is used as a method of determining eligibility for special education services. It is an interdisciplinary process that seeks to identify an "educationally disabling" condition, delineate other important factors that modify the student's learning abilities, and set learning goals and objectives in an IEP (see Chapter 34).

Psychological and educational tests are the mainstay of assessment for SLDs in school-age children. However, a complete medical, behavioral, educational, and social history also should be taken in order to consider confounding variables that may simulate or worsen SLD (Shapiro & Gallico, 1993). Simply looking at the discrepancy between potential and actual achievement can lead to misclassification of students' needs. Evaluators need to use procedures for assessment that provide more information than a simple statistic as an indicator of a student's abilities. The global standardized assessment tools are not sensitive enough to allow the instructional program to be tailored to ensure the student's academic growth. Standardized proficiency testing must be combined with authentic assessment, norm-referenced as well as criterion-referenced tests, informal assessment, and portfolio assessment to obtain the full picture of how the student with SLD is progressing. This permits connecting and applying this information to the content he or she is learning (Vacca et al., 2003). If this does not occur, inappropriate treatment recommendations can result. Labeling a test-taker as a "low achiever" does no service to the student. Well-documented strengths and challenges lead to a more serviceable IEP (Swanson, 1996).

The combination of assessment tools, such as those listed in Appendix E, is essential to a well-defined program of instruction and support services for a student with specific learning disabilities, but continued periodic assessment of progress in the class is also required. This periodic "snapshot" of achievement allows the effectiveness of the program to be evaluated and the instructional program to be adjusted. Although federal legislation no longer requires psychoeducational testing to be repeated every 3 years, periodic reassessment of cognitive and executive functions is warranted if the student is failing to progress. In addition, annual assessment of academic subjects is important to determine the progress the child has made and the effectiveness of the program.

INTERVENTION STRATEGIES

The primary goal of intervention is to facilitate the acquisition and expression of the knowledge needed for effective performance in the workplace. The objectives are to achieve academic competence, treat associated impairments, and prevent adverse mental health outcomes. This requires the cooperation of educators, health care professionals, and families. If children with specific reading disability are not provided with an intervention program composed of instruction in phonological awareness, sound–symbol relations, and contextual reading skills before the third grade, at least three quarters of these children will show little improvement in reading throughout their later school years (Shaywitz & Shaywitz, 2005). If given intensive remediation, however, improvement can occur (Lovett & Steinbach, 1997).

In addition to treating the core SLD, intervention strategies also need to focus on associated cognitive, attentional, perceptual, and sensory impairments. Immaturity, lack of motivation, and poor impulse control also must be considered in determining the child's needs for remediation (Bakker, 2006). Intervention must recognize the developmental changes that occur as the student ages. It must be sensitive to the changing demands of the curriculum, the typical developmental challenges faced by the child, and the effects of maturation and intervention on the academic abilities of the student. In addition, successful interventions must not be withdrawn prematurely.

Professionals continue to debate the most effective intervention strategies. A major consideration is whether to teach to the child's abilities (i.e., compensation/circumvention strategies) or to the disabilities (i.e., remedial strategies). Little evidence supports the superiority of one approach over the other. It is generally agreed, however, that there must be a combination of instructional and cognitive interventions (Alexander & Slinger-Constant, 2004).

Instructional and Other Types of Interventions

The following is a review of some interventions in reading, writing, mathematics, and other areas.

Reading   In 2000, the National Reading Panel released its report on scientific research-based reading instruction (National Institute of Child Health and Human Development, 2000). The panel identified the following six essential components to a sound reading program: 1) phonemic awareness; 2) phonics skills; 3) fluency, accuracy, speed, and expression; 4) reading comprehension strategies to enhance understanding; 5) teacher education; and 6) computer technology. Once decoding is unlocked, students are able to use these skills to build fluency. The focus can then shift to interventions that support and develop the expansion of a vocabulary (for general communication, usage, and technical use) and enhance the student's ability to comprehend the message of text.

Reading proficiency depends on phonological processing and alphabetical mapping. Phonics instruction, however, is different from phonological awareness training (Shaywitz, 2005). Clark and Uhry (1995) defined phonics as a low level of rote knowledge of the association between letters and sounds. As noted, phonological awareness includes higher-level metacognitive understandings of word boundaries within spoken sentences, of syllable boundaries in spoken words, and of how to isolate the phonemes and establish their location within syllables and words. Regardless of the method chosen, the major goal of reading instruction is to improve phonological awareness so that there is effective word recognition and comprehension of meaning. Reading activities focus on helping the child gain print awareness and become attuned to the sound characteristics of language (phoneme awareness) and letter–sound relationships (the alphabetic principle).

In elementary school, reading instruction includes methods designed to increase skills in acquiring vocabulary, using syntax, and understanding meaning (Alexander & Slinger-Constant, 2004; Maggart & Zintz, 1993; Schatschneider & Torgesen, 2004; Tierney & Readence, 2000). Many different approaches are proposed for the teaching of reading. Table 25.2 lists some of the techniques and the aspect of reading upon which they focus. No single model suffices for all children. In the final analysis, semantic, syntactic, and graphonemic systems must be united for successful reading (Singer & Ruddell, 1985).

Along with knowledge of phonics, a rapid sight vocabulary (words recognized on sight, without sounding them out phonetically) is essential to efficient reading. Different word recognition strategies include analysis of sound (phonics or phonetics), analysis for structure (visual configuration), and use of memory skills to recognize words as total entities (whole-word approach). Comprehension strategies center on

Table 25.2. Focuses and techniques for reading instruction

Focus	Examples
Explicit phonics training	Alphabetic Phonics (Cox, 1985)
	Orton-Gillingham (Gillingham & Stillman, 1997; Orton, 1937; Sheffield, 1991)
	Recipe for Reading (Traub & Bloom, 2000)
	Wilson Reading System (Wilson, 1988)
Sounds (oral-motor characteristics of speech)	Lindamood Phoneme Sequencing Program for Reading, Spelling, and Speech (LiPS; Lindamood & Lindamood, 1998)
Overlearning basic skills to increase skill level	Reading mastery
Comprehension	Project READ (Calfee & Henry, 1986)
Oral reading to increase comprehension by focusing on miscues and errors	Retrospective Miscue Analysis (Goodman & Marek, 1996)
	Word Study (Bear et al., 1996)
At-risk children	Reading Recovery (Clay, 1985)
	Success for All (Slavin et al., 1990)

developing the ability to draw meaning from text, often using a sequence of books that introduces words and concepts in a gradual progression.

Many students with a reading disability need an adjustment in the curriculum (Lewis, 1993). Some methods of teaching reading, such as Orton-Gillingham and Fernald (Denning, 1990; Silberberg, Iverson, & Goins, 1975), employ multisensory approaches (Birsh, 2005) for the remediation of difficulties in efficient sound–symbol processing. Other approaches include 1) whole language (reinforcing a spectrum of language arts; Edelsky, Atwerger, & Flores, 1991); 2) thematics (utilizing content areas conceptually; Lewis, 1993); 3) literature-based methods (using trade books to build on basal program skills); 4) individualized reading programs (using trade books and alternative literature forms to build personal reading; Fielding & Roller, 1992); 5) language experience (having students generate their own reading material; Tierney, Readence, & Dishner, 1995); and 6) functional skills (involving the use of materials involved in daily living—e.g., forms, notices, directions).

Teachers at all levels and in all types of classrooms can give students with a specific reading disability tools such as graphic organizers, anticipation guides, question/answer strategies, think-alouds, charting and outlining, or induced imagery schemata to help them retain the messages they get through their reading. The intent of these strategic reading methods is to provide the reader with ways to chunk or otherwise partition their reading material into segments that they can "digest" as they read in

order to expand the reading "diet." The goal of such instructional interventions is movement toward higher levels of critical thinking. By attaining these skills, the student can compete with peers in academic tasks that connect reading to other skills, such as writing and oral discussion (Tierney & Readence, 2000).

The demands of middle school, and the pressures of high school programs leading to the attainment of a diploma, can be trying for students with learning disabilities. As children move from the structure of elementary school to middle and high school, the demands of content reading become an additional burden. The early work of Gray (1925) and McCallister (1930), and subsequent follow-up studies (Moore et al., 1999, Moore, Readence, & Rickelman 1983) showed that the discrete skills of content reading and the related study skills needed for success in secondary education were divided into two approaches. One was a direct instructional approach that separated skills from content, and the other was a functional approach that embedded reading and study skills into the content.

In middle and high school, the reading process must connect with other skills needed for mastering content-related matter in subjects such as social studies, geography, higher-level mathematics, and sciences. Study, organizational, and problem-solving skills must blend with the processing skills involved in obtaining meaning from words, sentences, charts, maps, books, poetry, and dramatic or narrative literature. Meaning is easier to teach in the elementary and middle grades than in high school, when it may become buried in nuances of language, such as humor, sarcasm, and metaphor (Englert & Hiebert, 1984).

The expertise of middle and high school teachers is in the content they teach and not in the instructional mechanisms that help students organize, retrieve, and explain text related to that content. In addition, secondary school requires learning multiple content areas in discrete settings with several different teachers. Consequently, the student with a reading disability may become a "cumulative deficit" reader who makes progress but at a rate that is too slow to maintain adequate academic achievement. The content teacher, therefore, needs to understand the demands and organization of his or her content but also how students must organize that content from lessons so that they can use it in the many forms that secondary school demands (e.g., exams, research papers, debates).

Writing Students with dysgraphia have specific disabilities in processing and reporting information in written form. Writing is firmly connected to reading and spelling because comprehension and exposition of these skills are demonstrated through production of written symbols as indicators of understanding. Although writing is a representation of oral language, it also must convey meaning without the benefit of vocal intonation or stress. This makes additional demands on the writer.

Problems in writing may result from either an inability to manipulate a pen and paper to produce a legible representation of ideas or an inability to express oneself on paper. Word processors can assist children who have disabilities related to the manipulation of the writing implements (Bain, Bailet, & Moats, 2001). Remedial and instructional techniques helpful with problems of written expression include 1) the use of open-ended sentences (Mercer, Hughes, & Mercer, 1985); 2) probable passages (a strategy used to draw on a student's prior knowledge of a topic while incorporating writing into a basic reading lesson; Wood, 1984); 3) journal keeping (Beach & Anson, 1993; Taylor, 1991); 4) modified writing systems, using rebuses or other symbols (Newcomer, Nodine, & Barenbaum, 1988); and 5) newspapers and other print media to demonstrate various writing styles and organizational models.

Not to be forgotten is the connection of spelling to writing. The developmental stages of spelling need to be explored as teachers ap-

proach instruction that connects what is read to the written response of students. These stages include prephonemic, phonemic, transitional, and conventional spelling (Bear & Templeton, 1998). The International Reading Association and the National Association for the Education of Young Children (1998) issued a joint position statement that advocates a developmental approach to teaching writing as an outgrowth of the reading process. Students should be moved from the initial, prephonemic, and phonemic attempts at spelling toward correct, conventional spelling of English words. The process, however, should reflect an understanding of the developmental level and needs of the individual student.

Writing is also a sociocultural endeavor, representing a cognitive process learned through dialogic interactions, expressing the social and cultural perspectives of the student (Englert, 1992). The difficulties that a student with SLD may have with social perception and awareness of cultural aspects of personal development may influence the written product as well as the writing process.

Content area literacy calls for connections between reading and writing (Vacca et al., 2003). Study skills and organization of written materials so that they are retrievable for later use are both vital elements to the success of the student with SLD (Barr et al., 1991). Interventions in this area may call on students to share their writing with peers, and to examine the writing styles of others. Shared writing includes techniques such as Author's Chair (Graves & Hansen, 1983) and Dialogue Journals (Staton et al., 1988). Examination of style includes interventions such as Style Study (Caplan, 1987; Killgallon, 1997) and Reading/Writing Think Sheets (Raphael, Englert, & Kirschner, 1986).

Mathematics Students with SLD math have an inability to perform basic math operations (i.e., addition, subtraction, multiplication, division) or to apply those operations to daily situations. For some children with this disorder, a calculator may prove helpful as an aid. Often, however, the problem is in understanding the abstract concepts of mathematical usage. When students with dyscalculia have only written math problems to solve, the concepts remain vague. When functional applications (e.g., involving money or time) and manipulatives are used, however, the student can connect the concepts to their practical applications and demonstrate greater understanding

(Schwartz & Budd, 1983). Thus, teaching may focus on the use of money in fast-food restaurants (e.g., making change), grocery shopping (e.g., comparing prices per unit of weight), banking (e.g., balancing a checkbook, calculating interest), cooking (e.g., measurement), and transportation (e.g., reading, keeping to schedules).

Hutchinson (1992) and Montague (1992) demonstrated the effectiveness of an approach that emphasizes executive functions for solving mathematical word problems and complex operations (i.e., multiplication). This approach involves rehearsal, practice, and mastery of math skills in combination with corrective and positive feedback throughout the process of instruction. A metacognitive approach can give students with dyscalculia hope for greater success and facility in progressing to higher and more complex mathematical operations (Desoete, Roeyers, & Buysse, 2001; Keeler & Swanson, 2001).

For many students with mathematical disabilities, the more abstract levels of mathematics, such as algebra, geometry, and calculus, may remain mysteries forever; however, these students can still gain facility with basic mathematical facts used in daily life (Mercer & Pullen, 2004). Many schools teach students how and when to use calculators so that more complex problems can be simplified or homework checked for accuracy. In addition, computers are now common in school, and computer-assisted instruction in mathematics may provide opportunities for practice and reinforcement (Okolo, 1992).

Social Skills Training The maintenance of self-esteem and the development of social skills are very important in preventing adverse mental health outcomes in a child with SLD (Erlbaum & Vaughn, 2003; Gans, Kenny, & Ghany, 2003; Vaughn et al., 1998). The teacher can encourage this by giving the child special jobs in the classroom and by supporting participation in extracurricular activities such as sports, scouting, music, drama, arts and crafts, and so forth. Social skills training also can be provided in a group setting (using role-play techniques) and in summer camp programs.

Counseling Counseling may be required to treat underlying psychological disorders. This can be provided individually or in groups. Family-centered counseling also may be appropriate. Issues to be discussed may include homework, behavior management techniques, parental expectations, and the child's self-esteem. Families also should be provided a source of information about SLDs, support groups, and their legal rights and responsibilities in the education of their child.

Vocational Training and Career Education Career education should be an objective of educational programming beginning in the primary grades. Vocational training for students with SLDs begins with realistic counseling resulting from a comprehensive assessment of abilities and aptitudes. Without appropriately directed training, students may be unable to support themselves in an independent manner as adults (Michaels, 1994); also, if vocational rehabilitative services are delayed until adulthood, they are less likely to be effective (Dowdy, Smith, & Nowell, 1992). The design of these programs becomes part of the student's IEP as an individualized transition plan (ITP; see Chapter 34).

Vocational training, which usually begins in high school, consists of counseling, assessment, and training in the hands-on skills that future jobs require. The U.S. Department of Labor (1992) published competencies determined to be necessary for employment. These reports by the Secretary's Commission on Achieving Necessary Skills (SCANS) have been translated into curriculum areas that deemphasize specific job-related tasks while teaching general competencies that cross all job markets.

Even as adults, some individuals with SLDs have poor retention of verbal instructions and other problems that may interfere with effectiveness in their jobs. They also may be hesitant to ask questions and seek assistance. Social immaturity, clumsiness, and poor judgment may make social interactions more difficult. The skills taught in career education are those required to overcome these deficits and enhance success in the work environment, be it the classroom or the adult job market. Cooperation, respect, responsibility, teamwork, organization, and ways to seek information to solve one's problems are all part of career education (U.S. Department of Labor, 1992).

Medication Although SLDs cannot be "cured" through the use of medication, certain associated impairments that affect learning, such as ADHD (see Chapter 24) and behavior and emotional disorders, can be improved with the use of psychoactive drugs. If such drugs are used, their effectiveness must be monitored carefully. Medication should never be a substitute for sound educational programming.

Homework

The home and school should be able to function in partnership so that homework does not lead to tension among family members or misunderstanding of the teacher's intent in providing the home assignment. This may require training the parent to set up a workable system and schedule at home (Kay et al., 1994). Students with SLDs often feel that homework is an imposition, providing no personal fulfillment or advancement (Nicholls, McKenzie, & Shufro, 1994), so individualization and creative use of assignments is essential for homework to fulfill its reinforcing purpose. Homework should not supplement material that was not taught during the day (Alvermann & Phelps, 2005). Techniques to facilitate homework performance include parents' reading and reviewing difficult material with the child and teachers' minimizing the need for boring exercises, such as copying. Homework should be limited to a specific time allotment; for example, 10–20 minutes per day for children in kindergarten through second grade and 30–60 minutes per day for children in grades three through six. Ideally, homework should be completed in a specific area of the home that is quiet, organized, and stocked with needed supplies.

Periodic Reevaluations

The treatment programs for students with SLDs are complex, and many potential gaps exist. Furthermore, the child is a developing organism whose needs and abilities change from year to year. Therefore, ongoing monitoring is essential. The goal of periodic reassessments is to evaluate parent–child relationships, psychosocial issues, and academic progress. Reassessment is also an opportunity to convey new information to the family and ensure that it is obtaining appropriate resources. Finally, it is a time for retesting the child and revising the educational program. These reevaluations should occur yearly, usually in the spring, so that planning for the next school year can occur.

OUTCOME

Long-term outcome appears to depend less on the specific method used to help the student than on the severity of the SLD, the age at di-

agnosis and intervention, the IQ score, the presence of a comorbid condition, the socioeconomic status of the family, the child's motivation to learn, and the family support system (Satz et al.,1998). For example, children with comorbid conditions such as ADHD have a less optimistic outcome than individuals with an isolated SLD. By middle and secondary school, students with comorbid conditions may have acquired "learned helplessness," lacking confidence in their own ability to solve learning and social problems independently (Bryan, 1986). They also are at greater risk for making poor choices in their postsecondary education, employment, and independent living. In one study, during the years following high school, only 5% had professional- or managerial-level jobs (Brown, Aylward, & Keogh, 1996).

Adolescence is often a time when even children with SLDs who have learned to compensate for their disabilities may experience difficulty. Some children are able to compensate for organizational and study skills impairments during elementary school. Matters tend to deteriorate, however, during middle school when students encounter changing class schedules and the need for time management, organization of materials, and completion of multiple assignments and long-term projects (Shapiro & Gallico, 1993). In addition, the demands for sustained attention are greater as classes increase in duration and complexity. If intervention is not provided, these students may show dramatic worsening of behavior and academic performance in high school.

As adults, the outcome for most individuals with an isolated SLD is good (Kurzweil, 1992). Although they may never perform at grade level, most gain the academic skills required for everyday activities. Some students who do not achieve functional literacy during traditional education may still do so as young adults. Academic preparation of students with SLDs is permitting more and more students to pursue postsecondary education (Gajar, 1992; Shaw & Shaw, 1989). However, the average college student with developmental dyslexia reads only at about a tenth-grade level (Hughes & Smith, 1990; Mason & Mason, 2005). These students also read more slowly, make more spelling errors, and acquire less information from texts. They tend to have difficulty in writing essays, completing heavy reading assignments, scoring well on timed tests, and learning foreign languages (Denckla, 1993; Murray & Wren, 2003). Many colleges now offer adjustments to program loads and schedules as well as tutorial and other support services, which have permitted students with SLDs to complete college at an increasing rate (Brinckerhoff, Shaw, & McGuire, 1992; Durlak, Rose, & Bursuck, 1994; Scott, 1994; Vogel & Adelman, 1992).

SUMMARY

SLD is a disorder in which a healthy child with typical intelligence fails to learn adequately in one or more school subjects. The underlying cause of the most common of these disorders, specific reading disability, appears to be an impairment in phonological decoding. Neuroimaging and neuropathological studies in specific reading disability suggest developmental abnormalities in the temporal, parietal, and occipital lobes of the brain. There also appears to be a significant genetic component. Early detection of SLD is important because, untreated, the child may develop secondary emotional and behavior problems that hinder progress. If SLD is suspected, a psychoeducational evaluation should be performed to identify areas of strengths and challenge. Then the education team can develop an IEP and appropriate changes can be made. No one treatment method is best for all children, so a trial-and-error approach may be needed to find the most useful method. Career and vocational education should be integrated into the general educational program and included as an ITP within the IEP. Although the individual with SLD usually carries his or her learning impairment into adulthood, outcome is often good.

REFERENCES

Alarcon M., Defries J.C., Gillis Light J., et al. (1997). A twin study of mathematics disability. *Journal of Learning Disabilities, 30*, 617–623.

Alexander A.W., & Slinger-Constant A.M. (2004). Current status of treatments for dyslexia: Critical review. *Journal of Child Neurology, 19*, 744–758.

Alvermann, D.E., & Phelps, S.F. (2005). *Content reading and literacy: Succeeding in today's diverse classrooms* (4th ed.). Boston: Allyn & Bacon.

Bain, A.M., Bailet, L.L., & Moats, L.C. (2001). *Written language disorders: Theory into practice* (2nd ed.). Austin, TX: PRO-ED.

Bakker, D.J. (2006). Treatment of developmental dyslexia: A review. *Pediatric Rehabilitation, 9*, 3–13.

Barr, R., Kamil, M.L., Mosenthal, P.B., et al. (Eds.). (1991). *Handbook of reading research: Vol. II.* New York: Longman.

Beach, R., & Anson, C.M. (1993). Using peer-dialogue journals to foster response. In G. Newell & R.K. Durst (Eds.), *The role of discussion and writing in the teaching and learning of literature* (pp. 204–205). Norwood, MA: Christopher-Gordon Publishers.

Bear, D.R., Invernizzi. M., Templeton, S., et al. (1996). *Words their way: Word study for phonics, vocabulary and spelling instruction.* Upper Saddle River, NJ: Prentice Hall.

Bear, D.R., & Templeton, S. (1998). Explorations in developmental spelling: Foundations for learning and teaching phonics, spelling and vocabulary. *The Reading Teacher, 52*, 222–242.

Berninger, V.W., & Abbott, R.D. (1994). Redefining learning disabilities: Moving beyond aptitude—achievement discrepancies to failure to respond to validated treatment protocols. In G.R. Lyon (Ed.), *Frames of reference for the assessment of learning disabilities: New views on measurement issues* (pp. 163–183). Baltimore: Paul H. Brookes Publishing Co.

Birsh, J.R. (Ed.). (2005). *Multisensory teaching of basic language skills* (2nd ed.). Baltimore: Paul H. Brookes Publishing Co.

Brinckerhoff, L.C., Shaw, S.F., & McGuire, J.M. (1992). Promoting access, accommodations, and independence for college students with learning disabilities. *Journal of Learning Disabilities, 25*, 417–429.

Brown, F.R., Aylward, E., & Keogh, B.K. (Eds.). (1996). *Diagnosis and management of learning disabilities: An interdisciplinary lifespan approach* (3rd ed.). San Diego: Singular Publishing Group.

Bryan, T.H. (1986). Self-concept and attributions of the learning disabled. *Learning Disability Focus, 1*, 82–89.

Calfee, R., & Henry, M. (1986). Project READ: An inservice model for training classroom teachers in effective reading instruction. In J.V. Hoffman (Ed.), *Effective teaching of reading: Research and practice* (pp. 199–229). Newark, DE: International Reading Association.

Caplan, R. (1987). Style study. *The Quarterly, 7*, 10–14, and 29–31.

Casey, M.B., Cohen, M., Schuerholz, L.J., et al. (2000). Language-based cognitive functioning in parents of offspring with ADHD comorbid for Tourette syndrome or learning disability. *Developmental Neuropsychology, 17*, 85–110.

Clark, D.B., & Uhry, J.K. (1995). *Dyslexia: Theory and practice of remedial instruction* (2nd ed.). Timonium, MD: York Press.

Clay, M.M. (1985). *The early detection of reading difficulties: A diagnostic survey with recovery procedures.* Portsmouth, NH: Heinemann.

Coles, G. (1987). *The learning mystique: A critical look at learning disabilities.* New York: Fawcett.

Council for Exceptional Children. (2004, November). *CEC's IDEA reauthorization summary of significant issues.* Retrieved April 18, 2005 from http://www.cec.sped.org/law_res/doc

Cox, B.A. (1985). Alphabetic phonics: An organization and expansion of Orton-Gillingham. *Annals of Dyslexia, 35*, 187–198.

Cutting, L.E., Koth, L.W., & Denckla, M.B. (2000). How children with neurofibromatosis Type I differ from "typical" learning disability clinic attenders: Nonverbal learning disability revisited. *Developmental Neuropsychology, 17*, 29–47.

D'Angiulli, A., & Siegel, L. (2003). Cognitive functioning as measured by the WISC-R: Do children with learning disabilities have distinctive patterns of performance? *Journal of Learning Disabilities 36*, 48–58.

Dehaene, S., & Cohen, L. (1995). Towards an anatomical and functional model of number processing. *Math Cognition, 1*, 83–120.

Demonet, J.F., Taylor, M.J., & Chaix, Y. (2004). Developmental dyslexia. *The Lancet, 363,* 1451–1460.

Denckla, M.B. (1993). The child with developmental disabilities grown up: Adult residua of childhood disorders. *Neurology Clinics, 11,* 105–125.

Denning, E.M. (1990). *A comparison of nonoral and an oral method of teaching reading association skills to children with language learning disabilities.* Unpublished doctoral dissertation, The Johns Hopkins University, Baltimore.

Desoete, A., Roeyers, H., & Buysse, A. (2001). Metacognition and mathematical problem solving in grade 3. *Journal of Learning Disabilities, 34,* 435–449.

Dowdy, C.A., Smith, T.E.C., & Nowell, C.H. (1992). Learning disabilities and vocational rehabilitation. *Journal of Learning Disabilities, 25,* 442–447.

Durkin, D. (1989). *Teaching them to read.* Boston: Allyn & Bacon.

Durlak, C.M., Rose, E., & Bursuck, W.D. (1994). Preparing high school students with learning disabilities for the transition to postsecondary education: Teaching the skills of self-determination. *Journal of Learning Disabilities, 27,* 51–59.

Edelsky, C., Atwerger, B., & Flores, B. (1991). *Whole language: What's the difference?* Portsmouth, NH: Heinemann.

Eden G.F., Jones K.M., Cappell K., et al. (2004). Neuronal changes following remediation in adult developmental dyslexia. *Neuron, 44,* 411–422.

Englert, C.S. (1992). Writing instruction from a sociocultural perspective: The holistic, dialogic, and social enterprise of writing. *Journal of Learning Disabilities, 25,* 153–172.

Englert, C.S., & Hiebert, E.H. (1984). Children's developing awareness of text structure in expository material. *Journal of Educational Psychology, 76,* 65–74.

Erlbaum, B., & Vaughn, S. (2003). For which students with learning disabilities are self-concept interventions effective? *Journal of Learning Disabilities, 36,* 101–108.

Fielding, L., & Roller, C. (1992). Making difficult books accessible and easy books acceptable. *Reading Teacher, 45,* 678–685.

Fisher, S.E., & DeFries, J.C. (2002). Developmental dyslexia: Genetic dissection of a complex cognitive trait. *Nature Reviews: Neuroscience, 3,* 767–767

Fletcher, J.M., Shaywitz, S.E., Shankweiler, D., et al. (1994). Cognitive profiles of reading disability: Comparisons of discrepancy and low achievement definitions. *Journal of Educational Psychology, 86,* 6–23.

Flynn, J.M., & Rabar, M.H. (1994). Prevalence of reading failure in boys compared with girls. *Psychology in Schools, 31,* 66.

Francis, D.J., Fletcher, J.M., Stuebing, K.K., et al. (2005). Psychometric approaches to the identification of LD: IQ and achievement scores are not sufficient. *Journal of Learning Disabilities, 38,* 98–108.

Francis, D.J., Shaywitz, S.E., Stuebing, K.K., et al. (1996). Developmental lag versus deficit models of reading disability: A longitudinal, individual growth curves analysis. *Journal of Educational Psychology, 88,* 3–17.

Fuchs, D., Mock, D., Morgan, P.L., et al. (2003). Responsiveness-to-intervention: Definitions, evidence, and implications for the learning disabilities construct. *Learning Disabilities Research and Practice, 18,* 157–171.

Gajar, A. (1992). Adults with learning disabilities: Current and future research priorities. *Journal of Learning Disabilities, 25,* 507–519.

Gans A.M., Kenny, M.C., & Ghany, D.L. (2003). Comparing the self-concept of students with and without learning disabilities. *Journal of Learning Disabilities, 36,* 287–295.

Geary, D.C. (2004). Mathematics and learning disabilities. *Journal of Learning Disabilities, 37,* 4–15.

Gersten, R., Jordan, N.C., & Flojo, J.R. (2005). Early identification and interventions for students with mathematics difficulties. *Journal of Learning Disabilities, 38,* 293–304.

Gillingham, A., & Stillman, B.W. (1997). *The Gillingham manual: Remedial training for children with specific disabilities in reading, spelling, and penmanship* (8th ed.). Cambridge, MA: Educators Publishing Service.

Goodman, Y.M., & Marek, A.M. (1996). *Retrospecitve miscue analysis: Revaluing readers and reading.* Katonah, NY: Richard C. Owens.

Graves, D., & Hansen, J. (1983). The author's chair. *Language Arts, 60,* 176–183.

Gray, W.S. (1925). *Summary of investigations related to reading* (Supplementary Educational Monographs, No. 28). Chicago: University of Chicago Press.

Gregg, N., & Scott, S.S. (2000). Definition and documentation: Theory, measurement, and the courts. *Journal of Learning Disabilities, 33,* 5–13.

Hughes, C.A., & Smith, J.O. (1990). Cognitive and academic performance of college students with learning disabilities: A synthesis of the literature. *Learning Disabilities Quarterly, 13,* 66–79.

Hutchinson, N.L. (1992). The challenges of componential analysis: Cognitive and metacognitive instruction in mathematical problem solving. *Journal of Learning Disabilities, 25,* 249–252.

Individuals with Disabilities Education Act Amendments of 1997, PL 105-17, 20 U.S.C. §§ 1400 *et seq.*

Individuals with Disabilities Education Improvement Act of 2004, PL 108-446, 20 U.S.C. §§ 1400 *et seq.*

International Reading Association & National Association for the Education of Young Children. (1998). Learning to read and write: Developmentally appropriate practices for young children. *Young Children, 53,* 30–46.

Jordan, N.C., Hanich, L.B., & Kaplan, D. (2003). A longitudinal study of mathematical competencies in children with specific mathematics difficulties versus children with comorbid mathematics and reading difficulties. *Child Development, 74,* 834–850.

Kay, P.J., Fitzgerald, M., Paradee, C., et al. (1994). Making homework work at home: The parent's perspective. *Journal of Learning Disabilities, 27,* 550–561.

Keeler, M.K., & Swanson, H.L. (2001). Does strategy knowledge influence working memory in children with math disabilities? *Journal of Learning Disabilities, 34,* 418–434.

Killgallon, D. (1997). *Sentence composing for middle school: A worksheet on sentence variety and maturity.* Portsmouth, NH: Heinemann.

Kube, D.A., & Shapiro, B.K. (1996). Persistent school dysfunction: The impact of hidden morbidity and suboptimal therapy. *Clinical Pediatrics, 35,* 571–576.

Kurzweil, S.R. (1992). Developmental reading disorder: Predictors of outcome in adolescents who received early diagnosis and treatment. *Journal of Developmental and Behavioral Pediatrics, 13,* 399–404.

Lewis, M.E.B. (1993). *Thematic methods and strategies for learning disabled students.* San Diego: Singular Publishing Group.

Lindamood, P., & Lindamood, P.C. (1998). *Lindamood phoneme sequencing program for reading, spelling, and speech.* Austin, TX: PRO-ED.

Litt, J., Taylor, H.G., Klein, N., et al. (2005). Learning disabilities in children with very low birthweight: prevalence, neuropsychological correlates, and educational interventions. *Journal of Learning Disabilities, 38,* 130–141.

Lovett, M.W., & Steinbach, K.A. (1997). The effectiveness of remedial programs for reading disabled children of different ages: Does the benefit decrease for older children? *Learning Disability Quarterly, 20,* 189–210.

Lyon, G.R., Shaywitz S.E., & Shaywitz B.A. (2003). A definition of dyslexia. *Annals of Dyslexia, 53,* 1–14.

Maggart, Z.R., & Zintz, M. (1993). *The reading process: The teacher and the learner* (6th ed.). Dubuque, IA: William C. Brown.

Mann, V. (1994). Phonological skills and the prediction of early reading problems. In N.C. Jordan & J. Goldsmith-Phillips (Eds.), *Learning disabilities: New directions for assessment and intervention* (pp. 67–84). Needham Heights, MA: Allyn & Bacon.

Manor, O., Shalev, R., Joseph, A., et al. (2001). Arithmetic skills in kindergarten children with developmental language disorders. *European Pediatric Neurology Society, 5,* 71–77.

Marshall, R.M., Schafer, V.A., O'Donnell, L. et al. (1999). Arithmetic disabilities and ADHD subtypes: Implications for DSM-IV. *Journal of Learning Disabilities, 32,* 239–247.

Mason, A., & Mason, M. (2005). Understanding college students with learning disabilities. *Pediatric Clinics of North America, 52,* 61–70, viii.

Mazzocco, M.M.M. (2001). Math learning disability and math ld subtypes: Evidence from studies of Turner syndrome, fragile X syndrome, and neurofibromatosis type 1. *Journal of Learning Disabilities, 34,* 520–533.

McCallister, J.M. (1930). Guiding pupils' reading activities in the study of content subjects. *The Elementary School Journal, 31,* 271–284.

McKinlay, I., Ferguson, A., & Jolly, C. (1996). Ability and dependency in adolescents with severe learning disabilities. *Developmental Medicine and Child Neurology, 38,* 48–58.

McLean, J.F., & Hitch, G.J. (1999). Working memory impairments in children with specific arithmetic learning difficulties. *Journal of Experimental Child Psychology, 74*(3), 240–260.

Mercer, C.D., Hughes, C.A., & Mercer, A.R. (1985). Learning disabilities definitions used by state education departments. *Learning Disability Quarterly, 8,* 45–55.

Mercer, C.D., & Pullen P.C. (2004). *Students with learning disabilities* (6th ed.). Upper Saddle River, NJ: Merrill.

Michaels, C.A. (1994). *Transition strategies for persons with learning disabilities.* San Diego: Singular Publishing Group.

Montague, M. (1992). The effects of cognitive and metacognitive strategy instruction on the mathematical problem solving of middle school students with learning disabilities. *Journal of Learning Disabilities, 25,* 230–248.

Moore, D.W., Bean, T.W., Birdyshaw, D., et al. (1999). *Adolescent literacy: A position statement.* Newark, DE: International Reading Association

Moore, D.W., Readence, J.E., & Rickelman, R.J. (1983). An historical exploration of content area reading instruction. *Reading Research Quarterly, 18,* 419–438.

Murray, C., & Wren, C.T. (2003). Cognitive, academic, and attitudinal predictors of the grade point averages of college students. *Journal of Learning Disabilities, 36,* 407–415.

National Institute of Child Health and Human Development. (2000). *Report of the National Reading Panel: Teaching children to read. An evidence-based assessment of the scientific research literature on reading and its implications for reading instruction.* Retrieved January 8, 2002, from http://www.nichd.nih.gov/publications/nrp/smallbook.htm

Newcomer, P., Nodine, B., & Barenbaum, E. (1988). Teaching writing to exceptional children: Reaction and recommendations. *Exceptional Children, 54,* 559–564.

Nicholls, J.G., McKenzie, M., & Shufro, J. (1994). Schoolwork, homework, life's work: The experience of students with and without learning disabilities. *Journal of Learning Disabilities, 27,* 562–569.

Okolo, C.M. (1992). The effects of computer-based attribution retraining on the attributions, persistence, and mathematics computation of students with learning disabilities. *Journal of Learning Disabilities, 25,* 327–334.

Olitsky, S.E., & Nelson, L.B. (2003). Reading disorders in children. *Pediatric Clinics of North America, 50,* 213–224.

Orton, S.T. (1937). *Reading, writing, and speech problems in children* (a presentation of certain types of disorders in the development of the language faculty). New York: W.W. Norton.

Pennington, B.F. (1991). Genetics of learning disabilities. *Seminars in Neurology, 11,* 28–34.

Pennington, B.F., & Gilger, J.W. (1996). How is dyslexia transmitted? In C.H. Chase G.D. Rosen, & G.F. Sherman (Eds.), *Developmental dyslexia: Neural, cognitive, and genetic mechanisms* (pp. 41–61). Timonium, MD: York Press.

Pugh, K.R., Mencl, W.E., Jenner, A.R., et al. (2000). Functional neuroimaging studies of reading and reading disability (developmental dyslexia). *Mental Retardation and Developmental Disabilities Research Reviews, 6,* 207–213.

Raphael, T.E., Englert, C.S., & Kirschner, B.W. (1986). *The impact of text structure instruction and social context on students' comprehension and production of expository text* (Research Series No. 177). East Lansing: Michigan State University, Institute for Research on Teaching.

Reiss, A.L., & Freund, L. (1990). Fragile X syndrome. *Biological Psychiatry, 27,* 223–240.

Rock, E.E., Fessler, M.A., & Church, R.P. (1996). The concomitance of learning disabilities and emotional/behavioral disorders: A conceptual model. *Journal of Learning Disabilities, 30,* 245–265.

Rourke B.P., & Finlayson M.A.M. (1978). Neuropsychological significance of variations in patterns of academic performance: Verbal and visual–spatial abilities. *Journal of Abnormal Child Psychology, 6,* 121–123.

Sandak R., Mencl, W.E., Frost, S.J., et al. (2004). The neurobiological basis of skilled and impaired reading: recent findings and new directions. *Scientific Studies of Reading, 8,* 273–292.

Satz, P., Buka, S., Lipsitt, L., et al. (1998). The long-term prognosis of learning disabled children. In B.K. Shapiro, P.J. Accardo, & A.J. Capute (Eds.), *Specific reading disability: A view of the spectrum* (pp. 223–250). Timonium, MD: York Press.

Savage, R.C., & Wolcott, G.F. (Eds.). (1994). *Educational dimensions of acquired brain injury.* Austin, TX: PRO-ED.

Schatschneider, C., & Torgesen, J. (2004). Using our

current understanding of dyslexia to support early identification and intervention. *Journal of Child Neurology, 19,* 759–765.

Schulte, A.C., Conners, C.K., & Osborne, S.S. (1999). Linkages between attention deficit disorders and reading disability. In D.D. Duane (Ed.), *Reading and attention disorders: Neurobiological correlates* (pp. 161–184). Timonium, MD: York Press.

Schwartz, S.E., & Budd, D. (1983). Mathematics for handicapped learners: A functional approach for adolescents. In E. Meyer, G.A. Vergason, & B.P. Whelan (Eds.), *Promising practices for exceptional children: Curriculum implications* (pp. 321–340). Denver, CO: Love Publishing.

Scott, S.S. (1994). Determining reasonable academic adjustments for college students with learning disabilities. *Journal of Learning Disabilities, 27,* 403–412.

Sexson, S.B., & Madan-Swain, A. (1993). School reentry for the child with chronic illness. *Journal of Learning Disabilities, 26,* 115–125, 137.

Shalev, R.S. (2004). Developmental dyscalculia. *Journal of Child Neurology, 19,* 765–771.

Shalev, R.S., & Gross-Tsur, V. (2001). Developmental Dyscalculia. *Pediatric Neurology, 24,* 337–342.

Shalev, R.S., Manor O., & Gross-Tsur V. (2005). Developmental Dyscalculia: A prospective six-year study. *Developmental Medicine and Child Neurology, 47,* 121–125.

Shalev, R.S., Manor, O., Kerem, B., et al. (2001). Developmental dyscalculia is a familial learning disability. *Journal of Learning Disabilities, 34,* 59–65.

Shapiro, B.K. (1996). The prevalence of specific reading disability. *Mental Retardation and Developmental Disabilities Research Reviews, 2,* 10–13.

Shapiro, B.K., & Gallico, R.P. (1993). Learning disabilities. *Pediatric Clinics of North America, 40,* 491–505.

Shaw, S.F., & Shaw, S.R. (1989). Learning disabilities and college programming: A bibliography. *Journal of Postsecondary Education and Disability, 6,* 77–85.

Shaywitz, B.A., Fletcher, J.M., & Shaywitz, S.E. (1995). Defining and classifying learning disabilities and attention-deficit/hyperactivity disorder. *Journal of Child Neurology, 10*(Suppl.), S50–S57.

Shaywitz, B.A., Shaywitz, S.E., Blachman, B.A., et al. (2004). Development of left occipitotemporal systems for skilled reading in children after a phonolgically-based intervention. *Biological Psychiatry, 55,* 926–933.

Shaywitz, S.E. (2005). *Overcoming dyslexia: A new and complete science-based program for reading problems at any level.* New York. Vintage.

Shaywitz, S.E., Escobar, M.D., Shaywitz, B.A., et al. (1992). Evidence that dyslexia may represent the lower tail of a normal distribution of reading ability. *The New England Journal of Medicine, 326,* 145–150.

Shaywitz, S.E., & Shaywitz B.A. (2005). Dyslexia (specific reading disability). *Biological Psychiatry, 57,* 301–309.

Sheffield, B.B. (1991). The structured flexibility of Orton-Gillingham. *Annals of Dyslexia, 41,* 41–54.

Siegel, L.S. (1998). The discrepancy formula: Its use and abuse. In B.K. Shapiro, P.J. Accardo, & A.J. Capute (Eds.), *Specific reading disability: A view of the spectrum* (pp. 123–135). Timonium, MD: York Press.

Silberberg, N.E., Iverson, I.A., & Goins, J.T. (1975). Which reading method works best? *Journal of Learning Disabilities, 6,* 547–556.

Simos, P.G., Fletcher, J.M., Foorman, B.R., et al. (2002). Brain activation profiles during the early stages of reading acquisition. *Journal of Child Neurology, 17,* 159–163.

Singer, H., & Ruddell, R. (Eds.). (1985). *Theoretical models and processes or reading* (3rd ed.). Newark DE: International Reading Association.

Slavin, R.E., Madden, N.A., Dolan, L.J., et al. (1990). Success for All: A first year outcomes of a comprehensive plan for reforming urban education. *American Educational Research Journal, 27,* 255–278.

Staton, J., Shuy, R.W., Peyton, J.K., et al. (1988). *Dialogue journal communication: Classroom, linguistic, social and cognitive views.* Norwood, NJ: Ablex.

Swanson, H.L. (1996). Classification and dynamic assessment of children with learning disabilities. *Focus on Exceptional Children, 28,* 9.

Talcott, J.B., Witton, C., McLean, M.F., et al. (2000). From the cover: Dynamic sensory sensitivity and children's word decoding skills. *Proceedings of the National Academy of Sciences of the United States of America, 97,* 2952–2957.

Taylor, D.F. (1991). Literature letters and narrative response: Seventh and eighth graders write about their reading. In J. Feeley, D. Strickland, & S. Wepner (Eds.), *Process reading and writing: A literature-based approach* (pp. 164–178). New York: Teachers College Press.

Tierney, R.J., & Readence, J.E. (2000). *Reading strategies and practices: A compendium.* Boston: Allyn & Bacon.

Tierney, R.J., Readence, J.E., & Dishner, E.K. (1995). *Reading strategies and practices: A compendium.* Boston: Allyn & Bacon.

Traub, N., & Bloom, F. (2000). *Recipe for reading* (4th ed.). Cambridge, MA: Educators Publishing Service.

Turkeltaub, P.E., Gareau, L., Flowers D.L., et al. (2003). Development of neural mechanisms for reading. *Nature Neuroscience, 6,* 767–773.

U.S. Department of Education, National Center for Education Statistics. (2003). Table 52—Children 3 to 21 years old served in federally supported programs for the disabled, by type of disability: Selected years 1976–77 to 2001–2002. In *Digest of Education Statistics, 2003* (p. 72; NCES No. 2005-025). Washington, DC: U.S. Government Printing Office.

U.S. Department of Education, Office of Special Education Programs. (1991). *Youth with disabilities: How are they doing? The first comprehensive report from the National Longitudinal Transition Study of Special Education Students.* Menlo Park, CA: SRI International.

U.S. Department of Labor, Secretary's Commission on Achieving Necessary Skills (SCANS). (1992). *Learning a living: A blueprint for high performance. A SCANS report for AMERICA 2000.* Washington, DC: U.S. Government Printing Office.

Vacca, J.L., Vacca, R.T., Gove, M.K., et al. (2003). *Reading and learning to read* (5th ed.). Boston: Allyn & Bacon.

Vaughn, S., Elbaum, B.E., Schumm, J.S., et al. (1998). Social outcomes for students with and without learning disabilities in inclusive classrooms. *Journal of Learning Disabilities, 31,* 428–436.

Vaughn, S., & Fuchs, L.S. (2003). Redefining learning disabilities as inadequate response to instruction: The promise and potential problems. *Learning Disabilities Research & Practice, 18,* 137–146.

Vellutino F.R., Fletcher J.M., Snowling M.J., et al. (2004). Specific reading disability (dyslexia): What have we learned in the past four decades? *Journal of Child Psychology and Psychiatry, 45,* 2–40.

Vogel, S.A., & Adelman, P.B. (1992). The success of college students with learning disabilities: Factors related to educational attainment. *Journal of Learning Disabilities, 25,* 430–441.

Vukovic R.K., & Siegel, L.S. (2006). The double-deficit hypothesis: A comprehensive analysis of the evidence. *Journal of Learning Disabilities, 39,* 25–47.

Waber, D.P., Forbes, P.W., Wolff, P.H., et al. (2004). Neurodevelopmental characteristics of children with learning impairments classified according to the double-deficit hypothesis. *Journal of Learning Disabilities 37*(5), 451–461.

Wechsler, D. (1991). *Wechsler Intelligence Scale for Children–Third Edition (WISC-III).* San Antonio, TX: Harcourt Assessment.

Wechsler, D. (2003). *Wechsler Intelligence Scale for Children–Fourth Edition (WISC-IV).* San Antonio, TX: Harcourt Assessment.

Welsh, M.C., & Pennington, B.F. (1988). Assessing frontal lobe functioning in children: Views from developmental psychology. *Developmental Neuropsychology, 4,* 199–230.

Wilson, B.A. (1988). *Wilson Reading System program overview.* Millbury, MA: Wilson Language Training.

Wolf, M., & Bowers, P.G. (1999). The double-deficit hypothesis for the developmental dyslexias. *Journal of Educational Psychology, 91,* 415–438.

Wolf, M., Bowers, P.G., & Biddle, K. (2000). Naming-speed processes, timing, and reading: A conceptual review. *Journal of Learning Disabilities, 33,* 387–407.

Wood, K. (1984). Probable passages: A writing strategy. *The Reading Teacher, 37,* 496–499.

26

Cerebral Palsy

Louis Pellegrino

Upon completion of this chapter, the reader will

- Understand the definition and causes of cerebral palsy
- Understand how cerebral palsy is diagnosed
- Know the various types of cerebral palsy and their characteristics
- Know the sensory, cognitive, and medical problems commonly associated with cerebral palsy
- Understand the range of therapeutic options available to help children with cerebral palsy
- Be knowledgeable about the medical and functional prognoses for cerebral palsy

JAMAL

Jamal is a 15-month-old boy who was seen by his primary pediatrician for a routine well-child checkup. Jamal's mother expressed concern that her son was not yet walking. The pediatrician had documented some modest delays in motor development at Jamal's 12-month office visit but had attributed these delays to the fact that Jamal was born 3 months prematurely. Jamal's mother had delivered him vaginally following spontaneous onset of labor at 27 weeks' gestation. This spontaneous labor was probably caused by **chorioamnionitis,** an infection of the membranes surrounding the fetus. Jamal's birth weight was 1 pound, 10 ounces. He required ventilator support for 5 days, and at 2 weeks of age, an ultrasound study of the brain demonstrated a possible abnormality of the white matter of the brain.

As of his 12-month well-child checkup, Jamal had been sitting on his own for about 2 months. The pediatrician had explained to Jamal's mother that based on age adjusted for prematurity, Jamal began sitting at an adjusted age of 7 months. This was only slightly delayed compared with the expected age of sitting independently. Jamal's leg muscles were also a little stiff, and he sat slouched forward, but his pediatrician knew that many pre-

mature infants have mild, temporary abnormalities of muscle tone (known as transient **dystonia** of prematurity) that resolve by 15–18 months of age.

At this 15-month visit, Jamal was sitting well but still sat with a slouch. He could crawl stiffly on all fours but was not yet pulling up to a standing position. Jamal showed a pronounced tendency to keep his legs stiffly extended with his toes pointed and feet crossed at the ankles (scissoring). His pediatrician was concerned that Jamal was showing signs of cerebral palsy.

WHAT IS CEREBRAL PALSY?

Cerebral palsy is a developmental disability. As is the case with other developmental disabilities, cerebral palsy is defined on the basis of specific functional characteristics rather than on the basis of the diverse causes of the condition. The hallmark of cerebral palsy is a significant impairment of functional mobility that is associated with signs of neurological dysfunction. As the term *cerebral* implies, the locus of the dysfunction is the brain. Cerebral palsy is further distinguished from other motor impairment syndromes by the recognition that signature features of the condition are known to be associated with disturbances of the immature, or developing, brain. These disturbances most often occur during fetal development or in the perinatal period, but they may also occur during the first few years after birth. Whether the disturbances are a consequence of brain injury or relate to a genetically based problem with brain development, in all cases the presumption is that the processes resulting in the disturbance are time limited, or nonprogressive. Based on these observations, cerebral palsy may be defined as follows: Cerebral palsy is a disorder of movement and posture that is caused by a nonprogressive abnormality of the immature brain.

Modifications of this basic definition of cerebral palsy have recently been proposed that emphasize the complexity of the condition, including associated nonmotor impairments of sensation, cognition, communication, and behavior and associated medical conditions such as seizures (Bax et al., 2005). Although the neurological basis for cerebral palsy is considered nonprogressive, the functional consequences of the disorder can, in a sense, progress. For example, some children with more severe forms of cerebral palsy (e.g., spastic quadriplegia; see the Classifying the Subtypes of Cerebral Palsy section) are prone to develop orthopedic complications such as hip dislocation, scoliosis, and muscle contractures that may reduce their functional mobility over time (Liptak & Accardo, 2004).

WHAT CAUSES CEREBRAL PALSY?

Cerebral palsy is most often a consequence of brain injury, but in some cases may be due to genetically based problems with brain development (Nelson, 2002; O'Shea, 2002). Until the 1980s, it was thought that most cases of cerebral palsy resulted from "birth asphyxia" (hypoxic-ischemic encephalopathy; see Chapter 4), which has traditionally been defined as a disruption of blood flow (ischemia) and oxygen supply (hypoxia) to the brain as a consequence of problems encountered at the time of birth It is now clear, however, that true birth asphyxia is the cause of cerebral palsy in only a minority of cases (Hankins & Speer, 2003; Nelson & Grether, 1999; Pschirrer & Yeomans, 2000).

Prematurity-Related Cerebral Palsy

Jamal provides an example of cerebral palsy that is most likely related to complications of prematurity. Premature infants, especially those born prior to 28 weeks' gestations (or with a birth weight less than 1,500 grams), are recognized to be at increased risk for cerebral palsy. The overall prevalence of cerebral palsy is approximately 2.0–2.5 per 1,000 in the general population (Hagberg et al., 2001; Reddihough & Collins, 2003; Winter et al., 2002); premature infants represent 40%–50% of this group. Among infants born prior to 28 weeks, more than 12% will ultimately be diagnosed with cerebral palsy (Marlow et al., 2005; O'Shea, 2002; Vohr et al., 2005). The increased risk of cerebral palsy in the premature infants relates to a special vulnerability of the white matter of the brain (Volpe, 2003; see Chapter 9). The white matter contains neuronal processes (the "wiring" of the brain), some of which are involved in the control of movement and regulation of muscle tone (see discussion on corticospinal pathways in the Delayed Motor Development section). Disruption of these pathways can result in the signs and symptoms of cerebral palsy. (Recent research also suggests that disruption of brain white matter is associated with subtle but important associated disturbances in the neurons, or brain cells, that compose the "gray matter" of the brain. These disturbances may explain the learning and cognitive problems encountered in children with cerebral palsy [Volpe, 2005].) The two common causes of white matter injury in premature infants are periventricular leukomalacia (PVL) and intraventricular hemorrhage (IVH) (see Chapter 9). Immaturity of brain development predisposes premature infants to both of these conditions.

Cerebral Palsy in Full-Term Infants

A wide variety of prenatal, perinatal, and genetic factors have been highlighted as possible causes of cerebral palsy in full term-infants, including birth asphyxia, congenital brain malformations, coagulation abnormalities, complications related to multiple gestation and intrauterine infection/inflammation (Nelson, 2002). Compared with those born prematurely, children born at term who subsequently develop cerebral palsy are more often small for gestational age or have malformations inside and outside the central nervous system (CNS), suggesting a problem with early fetal development in some cases (Krageloh-Mann et al., 1995). In addition, if a full-term infant experiences severe birth asphyxia, he or she may develop cerebral palsy, especially the athetoid or dystonic types (see Classifying the Subtypes of Cerebral Palsy section), which reflects damage to deep brain structures (e.g., the basal ganglia). In the past, high bilirubin levels in the immediate postnatal period resulted in a condition called kernicterus, which also caused athetoid cerebral palsy. Although kernicterus is rare now in developed countries, more subtle bilirubin-induced neurologic dysfunction (BIND) continues to be a concern (Shapiro, 2005).

Infection and Cerebral Palsy

In both term and preterm infants, direct infection of the fetus by viruses (e.g., cytomegalovirus, rubella; see Chapter 6) and other infectious agents (e.g., toxoplasmosis, a parasitic infection) has long been a recognized cause of cerebral palsy. Although these types of infections are a fairly uncommon cause of cerebral palsy, there has been increasing recognition that chorioamnionitis, or maternal intrauterine infection, may play a key role in the genesis of cerebral palsy. Chorioamnionitis predisposes to premature delivery and may also have direct adverse effects on the fetal brain (Jacobsson, 2004; Yoon, Park, & Chaiworapongsa, 2003). Complex relationships likely exist between chorioamnionitis and other clinical entities that are thought to cause cerebral palsy. For example, placental infection may contribute to the development of hypoxic-ischemic encephalopathy/ birth asphyxia. Infection during pregnancy may also promote blood coagulation, leading to stroke-like events in the fetus (Leviton & Dammann, 2004; Nelson & Lynch, 2004). These relationships are currently the subject of intense investigation (Wu, 2002).

HOW IS CEREBRAL PALSY DIAGNOSED?

The diagnosis of cerebral palsy is based on the recognition of significant delays in motor development associated with signs of CNS dysfunction. Although newborns may have known risk factors for cerebral palsy (e.g., PVL), cerebral palsy cannot be diagnosed at birth. Children with more severe forms of cerebral palsy are usually diagnosed by 1 year of age; children with milder forms of cerebral palsy may not be diagnosed until 2 years of age (Aneja, 2004; Palmer, 2004; Russman & Ashwal, 2004).

Delayed Motor Development

Cerebral palsy is not the most common cause of delayed motor development. Children with motor delays in association with cognitive and learning disabilities far outnumber children with motor delays as a consequence of cerebral palsy (see Chapters 17 and 25). Cerebral palsy-related motor delay is distinguished by severity (children with cerebral palsy tend to have more severe motor delays) and by the presence of associated signs of upper motor neuron dysfunction.

Upper Motor Neuron Dysfunction in Cerebral Palsy

The upper motor neuron (UMN) system is not a discrete anatomical entity but refers collectively to the motor control systems based in the brain and spinal cord. The UMN system is distinguished from the lower motor neuron (LMN) system, which refers collectively to the peripheral nerves and the muscles that they innervate. The primary components of the UMN system are the **pyramidal tract** or **corticospinal pathways** and the **extrapyramidal system** (see Figure 26.1). These systems are differentially affected by disturbances to the developing brain depending on the timing and nature of these disturbances. Generically, UMN dysfunction is characterized by positive and negative signs. The positive signs refer to the presence of atypical neuromotor features, such as increased or decreased muscle tone, atypical reflex patterns, and involuntary movements. The negative signs refer to absent or deficient neuromotor functions, including poor motor control, poor balance, weakness, and easy fatigability. Virtually all children with cerebral palsy manifest the negative signs of UMN dysfunction to one degree or another. Significant problems with motor planning and motor control in particular are a hallmark of cerebral palsy, and tend to contribute most to deficits in functional mobility. The profile of positive signs tends to vary more from child to child and contributes to the classification of the subtypes of cerebral palsy (see Classifying the Subtypes of Cerebral Palsy).

Spasticity

Spasticity refers to a group of neuromotor signs that are seen in association with disturbances in the pyramidal component of the motor control system. The pyramidal system is composed of neurons that extend from the motor cortex to the brain stem and spinal cord. These corticospinal pathways directly control movement and also influence muscle tone and deep tendon reflexes (e.g., the familiar knee-jerk response) by inhibiting spinal cord mechanisms that control these processes. In the absence of normal corti-

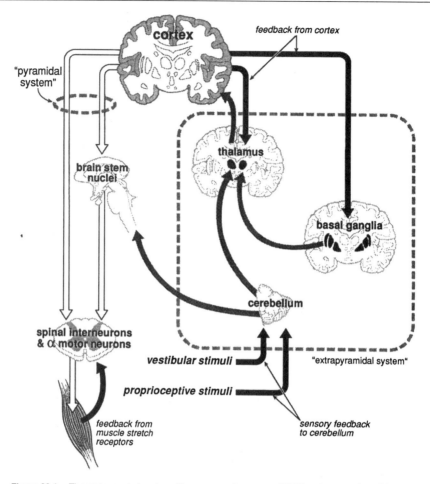

Figure 26.1. The motor control system. The upper motor neuron (UMN) system consists of the pyramidal and extrapyramidal systems. The pyramidal system connects the motor control center of the cortex to the brainstem and spinal cord and is responsible for the direct control of movement and muscle tone. The extrapyramidal system consists of deep brain structures (especially the basal ganglia and cerebellum) and works primarily by modifying and refining the output of the pyramidal system. The lower motor neuron (LMN) system consists of the muscles and the nerves that connect the muscles and the spinal cord, including the nerves that comprise the stretch reflex mechanism. (From Pellegrino, L., & Dormans, J.P. [1998]. Definitions, etiology, and epidemiology of cerebral palsy. In J.P. Dormans & L. Pellegrino [Eds.], *Caring for children with cerebral palsy: A team approach* [p. 10]. Baltimore: Paul H. Brookes Publishing Co.; reprinted by permission.)

cospinal inhibition, the spinal cord influences predominate, resulting in **spastic** hypertonicity (increased muscle tone) and exaggerated reflex responses, two of the hallmark features of spastic cerebral palsy. The clinical signs associated with spasticity are examples of release of inhibition phenomena, which characterize many forms of UMN disturbance.

Persistent Primitive Reflexes

Another example of release of inhibition phenomena relates to the abnormal persistence of primitive reflex patterns in some children with cerebral palsy. **Primitive reflexes** are called primitive because they are present in early life (in some cases, during intrauterine development) and because they are thought to be controlled by the primitive regions of the nervous system: the spinal cord, the labyrinths of the inner ear, lower brain areas, and the brain stem. Familiar examples of primitive reflexes include the suckling reflex and the hand-grasp reflex in the newborn. As the cortex matures, these reflexes are gradually suppressed and integrated into voluntary movement patterns. The process of integration is usually complete by 12 months of age. Because of a disturbance in normal maturation of corticospinal pathways in children with cerebral palsy, there is a tendency for these

Full-term Infant Resting Position

Asymmetrical Tonic Neck Reflex

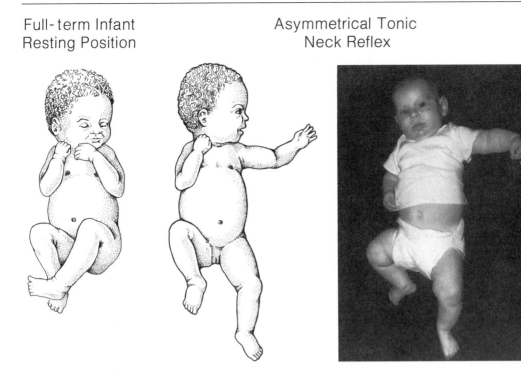

Figure 26.2. The asymmetric tone neck reflex. In the typical newborn infant, when the head is actively or passively turned to the side, the arm and leg on the same side will extend and the arm and leg on the opposite side will flex, resulting in a "fencing" posture. The opposite pattern occurs when the head is turn to the other side. In typically developing infants, the reflex fades (is integrated) by about 6 months of age and is never obligatory (the infant can break through the pattern with spontaneous movement, even in the newborn period). In children with cerebral palsy, the reflex tends to be more pronounced, persists beyond the expected age, and may be obligatory.

primitive reflex patterns to persist beyond early infancy. Among the primitive reflexes, the **asymmetric tone neck reflex** (Figure 26.2) and the **tonic labyrinthine response** (Figure 26.3) are particularly helpful in the diagnosis of cerebral palsy.

Involuntary Movements and Ataxia

Children who have cerebral palsy as a consequence of disturbances in the extrapyramidal system will sometimes exhibit atypical, involuntary movements, also know as **dyskinesias.** Rapid, random, jerky movements are known as **chorea**; slow, writhing movements are called **athetosis** (when seen together, these movements are called **choreoathetosis**). **Dystonia** refers to **rigid** posturing centered in the trunk and neck. **Ataxia** seen in association with cerebral palsy is characterized by abnormalities of voluntary movement involving balance and position of the trunk and limbs in space. For chil-

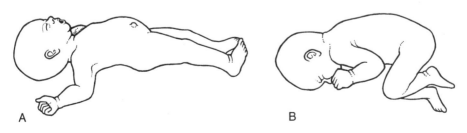

A   B

Figure 26.3. The tonic labyrinthine reflex. A) When the child is in the supine position with the head slightly extended, retraction of the shoulders and extension of the legs is observed. B) The opposite occurs when the infant is in the prone position with the head slightly flexed. In typically developing infants, the reflex pattern is barely evident in the newborn period; in children with cerebral palsy, the pattern may dominate posture and movement and may persist throughout life.

dren who can walk, this is noted most especially as a wide-based, unsteady gait. Difficulties with controlling the hand and arm during reaching (causing overshooting or past-pointing) and problems with the timing of motor movements are also seen.

Automatic Movement Reactions and the Development of Voluntary Control

As primitive reflexes diminish in intensity in the typically developing child, **postural reactions,** also known as **automatic movement reactions,** are developing (Figure 26.4). Some of the more important of these reactions include righting, equilibrium, and protective reactions, all of which enable the child to have more complex voluntary movement and better control of posture. These automatic movement responses serve a crucial supporting role in the development of specific motor milestones; delayed or absent development of these responses in children with cerebral palsy makes a significant contribution to their motor disability.

Walking and the Diagnosis of Cerebral Palsy

Many children with cerebral palsy first come to professional attention because of delayed walking. This developmental milestone has a powerful intrinsic meaning for parents and profes-

sionals alike. Most adults know that children begin walking at about 1 year of age, and there is an implicit understanding that a child's first steps mark the transition from infancy to toddlerhood. When a child does not make this transition at the expected time, it is more difficult to ignore than other delays in development. To walk, a child must be able to maintain an upright posture, move forward in a smoothly coordinated manner, and demonstrate protective responses for safety when falling. Even a child with the mildest form of cerebral palsy has difficulty attaining the continuous changes in muscle tone that are required for typical walking. The child's walk or gait is affected in many ways. Scissoring, the most common gait disturbance, occurs because of increased tone in the muscles that control adduction (movement toward the mid-line) and internal rotation of the hips. Toe walking results from an **equinus** position of the feet (Figure 26.5) and increased extensor tone in the legs. In children without cerebral palsy, a protective reaction called the parachute response develops by 10 months of age. This is manifest by forward extension of the arms when falling forward. Many children with cerebral palsy have delayed or absent development of this response, which makes walking inherently unsafe.

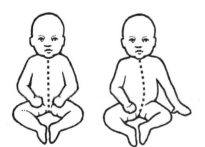

Figure 26.4. Automatic movement responses: the lateral prop reaction. At about 6 months of age, typically developing infants have already developed good postural control of the head and trunk (righting or equilibrium responses) and can stop themselves from falling forward when placed in sitting by extending their arms in front of them (forward prop response). By 6 months of age, most infants can also catch themselves when falling to the side by extending the arm on the same side (lateral prop response). This automatic movement reaction is critical for independent sitting and may be delayed or absent in children with cerebral palsy. (From Pellegrino, L., & Dormans, J.P. [1998]. Making the diagnosis of cerebral palsy. In J.P. Dormans & L. Pellegrino [Eds.], *Caring for children with cerebral palsy: A team approach* [p. 39]. Baltimore: Paul H. Brookes Publishing Co.; reprinted by permission.)

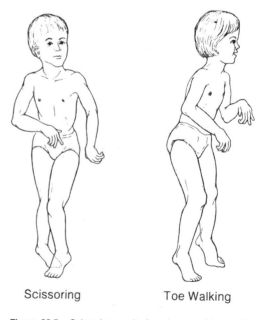

Scissoring   Toe Walking

Figure 26.5. Scissoring results from increased tone in the muscles on the inner aspect of the thigh that tend to pull the legs together and turn the legs inward. Toe walking is due to tightness of the calf muscles and Achilles tendon and increased extensor tone in the legs.

Classifying the Subtypes of Cerebral Palsy

Cerebral palsy is often classified according to the type of motor impairment that predominates (Figure 26.6; Koman, Smith, & Shilt, 2004), with spastic cerebral palsy being the most common type. Spastic cerebral palsy is further categorized according to the distribution of limbs involved. In **spastic hemiplegia,** one side of the body is more affected than the other; usually, the arm is more affected than the leg. Because the motor neurons that control one side of the body are located in the opposite cerebral cortex, a right-side hemiplegia implies damage to or dysfunction of the left side of the brain, and vice versa. In **spastic diplegia,** the legs are more affected than the arms. This is the type of cerebral palsy most frequently associated with prematurity (and is the type that Jamal exhibits in this chapter's case study). In **spastic quadriplegia,** all four limbs and usually the trunk and muscles that control the mouth, tongue, and pharynx are affected. The severity of the motor impairment in spastic quadriplegia implies wider cerebral dysfunction and worse outcome than for the other forms of spastic cerebral palsy. Individuals with spastic quadriplegia often have intellectual disability, seizures, sensory impairments, and medical complications.

Dyskinetic cerebral palsy (also known as extrapyramidal cerebral palsy) is characterized by abnormalities in muscle tone that involve the whole body. Changing patterns of tone from hour to hour and day to day are common. These children may exhibit rigid muscle tone while awake and normal or decreased tone while asleep. Involuntary movements are often present, although they are sometimes difficult to detect, and are the hallmark of this type of cerebral palsy. The term **athetoid cerebral palsy** characterizes a form of dyskinetic cerebral palsy associated with choreoathetosis. Similarly, **dystonic cerebral palsy** is associated with prominent involuntary posturing and dystonia.

Ataxic cerebral palsy is characterized by abnormalities of voluntary movement involving balance and position of the trunk and limbs in space (ataxia). Ataxic cerebral palsy may be associated with increased or decreased muscle tone.

The term **mixed cerebral palsy** is used when more than one type of motor pattern is present and should be used only when one pattern does not clearly predominate over another. The term *total body cerebral palsy* is sometimes used to emphasize that certain types of cerebral palsy (dyskinetic, ataxic, mixed, and spastic quadriplegia) involve the entire musculoskeletal system to a greater or lesser degree; other forms

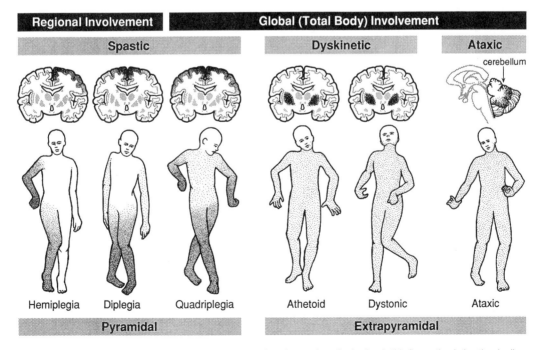

Figure 26.6. Different regions of the brain are affected in various forms of cerebral palsy. In this figure, the darker the shading, the more severe the involvement.

of spastic cerebral palsy (diplegia, hemiplegia) are localized to particular regions of the body.

Characterizing the Degree of Functional Disability Associated with Cerebral Palsy

Although there is some clinical utility in classifying cerebral palsy on the basis of neuromotor characteristics (e.g., spasticity, dyskinesias), there tends to be a great deal of functional variability within specific subtypes. For example, some children with spastic diplegia may be able to walk independently, whereas others depend on a wheelchair for mobility. A number of functional assessment systems have been developed to address this issue (Oeffinger et al., 2004; Palisano et al., 1997; see Table 26.1). These systems provide a means to classify individuals based on meaningful functional distinctions. Using this type of functional classification scheme is often helpful for planning therapeutic interventions and establishing goals for habilation (see the Habilitation section) and is more predictive of long-term functional outcome in comparison with the prognostic value of the traditional, impairment-focused classification scheme (Rosenbaum et al., 2002).

Table 26.1. Summary of Gross Motor Function Classification System (GMFCS)

Level	Age			
	< 2 years	2–4 years	4–6 years	6–12 years
I: Walks without restrictions	Sits well (hands free to play), crawls and pulls-to-stand; walks between 18 and 24 months without a device	Gets up and down from floor to standing without help; walking is preferred method of mobility	Walks indoors and outdoors; climbs stairs; starting to run/jump	Independent walking, running, jumping, but speed, balance, and coordination reduced
II: Walks without device; restricted community mobility	Sits but may need hands for balance; may creep or crawl; may pull-to-stand or cruise	Floor sits, but hard to keep both hands free; mobility by crawling, cruising, or walking with assistive device	Transfers with arm assist; walks without device at home, short distances outside; climbs stairs with railing; no running or jumping	Independent walking but limitations in challenging circumstances; minimal running, jumping
III: Walks with assistive device; limited community mobility	Sits with low back support; rolls and creeps	Floor sits, often W-sitting, needs help getting to sit; creeping and crawling primary means of mobility; limited assisted standing/walking	Sits in regular chair with pelvic support to allow free hands; walks with device on level surface; transported for long distances	Walks indoors or outdoors with assistive device; wheelchair mobility or transport for long distances
IV: Limited self-mobility; power mobility	Has head control, but needs trunk support for sitting; rolls to back, may roll to front	Needs hands to maintain sitting; adaptive equipment for sitting/standing; floor mobility only (rolling, creeping, or crawling without reciprocal leg movements)	Adaptive seating needed for maximum hand function; needs assistance for transfers; walks short distances with assistance; power mobility for long distances	Maintains function achieved by ages 4–6 or relies on power wheelchair for self-mobility
V: Self-mobility severely limited even with assistive devices	Limited voluntary control of movement; head and trunk control minimal; needs help to roll	Limited control of movement and posture; all areas of motor function are limited; adaptive equipment does not fully compensate functional limitations for sitting and standing; no independent mobility (requires transport); some children achieve very limited power mobility with extensive adaptations		

Source: Palisano, Rosenbaum, Walters, et al. (1997).

Establishing the Etiology of Cerebral Palsy

Diagnosis of the etiology, or cause, of cerebral palsy occurs in parallel with the process that establishes the disability or functional diagnosis of cerebral palsy itself (Ashwal et al., 2004). Establishing the etiology of cerebral palsy may have important implications for treatment, prognosis, and recurrence risk. Information gleaned from the medical history and physical examination is often critical in establishing etiology (e.g., knowing that a child was born prematurely and has signs of spastic diplegia strongly suggests the possibility of cerebral white matter injury). With regard to specialized diagnostic testing, brain imaging is especially helpful (Accardo, Kammann, & Hoon, 2004; Ancel et al., 2006). Ultrasonography is used for fetal and neonatal screening and can distinguish large malformations of the brain and abnormalities related to brain hemorrhage or injury (i.e., IVH, PVL). Computed tomography (CT) and especially magnetic resonance imaging (MRI) provide more detailed resolution of anatomical structures than ultrasound and may help to define the cause of cerebral palsy. Newer techniques—such as positron emission tomography (PET), functional magnetic resonance imaging (fMRI), **single photon emission computed tomography (SPECT),** and diffusion tensor imaging (DTI)—complement CT and MRI (primarily in the research setting) by providing information about brain metabolic function, which in some cases is abnormal even when brain structure appears to be normal (Davidson, Thomas, & Casey, 2003; Mohan, Chugani, & Chugani, 1999; Watts et al., 2003).

WHAT OTHER IMPAIRMENTS ARE ASSOCIATED WITH CEREBRAL PALSY?

All children with cerebral palsy have problems with movement and posture. Many also have other impairments associated with damage to the CNS. The most common associated disabilities are intellectual disability, visual impairments, hearing impairments, speech-language disorders, seizures, feeding and growth abnormalities, and behavior/emotional disorders.

Assessment of intellectual functioning in children with cerebral palsy may be difficult because most tests of cognition require motor or verbal responses. Even taking this into account, approximately one half of children with cerebral palsy have intellectual disability, and many of those with average intelligence exhibit some degree of learning disability (Nordmark, Hagglund, & Lagergren, 2001). There is a general correlation between physical and cognitive disability: Children with more severe forms of cerebral palsy are a greater risk for more significant intellectual disability.

Visual impairments are also common and diverse in children with cerebral palsy (Guzzetta, Mercuri, & Cioni, 2001). The premature infant may have severe visual impairment caused by retinopathy of prematurity (see Chapter 11). Nystagmus, or involuntary oscillating eye movements, may be present in the child with ataxia. Children with hemiplegia may present with homonomous hemianopsia, a condition causing loss of one part of the visual field. Strabismus, or squint, is seen in many children with cerebral palsy. Children with cerebral palsy are also more prone to hyperopia (farsightedness) than children without cerebral palsy are (Sobrado et al., 1999).

Hearing, speech, and language impairments are also common, occurring in about 30% of children with cerebral palsy. Children with congenital rubella or other intrauterine viral infections often have high-frequency hearing loss (see Chapter 12). Dyskinetic cerebral palsy is associated with articulation problems, as choreoathetosis affects tongue and vocal cord movements. Expressive or receptive language disorders are commonly observed among children with cerebral palsy who do not have intellectual disability and may be a harbinger of a learning disability, such as specific reading disability (see Chapter 25).

Approximately 40% of children with cerebral palsy also develop seizures (Nordmark et al., 2001). Children with more severe cognitive and physical disability are more prone to seizures, as are children whose cerebral palsy is a consequence of brain malformation, infection, or gray matter injury. Partial epilepsy (see Chapter 29) is the most common form of seizure activity in all children with cerebral palsy, and is especially common in children with hemiplegia who have seizures (Carlsson, Hagberg, & Olsson, 2003).

Feeding and growth difficulties are often present in children with cerebral palsy (Samson-Fang et al., 2002) and may be secondary to a variety of problems, including hypotonia, weak suck, poor coordination of the swallowing mechanism, tonic bite reflex, hyperactive gag reflex, and exaggerated tongue thrust. These problems may lead to poor nutrition and may require the use of alternative feeding methods, such as tube feeding (see Chapter 31). Medical problems related to poor gastrointestinal motility (including gastroesophageal reflux and constipation) tend to add to these difficulties. Poor nutrition and lack of weight-bearing activities also leads to **osteopenia,** or weak bones related to reduced bone mineral density, making children with cerebral palsy more prone to fractures. Bisphosphonates (drugs used to treat osteoporosis in older adults) have been shown to be effective for osteopenia is cerebral palsy (Henderson et al., 2002; Henderson et al., 2005).

Poor health in children with cerebral palsy significantly contributes to the societal and functional disadvantages they experience as a consequence of their disability (Liptak & Accardo, 2004; Samson-Fang et al., 2002). A comprehensive health plan implemented in the context of a well-defined "medical home" is a critical component to assuring that the health needs of the children are adequately addressed (Cooley & American Academy of Pediatrics Committee on Children with Disabilities, 2004).

WHAT CAN BE DONE TO HELP CHILDREN WITH CEREBRAL PALSY?

Habilitation

Cerebral palsy is a lifelong disability that has different functional implications at different stages of the life cycle. For families and professionals involved in the care of children with cerebral palsy, the ultimate goal of any treatment or intervention is to maximize functioning while minimizing any disability-related disadvantages. This is accomplished by recognizing the specific abilities and needs of the individual child as they occur within the context of his or her family and community. Habilitation is an intervention strategy that is family focused and community based. Ideally, it is conceived and implemented as a comprehensive program designed to facilitate adaptation to and participation in an increasing number and variety of societal environments, including home, school, clinic, child care, neighborhood, and day treatment programs (Pellegrino, 1995). The ultimate goal of intervention is to enhance participation in these environments and to afford access to new environments in a manner that is mutually satisfying for the individual and the community.

Early Intervention, School, and Therapy

For most children with cerebral palsy, the process of habilitation begins at home under the auspices of state-administered early intervention programs. These programs emphasize involvement of parents so that they can learn effective methods of working with their child (Guralnick, 1998). Programs are individualized according to the specific needs of the child and the family and while emphasizing home-based services may also provide consultative and center-based interventions (see Chapter 33).

For many children with cerebral palsy, entry into preschool represents the first major step into the wider community. Difficulties are often encountered in accommodating the physical, nutritional, and medical needs of these children at this stage. For school-age children, concerns regarding motor function and medical needs continue, but increased attention is focused on concerns related to learning disabilities, attention and behavior problems, intellectual disability, and sensory impairments. For many children, these comorbid conditions, rather than their motor disability, put them at greatest disadvantage relative to their peers.

Children with cerebral palsy have traditionally been segregated into classrooms with designations such as "multiply disabled" and "orthopedically impaired," sometimes without proper regard for their cognitive skills. The trend now, however, is toward inclusion in general education classrooms, which under ideal circumstances can accommodate the needs of children with a range of abilities. Inclusive environments require significant collaboration between the general and special education models and work best when a team of educators and paraprofessionals is associated with each classroom (see Chapter 34).

For children with cerebral palsy, therapy may come in many different forms. Most children receive traditional forms of speech, occupational, and physical therapy. The most common method of motor therapy for the young child with cerebral palsy is **neurodevelopmental therapy (NDT),** an approach employed by both occupational and physical therapists that is designed to provide the child with sensorimotor experiences that enhance the development of more typical movement patterns (see Chapter 37; Campbell, 2000). An individualized program of positioning, therapeutic handling, and play is developed for the child. Program goals include the normalization of tone and the improved control of movement during functional activities. Less traditional therapies, including **hippotherapy** (therapeutic horseback riding) and aquatic therapy (a variation of physical therapy performed in the water) are commonly employed therapeutic options that have mainly anecdotal support for efficacy (Meregillano, 2004). Most therapists utilize an eclectic mix of techniques in the pursuit of improved function and mobility based on the specific set of goals established for a specific child.

Recently, a promising technique known as constraint-induced therapy, or forced-use therapy, has been introduced to help children with hemiplegia cerebral palsy (Taub et al., 2004; Willis et al., 2002). The technique involves "constraining" the more functional arm or hand to force use of the less functional upper extremity. Randomized control trial suggests that the technique may be of significant benefit over traditional therapy alone (Taub et al., 2004).

Physical exercise is important to strengthen muscles and bones, enhance motor skills, and prevent contractures. In addition, the social and recreational aspects of organized physical activities can be highly beneficial (see Chapter 38). Many popular activities, including swimming, dancing, and horseback riding, can be modified so that children with cerebral palsy can participate. In addition, the Special Olympics has enabled thousands of children and young adults with intellectual disabilities to take part in various sporting events. The rewards of engaging in competitive sports are invaluable for enhancing self-esteem and providing a sense of belonging to a peer group. Parents and professionals should encourage all children to participate in whatever physical activities their interests, motivation, and capabilities allow (see Chapter 38).

Bracing, Splinting, and Positioning

Therapists make frequent use of braces and splints (referred to collectively as **orthotic** devices) and positioning devices as aids in the pursuit of functional goals for children with cerebral palsy. These devices are used to maintain adequate range of motion, prevent contractures at specific joints, provide stability, and control involuntary movements that interfere with function. One of the most commonly prescribed orthotics is a short leg brace, known as an ankle-foot **orthosis** (AFO). The AFO stabilizes the position of the foot and provides a consistent stretch to the Achilles tendon (see Chapter 37). A variety of splints may be used to improve hand function. For example, the resting hand splint is commonly used to hold the thumb in an abducted (away from the mid-line) position and the wrist in a neutral or slightly extended position. This helps the child keep his or her hand open, and tends to prevent the development of hand deformities (Figure 37.1). Another type of brace called a body splint is made of a flexible, porous material and controls abnormal tone and involuntary movements by stabilizing the trunk and limbs. Most pediatric braces and splints are custom-made from plastics that are molded directly on the child, so they must be monitored closely and modified as the child grows or changes abilities.

Positioning devices are used to promote skeletal alignment, to compensate for abnormal postures, or to prepare the child for independent mobility (Figure 26.7). Proper positioning geared to the age and functional status of the child is often a key intervention in addressing the tone and movement abnormalities associated with cerebral palsy. For children who must sit for extended periods or who use a wheelchair for mobility, a carefully designed seating system becomes an all-important component of their habilitation. Careful attention to functional seating may also have long-term benefits in the prevention of contractures and joint deformities related to spasticity (Myhr et al., 1995).

Adaptive Equipment

A wide variety of devices is available to aid mobility. For children who are ambulatory, crutches, walkers, and canes may help in the attainment of walking or in improvement of the quality and range of ambulation. The forearm, or Lofstrand, crutch is used in preference to the familiar under-the-arm crutch. A posterior walker (the child is positioned in front of the walker, rather than behind) with wheels is used in preference to a standard forward-position walker without wheels. Canes are used less commonly.

For children with limited walking skills, wheelchairs are essential for maximizing mobility and function. A wheelchair with a solid seat and back is usually recommended. Some children, however, have difficulty using this type of chair unless modifications are made. The addition of head and trunk supports or a tray may be needed for the child who lacks postural control

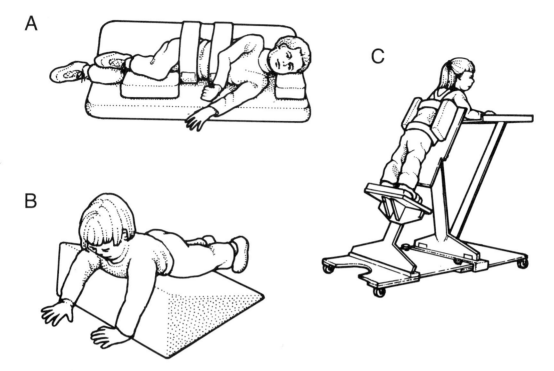

Figure 26.7. a) Child in sidelyer, b) child on prone wedge, and c) child in prone standing device.

due to low tone. The child with limited head control or with feeding difficulties may benefit from a high-backed chair that can be tilted back 10–15 degrees (Figure 26.8a). This helps to maintain the child's body and head in proper alignment.

Special seating cushions or custom-molded inserts that conform to the contours of the body can offer necessary support for the child with orthopedic deformities such as scoliosis. Motorized (power) wheelchairs can enhance the independence of children who are able to use them. Although these usually have an easily manipulated joystick for controlling both speed and direction (Figure 26.8b), other types of switches are available for children who cannot control their hand movements.

Special supportive strollers are an alternative to wheelchairs for mobility within the community or for the young child whose potential for ambulation has yet to be determined. These are lightweight and collapsible yet support the back and keep the hips properly aligned (Figure 26.8c).

Car seats are essential to the safety of all children who ride in automobiles. Several manufacturers offer adapted car seats that meet fed-eral safety guidelines as well as provide proper support for the child with cerebral palsy. Often these models include a base that allows the seat to be used as a stroller or a positioning chair outside of the car. Car beds and special straps are also available for children who have more severe disabilities or who require these special adaptations temporarily (e.g., following surgery).

Assistive Technology

Assistive technology devices are often an important part of the habilitation plan for children with cerebral palsy (see Chapter 36). The technology involved may be as simple as Velcro or as complex as a computer chip. Although it is often true that the simplest intervention is the best, it cannot be denied that the computer has become the hero of assistive technology. Computers can be used to control the environment, provide a lifeline with the outside world, enable a person to work at home, facilitate artificial speech and sight, and provide entertainment. The real potential of this technology to improve the quality of life for children with disabilities is just beginning to be realized. Enthusiasm for its use, however, is tempered by

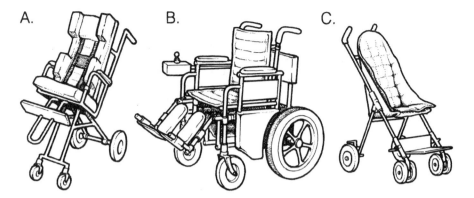

Figure 26.8. Wheelchairs. a) High-backed, tilting chair with lateral inserts and head supports. b) Motorized wheelchair with joystick control. c) Supportive collapsible stroller.

problems with access related to the cost and availability of durable hardware and well-designed software (see Chapter 36).

Managing Spasticity and Dystonia

The motor impairment associated with cerebral palsy is multifaceted, and the specific profile of skills and deficits varies greatly from child to child. The core impairment in all children with cerebral palsy, however, is a significant deficit in motor planning and motor control. Although this deficit is the primary target of therapy, it tends to be refractory to medical interventions. By contrast, specific manifestations of the UMN syndrome associated with cerebral palsy, namely spasticity and dystonia, are amenable to a variety of physical, pharmacologic, and surgical techniques. Spasticity and dystonia therefore represent tempting targets for intervention. A potential pitfall in targeting these symptoms is lack of sufficient care in establishing the connection between the impairments (spasticity or dystonia) and the disability (functional deficits). For some children, it is possible to significantly reduce spasticity or dystonia without improving (and in some cases even worsening) functional outcome. Consultation with experienced professionals who are intimately familiar with a child's particular pattern of skills and impairments is critical to the proper selection specific interventions.

The primary goals in treating spasticity and dystonia are to improve function, to prevent or postpone the musculoskeletal complications attendant to these conditions, and to ease the care of the child with significant muscle tightness. Different treatment options operate at different levels of the neuromotor apparatus (Figure 26.9); treatments may be used singly, sequentially, or simultaneously depending on the specific clinical circumstance. Because dystonia is caused by disturbances in the extrapyramidal component of the motor control system, pharmacological interventions for this condition must operate at the level of the CNS (brain and spinal cord). By contrast, the mechanisms that generate muscle spasticity operate from the level of the CNS down to the level of the muscle itself; a wider variety of therapeutic techniques are therefore available for targeting and modulating the effects of spasticity.

Casting   Tone-reducing, or inhibitive, casts are used in some centers as an adjunct to more traditional methods of managing spasticity (Law et al., 1991). The casts are made for arms or legs and can be designed either for immobilization or to be used during weight-bearing activities. Benefits of inhibitive casting include improved gait and weight bearing, increased range of motion, and improved functional hand use. Casts position the limbs so that spastic muscles are in lengthened positions, being gently stretched. Serial application of casts (serial casting) can allow the therapist to increase range of motion gradually when contractures are present. After maximal range and position have been achieved, a cast is worn intermittently to maintain the improvement. Casting is now most often used in conjunction with other therapeutic modalities, especially following use of botulinum toxin (Glanzman et al., 2004; Kay et al., 2004; Wasiak, Hoare, & Wallen, 2004).

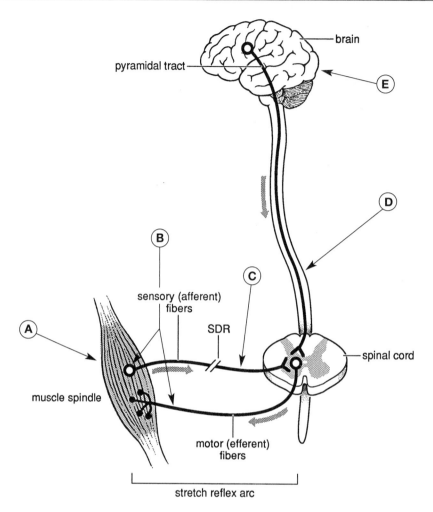

Figure 26.9. Levels of intervention for spasticity and dystonia. a) Inhibitive casting, physical therapy, exercise, and medications such as dantrolene directly affect tone at the muscle level. b) Nerve blocks, motor point blocks, and botulinum toxin work at the level of muscle and nerve entry into muscle. c) Selective dorsal rhizotomy reduces spasticity by interrupting the sensory component of the stretch reflex arc. d) Medications such as baclofen reduce spasticity at the level of the spinal cord. e) Medications for spasticity such as diazepam and medications for dystonia work at the level of the brain. (From Pellegrino, L., & Dormans, J.P. [1998]. Definitions, etiology, and epidemiology of cerebral palsy. In J.P. Dormans & L. Pellegrino [Eds.], *Caring for children with cerebral palsy: A team approach* [p. 46]. Baltimore: Paul H. Brookes Publishing Co.; adapted by permission.)

Nerve Blocks, Motor Point Blocks, and Botulinum Toxin Several injectable agents are available that can be used to target spasticity in particular muscle groups. Local anesthetic agents injected into the nerves that supply spastic muscles produce a temporary, reversible conduction block and are used for diagnostic purposes. Longer-lasting effects are achieved by injecting chemical agents, such as diluted alcohol or phenol, which denature muscle and nerve protein at the point of injection. Direct injections of denaturing agents into motor nerves, called **nerve blocks,** are some-

times used but carry the risk of sensory loss due to damaged sensory nerve fibers that are bundled together with motor fibers. A **motor point block** effectively interrupts the nerve supply at the entry site to a spastic muscle without compromising sensation. The main side effect of the procedure is localized pain that may persist for a few days after the injection. Inhibition of spasticity lasts for 4–6 months, and the procedure can be repeated after the initial effect has worn off. This temporary reduction of spasticity allows for more effective application of physical therapy to improve range of motion and function and may make it possible to postpone orthopedic surgery.

Injectable botulinum toxin (Botox) has been introduced as an alternative to motor point blocks and has largely supplanted alcohol and phenol in many clinical applications (Jefferson, 2004; Mooney, Koman, & Smith, 2003; Morton, Hankinson, & Nicholson, 2004; Pidcock, 2004). Botulinum toxin is produced by the bacterium that causes **botulism** and is among the most potent neurotoxins known. It works by blocking the nerve–muscle junction. When the toxin is absorbed into the general circulation (as with botulism), death may result from paralysis of respiratory muscles. Small quantities, however, can be safely injected directly into spastic muscles without significant spread of the toxin into the bloodstream. This results in weakening of the muscle and reduction of spasticity for 3–6 months (the antispastic effects of the injections dissipate over time). Although botulinum toxin is used mainly to treat spasticity in muscles of the limbs and trunk, novel uses, included injection of the salivary glands to reduce drooling (a common problem in many children with cerebral palsy) are now being reported (Jongerius et al., 2004). A large number of studies have demonstrated the efficacy and safety of botulinum toxin as a therapeutic modality in cerebral palsy (Jefferson, 2004; Mooney et al., 2003). Although clarification is still needed regarding the definition of clinical indications and outcomes, the use of injectable botulinum toxin has become a mainstay in the management of spasticity in cerebral palsy and has also found applications for specific types of dystonia (Gordon, 1999).

Oral and Intrathecal Medications

A variety of orally administered medications have been used to improve muscle tone in children with spasticity and rigidity (Krach, 2001). Although no drug has proved helpful for treating choreoathetosis, several drugs used in **Parkinson's disease,** including carbidopa-levodopa (Sinemet) and trihexyphenidyl (Artane), have been helpful for some children with dystonic cerebral palsy. The medications most commonly used to control spasticity and rigidity are diazepam (Valium), baclofen, and dantrolene (Dantrium). Diazepam and its derivative compounds, lorazepam (Ativan) and clonazepam (Klonopin), affect brain control of muscle tone, beginning within half an hour after ingestion and lasting about 4 hours. Withdrawal of these drugs should be gradual, as physical dependency can develop. Side effects include drowsiness and excessive drooling, which may interfere with feeding and speech.

Baclofen has been most commonly used to treat adults with multiple sclerosis and traumatic damage to the spinal cord. Drowsiness, nausea, headache, and low blood pressure are the most common side effects of the oral form of the medication in children with cerebral palsy. About 10% of children treated with baclofen experience side effects unpleasant enough to necessitate discontinuation of the medication. Care must be taken when stopping the medication to gradually taper it, as rapid withdrawal can lead to severe side effects, including hallucinations.

Dantrolene works on muscle cells directly, as a calcium channel blocker, to inhibit their contraction. It is usually given two to three times daily. Side effects include drowsiness, muscle weakness, and increased drooling. A rare side effect of this drug is severe liver damage, so liver function tests should be performed periodically.

Although a variety of additional medications are becoming available for the treatment of spasticity in children with cerebral palsy, most cause problematic side effects similar to those described for diazepam, baclofen, and dantrolene, and none are clearly superior to these medications (Krach, 2001).

Intrathecal baclofen therapy is a newer therapeutic modality that allows for the direct delivery of antispasticity medication (baclofen) into the spinal fluid (intrathecal) space, where it can inhibit motor nerve conduction at the level of the spinal cord (Disabato & Ritchie, 2003; Fitzgerald, Tsegaye, & Vloeberghs, 2004; Tilton, 2004). A disk-shaped pump is placed beneath the skin of the abdomen, and a catheter is tunneled below the skin around to the back, where it is inserted through the lumbar spine into the intrathecal space. The intrathecal medication most often used is baclofen, which is stored in a reservoir in the disk that can be refilled with a needle inserted into the reservoir through the skin. The medication is delivered at a continuous rate that is computer controlled and adjustable. Because the drug is delivered directly to its site of action (the cerebrospinal fluid), much lower dosage may be used to achieve benefit, with a reduced risk of side effects. Improvements in lower extremity, upper extremity, and even oral-motor function have been observed. The main benefit of the method is dramatic reduction in spasticity and adjustable dosing (Fitzgerald et al., 2004). The main disadvantages are fairly common although usually manageable side effects, including hypotonia (low muscle tone), increased seizures in individuals with known epilepsy, sleepiness, and nausea/vomiting (Gilmartin et al., 2000). Complications related to mechanical failures and infection and the need for intensive and reliable medical follow-up are also significant concerns (Murphy, Irwin, & Hoff, 2002).

Selective Dorsal Rhizotomy

Selective posterior rhizotomy is a neurosurgical procedure that reduces spasticity by interrupting the sensory, or afferent, component of the deep tendon (or stretch) reflex. This reflex mechanism is exaggerated in children with spastic forms of cerebral palsy. The surgery reduces spasticity permanently in the legs but not in the arms, so its use is confined mainly to children with spastic diplegia. Uncertainties exist regarding long-term functional outcomes in children who undergo this procedure (Koman et al., 2004).

Another neurosurgical procedure currently under investigation, deep brain stimulation (DBS), has been proposed as a method to reduce choreoathetosis and dystonia associated with some forms of extrapyramidal cerebral palsy. Initial results are promising, but DBS is still in its infancy, and information is lacking regarding its use in children (Krauss et al., 2003).

Managing the Musculoskeletal Complications of Cerebral Palsy

Because of the abnormal or asymmetrical distribution of muscle tone, children who have cerebral palsy are susceptible to the development of joint deformities. The most common of these result from permanent shortening or contracture of one or more groups of muscles around a joint, which limits joint mobility. Orthopedic surgery is done to increase the range of motion by lengthening a tendon, by cutting through muscle or tendon (release), or by moving the point of attachment of a tendon on bone. For example, a partial release or transfer of the hip adductor muscles may improve the child's ability to sit and walk and may lessen the chances of a hip dislocation (Hagglund et al., 2005; Stott, Piedrahita, & American Academy for Cerebral Palsy and Developmental Medicine, 2004). A partial hamstring release, involving the lengthening or transfer of muscles around the knee, also may facilitate sitting and walking. A lengthening of the Achilles tendon at the ankle improves walking (Figure 26.10).

More complicated orthopedic procedures may be required for correction of a dislocated hip. If this is diagnosed when there is a partial dislocation (called **subluxation**), release of the hip adductor muscles alone can be effective (Figure 26.11). If the head of the femur is dislocated more than one third to one half of the way out of a hip joint socket, a more complex procedure, a varus derotational osteotomy, may be necessary. In this operation, the angle of the femur (the thigh bone) is changed surgically to place the head of the femur back into the hip socket (Figure 26.12). In some cases, the hip socket also must be reshaped to ensure that the hip joint remains functional. Sometimes muscle releases or lengthening are performed at the same time as these bony procedures.

For ambulatory children with cerebral palsy, deciding which type of surgery is most

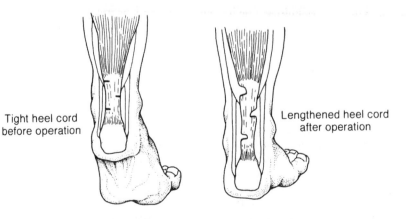

Tight heel cord before operation

Lengthened heel cord after operation

Figure 26.10. Achilles tendon lengthening operation. When the heel cord is tight, the child walks on his or her toes. Surgery lengthens the heel cord and permits a more flat-footed gait.

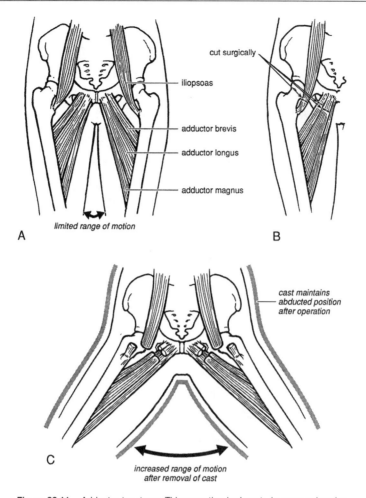

cut surgically

iliopsoas

adductor brevis

adductor longus

adductor magnus

limited range of motion

A

B

cast maintains
abducted position
after operation

C

increased range of motion
after removal of cast

Figure 26.11. Adductor tenotomy. This operation is done to improve scissoring (Figure 26.5) and to prevent hip dislocation caused by contractures of the adductor muscles in the thigh (A). In this procedure, the iliopsoas, adductor brevis, and adductor longus muscles are cut, leaving the adductor magnus intact (B). The child is then placed in a cast for 6–8 weeks to maintain a more open (abducted) position (C). The muscles eventually grow together in a lengthened position, allowing improved sitting and/or walking.

likely to improve function is a complex issue. Computerized gait analysis conducted prior to surgical intervention has become increasingly common as an aid in the decision-making process. Precise measurements obtained through motion analysis, force plates, and electromyography offer detailed information relating to specific abnormalities at each lower extremity joint as well as the muscle activity that controls motion through all phases of the gait (Cook et al., 2003). Such precise definition is not possible through clinical observation alone. Preoperative gait analysis helps to determine exactly which procedures are likely to be successful.

Postoperative analysis can provide an objective measure of outcome.

In addition to treating contractures and dislocations, orthopedic surgeons also are involved in the care of scoliosis, a complication of both spastic and nonspastic forms of cerebral palsy. If untreated, a spinal curvature can interfere with sitting, walking, and self-care skills. If severe enough, it also can affect lung capacity and respiratory efforts. Treatment of significant scoliosis ranges from a molded plastic jacket or a chair insert to invasive surgery to straighten the spine as much as possible. This surgery involves using rods and wires to hold the spine in

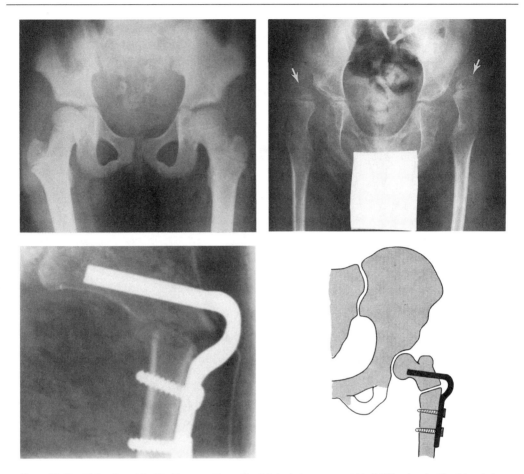

Figure 26.12.　Dislocation of the hip. The upper X rays (frontal view) show a normal hip (left X ray) and a hip dislocated on both sides (right X ray). The arrows indicate the points of dislocation. The lower pictures show the results of a varus derotational osteotomy to correct the left-hip dislocation. The femur has been cut and realigned so that it now fits into the hip socket. Pins, which are later removed, hold the bone in place until it heals.

an improved alignment while bone graft material fuses the spine in position (Figure 26.13).

OUTCOME

Life Expectancy

Although most children with cerebral palsy will live to adulthood, their projected life expectancy is somewhat less than that of the general population (Hemming et al., 2005; Katz, 2003). Outcome varies for each type of cerebral palsy. A child with mild left hemiplegia probably will have a typical life span, whereas a child with spastic quadriplegia may not live beyond age 40 (Strauss & Shavelle, 2001). Children with very severe impairments, measured in terms of functional characteristics, have the poorest outcome. For example, children who cannot lift their

heads and are fed via gastrostomy tube may not survive to adulthood (Strauss, Shavelle, & Anderson, 1998). Excess mortality for people with cerebral palsy may also be due to factors not directly connected with the cerebral palsy itself. Rates of mortality due to breast cancer, brain tumors, circulatory and digestive diseases, and accidents are higher for people with cerebral palsy than for the general population, suggesting that inadequate medical surveillance and psychosocial issues may play roles in excess mortality (Cooley & American Academy of Pediatrics, 2004; Strauss, Cable, & Shavelle, 1999).

Walking

When a child is first diagnosed with cerebral palsy, one of the first questions that arises in the minds of parents is whether their child will

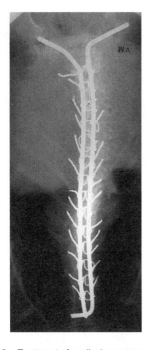

Figure 26.13. Treatment of scoliosis may require spinal fusion. This X ray shows improved scoliosis following a Luque procedure. During this surgery, the position of the spine is improved using metal hooks, rods, and wires while bone graft material fuses the spine in position.

eventually be able to walk. In addressing this question, it is important to recognize that "walking" can refer to several levels of ability. A child may be able to walk independently or may need crutches or a walker. A child may be able to walk long distances (community ambulation), short distances only (household ambulation), or only in the context of therapy (exercise ambulation). In general, children with better motor skills at a younger age (e.g., being able to sit and pull-to-stand before 2 years of age) have a better prognosis for walking than those with less well-developed skills. Recent research has provided greater specificity to this observation. For example, the previously described Gross Motor Function Classification System (GMFCS) can be used to estimate prognosis for walking (Rosenbaum et al., 2002; Wood & Rosenbaum, 2000). Children at any given level within the classification scheme tend to stay at that same level. In general, children at GMFCS Level of I or II will have a good prognosis for some degree of independent walking, children at Levels III and IV with have a variable prognosis for walking with some form of assistance, and children at Level V have a poor prognosis for any type of walking. Precise probability curves for ambulation have been published that allow even more

exact predictions of ambulatory potential based on motor functioning at 2½ years of age (Wu et al., 2004). For example, using these curves it can be predicted that a child who is able to roll, sit, and pull-to-stand at 2½ years of age has a greater than 70% probability of being able to engage in some form of ambulation at age 7 years. By contrast, a child who can roll but cannot sit or pull-to-stand at 2½ years has approximately a 25% chance of walking and would most likely do this with the help of an **assistive device.**

Societal Independence

The ability to participate independently and effectively in a variety of societal settings is a complex function of a child's profile of abilities and disabilities but is also affected by environmental factors (e.g., family, neighborhood, economic) and by a child's health status (Liptak & Accardo, 2004). Motor skills and mobility may not be the primary determinant of societal independence. When asked, parents often identify communication and socialization as the functional areas of greatest concern to them. A child's ability to successfully participate in society is probably more strongly related to cognitive and interpersonal strengths than to physical ability.

Although about half of the individuals who have cerebral palsy have average intelligence, most of these individuals still have difficulty leading completely typical lives (Murphy, Molnar, & Lankasky, 1995). Studies suggest that employability is not related solely to the degree of disability but to a variety of other factors including family support, quality of educational programs, and the availability of community-based training and technical support (Russman & Gage, 1989). In a study of young adults with cerebral palsy (van der Dussen et al., 2001), 75% were fully independent with activities of daily living, 90% moved independently indoors, and 70% moved independently outdoors. The study also found that 77.5% of these individuals had adequate communication for telephone conversation, 30% lived with their parents, 12.5% lived with a partner, and 32.5% lived alone. In addition, 53% had some form of secondary education, but only 36.3% had paid employment. It is hoped that these figures will improve as a result of federal mandates (e.g., the Americans with Disabilities Act [ADA] of 1990, PL 101-336), which define the rights of people with disabilities and are making inroads into societal perceptions of disability. Once society recognizes that functional outcomes are related as much to societal conditions as they are to the characteristics of a particular child with a disability, society's perception of outcome will undergo a major shift. Ultimately, strengthening supports to families (Raina et al., 2005) improving schools, increasing opportunities for employment, and changing attitudes about disabilities in society at large may do as much for children with cerebral palsy as traditional therapy and medical interventions.

SUMMARY

Cerebral palsy is a developmental disability that results from damage to or dysfunction of the developing brain. The impairments associated with cerebral palsy are nonprogressive but permanent. Varying degrees of ability related to functional mobility, daily living skills, and communication/socialization skills result from these impairments. Habilitation is an interdisciplinary strategy that seeks to maximize function and minimize the disadvantage a person experiences as a consequence of disability or societal circumstances. Efforts founded on the principles articulated in the ADA will create new opportunities for greater participation and enhanced quality of life for people with cerebral palsy.

REFERENCES

Accardo, J., Kammann, H., & Hoon, A.H., Jr. (2004). Neuroimaging in cerebral palsy. *The Journal of Pediatrics, 145*(2, Suppl.), S19–S27.

Americans with Disabilities Act (ADA) of 1990, PL 101-336, 42 U.S.C. §§ 12101 *et seq.*

Ancel, P.Y., Livinec, F., Larroque, B., et al. (2006). Cerebral palsy among very preterm children in relation to gestational age and neonatal ultrasound abnormalities: The EPIPAGE cohort study. *Pediatrics, 117*(3), 828–835.

Aneja, S. (2004). Evaluation of a child with cerebral palsy. *Indian Journal of Pediatrics, 71*(7), 627–634.

Ashwal, S., Russman, B.S., Blasco, P.A., et al. (2004). Practice parameter: Diagnostic assessment of the child with cerebral palsy—report of the Quality Standards Subcommittee of the American Academy of Neurology and the Practice Committee of the Child Neurology Society. *Neurology, 62*(6), 851–863.

Bax, M., Goldstein, M., Rosenbaum, P., et al. (2005). Proposed definition and classification of cerebral palsy, April 2005. *Developmental Medicine and Child Neurology, 47*(8), 571–576.

Campbell, S. (Ed.). (2000). *Physical therapy for children* (2nd ed.). Philadelphia: W.B. Saunders.

Carlsson, M., Hagberg, G., & Olsson, I. (2003). Clinical and aetiological aspects of epilepsy in children with cerebral palsy. *Developmental Medicine and Child Neurology, 45*(6), 371–376.

Cook, R.E., Schneider, I., Hazlewood, M.E., et al. (2003). Gait analysis alters decision-making in cerebral palsy. *Journal of Pediatric Orthopedics, 23*(3), 292–295.

Cooley, W.C., & American Academy of Pediatrics Committee on Children with Disabilities. (2004). Providing a primary care medical home for children and youth with cerebral palsy. *Pediatrics, 114*(4), 1106–1113.

Davidson, M.C., Thomas, K.M., & Casey, B.J. (2003). Imaging the developing brain with fMRI. *Mental Retardation and Developmental Disabilities Research Reviews, 9*(3), 161–167.

Disabato, J., & Ritchie, A. (2003). Intrathecal baclofen for the treatment of spasticity of cerebral origin. *Journal for Specialists in Pediatric Nursing, 8*(1), 31–34.

Fitzgerald, J.J., Tsegaye, M., & Vloeberghs, M.H. (2004). Treatment of childhood spasticity of cerebral origin with intrathecal baclofen: A series of 52 cases. *British Journal of Neurosurgery, 18*(3), 240–245.

Gilmartin, R., Bruce, D., Storrs, B.B., et al. (2000). Intrathecal baclofen for management of spastic cerebral palsy: Multicenter trial. *Journal of Child Neurology, 15*(2), 71–77.

Glanzman, A.M., Kim, H., Swaminathan, K., et al. (2004). Efficacy of botulinum toxin A, serial casting, and combined treatment for spastic equinus: A retrospective analysis. *Developmental Medicine and Child Neurology, 46*(12), 807–811.

Gordon, N. (1999). The role of botulinus toxin type A in treatment—with special reference to children. *Brain & Development, 21*(3), 147–151.

Guralnick, M.J. (1998). Effectiveness of early intervention for vulnerable children: A developmental perspective. *American Journal of Mental Retardation, 102*(4), 319–345.

Guzzetta, A., Mercuri, E., & Cioni, G. (2001). Visual disorders in children with brain lesions: 2. Visual impairment associated with cerebral palsy. *European Journal of Paediatric Neurology, 5*(3), 115–119.

Hagberg, B., Hagberg, G., Beckung, E., et al. (2001). Changing panorama of cerebral palsy in Sweden. VIII. Prevalence and origin in the birth year period 1991–94. *Acta Paediatrica, 90*(3), 271–277.

Hagglund, G., Andersson, S., Duppe, H., et al. (2005). Prevention of dislocation of the hip in children with cerebral palsy: The first ten years of a population-based prevention programme. *Journal of Bone and Joint Surgery: British Volume, 87* (1), 95–101.

Hankins, G.D., & Speer, M. (2003). Defining the pathogenesis and pathophysiology of neonatal encephalopathy and cerebral palsy. *Obstetrics and Gynecology, 102*(3), 628–636.

Hemming, K., Hutton, J.L., Colver, A., et al. (2005). Regional variation in survival of people with cerebral palsy in the United Kingdom. *Pediatrics, 116*(6), 1383–1390.

Henderson, R.C., Kairalla, J.A., Barrington, J.W., et al. (2005). Longitudinal changes in bone density in children and adolescents with moderate to severe cerebral palsy. *The Journal of Pediatrics, 146*(6), 769–775.

Henderson, R.C., Lark, R.K., Kecskemethy, H.H., et al. (2002). Bisphosphonates to treat osteopenia in children with quadriplegic cerebral palsy: A randomized, placebo-controlled clinical trial. *The Journal of Pediatrics, 141*(5), 644–651.

Jacobsson, B. (2004). Infectious and inflammatory mechanisms in preterm birth and cerebral palsy. *European Journal of Obstetrics, Gynecology, and Reproductive Biology, 115*(2), 159–160.

Jefferson, R.J. (2004). Botulinum toxin in the management of cerebral palsy. *Developmental Medicine and Child Neurology, 46*(7), 491–499.

Jongerius, P.H., van den Hoogen, F.J., van Limbeek, J., et al. (2004). Effect of botulinum toxin in the treatment of drooling: A controlled clinical trial. *Pediatrics, 114*(3), 620–627.

Katz, R.T. (2003). Life expectancy for children with cerebral palsy and mental retardation: Implications for life care planning. *Neurorehabilitation, 18*(3), 261–270.

Kay, R.M., Rethlefsen, S.A., Fern-Buneo, A., et al. (2004). Botulinum toxin as an adjunct to serial casting treatment in children with cerebral palsy. *Journal of Bone and Joint Surgery: American Volume, 86-A*(11), 2377–2384.

Koman, L.A., Smith, B.P., & Shilt, J.S. (2004). Cerebral palsy. *The Lancet, 363*(9421), 1619–1631.

Krach, L.E. (2001). Pharmacotherapy of spasticity: Oral medications and intrathecal baclofen. *Journal of Child Neurology, 16*(1), 31–36.

Krageloh-Mann, I., Petersen, D., Hagberg, G., et al. (1995). Bilateral spastic cerebral palsy: MRI pathology and origin. Analysis from a representative series of 56 cases. *Developmental Medicine and Child Neurology, 37*, 379–397.

Krauss, J.K., Loher, T.J., Weigel, R., et al. (2003). Chronic stimulation of the globus pallidus internus for treatment of non-dYT1 generalized dystonia and choreoathetosis: 2-year follow up. *Journal of Neurosurgery, 98*(4), 785–792.

Law, M., Cadman, D., Rosenbaum, P., et al. (1991). Neurodevelopmental therapy and upper-extremity inhibitive casting for children with cerebral palsy. *Developmental Medicine and Child Neurology, 33*(5), 379–387.

Leviton, A., & Dammann, O. (2004). Coagulation, inflammation, and the risk of neonatal white matter damage. *Pediatric Research, 55*(4), 541–545.

Liptak, G.S., & Accardo, P.J. (2004). Health and social outcomes of children with cerebral palsy. *The Journal of Pediatrics, 145*(2, Suppl.), S36–S41.

Marlow, N., Wolke, D., Bracewell, M.A., et al. (2005). Neurologic and developmental disability at six years of age after extremely preterm birth. *The New England Journal of Medicine, 352*(1), 9–19.

Meregillano, G. (2004). Hippotherapy. *Physical Medicine and Rehabilitation Clinics of North America, 15*(4), 843–854.

Mohan, K.K., Chugani, D.C., & Chugani, H.T. (1999). Positron emission tomography in pediatric neurology. *Seminars in Pediatric Neurology, 6*(2), 111–119.

Mooney, J.F., Koman, L.A., & Smith, B.P. (2003). Pharmacologic management of spasticity in cerebral palsy. *Journal of Pediatric Orthopedics, 23*(5), 679–686.

Morton, R.E., Hankinson, J., & Nicholson, J. (2004). Botulinum toxin for cerebral palsy: Where are we now? *Archives of Disease in Childhood, 89*(12), 1133–1137.

Murphy, K., Molnar, G., & Lankasky, K. (1995). Medical and functional status of adults with cerebral palsy. *Developmental Medicine and Child Neurology, 37*, 1075–1084.

Murphy, N.A., Irwin, M.C., & Hoff, C. (2002). Intrathecal baclofen therapy in children with cerebral palsy:

Efficacy and complications. *Archives of Physical Medicine and Rehabilitation, 83*(12), 1721–1725.

Myhr, U., von Wendt, L., Norrlin, S., et al. (1995). Five-year follow-up of functional sitting position in children with cerebral palsy. *Developmental Medicine and Child Neurology, 37*(7), 587–596.

Nelson, K.B. (2002). The epidemiology of cerebral palsy in term infants. *Mental Retardation and Developmental Disabilities Research Reviews, 8*(3), 146–150.

Nelson, K.B., & Grether, J.K. (1999). Causes of cerebral palsy. *Current Opinion in Pediatrics, 11*(6), 487–491.

Nelson, K.B., & Lynch, J.K. (2004). Stroke in newborn infants. *The Lancet Neurology, 3*(3), 150–158.

Nordmark, E., Hagglund, G., & Lagergren, J. (2001). Cerebral palsy in southern Sweden II. Gross motor function and disabilities. *Acta Paediatrica, 90*(11), 1277–1282.

Oeffinger, D.J., Tylkowski, C.M., Rayens, M.K., et al. (2004). Gross Motor Function Classification System and outcome tools for assessing ambulatory cerebral palsy: A multicenter study. *Developmental Medicine and Child Neurology, 46*(5), 311–319.

O'Shea, T.M. (2002). Cerebral palsy in very preterm infants: New epidemiological insights. *Mental Retardation and Developmental Disabilities Research Reviews, 8*(3), 135–145.

Palisano, R., Rosenbaum, P., Walter, S., et al. (1997). Development and reliability of a system to classify gross motor function in children with cerebral palsy. *Developmental Medicine and Child Neurology, 39*(4), 214–223.

Palmer, F.B. (2004). Strategies for the early diagnosis of cerebral palsy. *The Journal of Pediatrics, 145*(2, Suppl.), S8–S11.

Pellegrino, L. (1995). Cerebral palsy: A paradigm for developmental disabilities. *Developmental Medicine and Child Neurology, 37*, 834–839.

Pidcock, F.S. (2004). The emerging role of therapeutic botulinum toxin in the treatment of cerebral palsy. *The Journal of Pediatrics, 145*(2, Suppl.), S33–35.

Pschirrer, E.R., & Yeomans, E.R. (2000). Does asphyxia cause cerebral palsy? *Seminars in Perinatology, 24*(3), 215–220.

Raina, P., O'Donnell, M., Rosenbaum, P., et al. (2005). The health and well-being of caregivers of children with cerebral palsy. *Pediatrics, 115*(6), e626–e636.

Reddihough, D.S., & Collins, K.J. (2003). The epidemiology and causes of cerebral palsy. *Australian Journal of Physiotherapy, 49*(1), 7–12.

Rosenbaum, P.L., Walter, S.D., Hanna, S.E., et al. (2002). Prognosis for gross motor function in cerebral palsy: Creation of motor development curves. *Journal of the American Medical Association, 288*(11), 1357–1363.

Russman, B., & Gage, J. (1989). Cerebral palsy. *Current Problems in Pediatrics, 19*, 65–111.

Russman, B.S., & Ashwal, S. (2004). Evaluation of the child with cerebral palsy. *Seminars in Pediatric Neurology, 11*(1), 47–57.

Samson-Fang, L., Fung, E., Stallings, V.A., et al. (2002). Relationship of nutritional status to health and societal participation in children with cerebral palsy. *The Journal of Pediatrics, 141*(5), 637–643.

Shapiro, S.M. (2005). Definition of the clinical spectrum of kernicterus and bilirubin-induced neurologic dysfunction (BIND). *Journal of Perinatology, 25*, 54–59.

Sobrado, P., Suarez, J., Garcia-Sanchez, F.A., (1999). Refractive errors in children with cerebral palsy, psychomotor retardation, and other non-cerebral palsy neuromotor disabilities. *Developmental Medicine and Child Neurology, 41*(6), 396–403.

Stott, N.S., Piedrahita, L., & American Academy for Cerebral Palsy and Developmental Medicine. (2004). Effects of surgical adductor releases for hip subluxation in cerebral palsy: An AACPDM evidence report. *Developmental Medicine and Child Neurology, 46*(9), 628–645.

Strauss, D., Cable, W., & Shavelle, R. (1999). Causes of excess mortality in cerebral palsy. *Developmental Medicine and Child Neurology, 41*(9), 580–585.

Strauss, D., & Shavelle, R. (2001). Life expectancy in cerebral palsy. *Archives of Disease in Childhood, 85*(5), 442.

Strauss, D.J., Shavelle, R.M., & Anderson, T.W. (1998). Life expectancy of children with cerebral palsy. *Pediatric Neurology, 18*(2), 143–149.

Taub, E., Ramey, S.L., DeLuca, S., et al. (2004). Efficacy of constraint-induced movement therapy for children with cerebral palsy with asymmetric motor impairment. *Pediatrics, 113*(2), 305–312.

Tilton, A.H. (2004). Management of spasticity in children with cerebral palsy. *Seminars in Pediatric Neurology, 11*(1), 58–65.

van der Dussen, L., Nieuwstraten, W., Roebroeck, M., et al. (2001). Functional level of young adults with cerebral palsy. *Clinical Rehabilitation, 15*, 84–91.

Vohr, B.R., Msall, M.E., Wilson, D., et al. (2005). Spectrum of gross motor function in extremely low birth weight children with cerebral palsy at 18 months of age. *Pediatrics, 116*(1), 123–129.

Volpe, J.J. (2003). Cerebral white matter injury of the premature infant—more common than you think. *Pediatrics, 112*(1, Pt. 1), 176–180.

Volpe, J.J. (2005). Encephalopathy of prematurity includes neuronal abnormalities. *Pediatrics, 116*(1), 221–225.

Wasiak, J., Hoare, B., & Wallen, M. (2004). Botulinum toxin A as an adjunct to treatment in the management of the upper limb in children with spastic cerebral palsy. *Cochrane Database of Systematic Reviews, 4*, CD003469.

Watts, R., Liston, C., Niogi, S., et al. (2003). Fiber tracking using magnetic resonance diffusion tensor imaging and its applications to human brain development. *Mental Retardation and Developmental Disabilities Research Reviews, 9*(3), 168–177.

Willis, J.K., Morello, A., Davie, A., et al. (2002). Forced use treatment of childhood hemiparesis. *Pediatrics, 110*(1, Pt. 1), 94–96.

Winter, S., Autry, A., Boyle, C., et al. (2002). Trends in the prevalence of cerebral palsy in a population-based study. *Pediatrics, 110*(6), 1220–1225.

Wood, E., & Rosenbaum, P. (2000). The gross motor function classification system for cerebral palsy: a study of reliability and stability over time. *Developmental Medicine and Child Neurology, 42*(5), 292–296.

Wu, Y.W. (2002). Systematic review of chorioamnionitis and cerebral palsy. *Mental Retardation and Developmental Disabilities Research Reviews, 8*(1), 25–29.

Wu, Y.W., Day, S.M., Strauss, D.J., et al. (2004). Prognosis for ambulation in cerebral palsy: A population-based study. *Pediatrics, 114*(5), 1264–1271.

Yoon, B.H., Park, C.W., & Chaiworapongsa, T. (2003). Intrauterine infection and the development of cerebral palsy. *BJOG: An International Journal of Obstetrics and Gynaecology, 110*(Suppl. 20), 124–127.

27 Movement Disorders

W. Bryan Burnette and Harvey S. Singer

Upon completion of this chapter, the reader should be able to

- Define and recognize different types of movement disorders that occur in children
- Understand treatment approaches to and outcomes of several common movement disorders in children
- Recognize certain normal behaviors that are frequently mistaken for movement disorders

---

Movement disorders are common in childhood, with certain types occurring in more than 10% of school-age children (Kurlan et al., 2001). They may occur as a primary disorder or secondary to other disorders of the nervous system such as cerebral palsy or traumatic brain injury. Movement disorders may be mistaken for other episodic disorders that are common in childhood, such as seizures. Furthermore, movements that are within the range of typical childhood behaviors may be misdiagnosed as abnormal, leading to unnecessary testing.

REGGIE

At 7 years of age, Reggie's parents began to notice that he would intermittently tilt his head to the left or right with a sudden, quick motion. Within a few months, they observed the gradual onset of episodic movements, including eye blinking, shoulder shrugging, and twitching at the corner of his mouth. The movements gradually subsided, but Reggie began to frequently clear his throat for no apparent reason. He was seen by his pediatrician, who examined his oropharynx and sent a rapid test for streptococcal infection. His physical examination was normal, and the strep test was negative. The movements and sounds were increased by stress, anxiety, and fatigue, and they seemed better when he was concentrating on other activities. When asked to suppress the throat clearing or the movements, Reggie could do so only briefly.

Reggie's movements were noticed by his teachers and classmates at school, causing hurtful comments from peers and his withdrawal from social activities. More than 1 year after the movements began, Reggie was referred to a child neurologist, who observed Reggie's **tics.** The neurologic examination was otherwise normal. Reggie was diagnosed with Tourette syndrome and started on therapy with clonidine. After a number of dose adjustments, his tics improved. At 9 years of age, Reggie now has many friends in his peer group and is doing well in school.

DEFINITION AND CLASSIFICATION OF MOVEMENT DISORDERS

Movement disorders consist of either 1) a loss or poverty of movement (akinesia) or slowness (bradykinesia) of movement that is not associated with weakness or paralysis, or 2) an excess of abnormal involuntary movements (dyskinesia). Various systems exist for classifying movement disorders. In one approach, disorders are categorized on the basis of whether they are **paroxysmal** (occurring in episodes of sudden onset); transient developmental phenomena (resolving in early childhood); secondary to a noninherited, static injury; or a manifestation of a hereditary or metabolic disorder. Using this system, there is the potential for overlap among categories. For example, tics may occur as a paroxysmal disorder, may be a transient developmental phenomenon, or may be due to a static injury. In another approach, the movement disorder is categorized by the predominant abnormal movement involved.

This chapter uses a combined approach, beginning with a discussion of the common paroxysmal disorders, followed by a description of disorders with specific movements. In each section, an abnormal movement is defined, and examples of disorders in which the movement occurs are discussed. Epidemiology, pathophysiology, genetics, clinical course, and treatment options are presented. This chapter focuses on those disorders likely to be encountered by teachers, therapists, and clinicians. Because of the diverse nature of childhood movement disorders, treatment and outcomes are discussed within each section.

PAROXYSMAL MOVEMENT DISORDERS

Paroxysmal movement disorders, particularly tic disorders, are a relatively common source of referrals to child neurologists. Diagnosis is made by observation, either directly or via videotape, by an experienced clinician. Epilepsy is the other episodic disorder associated with abnormal movements. Seizures may be distinguished from movement disorders on the basis of the types of movements, the presence or absence of alterations in level of awareness, and the presence or absence of abnormalities on electroencephalograms (EEGs). These differences are not universal, however, and distinguishing one problem from the other requires a systematic approach. This distinction is vital, because the treatments for and outcomes of the two types of disorders may be quite different.

Tics

Definition Tics are involuntary, sudden, rapid, repetitive, nonrhythmic movements or vocalizations. They are manifested in a variety of forms, with different durations and degrees of complexity. Simple motor tics are brief, rapid movements that often involve only one muscle group (e.g., eye blink, head jerk, shoulder shrug). Complex motor tics are abrupt movements that involve either a cluster of simple movements or a more coordinated sequence of movements. Complex motor tics may be nonpurposeful (e.g., facial or body contortions) or appear to be more purposeful but actually serve no purpose (e.g., touching, smelling,

jumping, obscene gestures). Simple vocal tics include such sounds as grunting, barking, yelping, and throat clearing. Complex vocalizations may include syllables, phrases, echolalia (repeating the words of others), palilalia (repeating one's own words), or coprolalia (obscene words).

Tic disorders are relatively common in childhood and adolescence, occurring with an estimated prevalence of 6%–12% (Kurlan et al., 2001). The peak prevalence occurs between ages 9–11 years (Snider et al., 2002). Tics are more common in males by a ratio of 3 to 1 and have a higher incidence in winter than in spring (Snider et al., 2002). They are more common in children with attention-deficit/hyperactivity disorder (ADHD; Spencer et al., 1999) and in children who attend special education classes (Kurlan et al., 2001).

Causes Tics may occur as a primary inherited disorder or as a secondary phenomenon that is associated with infection (Northam & Singer, 1991), stroke (Kwak & Jankovic, 2002), head trauma (Krauss & Jankovic, 1997), surgery (Singer et al., 1997), adverse reaction to a medication (Singer, 1981) or toxin (Ko et al., 2004), or as a feature of other sporadic or inherited diseases (Jankovic & Ashizawa, 1995).

Examples Paroxysmal movement disorders include transient tic disorder, chronic tic disorder, Tourette syndrome (TS), and pediatric autoimmune neuropsychiatric disorders associated with streptococcal infection (PANDAS). Each is detailed next.

By definition, transient tic disorder is present for less than 12 months (Singer, 2005). Symptoms may include both motor and vocal tics, which are usually relatively mild. Many cases of transient tic disorder never come to medical attention, so the true incidence of the disorder is difficult to estimate.

Chronic tic disorder can consist of solely motor tics or, less commonly, vocal tics. Symptoms must be present for longer than 12 months. Other features, including treatment, are similar to those in TS, as discussed in the following section.

TS is a chronic, primary tic disorder, characterized by multiple motor tics and at least one vocal tic (Singer, 2005). Current diagnostic criteria also require that symptoms begin by 21 years of age, last for longer than 1 year, and are not secondary to a drug, infection or other disorder. Tics should be diagnosed by a knowledgeable individual (The Tourette Syndrome

Classification Study Group, 1993). TS occurs with a prevalence of 1–10 in 1,000 children and adolescents (Kurlan et al., 2001). The disorder usually presents with onset of motor tics at 6–7 years of age, with later onset of vocal tics. Early in the course, it is often misdiagnosed as asthma or allergies because the child has a chronic cough or throat clearing or has dermatitis because of frequent scratching (Jankovic & Sekula, 1998). Coprolalia, one of the more easily recognized and distressing symptoms of TS, occurs in only 10% of patients (Goldenberg, Brown, & Weiner, 1994). As with other tic disorders, the frequency, quality, and severity of tics waxes and wanes over time.

The etiology of TS is incompletely understood. Strong concordance in monozygotic twins suggests that it is an inherited disorder (Price et al., 1985), but the pattern of inheritance is unclear. Extensive studies have failed to identify a single gene or set of genes responsible for the syndrome. The anatomic substrate underlying TS is believed to involve neuronal circuits that communicate among the prefrontal cerebral cortex, the basal ganglia, and the thalamus (Berardelli et al., 2003). Regional abnormalities in the function of various neurotransmitters within these areas of the brain have been hypothesized to play a role in the disorder. In particular, dopamine has been implicated by evidence from various anatomic and neurochemical studies (Wolf et al., 1996) and by the response of TS to certain medications that modify dopamine activity in the brain.

TS is frequently associated with behavioral abnormalities, particularly obsessive-compulsive behaviors (Robertson, Trimble, & Lees, 1989) and ADHD (Coffey & Park, 1997). These comorbidities are often more disabling than the tics themselves. Obsessive-compulsive behaviors occur in 20%–60% of children with TS. They are more common in this population than full-spectrum obsessive-compulsive disorder (OCD), the diagnosis of which requires a major impact on daily activities or symptoms for greater than 1 hour per day. In children with TS, obsessive-compulsive behaviors often manifest as self-injurious activities such as biting, scratching, or hitting (Jankovic & Sekula, 1998). ADHD affects approximately half of children with TS (Comings & Comings, 1987) and usually presents 2–3 years before the onset of tics. The coexistence of ADHD in children with TS increases the degree of functional impairment (Abwender et al., 1996).

PANDAS is the name given to a clinical entity initially described in 1998 (Swedo et al., 1998), the existence of which is still debated (Kurlan & Kaplan, 2004). The concept of PANDAS initially derived from the observation that certain children with tic disorders, OCD, or both had acute exacerbations of their symptoms around the time of an infection with Group A beta-hemolytic *streptococcus* (GABHS). The proposed etiology of PANDAS is similar to that of Sydenham's chorea (Husby et al., 1976), in that infection stimulates the production of antibodies against portions of GABHS that cross-react to neuronal antigens within the basal ganglia and cause symptoms. Although a limited study of immunomodulatory therapy for children diagnosed with PANDAS supported this hypothesis (Perlmutter et al., 1999), attempts to differentiate the antibody profiles of affected children from those of various control groups (Church, Dale, & Giovannoni, 2004) and to reproduce PANDAS in an animal model (Loiselle et al., 2004) have produced mixed results. Because symptoms fluctuate in both tic disorders and OCD, association of GABHS infection with the onset or exacerbation of symptoms is difficult to establish, and prospective epidemiologic studies have failed to uniformly show such a link between GABHS infection and tics or OCD (Perrin et al., 2004).

Treatment   Although there is no cure for tic disorders, a variety of medications are effective in suppressing tics. Rather than focusing on the complete elimination of tics (which may not be possible or may require drug dosages with significant side effects), therapy is directed at achieving a degree of control that minimizes impairment and addresses comorbidities. For mild tics, medications such as clonidine (Catapres) (Gaffney et al., 2002), guanfacine (Tenex) (Scahill et al., 2001), baclofen (Singer et al., 2001), and clonazepam (Klonopin) (Gonce & Barbeau, 1977) are generally effective (see Appendix C). More severe tics are treated with agents that act on dopamine receptors within the brain, such as the classic neuroleptics pimozide (Orap), fluphenazine (Prolixin), or haloperidol (Haldol). Newer, or atypical, neuroleptics, such as risperidone (Risperdal) (Gilbert et al., 2004), olanzapine (Zyprexa) (Stephens, Bassel, & Sandor, 2004), ziprasidone (Geodon) (Sallee et al., 2000), and quetiapine (Seroquel) (Mukaddes & Abali, 2003), effectively suppress tics with fewer side effects than the classic neuroleptics. Botulinum toxin (Botox) has been successfully used in the treatment of motor and vocal tics in small numbers of patients (Trimble et al., 1998) but is not yet in widespread use.

Various behavioral therapies have been proposed as treatment for TS, but few have been adequately assessed (Bergin et al., 1998). Adjustments in the school environment, however, may improve motivation and self-esteem in children with TS (Marras et al., 2001).

Coexistent obsessive-compulsive behaviors are treated with selective serotonin reuptake inhibitors, such as fluoxetine (Prozac), sertraline (Zoloft), and fluvoxamine (Luvox). These medications are effective, well-tolerated (Flament & Bisserbe, 1997), and do not exacerbate tics. ADHD is managed with stimulant medications, such as methylphenidate (Ritalin, Concerta, Metadate CD, Focalin), dextroamphetamine, or mixed amphetamine salts (Adderall); with the nonstimulant atomoxetine (Strattera); or with alpha-adrenergic agonists such as clonidine or guanfacine (Tourette's Syndrome Study Group, 2002). Prior concerns about stimulants exacerbating tics appear to be unfounded (Kurlan, 2003).

Although the severity of tics in TS waxes and wanes, long-term studies reveal that the maximum severity occurs at 8–12 years of age, followed by a steady improvement in symptoms in adolescence (Leckman et al., 1998). By ages 18–24 years, more than 70% of individuals with TS subjectively report either a substantial decrease or complete cessation of tics (Erenberg, Cruse, & Rothner, 1987). When a group of 58 adults diagnosed with TS in childhood or adolescence were assessed objectively, however, 90% continued to have tics, even though the majority subjectively reported to the contrary (Pappert et al., 2003). Severity of tics early in the course does not predict later severity (Leckman et al., 1998). Comorbid behavioral disturbances increase the degree of impairment, regardless of tic severity (Channon et al., 2003).

Stereotypies

Stereotypies are involuntary, patterned, purposeless, repetitive, rhythmic movements (e.g., recurrent arm flapping, handwaving/rotating, finger wiggling, body rocking, leg shaking, and mouth opening). Stereotypic movements have been inaccurately assumed to be strictly associated with intellectual disability, autism spectrum disorders, schizophrenia, **tardive dyskinesia,** and neurodegenerative diseases. These

movements need to be differentiated from other conditions such as habits, mannerisms, compulsions, and complex motor tics (Mahone et al., 2004). Pharmacotherapy is generally not beneficial, whereas habit reversal behavior management therapy may diminish movements (Miller et al., 2006).

DISORDERS ASSOCIATED WITH SPECIFIC MOVEMENT ABNORMALITIES

Choreoathetosis

Definition *Chorea* is the term given to flowing, continuous, unsustained, rapid, random, abrupt, irregular, nonstereotyped movements that are usually bilateral and affect all parts of the body (face, trunk, and limbs) (O'Brien, 1998). The timing, direction, and distribution of movements vary from moment to moment. In contrast, athetosis describes slower, often continuous, more writhing activities that predominantly involve the distal extremities (legs), with a rotatory component about the long axis of the limb that is often accompanied by spooning or hyperextension and flexion of the digits. In addition, the neck, face, and trunk are frequently involved, and dysarthria is characteristic. Because chorea and athetosis usually overlap in children, *choreoathetosis* is the commonly utilized term.

Causes In childhood, the most common causes of chorea are cerebral palsy, drug-induced chorea, and Sydenham's chorea. Choreoathetosis in the setting of cerebral palsy is discussed in Chapter 26. Chorea may be a side effect of medications, especially dopamine antagonists (Janavs & Aminoff, 1998). Chorea also may occur secondary to the use of antiepileptic drugs, such as phenytoin (Dilantin) and ethosuximide (Zarontin); oral contraceptives; or stimulants used in the treatment of ADHD.

Dystonia

Definition Dystonia involves the simultaneous contraction of both agonist and antagonist muscles, resulting in a distorted posture of the face, limbs, or trunk. A balanced contracture produces a fixed posture, whereas one that is unbalanced causes a slow movement of a body part that often ends in a fixed extreme posture. Torticollis (wry neck) is a sustained deviation of the head toward one side. The term *torticollis* describes a lateral head movement, whereas antecollis and retrocollis indicate forward or backward movements, respectively. Dystonic movements may occur spontaneously or may be precipitated or made worse by posture or voluntary movement. Factors that tend to make dystonia worse include stress, fatigue, or startle, whereas sleep or distraction may lead to improvement. A *geste antagoniste*, or sensory trick, such as touching an affected body part, may also improve symptoms of dystonia.

Dystonia is classified on the basis of the body parts involved, age of onset, and etiology or genetic defect (Fahn, Bressman, & Marsden, 1998). Focal dystonia involves a single body region. Examples include blepharospasm (involuntary tight closure of the eyelids associated with excessive blinking), torticollis, graphospasm ("writer's cramp"), or foot twisting. Segmental dystonia affects contiguous body regions (e.g., torticollis and writer's cramp). Multifocal dystonia affects noncontiguous regions (e.g., an arm and a leg). Generalized dystonia involves both legs and at least one other body region. Early onset dystonia, which begins before 28 years of age, typically starts in a limb and tends to become generalized; late onset dystonia starts after age 28 years, usually begins in the head, neck, or an arm, and tends to spread regionally rather than becoming generalized.

Causes Primary dystonias lack other neurological deficits and are distinguished from secondary dystonias by the absence of birth injury, stroke, or drug reaction. Advances in molecular physiology and genetics have led to the discovery of specific etiologies for these disorders, a group of which have been labeled DYT 1-13 after the involved genes. The overall prevalence of childhood dystonia is unknown, but generalized dystonia has a prevalence of approximately 1.4 per 100,000.

Examples Dopa-responsive dystonia (DRD, DYT5) is a childhood-onset primary generalized dystonia. Most cases are accounted for by various mutations in the gene encoding the enzyme guanosine triphosphate cyclohydrolase I (GCH-I) on chromosome 14 (Ichinose et al., 1994), although some cases are associated with abnormalities in the enzyme tyrosine hydroxylase (TH). DRD due to GCH-I is usually transmitted in an autosomal dominant pattern with a penetrance (the proportion of carriers of

the mutation who develop the disease) of approximately 30% (Nygaard et al., 1990). Penetrance is higher in females, leading to a female predominance of the disorder. New mutations are common, and a significant proportion of patients with DRD have no known mutation (Furukawa & Kish, 1999).

There is considerable variability in the manifestations of DRD, but a common presentation is that of a child 5–6 years of age with abnormal posturing of a single leg or foot, leading to a gait disturbance. Posturing gradually worsens over the course of 10–15 years, spreading to involve all extremities in an asymmetric fashion (Segawa, Nomura, & Nishiyama, 2003). More than half of the patients demonstrate diurnal fluctuation, with symptoms worsening through the day and improving in the morning after sleep. Patients commonly have brisk tendon reflexes on examination and may show an extensor plantar response (Babinski sign) without true spasticity. A variant form of DRD is associated with familial spastic paraparesis, a hereditary disorder that manifests as slowly progressive lower extremity weakness and spasticity (Furukawa et al., 2001). DRD may also present with parkinsonian features, such as bradykinesia (slowed movements), rigidity, masked facies, and postural instability. These findings may lead to an incorrect diagnosis of juvenile Parkinson's disease (JPD), a disorder in which rigidity is also a prominent feature. JPD can be distinguished clinically from DRD in that it lacks the diurnal symptom fluctuations characteristic of DRD. The progression of symptoms of DRD tends to slow over time, with most individuals reaching a plateau in the fourth decade of life. The hallmark of DRD is a dramatic and sustained response to levodopa. Patients with later symptom onset may require larger doses to produce a desirable clinical response (Furukawa et al., 1998). A good response to the anticholinergic medication trihexyphenidyl (Artane) has also been reported (Jarman et al., 1997). A number of tests have been developed to diagnose DRD, including genetic testing; measurement of cerebrospinal fluid levels of biopterin, neopterin, or neurotransmitter metabolites; and phenylalanine loading.

Idiopathic torsion dystonia (ITD)—also known as primary torsion dystonia, dystonia musculorum deformans, or Oppenheim's dystonia—is a childhood-onset primary generalized dystonia associated with a known genetic defect. It is transmitted in an autosomal dominant pattern with a penetrance of about 30%–

40% (Risch et al., 1990). This leads to considerable variability in the severity of the disorder among patients, even within the same family. In 90% of Ashkenazi Jews, and in 50%–60% of other populations, ITD results from a deletion in the DYT1 gene. DYT1, located on chromosome 9q34.1, encodes the protein torsin A. The function of torsin A is unknown, but evidence suggests that it has a role in intracellular trafficking and may be important in the transport of vesicles to the presynaptic terminal (Breakefield, Kamm, & Hanson, 2001). The prevalence of the DYT1 gene defect is 1 in 2,000 in Jews of Ashkenazi ancestry (Risch et al., 1995). Symptoms usually begin around 9–12 years of age with action-induced dystonia in a limb, most often a leg. In the majority of individuals, dystonia generalizes over about 5 years. Patients with earlier onset and onset in a lower extremity tend to be more severely affected and frequently lose the ability to walk independently. Diagnosis is made by commercially available genetic testing for the deletion in the DYT1 gene in an individual with a consistent clinical presentation.

Treatment No pharmacologic therapy has consistently shown efficacy in idiopathic torsion dystonia. A trial of levodopa is often given before confirmation of the genetic abnormality, as this medication is highly effective in the treatment of DRD. Medications used to treat ITD include anticholinergic medications, baclofen, clonazepam, and botulinum toxin. Improvement with deep brain stimulation of the globus pallidus in a small number of individuals has also been reported (Coubes et al., 2000).

Tremor

Definition Tremor is a rhythmic, regular oscillation of one or more body parts produced by alternating or synchronous contractions of opposing muscles. Tremors are categorized according to whether they occur at rest, with the affected body part in complete repose and fully supported, or with action. The most common is physiologic tremor, which occurs in all people, and is usually barely detectable. It is a low-amplitude, short-duration postural tremor that has a frequency of less than 6 Hz in childhood, increasing to around 12 Hz by adolescence, and decreasing to approximately 6 Hz after age 70 (Young et al., 1975). Resting tremor is usually seen in Parkinsonism, which is rare in childhood. Resting tremor can occur in dopa-responsive dystonia, JPD, brain tumors, as a drug effect, and in a number of neurodegenerative disorders.

Causes A number of factors can enhance physiologic tremor, including anxiety, hyperthyroidism, and stimulants. Physiologic tremor rarely interferes with activities of daily living and is not a pathologic condition. Physiologic tremor requires no specific therapy other than, if possible, removal or avoidance of the inciting factor. Other causes of tremor are discussed separately in sections devoted to specific disorders.

Example Essential tremor (ET) is the most common movement disorder in adults. It is much less common in children, with the mean age of onset being 8 years but with cases reported as early as 2 years (Louis, Dure, & Pullman, 2001). It has a male predominance in children. Although several lines of evidence support the hypothesis that ET is a genetic disorder, the finding of only a 60% concordance rate in monozygotic twins (Tanner et al., 2001) suggests an additional role for environmental factors in its pathogenesis. No structural or biochemical abnormalities have been described, although the cerebellum has been proposed as a site of involvement (Bucher et al., 1997). ET usually presents as a gradual-onset postural tremor of the upper extremities, which is exacerbated by stress or anxiety. Affected children frequently develop a kinetic tremor, which may interfere with activities such as writing or eating with utensils. In contrast to adults with ET, in whom other neurologic abnormalities such as mild impairments in gait and cognition have been described (Lombardi et al., 2001), no other associated signs occur in children.

Treatment The diagnosis of ET is made on clinical grounds. A tremor resembling ET may be caused by a variety of metabolic disturbances, infections, and other conditions; these should be ruled out before treatment for ET occurs. ET may cause significant functional or social impairment. Pharmacologic therapy should be considered in such cases, but in general, medications used have only modest efficacy in controlling tremor. These include the antiepileptic drug primidone (Mysoline) and the beta blocker propranolol (Inderal). Other antiepileptic drugs, such as gabapentin (Neurontin), topiramate (Topamax), and clonazepam (Klonopin) are also given, but evidence to support their use is limited. Botulinum toxin has been used (Warrick et al., 2000; Wissel et al., 1997) but may cause undesired muscle weakness in the hands.

Myoclonus

Definition Myoclonus describes sudden, brief muscle contractions that produce a simple, quick movement. Jerks may be random and unpredictable, or rarely, repetitive and rhythmic. Myoclonus may occur spontaneously, with voluntary movement (action myoclonus), or in response to a stimulus (stimulus-sensitive or reflex myoclonus). Action myoclonus may be particularly disabling.

Myoclonus is classified clinically on the basis of body parts affected (i.e., focal, segmental, multifocal, or generalized), relation to activity (e.g., action myoclonus), or etiology. Myoclonus may also be classified by the site of origin within the nervous system (i.e., cortex, thalamus, brainstem, spinal cord).

Causes Myoclonus may occur as a normal physiologic phenomenon, may occur in association with epilepsy (see Chapter 29), or may be nonepileptic. Many of these disorders are associated with severe disability and significant morbidity.

Example Essential myoclonus is characterized by jerking that may be focal, segmental, or generalized; is exacerbated by stress or by action; and involves the face, trunk, and proximal limbs. Symptoms begin in the first two decades of life, and there is no gender predominance. The disorder may occur sporadically, or it may be inherited in an autosomal dominant pattern. Diagnosis is based on the clinical characteristics and the absence of other associated neurologic abnormalities. Clonazepam is particularly useful for decreasing both the abnormal movements and associated anxiety.

Treatment Pharmacologic treatment of myoclonus should be considered for children who experience disruption in activities of daily living or impairment in social interactions. Treatment of symptomatic myoclonus, when possible, is directed at the underlying cause. Many forms of myoclonus are effectively treated with antiepileptic drugs, such as benzodiazepines (clonazepam [Klonopin], valproate (Depakote), levetiracetam (Keppra), or primidone, regardless of whether the movements are related to epilepsy.

NORMAL MOVEMENTS OFTEN MISTAKENLY CONSIDERED ABNORMAL

There are a number of movements observed in otherwise typically developing children that are a part of normal development. These movements may cause concern to parents and may lead to evaluation by a pediatrician or child neurologist. It is important that the movements be recognized as normal variants in order to provide reassurance to families and to avoid unnecessary testing. The list of phenomena described next is by no means exhaustive, but it gives the reader an idea of the wide variety of normal movements in children.

Habits are part of a repertoire of coordinated movements seen in otherwise typically developing children (e.g., thumb sucking and body rocking in the young child, nail biting and foot tapping in older children). These activities tend to increase during periods of anxiety, stress, fatigue, or boredom.

Mannerisms are gestures or individual flourishes/embellishments that are added to a normal activity (e.g., a baseball player's routine while awaiting a pitch). These movements, which are unique to the individual, are rarely repetitive, do not appear in clusters, are of brief duration, and are less complex than stereotypies.

Periodic head nodding, consisting of repetitive flexion of the neck, can be seen in otherwise typically developing young children (Hottinger-Blanc, Ziegler, & Deonna, 2002). Movements may be vertical (yes-yes), horizontal (no-no), or oblique and may occur when children are sitting or standing. In many cases, the movements resolve within a few months but may persist as a stereotypy. Head nodding may also occur with other stereotypies, and in children with a family history of ET (DiMario, 2000). Development is typical in these children. Head nodding should be distinguished from the "bobble-head doll" syndrome, which presents in infants and young children as intermittent jerky head movements, resembling those of a doll's head perched atop a spring, with a frequency ranging from two to three cycles per second. This syndrome is often associated with cysts or dilatation of the third ventricle seen on neuroimaging. Movements usually resolve after surgical treatment (Hagebeuk et al., 2005).

Shuddering (shivering) is characterized by flexion of the head, elbows, trunk and knees with adduction of the arms and legs. Parents describe their child as having a chill.

SUMMARY

Movement disorders are common in childhood, occurring with a frequency comparable to seizures. They are quite heterogeneous in terms of etiology, manifestations, and outcomes. In contrast to epilepsy, no single, universally accepted classification scheme exists for movement disorders. They may be categorized on the basis of the nature of the disorder (paroxysmal, transient, due to a static injury, or related to a metabolic disorder), or by the type of abnormal movements observed (tics, choreoathetosis, dystonia, tremor, or myoclonus). Many movements observed in children are typical developmental phenomena. Movement disorders are unique in that they require direct observation by an experienced clinician in order to be appropriately identified and treated. Effective therapies are available for many childhood movement disorders (e.g., tic disorders, DRD), and many disorders improve or remit spontaneously over time. Nevertheless, significant functional or psychosocial impairment may occur in the absence of appropriate diagnosis and management.

REFERENCES

Abwender, D.A., Como, P.G., Kurlan, R., et al. (1996). School problems in Tourette's syndrome. *Archives of Neurology, 53*, 509–511.

Berardelli, A., Curra, A., Fabbrini, G., et al. (2003). Pathophysiology of tics and Tourette syndrome. *Journal of Neurology, 250*, 781–787.

Bergin, A., Waranch, H.R., Brown, J., et al. (1998). Relaxation therapy in Tourette syndrome: A pilot study. *Pediatric Neurology, 18*, 136–142.

Breakefield, X.O., Kamm, C., & Hanson, P.I. (2001). Torsin A: Movement at many levels. *Neuron, 31*, 9–12.

Bucher, S.F., Seelos, K.C., Dodel, R.C., et al. (1997). Activation mapping in essential tremor with functional magnetic resonance imaging. *Annals of Neurology, 41*, 32–40.

Channon, S., Crawford, S., Vakili, K., et al. (2003). Real-life-type problem solving in Tourette syndrome. *Cognitive and Behavioral Neurology, 16*, 3–15.

Church, A.J., Dale, R.C., & Giovannoni, G. (2004). Anti-basal ganglia antibodies: A possible diagnostic utility in idiopathic movement disorders? *Archives of Disease in Childhood, 89*, 611–614.

Coffey, B.J., & Park, K.S. (1997). Behavioral and emotional aspects of Tourette syndrome. *Neurologic Clinics, 15*, 277–289.

Comings, D.E., & Comings, B.G. (1987). A controlled study of Tourette syndrome: I. Attention-deficit disorder, learning disorders, and school problems. *American Journal of Human Genetics, 41*, 701–741.

Coubes, P., Roubertie, A., Vayssiere, N., et al. (2000). Treatment of DYT1-generalised dystonia by stimula-tion of the internal globus pallidus. *The Lancet, 355*, 2220–2221.

DiMario, F.J., Jr. (2000). Childhood head tremor. *Journal of Child Neurology, 15*, 22–25.

Egger, J., Grossmann, G., & Auchterlonie, I.A. (2003). Benign sleep myoclonus in infancy mistaken for epilepsy. *British Medical Journal, 326*, 975–976.

Erenberg, G., Cruse, R.P., & Rothner, A.D. (1987). The natural history of Tourette syndrome: A follow-up study. *Annals of Neurology, 22*, 383–385.

Fahn, S., Bressman, S.B., & Marsden, C.D. (1998). Classification of dystonia. *Advances in Neurology, 78*, 1–10.

Flament, M.F., & Bisserbe, J.C. (1997). Pharmacologic treatment of obsessive-compulsive disorder: Comparative studies. *Journal of Clinical Psychiatry, 58*(Suppl. 12), 18–22.

Furukawa, Y., Graf, W.D., Wong, H., et al. (2001). Dopa-responsive dystonia simulating spastic paraplegia due to tyrosine hydroxylase (TH) gene mutations. *Neurology, 56*, 260–263.

Furukawa, Y., & Kish, S.J. (1999). Dopa-responsive dystonia: Recent advances and remaining issues to be addressed. *Movement Disorders, 14*, 709–715.

Furukawa, Y., Shimadzu, M., Hornykiewicz, O., et al. (1998). Molecular and biochemical aspects of hereditary progressive and dopa-responsive dystonia. *Advances in Neurology, 78*, 267–282.

Gaffney, G.R., Perry, P.J., Lund, B.C., et al. (2002). Risperidone versus clonidine in the treatment of children and adolescents with Tourette's syndrome. *Journal of the American Academy of Child and Adolescent Psychiatry, 41*, 330–336.

Gilbert, D.L., Batterson, J.R., Sethuraman, G., et al. (2004). Tic reduction with risperidone versus pimozide in a randomized, double-blind, crossover trial. *Journal of the American Academy of Child and Adolescent Psychiatry, 43*, 206–214.

Goldenberg, J.N., Brown, S.B., & Weiner, W.J. (1994). Coprolalia in younger patients with Gilles de la Tourette syndrome. *Movement Disorders, 9*, 622–625.

Gonce, M., & Barbeau, A. (1977). Seven cases of Gilles de la Tourette's syndrome: Partial relief with clonazepam: A pilot study. *The Canadian Journal of Neurological Sciences, 4*, 279–283.

Hagebeuk, E.E., Kloet, A., Grotenhuis, J.A., et al. (2005). Bobble-head doll syndrome successfully treated with an endoscopic ventriculocystocisternostomy. *Journal of Neurosurgery, 103*(3, Suppl.), 253–259.

Hottinger-Blanc, P.M., Ziegler, A.L., & Deonna, T. (2002). A special type of head stereotypies in children with developmental (?cerebellar) disorder: Description of 8 cases and literature review. *European Journal of Paediatric Neurology, 6*, 143–152.

Husby, G., van de Rijn, I., Zabriskie, J.B., et al. (1976). Antibodies reacting with cytoplasm of subthalamic and caudate nuclei neurons in chorea and acute rheumatic fever. *The Journal of Experimental Medicine, 144*, 1094–1110.

Ichinose, H., Ohye, T., Takahashi, E., et al. (1994). Hereditary progressive dystonia with marked diurnal fluctuation caused by mutations in the GTP cyclohydrolase I gene. *Nature Genetics, 8*, 236–242.

Janavs, J.L., & Aminoff, M.J. (1998). Dystonia and chorea in acquired systemic disorders. *Journal of Neurology, Neurosurgery, and Psychiatry, 65*, 436–445.

Jankovic, J., & Ashizawa, T. (1995). Tourettism associated with Huntington's disease. *Movement Disorders, 10*, 103–105.

Jankovic, J., & Sekula, S. (1998). Dermatological manifestations of Tourette syndrome and obsessive-compulsive disorder. *Archives of Dermatology, 134,* 113–114.

Jarman, P.R., Bandmann, O., Marsden, C.D., et al. (1997). GTP cyclohydrolase I mutations in patients with dystonia responsive to anticholinergic drugs. *Journal of Neurology Neurosurgery, and Psychiatry, 63,* 304–308.

Ko, S., Ahn, T., Kim, J., et al. (2004). A case of adult onset tic disorder following carbon monoxide intoxication. *The Canadian Journal of Neurological Sciences, 31,* 268–270.

Krauss, J., & Jankovic, J. (1997). Tics secondary to craniocerebral trauma. *Movement Disorders, 12,* 776–782.

Kurlan, R. (2003). Tourette's syndrome: Are stimulants safe? *Current Neurology and Neuroscience Reports, 3,* 285–288.

Kurlan, R., & Kaplan, E.L. (2004). The pediatric autoimmune neuropsychiatric disorders associated with streptococcal infection (PANDAS) etiology for tics and obsessive-compulsive symptoms: Hypothesis or entity? Practical considerations for the clinician. *Pediatrics, 113,* 883–886.

Kurlan, R., McDermott, M.P., Deeley, C., et al. (2001). Prevalence of tics in schoolchildren and association with placement in special education. *Neurology, 57,* 1383–1388.

Kwak, C.H., & Jankovic, J. (2002). Tourettism and dystonia after subcortical stroke. *Movements Disorders, 17,* 821–825.

Leckman, J.F., Zhang, H., Vitale, A., et al. (1998). Course of tic severity in Tourette syndrome: The first two decades. *Pediatrics, 102,* 14–19.

Loiselle, C.R., Lee, O., Moran, T.H., et al. (2004). Striatal microinfusion of Tourette syndrome and PANDAS sera: Failure to induce behavioral changes. *Movement Disorders, 19,* 390–396.

Lombardi, W.J., Woolston, D.J., Roberts, J.W., et al. (2001). Cognitive deficits in patients with essential tremor. *Neurology, 57,* 785–790.

Louis, E.D., Dure, L.S., & Pullman, S. (2001). Essential tremor in childhood: A series of nineteen cases. *Movement Disorders, 16,* 921–923.

Mahone, E.M., Bridges, D., Prahme, C., et al. (2004). Repetitive arm and hand movements (complex motor stereotypies) in children. *The Journal of Pediatrics, 145,* 391–395.

Marras, C., Andrews, D., Sime, E., et al. (2001). Botulinum toxin for simple motor tics: A randomized, double-blind, controlled clinical trial. *Neurology, 56,* 605–610.

Miller, J.M., Singer, H.S., Waranch, H.R., et al. (2006). Behavioral therapy for treatment of stereotypic movements in non-autistic children. *Journal of Child Neurology, 21,* 119–125.

Mukaddes, N.M., & Abali, O. (2003). Quetiapine treatment of children and adolescents with Tourette's disorder. *Journal of Child and Adolescent Psychopharmacology, 13,* 295–299.

Northam, R.S., & Singer, H.S. (1991). Postencephalitic acquired Tourette-like syndrome in a child. *Neurology, 41,* 592–593.

Nygaard, T.G., Trugman, J.M., deYebenes, J.G., et al. (1990). Dopa-responsive dystonia: The spectrum of clinical manifestations in a large North American family. *Neurology, 40,* 66–69.

O'Brien, C.F. (1998). Chorea. In J. Jankovic & E. Tolosa (Eds.), *Parkinson's disease and movement disorders* (pp. 357–364). Philadelphia: Lippincott, Williams & Wilkins.

Pappert, E.J., Goetz, C.G., Louis, E.D., et al. (2003). Objective assessments of longitudinal outcome in Gilles de la Tourette's syndrome. *Neurology, 61,* 936–940.

Perlmutter, S.J., Leitman, S.F., Garvey, M.A. (1999). Therapeutic plasma exchange and intravenous immunoglobulin for obsessive-compulsive disorder and tic disorders in childhood. *The Lancet, 354,* 1153–1158.

Perrin, E.M., Murphy, M.L., Casey, J.R., et al. (2004). Does group A beta-hemolytic streptococcal infection increase risk for behavioral and neuropsychiatric symptoms in children? *Archives of Pediatrics & Adolescent Medicine, 158,* 848–856.

Price, R.A., Kidd, K.K., Cohen, D.J., et al. (1985). A twin study of Tourette syndrome. *Archives of General Psychiatry, 42,* 815–820.

Risch, N.J., Bressman, S.B., deLeon, D., et al. (1990). Segregation analysis of idiopathic torsion dystonia in Ashkenazi Jews suggests autosomal dominant inheritance. *American Journal of Human Genetics, 46,* 533–538.

Risch, N., de Leon, D., Ozelius, L., et al. (1995). Genetic analysis of idiopathic torsion dystonia in Ashkenazi Jews and their recent descent from a small founder population. *Nature Genetics, 9,* 152–159.

Robertson, M.M., Trimble, M.R., & Lees, A.J. (1989). Self-injurious behaviour and the Gilles de la Tourette syndrome: A clinical study and review of the literature. *Psychological Medicine, 19,* 611–625.

Sallee, F.R., Kurlan, R., Goetz, C.G., et al. (2000). Ziprasidone treatment of children and adolescents with Tourette's syndrome: A pilot study. *Journal of the American Academy of Child and Adolescent Psychiatry, 39,* 292–299.

Scahill, L., Chappell, P.B., Kim, Y.S., et al. (2001). A placebo-controlled study of guanfacine in the treatment of children with tic disorders and attention deficit hyperactivity disorder. *The American Journal of Psychiatry, 158,* 1067–1074.

Segawa, M., Nomura, Y., & Nishiyama, N. (2003). Autosomal dominant guanosine triphosphate cyclohydrolase I deficiency (Segawa disease). *Annals of Neurology, 54*(Suppl. 6), S32–S45.

Singer, H.S. (2005). Tourette's syndrome: From behaviour to biology. *The Lancet Neurology, 4,* 149–159.

Singer, H.S., Dela Cruz, P.S., Abrams, M.T., et al. (1997). A Tourette-like syndrome following cardiopulmonary bypass and hypothermia: MRI volumetric measurements. *Movement Disorders, 12,* 588–592.

Singer, H.S., Wendlandt, J., Krieger, M., et al. (2001). Baclofen treatment in Tourette syndrome: A double-blind, placebo-controlled, crossover trial. *Neurology, 56,* 599–604.

Singer, W.D. (1981). Transient Gilles de la Tourette syndrome after chronic neuroleptic withdrawal. *Developmental Medicine and Child Neurology, 23,* 518–521.

Snider, L., Seligman, L., Ketchen, B., et al. (2002). Tics and problem behaviors in schoolchildren: Prevalence, characterization, and associations. *Pediatrics, 110,* 331–336.

Spencer, T., Biederman, M., Coffey, B., et al. (1999). The 4-year course of tic disorders in boys with attention-deficit/hyperactivity disorder. *Archives of General Psychiatry, 56,* 842–847.

Stephens, R.J., Bassel, C., & Sandor, P. (2004). Olanzapine in the treatment of aggression and tics in children with Tourette's syndrome—a pilot study. *Journal of Child and Adolescent Psychopharmacology, 14,* 255–266.

Swedo, S.E., Leonard, H.L., Garvey, M., et al. (1998). Pediatric autoimmune neuropsychiatric disorders associated with streptococcal infections: Clinical description of the first 50 cases. *The American Journal of Psychiatry, 155,* 264–271.

Tanner, C.M., Goldman, S.M., Lyons, K.E., et al. (2001). Essential tremor in twins: an assessment of genetic vs. environmental determinants of etiology. *Neurology, 57* 1389–1391.

The Tourette Syndrome Classification Study Group. (1993). Definitions and classification of tic disorders. *Archives of Neurology, 50,* 1013–1016.

Tourette's Syndrome Study Group. (2002). Treatment of ADHD in children with tics: A randomized controlled trial. *Neurology, 58,* 527–536.

Trimble, M.R., Whurr, R., Brookes, G., et al. (1998). Vocal tics in Gilles de la Tourette syndrome treated with botulinum toxin injections. *Movement Disorders, 13,* 617–619.

Warrick, P., Dromey, C., Irish, J.C., et al. (2000). Botulinum toxin for essential tremor of the voice with multiple anatomical sites of tremor: A crossover design study of unilateral versus bilateral injection. *Laryngoscope, 110,* 1366–1374.

Wissel, J., Masuhr, F., Schelosky, L., et al. (1997). Quantitative assessment of botulinum toxin treatment in 43 patients with head tremor. *Movement Disorders, 12,* 722–726.

Wolf, S.S., Jones, D.W., Knable, M.B., et al. (1996). Tourette syndrome: prediction of phenotypic variation in monozygotic twins by caudate nucleus D2 receptor binding. *Science, 273,* 1225–1227.

Young, R.R., Growdon, J.H., & Shahani, B.T. (1975). Beta-adrenergic mechanisms in action tremor. *The New England Journal of Medicine, 293,* 950–953.

28 Neural Tube Defects

Gregory S. Liptak

Upon completion of this chapter, the reader will

- Be able to define the term *neural tube defects* and its various subtypes
- Know the occurrence and multifactorial causes of neural tube defects
- Understand the impact of meningomyelocele on body structures, on functions, and on the child's activities and participation
- Understand strategies for intervention, the need for multidisciplinary care, and goals for independence

Neural tube defects (NTDs) are a group of malformations of the spinal cord, brain, and vertebrae. The three major NTDs are encephalocele, anencephaly, and spina bifida. Encephalocele is a malformation of the skull that allows a portion of the brain, that is usually malformed, to protrude. The vast majority of encephaloceles occur in the occipital, or back, region of the brain. Affected children often have intellectual disability, hydrocephalus (excess fluid in the cavities of the brain), spastic legs, and/or seizures. Encephaloceles also occur in the frontal area, such as the forehead, and may even appear as a mass in the nose or orbit (eye socket). The following factors are associated with a better outcome in children with encephaloceles: 1) no associated abnormalities of the brain (e.g., hydrocephalus, abnormal cell migration), 2) no other physical abnormalities, 3) frontal rather than occipital location, 4) head circumference in the normal range (rather than too small or too large), and 5) less brain tissue in the sac. Anencephaly is an even more severe congenital malformation of the skull and brain in which no neural development occurs above the brainstem (the most primitive part of the brain). About half of fetuses with anencephaly are spontaneously aborted; those who are live born rarely survive infancy.

The most common NTD is spina bifida, which is a split of the vertebral arches. This split may be isolated to the bone or occur with a protruding meningeal sac that may contain a portion of the spinal cord. The most common form of spina bifida, spina bifida occulta, is also the most benign. Approximately 10% of the general population has this hidden separation of the vertebral arches. Individuals with spina bifida occulta do not have 1) abnormalities visible on their back, 2) a sac or protruding spinal cord, or 3) any symptoms.

A form of spina bifida not to be confused with spina bifida occulta is occult spinal dysraphism (OSD). In this condition the infant is born with a visible abnormality on the lower back. This may be a birthmark (especially a reddish area called a **hemangioma** or a flame nevus), tufts of hair, a dermal sinus (opening in the skin), or a small lump (containing a fatty benign tumor, called a **lipoma**) (Guggisberg et al., 2004; Tubbs et al., 2003). Although many otherwise typically developing infants are born with a small, mid-line sacral dimple, if the dimple is not in the middle, is above the sacral region, is large, or does not have a visible bottom, it, too, may be associated with OSD. In OSD, the underlying spinal cord may be connected to the surface through a sinus (opening) that exposes it to bacteria, thereby increasing the risk of infection, especially meningitis. The spinal cord itself may be tied down (tethered) to surrounding tissue, or it may be split (diastematomyelia or diplomyelia; Kumar et al., 2002). These defects can lead to subsequent neurological damage as the child grows. Therefore, infants who have these stigmata should have an evaluation of the underlying soft tissue and spinal cord. This can be accomplished by ultrasound or magnetic resonance imaging (MRI) scan. Most clinicians believe that surgical treatment to correct the OSD should be performed early, even in asymptomatic infants, to prevent progressive neurological damage (Kang et al., 2003).

Some individuals are born with an exposed membranous sac covering the spinal cord, called a meningocele. In this form of spina bifida, the spinal cord itself is not entrapped, and these children usually have no symptoms. When the sac is associated with a malformed spinal cord, the condition is called meningomyelocele (or myelomeningocele). This disorder, often simply referred to as "spina bifida," is associated with a complex array of symptoms that includes paralysis, sensory loss below the lesion of the spinal abnormality, and hydrocephalus. Most meningomyeloceles are open, and a portion of the spinal cord is visible at birth as an open sac overlying part of the vertebral column. Children with meningomyelocele typically have associated abnormalities of the brain, including abnormal migration of neurons (Bartonek & Saraste, 2001). These abnormalities may manifest clinically as difficulties with learning. Because of its profound effects on multiple body systems, meningomyelocele has been called the most complex congenital malformation compatible with life.

This chapter focuses on meningomyelocele. It discusses the effects of the condition on psychosocial and cognitive development, approaches to treatment, and the psychological and economic stress that can affect families of children with this disorder.

PREVALENCE OF NEURAL TUBE DEFECTS

The prevalence of NTDs varies among countries. In the United States, meningomyelocele occurs in approximately 60 in 100,000 births; encephalocele, in 10 of 100,000 births; and anencephaly, in 20 of 100,000 births (Rader & Schneeman, 2006; Williams et al., 2005). In Wales and Ireland, the prevalence is three to four times higher; in Africa it is much lower (Rankin et al., 2000). This variability is a reflection of genetic influences in certain ethnic groups as well as environmental factors. Females are affected three to seven times as frequently as males, except for sacral-level NTDs, in which the occurrence is equal (Hall et al., 1988). The incidence also increases with maternal age and with lower socioeconomic status.

The prevalence of NTDs is falling worldwide as a result of a number of factors. Developed countries are now using maternal serum testing to screen prenatally for NTDs (Feldkamp, Friedrichs, & Carey, 2002). Approximately half of couples, upon learning that they are carrying an affected fetus, choose to terminate the pregnancy, although this varies according to religion and ethic background (Forrester & Merz, 2000). A number of countries, including the United States, now enrich flour with folic acid, and obstetricians generally recommend folic acid supplementation during pregnancy because of its association with a decreased risk of NTDs. Although prevalence at birth has decreased, survival due to improved medical care has increased. This has resulted in an increased population of adolescents and adults with meningomyelocele (Dillon et al., 2000). Thus, improving the transition of these individuals from adolescence to adulthood and ensuring the availability of adult services has become more important.

THE ORIGIN OF NEURAL TUBE DEFECTS

The malformation causing NTDs occurs by 26 days after fertilization of the egg during the period of neurulation (Figure 28.1; Copp, Fleming, & Greene, 1998), the first step in the formation of the central nervous system (CNS; see Chapter 13). During this time, the neural groove folds over to become the neural tube, which develops into the spinal cord and vertebral arches. During this process, if a portion of the neural groove does not close completely, a NTD results, and the spinal cord is malformed. Although the mechanism of neural tube closure is not fully understood, it does not simply work like a zipper but has multiple sites of closure. Each of these sites may be under separate genetic control, with differential sensitivity to environmental factors as well (Gos & Szpecht, 2002).

The causes of NTDs remain uncertain. Both environmental and genetic factors play a role, and they interact with each other in complex ways (Hall & Solehdin 1998). Several candidate genes have been identified in human studies as increasing the risk for NTDs (Boyles, Hammock, & Speer, 2005). Some of these are associated with the metabolism of folic acid. For example, abnormalities of 5,10-methylene tetrahydrofolate reductase (MTHFR), an en-

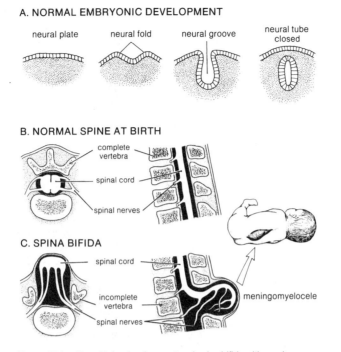

A. NORMAL EMBRYONIC DEVELOPMENT

neural plate   neural fold   neural groove   neural tube closed

B. NORMAL SPINE AT BIRTH

complete vertebra
spinal cord
spinal nerves

C. SPINA BIFIDA

spinal cord
incomplete vertebra
spinal nerves
meningomyelocele

Figure 28.1.   Neural tube development and spina bifida with meningomyelocele. A) The typical formation of the neural tube (i.e., the precursor of the spinal column) during the first month of gestation. B) Complete closure of the neural groove has occurred, and the vertebral column and spinal cord appear normal in the cross-section on the left and in the longitudinal section on the right. C) Incomplete closure of an area of the spine is called spina bifida and may be accompanied by a meningomyelocele, a sac-like abnormality of the spinal cord. As nerves do not normally form below this malformation, the child is paralyzed below (or caudal to) that point.

zyme involved in the conversion of the amino acid homocysteine to methionine, predispose humans to NTDs. Supplementation with its co-factor, folic acid (also called folate), reduces the risk of NTDs in affected families (Charles et al., 2005; Shurtleff, 2004). Abnormalities in the candidate genes identified thus far, however, account for only a small percentage of NTDs in humans (Boyles et al., 2005). Other conditions that have been associated with the development of NTDs include 1) chromosomal disorders (aneuploides—especially trisomy 13 and 18—see Appendix B, as well as chromosomal deletions and duplications; Lynch, 2005), 2) maternal exposure to the antiepileptic drugs valproic acid (Depakene, Depakote) and carbamazepine (Tegretol) and to the acne medication isotretinoin (Accutane; Ornoy, 2006), 3) excessive maternal use of alcohol, 4) maternal exposure to hyperthermia (e.g., the use of saunas, high fever; Suarez, Felkner, & Hendricks, 2004), and 5) maternal diabetes (Chen, 2005). Maternal obe-

sity has also been associated with the development of NTDs in offspring. For example, the risk of having a child with spina bifida is doubled if the body mass index (BMI; see Chapter 10) is greater than 29 kilograms per meters squared (normal is less than 25). Risks have also been found to vary by ethnicity and gender of the child. For example, obese Latina women who have daughters are eight times more likely to have a child with meningomyelocele than nonobese Caucasian women who have sons (Shaw et al., 2003).

It is unclear whether the neural damage in NTDs results simply from the malformed spinal cord or from a combination of malformation and the inflammatory effects of chronic exposure of the open cord to amniotic fluid. Studies in sheep (Meuli et al., 1995) suggest that closing an open lesion in the back results in less neural damage. Experimental trials of prenatal surgery have been performed in human fetuses that were diagnosed prenatally with meningomyelocele. The results of these studies indicate that prenatal surgery does not improve leg or bladder function. Infants born after prenatal surgery, however, have less severe Chiari II malformations (discussed later) and resultant hydrocephalus and have less need for ventricular shunting (Bruner & Tulipan, 2005; Sutton & Adzick 2004). The failure of prenatal surgery to improve neurological functioning of the legs and bladder suggests either that inflammation of exposed tissue is not an important factor or that the surgery is currently being performed too late to prevent this damage from occurring. Premature delivery of the infant and maternal complications (bleeding and infection) remain major risks with this procedure. The risks and benefits of prenatal surgery have not been sufficiently evaluated to consider the surgery as standard medical practice (Bannister, 2000). A multicenter controlled clinical trial is being conducted in the United States to evaluate the effects of prenatal surgery (National Institute of Child Health and Human Development, 2004).

PREVENTION OF NEURAL TUBE DEFECTS USING FOLIC ACID SUPPLEMENTATION

Although this chapter focuses on the treatment of children with meningomyelocele, it is important to recognize that prevention is possible based on the strong link between NTDs and folic acid deficiency. Couples who have had one child with an NTD have a recurrence risk about 30 times higher (i.e., 3 in 100) than that of the general population. If these women take folic acid (4 milligrams per day) at or before conception and continue this supplementation for the first 3 months of the pregnancy, their recurrence risk is reduced by 70% (MRC Vitamin Study Research Group, 1991). Women who have an NTD or have a first-degree relative with an NTD also should take 4 milligrams per day from around the time of conception.

Studies also have shown that daily supplemental doses of folic acid can reduce the occurrence of new cases of NTDs in the general population by 50% or more (De Villarreal et al., 2002; Gucciardi et al., 2002; Persad et al., 2002) As a result, it is now recommended that all women who are contemplating a pregnancy take 0.4 milligrams (400 micrograms) of supplemental folic acid per day while they are trying to conceive and during the first 12 weeks of pregnancy (American Academy of Pediatrics,

Committee on Genetics, 1999; Manning, Jennings, & Madsen, 2000). Supplementation with folate can also decrease the occurrence of cleft lip and palate (van Rooij et al., 2004). Yet, only about one third of women who are planning a pregnancy take folic acid around the time of conception (Schader & Corwin, 1999), and half of all pregnancies in the United States are unplanned (Centers for Disease Control and Prevention [CDC], 2000). To address this problem, since 1998 certain food staples in the United States (e.g., bread, flour) have been made with grain fortified with folic acid (Honein et al., 2001). The incidence in the United States in 1995–1996 (including prenatal occurrences), prior to supplementation, was 6.4 per 100,000; in 1999–2000, after supplementation, it was 4.1 per 100,000 (CDC, 2004). The amount of folic acid in a typical diet, even with this fortification, however, is not optimally sufficient to prevent NTDs, so individual supplements are important in women of childbearing age. Folic acid supplementation has little effect on certain types of NTDs, however, including lipomyelomeningocele (McNeely & Howes, 2004).

PRENATAL DIAGNOSIS

NTDs can be diagnosed prenatally by several methods (see Chapter 7; Main & Mennuti, 1986). Most obstetricians first measure levels of alpha-fetoprotein (AFP) in the mother's serum during the 16th–18th week of pregnancy (Bahado-Singh, 2004). AFP is a chemical typically found in the fetal spinal fluid, brain, and spinal cord. In the presence of an open meningomyelocele, encephalocele, or anencephaly, AFP leaks from the open spine into the amniotic fluid, then into the maternal circulation, where it can be detected in minute amounts. Because other conditions in both mother and fetus can lead to elevated AFP levels, maternal serum AFP (MSAFP) is used only as a screening test for NTDs. After a positive AFP screen has been obtained, a high-resolution ultrasound is used to detect specific abnormalities of the fetal head and back consistent with an NTD (Babcock, 1995; Norem et al., 2005). Correct interpretation of the ultrasound depends a great deal on the training and experience of the radiologist conducting the study (Bruner et al., 2004). If a NTD is suspected after the ultrasound, amniocentesis is performed. The levels of two substances in the amniotic fluid, AFP and an enzyme specific for NTDs called acetylcholinesterase

(ACH) that can be found in fetal cerebrospinal fluid (CSF), are then measured. The combination of elevated levels of AFP and ACH with abnormal ultrasonographic findings makes the diagnosis of an NTD in the fetus quite certain. Chromosomal analysis of the amniotic fluid is also performed to rule out syndromes (e.g., trisomy 13) that are associated with NTDs. Even if a family is not considering a therapeutic abortion if a NTD is detected, obtaining a prenatal diagnosis can help the parents plan for the special needs of their child. For example, they may opt to deliver their child via cesarean section at a center with a neonatal intensive care unit and to have the back lesion closed early, precautions that some believe may decrease the severity of paralysis (Liu et al., 1999).

TREATMENT OF MENINGOMYELOCELE IN THE NEWBORN PERIOD

When an infant is born with meningomyelocele, the first two priorities are to prevent spinal cord infection and to protect exposed spinal nerves and associated structures from physical injury. Both of these goals can be accomplished by the surgical closure of the defect within the first few days of life. In addition, a ventricular shunting procedure is often required shortly after the back closure to prevent CSF (which can no longer leak from an open meningomyelocele) from accumulating and causing progressive hydrocephalus (Tuli et al., 2003).

PRIMARY NEUROLOGICAL IMPAIRMENTS IN CHILDREN WITH MENINGOMYELOCELE

The malformation leading to meningomyelocele affects the entire CNS (Dahl et al., 1995). Table 28.1 lists some of the brain abnormalities commonly found in children with meningomyelocele. These include multiple disorders of the cranial nerve nuclei (e.g., the visual gaze centers of the brain can be affected, leading to strabismus); excessive fluid or splitting of the spinal cord above the primary lesion, resulting in additional motor impairment; and scattered changes in the brain's cortex from migration defects that are associated with cognitive impairments. The primary neurological abnormalities, however, are paralysis, loss of sensation, learning disabilities, and the Chiari II malformation with associated hydrocephalus.

Table 28.1. Malformations of the brain frequently seen in children with meningomyelocele

Malformation	Prevalence (%)
Dysplasia of cerebral cortex	92
Displaced nerve cells	44
Small gyri with abnormal layers	40
Abnormalities of layers	24
Profound primitive development	24
Small gyri with normal layers	12
Malformations of the brainstem	76
Malformations of the cerebellum	72

Source: Gilbert et al. (1986).

Paralysis and Loss of Sensation

The extent of motor paralysis and sensory loss in meningomyelocele depends on the location of the defect in the spinal cord (Figures 28.2 and 28.3), as sensory and motor function below that point are typically impaired. Factors such as ventriculitis (infection of the cerebral ventri-

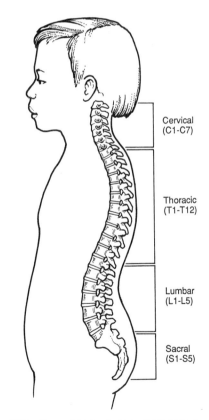

Figure 28.2. The vertebral column is divided into 7 neck (cervical), 12 chest (thoracic), 5 back (lumbar), and 5 lower-back (sacral) vertebrae. Meningomyelocele most commonly affects the thoracolumbar region.

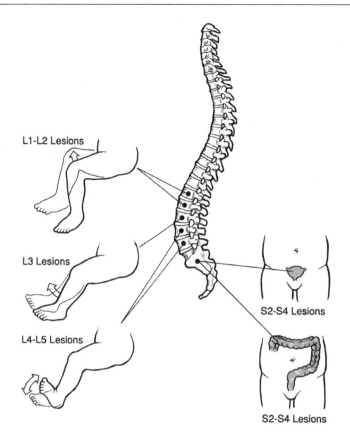

Figure 28.3. Diagram showing where movement, sensation, and bladder and bowel function are usually controlled in the spinal cord. Meningomyelocele at these levels usually prevents typical functioning at and below the levels shown.

cles), multiple episodes of shunt failure, joint contractures, previous surgeries, obesity, and types of bracing also affect ambulation. All individuals with meningomyelocele experience some loss of sensation. The loss of motor and sensory function is not always symmetrical; one side may have better motor function or sensation than the other (Figure 28.4).

Chiari Malformation and Hydrocephalus

Almost all children with meningomyelocele above the sacral level have a Chiari type II malformation of the brain (Stevenson, 2004). In this abnormality, the brainstem and part of the cerebellum are displaced downward toward the neck, rather than remaining within the skull (Figure 28.5), as if the spinal cord had been pulled downward prior to birth. Symptoms and signs of spinal cord compression from the malformation include difficulty swallowing, chok-

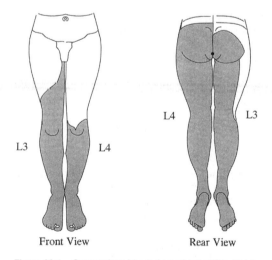

Figure 28.4. Sensory loss (shaded areas) in a child with L3- to L4-level meningomyelocele. The back of legs has more loss than the front. Asymmetry of sensory or motor loss is common; sensory loss may not completely correlate with loss of motor function.

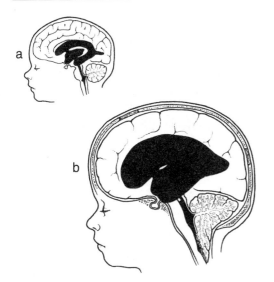

Figure 28.5. a) The typical brain, with ventricles of normal size (shaded area). b) In the Chiari II malformation and hydrocephalus (shaded area), the brainstem and part of the cerebellum are displaced downward toward the neck region, which can cause symptoms such as difficulty swallowing and hoarseness.

ing, hoarseness, breath-holding spells, apnea (periodic brief respiratory arrests), disordered breathing during sleep, stiffness in the arms, and opisthotonos (holding the head arched backward). If symptoms of compression develop, they can be treated surgically by a decompression procedure, in which the lower back of the skull and the arches of some of the cervical (neck) vertebral bodies are removed to provide additional space for the brainstem. This provides short-term benefit, but the long-term effectiveness remains uncertain. Children with more severe symptoms (e.g., vocal cord paralysis) and children who have been symptomatic for a longer period (e.g., months) have poorer outcomes following decompressive surgery.

Disordered breathing during sleep occurs frequently in individuals with meningomyelocele and has been called the "missed diagnosis." It may be the result of obstructive sleep apnea, central apnea, or central hypoventilation (Kirk et al., 1999). Disordered sleep can cause children to be tired during the day, interfering with their ability to function in school. A formal sleep study can help differentiate among the various problems that can cause disordered breathing during sleep. The treatment depends on the nature of the breathing disorder identified by this study. For example, tonsillectomy with adenoidectomy may help if the upper airway is obstructed. If there is an underlying central apnea,

surgery to provide posterior fossa decompression of the Chiari II malformation may be performed, although this is not always effective. A significant proportion of children with severe breathing disorders that do not respond to the above measures will require continuous positive airway pressure (CPAP) or bilevel positive airway pressure (BiPAP) during sleep (the BiPAP machine fits over the child's face and monitors the child's breathing electronically, providing a higher pressure during inhalation and a lower pressure during exhalation) or even tracheostomy with mechanical ventilation.

Hydrocephalus (Table 28.2) occurs in 60%–95% of children with meningomyelocele and is most common in thoracolumbar lesions (Tuli et al., 2003). Hydrocephalus develops as a result of an abnormal CSF flow pattern, leading to an enlargement of the ventricular system of the brain. It can be diagnosed by neuroimaging studies: ultrasonography in the prenatal period and in infancy, and computed tomography (CT) or MRI in older children.

Hydrocephalus is treated with a surgically implanted shunt. Shunting diverts CSF from the enlarged ventricular system to another place in the body where it can be better absorbed. The most common type, a **ventriculoperitoneal shunt,** drains fluid into the child's abdominal cavity (Figure 28.6). Shunts to the pleural space (surrounding the lungs) may be used as an alternative.

Neither of these types of shunts necessitates prophylactic antibiotics prior to dental procedures. Shunts to the atrium of the heart, however, do require antibiotic prophylaxis and can result in inflammation of the kidney (nephritis) and chronic embolization to the lungs. As a result, ventriculo-atrial shunts are rarely used now. In infants, a ventriculo-subgaleal shunt may be implanted, draining CSF from the ventricles to the scalp (Tubbs et al., 2003).

Shunts can become blocked or infected, especially during the first year of life. By 2–3 years of age, approximately half of the shunts inserted have failed and been replaced surgically (Tuli et al., 2003). In infants, signs of a blocked shunt include excessive head growth and a tense anterior fontanel ("soft spot") on the forehead. In all children, a blocked shunt may result in symptoms of lethargy, headache, vomiting, and irritability. The increased intracranial pressure can also lead to paralysis of the sixth cranial nerve (VI), with resultant strabismus and double vision, or to paralysis of upward gaze (the inability to look upward). A child with an infected

Table 28.2. Degree of paralysis in meningomyelocele and functional implications

Degree of paralysis	Hydro-cephalus (%)	Effect on movement	Mobility status	
			Childhood	Adulthood
Thoracic (T1–T12) or high lumbar (L1, L2)	90	Paralysis affects the legs and hips; causes variable weakness and sensory loss in the abdomen and lower body region	Will require extensive orthosis like para-podium, reciprocal gait orthosis, or HKAFO[a]	Typically use wheel-chairs; community ambulation rare
Lumbar (L3, L4)	80	Hips flex and knees extend; ankles and toes are paralyzed	Will ambulate with less extensive orthotics, using crutches	Most use wheel-chairs; community ambulation is uncommon
Low lumbar (L5)	65	Hips flex, knees extend and ankles flex; weak or absent ankle extension, toe flexion, and hip extension	Will ambulate with minimal or no bracing, with or without crutches	Most continue to be community ambulators
Sacral (S1–S4)	40	Mild weakness of ankles and/or toes	Will ambulate with minimal or no bracing, without crutches	Most continue to be community ambulators

From Charney, E.B. (1997). Myelomeningocele. In M.W. Schwartz et al. (Eds.), *Pediatric primary care: A problem-oriented approach* (3rd ed., p. 812). St. Louis: Mosby; adapted by permission.

[a]HKAFO, hip-knee-ankle-foot orthosis.

shunt can display symptoms similar to those seen in shunt blockage but will also have a fever and an elevated white blood cell count. Signs and symptoms of a blocked shunt can mimic those of a tethered cord or Chiari malformation. Therefore, whenever a child with a meningomyelocele develops new neurological symptoms, especially deterioration of physical or cognitive function, a blocked or infected shunt should be investigated. More subtle symptoms of a partial shunt failure include a change in personality, decline in school performance, or weakness of the arms or legs (Matson et al., 2005).

Early recognition of shunt failure or infection is critical, as both complications can be life threatening. A child who develops new neurological symptoms should be evaluated immediately for shunt failure. If a blocked shunt is suspected, the physician may order a neuroimaging study (CT or MRI) to determine if the ventricles have increased in size as well as radiographs of the shunt system (shunt series) to determine if the tubing is broken or kinked. If the shunt is found to be obstructed, the blocked portion will be replaced surgically with a new catheter and/or valve.

If the shunt is infected, the child also needs to receive intravenous antibiotics. In addition, it may be necessary to remove the infected

shunt surgically and, after antibiotic treatment, replace it with a new one. It is important to emphasize that the individual with hydrocephalus almost always requires a working shunt throughout his or her life. In some children, however, a new surgical procedure called endoscopic third ventriculostomy may obviate the need for ventricular shunts. This technique involves placing a hole in the floor of one of the ventricles to drain CSF within the brain. Its safety and effectiveness in the treatment of children with hydrocephalus associated with NTDs is still uncertain (Marlin, 2004).

ASSOCIATED IMPAIRMENTS AND MEDICAL COMPLICATIONS

Meningomyelocele, hydrocephalus, and the associated malformations of the brain lead to developmental disabilities and place the child at risk for a number of medical complications (Verhoef et al., 2004). These associated disabilities include mobility impairment, cognitive impairments, seizure disorders, fine motor impairments, and visual impairment. Medical complications include musculoskeletal abnormalities, spinal curvatures and humps, urinary and bowel dysfunction, skin sores, weight and stature abnormalities, sexual issues such as dysfunction,

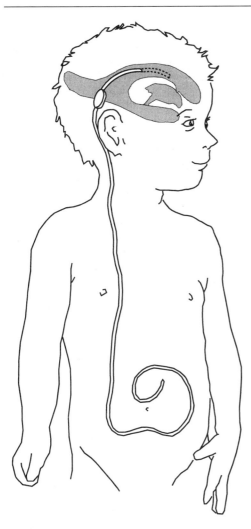

Figure 28.6. Ventriculoperitoneal shunt, which has been placed for hydrocephalus. A plastic tube is inserted into one of the lateral ventricles and connected to a one-way valve. Another tube runs under the skin from the valve to the abdominal cavity. Enough extra tubing is left in the abdomen to uncoil as the child grows.

Children with sacral lesions generally learn to walk well by 2 or 3 years of age with bracing at the ankles or no bracing at all. Children with mid-lumbar (L3) paralysis often require crutches and bracing up to the hip (Table 28.2). Children with thoracic or high lumbar (L1 and L2) paralysis may eventually stand upright and walk but only with support of the hips, knees, and ankles. This support may be provided by extensive bracing and/or mobility devices such as a parapodium, a reciprocal gait orthosis, or a hip-knee-ankle-foot orthosis (HKAFO) used in combination with crutches or a walker.

As children with L3 and L4 lesions approach adolescence and their center of gravity and relative strength change, most will rely increasingly on wheelchairs for mobility (Table 28.2; Norrlin et al., 2003; van den Berg-Emons et al., 2001). Because most children with meningomyelocele will not become effective community ambulators, the supplemental or primary use of a wheelchair should be considered at least by early adolescence as it offers the advantages of speed, efficiency, and attractiveness.

Cognitive Impairments

Approximately three quarters of children with meningomyelocele have IQ scores that fall within the average range (Barf et al., 2004). Most of the remaining one quarter have mild intellectual disability. The few children with meningomyelocele who have severe intellectual disability usually have had a complicating brain infection resulting from an infected shunt or severe prenatal hydrocephalus.

Although the majority of children with meningomyelocele have typical intellectual function, they tend to show significant impairments in perceptual skills, organizational abilities, attention span, speed of motor response, memory, and hand function (Snow, 1994). By school age, many children with meningomyelocele and hydrocephalus are diagnosed with a nonverbal learning disability (see Chapter 25). These children typically have better reading than math skills. In addition to the learning disability, they often have impairments in executive function that have an impact on education, social, and self-help skills. Executive function skills include the ability to plan, initiate, sequence, sustain, inhibit competing responses, and pace work (Burmeister et al., 2005). For example, the child may know the steps involved in self-catheterization but may have difficulty planning and carrying out the process. Also,

and allergy to latex. Many of these disabilities and medical complications can be prevented or their impact lessened by meticulous clinical care and monitoring by the family, the child, and health care professionals.

Mobility Impairments

The higher the level of the meningomyelocele and the greater the muscle weakness, the more ambulation will be impaired. Even children with low-level lesions (L4 and below), however, are likely to have significant impairment in mobility. Many infants with meningomyelocele have delayed rolling, sitting, and walking skills.

disorders of the cerebellum have been associated with cognitive problems, including impairments in executive function, visual-spatial function, expressive language, verbal memory and modulation of affect (Barnes, Dennis, & Hetherington, 2004; Iddon et al., 2004). In addition, many children with meningomyelocele have attention-deficit/hyperactivity disorder; about one third of these children respond to stimulant medication (see Chapter 24). Half of the adolescents who had spina bifida with hydrocephalus required special intervention for secondary education, compared with only 8% for those with spina bifida without hydrocephalus (Barf et al., 2004).

Because children with meningomyelocele are at increased risk for multiple developmental disabilities, they should be referred to an early intervention program in infancy (see Chapter 33). This should be followed by a formal psychoeducational evaluation prior to school entry to identify strengths and weaknesses and to develop an individualized education program (IEP; see Chapter 34).

Seizure Disorders

Approximately 15% of individuals with meningomyelocele develop a seizure disorder (Battaglia et al., 2004). The seizures usually are generalized **tonic-clonic** and respond well to antiepileptic medication (see Chapter 29). If a new type of seizure develops or if seizure frequency increases, however, a blocked shunt or shunt infection should be suspected and investigated.

Visual Impairments

Strabismus is present in about 20% of children with meningomyelocele and often requires surgical correction (Verhoef et al., 2004). Visual impairments can result from abnormalities of the visual gaze center in the brain or from increased intracranial pressure caused by a malfunctioning ventricular shunt (see Chapter 11).

Musculoskeletal Abnormalities

With partial or total paralysis, muscle imbalances and lack of mobility may lead to deformities around joints (Dias, 2004). This can occur even prior to birth. For example, children with meningomyelocele may be born with a clubfoot (see Chapter 14) or a calcaneus deformity as a result of the foot being pressed against the uter-ine wall and becoming stuck in one position. Treatment of clubfoot involves serial casting during the first 3–4 months of life to gradually straighten the deformity. Corrective surgery can then follow at 4 months to 1 year of age (Flynn et al., 2004). Other ankle and foot deformities may require surgical intervention to facilitate proper foot placement in shoes. Bracing is used to help maintain proper positioning of joints and should be monitored to minimize the occurrence of skin breakdown over bony prominences (e.g., **decubitus ulcers** of the ankle or buttocks).

Muscle imbalance and lack of movement also can lead to hip deformities. Surgical correction is controversial and may be appropriate only for those children with low lumbar paralysis who have the potential for functional ambulation (Lorente et al., 2005). The goals of orthopedic treatment are to maintain alignment and range of motion, stabilize the spine and extremities, maximize function, provide comfort, and protect the skin. Loss of muscle strength and inactivity predispose affected children to fractures. These pathological fractures may also occur after orthopedic surgery, especially following prolonged casting. All individuals with spina bifida should receive adequate calcium and vitamin D in order to minimize osteoporosis and the susceptibility to pathological fractures. This is especially true if the child is taking antiepileptic drugs that interfere with calcium and vitamin D metabolism. In addition, weight-bearing activities should be encouraged whenever possible. Following surgical procedures, steps should be taken to prevent deep vein thrombosis, which predisposes the individual to pulmonary emboli. Lastly, as individuals with spina bifida age, they may develop arthritis of the hips or knees secondary to abnormal sensation and gait (Nagarkatti, Banta, & Thomson, 2000).

Spinal Curvatures and Humps Almost 90% of children with a meningomyelocele above the sacral level have spinal curvatures and/or humps (Trivedi et al., 2002). These deformities include **scoliosis** (a spinal curvature), **kyphosis** (a spinal hump; Figure 28.7), and **kyphoscoliosis** (a combination of both conditions). Scoliosis and kyphosis may be present before birth (congenital) or develop later in childhood (acquired). If untreated, spinal deformities may eventually interfere with sitting and walking and even decrease lung capacity. Scoliosis greater than 25 degrees is treated with an orthotic support (a molded plastic shield-like

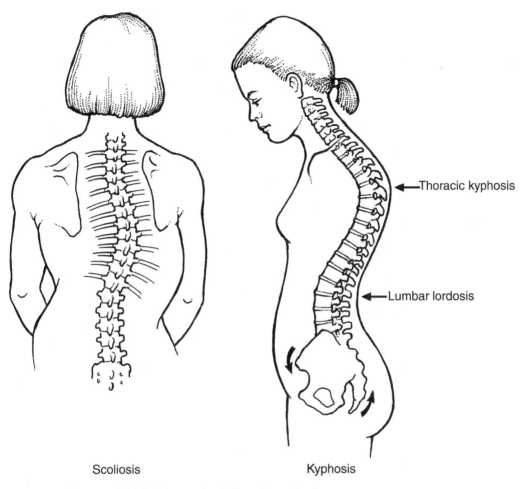

Scoliosis   Kyphosis

Figure 28.7. Common spinal deformities associated with meningomyelocele.

orthotic jacket). Despite this, the curvature often progresses, and surgery may be necessary (Parisini et al., 2002). Surgical correction involves a spinal fusion with bone grafts. This often requires two surgical procedures, one through the front and one from the back. The procedures use metal rods (internal fixation) and wires (Luque procedure; Figure 26.13) for stabilization of the spinal column. The two-stage procedure has been successfully replaced by a single frontal (anterior) approach in some children whose curve is less than 75 degrees in the absence of abnormalities of the spinal cord. Children with congenital rather than developmental scoliosis or kyphosis generally respond poorly to orthotic treatment and require spinal fusion at younger ages.

Kyphosis is usually located in the thoracic spine and may measure as much as 80 to 90 degrees at birth. The hump on the spine may be rigid and worsen over time. Surgical removal of the deformity is accomplished by an operation called a kyphectomy. This procedure has a high rate of complications and recurrences in infancy, but when performed in school-age children, it has been quite effective (Niall et al., 2004).

Some evidence indicates that tethering of the spinal cord (discussed later) may lead to rapidly progressive scoliosis. Surgery to untether the cord may halt or even reverse the progression of the curve in individuals whose curves are less than 50 degrees at the time of surgery (Pierz et al., 2000). In addition, a significant number of individuals with spina bifida will have an abnormal fluid collection in the spinal cord or even thinning (hypoplasia) of the cord (Moskowitz et al., 1998). Because spinal surgery fuses the bones of the spine, making subsequent neurological surgery especially challenging, many centers obtain an MRI scan of the spine on all individuals prior to surgery for kyphosis or scoliosis. In this way, they can identify tethering or cavities in the spinal cord that might require surgery prior to the orthopedic procedure.

Urinary Dysfunction

Because the bladder, the urinary outlet (**urethra**), and rectum are all controlled by nerves that leave the spinal cord in the lower sacrum (Figure 28.3), bladder and bowel dysfunction are present in virtually all children with meningomyelocele. Even children with sacral lesions and normal leg movement typically have bladder and bowel problems. In addition, these children have a higher incidence of malformations of the kidneys, including horseshoe kidney and absent kidney.

The bladder has two major functions: 1) to store urine that has been produced by the kidneys, and 2) to empty the urine once the bladder is full. Children with meningomyelocele often have difficulty with both functions and are consequently incontinent. In addition, the inability to completely empty the bladder of urine may predispose the child to infections of the bladder and/or kidneys. The combination of a tight bladder outlet and increased tone in the bladder also may produce kidney damage over time (Hopps & Kropp, 2003; Snodgrass & Adams, 2004).

To detect early structural damage, the urinary tract is imaged using ultrasonography at regular intervals beginning in infancy. Ultrasound examination permits detection of malformations and abnormal functioning of the bladder and urinary outlet. Bladder function also may be evaluated using a cystometrogram (urodynamics), a procedure in which fluid is injected into the bladder and pressure is measured. If elevated pressure is found, it must be reduced to avoid permanent kidney damage. Reducing bladder pressure is accomplished by using daily intermittent catheterization (CIC) (Hopps & Kropp, 2003). In CIC, the individual or his or her parents are taught to insert a clean, but not sterile, catheter (tube) through the urethra and into the bladder. This commonly is done at least four times per day to drain urine. When CIC is performed correctly, urine does not accumulate, become infected, or flow back into the kidneys. In some infants, however, this is not successful and a surgical procedure called a **vesicostomy** is performed. Here an opening through the abdominal wall and into the bladder is produced, allowing urine to drain directly

into the diaper. When the child is older, the vesicostomy typically is closed surgically and he or she begins a CIC program.

In addition to assessing bladder pressure, the infant is monitored for the occurrence of urinary infections, which occur in at least half of individuals with meningomyelocele. If these happen frequently, long-term prophylactic oral antibiotics such as cephalexin (Keflex) or trimethoprim/sulfamethoxazole (Bactrim or Septra) may be given to prevent infections. Alternatively, antibiotics can be instilled directly into the bladder through the catheter.

Attempts to achieve urinary continence are generally begun at 3–4 years of age. In addition, medications may be used: Oxybutynin chloride (Ditropan) can be given orally or instilled into the bladder to diminish bladder wall contractions, and pseudoephedrine (Sudafed) or imipramine (Tofranil) may be given orally to enhance storage of urine. About 70% of children who receive a combination of CIC and medications achieve continence during elementary school.

If CIC and medication are unsuccessful in producing continence, a surgical intervention may be undertaken. In the past, a silicone-like material was injected around the urethra using an endoscope; however, its long-term effectiveness has been questioned (Block, Cooper, & Hawtrey, 2003; Halachmi et al., 2004). Another approach is a bladder augmentation procedure, in which the bladder capacity is increased using a flap of bowel or stomach. A third procedure is an appendicovesicostomy, in which the appendix is used to connect the bladder to the abdominal wall, permitting catheterization through the appendix. These approaches may be used in combination.

"Volitional" voiding is also possible using an artificial urinary sphincter that surrounds the urethra and stays closed to prevent leakage of urine. A bulb mechanism is placed in the scrotum or labia majora; when it is squeezed, fluid drains out of the artificial sphincter allowing urine to drain from the bladder. Complications such as erosion of the skin around the bulb and poor adherence leading to over distension of the bladder and resultant kidney damage are common with this procedure (Kryger et al., 1999). Yet, for a select group of highly motivated individuals, the artificial sphincter can permit volitional voiding.

Finally, as the risk of bladder cancer is increased, adults with meningomyelocele probably should be monitored annually with endoscopy of the bladder and cytological analysis of the cells from the urine (Game et al., 2006).

Bowel Dysfunction

Bowel problems in children with meningomyelocele are related to uncoordinated propulsive action of the intestines, ineffectual function of the anus, and lack of rectal sensation. Constipation is common and may be interspersed with periods of overflow diarrhea. Lack of sensation and failure of anal function also lead to soiling that can be socially devastating. In individuals with typical bowel function, the rectal sampling reflex can discriminate between gas, liquid stool, and solid stool. Absence of this reflex in children with meningomyelocele worsens continence.

Attempts at bowel management can begin as soon as the child starts eating solids by encouraging foods that are high in fiber. Between $2\frac{1}{2}$ and 4 years of age, timed potty sitting can be tried after every meal to take advantage of the postfeeding gastrocolic (propulsive) reflex. If bowel control has not been achieved after several months, parents may be instructed to administer one or more of the following medications that will facilitate more complete bowel emptying: 1) a daily laxative such as lactulose (a complex sugar), MiraLax (an agent that keeps water in the stool), or senna (e.g., Senokot); 2) a fiber supplement such as psyllium (e.g., Metamucil); or 3) a nightly rectal suppository such as bisacodyl (e.g., Dulcolax), or daily enemas using saline.

Two surgical procedures—one that connects the appendix to the colon (Malone procedure) and another that provides a direct connection between the abdominal wall and the colon (cecostomy)—allow irrigation of the colon on a regular basis (antegrade [forward-flowing] colonic enema, or ACE). The cecostomy can be performed either in the operating room or in an interventional radiology suite. These approaches have been shown to be successful in children for whom more conventional bowel techniques have failed (Aksnes et al., 2002; Leibold, Ekmark, & Adams, 2000). There is a newer ACE procedure in which a surgical hole is placed on the left side of the abdomen; irrigation fluids can be inserted into the descending colon, which allows more rapid washout of stool (Ahn, Han, & Choi, 2004; Kim et al., 2006). Its long-term use, however, has not been established.

For a select group of older children with low-level (sacral) meningomyeloceles who have rectal sensation, biofeedback training may be used to improve rectal function (Aslan & Kogan, 2002). In this training technique, children use a balloon pressure transducer connected to a visible pressure monitor to optimize rectal function, including coordinating efforts to expulse stool.

Skin Sores

Skin sores or decubitus ulcers frequently occur in children with meningomyelocele, whose weight-bearing surfaces (e.g., feet, buttocks) are not sensitive to pain. These children may sustain injuries that they do not feel, often resulting in a skin sore. This problem becomes more frequent during adolescence and, if not caught early, the decubitus ulcer may require prolonged hospitalizations for debridement (removal of dead tissue), plastic surgery, and intravenous antibiotics. Therefore, the best treatment is prevention. Certain reasonable rules should be followed: 1) Examine insensate skin regularly to detect small sores, 2) replace tight-fitting shoes or braces, 3) avoid hot baths, 4) give the child protective foot covering for swimming, 5) do not let the young child crawl about on rough or hot surfaces, and 6) ensure that wheelchair cushions continue to be protective.

For children in wheelchairs, pressure sores on the buttocks or coccyx (tail bone) can be prevented by modifying the wheelchair with an adaptive seating system. Individuals can minimize prolonged pressure by performing regular wheelchair pushups to relieve pressure and by frequently changing position (Samaniego, 2002). Small skin sores should be treated by alleviating pressure and using saline-soaked dressings or artificial skin preparations such as Tegaderm or Vigilon. If ulcers do not heal in a reasonable time, an underlying infection may be present, requiring surgical debridement and intravenous antibiotic treatment. Many new coverings and techniques, such as vacuum assisted closure, have been tried to heal pressure ulcers. The most important rule, however, is that the only thing that should not be placed on a pressure sore is the child!

Weight and Stature Abnormalities

Children with meningomyelocele, particularly those with thoracic to L2 lesions, are at increased risk for obesity (Littlewood et al., 2003). About two thirds of these children are significantly overweight. Attention should be directed at increasing involvement in physical activities such as aerobic conditioning (e.g., wheelchair sports) and strength training (e.g., lifting free weights) (Widman, McDonald, & Abresch, 2006). Exercise should be combined with dietary restrictions of sweets and fats, especially because individuals who have paraplegia need fewer calories to grow and maintain normal weight. Affected children also are likely to have short stature. This results from a combination of failure of growth of the legs, spinal curves, and, occasionally, a deficiency of growth hormone (Hochhaus, Butenandt, & Ring-Mrozik, 1999). Long-term treatment of select individuals with recombinant human growth hormone may lead to more normal final adult stature (Rotenstein & Bass, 2004).

Sexual Issues

Although three quarters of adult males with meningomyelocele can have erections, most do not have control of them (Game et al., 2006). Penile implants, injection or application of prostaglandin prior to coitus (Kim & McVary, 1995), the use of vacuum devices (Chen et al., 1995), and sildenafil (Viagra) (Palmer, Kaplan, & Firlit, 1999) can help males achieve volitional erections that allow intercourse. There may be the additional problem of retrograde ejaculation, in which the semen is discharged into the bladder. Despite this, two thirds of males with spina bifida have sufficient sperm in their ejaculate to permit fatherhood using artificial insemination or in vitro fertilization (Hultling et al., 2000). Although there are many sexual and reproductive health issues relating to meningomyclocele, in a survey of young adults with spina bifida, 95% stated they had inadequate knowledge about these problems (Sawyer & Roberts, 1999).

Females with meningomyelocele have normal fertility and, if sexually active, should use the same precautions to avoid pregnancy and sexually transmitted diseases as the general population. Although many of these women are able to experience orgasm during sexual intercourse, they usually have decreased genital sensation and less sexually stimulated lubrication. As a result, frequent intercourse without adequate lubrication can lead to vaginal sores. Precocious puberty (e.g., breast development 1–2 years before usual) is a common occurrence in females who have meningomyelocele with hydrocephalus due to a disorder of the hypothalamus (a part of the brain that controls certain endocrine hormones). This can be treated with leuprolide (Lupron), a synthetic sex hormone that can slow sexual development (Trollmann et al., 1998). Women with meningomyelocele who become pregnant benefit from close monitoring during gestation. Problems such as recurrent urinary tract infections, persistent decubitus ulcers, back pain or slipped disk, and difficult vaginal delivery secondary to hip contractures may occur. Although these are concerns, it is important to note that most women with meningomyelocele have good pregnancy outcomes with relatively few complications (Arata et al., 2000). Sexual abuse of women and female teens who have spina bifida appears to be more common than that found in the general population (Woodhouse, 2005).

Allergy to Latex

More than half of all children with meningomyelocele develop an allergy to latex in childhood (Cremer et al., 2002). Although the reason for this is unclear, the allergy seems to be more common in children who have had frequent surgical procedures. The risk of allergy increases as the child gets older (Mazon et al., 2000). This allergic reaction can be life threatening. Latex allergy can be diagnosed by a clear history of an allergic reaction to latex, by skin testing, or by immunoassay blood testing (Nieto et al., 2000). As a result of the high incidence of allergy to latex in these children, all surgical procedures, including dental procedures, should occur in latex-free settings. Early contact of the infant with latex should be avoided, if possible, in an effort to prevent the development of allergy. Catheterization should be performed with nonlatex catheters, and nonlatex gloves should be used during care. Toys that contain significant amounts of latex, such as balloons and rubber balls, should be avoided, as should latex products that come into contact with the skin, such as Band-Aids and Ace wraps.

Neurological Deterioration

If a child's strength, bowel and bladder function, or daily living skills deteriorate, a cause must be sought. The origin of the deterioration may be a malfunctioning or blocked ventricular shunt; a tethered spinal cord; or, rarely, swelling in (syrinx, syringomyelia, or hydromyelia) or splitting (diastematomyelia or diplomyelia) of the spinal cord. A tethered spinal cord may result from 1) scarring at the site of the initial surgery to close the back, 2) scoliosis, or 3) the pressure of a lipoma. Pressure or stretch on the tethered cord leads to poor circulation and diminished motor functioning. The Chiari II malformation may become symptomatic, too, leading to difficulty swallowing, hoarseness, weakness of the arms, or difficulty with respiration.

All children who present with neurological deterioration first should be evaluated for structure and function of the ventricular shunt. This involves imaging of the head (e.g., CT, MRI) with or without plain radiographic imaging of the shunt from head to abdomen (to look for a break in the tubing). In addition, the posterior fossa and spinal cord should be evaluated by cranial MRI with flow (to look for Chiari II malformation and to look for tethered, swollen, or split cord, respectively; Levy, 1999) and spinal MRI. If identified early, each of these problems can be addressed successfully. A blocked shunt can be replaced, a tethered cord released, a lipoma removed, and a posterior fossa decompressed. Treatment of syringomyelia (syrinx or hydromyelia), however, is more controversial and often less rewarding (Piatt, 2004).

EDUCATIONAL PROGRAMS

Referral to an early intervention program should occur by 6 months of age (see Chapter 33). Sensorimotor assessment during the child's first year should include evaluations of range of motion of joints, muscle tone, strength and bulk, sensation, movement skills, postural control, and sensory integration skills. Treatment should focus on maintaining range of motion, enhancing strength, and moving toward standing and ambulation. Because of the considerable variability in the degree of motor delay among these children, individualized intervention plans must be developed. Adaptive equipment should be provided as needed (Chapter 36).

As the child moves toward school entry, it is important to perform psychoeducational testing. This permits the identification of the child's cognitive strengths and challenges, the development or realistic expectations that will optimize the child's learning, and the planning of an IEP for school. Physical therapy should be provided as part of the school program. Yearly reassessments will permit modification of the program based on the child's changing needs (see Chapter 34; Thompson, 1997).

PSYCHOSOCIAL ISSUES FOR THE CHILD

During the preschool years, the achievement of independence may be thwarted by problems with mobility and bladder and bowel control. A sense of industry that develops in the school-age child may be reduced by the child's learning impairments as well as by his or her inability to compete with peers in sports. Difficulty in the school environment may exacerbate a preexisting poor self-image that many of these children have as a result of their physical disabilities. The feeling of being different can impair the establishment of peer relationships in both school and community. The child's self-esteem also may be lowered if he or she must continue to wear diapers or care for an ostomy (Moore, Kogan, & Parekh, 2004).

Teens with spina bifida tend to be more socially immature and passive, more socially isolated, less independent, and less physically active (Holmbeck et al., 2003). During adolescence, lower self-esteem may relate to a poor body image and difficulty in dealing with sexual changes and feelings. Positive self-image has been linked to factors such as higher socioeconomic status (Holmbeck et al, 2003) and the presence of social support (Antle, 2004). Problems for the young adult with meningomyelocele may include increasing social isolation, a realization that the disability is permanent, and sexual dysfunction. Social outcomes, such as behavior problems, do not necessarily relate to the severity of physical impairment but are interrelated with functional status, such as scholastic achievement (Hommeyer et al., 1999). Helping a child cope with a disability requires 1) insight into the issues faced by the child, such as the developmental stages of Erikson (1959); 2) knowledge of the strengths and weaknesses of the child, such as temperament (children with spina bifida may have a pattern of temperament different from that of other children (Vachha & Adams, 2005) and social skills; 3) a strategy for dealing with the issues (e.g., behavior supports); and 4) support to carry out the strategies. Children require encouragement and support from adults. This assumes that families have sufficient financial and emotional resources to cope with their child's condition, which is not always the case. Efforts should be made to maximize the child's self-management, allowing the child to be as independent as possible in his or her own care. Providing safe, structured opportunities to learn socialization (e.g., arranging trips to the movies, the mall, and fast-food restaurants with friends) can be helpful in boosting an adolescent's self-esteem.

Some studies have found a higher-than-expected rate of depression in individuals with meningomyelocele. Medical problems such as an adverse reaction to medication, problems with the ventricular shunt, and infections, however, can cause similar symptoms and must be ruled out. Many individuals with meningomyelocele develop learned helplessness; they feel that unpleasant or aversive stimuli cannot be controlled. As a result, they cease trying to remedy an aversive circumstance, even if they are capable of exerting some influence. This contributes to depressive feelings. Depression should be recognized and brought to the attention of an appropriate professional. A multimodal approach including counseling, exercise programs, and medications (especially selective serotonin reuptake inhibitors) is usually effective.

INTERDISCIPLINARY MANAGEMENT

The goals of therapy are to improve functioning and independence and to prevent or correct secondary physical or emotional problems. This generally involves surgical interventions, adaptive equipment, special education services, and psychosocial support for the child and family (see Chapter 40). As a result of the complexity of the resultant disabilities, an interdisciplinary approach to treating the child with meningomyelocele is essential (McDonald, 1995). The team of health care professionals should include a physician (e.g., neurodevelopmental pediatrician, pediatric neurologist, physiatrist) with particular interest and expertise in the care of meningomyelocele; a nurse specialist; physical and occupational therapists; a social worker; consulting orthopedic, urological, and neurosurgeons; and an orthotist. Other team members or consultants may include a psychologist, plastic surgeon, dentist, special educator, speech-language pathologist, genetic counselor, and financial counselor. The services that the child needs and receives should be coordinated by a designated service coordinator (or case manager). Efforts should be made to empower the child and family by involving them in the design of a management plan that is both appropriate and realistic.

The successful development of the child with meningomyelocele is largely dependent on how well the family is able to meet the needs of the child. This requires emotional and behavioral supports, realistic expectations, special education services, and coordinated community services. The care of a child with meningomyelocele is expensive. Direct medical expenses have been estimated to total more than $100,000 over the individual's lifetime (Waitzman, Romano, & Scheffler, 1994); indirect costs, such as loss of parental income and decreased productivity of the affected individual, are estimated to total $250,000 over the life span (CDC, 1990). Therefore, one of the priorities of care is to provide financial counseling to families.

OUTCOME

The survival rate of children with meningomyelocele has improved dramatically in the past 50 years. In the 1950s survival to adulthood was less than 10% (Dunne & Shurtleff, 1986); in the 1990s, about 85% of children with meningomyelocele survived to adulthood (Davis et al., 2005) This improved survival has resulted from many factors, including the use of ventriculoperitoneal shunts to control hydrocephalus and the prevention of kidney damage by CIC and urological surgery.

Outcome data for adults are incomplete, and the population is quite heterogeneous. In one center, Hunt (1990, 1999; Hunt & Oakeshott, 2003) found that half the individuals with meningomyelocele were able to walk 50 yards or more in adulthood. Half also were able to maintain urinary and bowel continence. Overall, 12% had minimal disabilities, with average IQ scores, community ambulation, and well-managed continence; 52% had moderate disability with borderline IQ scores, the ability to attend to toilet needs independently, and the ability to use and transfer from a wheelchair. Severe disability involving intellectual disability, incontinence, and dependence for most self-help skills was found in 37% of the individuals and was most related to a history of shunt infections or shunt failure. Adults with hydrocephalus have persistent learning disabilities, including executive dysfunction (Barnes et al., 2004; Iddon et al., 2004). Verhoef et al. (2004) found that pain was common in adults with spina bifida; males frequently had problems with sexual function. About 15% of adults in their study had problems with pressure sores.

SUMMARY

In meningomyelocele, an overlying sac protruding from the spine contains a malformed spinal cord and leads to the most complex birth defect compatible with life. Paralysis and loss of sensation occur below the level of the spinal cord defect, usually associated with hydrocephalus. Numerous disabilities arise as a consequence of this condition, including paralysis, musculoskeletal abnormalities, bowel and bladder incontinence, impotence, obesity, and cognitive impairments, including nonverbal learning disorders. Meningomyelocele, however, should be considered a nonprogressive condition, and any deterioration in function should lead to a search for a treatable cause, such as a blocked ventricular shunt or a tethered spinal cord. Advances in surgical and medical care have enhanced the survival and physical well-being of individuals with meningomyelocele but have not completely corrected the associated impairments. To help an individual with meningomyelocele reach his or her potential, professionals must advocate for the child and family in the areas of education and psychosocial adjustment while providing integrated, high-quality health care.

REFERENCES

Ahn, S.M., Han, S.W., & Choi, S.H. (2004, July). The results of antegrade continence enema using a retubularized sigmoidostomy. *Pediatric Surgery International*, 488–491.

Aksnes, G., Diseth, T.H., Helseth, A., et al. (2002). Appendicostomy for antegrade enema: Effects on somatic and psychosocial functioning in children with meningomyelocele. *Pediatrics, 109*, 484–489.

American Academy of Pediatrics, Committee on Genetics. (1999). Folic acid for the prevention of neural tube defects. *Pediatrics, 104*, 325–327.

Antle, B.J. (2004, August). Factors associated with self-worth in young people with physical disabilities. *Health & Social Work*, 167–175.

Arata, M., Grover, S., Dunne, K., et al. (2000). Pregnancy outcome and complications in women with spina bifida. *The Journal of Reproductive Medicine, 45*, 743–748.

Aslan, A.R., & Kogan, B.A. (2002). Conservative management in neurogenic bladder dysfunction. *Current Opinion in Urology, 12*, 473–477.

Babcock, C.J. (1995). Ultrasound evaluation of prenatal and neonatal spina bifida. *Neurosurgery Clinics of North America, 6*, 203–218.

Bahado-Singh, R.O., & Sutton-Riley, J. (2004). Bio-chemical screening for congenital defects. *Obstetrics and Gynecology Clinics of North America, 31*, 857–72, xi.

Bannister, C.M., Russell, S.A., Rimmer, S., et al. (2000). Can prognostic indicators be identified in a fetus with an encephalocele? *European Journal of Pediatric Surgery, 10*(Suppl. 1), 20–23.

Barf, H.A., Verhoef, M., Post, M.W., et al. (2004). Educational career and predictors of type of education in young adults with spina bifida. *International Journal of Rehabilitation Research, 27*(1), 45–52.

Barnes, M., Dennis, M., & Hetherington, R. (2004, September). Reading and writing skills in young adults with spina bifida and hydrocephalus. *Journal of the International Neuropsychological Society*, 655–663.

Bartonek, A., & Saraste, H. (2001). Factors influencing ambulation in myelomeningocele: A cross-sectional study. *Developmental Medicine and Child Neurology, 43*, 253–260.

Battaglia, D., Acquafondata, C., Lettori, D., et al. (2004). Observation of continuous spike-waves during slow sleep in children with myelomeningocele. *Child's Nervous System, 20*, 462–467.

Block, C.A., Cooper, C.S., & Hawtrey, C.E. (2003, January). Long-term efficacy of periurethral collagen injection for the treatment of urinary incontinence secondary to myelomeningocele. *The Journal of Urology*, 327–329.

Boyles, A.L., Hammock, P., & Speer, M.C. (2005). Candidate gene analysis in human neural tube defects. *American Journal of Medical Genetics, Part C: Seminars in Medical Genetics, 135*, 9–23.

Bruner, J.P., & Tulipan, N. (2005). Intrauterine repair of spina bifida. *Clinics in Obstetrics and Gynecology, 48*, 942–955.

Bruner, J.P., Tulipan, N., Dabrowiak, M.E., et al. (2004). Upper level of the spina bifida defect: How good are we? *Ultrasound in Obstetrics & Gynecology*, 612–617.

Burmeister, R., Hannay, H.J., Copeland, K., et al. (2005). Attention problems and executive functions in children with spina bifida and hydrocephalus. *Child Neuropsychology: A Journal on Normal and Abnormal Development in Childhood and Adolescence, 11*, 265–283.

Centers for Disease Control and Prevention. (1990). Economic burden of spina bifida: United States, 1980–1990. *Morbidity and Mortality Weekly Report, 38*(15), 264–267.

Centers for Disease Control and Prevention. (2000). Folate status in women of childbearing age—United States, 1999. *Morbidity and Mortality Weekly Report, 49*(42), 962–965.

Centers for Disease Control and Prevention. (2004). Spina bifida and anencephaly before and after folic acid mandate—United States, 1995–1996 and 1999–2000 (2004, May 7). *Morbidity and Mortality Weekly Report, 362*–365.

Charles, D.H., Ness, A.R., Campbell, D., et al. (2005). Folic acid supplements in pregnancy and birth outcome: Re-analysis of a large randomised controlled trial and update of Cochrane review. *Paediatric and Perinatal Epidemiology, 19*, 112–124.

Chen, C.P. (2005). Maternal diabetes and neural tube defects: prenatal diagnosis of lumbosacral myelomeningocele, ventriculomegaly, Arnold-Chiari malformation and foot deformities in a pregnancy with poor maternal metabolic control, and review of the literature. *Genetic Counseling, 16*, 313–316.

Chen, J., Godschalk, M.F., Katz, P.G., et al. (1995).

Combining intracavernous injection and external vacuum as treatment for erectile dysfunction. *The Journal of Urology, 153,* 1476–1477.

Cremer, R., Kleine-Diepenbruck, U., Hering, F., et al. (2002). Reduction of latex sensitisation in spina bifida patients by a primary prophylaxis programme (five years experience). *European Journal of Pediatric Surgery, 12*(Suppl.), S19–S21.

Copp, A.J., Fleming, A., & Greene, N.D.E. (1998). Embryonic mechanisms underlying the prevention of neural tube defects. *Mental Retardation and Developmental Disabilities Research Reviews, 4,* 264–268.

Dahl, M., Ahlsten, G., Carlson, H., et al. (1995). Neurological dysfunction above cele level in children with spina bifida cystica: A prospective study to three years. *Developmental Medicine and Child Neurology, 37,* 30–40.

Davis, B.E., Dillon, C.M., Shurtleff, D.B., et al. (2005). Long term survival of patients with myelomeningocele. *Pediatric Neurosurgery, 41,* 186–191.

De Villarreal, L.M., Perez, J.Z., Vasquez, P.A., et al. (2002). Decline of neural tube defects after a folic acid campaign in Neuvo Leon, Mexico. *Teratology, 66*(5), 249–256.

Dias, L. (2004). Orthopaedic care in spina bifida: Past, present, and future. *Developmental Medicine and Child Neurology, 46,* 579.

Dillon, C.M., Davis, B.E., Duguay, S., et al. (2000). Longevity of patients born with myelomeningocele. *European Journal of Pediatric Surgery, 10*(Suppl. 1), 33–34.

Dunne, K.B., & Shurtleff, D.B. (1986). The adult with meningomyelocele: A preliminary report. In R.L. McLaurin (Ed.), *Spina bifida* (pp. 38–51). New York: Praeger.

Erikson, E.H. (1959). Identity and the life cycle. *Psychological Issues, 1,* 1–171.

Feldkamp, M., Friedrichs, M., & Carey, J.C. (2002). Decreasing prevalence of neural tube defects in Utah, 1985–2000. *Teratology, 66*(Suppl. 1), S23–S28.

Flynn, J.M., Herrera-Soto, J.A., Ramirez, N.F., et al. (2004). Clubfoot release in myelodysplasia. *Journal of Pediatric Orthopaedics B, 13,* 259–262.

Forrester, M.B., & Merz, R.D. (2000). Prenatal diagnosis and elective termination of neural tube defects in Hawaii, 1986–1997. *Fetal Diagnosis and Therapy, 15,* 146–151.

Game, X., Moscovici, J., Game, L., et al. (2006). Evaluation of sexual function in young men with spina bifida and myelomeningocele using the International Index of Erectile Function. *Urology, 67,* 566–570.

Gilbert, J.N., Jones, K.L., Rorke, L.B., et al. (1986). Central nervous system anomalies associated with meningomyelocele, hydrocephalus, and the Arnold-Chiari malformation: Reappraisal of theories regarding the pathogenesis of posterior neural tube closure defects. *Neurosurgery, 18,* 559–564.

Gos, M., Jr., & Szpecht-Potocka, A. (2002). Genetic basis of neural tube defects. II. Genes correlated with folate and methionine metabolism. *Journal of Applied Genetics, 43,* 511–524.

Gucciardi, E., Pietrusiak, M.A., Reynolds, D.L., et al. (2002). Incidence of neural tube defects in Ontario, 1986–1999. *Canadian Medical Association Journal, 167,* 237–240.

Guggisberg, D., Hadj-Rabia, S., Viney, C., et al. (2004). Skin markers of occult spinal dysraphism in children: A review of 54 cases. *Archives of Dermatology, 140,* 1109–1115.

Halachmi, S., Farhat, W., Metcalfe, P., et al. (2004, March). Efficacy of polydimethylsiloxane injection to the bladder neck and leaking diverting stoma for urinary continence. *The Journal of Urology,* 1287–1290.

Hall, J.G., Friedman, J.M., Kenna, B.A., et al. (1988). Clinical, genetic, and epidemiological factors in neural tube defects. *American Journal of Human Genetics, 43,* 827–837.

Hall, J.G., & Solehdin, F. (1998). Genetics of neural tube defects. *Mental Retardation and Developmental Disabilities Research Reviews, 4,* 269–281.

Hochhaus, F., Butenandt, O., & Ring-Mrozik, E.J. (1999). One-year treatment with recombinant human growth hormone of children with meningomyelocele and growth hormone deficiency: A comparison of supine length and arm span. *Journal of Pediatric Endocrinology and Metabolism, 12,* 153–159.

Holmbeck, G.N., Westhoven, V.C., Phillips, W.S., et al. (2003, August). A multimethod, multi-informant, and multidimensional perspective on psychosocial adjustment in preadolescents with spina bifida. *Journal of Consulting and Clinical Psychology,* 782–796.

Hommeyer, J.S., Holmbeck, G.N., Wills, K.E., et al. (1999). Condition severity and psychosocial functioning in pre-adolescents with spina bifida: Disentangling proximal functional status and distal adjustment outcomes. *Journal of Pediatric Psychology, 24,* 499–509.

Honein, M.A., Paulozzi, L.J., Mathews, M.S., et al. (2001). Impact of folic acid fortification of the US food supply on the occurrence of neural tube defects. *Journal of the American Medical Association, 285,* 2981–2986.

Hopps, C.V., & Kropp, K.A. (2003). Preservation of renal function in children with myelomeningocele managed with basic newborn evaluation and close follow up. *Journal of Urology, 169,* 305–308.

Hultling, C., Levi, R., Amark, S.P., et al. (2000). Semen retrieval and analysis in men with myelomeningocele. *Developmental Medicine and Child Neurology, 42*(10), 681–684.

Hunt, G.M. (1990). Open spina bifida: Outcome for a complete cohort treated unselectively and followed into adulthood. *Developmental Medicine and Child Neurology, 32,* 108–118.

Hunt, G.M. (1999). The Casey Holter lecture: Nonselective intervention in newborn babies with open spina bifida: The outcome 30 years on for the complete cohort. *European Journal of Pediatric Surgery, 9*(Suppl. 1), 5–8.

Hunt, G.M., & Oakeshott, P. (2003). Outcome in people with spina bifida at age 35: Prospective community based cohort study. *BMJ, 326,* 1365–1366.

Iddon, J.L., Morgan, D.J., Loveday, C., et al. (2004, August). Neuropsychological profile of young adults with spina bifida with or without hydrocephalus. *Journal of Neurology, Neurosurgery, and Psychiatry,* 1112–1118.

Kang, J.K., Lee, K.S., Jeun, S.S., et al. (2003, January). Role of surgery for maintaining urological function and prevention of retethering in the treatment of lipomeningomyelocele: Experience recorded in 75 lipomeningomyelocele patients. *Child's Nervous System,* 23–29.

Kim, E.D., & McVary, K.T. (1995). Topical prostaglandin-E1 for the treatment of erectile dysfunction. *The Journal of Urology, 153,* 1828–1830.

Kim, S.M., Han, S.W., & Choi, S.H. (2006). Left colonic antegrade continence enema: Experience gained from 19 cases. *Journal of Pediatric Surgery, 41,* 1750–1754.

Kirk, V.G., Morielli, A., & Brouillette, R.T. (1999). Sleep-disordered breathing in patients with myelomeningocele: The missed diagnosis. *Developmental Medicine and Child Neurology, 41,* 40–43.

Kryger, J.V., Spencer Barthold, J., & Fleming, P., et al. (1999). The outcome of artificial urinary sphincter placement after a mean 15-year follow-up in a paediatric population. *BJU International, 83,* 1026–1031.

Kumar, R., Bansal, K.K., & Chhabra, D.K. (2002). Occurrence of split cord malformation in meningomyelocele: Complex spina bifida. *Pediatric Neurosurgery, 36,* 119–127.

Leibold, S., Ekmark, E., & Adams, R.C. (2000). Decision-making for a successful bowel continence program. *European Journal of Pediatric Surgery, 10*(Suppl. 1), 26–30.

Levy, L.M. (1999). MR imaging of cerebrospinal fluid flow and spinal cord motion in neurologic disorders of the spine. *Magnetic Resonance Imaging Clinics of North America, 7,* 573–587.

Littlewood, R.A., Trocki, O., Shepherd, R.W., et al. (2003). Resting energy expenditure and body composition in children with myelomeningocele. *Pediatric Rehabilitation, 6,* 31–37.

Liu, S.L., Shurtleff, D.B., Ellenbogen, R.G., et al. (1999). 19-year follow-up of fetal myelomeningocele brought to term. *European Journal of Pediatric Surgery, 9*(Suppl. 1), 12–14.

Lorente Molto, F.J., & Martinez, G.I. (2005). Retrospective review of L3 myelomeningocele in three age groups: Should posterolateral iliopsoas transfer still be indicated to stabilize the hip? *Journal of Pediatric Orthopaedics B, 14,* 177–184.

Lynch, S.A. (2005). Non-multifactorial neural tube defects. *American Journal of Medical Genetics, C, Seminars in Medical Genetics, 135,* 69–76.

Main, D.M., & Mennuti, M.T. (1986). Neural tube defects: Issues in prenatal diagnosis and counselling. *Obstetrics and Gynecology, 67,* 1–16.

Manning, S.M., Jennings, R., & Madsen, J.R. (2000). Pathophysiology, prevention and potential treatment of neural tube defects. *Mental Retardation and Developmental Disabilities Research Reviews, 6,* 6–14.

Marlin, A.E. (2004, February). Management of hydrocephalus in the patient with myelomeningocele: An argument against third ventriculostomy. *Neurosurgical Focus,* E4.

Matson, M.A., Mahone, E.M., & Zabel, T.A. (2005). Serial neuropsychological assessment and evidence of shunt malfunction in spina bifida: A longitudinal case study. *Child Neuropsychology, 11,* 315–332.

Mazon, A., Nieto, A., Linana, J.J., et al. (2000). Latex sensitization in children with spina bifida: Follow-up comparative study after two years. *Annals of Allergy, Asthma and Immunology, 84,* 207–210.

McDonald, C.M. (1995). Rehabilitation of children with spinal dysraphism. *Neurosurgery Clinics of North America, 6,* 393.

McNeely, P.D., & Howes, W.J. (2004, February). Ineffectiveness of dietary folic acid supplementation on the incidence of lipomyelomeningocele: Pathogenetic implications. *Journal of Neurosurgery,* 98–100.

Meuli, M., Meuli-Simmen, C., Hutchins G.M., et al. (1995). In utero surgery rescues neurological function at birth in sheep with spina bifida. *Nature Medicine, 1,* 142–147.

Moore, C., Kogan, B.A., & Parekh, A. (2004, April). Impact of urinary incontinence on self-concept in children with spina bifida. *The Journal of Urology,* 1659–1662.

Moskowitz, D., Shurtleff, D.B., Weinberger, E., et al. (1998). Anatomy of the spinal cord in patients with meningomyelocele with and without hypoplasia or hydromyelia. *European Journal of Pediatric Surgery, 8*(Suppl. 1), 18–21.

MRC Vitamin Study Research Group. (1991). Prevention of neural tube defects: Results of the Medical Research Council Vitamin Study. *The Lancet, 338,* 131–137.

Nagarkatti, D.G., Banta, J.V., & Thomson, J.D. (2000). Charcot arthropathy in spina bifida. *Journal of Pediatric Orthopedics, 20,* 82–87.

National Institute of Child Health and Human Development. (2004). *Management of Myelomeningocele Study (MOMS).* Retrieved February 7, 2007, from http://www.spinabifidamoms.com/english/overview.html

Niall, D.M., Dowling, F.E., Fogarty, E.E., et al. (2004). Kyphectomy in children with myelomeningocele: A long-term outcome study. *Journal of Pediatric Orthopaedics, 24,* 37–44.

Nieto, A., Mazon, A., Estornell, F., et al. (2000). The search of latex sensitization in spina bifida: Diagnostic approach. *Clinical and Experimental Allergy, 30,* 264–269.

Norem, C.T., Schoen, E.J., Walton, D.L., et al. (2005). Routine ultrasonography compared with maternal serum alpha-fetoprotein for neural tube defect screening. *Obstetrics and Gynecology, 106,* 747–752.

Norrlin, S., Strinnholm, M., Carlsson, M., et al. (2003). Factors of significance for mobility in children with myelomeningocele. *Acta Paediatrica, 92,* 204–210.

Ornoy, A. (2006). Neuroteratogens in man: An overview with special emphasis on the teratogenicity of antiepileptic drugs in pregnancy. *Reproductive Toxicology, 22,* 214–226.

Palmer, J.S., Kaplan, W.E., & Firlit, C.F. (1999). Erectile dysfunction in spina bifida is treatable. *The Lancet, 354,* 125–126.

Parisini, P., Greggi, T., Di, S.M., et al. (2002). Surgical treatment of scoliosis in myelomeningocele. *Studies in Health Technology and Informatics, 91,* 442–447.

Persad, V.L., Van den Hof, M.C., Dubé, J.M., et al. (2002). Incidence of open neural tube defects in Nova Scotia after folic acid fortification. *Canadian Medical Association Journal, 167,* 241–245.

Piatt, J.H., Jr. (2004). Syringomyelia complicating myelomeningocele: Review of the evidence. *Journal of Neurosurgery, 100,* 101–109.

Pierz, K., Banta, J., Thomson, J., et al. (2000). The effect of tethered cord release on scoliosis in myelomeningocele. *Journal of Pediatric Orthopedics, 20,* 362–365.

Rader, J.I., & Schneeman, B.O. (2006). Prevalence of neural tube defects, folate status, and folate fortification of enriched cereal-grain products in the United States. *Pediatrics, 117,* 1394–1399.

Rankin, J., Glinianaia, S., Brown, R., et al. (2000). The changing prevalence of neural tube defects: A population-based study in the north of England, 1984–96. Northern Congenital Abnormality Survey Steering Group. *Paediatric and Perinatal Epidemiology, 14,* 104–110.

Rotenstein, D., & Bass, A.N. (2004). Treatment to near adult statue of patients with myelomeningocele with recombinant human growth hormone. *Journal of Pediatric Endocrinology & Metabolism, 17,* 1195–1200.

Samaniego, I. (2002). Developing a skin care pathway for pediatrics. *Dermatology Nursing/Dermatology Nurses' Association, 14,* 393–396.

Sawyer, S.M., & Roberts, K.V. (1999). Sexual and reproductive health in young people with spina bifida. *Developmental Medicine and Child Neurology, 41,* 671–675.

Schader, I., & Corwin, P. (1999). How many pregnant women in Christchurch are using folic acid supplements in early pregnancy? *The New Zealand Medical Journal, 112,* 463–465.

Shaw, G.M., Quach, T., Nelson, V., et al. (2003). Neural tube defects associated with maternal periconceptional dietary intake of simple sugars and glycemic index. *The American Journal of Clinical Nutrition, 78,* 972–978.

Shurtleff, D.B. (2004). Epidemiology of neural tube defects and folic acid. *Cerebrospinal Fluid Research, 1,* 5.

Snodgrass, W.T., & Adams, R. (2004). Initial urologic management of myelomeningocele. *The Urologic Clinics of North America, 31,* 427–434, viii.

Snow, J.H. (1994). Memory functions for children with spina bifida: Assessment in rehabilitation and exceptionality. *Pediatrics, 1,* 20–27.

Stevenson, K.L. (2004). Chiari Type II malformation: past, present, and future. *Neurosurgical Focus, 16,* E5.

Suarez, L., Felkner, M., & Hendricks, K. (2004). The effect of fever, febrile illnesses, and heat exposures on the risk of neural tube defects in a Texas–Mexico border population. *Birth Defects Research, Part A: Clinical and Molecular Teratology, 70,* 815–819.

Sutton, L.N., & Adzick, N.S. (2004). Fetal surgery for myelomeningocele. *Clinical Neurosurgery, 51,* 155–162.

Thompson, S. (1997). *The source for nonverbal learning disorders.* East Moline, IL: LinguiSystems.

Trivedi, J., Thomson, J.D., Slakey, J.B., et al. (2002). Clinical and radiographic predictors of scoliosis in patients with myelomeningocele. *The Journal of Bone and Joint Surgery, American Volume, 84-A,* 1389–1394.

Trollmann, R., Strehl, E., & Dorr, H.G. (1998). Precocious puberty in children with myelomeningocele: Treatment with gonadotropin-releasing hormone analogues. *Developmental Medicine and Child Neurology, 40,* 38–43.

Tubbs, R.S., Smyth, M.D., Wellons, J.C., III, et al. (2003). Alternative uses for the subgaleal shunt in pediatric neurosurgery. *Pediatric Neurosurgery, 39,* 22–24.

Tuli, S., Drake, J., & Lamberti-Pasculli, M. (2003). Long-term outcome of hydrocephalus management in myelomeningoceles. *Child's Nervous System, 19,* 286–291.

Vachha, B., & Adams, R.C. (2005). Memory and selective learning in children with spina bifida-myelomeningocele and shunted hydrocephalus: A preliminary study. *Cerebrospinal Fluid Research, 2,* 10.

van den Berg-Emons, H.J., Bussmann, J.B., Brobbel, A.S., et al. (2001). Everyday physical activity in adolescents and young adults with meningomyelocele as measured with a novel activity monitor. *Journal of Pediatrics, 139,* 880–886.

van Rooij, I.A., Ocke, M.C., Straatman, H., et al. (2004). Periconceptional folate intake by supplement and food reduces the risk of nonsyndromic cleft lip with or without cleft palate. *Preventive Medicine, 39,* 689–694.

Verhoef, M., Barf, H.A., Post, M.W., et al. (2004, June). Secondary impairments in young adults with spina bifida. *Developmental Medicine and Child Neurology,* 420–427.

Waitzman, N.J., Romano, P.S., & Scheffler, R.M. (1994). Estimates of the economic costs of birth defects. *Inquiry, 31,* 188–205.

Widman, L.M., McDonald, C.M., & Abresch, R.T. (2006). Effectiveness of an upper extremity exercise device integrated with computer gaming for aerobic training in adolescents with spinal cord dysfunction. *Journal of Spinal Cord Medicine, 29,* 363–370.

Williams, L.J., Rasmussen, S.A., Flores, A., et al. (2005). Decline in the prevalence of spina bifida and anencephaly by race/ethnicity: 1995–2002. *Pediatrics, 116,* 580–586.

Woodhouse, C.R. (2005). Myelomeningocele in young adults. *BJU International, 95,* 223–230.

29 Epilepsy

Steven L. Weinstein and William Davis Gaillard

Upon completion of this chapter, the reader will

- Understand the basis and causes of seizures
- Know how to recognize the manifestations of seizures
- Be able to distinguish seizures from other paroxysmal events
- Understand what is involved in the medical evaluation and therapy of seizure disorders
- Understand how to respond to family concerns

Seizures are brief, stereotyped, generally unpredictable neurological events that are commonly followed by a confused state. They occur frequently in childhood, with as many as 1 in 10 children having at least one event (Hauser, 1994; Kurtz, Tookey, Ros, et al., 1998). During the first years of life, the most common cause of an isolated seizure is a fever. Other seizures may be precipitated by acute illness (e.g., a metabolic disturbance, toxin ingestion), central nervous system (CNS) infection (e.g., meningitis, encephalitis), or traumatic brain injury (TBI) (Huang, Chang, et al., 1998). These isolated provoked seizures must be distinguished from the condition of unprovoked recurrent seizures, termed epilepsy.

JUANITA

Juanita's first seizure was a generalized **tonic-clonic seizure.** It was not associated with fever and occurred when she was 5 years old. A second seizure happened 2 weeks later. No immediate precipitant or neurological abnormality could be found. Juanita's electroencephalogram (EEG) was abnormal, showing focal spike and sharp waves. She was given carbamazepine (Tegretol) to control the seizures, but despite adequate levels of the medication, her seizures continued. Her family had difficulty coping with the problem, and they found it hard to give her the support and encouragement she needed. Juanita felt ostracized at school; she was self-conscious about her disability

and reticent about developing new friendships. Valproate (Depakote) was soon added to the carbamazepine therapy, and her seizures became less frequent. Juanita's pediatrician had difficulty achieving the desired drug level. Sometimes her medication levels were too high and Juanita was lethargic; at other times the medication levels were too low and she had seizures. Finally, the right dosage was obtained and her seizures came under good control. When emotional problems for Juanita and her family persisted, they were referred to a social worker for family counseling. Juanita began to feel better about herself. Her parents developed ways of coping with her illness and began to handle the situation more effectively. At 8 years of age, Juanita is doing well in school. She now attends Brownie Girl Scouts and dancing classes; although still shy, she is making friends.

Epilepsy is a common medical condition that occurs with increased frequency in children with developmental disabilities (see Chapter 16). This is especially the case in cerebral palsy; autism spectrum disorders (ASDs), neurocutaneous disorders (e.g., tuberous sclerosis), inborn errors of metabolism, and progressive neurologic disorders (e.g., Tay-Sachs disease) (Ballaban-Gil & Tuchman, 2000; Murphy, Trevathan, Yeargin-Allsopp, et al., 1995). In these circumstances, epilepsy is another manifestation of a brain abnormality and may complicate the care and needs of the child. Epilepsy itself can contribute to impaired cognitive function, as can side effects of antiepileptic drugs (AEDs). Children with epilepsy also have a high incidence of attention-deficit/hyperactivity disorder, learning disabilities, anxiety disorders, and depression. The prevalence of these conditions is greater than in other chronic diseases of childhood, such as asthma and diabetes.

Learning and behavioral disorders are often present at the onset of epilepsy (Austin, Harezlak, Dunn, et al., 2001). This observation provides evidence that learning disabilities, behavioral disorders, and epilepsy are different manifestations of the same underlying brain dysfunction.

EPILEPSY DEFINITIONS, CAUSES, AND CONSEQUENCES

The word *epilepsy* is derived from a Greek word meaning "take hold of" or "seize" (Reynolds, 2000). Epilepsy is defined as a condition involving two unprovoked seizures separated by 24 hours. The term does not define severity or prognosis. The word *seizure* is not synonymous with epilepsy, and a single seizure does not qualify an individual for the diagnosis of epilepsy. The circumstances surrounding a first-time single seizure may be unique or have occurred during a specific developmental window such that it is unlikely to recur. Examples of this include a single **febrile** seizure in the preschool-age child, a convulsion that follows a faint, and a seizure following minor head trauma. In contrast, epilepsy may be an expression of a chronic neurological condition of which one manifestation is recurrent seizures.

For most children, epilepsy is a self-limited condition that resolves over several years. For some children, however, epilepsy is a chronic condition characterized by recurrent seizures that is an expression of an underlying brain abnormality. A seizure involves the abnormal, excessive, and concurrent firing of a large population of cortical neurons. This results in the interruption of usual brain-generated electrical signals, leading to an abrupt change in the person's behavior. The abnormal brain activity spreads to adjacent brain areas over the ensuing seconds to minutes. This is accompanied by behavioral changes followed by a relatively rapid end and return to baseline (Shorvon, 2000). This evolution is useful in differentiating seizures from nonepileptic paroxysmal events—spells such as fainting that abruptly interrupt the child's behavior but are not seizures. This

distinction is important because the causes of and treatments for each are different (Reynolds, 2000).

Several factors modulate the predisposition for seizures and the threshold at which they occur. An acute brain insult has the potential to trigger a seizure in anyone, but not everyone will have a seizure when presented with the same insult. This differing susceptibility reflects genetic and acquired factors that affect structural and chemical brain interactions (Briellmann, Jackson, Torn-Broers, et al., 2001; Frucht, Quigg, Schwaner, et al., 2000; Prasad, Prasad, Stafstrom, et al., 1999).

The age of the child, reflecting the stage of brain development, also influences the **seizure threshold** (Moshe, 2000). This explains why some children appear to grow into or outgrow epilepsy (Sillanpaa, 2000). It also indicates why some types of seizures are only seen during certain age windows (e.g., neonatal period, adolescence). Not only does the brain undergo obvious alterations in structure over time (Gage, 2002), but there are also changes in brain chemistry. This affects which neurotransmitters are released and how other cells respond to them (Kriegstein, Owens, Avoli, et al., 1999). Alterations in typical brain development, structure, or chemistry can affect the subsequent cascade of brain maturation and predispose the child to epilepsy (Lowenstein & Alldredge, 1998). Reparative mechanisms following certain brain injuries can also lead to the formation of abnormal neuronal networks that may generate seizure activity (Cole, 2000). (See Chapter 30 for a discussion of seizures following TBI.)

Seizures are ultimately a disorder of neuronal transmission and brain network interactions. The factors that predispose a child to have seizures are poorly understood but include 1) injury to brain cells that make them dysfunctional, as occurs in TBI or brain tumors; 2) disruption of brain cell circuits, as occurs in tuberous sclerosis and cerebral dysplasia; and 3) alterations in intrinsic brain cell excitability, as occurs in many inherited forms of epilepsy such as severe myoclonic epilepsy and autosomal dominant nocturnal frontal lobe epilepsy. Both the environment and intrinsic qualities of a specific neuron influence its behavior. As there are many connections between individual neurons, the likelihood of any given neuron being recruited to fire is the result of the summation of excitatory and inhibitory influences of neighboring neurons (Kandel, Schwartz, Jessell, et al., 2000).

Seizures are commonly viewed as disorders of excessive excitatory neurotransmitter activity or diminished inhibitory transmission. During a seizure, a network of brain cells begins to fire abnormally, producing excessively synchronous discharges. At times, this occurs with the simultaneous involvement or subsequent recruitment of an increasingly larger population of surrounding cortical neurons. The abnormal firing continues until it is extinguished by inhibitory neurochemical influences or until the excitatory neurochemicals are depleted. The seizure usually subsides in seconds to minutes, but in some instances it will not stop spontaneously, a condition termed *status epilepticus.*

The initial **ictal** (seizure) activity produces signs and symptoms typical of the function of the brain area from which it arises. For example, in a simple partial seizure there may be unusual sensations, called an aura (originating from the mesial temporal lobe), abnormal motor activity, such as jerking of fingers or hand (involving the primary motor cortex of the frontal lobe), or abnormal posture (propogation of the seizure through the basal ganglia). Once the electrical discharge extends beyond the original site to involve brain structures that are necessary to sustain consciousness (e.g., limbic system), the clinical expression changes and becomes a complex partial seizure. There is a progressive alteration of consciousness that is frequently associated with automatisms such as staring, fumbling, or picking at clothing. If the entire brain becomes involved, with bilateral motor activity, the result is a generalized tonic-clonic seizure (Risinger, 2000). The ability of the brain to confine the abnormal electrical discharge to a limited area and its capacity to extinguish the seizure explain the limited spread and duration of most seizures. When these mechanisms fail, seizures may become prolonged. Status epilepticus seizures are those that last longer than 15–30 minutes. Because most seizures are brief and self-limited they do not require urgent medical attention; the exception is status epilepticus (see later discussion).

There is much debate about the potential adverse effects of clinical seizures on brain structure and function (Camfield, 1997; Wasterlain, 1997). In tonic-clonic seizures, although the frequently observed cyanosis (blueness of the lips and face from inefficient breathing and shunting of oxygenated blood to the brain) is the most frightening feature, the neurochemical changes in the brain during the seizure are of the greatest concern to physicians. The overex-

citation of neurons during a seizure leads to the release of excitatory neurotransmitters, such as glutamate. This release can lead to cell death, increasing the likelihood of future seizures, and possibly leading to progressive cognitive and behavioral impairments. For example, children who have had multiple focal and prolonged febrile seizures during early childhood are more likely to develop complex partial seizures in adolescence. This condition, termed mesial temporal sclerosis, results from damage to the hippocampus, a critical center for memory and new learning (Berg, Shinnar, Levy, et al., 2000). It is important to note that the vast majority of children who have experienced febrile seizures do not sustain brain injury or develop epilepsy later in life.

Some experts argue that the epileptic focus in the brain is caused by recurrent seizures; others hold that a preexisting brain abnormality causes both the seizures and associated neurological and behavioral disturbances. There is evidence that some forms of epilepsy result in progressive structural and functional brain injury (Gaillard, Kopylev, Weinstein, et al., 2002; Liu, Lemieux, Bell, et al., 2003). Unfortunately, most AEDs do not protect the brain from the process of pathological reorganization that can form an epileptic focus in the brain (Shinnar & Berg, 1994). A number of seizure types (e.g., benign **rolandic epilepsy,** absence seizures) do not appear to be associated with brain injury.

CLASSIFICATION OF EPILEPSY AND EPILEPSY SYNDROMES

The epilepsies are commonly categorized as having either an apparently generalized onset (simultaneously involving widely spread cortical regions over both brain hemispheres) or a partial onset (starting in one limited brain region, with variable degrees of spread). Epilepsy syndromes, which form another category, are classified based on the clinical appearance of the seizures, the EEG, and the age of onset. This classification is important in both guiding the diagnostic evaluation and prescribing appropriate therapy. Yet, confusion may arise in classifying epilepsy for a number of reasons: 1) the onset of the seizure is often not observed or remembered; 2) the seizure spread is rapid, and the focal signs may be lost among the associated dramatic behaviors; and 3) observers may be so overwhelmed by the experience that they do not recognize the subtleties of the seizure presentation. Fortunately, the nature of the seizure onset can often be inferred by the interictal (between-seizure) EEG pattern (Panayiotopoulos, 1999). The different seizure types are discussed next.

Seizures with Primarily Altered Consciousness

Primarily Generalized Seizures Primarily generalized seizures account for more than 35% of pediatric epileptic disorders. These seizures do not have a recognizable focus of onset; instead, large areas of each cortex appear to be simultaneously affected. During a generalized seizure, the child may have decreased motor activity (e.g., absence seizures) or vigorous abnormal motor behaviors (e.g., myoclonic, atonic, and tonic-clonic seizures). The underlying cause is often genetic, and when it results from neurochemical or receptor alterations in cortical neurons it is called a channelopathy (Noebels, 2003).

Absence Seizures Absence seizures (previously called petit mal seizures; Table 29.1) are among the most benign seizure types. They appear to arise simultaneously in broad regions of the brain and are mediated through the thalamus. The onset is usually between 3 and 12 years of age. They are characterized by a brief (usually less than 30 seconds) behavioral arrest with impaired consciousness. During this time, a characteristic 3-hertz spike and wave discharge occurs on EEG. Unlike most other seizures, there is no postictal (time immediately following a seizure) period of confusion prior to the restoration of full awareness. The child may continue to perform a simple activity, such as walking or looking at something, but he or she is unable to rapidly respond to a novel task, such as reading. Rarely is the behavior arrest just a

motionless blank stare; there is usually a glazed eye appearance, associated eye blinks, and/or changes in head and extremity tone. Unlike simple daydreaming, absence seizures cannot be interrupted by verbal or tactile (touch) stimulation (Loiseau, 1992). Untreated, these episodes can occur hundreds of times during the day and may significantly interfere with learning. In addition, absence seizures can be a physical hazard as the child may sustain injury by continuing to walk, unaware, into a busy street or down steps. If absence seizures last longer (more than 30 seconds) or are associated with prominent motor activity, they may be but one aspect of an epilepsy syndrome, such as juvenile myoclonic epilepsy (JME) or atypical absence epilepsy. Absence epilepsy may evolve to include generalized tonic-clonic seizures, especially in adolescence (Mayville, Fakhoury, Abou-Khalil, et al., 2000).

Partial Seizures Partial seizures are the most common type of seizure disorder in childhood, accounting for almost 60% of all cases (Eriksson & Koivikko, 1997). Partial seizures may arise not only in the motor control centers of the brain but also in areas involved in sensory, behavioral, and cognitive functions (Figure 29.1). These seizures often start with an aura and/or an abrupt and unprovoked alteration in behavior. Given that most children will have a single cortical region of seizure onset, the specific feelings/behaviors will occur with little variation from one episode to another.

When the electrical event is limited to a small region of one hemisphere, with maintenance of normal alertness, it is categorized as a simple seizure. If the event is merely sensory in nature, it is called an aura. If the seizure spreads and alters consciousness, it is called a complex partial seizure (previously called psychomotor seizure). This type of seizure may occur with or without subsequent secondary generalization into a tonic-clonic motor seizure.

The signs and symptoms of complex partial seizures are the result of the brain's impaired ability to rapidly plan motor activities and process environmental stimuli; these signs also provide clues to the region of seizure onset (Risinger, 2000). During a complex partial seizure, the abnormal electrical disturbance in the brain causes the child's movements to become purposeless and slowed. Frequently this is accompanied by motor automatisms including eye blinking, lip smacking, facial grimacing, groaning, chewing, and unbuttoning and buttoning of clothing. In addition, depending on the site

Table 29.1. Comparison of complex partial seizures and absence seizures

	Complex partial	Absence
Incidence	Common	Uncommon
Duration	30 seconds to 5 minutes	Less than 30 seconds
Frequency of occurrence	Occasional	Multiple times daily
Aura	Yes	No
Consciousness	Partial amnesia and confusion	Immediate return to consciousness
Electroencephalogram (EEG) pattern	Focal	Generalized

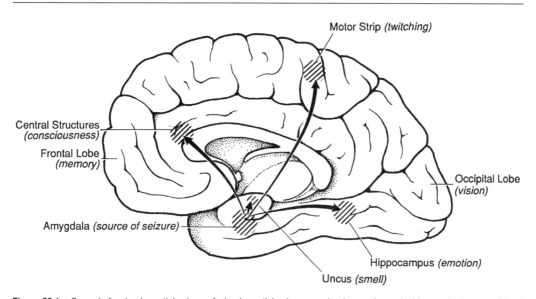

Figure 29.1. Spread of a simple partial seizure. A simple partial seizure may begin anywhere—in this case in the amygdala of the temporal lobe. The intial feature may be the child's smelling an unusual odor. The seizure may stop there or project out to the hippocampus, which might trigger feelings of fearfulness or abdominal queasiness. Memory and visual perception may be affected if the frontal or occipital lobe is involved. The seizure might ultimately extend to the motor strip, resulting in twitching of a limb, which may spread to other limbs or to central structures (causing loss of consiousness), thus becoming a complex partial seizure. Finally, the seizure may cross the corpus callosum to the other cerebral hemisphere and thus be converted from a partial to a generalized seizure.

of seizure onset, the child may appear agitated. These seizures tend to occur during sleep and can be misinterpreted as night terrors. When they happen during the day, the child may strike out at someone who comes too close during the seizure or postictal period. This is not a directed activity but the result of the child's confused state.

Seizures with Prominent Motor Manifestations

Seizures with prominent motor manifestations, like seizures that primarily alter consciousness, can arise focally (partial seizure) or diffusely (primarily generalized seizure) and can be either brief or prolonged.

Myoclonic and Atonic Seizures The briefest types of seizures with motor components are myoclonic and atonic seizures. Myoclonic seizures are lightning motor attacks, with sudden flexion or bending backward of the upper torso and head. Some of these seizures are subtle, with just head nodding, whereas others appear to abruptly pull the child over. Myoclonic seizures, atonic seizures (which involve loss of muscle tone), and any other type of seizure that leads to an abrupt loss of posture com-

pose a group called drop seizures. Consciousness is usually impaired during these events, and the child makes no attempt to protect him- or herself during the fall. As a result, there is a risk of the head striking the ground. Children with these kinds of seizures should wear a protective helmet throughout the day. Following these brief seizures, the child immediately regains consciousness, often crying, seemingly not in pain but upset by the sudden disruption.

Tonic-Clonic Seizures The tonic-clonic seizure is the most frightening seizure to observe; it is what the public generally calls a grand mal seizure (Shorvon, 2000). It may arise focally and then secondarily generalize (a partial seizure), or it may arise diffusely from both hemispheres (a primary generalized seizure). Clonic motor activity (repetitive jerking occurring at a regular rate) and tonic motor activity (sustained stiffening) often occur within the same seizure. On occasion a clonic seizure may spread from one portion of the brain to a contiguous area, producing a spread of the shaking to other body parts (called a Jacksonian seizure). Tonic seizures may also start in one area of the body (a partial seizure), or they may occur bilaterally, involving the trunk and extremities (a generalized seizure). If focal in onset, tonic or clonic seizures can be followed by a period of weakness on the body side that was first affected (called Todd's paralysis). This may be misinterpreted as a stroke by parents and health care providers (Szabo & Luders, 2000). Tonic-clonic seizures account for about one quarter of seizures in individuals of any age (Kotagal, 2000). During the seizure, observers frequently hear raspy breathing or see no breathing effort at all and may mistakenly assume that the tongue has been swallowed. Tonic-clonic seizures are often associated with an unusual cry, cyanosis, and incontinence. A period of sleep is required for recovery, and the individual usually has no memory of the event.

Status Epilepticus Although prolonged seizures (status epilepticus) occur infrequently with any seizure type, they deserve special consideration. Such seizures have the potential to be life threatening and/or to lead to permanent pathological changes within the brain's structural organization. Status epilepticus is defined as a "single seizure or cluster of seizures that is sufficiently prolonged or repeated at sufficiently brief intervals to produce an unvarying and enduring epileptic condition" (Gastaut, 1982). Although this definition does not establish a precise duration, most clinicians consider 15–30 minutes of continuous seizing or repetitive seizures without a full return of consciousness to represent status epilepticus (Lowenstein, 1999). There is evidence from animal models that irreversible changes in brain structure may occur as a result of status epilepticus (Fujikawa, Shinmei, Cai, et al., 2000). Death is a rare consequence (Lhatoo, Johnson, Goodridge, et al., 2001). Status epilepticus is a medical emergency and requires immediate diagnostic and therapeutic intervention. In the emergency room, the physician will evaluate the child to exclude acute causes for the prolonged seizure and use intravenous medication to stop the seizure. Frequently, a follow-up visit to a neurologist is indicated to exclude other underlying chronic disorders that could precipitate future episodes of status epilepticus.

Epilepsy Syndromes

Epilepsy syndromes are seizure disorders characterized by specific clinical features and characteristic EEG findings. A group of signs, symptoms, diagnostic tests, and historic information defines an epilepsy syndrome. These include 1) age, 2) neurological signs and symptoms,

3) clinical course, and 4) characteristic EEG findings and may involve 5) a genetic component (Wolf, 1994). Examples of epilepsy syndromes are described next.

Benign Partial Seizures Typically benign partial seizures have their onset around the age of school entry and disappear by adolescence (Okumura, Hayakawa, Kato, et al., 2000). They usually have a characteristic EEG, and neuroimaging studies (magnetic resonance imaging [MRI] scan) are always normal. They demonstrate a strong genetic influence, with 30%–40% of near relatives having seizures (Neubauer, 2000). Usually these syndromes are unassociated with long-term sequelae (Fejerman, Caraballo, Tenembaum, et al., 2000).

Rolandic epilepsy is the most common benign epilepsy syndrome of childhood. The seizures typically start in the region of the cortex that controls tongue, face, and hand movements; they most commonly occur at sleep onset or at arousal. When starting in sleep, the partial onset is unobserved, so children may appear to have generalized tonic-clonic seizures (Lerman, 1992).

Other benign partial seizures arise from the occipital lobe and frequently are associated with visual disturbances. They can occasionally be triggered by entering or leaving a well-lit room. At night these seizures can simulate a migraine-like event, with vomiting and severe headache (Caraballo, Cersosimo, Medina, et al., 2000).

Infantile Spasms and Myoclonic Epilepsy Syndromes Myoclonic epilepsy is often a reflection of a serious underlying disease (e.g., Tay-Sachs disease). The exception is a rare, transient, benign form of myoclonic epilepsy that occurs early in infancy, is responsive to AEDs, and does not lead to long-term cognitive impairments (Lin, Itomi, Takada, et al., 1998). Myoclonic epilepsy is strongly associated with a family history of epilepsy and has an EEG pattern that shows spike and polyspike and wave discharges.

Infantile spasms are characterized by serial brief flexor (head, arms, and hip) or extensor (arms and trunk) seizures, EEG abnormalities, and intellectual disability. Its onset is typically between 4 and 8 months of age, and it is difficult to control with AEDs (Shields, 2000). The seizures occur in flurries that typically occur upon arousal from sleep but may happen sporadically throughout wakefulness. They can occur in combination with altered consciousness as a part of a complex partial seizure (Kubota, Aso, Negoro, et al., 1999). The affected infant is generally lethargic, has poor visual fixation, and shows a plateauing or loss of developmental milestones.

More than three quarters of these infants have a defined underlying disorder (Trasmonte & Barron, 1998) such as tuberous sclerosis (see Appendix B), other brain malformations and dysplasia (e.g., lissencephaly, Aicardi syndrome; see Appendix B), genetic syndromes (e.g., Down syndrome; see Chapter 18), and inherited metabolic disorders (e.g., phenylketonuria, nonketotic hyperglycinemia, biotinidase deficiency; see Appendix B). Perinatal events causing brain injury, such as birth asphyxia and congenital infections (e.g., cytomegalovirus; see Chapter 6), also can predispose the infant to the development of infantile spasms. This epilepsy frequently evolves into Lennox-Gastaut syndrome in early childhood.

A small percentage of infants have cryptogenic infantile spasms (i.e., spasms with no identifiable etiology). These children respond rapidly to therapy, do not develop Lennox-Gastaut syndrome, have typical development prior to spasm onset, and can have a fair developmental outcome. The EEGs of both spasm groups show a characteristic and markedly disorganized EEG pattern called hypsarrhythmia.

Medical therapy aims to both normalize the EEG pattern and prevent further seizures. Treatment with adrenocorticotropic hormone (ACTH) is effective (Riikonen, 2000). AEDs have also been used as therapy, including valproate (Depakene, Depakote), phenobarbital (Luminal), lamotrigine (Lamictal), topiramate (Topamax), clonazepam (Klonopin), and pyridoxine (vitamin B$_6$) (Ito, 1998). A new AED, vigabatrin (Sabril), has also been found to be helpful in controlling infantile spasms, especially those associated with tuberous sclerosis (Jambaque, Chiron, Dumas, et al., 2000). The Food and Drug Administration (FDA) has not approved this drug for use in the United States because of its potential for retinal toxicity (Harding, Wild, Robertson, et al., 2000). In rare instances of infantile spasms, a single seizure focus can be identified and surgically removed, "curing" the condition (Shields, Shewmon, Peacock, et al., 1999).

Juvenile myoclonic epilepsy (JME) commonly begins during later adolescence as morning myoclonus. Medical attention for JME is frequently not sought until the teen or young adult has experienced a generalized tonic-clonic seizure following sleep deprivation, photic pre-

cipitation, or alcohol ingestion (Pedersen & Petersen, 1998). JME is a "benign" genetic disorder and is not associated with intellectual disability. The diagnosis of JME is problematic. It is frequently underrecognized, leading to treatment with the wrong AED. Drugs used to treat generalized rather than partial seizures are indicated in JME (Montalenti, Imperiale, Rovera, et al., 2001; Wallace 1998). Once diagnosed, the patient requires lifelong treatment with an AED.

Atypical absence epilepsy syndromes are classified as a form of childhood absence epilepsy, but these syndromes have a worse prognosis (Wolf, 1992) than typical absence seizures. These seizure types may also be present in Lennox-Gastaut and Landau-Kleffner syndromes (see the discussion that follows). The onset of atypical absence epilepsy syndromes is either in childhood or adolescence. Beyond the brief staring spells that are typical of absence seizures, these syndromes may be associated with generalized tonic-clonic seizures or with prominent myoclonus.

Lennox-Gastaut syndrome, which often evolves from infantile spasms, is associated with intellectual disability and behavioral disturbances. Unlike other epilepsies, this syndrome is characterized by multiple types of seizures that occur throughout the day (Rantala & Putkonen, 1999). The seizure pattern encompasses tonic seizures during sleep, and absence/atypical absence, drop (including myoclonic), tonic-clonic, and complex partial seizures during awake hours. The EEG has a characteristic pattern, and there is abundant epileptiform activity during sleep. Treatment of Lennox-Gastaut syndrome is difficult, and both seizures and EEG resolution appear to be necessary for improved cognitive and behavioral outcomes.

Landau-Kleffner syndrome, or acquired epileptic aphasia, is characterized by a progressive encephalopathy, the hallmark of which is loss of language skills. The disorder is manifested by an auditory agnosia (inability to distinguish different sounds), language regression (or, rarely, the inability to attain language skills), and behavioral disturbances that include inattention. Occasionally the clinical picture resembles an ASD (see Chapter 23; Tuchman, 1997). Clinically evident seizures may be infrequent or absent, but when the child is asleep, the EEG pattern shows continuous abnormal epileptiform activity that obscures the normal sleep pattern (Rossi, Parmeggiani, Posar, et al., 1999). As with Lennox-Gastaut syndrome, treatment is difficult. EEG normalization and seizure control seem to be necessary for improved outcome, and steroid medication may be useful. The syndrome is important as it may serve as a model for a treatable form of autism.

Febrile Seizures

Febrile seizures are the most commonly witnessed seizures during childhood. Because they are provoked by fever, they are not considered an epilepsy syndrome. They occur in approximately 5% of all children who are between the ages of 6 months and 5 years; they rarely appear at an older age (Nelson & Ellenberg, 1978) (Figure 29.2). Febrile convulsions are generally seen with temperature elevations above 39 degrees Celsius (102 degrees Fahrenheit). Those seizures that occur with lower temperatures are associated with an increased risk of subsequent febrile seizures (Berg, Darefsky, Holford, et al., 1998). Upper respiratory illnesses, middle-ear infections, gastroenteritis, immunizations, and viruses associated with skin rashes (e.g., roseola) are known precipitants. Greater than 80% of all febrile seizures are brief, symmetric tonic or clonic-tonic events that occur once during an illness. These are called simple febrile seizures; in contrast, complex febrile seizures are prolonged, focal, and/or recurrent during a single illness (Hirtz, 1997). Complex febrile seizures are frequently of unknown cause, but a more aggressive evaluation than for simple febrile seizures may be undertaken to exclude a chronic encephalopthy or an acute CNS infection (e.g., meningitis, encephalitis).

After the first fever-provoked seizure, the risk of subsequent febrile seizures is 30%–50%, depending upon the child's age at the time of the first seizure, a family history of febrile convulsions, and the intensity of the fever (Berg, Shinnar, Hauser, et al., 1992). The risk of developing epilepsy (recurrent seizures) by school age in a typically developing child is 1% following simple febrile seizures and 2%–3% following complex febrile seizures (Nelson & Ellenberg, 1976). The risk of developing epilepsy by adulthood may be somewhat higher (Berg & Shinnar, 1996). The risk of future epilepsy is increased in a child with a preexisting developmental disability (e.g., intellectual disability, see Chapter 17; cerebral palsy, see Chapter 26) or with a family history of epilepsy (Nelson & Ellenberg, 1976). As many as 30%–50% of adults with intractable epilepsy resulting from mesial temporal sclerosis have a history of febrile seizures (Bower, Kilpatrick, Vogrin, et al., 2000). Risk of future febrile convulsions should not influence the decision to treat (or not treat) with AEDs after a seizure. Although medications may prevent subsequent febrile seizures, AEDs do not prevent the development of future epilepsy (Knudsen, 2000).

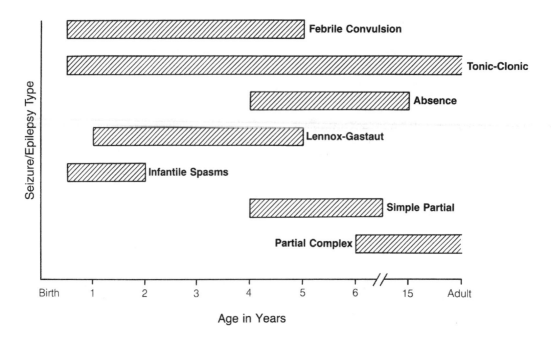

Figure 29.2. Common ages of occurrence of various types of seizures.

Conditions that Mimic Epilepsy

Not all paroxysmal events are epilepsy. A generalization is that if a behavior can be triggered, interrupted, or modified by external stimuli, then it probably is not a seizure. Examples include sleep disorders, movement disorders (see Chapter 27) (Greene, Kang, Fahn, et al., 1995), behavior disturbances, syncope (fainting) (Ilhan, Tuncer, et al., 1999), migraine (Andermann & Zifkin, 1998; Hernandez-Latorre & Roig, 2000), pseudoseizures (Bye, Kok, et al. 2000), and systemic disorders such as gastroesophageal reflux (Werlin, D'Souza, Hogan, et al., 1980). Exceptions to this rule include **parasomnias** (e.g., night terrors, sleep walking), febrile-induced seizures and abnormal shaking in infancy (Tal, Even, Kugelman, et al., 1997), hypotonic-hyporesponsive spells after vaccines (DuVernoy & Braun, 2000), and reflex epilepsy in older children (e.g., induced by flickering lights or causing other specific sensory changes). A sampling of these disorders is discussed next.

Sleep Disorders   Most motor events during sleep are a part of normal sleep activity. These include the random jerks of the extremities or eyes (rapid eye movement) that occur during active sleep when the child is dreaming. More pronounced jerking occurs at sleep onset and may awaken the child or anyone sleeping in the same bed. Benign **sleep myoclonus** of infancy, an uncommon symmetric and pronounced jerking of extremities that resembles a generalized clonic seizure, can occur in newborns and infants during sleep but ceases on arousal (Pachatz, Fusco, Vigevano, et al., 1999). The EEG is normal during this behavior, which stops by a few months of age with no long-term consequences.

Other, more complex motor behaviors may occur 1–2 hours after sleep onset or occasionally upon arousal. These parasomnias include night terrors, sleep talking, sleepwalking, and teeth grinding (Laberge, Tremblay, Vitaro, et al., 2000). Rarely, nocturnal frontal lobe seizures are misinterpreted as a parasomnia because they may be bizarre; a video EEG recording is required to distinguish between the two (Lombroso, 2000; Zucconi, Oldani, Ferini-Strambi, et al., 1997). During a parasomnia, the eyes are open and the child appears to be awake, but the EEG shows a normal sleep rhythm. These parasomnia episodes may last as long as 15–30 minutes, a duration that is much longer than typical seizures, and the parent may be unable to end the spell or rouse the child during

this time. Rarely, treatment with medication such as diazepam (Valium) is necessary if the behavior is significantly disruptive to family life.

Behavior Disorders   Behaviors associated with apparent altered consciousness can occur during sleep or wakefulness and may simulate seizures. Brief staring spells (daydreaming or "spacing out") are most commonly a sign of inattention than of seizure activity. They rarely interrupt an active behavior, and they lack the subtle motor changes seen with absence or complex partial seizures (Bye, Kok, Ferenschild, et al., 2000).

Temper tantrums and rage attacks may also resemble seizures (Gordon, 1999). During these episodes the child cries, yells, throws him- or herself on the floor, and lashes out at nearby people. Occasionally sweating, paleness, and dilated pupils, as well as post-event sleepiness, can be observed. Tantrums can be distinguished from seizures by the presence of a behavioral provocation, the absence of stereotypic behaviors that occur consistently with each event, and the presence of movements that are either directed at a person or too coordinated or rapid to occur during the confused state of a seizure.

Breath-holding spells are a common nonepileptic cause of loss of consciousness that can be confused with seizures in infants age 6–18 months. Breath-holding episodes are precipitated by unexpected pain, anger, or frustration. This leads to prolonged crying and the eventual arrest of breathing. This breath holding may last close to a minute and may be associated with blueness of the lips, back arching, and loss of consciousness (Breningstall, 1996). The breath-holding spell ends with a sudden gasping for breath and rapid neurological recovery. Prolonged episodes can be associated with brief generalized convulsive movements followed by lethargy (Kuhle, Tiefenthaler, Seidl, et al., 2000). It is usually inappropriate to treat breath-holding spells with AEDs; there is evidence that treatment with iron supplements decreases the number of spells, especially if the child is anemic (Mocan, Yildiran, Orhan, et al., 1999).

DIAGNOSIS AND EVALUATION OF SEIZURE DISORDERS

The evaluation of a child who has experienced a first seizure involves obtaining 1) a description of the seizure that includes the sleep–wake status of the child, 2) initial signs/symptoms and their evolution over time, and 3) postictal status with any transient neurological impairments following the seizure. Predisposing factors also should be explored such as 1) behavioral changes the day prior to the event; 2) sleep activity the prior evening and morning; and 3) exposure to precipitants such as an acute infection, trauma, or drugs (illicit, prescribed, or accidentally ingested). A physical and neurological examination is performed to identify the presence of an acute illness or evidence suggestive of a chronic neurological disorder.

If the child is well and has fully recovered from the seizure, then additional studies are unlikely to be revealing or helpful in deciding therapy. Some physicians may choose to pursue further medical evaluations in order to a rule out possible underlying disorders, to alleviate parental anxiety, and/or to address medical and legal concerns. Typically this evaluation includes determinations of blood glucose and electrolytes (especially if the child is younger than 2 years), an EEG, and a brain imaging study such as computed tomography (CT) or MRI (preferred) (Berg, Testa, Levy, et al., 2000). A complete blood count or lumbar puncture is unhelpful unless one is evaluating a child with febrile seizures or if a CNS infection is a concern. Certainly if the child continues to have neurological impairments after the seizure, these tests should be performed to exclude a significant underlying disease. Under these circumstances screening tests may be considered for inborn errors of metabolism (e.g., plasma amino acids, urinary organic acids). Once seizures recur, fulfilling the criteria for epilepsy, evaluation is warranted to detect an underlying condition that may be treatable (Hirtz, Ashwal, Berg, et al., 2000). Antiepileptic medication is usually not recommended until a second unprovoked seizure has occurred (Hirtz, Berg, Donley, et al., 2003).

Electroencephalogram

The EEG is most often performed during an interictal period (between seizures) to demonstrate disturbances in brain electrical activity that are typically found in individuals with a seizure disorder (Fisch, 1999). In this study, electrodes are pasted on the head at set points to record voltage changes generated by neuronal networks in the cortex below the electrodes. Brain wave patterns on the EEG may indicate either nonspecific widespread abnormalities, suggestive of a diffuse brain dysfunction (encephalopathy), or specific findings (spikes and

sharp waves) indicative of a specific epileptic disorder or syndrome. Occasionally a seizure is captured or induced during the EEG recording.

From the clinical descriptions of the seizures and the EEG profile, a specific seizure type can often be defined. It is important to obtain the EEG both during wakefulness (to identify encephalopathy) and in light sleep (to find epileptiform abnormalities) (Fountain, Kim, Lee, et al., 1998). Hyperventilation and photic stimulation (with strobe lights) may also be performed to elicit EEG patterns found in certain absence, other generalized and complex partial seizure syndromes (Hennessy & Binnie, 2000). When the nature of the suspected seizure remains unclear, prolonged (1–7 days) EEG monitoring with continuous video telemetry is performed to characterize the events and distinguish absence from complex partial seizures (Bye et al., 2000).

If nothing is known about the patient other than that an unprovoked seizure has occurred, the risk of the child's having a second seizure can be estimated as 30%–55%. The presence of an abnormal EEG with spikes following this first seizure increases that recurrence risk to 40%–70%, whereas the presence of a normal EEG is associated with a recurrence risk of 20%–40% (Shinnar, Berg, Moshe, et al., 1996).

The EEG also establishes a baseline that can be used to assess electrographic deterioration in the event that the seizure heralds a progressive neurological disorder (Gilbert & Buncher, 2000). Focal abnormalities on EEG may suggest the site of seizure onset, allowing the area of interest to be studied using neuroimaging techniques. Not only does the EEG characterize the seizure type or syndrome, but it is also helpful in predicting the future course of the disorder and in choosing an AED for treatment.

The interictal spikes rarely disappear, even when the child's seizures are under good control with an AED (Andersson, Braathen, Persson, et al., 1997). Absence epilepsies represent a particular challenge because the electrographic abnormality may persist, even though parents report that the episodes have disappeared (Appleton & Beirne, 1996). Only in rare epilepsy syndromes (e.g., Landau-Kleffner syndrome, infantile spasms) does the neurologist treat the between-seizure spikes. Therefore, there is usually no medical reason to routinely follow the EEG in a child who is seizure free. If the seizures are increasing or are changing in nature or if the underlying condition is worsening, a follow-up

EEG may be helpful. The decision to discontinue AEDs may provide another reason to perform a repeat EEG. If the EEG continues to demonstrate severe abnormalities of background activity and abundant spikes and waves, then the recurrence risk of a seizure following drug withdrawal is substantial (Andersson et al., 1997). In contrast, if the EEG has totally normalized, the chances for recurrence are far less.

Prolonged video EEG may also be utilized during a presurgical assessment (Jayakar, 1999) in children whose epilepsy is refractory to medical therapy. This technique precisely defines the site of seizure onset and maps normal brain functions in the area to be removed during surgery.

Brain Imaging Techniques

Several imaging methods are available to evaluate brain structure and function in childhood epilepsy: CT, MRI, magnetic resonance spectroscopy (MRS), positron emission tomography (PET), single photon emission computed tomography (SPECT), and magneto-electro-encephalography (MEG).

CT uses X rays and has limited anatomic detail, but is readily available and is useful in emergency situations to exclude large structural lesions, calcifications (from congenital infections), or blood from trauma. MRI uses the intrinsic magnetic characteristics of the molecules of the brain, rather than X rays, to produce images. MRI has superior anatomic resolution and detail compared with CT and is the imaging method of choice to identify brain abnormalities that can cause epilepsy (Berg, Testa, Levy, et al., 2000; Hirtz, Ashwal, Berg, et al., 2000). CT and MRI examine brain structure, whereas the other brain imaging studies listed focus on abnormalities in brain blood flow and metabolism. PET and SPECT scans require injection of small amounts of radioactive material and are restricted to evaluating children for epilepsy surgery. PET is less readily available than SPECT. PET images reveal metabolic activity of the brain, and SPECT maps blood flow to brain areas. These two techniques can assist in localizing a seizure focus by identifying areas of the brain that have decreased glucose consumption between seizures (PET) and increased blood flow during a seizure (SPECT) (Gaillard, 2000). The techniques can also help to examine neurotransmitter function and identify abnormalities in neurotransmitter receptors that occur in certain types of epilepsy.

Other rapidly developing technologies, including MRS, functional MRI (fMRI), and magnetoencephalography (MEG), have the potential to demonstrate brain activity without the need for radioactive tracers (Gaillard, Bookheimer, Cohen, et al., 2000). MRS, which can be done as part of a routine MRI scan, is being used to identify certain metabolic derangements in the brain that can cause seizures, as those that occur in mitochondrial disorders and other inborn errors of metabolism. fMRI is used to map the location of specific brain functions (e.g., language, motor cortex) by detecting changes in the MR signal elicited by changes in blood flow that occur during activities such as reading or moving fingers. MEG is another modality that permits a window on brain function by measuring magnetic activity of the cortex to produce three-dimensional localization of a seizure focus, which may be helpful in planning epilepsy surgery (Ebersole, 1999).

TREATMENT OF EPILEPSY

Intervention During a Seizure

The need for intervention during a seizure by parents or professionals depends on the seizure type and duration. Repeated absence seizures require no immediate action. Prolonged complex partial seizures require intervention after 10–15 minutes. Tonic-clonic seizures require simple, common-sense first aid procedures (Berg, Shinnar, Hauser, et al., 2001). The child should be placed on the floor or a bed and turned to one side to prevent choking or aspirating of vomitus. The child should not be tightly restrained. Clothing should be loosened around the neck. Fingers, tongue blades, spoons, or other instruments should not be inserted between the child's teeth to prevent "swallowing of the tongue," which is physically impossible. Cardiopulmonary resuscitation efforts should generally be avoided because they are unnecessary and can lead to the "rescuer" suffering bitten fingers and the child sustaining loosened teeth and vomiting and/or aspirating the vomit.

Normally, emergency medical services (i.e., 911 in most locations of the United States) need to be called only if the seizure lasts more than 5–10 minutes, which is uncommon in children. The Epilepsy Foundation (n.d.) suggests that an ambulance be called if 1) the child is not known to have had prior seizures, 2) the child has an intercurrent illness, 3) a second seizure

occurs, or 4) consciousness is not regained following the seizure. If the seizure occurs with
fever or trauma, urgent care should be sought.
Otherwise, the child should be attended until
fully awake and alert and then allowed to nap.
The child often needs reassurance and comfort-
ing and should be encouraged to resume activities after recovering fully. Parents should be notified and the details of the seizure explained. It
is ideal to have a treatment plan in the school
nurse's office outlining these interventions in
advance of a seizure occurring in a child with
epilepsy and to have a similar plan available to
adults caring for the child in other environments (e.g., child care, sport or community activities, summer camp).

Medical Treatment with Antiepileptic Drugs

AEDs manipulate neurotransmitter activity and
ionic channels, influencing seizure activity (Rogawski & Loscher, 2004). The decision to treat
a child who has seizures with an AED requires a
balancing of potential benefits and risks. The
first consideration is making a correct diagnosis. Diagnostic studies may assist in clarifying
the nature of the spell and the recurrence risk.
Ultimately the decision to treat or not depends
on the parents' and physician's assessment of
the risk of seizures (biological and social) versus
the risk associated with the AED (Greenwood
& Tennison, 1999; Hirtz, Berg, Donley, et al.,
2003). This includes considering whether the
recurrence risk is high and whether seizure control will alter the biological outcome. For these
reasons, treatment is usually instituted only after
a second unprovoked seizure (Hirtz, Berg, et al.,
2003).

The optimal AED should prevent all seizures from occurring without producing side
effects (Fisher, Vickrey, Gibson, et al., 2000a).
At the most, one dose each day should be required, and the AED should improve or cure
the underlying disorder. Unfortunately, present
therapies do not meet these criteria. As a rule,
multiple doses of medication are required to
keep peak blood AED levels from becoming too
high and producing toxic effects while keeping
trough levels high enough to prevent seizures
from occurring. Current AEDs do not improve
the underlying condition that causes the seizures.

The definition of successful seizure control often differs among children, their parents,
other caregivers, and physicians. Children gen-

erally do not like taking the medication or having side effects, so they want fewer and lower
doses of AED. Teachers and parents want the
children to be seizure free and without medication side effects, so that they can concentrate
and learn. There must also be agreement between parent and physician as to whether the
desired outcome is seizure freedom or a substantial reduction in seizure activity, as this decision may affect the medication regimen or the
choice of performing surgery.

Mechanisms, Selection, and Use of Antiepileptic Drugs
AEDs work by inter-
fering with the physiological mechanisms that
lead to seizures (Rogawski & Loscher, 2004).
There are numerous channels on neurons that
allow the flow of ions (e.g., calcium, potassium,
sodium) into and out of cells. These channels
are opened and closed by excitatory (glutamate)
and inhibitory (gamma aminobutyric acid, or
GABA) neurotransmitters that are released
from nearby cells. The older AEDs (e.g., phenytoin [Dilantin], carbamazepine [Tegretol]) block
the high-frequency voltage-dependent sodium
channels. Several newer AEDs (e.g., felbamate
[Felbatol], lamotrigine) block this channel but
also inhibit excitatory neurotransmission. Other
AEDs (e.g., valproate [Depakene, Depakote],
topiramate) have even a wider range of potential mechanisms. Valproate blocks voltage-
dependent sodium channels and calcium cur-
rents while also influencing GABA transmission.
Topiramate blocks sodium channels, opens chloride channels, and interferes with glutamate
transmission. Other AEDs (e.g., barbiturates
[phenobarbitol], benzodiazepines [Valium], vigabatrin [Sabril], tiagabine [Gabitril], gabapentin
[Neurontin]) primarily increase inhibitory mechanisms mediated by the neurotransmitter GABA.
The mechanism of action of some drugs (e.g.,
levetiracetam [Keppra]) is not fully understood.
This raises the possibility that additional mechanisms of action of AEDs are yet to be discovered (Moshe, 2000).

AEDs are probably best utilized as single
therapy (Guberman, 1998). Use of multiple
drugs carries the potential for biochemical interactions. One drug may increase or decrease
the metabolism of the other in the child's body
or brain, possibly decreasing efficacy and/or increasing side effects. Drug interactions also can
occur with medications taken for other conditions, and certain foods (e.g., grapefruit) can affect the metabolism of some drugs. In severe
epilepsy that is unresponsive to a single medica-

tion, an additional drug may be required (Leppik, 2000).

After an assessment of the risks and benefits of using an AED, the specific medication or group of medications is chosen based on the seizure type, age of the child, specific epilepsy disorder, and potential side effects (Bourgeois, 2000). Once a particular drug is selected, additional choices remain: generic versus brand-name drug, capsule versus liquid, and so forth. The generic drug (if available) will be cheaper, but it may not have the same formulation, resulting in less predictable absorption and metabolism (Besag, 2000). AEDs may be packaged in many forms: a syrup (rapidly absorbed but with quickly disappearing effects), sprinkles (easily administered, delayed in absorption, and longer lasting), and sustained-release pills/capsules (easier to take, as fewer doses per day are required, but must be swallowed). Sprinkles and sustained-release pills/capsules can potentially be more effective in controlling seizures by maintaining a more stable blood level of the medication throughout the day. Care must be taken when switching from one formulation of a drug to another, as it cannot be assumed that drug levels and seizure control will remain stable.

Before 1993, the most commonly used AEDs were phenobarbital, phenytoin, carbamazepine, ethosuximide (Zarontin), and valproate. Since 1993, nine new AEDs have been approved by the FDA (but not all have been studied in children, and fewer have been tested in infants): felbamate, gabapentin, lamotrigine, levetiracetam, oxcarbazepine (Trileptal), tiagabine, topiramate, zonisamide (Zonegran), and pregabalin (Lyrica). In addition, new sustained-release formulations of two older drugs have decreased their toxicity: carbamazepine (Tegretol XR, Carbatrol) and valproate (Depakote ER). Intravenous drugs used to treat status epilepticus have undergone reformulation (e.g., fosphyenytoin [Cerebyx], which is closely related to phenytoin), and there is now a rectal gel preparation of diazepam (Diastat). These newer medications have increased both the options and the complexity of AED therapy. The major advantage of the new drugs is that they may be more specific in their action. As a result they can theoretically be more effective at a lower dosage and have fewer side effects. (See Appendix C for more information on AED preparations available, dosages, and side effects.)

Most AEDs do not work solely on the neurons that trigger seizures. They alter neuro-chemistry diffusely throughout the brain. Some AEDs may also be prescribed for conditions that affect behavior and emotions: mood disorders (carbamazepine, valproate, lamotringene), aggression and pain (carbamazepine, gabapentin), and migraines (valproate, topiramate) (Backonja, 2000; Mitchell, Zhou, Chavez, et al., 1993; Nemeroff, 2000).

Side Effects of Antiepileptic Drugs

The most common side effects of AEDs involve motor and cognitive aspects of brain function. They include sleepiness, decreased attention and memory, dysphasia (difficulty producing speech), ataxia (unstable gait), and diplopia (double vision). These side effects may occur transiently when a new drug is started or dosage is increased, or they may persist and require the discontinuation of the medication.

There is an additional concern that AEDs may have an adverse effect on learning that may persist long after the drug has been discontinued. This issue was raised by a study of phenobarbital in children with febrile seizures (Farwell, Lee, Hirtz, et al., 1990), in which children were found to have cognitive impairments that persisted for 6 months after drug cessation. Topiramate and zonisimide may also lead to impaired cognition. Virtually all AEDs, especially at high dosages, have the potential to cause cognitive impairments during treatment, but long-term effects, especially of the newer medications, have not been studied to date (Kwan & Brodie, 2001; Loring & Meador, 2004).

Medication administration requires gastrointestinal absorption, dissolution in the blood, and eventual exposure of other body organs to the drug. As a result, side effects of AEDs can involve many organs in addition to the brain. There can be gastrointestinal irritation (e.g., stomach discomfort), bone marrow suppression (leading to low white and red blood cell counts), liver dysfunction (e.g., as revealed by elevated liver function tests), kidney stones, pancreatitis, cardiac arrhythmia or decreased heart contractility, and dermatological changes (e.g., hair loss, coarsening of facial features, gum overgrowth, skin changes). Certain AEDs taken during pregnancy can increase the risk of having a child with a neural tube defect or other birth defects (see Chapter 2). Other side effects are hormonal/metabolic in nature and are more common with long-term therapy. These include abnormal calcium and vitamin D metabolism (see Chapter 10) that may be severe enough to increase the risk of bone fractures or rickets;

weight gain or loss; in females, polycystic ovaries, leading to impaired fertility; and decreased thyroid hormone level.

Many of the medication side effects are dosage related, so decreasing the prescribed amount of an AED can lead to elimination of adverse effects. Sometimes the side effects are independent of dosage and probably reflect genetic differences in the metabolism or sensitivity of the patient to the drug. In these instances, if the side effects are severe, the AED should be stopped (Harden 2000).

The *Physician's Desk Reference (PDR)* manual on prescription drugs (published annually by Medical Economics Company), and the package inserts from medications, typically list 2–3 pages of potential side effects for each AED. When an AED is being selected, it is reasonable to decide which of the more common side effects the child and family is willing to consider tolerating. If there are significant side effects, it is fairly straightforward to change medications, as several alternatives are available.

Determining Dosage of Antiepileptic Drugs
The usual approach in determining AED dosage is to use the lowest dosage that is effective in controlling the seizures and does not produce unacceptable side effects. This is achieved by starting at a low dosage of a single AED and gradually increasing it as necessary. Some practitioners aim to achieve a blood level within a particular range. This therapeutic range represents a blood level that will have the desired effect—seizure control—without toxicity for most children. These published norms may not always be useful in decision making for the individual child. Some children can either achieve seizure control or have side effects with levels below this range. Similarly, other children require dosages above the therapeutic range to control their seizures, yet these children may never experience side effects.

How quickly the drug dosage is increased after it is first started depends on the severity and frequency of the seizures as well as the metabolism of the medication. The newer AEDs appear to have fewer side effects overall but, if increased rapidly, can still produce side effects or toxicity significant enough to require their discontinuation. This is an argument for a gradual increase in dosage of a new medication.

Monitoring Drug Therapy
After starting an AED, parents and physicians need to be attuned to changes in the child's well-being. Some practitioners require routine blood tests, including drug levels, complete blood counts, and liver function tests. They argue that this monitoring will provide early evidence of toxicity, demonstrate compliance, and provide information on how rapidly a child metabolizes a medication (Glauser & Pippenger, 2000). Other physicians suggest that routine blood studies are not necessary (Camfield & Camfield, 2000). They note that if the patient is clinically doing well, any blood abnormality is likely to be incidental and will resolve spontaneously. They feel that finding an abnormal level only leads to parental anxiety and child discomfort. Although there is controversy about the importance of routine testing, there is general agreement that these blood tests should be obtained if there are breakthrough seizures (seizures while on AEDs) or clinical signs of drug toxicity.

Deciding When Drug Therapy Should Be Started
Drug therapy is usually started only when a child is diagnosed with epilepsy. An AED is usually not started at the time of the first seizure, and, in the case of febrile seizures, it may never be started despite multiple seizure episodes (Hirtz, Berg, Donley, et al., 2003). There is no evidence that a delay in therapy until epilepsy is confirmed affects the risk of brain injury, long-term prognosis, or efficacy of AED therapy (Hirtz, Berg, Donley, et al., 2003). Issues such as the ability to drive, safety (e.g., preventing traumatic falls from drop seizures), social stigma (e.g., dealing with incontinence following a seizure), parental fear (e.g., of a seizure resulting in injury or death) and medical risk of a seizure in some chronic diseases (congenital heart disease, metabolic disorders, and sickle cell disease) may influence that decision.

Deciding When Drug Therapy Can Be Stopped
In the past, AED treatment was prescribed for life. There are, however, significant concerns regarding the long-term use of AEDs, including 1) potential teratogenicity during pregnancy; 2) establishment of a poor self-image of being chronically ill; and 3) cost in time and money for medications, doctor's visits, and laboratory monitoring. Now every attempt is made to stop the drug after a seizure-free interval. Overall, after an individual has been seizure free for 2 years, the risk of seizure recurrence after medication is stopped is about 25%–35% (Caviedes & Herranz, 1998). The risk is higher in children with 1) developmental disabilities, 2) identified structural brain abnormalities, 3) requirement for more than one AED to achieve seizure control, and 4) onset of epilepsy during

adolescence. The EEG is often helpful in deciding whether to stop therapy. The presence of a normal EEG suggests that it is safe to stop AEDs, whereas an abnormal EEG points to increased uncertainty for seizure recurrence if AEDs are stopped.

Other Antiepileptic Therapies

A number of antiepileptic therapies do not rely on medication. Some are old therapies that have recently regained favor based on new research findings (e.g., ketogenic diet, epilepsy surgery). Others are preventive approaches involving vitamin and mineral supplementation and lifestyle changes that have been found to be helpful. In addition, there are alternative therapies that have not been tested scientifically and should be viewed with skepticism. Finally, there is the promise of new approaches to treating seizures in the future. These various therapies are briefly discussed in the section that follows.

Ketogenic Diet The ketogenic diet represents an alternative method to treat epilepsy for some patients. Although controlled studies are lacking, the existing studies indicate that 56% of individuals with epilepsy have a reduction in seizures while on a ketogenic diet, and 16% stop seizing completely (Hemingway, Freeman, Pilas, et al., 2001). The mechanism of action of the diet is unknown but appears to be associated with utilizing fat rather than carbohydrates for cellular energy. To be effective, the ketogenic diet requires weighing and calculating the amounts of nutrients in all foods the child eats. The sugars/carbohydrates from any medications must also be considered in the calculations. In addition, the urine must be monitored to assure adequate spillage of ketones (from which the diet gets its name), a byproduct of fat metabolism. The ketogenic diet is severely restrictive and not very tasty. Side effects include metabolic acidosis, electrolyte disturbances, uric acid kidney stones, diarrhea/vomiting, constipation, and failure to thrive. The diet, similar to AED therapy, can be stopped after the child has a period of being seizure free. It is rarely tolerated for more than a year or two because of the side effects.

Surgical Interventions The only "cure" for epilepsy is surgical removal of the seizure focus. This has been most successfully accomplished in complex partial seizures arising from the mesial temporal lobe (Wiebe, Blume,

Girvin, et al., 2001). It has also been used in well-defined structural abnormalities such as a tumor, vascular malformation, or focal cortical dysplasia. When there are multiple foci in one side of the brain, another operation can be used, hemispherectomy. This procedure involves the removal of most of one side of the brain. It is used most often in uncontrollable seizures resulting from progressive unilateral disorders, such as Rasmussen encephalitis, Sturge-Weber syndrome, hemispheric dysplasia, or stroke (porencephaly) (see Appendix B).

In addition to these "curative" surgical procedures, palliative surgical interventions are also available. One example is corpus callosotomy (cutting of the corpus collosum, which connects the two hemispheres) for treating drop seizures. A second is electrical stimulation of the vagus nerve or, rarely, the thalamus for intractable mixed seizures that have an onset that cannot be localized to one area or one hemisphere.

Uncommon complications of surgical interventions include bleeding, infection, and harm to the eloquent (speech), memory, or motor cortex. The decision to perform surgery generally follows the failure of the child's seizures to respond to AEDs. Determining how many drugs should be tried without success before considering surgery is difficult. After the third or fourth drug failure the likelihood of completely controlling the seizures with medication is estimated to be only 10% (Bourgeois, 2000). The timing of surgery is not only driven by how frequent and how severe the seizures are but also by the seizures' impact on the child's life and family dynamics.

Nonspecific Interventions There are also certain nonspecific interventions that might be used to decrease seizure occurrence. These include ensuring that the child obtains regular, reasonable amounts of sleep and avoids sedative medications. These strategies help because many forms of epilepsy are exacerbated by drowsiness. Infection and/or fever can also trigger seizures, so appropriate hand washing, avoidance of contact with people who have viral illnesses, and aggressive fever control should be undertaken. Finally, it is important to identify and avoid or alter specific triggers that provoke seizures. The most common of these are the ovulatory cycle in females and flashing lights for the child with photic-induced seizures. In deciding whether a potential trigger is really a precipitant, it must be remembered how many times that event has occurred without precipitating a seizure.

Vitamins and Minerals For the child with seizures, supplementation with a multivitamin containing calcium may be useful in preventing osteoporosis. For females of childbearing age who are taking valproate, folate supplementation is also recommended. Megadoses of the B and E vitamins or supplemental carnitine are not indicated for the typical child with epilepsy (Baxter, 1999). In fact, high dosages of supplemental vitamins and minerals may be harmful, except in rare cases of pyridoxine dependency/deficiency, which require moderate dosages of vitamin B_6. Certain rare inborn errors of metabolism that are associated with seizure disorders are treated with a combination of vitamins and nutritional supplements (see Chapter 20).

Complementary and Alternative Medicine Various homeopathic and herbal remedies have been touted to treat epilepsy, but none have been shown to be effective in controlled clinical trials (Danesi & Adetunji, 1994). These interventions, although often labeled "natural," are not necessarily harmless. When considering the use of complementary and alternative medicine, the remedy should not 1) carry a significant risk of increasing seizure activity; 2) compromise any therapy already in place, such as AEDs; 3) be harmful to the child's general health; or 4) be costly.

Future Therapeutic Approaches A number of research therapies may prove useful in the future. In animal studies reservoirs are being implanted into areas of the brain affected by seizures, permitting AEDs to be infused directly into the seizure focus (Stein, Eder, Blum, et al., 2000). Electrical stimulators are being implanted into the thalamus to alter the pathways that lead from this organ to broad regions of the cerebral cortex or over the seizure focus to abort seizures (Velasco, Velasco, Velasco, et al., 2000). The use of transcranial magnetic brain stimulation is also being tested (Theodore & Gaillard, 2002; Ziemann, Steinhoff, Tergau, et al., 1998). In the future, medical intervention is likely to shift from treating the symptom (seizures) of the brain disorder to treating the underlying abnormality. Gene therapy may allow the introduction of new genes into patients with specific mutations (e.g., channelopathies) that lead to epilepsy. Agents may be developed that are given immediately after a brain injury to interrupt abnormal reorganization of neural networks. Stem cell implantation into the brain, with the provision of appropriate growth factors, may allow the replacement of destroyed neural networks. Finally, microchip implantation may permit the creation of a "bionic" part of the brain that assumes those functions lost in the seizure focus.

MULTIDISCIPLINARY NEEDS AND INTERVENTION

The care of the child with epilepsy involves more than just medical or surgical treatment of the seizures. Education, psychosocial support, and involvement of the entire family are all critical to effective management for the child (Kwong, Wong, So, et al., 2000). For these reasons, it is wise to have a comprehensive epilepsy center follow a child with seizures that are difficult to control. These multidisciplinary clinics are staffed with by a team of neurologists, psychiatrists, psychologists, nurses, social workers, and other health care professionals working together. For families living at a distance from an epilepsy center, the center's staff can work with the local pediatrician as consultants in helping to ensure optimal seizure control.

Educational Programs

From an educational perspective, the student's basic needs are dictated by his or her cognitive and learning abilities (Bulteau, Jambaque, Viguier, et al., 2000). Teachers must be alert for signs of difficulty attributable to seizures or side effects from AEDs. The child with absence seizures who suddenly begins to do poorly in class may have unrecognized increased seizure activity. Alternatively, new or worsening school problems may develop as a result of side effects from an increased AED dosage or a switch to a new medication (Fisher, Vickrey, Gibson, et al., 2000b). Behavioral side effects may include fatigue, inattention, irritability, and aggression. Teachers and parents must be alert to these signs, for they may indicate the need to check drug levels or to change the AED dosage schedule. Alternatively, these nonspecific features may point to intercurrent illness, peer problems, new learning difficulties, or the need to reevaluate the entire educational program. Children with epilepsy are covered by the Individuals with Disabilities Education Improvement Act of 2004 (PL 108-446) under "other health impairments" and can receive special education and related services (see Chapter 34).

There are also the psychological side effects of a child having a seizure in class. For example, bowel and bladder incontinence during a tonic-clonic seizure may cause the child intense embarrassment. For the child whose seizures are under good control and who has no known daytime seizures, there is no reason to discuss his or her epilepsy with the class. This will simply identify the child as being different and subject to being stigmatized. Parents who are worried about a seizure occurring in class may request a classroom discussion about epilepsy. This can be done without identifying the specific child (Coleman & Fielder, 1999). Conversely, if the student is likely to have seizures in the classroom, the best approach is anticipatory education of classmates about seizures so that they know what to expect and can be helpful. A towel and a fresh change of clothing can be kept in the nurse's office for children who have poorly controlled tonic-clonic seizures that are associated with incontinence.

Psychosocial Issues

Seizures have a significant impact on the child and his or her family (Fisher, Vickrey, et al., 2000a; Fisher, Vickrey, et al., 2000b). Although most children have infrequent seizures and the total time of ictal activity is a tiny fraction of their lives, the disorder and its treatment may become all consuming for the family. The uncertainty of when the seizure will strike next may be what causes such distress. The child with epilepsy must be educated about the cause of the seizures. Even if seizures become rare after achieving proper medication dosage, full discussion is appropriate.

The social stigma attached to epilepsy may need to be addressed with the child and family (Schoenfeld, Seidenberg, Woodward, et al., 1999). Surveys find that the self-perception of a person with epilepsy is far worse than how others see this person (Arnston, Droge, et al., 1986). Some children with epilepsy have low self-esteem and depression, leading to absenteeism in school and overdependence on their parents. Unfortunately, these self-esteem concerns and parental overprotection can lead to social isolation. When this is combined with subtle impairments in memory or learning, school failure may result. Although the seizures themselves or the social reaction to them are major concerns for families, it is actually the as-

sociated brain dysfunction—cognitive, behavioral, and motor impairment—that is more problematic. Unlike a seizure, which is a time-limited episode, these deficits are persistent and affect daily functioning.

The issue of sports has been controversial (Steinhoff, Neususs, Thegeder, et al., 1996). At one time, children with epilepsy were precluded from participation in many sports; now it is thought that most sports are permissible once seizures are well controlled (Nakken, 1999) (see Chapter 34). Most clinicians continue to recommend that children with epilepsy avoid heavy contact sports such as tackle football as well as unusually dangerous activities such as rock climbing and scuba diving. Of course, routine safety precautions recommended for all children should be taken.

Similarly, family vacations and camping trips need not be curtailed in the child with well-controlled seizures. Excessive fatigue should be avoided, as it may precipitate a seizure, and the family should travel with an adequate supply of the AED and a written prescription or the doctor's and pharmacist's telephone numbers in case the medicine is misplaced or stolen. The decision for the child to wear a medical identification bracelet or necklace optimally should be made with the child's assent; its value is considerably diminished if it is felt to be stigmatizing.

The family structure and routine should be kept intact as much as possible, and it is important not to overprotect the child. Care should be taken to use common sense precautions, especially if the seizures are poorly controlled. These include having the child take showers rather than baths (unless attended), having him or her not lock the bathroom door, and supervising the child when he or she is working near a stove or on a ladder. When using a babysitter, parents need to provide careful instruction for seizure recognition, first aid, and a plan of action if a seizure occurs.

There may also be significant financial issues for the family regarding the cost of medications, doctor visits, laboratory tests, hospitalizations, and time off work (Begley, Famulari, Annegers, et al., 2000). (See Chapter 42 for a discussion of health care financing and different funding options for families.) Families may have to make decisions as to where they can live and what jobs they can accept based on their concerns for the care of their children. As the child moves toward adulthood, independence should be encouraged as much as possible (see Chapter

41). This includes fostering independent living, driving (only when seizure free for 3–12 months, depending on state regulations), and the pursuit of appropriate job opportunities; addressing concerns about insurance; and dealing with altered fertility rate and potential teratogenic effects of AEDs.

Advocacy

Organizations such as the American Epilepsy Society, the Epilepsy Foundation, and the International League Against Epilepsy; numerous other societies and medical centers across the world; and self-help groups advocate for acceptance of individuals with epilepsy in society. Governments are lobbied, businesses and school personnel educated, and children and families counseled in order to provide the needed resources for children with epilepsy (see Appendix D).

OUTCOME

Most children with seizure disorders have typical intelligence scores (Dodson, 2001). There has been controversy as to whether repeated seizures or chronic AED treatment can lead to subtle brain injury, limiting the child's potential over time. Repeated IQ tests have not shown a decline in intellectual abilities, unless the child is overmedicated, is exposed to certain AEDs that carry higher risk of cognitive impairment, or has had a very prolonged episode of status epilepticus.

Prognosis mostly depends on the seizure type and the underlying brain pathology. For example, the average IQ score for children with absence seizures is in the normal range, whereas children with Lennox-Gastaut syndrome have intellectual disability. Prognosis depends not solely on intelligence but also on how the child and family handle this chronic illness. If the seizures come under control easily and drug side effects are few, the family is likely to cope well. If the seizures prove resistant to treatment and drug side effects are many, these stresses may interfere with the functioning of both the child and family.

If psychosocial issues and subtle impairments in memory and learning are approached in an effective manner, the prognosis is generally good. As most seizures remit during childhood, it is critical to encourage each child to achieve his or her maximal potential. For those whose epilepsy is but one feature of a multiple disability disorder, the eventual outcome is more commonly a function of the other disabilities than of the seizures.

About 70%–80% of children with epilepsy achieve control of their seizures with the first or second AED tried. Two thirds remain seizure free during a 5-year follow-up period, and almost the same percentage can be successfully weaned from their AED after 2 years of being seizure free (MacDonald, Johnson, Goodridge, et al., 2000). These generalizations are somewhat misleading because they may not include all of the childhood seizure syndromes. These statements also overrepresent the more severe cases that are followed in epilepsy clinics, and the statistics do not deal with medication compliance issues or provide long-term follow-up (across several decades). Finally, epilepsy is not a homogeneous disorder; even within families with a genetic form of epilepsy, there is variability of seizure expression.

SUMMARY

Epilepsy is a chronic neurological condition that involves recurrent seizures as an expression of an underlying brain abnormality. The seizures themselves are manifestations of abnormal electrical discharges within the brain. Generalized seizures include those classified as tonic-clonic, absence, myoclonic, and atonic. Partial seizures are defined as simple or complex, depending on whether there is loss of consciousness or secondarily generalized. Seizures may occur singly or in combination and may start in the newborn period, in infancy, or in later childhood. For about half of affected children, the seizures are an isolated disability. Most can be controlled by a single AED, and these children can lead quite typical lives. For a child with multiple disabilities, the prognosis is generally more a function of the other disabilities than of the seizures. Key problems in our understanding of the condition include difficulty in predicting outcome, not knowing whether recurrent seizures cause biologic harm, problems in using medications to prevent subsequent seizures without eliciting toxicity, and deciding when it is safe to discontinue medications.

REFERENCES

Andermann, F., & Zifkin, B. (1998). The benign occipital epilepsies of childhood: An overview of the idiopathic syndromes and of the relationship to migraine. *Epilepsia, 39*(Suppl. 4), S9–S23.

Andersson, T., Braathen, G., Persson, A., et al. (1997). A comparison between one and three years of treatment in uncomplicated childhood epilepsy: A prospective study. II. The EEG as predictor of outcome after withdrawal of treatment. *Epilepsia, 38*(2), 225–232.

Appleton, R.E., & Beirne, M. (1996). Absence epilepsy in children: The role of EEG in monitoring response to treatment. *Seizure, 5*(2), 147–148.

Arnston, P., Droge, D., et al. (1986). The perceived psychosocial consequences of having epilepsy. In S. Whitman & B.P. Herman (Eds.), *Psychopathology in epilepsy: Social dimensions* (pp. 143–161). New York, Oxford University Press.

Austin, J.K., Harezlak, J., Dunn, D.W., et al. (2001). Behavior problems in children before first recognized seizures. *Pediatrics, 107*(1), 115–122.

Backonja, M.M. (2000). Anticonvulsants (antineuropathics) for neuropathic pain syndromes. *The Clinical Journal of Pain, 16*(2, Suppl.), S67–S72.

Ballaban-Gil, K., & Tuchman, R. (2000). Epilepsy and epileptiform EEG: Association with autism and language disorders. *Mental Retardation and Developmental Disabilities Research Reviews, 6*(4), 300–308.

Baxter, P. (1999). Epidemiology of pyridoxine dependent and pyridoxine responsive seizures in the UK. *Archives of Disease in Childhood, 81*(5), 431–433.

Begley, C.E., Famulari, M., Annegers, J.F., et al. (2000). The cost of epilepsy in the United States: An estimate from population-based clinical and survey data. *Epilepsia, 41*(3), 342–351.

Berg, A.T., Darefsky, A.S., Holford, T.R., et al. (1998). Seizures with fever after unprovoked seizures: An analysis in children followed from the time of a first febrile seizure. *Epilepsia, 39*(1), 77–80.

Berg, A.T., & Shinnar, S. (1996). Unprovoked seizures in children with febrile seizures: Short-term outcome. *Neurology, 47*(2), 562–568.

Berg, A.T., Shinnar, S., Hauser, W.A., et al. (1992). A prospective study of recurrent febrile seizures. *The New England Journal of Medicine, 327*(16), 1122–1127.

Berg, A.T., Shinnar, S., Levy, S.R., et al. (2000). How well can epilepsy syndromes be identified at diagnosis? A reassessment 2 years after initial diagnosis. *Epilepsia 41*(10), 1269–1275.

Berg, A.T., Shinnar, S., Levy, S.R., et al. (2001). Defining early seizure outcomes in pediatric epilepsy: The good, the bad and the in-between. *Epilepsy Research, 43*(1), 75–84.

Berg, A.T., Testa, F.M., Levy, S.R., et al. (2000). Neuroimaging in children with newly diagnosed epilepsy: A community-based study. *Pediatrics, 106*(3), 527–532.

Besag, F.M. (2000). Is generic prescribing acceptable in epilepsy? *Drug Safety, 23*(3), 173–182.

Bourgeois, B. (2000, December). *Presidential symposium.* Annual meeting of the American Epilepsy Society, Los Angeles.

Bower, S.P., Kilpatrick, C.J., Vogrin, S.J., et al. (2000). Degree of hippocampal atrophy is not related to a history of febrile seizures in patients with proved hippocampal sclerosis. *Journal of Neurology, Neurosurgery, and Psychiatry, 69*(6), 733–738.

Breningstall, G.N. (1996). Breath-holding spells. *Pediatric Neurology, 14*(2), 91–97.

Briellmann, R.S., Jackson, G.D., Torn-Broers, Y., et al. (2001). Causes of epilepsies: Insights from discordant monozygotic twins. *Annals of Neurology, 49*(1), 45–52.

Bulteau, C., Jambaque, I., Viguier, D., et al. (2000). Epileptic syndromes, cognitive assessment and school placement: A study of 251 children. *Developmental Medicine and Child Neurology, 42*(5), 319–327.

Bye, A.M., Kok, D.J., Ferenschild, F.T., et al. (2000). Paroxysmal non-epileptic events in children: A retrospective study over a period of 10 years. *Journal of Paediatrics and Child Health, 36*(3), 244–248.

Camfield, P.R. (1997). Recurrent seizures in the developing brain are not harmful. *Epilepsia, 38*(6), 735–737.

Camfield, P.R., & Camfield, C.S. (2000). Treatment of children with "ordinary" epilepsy. *Epileptic Disorders, 2*(1), 45–51.

Caraballo, R., Cersosimo, R., Medina, C., et al. (2000). Panayiotopoulos-type benign childhood occipital epilepsy: A prospective study. *Neurology, 55*(8), 1096–1100.

Caviedes, B.E., & Herranz, J.L. (1998). Seizure recurrence and risk factors after withdrawal of chronic antiepileptic therapy in children. *Seizure, 7*(2), 107–714.

Cole, A.J. (2000). Is epilepsy a progressive disease? The neurobiological consequences of epilepsy. *Epilepsia, 41*(Suppl. 2), S13–S22.

Coleman, H., & Fielder, A. (1999). Epilepsy education in schools. *Paediatric Nursing, 11*(9), 29–32.

Danesi, M.A., & Adetunji, J.B. (1994). Use of alternative medicine by patients with epilepsy: A survey of 265 epileptic patients in a developing country. *Epilepsia, 35*(2), 344–351.

Dodson, W.E. (2001). Epilepsy, cerebral palsy, and IQ. In J.M. Pellock, W.E. Dodson, & B.F.D. Bourgois (Eds.), *Pediatric epilepsy and therapy* (pp. 613–627). New York: Demos Medical.

DuVernoy, T.S., & Braun, M.M. (2000). Hypotonic-hyporesponsive episodes reported to the Vaccine Adverse Event Reporting System (VAERS), 1996–1998. *Pediatrics, 106*(4), E52.

Ebersole, J.S. (1999). Non-invasive pre-surgical evaluation with EEG/MEG source analysis. *Electroencephalography and Clinical Neurophysiology Supplement, 50,* 167–174.

Epilepsy Foundation. (n.d.). *Is an emergency room visit needed?* Retrieved February 28, 2006, from http://www.epilepsyfoundation.org/answerplace/Medical/firstaid/seizureer.cfm

Eriksson, K.J., & Koivikko, M.J. (1997). Prevalence, classification, and severity of epilepsy and epileptic syndromes in children. *Epilepsia, 38*(12), 1275–1282.

Farwell, J.R., Lee, Y.J., Hirtz, D.G., et al. (1990). Phenobarbital for febrile seizures—effects on intelligence and on seizure recurrence. *The New England Journal of Medicine, 322*(6), 364–369.

Fejerman, N., Caraballo, R., Tenembaum, S.N., et al. (2000). Atypical evolutions of benign localization-related epilepsies in children: Are they predictable? *Epilepsia, 41*(4), 380–390.

Fisch, B.J. (1999). *Fisch and Spehlmann's EEG primer: Basic principles of digital and analog EEG.* New York: Elsevier Science.

Fisher, R.S., Vickrey, B.G., Gibson, P., et al. (2000a). The impact of epilepsy from the patient's perspective I: Descriptions and subjective perceptions. *Epilepsy Research, 41*(1), 39–51.

Fisher, R.S., Vickrey, B.G., Gibson, P., et al. (2000b). The impact of epilepsy from the patient's perspective II: Views about therapy and health care. *Epilepsy Research, 41*(1), 53–61.

Fountain, N.B., Kim, J.S., & Lee, S.I. (1998). Sleep deprivation activates epileptiform discharges independent of the activating effects of sleep. *Journal of Clinical Neurophysiology, 15*(1), 69–75.

Frucht, M.M., Quigg, M., Schwaner, C., et al. (2000). Distribution of seizure precipitants among epilepsy syndromes. *Epilepsia, 41*(12), 1534–1539.

Fujikawa, D.G., Shinmei, S.S., Cai, B., et al. (2000). Seizure-induced neuronal necrosis: Implications for programmed cell death mechanisms. *Epilepsia, 41* (Suppl. 6), S9–S13.

Gage, F.H. (2002). Neurogenesis in the adult brain. *The Journal of Neuroscience, 22*(3), 612–613.

Gaillard, W., Bookheimer, S.Y., & Cohen, M. (2000). The use of fMRI in neocortical epilepsy. In P.D. Williamson, A.M. Siegel, V.M. Thadani, et al. (Eds.), *Advances in neurology, 84: Neocortical epilepsy* (pp. 391–404). Philadelphia: Lippincott, Williams & Wilkins.

Gaillard, W.D. (2000). Structural and functional imaging in children with partial epilepsy. *Mental Retardation and Developmental Disabilities Research Reviews, 6*(3), 220–226.

Gaillard, W.D., Kopylev, L., Weinstein, S., et al. (2002). Low incidence of abnormal (18)FDG-PET in children with new-onset partial epilepsy: A prospective study. *Neurology, 58*(5), 717–722.

Gastaut, H. (1982). Classification of status epilepticus. In A.V. Delgado-Escueta, R.J. Porter, & C.G. Wasterlain (Eds.), *Status epilepticus: Mechanisms of brain damage and treatment.* New York: Raven Press.

Gilbert, D.L., & Buncher, C.R. (2000). An EEG should not be obtained routinely after first unprovoked seizure in childhood. *Neurology, 54*(3), 635–641.

Glauser, T.A., & Pippenger, C.E. (2000). Controversies in blood-level monitoring: Reexamining its role in the treatment of epilepsy. *Epilepsia, 41*(Suppl. 8), S6–S15.

Gordon, N. (1999). Episodic dyscontrol syndrome. *Developmental Medicine and Child Neurology, 41*(11), 786–788.

Greene, P., Kang, U.J., Fahn, S., et al. (1995). Spread of symptoms in idiopathic torsion dystonia. *Movement Disorders, 10*(2), 143–152.

Greenwood, R.S., & Tennison, M.B. (1999). When to start and stop anticonvulsant therapy in children. *Archives of Neurology, 56*(9), 1073–1077.

Guberman, A. (1998). Monotherapy or polytherapy for epilepsy? *The Canadian Journal of Neurological Science, 25*(4), S3–S8.

Harden, C.L. (2000). Therapeutic safety monitoring: What to look for and when to look for it. *Epilepsia, 41* (Suppl. 8), S37–S44.

Harding, G.F., Wild, J.M., Robertson, K.A., et al. (2000). Electro-oculography, electroretinography, visual evoked potentials, and multifocal electroretinography in patients with vigabatrin-attributed visual field constriction. *Epilepsia, 41*(11), 1420–1431.

Hauser, W.A. (1994). The prevalence and incidence of convulsive disorders in children. *Epilepsia, 35*(Suppl. 2), S1–S6.

Hemingway, C., Freeman, J.M., Pilas, D.J., et al. (2001). The ketogenic diet: A 3- to 6-year follow-up of 150 children enrolled prospectively. *Pediatrics, 108*(4), 898–905.

Hennessy, M.J., & Binnie, C.D. (2000). Photogenic partial seizures. *Epilepsia, 41*(1), 59–64.

Hernandez-Latorre, M.A., & Roig, M. (2000). Natural history of migraine in childhood. *Cephalalgia, 20*(6), 573–579.

Hirtz, D., Ashwal, S., Berg, A., et al. (2000). Practice parameter: Evaluating a first nonfebrile seizure in children: Report of the quality standards subcommittee of the American Academy of Neurology, The Child Neurology Society, and The American Epilepsy Society. *Neurology, 55*(5), 616–623.

Hirtz, D., Berg, A., Donley, D., et al. (2003). Practice parameter: Treatment of the child with a first unprovoked seizure: Report of the Quality Standards Subcommittee of the American Academy of Neurology and the Practice Committee of the Child Neurology Society. *Neurology, 60*(2), 166–175.

Hirtz, D.G. (1997). Febrile seizures. *Pediatrics in Review, 18*(1), 5–8; quiz, 9.

Huang, C.C., Chang, Y.C., et al. (1998). Acute symptomatic seizure disorders in young children—a population study in southern Taiwan. *Epilepsia, 39*(9), 960–964.

Ilhan, A., Tuncer, C., et al. (1999). Jervell and Lange-Nielsen syndrome: Neurologic and cardiologic evaluation. *Pediatric Neurology, 21*(5), 809–813.

Individuals with Disabilities Education Improvement Act of 2004, PL 108-446, 20 U.S.C. §§ 1400 *et seq.*

Ito, M. (1998). Antiepileptic drug treatment of West syndrome. *Epilepsia, 39*(Suppl. 5), 38–41.

Jambaque, I., Chiron, C., Dumas, C., et al. (2000). Mental and behavioural outcome of infantile epilepsy treated by vigabatrin in tuberous sclerosis patients. *Epilepsy Research, 38*(2–3), 151–160.

Jayakar, P. (1999). Invasive EEG monitoring in children: Wen, where, and what? *Journal of Clinical Neurophysiology, 16*(5), 408–418.

Kandel, E.R., Schwartz, J.H., Jessell, T.M., et al. (Eds.). (2000). *Principles of neural science.* New York: McGraw-Hill.

Knudsen, F.U. (2000). Febrile seizures: Treatment and prognosis. *Epilepsia, 41*(1), 2–9.

Kotagal, P. (2000). Tonic-clonic seizures. In H.O. Luders & S. Noachtar (Eds.), *Epileptic seizures: Pathophysiology and clinical semiology* (pp. 425–432). New York: Churchill Livingstone.

Kriegstein, A.R., Owens, D.F., Avoli, M., et al. (1999). Ontogeny of channels, transmitters and epileptogenesis. *Advances in Neurology, 79*, 145–159.

Kubota, T., Aso, K., Negoro, T., et al. (1999). Epileptic spasms preceded by partial seizures with a close temporal association. *Epilepsia, 40*(11), 1572–1579.

Kuhle, S., Tiefenthaler, M., Seidl, R., et al. (2000). Prolonged generalized epileptic seizures triggered by breath-holding spells. *Pediatric Neurology, 23*(3), 271–273.

Kurtz, Z., Tookey, P., Ros, E., et al. (1998). Epilepsy in young people: 23 year follow up of the British national child development study. *British Medical Journal, 316* (7128), 339–342.

Kwan, P., & Brodie, M.J. (2001). Neuropsychological effects of epilepsy and antiepileptic drugs. *The Lancet, 357*(9251), 216–222.

Kwong, K.L., Wong, S.N., So, K.T., et al. (2000). Parental perception, worries and needs in children with epilepsy. *Acta Paediatrica, 89*(5), 593–596.

Laberge, L., Tremblay, R.E., Vitaro, F., et al. (2000). Development of parasomnias from childhood to early adolescence. *Pediatrics, 106*(1, Pt. 1), 67–74.

Leppik, I.E. (2000). Monotherapy and polypharmacy. *Neurology, 55*(11, Suppl. 3), S25–S29.

Lerman, P. (1992). Benign partial epilepsy with centrotemporal spikes. In J. Roger, M. Bureau, C. Dravet, et al. (Eds.), *Epileptic syndromes in infancy, childhood and adolescence* (pp. 189–200). London: John Libbey & Co. Ltd.

Lhatoo, S. D., Johnson, A.L., Goodridge, D.M., et al.

(2001). Mortality in epilepsy in the first 11 to 14 years after diagnosis: Multivariate analysis of a long-term, prospective, population-based cohort. *Annals of Neurology, 49*(3), 336–344.

Lin, Y., Itomi, K., Takada, H., et al. (1998). Benign myoclonic epilepsy in infants: video-EEG features and long-term follow-up. *Neuropediatrics, 29*(5), 268–271.

Liu, R.S., Lemieux, L., Bell, G.S., et al. (2003). Progressive neocortical damage in epilepsy. *Annals of Neurology, 53*(3), 312–324.

Loiseau, P. (1992). Childhood absence epilepsy. In J. Roger, M. Bureau, C. Dravet, et al. (Eds.), *Epileptic syndromes in infancy, childhood and adolescence* (pp. 135–150). London: John Libbey & Co. Ltd.

Lombroso, C.T. (2000). Pavor nocturnus of proven epileptic origin. *Epilepsia, 41*(9), 1221–1226.

Loring, D.W., & Meador, K.J. (2004). Cognitive side effects of antiepileptic drugs in children. *Neurology, 62*(6), 872–877.

Lowenstein, D.H. (1999). Status epilepticus: An overview of the clinical problem. *Epilepsia, 40*(Suppl. 1), S3–S8; discussion, S21–S22.

Lowenstein, D.H., & Alldredge, B.K. (1998). Status epilepticus. *The New England Journal of Medicine, 338*(14), 970–976.

MacDonald, B.K., Johnson, A.L., Goodridge, D.M., et al. (2000). Factors predicting prognosis of epilepsy after presentation with seizures. *Annals of Neurology, 48*(6), 833–841.

Mayville, C., Fakhoury, T., Abou-Khalil, et al. (2000). Absence seizures with evolution into generalized tonic-clonic activity: clinical and EEG features. *Epilepsia, 41*(4), 391–394.

Mitchell, W.G., Zhou, Y., Chavez, J.M., et al. (1993). Effects of antiepileptic drugs on reaction time, attention, and impulsivity in children. *Pediatrics, 91*(1), 101–105.

Mocan, H., Yildiran, A., Orhan, F., et al. (1999). Breath holding spells in 91 children and response to treatment with iron. *Archives of Disease in Childhood, 81*(3), 261–262.

Montalenti, E., Imperiale, D., Rovera, A., et al. (2001). Clinical features, EEG findings and diagnostic pitfalls in juvenile myoclonic epilepsy: A series of 63 patients. *Journal of Neurological Sciences, 184*(1), 65–70.

Moshe, S.L. (2000). Seizures early in life. *Neurology, 55*(5, Suppl. 1), S15–S20; discussion, S54–S58.

Murphy, C.C., Trevathan, E., Yeargin-Allsopp, M., et al. (1995). Prevalence of epilepsy and epileptic seizures in 10-year-old children: Results from the Metropolitan Atlanta Developmental Disabilities Study. *Epilepsia, 36*(9), 866–872.

Nakken, K.O. (1999). Physical exercise in outpatients with epilepsy. *Epilepsia, 40*(5), 643–651.

Nelson, K.B., & Ellenberg, J.H. (1976). Predictors of epilepsy in children who have experienced febrile seizures. *The New England Journal of Medicine, 295*(19), 1029–1033.

Nelson, K.B., & Ellenberg, J.H. (1978). Prognosis in children with febrile seizures. *Pediatrics, 61*(5), 720–727.

Nemeroff, C.B. (2000). An ever-increasing pharmacopoeia for the management of patients with bipolar disorder. *The Journal of Clinical Psychiatry, 61*(Supp. 13), 19–25.

Neubauer, B.A. (2000). The genetics of rolandic epilepsy. *Epilepsia, 41*(8), 1061–1062.

Noebels, J.L. (2003). The biology of epilepsy genes. *Annual Review of Neuroscience, 26*, 599–625.

Okumura, A., Hayakawa, F., Kato, T., et al. (2000). Early recognition of benign partial epilepsy in infancy. *Epilepsia, 41*(6), 714–717.

Pachatz, C., Fusco, L., Vigevano, F., et al. (1999). Benign myoclonus of early infancy. *Epileptic Disorders, 1*(1), 57–61.

Panayiotopoulos, C.P. (1999). *Current problems in epilepsy series: Vol. 15. Benign childhood partial seizures and related epileptic syndromes.* London: John Libbey & Co. Ltd.

Pedersen, S.B., & Petersen, K.A. (1998). Juvenile myoclonic epilepsy: Clinical and EEG features. *Acta Neurologica Scandinavica, 97*(3), 160–163.

Prasad, A. N., Prasad, C., Stafstrom, C.E., et al. (1999). Recent advances in the genetics of epilepsy: Insights from human and animal studies. *Epilepsia, 40*(10), 1329–1352.

Rantala, H., & Putkonen, T. (1999). Occurrence, outcome, and prognostic factors of infantile spasms and Lennox-Gastaut syndrome. *Epilepsia, 40*(3), 286–289.

Reynolds, E.H. (2000). The ILAE/IBE/WHO Global Campaign against Epilepsy: Bringing Epilepsy "Out of the Shadows." *Epilepsy & Behavior, 1*(4), S3–S8.

Riikonen, R.S. (2000). Steroids or vigabatrin in the treatment of infantile spasms? *Pediatric Neurology, 23* (5), 403–408.

Risinger, M.W. (2000). Noninvasive ictal electroencephalography in humans. In H.O. Luders & S. Noachtar (Eds.), *Epileptic seizures: Pathophysiology and clinical semiology* (pp. 32–48). New York: Churchill Livingstone.

Rogawski, M.A., & Loscher, W. (2004). The neurobiology of antiepileptic drugs. *Nature Reviews Neuroscience, 5*(7), 553–564.

Rossi, P.G., Parmeggiani, A., Posar, A., et al. (1999). Landau-Kleffner syndrome (LKS): Long-term follow-up and links with electrical status epilepticus during sleep (ESES). *Brain & Development, 21*(2), 90–98.

Schoenfeld, J.,Seidenberg, M., Woodward, A., et al. (1999). Neuropsychological and behavioral status of children with complex partial seizures. *Developmental Medicine and Child Neurology, 41*(11), 724–731.

Shields, W.D. (2000). Catastrophic epilepsy in childhood. *Epilepsia, 41*(Suppl. 2), S2–S6.

Shields, W.D., Shewmon, D.A., Peacock, D.M., et al. (1999). Surgery for the treatment of medically intractable infantile spasms: A cautionary case. *Epilepsia, 40*(9), 1305–1308.

Shinnar, S., & Berg, A.T. (1994). Does antiepileptic drug therapy alter the prognosis of childhood seizures and prevent the development of chronic epilepsy? *Seminars in Pediatric Neurology, 1*(2), 111–117.

Shinnar, S., Berg, A.T., Moshe, S.L., et al. (1996). The risk of seizure recurrence after a first unprovoked afebrile seizure in childhood: An extended follow-up. *Pediatrics, 98*(2, Pt. 1), 216–225.

Shorvon, S. (2000). *Handbook of epilepsy treatment.* Malden, MA: Blackwell Science.

Sillanpaa, M. (2000). Long-term outcome of epilepsy. *Epileptic Disorders, 2*(2), 79–88.

Stein, A.G., Eder, H.G., Blum, D.E., et al. (2000). An automated drug delivery system for focal epilepsy. *Epilepsy Research, 39*(2), 103–114.

Steinhoff, B.J., Neususs, K., Thegeder, H., et al. (1996). Leisure time activity and physical fitness in patients with epilepsy. *Epilepsia, 37*(12), 1221–1227.

Szabo, C.A., & Luders, H.O. (2000). Todd's paralysis and postictal aphasia. In H.O. Luders & S. Noachtar (Eds.), *Epileptic seizures: Pathophysiology and clinical semiology* (pp. 652–657). New York: Churchill Livingstone.

Tal, Y., Even, L., Kugelman, A., et al. (1997). The clinical significance of rigors in febrile children. *European Journal of Pediatrics, 156*(6), 457–459.

Theodore, W.H., & Gaillard, W.D. (2002). Neuroimaging and the progression of epilepsy. *Progress in Brain Research, 135,* 305–313.

Trasmonte, J.V., & Barron, T.F. (1998). Infantile spasms: A proposal for a staged evaluation. *Pediatric Neurology, 19*(5), 368–371.

Tuchman, R.F. (1997). Acquired epileptiform aphasia. *Seminars in Pediatric Neurology, 4*(2), 93–101.

Velasco, A.L., Velasco, M., Velasco, F., et al. (2000). Subacute and chronic electrical stimulation of the hippocampus on intractable temporal lobe seizures: Preliminary report. *Archives of Medical Research, 31*(3), 316–328.

Wallace, S.J. (1998). Myoclonus and epilepsy in childhood: A review of treatment with valproate, ethosuximide, lamotrigine and zonisamide. *Epilepsy Research, 29*(2), 147–154.

Wasterlain, C.G. (1997). Recurrent seizures in the developing brain are harmful. *Epilepsia, 38*(6), 728–734.

Werlin, S.L., D'Souza, B.J., Hogan, W.J., et al. (1980). Sandifer syndrome: An unappreciated clinical entity. *Developmental Medicine and Child Neurology, 22*(3), 374–378.

Wiebe, S., Blume, W.T., Girvin, J.P., et al. (2001). A randomized, controlled trial of surgery for temporal-lobe epilepsy. *The New England Journal of Medicine, 345*(5), 311–318.

Wolf, P. (1992). Epilepsy with grand mal on awakening. In J. Roger, M. Bureau, C. Dravet, et al. (Eds.), *Epileptic syndromes in infancy, childhood and adolescence* (pp. 329–342). London: John Libbey & Co. Ltd.

Wolf, P. (1994). *Epileptic seizures and syndromes.* London: John Libbey & Co. Ltd.

Ziemann, U., Steinhoff, B.J., Tergau, F., et al. (1998). Transcranial magnetic stimulation: Its current role in epilepsy research. *Epilepsy Research, 30*(1), 11–30.

Zucconi, M., Oldani, A., Ferini-Strambi, L., et al. (1997). Nocturnal paroxysmal arousals with motor behaviors during sleep: Frontal lobe epilepsy or parasomnia? *Journal of Clinical Neurophysiology, 14*(6), 513–522.

30 Traumatic Brain Injury

Linda J. Michaud, Ann-Christine Duhaime,
Shari L. Wade, Jeffrey P. Rabin, Dorothy O. Jones, and Mary F. Lazar

---

Upon completion of this chapter, the reader will

- Know the major causes of traumatic brain injury in children
- Be able to distinguish among mild, moderate, and severe traumatic brain injury
- Be able to identify prognostic factors for traumatic brain injury in children
- Understand the long-term effects of the injury on the child and family
- Be able to identify preventive means to reduce the incidence of traumatic brain injury

---

Most head trauma in children is minor and not associated with persisting impairments (Thiessen & Woolridge, 2006). However, severe head injury (with associated brain injury) occurs with sufficient frequency to make it the most common cause of acquired disability in childhood (Ducrocq et al., 2006). Even when obvious physical complications are minimal, neuropsychological impairments may lead to chronic academic, behavior, and interpersonal difficulties that pose an enormous challenge to the child, family, and society. Effective acute management and long-term rehabilitation are vital after traumatic brain injury (TBI) in order to optimize the child's outcome (National Institutes of Health [NIH] Consensus Development Panel, 1999). The best approach to TBI, however, is prevention.

ETHAN

Ethan was 7 years old when he was hit by a car while riding his bicycle without a helmet. Minutes after the collision, emergency medical services arrived and found him unresponsive and with an abnormal flexion motor response. A cranial computed tomography (CT) scan performed on admission to the hospital showed a large **subdural hematoma** over the left frontal, temporal, and parietal lobes. There were no other injuries. Ethan was taken to the operating room within an hour, and the neuro-

surgeon removed the hematoma and placed an intracranial pressure monitor in him. Ethan was found to have elevated intracranial pressure that was eventually reduced with mannitol and placement of a ventriculostomy.

Ethan remained unresponsive for 10 weeks but then began to follow the command, "Move your hand," by opening his left hand. He also followed objects placed in his field of vision but did not speak. He was transferred to the neurorehabilitation service, where he received physical, occupational, and speech-language therapy twice daily. Gradually, over the next 12 weeks, his motor control improved, although he had spasticity on the right side of his body. He began to walk with an ankle-foot orthosis (brace) and was able to complete self-care activities independently, primarily using his left arm, with some assistance from the right. Communication remained a major problem, as both expressive and receptive language impairments were evident. Cognitive testing (Wechsler Intelligence Scale for Children–Fourth Edition) revealed persisting impairments, with scores on both verbal and performance subtests more than 2 standard deviations below the norms.

Ethan was eventually discharged and enrolled in an outpatient rehabilitation program, in which he received physical and occupational therapy weekly and speech-language therapy three times weekly. Three months later, he returned to school

461

in a self-contained class for children with communication disorders; he also received physical and occupational therapy.

At 1-year follow-up, Ethan's right hand functioning had gradually improved, but he continued to prefer using his left hand. Both expressive and receptive language skills had significantly increased. His individualized education program (IEP; see Chapter 34) for the next school year included continued placement in a class for children with communication disorders, with participation in a general education third-grade class for 20% of the day. He continued to receive physical and occupational therapies. Ethan was not able to keep up with his old friends but was making new ones. It is likely that he will continue to have disabilities, but he will also continue to gain new skills and knowledge that should help him cope with his disabilities.

INCIDENCE OF HEAD INJURIES

Each year, approximately 1 in 25 children receive medical attention because of a head injury (Ducrocq et al., 2006; Schneier et al., 2006). These injuries range from confined areas of scalp or skull trauma to more diffuse and severe brain damage. TBI, defined as trauma sufficient to result in a change in level of consciousness and/or an anatomical abnormality of the brain, occurs in approximately 1 in 500 children per year (Centers for Disease Control and Prevention, 2006; Schneier et al., 2006). Head injuries most commonly occur in the spring and summer, on weekends, and in the afternoons, when children are most likely to be outside playing or riding in cars. Although TBI can occur at any age, there are two stages in a child's life when the risk is notably higher. The first is from birth until 5 years, when cognitive and motor functions are most actively developing, and the second is in adolescence, when peer approval, impulsivity, and a sense of immortality increase risk-taking behaviors (Luerssen, Klauber, & Marshall, 1988; Parslow et al., 2005).

CAUSES OF TRAUMATIC BRAIN INJURY

Common causes of TBI include falls from heights; sports- and recreation-related injuries; motor vehicle crashes; and assaults, including child abuse. The frequency of these types of brain injuries varies with age. Young children are more likely to sustain brain injuries as a result of falls, whereas teenagers are more often involved in motor vehicle crashes. The frequency of gunshot wounds to the head has increased dramatically in children living in urban areas (Sheehan et al., 1997).

Certain psychosocial factors may increase the risk of childhood head trauma. Children with a conduct disorder or hyperactive-impulsive behavior (as seen in children with attention-deficit/hyperactivity disorder [ADHD]) may act in a dangerous manner, although hyperactive behavior itself does not necessarily increase the risk of injury (Byrne et al., 2003; Gerring et al., 1998). Adolescents who are severely depressed may attempt suicide. In addition, head injury from child abuse occurs more commonly in children who were born prematurely, who have a preexisting developmental disability, who were born to young parents, and who live with unstable family dynamics (Keenan, Runyan, & Nocera, 2006).

TYPES OF BRAIN INJURIES

The type of brain injury that a child sustains depends primarily on the nature of the force that caused the injury and the severity of the insult. Head trauma can be caused by both **impact** and **inertial** forces. Impact or contact forces occur when the head strikes a surface or is struck by a moving object. Impact forces can result in scalp injuries, skull fractures, focal brain bruises (**contusions**), or blood collections beneath the skull (i.e., **epidural hematomas**). Inertial forces occur when the brain undergoes violent motion inside the skull, which tears the nerve fibers and blood vessels. The severity of injuries caused by inertial forces depends on the magnitude and the direction of the motion. Angular acceleration/deceleration forces, such as those that might occur in a high-speed motor vehicle crash, cause much more serious damage than do straight-line (translational) forces, such as those that might occur in a fall. Injuries caused by inertial forces range from relatively mild **concussions** to more serious injuries, such as **diffuse axonal injuries (DAIs)** and subdural hematomas. Most clinical brain injuries include both impact and inertial components, with several injury types occurring simultaneously.

INFLICTED BRAIN INJURY

Though most brain injuries are unintentional, inflicted injuries (i.e., due to physical abuse) do occur and pose special problems for the practitioner. Manner of presentation and injury types are helpful in diagnosing inflicted TBI (Keenan et al., 2004). Inflicted injuries are most commonly seen in children younger than 3 years of age and are the leading cause of traumatic death in infancy (McCabe & Donahue, 2000). Reece and Sege (2000) found that confirmed abuse accounted for 19% of hospital admissions for head injury in children younger than 6½ years old and for 33% of those younger than 3 years old. The term *shaken baby syndrome* is frequently used to describe this type of injury. Some suggest that the use of the term *shaken impact syndrome* better reflects the fact that when the child is shaken, the head usually hits a surface such as a bed, floor, or wall (Salehi-Had et al., 2006). Because of uncertainty about the exact mechanism, the term *inflicted injury* is probably the most useful for this class of injuries.

Clues that the injury might have been inflicted rather than unintentional include a history that is inconsistent with the injuries or a delay in reporting the injury and seeking medical attention. For example, a fall from a low height (less than 4 feet) or from an infant swing or trivial forces encountered in childhood play are rarely sufficient to cause a significant head injury (Duhaime et al., 1998). Whereas small surface hemorrhages may occur from these mechanisms, the primary injury to the brain is usually minor.

Certain injuries can alert the practitioner that the trauma may have been inflicted. These include complex skull fractures, subdural hematomas, and subarachnoid hemorrhage. Retinal hemorrhages, although not diagnostic, are strongly suggestive of abuse (Reece & Sege, 2000). The abused child may also show signs of previous injuries, including bone fractures and bruises that are in different stages of the healing process. Ewing-Cobbs et al. (1998) reported that 45% of children with inflicted head injuries showed signs of prior head injuries, even when the children were as young as 6 weeks old.

Children with inflicted brain injuries are more likely to die than those with unintentional injuries. Seizures are also more common in this group, being seen in up to 70% (Duhaime et al., 1998). Those children who survive have poorer recovery, with greater motor, cognitive, and visual impairment (Michaud, 2003).

DETECTING SIGNIFICANT BRAIN INJURY

Most head trauma is minor and does not require treatment or result in significant consequences. But how does a caregiver know whether head trauma warrants treatment? Generally speaking, if a child hits his or her head and does not lose consciousness, has no visible bump or bruise, and remains awake, alert, and without symptoms, he or she can be observed. Medical evaluation (a visit to a physician or the emergency room) is needed, however, if the child becomes lethargic, confused, or irritable; has a severe headache; demonstrates acute impairments in speech, vision, or movements of the arms or legs; has significant bleeding or a large bump or other abnormality of the surface of the head; or vomits repeatedly. Some children will have a seizure shortly after a head injury; this does not necessarily mean that the injury is severe, but it usually warrants evaluation.

If the child is momentarily unconscious and then resumes activities, he or she may have a mild concussion. If there has been more than a momentary loss of consciousness or confusion, the child should be taken to the emergency room, where a neurological examination will be performed. A brain imaging study may be performed to determine whether there is significant brain injury. If there are no abnormal neurological or radiological findings, the child may then be sent home. Parents will be given instructions to make sure the child can be roused from sleep, is not confused, and develops no new neurological symptoms.

If the child remains unconscious for more than a few minutes, 911 should be called. If, upon arrival at the hospital, the child is still unconscious, he or she will be stabilized in the emergency room and then usually transferred to the intensive care unit. Immediate coma after head trauma is the result of primary injury to neural pathways. There may be worsening in the subsequent 24 hours as a consequence of secondary hemorrhaging or brain swelling.

SEVERITY OF BRAIN INJURY

The duration and severity of coma indicate the seriousness of a brain injury. The most frequently used scale for coma severity is the Glasgow Coma Scale (GCS) (Table 30.1; Brain Trauma Foundation, American Association of Neurological Surgeons, & Joint Section on Neurotrauma and Critical Care, 2000; Jennett et al., 1977). Although this scale was devised for use in adults and can be difficult to apply to very young children, it remains the most useful method available for classifying severe brain injuries in the early period after trauma. Using this scale within the first 6 hours after injury

Table 30.1. Glasgow Coma Scale (GCS)

Response	Score
Eye opening	
Spontaneous	4
To speech	3
To pain	2
Nil	1
Best motor response	
Obeys	6
Localizes	5
Withdraws	4
Abnormal flexion	3
Extensor response	2
Nil	1
Verbal response	
Oriented	5
Confused conversation	4
Inappropriate words	3
Incomprehensible sounds	2
Nil	1

From Jennett, B., Teasdale, G., Galbraith, S., et al. (1977). Severe head injuries in three countries. *Journal of Neurology, Neurosurgery, and Psychiatry, 40,* 293; reprinted by permission of BMJ Publishing Group.

and after initial resuscitation, the trauma team assigns the child a score based on the degree and quality of movement, vocalization, and eye opening. Individuals receive a score between 3 and 15. The highest score is 15, representing the least severe brain injury. An individual with a score of 3 has no eye opening, movement, or verbal response and is in deep coma. An individual who looks about, moves limbs in response to requests, and is oriented to the environment receives a score of 15. Someone who opens his or her eyes when physically prodded, withdraws a limb that is touched, and makes only incomprehensible sounds receives a score of 8. Age-appropriate scales for infants have been developed and may be helpful in preverbal children (Durham et al., 2000). Severe brain injury is defined as a score of 8 or less. Scores of 9–12 reflect moderate brain injury, and scores of 13–15 reflect minor brain injury. Fatality rate after severe brain injury is between 20% and 40% (Feickert, Drommer, & Heyer, 1999; Sills, Libby, & Orton, 2005).

Another tool to assess the severity of brain injury is the duration of posttraumatic amnesia (PTA), which includes the period of coma and the subsequent time during which the individual with TBI is unable to store and remember new events. According to this classification, the duration of PTA in mild head injuries is less than 1 hour, in moderate brain injuries is 1–24 hours, and in severe injuries is greater than 24 hours (Zafonte et al., 1997). Duration of PTA in children can be reliably and validly measured using the Children's Orientation and Amnesia Test (COAT; Ewing-Cobbs et al., 1990).

TREATMENT

Approaches to therapy depend on the stage of recovery from coma and associated medical and physical problems. Treatment can be divided into an acute medical phase and a rehabilitative phase. Initial rehabilitation, which may last for weeks to months, is often provided in an inpatient setting after severe injury. Subsequent outpatient rehabilitation can be provided in a hospital, rehabilitation center, or school.

The societal and financial costs of brain injury in children are monumental. Each year the cost of acute and rehabilitative care for new cases of TBI totals more than $9 billion (NIH Consensus Development Panel, 1999). Jaffe et al. (1993) found that the median cost of acute and rehabilitative care for a child with severe brain injury was more than $50,000. When the costs of rehospitalizations and/or long-term care, outpatient rehabilitation, medical equipment, provision of special education services, and loss of future earnings are added, the figure is vastly greater. Unfortunately, due to caps on insurance policies, rehabilitative services are often time limited. Furthermore, schools may be ill prepared to care for these children, who may have complex neuropsychological impairments. These problems can adversely affect recovery and outcome.

Acute Medical Treatment

Each year more than 500,000 children are seen in emergency rooms nationwide following head trauma (Schutzman et al., 2001). The majority of these visits are for minor head trauma. Until the late 1990s, there had been no consensus on the best management for these children (Savitsky & Votey, 2000). Less than 0.02% (1 in 5,000) of children older than 2 years of age with minor closed head injury and no loss of consciousness develop intracranial bleeding that requires medical or surgical intervention (Schutzman & Greenes, 2001). When the injury is associated with a brief loss of consciousness, this figure increases to 2%–5% (American Academy of Pediatrics [AAP], Committee on Quality Improvement, & American Academy of Family Physicians [AAFP], Commission on Clinical Policies and Research, 1999). In infants this figure is even higher at 3%–6% (Schutzman et al., 2001). Beginning in 1999, guidelines for both infants and older children were developed by experts in the field to aid in the evaluation and management of children with minor head trauma (AAP & AAFP, 1999; Schutzman et al., 2001).

The occurrence of seizures immediately after the injury or within the first few days after a brain injury is rather common, even in children with only mild concussions. Young children are particularly susceptible to early seizures, whereas older children and adults are prone to late posttraumatic seizures (Statler et al., 2006). Less than 2% of children with early seizures will subsequently develop a seizure disorder (Asikainen et al., 1999a). Factors that increase this risk include bleeding into the brain and penetrating injury that may cause the formation of scar tissue. Antiepileptic medication may be given preventively for a week after the injury, but prolonged treatment is generally used only if the child develops recurrent seizure activity (see Chapter 29).

Rehabilitation

Rehabilitation aims to 1) avert complications that arise from immobilization, disuse, and neurological dysfunction; 2) augment the use of abilities regained as a result of recovery from coma; 3) teach adaptive compensation for impaired or lost function; and 4) alleviate the effect of chronic disability on the process of growth and development (NIH Consensus Development Panel, 1999). Rehabilitation begins almost immediately after vital signs have been stabilized, often while the child is still in coma.

Acute rehabilitative care following TBI aims to limit secondary musculoskeletal damage by passive range-of-motion exercises, positioning, and splinting of limbs. These efforts can help to prevent the later development of contractures, which could interfere with seating, ambulation, and participation in daily activities. Other important acute rehabilitative measures include changing body position and caring for the skin to prevent the development of pressure sores. In addition, adequate nutrition promotes wound healing. These measures, taken together, appear to shorten hospitalization and improve outcome.

Evaluating and Treating Functional Impairments As the child begins to recover

from coma, physical, cognitive, and emotional problems may become evident (Savage et al., 2005). The nature and severity of functional impairments will determine the rehabilitative strategies. Severe DAI is likely to result in impairment in all areas of functioning, whereas focal damage may result in more localized abnormalities. Interdisciplinary services typically include medical, nutritional, physical, occupational, speech-language, and recreational therapies, as well as rehabilitation nursing, psychological, special education, and social services. Services are discussed in relation to the specific impairments that they are intended to remediate.

Addressing Motor Impairments The site(s) of brain injury determines the type of motor dysfunction that follows. Spasticity, rigidity, and ataxia/tremor are the most common motor abnormalities, indicating damage to the corticospinal (pyramidal) tract, basal ganglia, and cerebellum (see Chapter 13).

Medication and surgery have had varying success in treating motor impairments. As of 2007, there is no effective medical or surgical approach to treating ataxia. Tremor may respond to propranolol. Useful medications to treat spasticity and rigidity include those that are used to treat spastic cerebral palsy: baclofen (Lioresal), dantrolene (Dantrium), and diazepam (Valium) (Chapter 26). Baclofen can be administered intrathecally (into the spinal fluid) as well as orally (Rawlins et al., 2004).

Management of spasticity may also include nerve blocks, such as botulinum toxin A (Botox). The effects of botulinum toxin A last for several months, but repeated injections are required if spasticity persists. Intramuscular injections of botulinum toxin A appear safe and effective in reducing localized spasticity in children (van Rhijn, Molenaers, & Ceulemans, 2005). Serial casting may be used to correct a limb deformity in some cases of spasticity, and are often applied following botulinum toxin A injections to facilitate muscle lengthening.

Orthopedic surgery may be required in some cases. Long-term contractures or dislocations may need to be treated by performing tendon releases, femoral osteotomies, or scoliosis surgery (see Chapter 26).

Medical and surgical approaches may be helpful, but they offer no cure. The child may continue to have motor impairments that interfere with the ability to ambulate and to participate in self-care skills. Furthermore, cognitive and visual-perceptual impairments may exacerbate motor impairments. Active physical and occupational therapy is needed to assist the child in regaining motor function. Exercises and activities are designed to increase strength, balance, and coordination; to reduce spasticity; and to prevent contractures and dislocations. The child may need to relearn how to walk and may require orthoses, crutches, walkers, or a wheelchair (see Chapter 36). The importance of addressing these issues cannot be overstated because long-term outcome following TBI in the school-age years is highly correlated with the degree of mobility (Haley et al., 2003) and ability to self-feed (Strauss, Shavelle, & Anderson, 1998).

Managing Feeding Disorders Feeding disorders often accompany motor impairments (Morgan et al., 2003). Food intake may decrease if the child is unable to communicate hunger, if the ability to obtain food or to eat is compromised because of impaired motor skills, if there are problems with swallowing or gastroesophageal reflux, or if there are impairments in smell or taste.

Nutritional treatment during coma may involve intravenous hyperalimentation (see Chapter 10). Even after coma has resolved, children who are unable to take in sufficient sustenance by mouth will require temporary or long-term nasogastric or gastrostomy tube-feedings (see Chapter 31) with high-calorie formulas.

A number of rehabilitation therapies also are involved in treating feeding disorders. An occupational therapist may work on proper positioning for feeding. A speech-language pathologist may use desensitization techniques; may stimulate the swallowing reflex; may treat re-emergence of primitive reflexes; and may facilitate tongue, lip, and jaw control to improve swallowing. Nutritionists provide advice concerning the textures, taste, temperature, and caloric density of the food (see Chapter 10). Finally, medication to control reflux may improve the child's ability to eat and gain weight (see Chapter 31).

Managing Sensory Impairments Vision and hearing can both be affected by TBI. The most common visual complication is diplopia (i.e., double vision), caused by eye muscle palsy (Kapoor & Ciuffreda, 2002). Nystagmus, caused by injury to the cerebellum, is also quite common among children with severe TBI. Less commonly, a crush injury (e.g., blunt object)

may damage an eye or a missile injury (e.g., gunshot) may sever a portion of the visual pathway; both types of injury cause irreversible damage. Injury affecting the visual pathway may result in cuts in the visual fields. Finally, a TBI accompanied by severe brain swelling can result in a stroke or cortical blindness. Cortical blindness involves an abnormality in the visual cortex but not the eye itself, and partial or complete recovery can occur (see Chapter 11). As a result of these problems, vision testing should be included in the evaluation after recovery from coma.

Sensorineural hearing loss after TBI most commonly results from a fracture of the temporal bone and is usually unilateral (Roizen, 1999). Transverse fractures can affect the cochlea and result in sensorineural hearing loss. Longitudinal fractures involving the middle-ear structures are associated with a conductive hearing loss. Formal hearing assessment should be conducted following severe TBI because of the frequency with which hearing loss occurs. Because involvement is usually unilateral, deafness does not generally result. Even a mild hearing loss, however, should be identified and corrected with amplification if indicated so that the child can benefit maximally from all of his or her senses when working toward recovery (see Chapter 12). Auditory brainstem responses in minimally responsive patients can assist with prognosis. Testing for central auditory processing may be beneficial for children older than 5 years of age to assist with school planning.

Managing Communication Impairments If the left hemisphere of the brain is damaged, speech and language impairments are likely. Language disorders may be expressive, receptive, or mixed. Dysarthria and dysphasia are the most common expressive language problems seen in children with TBI (see Chapter 22). Receptive language impairments most commonly involve auditory-perceptual problems. Recovery of speech motor function often is more complete than recovery of receptive language abilities (Catroppa & Anderson, 2004). Usually when language is disordered, cognition also is affected (Johnson et al., 2006). In addition, problems in communication are often accompanied by impairments in social cognition and skills. Specifically, children with TBI may communicate a lot of tangentially related information without adequately summarizing what they are trying to say (Chapman et al., 2004). As a result, peers may become frustrated or disengaged. Intervention by a speech-language pathologist is directed at improving the speech disorder and the language as well as associated cognitive and social impairments. Initially, this involves using simple commands and discussing uncomplicated topics related to the surroundings. The speech-language pathologist will also help to train the nursing staff and parents to use simple commands and, if needed, alternate means of communication.

Addressing Cognitive Impairments

Recovery of cognitive functioning is typically not as complete as recovery of motor functioning following severe TBI (Anderson et al., 2004; Massagli, Michaud, & Rivara, 1996). Furthermore, children who are preschoolers at the time of injury may have delayed manifestation of cognitive impairments, showing difficulty handling more complex tasks as they get older (Anderson et al., 2005; Meekes, Jennekens-Schinkel, & van Schooneveld, 2006).

Investigations of mild TBI in children have demonstrated no significant long-term adverse consequences on cognitive functioning (Carroll et al., 2004; Yeates et al., 2002). Studies of children who have sustained moderate to severe TBI, however, document significant cognitive impairments (Campbell et al., 2004). Intellectual and neuropsychological impairment is increased with greater severity of injury (Jaffe et al., 1993). The cognitive sequelae most often associated with pediatric TBI are lowered performance on visuospatial and visual-motor tasks as compared with performance on verbal tasks; problems with attention, learning, and memory (Anderson, Catroppa, Rosenfeld, et al., 2000); and diminished speed of information processing (Massagli, Jaffe, et al., 1996). Impairments in executive function, including judgment, problem solving, reasoning, and organizational skills, have also been demonstrated (Anderson & Catroppa, 2005). Cognitive and learning profiles following TBI can vary tremendously. Often global intelligence and preinjury academic skills remain intact while attention, short-term memory, and new learning are impaired (Ylvisaker et al., 2001).

To identify impairments, neuropsychologists evaluate children using measures of intelligence as well as assessments of more discrete and/or subtle impairments in cognition that typically result from significant brain injury. This assessment involves a series of standardized tests that measure concept formation, reasoning, adaptive problem-solving skills, language, memory, concentration, visuospatial skills,

sensory-perceptual and sensorimotor abilities, and academic performance. Results of such evaluations are used in planning appropriate rehabilitation programs and educational curricula (Ylvisaker et al., 2001).

Performance on cognitive tasks varies in different settings. In a typical neuropsychological evaluation, the examiner meets individually with the child in a quiet room under very structured conditions. Because this situation is unlike the typical classroom with its many distractions, these tests alone may not accurately represent the child's ability to function in a general classroom setting. For this reason, it is recommended that such evaluations be augmented by contextual assessments (Telzrow, 1991) as well as by functional assessment measures (Anderson et al., 2006).

Impairments in intellectual and neuropsychological functioning are generally proportional to the severity of the injury (Jaffe et al., 1993). Although significant recovery occurs during the first 6 months to 1 year after severe injury in children, the recovery rate slows subsequently (Taylor et al., 1999). Cognitive recovery is also influenced by other factors such as the home environment and family resources (Keenan et al., 2006). Much remains to be learned about the role of rehabilitative and educational interventions in influencing the rate and extent of recovery of specific cognitive functions.

Interventions to address cognitive impairments may be useful even during the inpatient phase of management. Multidisciplinary cognitive remediation may use a combination of memory training exercises (psychology), language therapy (speech-language pathology), and educational programming (special education). The strategy is to improve areas of impairment and encourage the development of compensatory techniques, such as the use of assistive technology (including computer-assisted learning) (Gillette & DePompei, 2004). Impairments in communication and cognition often are the main deterrents to successful reintegration into the home, school, and community environments. Social inclusion (i.e., full, meaningful inclusion in the social fabric of the culture) should be a major goal of provision of assistive technology for children with impairments after TBI.

Identifying and remediating cognitive problems following TBI can be complicated by a variety of factors, including preinjury problems with learning, attention, and behavior and limited follow-up after acute hospitalization. As a result, parents and teachers may have difficulty distinguishing new problems arising from the TBI from preexisting difficulties. In addition, children may initially appear to be unaffected, but then display emerging deficits as the demands for abstract thinking and new learning increase (see Ylviskaker, Adelson, et al., 2005). As a result, both parents and teachers need to be educated about the importance of monitoring the child's progress over time.

Modifying the Academic Environment Research has consistently documented that children who have sustained a moderate to severe TBI tend to experience academic problems. Although these difficulties may be demonstrated in a particular area, such as reading or math, impairments in attention, problem solving, and speed of information processing more typically compromise all academic performance (Hawley et al., 2004). Standardized school achievement tests are not able to detect subtle learning disabilities and should not be used in place of the more comprehensive individual neuropsychological evaluation (Ewing-Cobbs et al., 1998). It is important to recognize that a child with a mild to moderate head injury may appear to be unaffected initially. It is possible for a child to score typically when tested at a young age and subsequently develop learning difficulties as she or he reaches adolescence. Thus, repeat testing may be required as the young child grows to determine whether the child has subtle impairments in domains that could not be tested at the age of injury.

Following moderate or severe TBI, the child often requires modifications to the general education curriculum, ranging from self-contained, special education classes to assistance in a resource room or in the classroom. Focused instruction based on each child's specific skills or impairments is most useful, especially when the instruction is both highly structured and motivating with feedback and correction. Strategies such as appropriate pacing, practice and review, organizational support, and errorless learning can be successful strategies for addressing deficits in attention, organization, and memory following TBI. Other strategies include having a consistent and structured daily routine. In addition, physical, occupational, and/or speech-language therapy may be provided as part of the child's IEP (see Chapter 34). Parent and teacher communication is vital for the student's success. Consistency between the home and school settings is desirable.

TBI is recognized as a specific category of disability within special education, as mandated by the Individuals with Disabilities Education Act (IDEA) of 1990 (PL 101-476), its 1997 (IDEA '97; PL 105-17) amendments, and its 2004 reauthorization (IDEA 2004; PL 108-446). There was a lag between the passage of this legislation and its actual implementation, and the definition of brain injury has not been interpreted consistently on a state-by-state basis. Many children who should be receiving special services following TBI are not, and those who do receive services are often misclassified (Taylor et al., 2003). Because there are so few children with TBI in any given school and so many school systems lack adequate resources (e.g., funding, school personnel with training in TBI), these children often receive inadequate educational programming (Carney & Schoenbrodt, 1994; Glang et al., 2004; Ylvisaker et al., 2001). Teachers often receive little information about brain injury during their training and may underestimate the effects of TBI on memory, learning, and emotional regulation. In a survey of 71 educators from 17 school districts in Cincinnati, teachers ranked their comfort level with TBI as 24th among 25 special needs conditions (Malone, personal communication). Children with learning or behavior problems that predated their injury pose particular problems for placement and programming. Although children with TBI may be identified as having behavior disorders (Michaud et al., 1993) or learning problems, their patterns of cognitive impairment are actually quite different from those seen in children with ADHD or specific learning disability. Unlike both of those disorders, two hallmarks of TBI are highly variable performance within and across academic subjects and continued change over time. Depending on the time since the injury, recovery may still be proceeding rapidly, with abilities changing from month to month. As a result, an appropriate educational approach in September may be outdated by November. Thus, flexibility and innovative approaches are needed to teach the child who is recovering from TBI. Above all, careful management of school reentry and long-term monitoring are essential in facilitating a successful academic outcome.

Mitigating Psychobehavioral Impairments Changes in personality and behavior also often follow severe TBI (Yeates & Taylor, 2005). Behavioral outcomes after mild to moderate injuries seem to be more varied (Dahl, von Wendt, & Emanuelson, 2006; Thompson

& Irby, 2003). Injuries to certain areas of the brain, specifically the thalamus and basal ganglia, are particularly associated with the development of secondary attentional and memory difficulties (Levin & Hanten, 2005).

Even with adequate cognitive functioning, significant behavior challenges can be expected (Bloom et al., 2001). Changes may include inattention, increased or decreased activity, impulsivity, irritability, lowered frustration tolerance, emotional lability, apathy, aggression, and/or social withdrawal (Max et al., 2005). As a result of these behavioral issues, children with TBI often develop problems with peer relationships. Treatment for behavior problems may include counseling, behavior management, medication, or a combination of these approaches (Bates, 2006; Ylvisaker, Turkstra, & Coelho, 2005). Feeney and Ylvisaker (2006) provided evidence for the efficacy of a model incorporating environmental supports, antecedent behavioral controls, and ongoing scaffolding by parents and school personnel to support the child's functioning. These behavioral problems also have a profound impact on other family members that must be considered by the rehabilitation team.

Addressing Social and Family Difficulties
The effects of severe TBI on the family can be enormous (Montgomery et al., 2002). In many ways, they are similar to the challenges faced by all families of children newly diagnosed with a developmental disability (see Chapter 40). Parents of children with TBI, in addition, may face overwhelming feelings of guilt and remorse, particularly if the child was in the parents' care when the injury occurred or if the parents feel otherwise responsible. Siblings also may feel guilty that they were left unharmed or did not protect their brother or sister. In addition, prolonged hospitalization and rehabilitation can place a heavy financial burden on the family. One parent may be forced to take a leave of absence from work to be with the child. This loss of income, combined with the additional costs of modifying a home or providing outpatient rehabilitation, can have a devastating effect on family finances.

Even after less severe TBI, psychosocial problems may develop (Watts & Perlesz, 1999). The family may rush to put the experience behind them and thus deny or ignore mild but persistent impairments, especially if the child appears to have recovered well. This can lead parents (and teachers) to expect normal achievement from the child, even if subtle cognitive impairments persist. If these impairments go undetected, they can lead to frustration, behavior problems, and poor learning (Warschausky, Kewman, & Kay, 1999).

Studies have shown that the family's preinjury level of functioning is predictive of family functioning 1 and 3 years after the child's TBI (Rivara et al., 1994). Other factors such as interpersonal stresses and resources, parental coping, and demographic characteristics also contribute to parental and family adaptation over time (Wade et al., 2004; Yeates et al., 2002). Not surprisingly, families with fewer supports and resources prior to the injury have greater difficulties adjusting afterward. Family adaptation has also been linked to the child's recovery, underscoring the importance of facilitating family adjustment (Taylor et al., 1999). These investigations strongly support the need to identify families at risk very early in the rehabilitation process. Families can be assisted by individual and family counseling, by participation in support groups, and by information and support from teachers and health professionals. In addition, families may need ongoing service coordination, especially if they are having difficulty gaining access to resources (Aitken et al., 2005).

Fostering Vocational Endeavors
TBI may have a major effect on the child's vocational development and outcome. In one follow-up study of Finnish adults who had sustained severe TBI during their preschool years, only one fourth were able to work full time, although half had achieved average school performance (Nybo & Koskiniemi, 1999). In these adults, vocational success was associated with better scores on tests involving speed, memory, and executive function. The Finnish investigators also found that the individual's sense of identity was a major predictor of the capability to care for oneself in adulthood. Asikainen, Kaste, and Sarna (1999b) also found that adults who suffered a severe TBI before 8 years of age were less often independently employed than their counterparts who were older at the time of the severe TBI. This age association was not seen with mild or moderate head injuries (Verger et al., 2000). Vocational services for children and adolescents with TBI have generally not been provided through either the medical rehabilitation or educational systems. IDEA '97 mandated provision of transition services that include vocational evaluation and training for students with disabilities, beginning no later than age 14. This legislation was certainly a step in the right direction in aiding children with disabilities, including those with TBI, to

achieve the ability to work and live independently in adulthood (see Chapter 41). More recently, IDEA 2004 stated that transition planning should become part of the IEP by age 16. Experts say that best practice is to begin planning for transition from school to adult life by age 14. Many states allow students with TBI to defer high school graduation, up to the age of 22 years, which can facilitate postsecondary placement by allowing other community resources to begin to work with the student on such goals as college or vocational training.

OUTCOME

Almost 95% of children admitted to a hospital following a TBI survive. For these children, a number of factors have been identified as predictors of outcome: GCS scores, duration of coma, duration of PTA, type of brain injury, age at injury, and preinjury functional level (Chung et al., 2006; Taylor & Alden, 1997).

Lower GCS scores generally indicate greater severity of TBI and a poorer outcome (Johnson et al., 2006; Michaud et al., 1992). As in the case of Ethan, the duration of unresponsiveness (i.e., not following commands) is a major index of the severity of the TBI (Massagli, Michaud, et al., 1996). Children who become responsive within 6 weeks have a good prognosis for recovery. When duration of unresponsiveness is between 6 weeks and 3 months, outcome is variable; and when the duration is longer than 3 months, prognosis for recovery of functioning is generally poor (Brink & Hoffer, 1978). Those children who do recover motor functioning after a prolonged period of unresponsiveness generally have impairments in cognitive functioning and changes in personality.

The duration of PTA is also a prognostic indicator (Wilde et al., 2006). Longer duration of PTA indicates more severe TBI and is associated with worse outcome.

The type of brain injury also is important in determining outcome. Children with focal lesions in addition to DAI have been observed to have poorer outcomes than those with only DAI (Paterakis et al., 2000). Outcomes are usually good for children who have epidural hematomas but poor for those with subdural hematomas (Rocchi et al., 2005). Injuries resulting in multiple organ damage also carry a poorer prognosis, as the associated oxygen deprivation and low blood pressure may cause secondary hypoxic-ischemic injury to the brain. As previously noted, younger children with brain injuries due to physical abuse (e.g., shaken impact syndrome) have significantly worse cognitive and motor outcomes than age-matched children with brain injury from other causes (e.g., motor vehicle crashes) (Newton & Vandeven, 2005).

The impact of age is complex, and the results of different studies have been inconsistent. In some studies, poorer outcomes have been observed in children who are quite young at the time of injury (Verger et al., 2000). In other studies, however, outcome has been found to be unrelated to age at the time of injury (Barlow et al., 2004, 2005). Researchers have distinguished among TBI severity: young children with severe TBI do worse than their adult counterparts, whereas adults and young children with moderate and mild TBI fare equally well (Anderson, Catroppa, Morse, et al., 2000). Contrasting findings may reflect the fact that different areas of functional outcome were being assessed. The brain of the young child may have a greater degree of plasticity (see Chapter 13) than that of the older child or adult. Yet, this advantage may be offset by the fact that brain injury impairs new learning more than the retention of prior information. The young child has had less time to develop learning strategies and to store knowledge before the injury and therefore may experience greater impairment in cognitive functioning. Recent findings support a "double-hazard" model, with injuries that are both early and severe resulting in the least recovery (Anderson, Catroppa, Morse, et al., 2005).

Finally, one must consider any preexisting developmental disability in predicting outcome. If ADHD or intellectual disability is evident in a child after recovery from TBI, it is important to know whether this predated the injury. Cognitive impairments following an injury should be compared with any preexisting intelligence test scores. In one study, children with ongoing problems following mild TBI were found to be more likely to have premorbid neurological or psychiatric problems, family stressors, or learning difficulty or to have had a previous head injury (Ponsford et al., 1999). Another large study conducted in England suggests that these cognitive impairments seen in some children with multiple mild head injuries are related more to social and personal factors than to the head injury itself (Bijur, Haslum, & Golding, 1996).

PREVENTION

Most childhood head trauma is preventable (MacKenzie, 2000). Because a number of factors contribute to the risk of injury, however, no single intervention will be completely effective. Rather, specific preventive strategies must be employed for each major category of TBI (i.e., motor vehicle crashes, including those associated with pedestrian and bicycle injuries; assaults and abuse; household incidents, including falls and near-drownings; sports- and recreation-related injuries; and suicide attempts) (Chorley, 1998; Mello et al., 2005; Murray et al., 2000). Prevention also is important in children who have already sustained TBI, as the effect of subsequent injury is cumulative. Persistent neurological impairments that result in impulsivity or hyperactivity place these children at high risk for additional injury.

Laws in all states requiring restraint of children who are passengers in motor vehicles have been highly (but not completely) effective in lowering the frequency and severity of TBI (Elliott et al., 2006). Passive restraints such as airbags have also been found to be effective. When small children are seated in the front seat, however, airbag deployment can lead to injury and even death (Newgard & Lewis, 2005), emphasizing the importance of placing children in approved, properly placed car seats or restraints in the back seat. Belt-positioning booster seats have been shown to add safety benefits compared with seat belts for children ages 4–7 years (Durbin, Elliott, & Winston, 2003). The number of motor vehicle crashes in which teenagers sustain brain injuries continues to be too high. Education about the risks of drinking and driving has had some impact. Many experts believe, however, that further effective prevention efforts must include nighttime curfews and other graduated licensing measures, delaying licensure to 17 years of age, eliminating driver education courses that allow teenagers to obtain their licenses at younger ages, and random breath testing for alcohol (Durbin, 1999).

Efforts also should be supported to improve pedestrian safety. Although children can improve street-crossing skills somewhat with training, children younger than 11–12 years of age have developmental limitations in their ability to assess distances and speeds and negotiate traffic safely (Christoffel et al., 1996). Reducing the speed of traffic, separating pedestrians from traffic, and enforcing laws that govern motor vehicle–pedestrian interactions have been recommended as community strategies to reduce childhood pedestrian injuries (Rivara et al., 1994).

Bicycle helmets have been found to reduce the risk of TBI due to bicycle-related trauma by 88%, and their use should be strongly promoted (Lee, Schofer, & Koppelman, 2005; Miller, Binns, & Christoffel, 1996). Researchers at the National Center for Injury Prevention and Control reported that if all children were to wear bicycle helmets when riding, as many as 184 deaths and 116,000 head injuries might be prevented each year (Sosin et al., 1996). Individuals riding on motorcycles, as well as those who participate in contact sports (e.g., football, hockey) and certain recreational activities (e.g., horseback riding, rollerblading, skateboarding) should also wear adequate head protection.

Falls could be reduced through measures such as maximizing safety of playground surfaces and reducing the height of playground equipment and increasing house safety by placing bars on windows. Use of infant walkers increases exposure to household hazards such as stairs and should be discouraged (Shields & Smith, 2006).

Although assaults and physical abuse theoretically represent entirely preventable causes of childhood TBI, society is making little progress in preventing them. Programs that provide in-home support and teaching of parenting skills to young mothers have been used in an attempt to decrease the risk of child abuse (Vandeven & Newton 2006).

Most suicides in children also are preventable. A suicide attempt in a child is usually an impulsive act, a cry for help. If caregivers are attuned to recognize signs of depression, drug abuse, or other problems leading to this gesture, many suicide attempts could be prevented. Parent and teacher awareness needs to improve in this area. Reduced availability of firearms to children and adolescents could also reduce pediatric suicide (and homicide) rates (Senturia, Christoffel, & Donovan, 1996). Gun control legislation represents one important attempt to limit access to lethal weapons, but enactment has proven a political minefield (Christoffel, 1995).

Finally, parents, teachers, and community groups need to be educated regarding the appropriate restraint of children in motor vehicles; safe pedestrian behavior; use of helmets for appropriate activities; and the prevention of falls from heights, playground injuries, pool drownings, and sports injuries.

SUMMARY

Head trauma is a common childhood event, and the spectrum of consequences is broad. Depending on the severity, type, and location of the injury, outcome may range from complete recovery to severe functional disability. Persistent motor, communication, cognitive, behavior, and sensory impairments may result from TBI. Restoration of function in affected areas is the goal of rehabilitation and requires the participation of multiple medical specialists, allied health professionals, and educators. Although treatment is important, most head injuries in children are preventable. Injury prevention programs must be supported if there is to be a significant decrease in TBI in the future.

REFERENCES

Aitken, M.E., Korehbandi, P., Parnell, D., et al. (2005). Experiences from the development of a comprehensive family support program for pediatric trauma and rehabilitation patients. *Archives of Physical Medicine and Rehabilitation, 86*(1), 175–179.

American Academy of Pediatrics, Committee on Quality Improvement, & American Academy of Family Physicians, Commission on Clinical Policies and Research. (1999). The management of minor closed head injury in children. *Pediatrics, 104*, 1407–1415.

Anderson, V., & Catroppa C. (2005). Recovery of executive skills following paediatric traumatic brain injury (TBI): A 2 year follow-up. *Brain Injury, 19*(6), 459–470.

Anderson, V., Catroppa, C., Morse, S., et al. (2000). Recovery of intellectual ability following traumatic brain injury in childhood: Impact of injury severity and age at injury. *Pediatric Neurosurgery, 32*, 282–290.

Anderson, V., Catroppa, C., Morse, S., et al. (2005). Functional plasticity or vulnerability after early brain injury? *Pediatrics, 116*(6), 1374–1382.

Anderson, V.A., Catroppa, C., Dudgeon, P., et al. (2006). Advances in postacute rehabilitation after childhood-acquired brain injury: A focus on cognitive, behavioral, and social domains. *American Journal of Physical Medicine and Rehabilitation, 85*(9), 767–778.

Anderson, V.A., Catroppa, C., Rosenfeld, J., et al. (2000). Recovery of memory function following traumatic brain injury in pre-school children. *Brain Injury, 14*, 679–692.

Anderson, V.A., Morse, S.A., Catroppa, C., et al. (2004). Thirty month outcome from early childhood head injury: A prospective analysis of neurobehavioural recovery. *Brain, 127*(Pt. 12), 2608–2620. Epub 2004 Nov 10.

Annegers, J.F. (1998). A population based study of seizures after traumatic brain injuries. *The New England Journal of Medicine, 338*, 20–24.

Asikainen, I., Kaste, M., & Sarna, S. (1999a). Early and late posttraumatic seizures in traumatic brain injury rehabilitation patients: Brain injury factors causing late seizures and influence of seizures on long-term outcome. *Epilepsia, 40*(5), 584–589.

Asikainen, I., Kaste, M., & Sarna, S. (1999b). Patients with traumatic brain injury referred to a rehabilitation and re-employment programme: Social and professional outcome for 508 Finnish patients 5 or more years after injury. *Brain Injury, 10*, 883–899.

Barlow, K., Thompson, E., Johnson, D., et al. (2004). The neurological outcome of non-accidental head injury. *Pediatric Rehabilitation, 7*(3), 195–203.

Barlow, K.M., Thomson, E., Johnson, D., et al. (2005). Late neurologic and cognitive sequelae of inflicted traumatic brain injury in infancy. *Pediatrics, 116*(2), e174–e185.

Bates, G. (2006). Medication in the treatment of the behavioural sequelae of traumatic brain injury. *Developmental Medicine and Child Neurology, 48*(8), 697–701. Review.

Ben Abraham, R., Lahat, E., Sheinman, G., et al. (2000). Metabolic and clinical markers of prognosis in the era of CT imaging in children with acute epidural hematomas. *Pediatric Neurosurgery, 33*, 70–75.

Biagas, K.V., & Gaeta, M.L. (1998). Treatment of traumatic brain injury with hypothermia. *Current Opinion in Pediatrics, 10*, 271–277.

Bigler, E.D. (1999). Neuroimaging in pediatric traumatic head injury: Diagnostic considerations and relationships to neurobehavioral outcome. *The Journal of Head Trauma Rehabilitation, 14*, 406–423.

Bijur, P.E., Haslum, M., & Golding, J. (1996). Cognitive outcomes of multiple mild head injuries in children. *Journal of Developmental and Behavioral Pediatrics, 17*, 143–148.

Bloom, D.R., Levin, H.S., Ewing-Cobbs, L., et al. (2001). Lifetime and novel psychiatric disorders after pediatric traumatic brain injury. *Journal of the American Academy of Child and Adolescent Psychiatry, 40*(5), 572–579.

Brain Trauma Foundation, American Association of Neurological Surgeons, & Joint Section on Neurotrauma and Critical Care. (2000). Glasgow Coma Scale score. *Journal of Neurotrauma, 17*(6–7), 573–581.

Brink, J.D., & Hoffer, M.M. (1978). Rehabilitation of brain injured children. *Orthopedic Clinics of North America, 9*, 451–454.

Byrne, J.M., Bawden, H.N., Beattie, T., et al. (2003). Risk for injury in preschoolers: Relationship to attention deficit hyperactivity disorder. *Child Neuropsychology, 9*(2), 142–151.

Campbell, C.G., Kuehn, S.M., Richards, P.M., et al. (2004). Medical and cognitive outcome in children with traumatic brain injury. *The Canadian Journal of Neurological Sciences, 31*(2), 213–219.

Cantu, R.C. (2003). Recurrent athletic head injury: Risks and when to retire. *Clinics in Sports Medicine, 22*, 593–603.

Carney, J., & Schoenbrodt, L. (1994). Educational implications of traumatic brain injury. *Pediatric Annals, 23*, 47–52.

Carroll, L.J., Cassidy, J.D., Peloso, P.M., et al. (2004). Prognosis for mild traumatic brain injury: Results of the WHO Collaborating Centre Task Force on Mild Traumatic Brain Injury. *Journal of Rehabilitation Medicine, 43*(Suppl.), 84–105. Review.

Catroppa, C., & Anderson, V. (2004). Recovery and predictors of language skills two years following pediatric traumatic brain injury. *Brain and Language, 88*(1), 68–78.

Centers for Disease Control and Prevention. (2006). Incidence rates of hospitalization related to traumatic brain injury—12 states, 2002. *Morbidity and Mortality Weekly Report, 55*(8), 201–204.

Chapman, S.B. Sparks, G., Levin, H.S., et al. (2004). Discourse macrolevel processing after severe pediatric traumatic brain injury. *Developmental Neuropsychology, 25,* 37–60.

Chorley, J.N. (1998). Sports-related head injuries. *Current Opinion in Pediatrics, 10,* 350–355.

Chung, C.Y., Chen, C.L., Cheng, P.T., (2006). Critical score of Glasgow Coma Scale for pediatric traumatic brain injury. *Pediatric Neurology, 34*(5), 379–387.

Christoffel, K.K. (1995). The "guns" debate. *Pediatrics, 95,* 619.

Christoffel, K.K., Donovan, M., Schofer, J., et al. (1996). Psychosocial factors in childhood pedestrian injury: A matched case-control study. *Pediatrics, 97,* 33–42.

Dahl, E., von Wendt, L., & Emanuelson, I. (2006). A prospective, population-based, follow-up study of mild traumatic brain injury in children. *Injury, 37*(5), 402–409. Epub 2005 Dec 20.

Ducrocq, S.C., Meyer, P.G., Orliaguet, G.A., et al. (2006). Epidemiology and early predictive factors of mortality and outcome in children with traumatic severe brain injury: Experience of a French pediatric trauma center. *Pediatric Critical Care Medicine, 7*(5), 461–467.

Duhaime, A.C., Christian, C.W., Rorke, L.B., et al. (1998). Nonaccidental head injury in infants—the "shaken-baby syndrome." *The New England Journal of Medicine, 338*(25), 1822–1829.

Durbin, D.R. (1999). Preventing motor vehicle injuries. *Current Opinion in Pediatrics, 11,* 583–587.

Durbin, D.R., Elliott, M.R., & Winston, F.K. (2003). Belt-positioning booster seats and reduction in risk of injury among children in vehicle crashes. *Journal of the American Medical Association, 289,* 2835–2840.

Durham, S.R., Clancy, R.R., Leuthardt, E., et al. (2000). CHOP infant coma scale ("Infant Face Scale"): A novel coma scale for children less than two years of age. *Journal of Neurotrauma, 17,* 729–737.

Elliott, M.R., Kallan, M.J., Durbin, D.R., et al. (2006). Effectiveness of child safety seats vs. seat belts in reducing risk for death in children in passenger vehicle crashes. *Archives of Pediatrics and Adolescent Medicine, 160*(6), 617–21. Erratum, *Archives of Pediatrics and Adolescent Medicine, 160*(9), 952.

Ewing-Cobbs, L., Fletcher, J.M., Levin, H.S., et al. (1998). Academic achievement and academic placement following traumatic brain injury in children and adolescents: A two year longitudinal study. *Journal of Clinical and Experimental Neuropsychology, 20,* 769–781.

Ewing-Cobbs, L., Levin, H.S., Fletcher, J.M., et al. (1990). The Children's Orientation and Amnesia Test: Relationship to severity of acute head injury and to recovery of memory. *Neurosurgery, 27,* 683–691.

Feeney, T., & Ylvisaker, M. (2006). Context-sensitive cognitive-behavioural supports for young children with TBI: A replication study. *Brain Injury, 20*(6), 629–645.

Feickert, H.J., Drommer, S., & Heyer, R. (1999). Severe head injury in children: impact of risk factors on outcome. *The Journal of Trauma, 47*(1), 33–38.

Felderhoff-Mueser, U., & Ikonomidou, C. (2000). Mechanisms of neurodegeneration after paediatric brain injury. *Current Opinion in Neurology, 13,* 1–5.

Gerring, J.P., Brady, K.D., Chen, A., et al. (1998). Premorbid prevalence of ADHD and development of secondary ADHD after closed head injury. *Journal of the American Academy of Child and Adolescent Psychiatry, 37,* 647–654.

Glang, A., Tyler, J., Pearson, S., et al. (2004). Improving educational services for students with TBI through statewide consulting teams. *NeuroRehabilitation, 19*(3), 219–231. Review.

Gillette, Y., & DePompei, R. (2004). The potential of electronic organizers as a tool in the cognitive rehabilitation of young people. *NeuroRehabilitation, 19*(3), 233–243. Review.

Grasso, S.N., & Keller, M.S. (1998). Diagnostic imaging in pediatric trauma. *Current Opinion in Pediatrics, 10,* 299–302.

Gruskin, K.D., & Schutzman, S.A. (1999). Head trauma in children younger than 2 years: Are there predictors for complications? *Archives of Pediatric and Adolescent Medicine, 153,* 15–20.

Hagen, C., Malkmus, D., & Durham, P. (1979). Levels of cognitive functioning. In *Rehabilitation of the head injured adult: Comprehensive physical management.* Downey, CA: Professional Staff Association of Ranchos Los Amigos Hospital.

Haley, S.M., Dumas, H.M., Rabin, J.P., et al. (2003). Early recovery of walking in children and youths after traumatic brain injury. *Developmental Medicine and Child Neurology, 45,* 671–675.

Hawley, C.A., Ward, A.B., Magnay, A.R., et al. (2004). Return to school after brain injury. *Archives of Disease in Childhood, 89*(2), 136–142.

Homer, C.J., & Kleinman, L. (1999). Technical report: Minor head injury in children. *Pediatrics, 104,* e78.

Individuals with Disabilities Education Act Amendments of 1997, PL 105-17, 20 U.S.C. §§ 1400 *et seq.*

Individuals with Disabilities Education Act (IDEA) of 1990, PL 101-476, 20 U.S.C. §§ 1400 *et seq.*

Individuals with Disabilities Education Improvement Act of 2004, PL 108-446, 20 U.S.C. §§ 1400 *et seq.*

Jaffe, K.M., Massagli, T.L., Martin, K.M,. et al. (1993). Pediatric traumatic brain injury: Acute and rehabilitation costs. *Archives of Physical Medicine and Rehabilitation, 74,* 681–686.

Jennett, B., Teasdale, G., Galbraith, S., et al. (1977). Severe head injuries in three countries. *Journal of Neurology, Neurosurgery, and Psychiatry, 40,* 291–298.

Johnson, P., Thomas-Stonell, N., Rumney, P., et al. (2006). Long-term outcomes of pediatric acquired brain injury. *Brain and Cognition, 60*(2), 205–206.

Kapoor, N., & Ciuffreda, K.J. (2002). Vision disturbances following traumatic brain injury. *Current Treatment Options in Neurology, 4*(4), 271–280.

Keenan, H.T., Runyan, D.K., Marshall, S.W., et al. (2004). A population-based comparison of clinical and outcome characteristics of young children with serious inflicted and noninflicted traumatic brain injury. *Pediatrics, 114,* 633–639.

Keenan, H.T., Runyan, D.K., & Nocera, M. (2006). Longitudinal follow-up of families and young children with traumatic brain injury. *Pediatrics, 117*(4), 1291–1297.

Khanna, S., Davis, D., Peterson, B., et al. (2000). Use of hypertonic saline in the treatment of severe refractory posttraumatic intracranial hypertension in pediatric traumatic brain injury. *Critical Care Medicine, 28,* 1144–1151.

Koc, R.K., Akdemir, H., Oktem, I.S., et al. (1997). Acute subdural hematoma: Outcome and outcome prediction. *Neurosurgical Review, 20*(4), 239–244.

Lam, W.H., & MacKersie, A. (1999). Paediatric head injury: Incidence, aetiology and management. *Paediatric Anaesthesia, 9*(5), 377–385.

Lavelle, J.M., & Shaw, K.N. (1998). Evaluation of head injury in a pediatric emergency department: Pretrauma and posttrauma system. *Archives of Pediatrics and Adolescent Medicine, 152,* 1220–1224.

Lee, E.J., Hung, Y.C., Wang, L.C., et al. (1998). Factors influencing the functional outcome of patients with acute epidural hematomas: Analysis of 200 patients undergoing surgery. *The Journal of Trauma, 45,* 946–952.

Lee, B.H., Schofer, J.L., & Koppelman, F.S. (2005). Bicycle safety helmet legislation and bicycle-related non-fatal injuries in California. *Accident: Analysis and Prevention, 37*(1), 93–102.

Levin, H.S., & Hanten, G. (2005). Executive functions after traumatic brain injury in children. *Pediatric Neurology, 33*(2), 79–93. Review.

Luerssen, T.G., Klauber, M.R., & Marshall, L.F. (1988). Outcome from head injury related to patient's age: A longitudinal prospective study of adult and pediatric head injury. *Journal of Neurosurgery, 68,* 409–416.

MacKenzie, E.J. (2000). Epidemiology of injuries: Current trends and future challenges. *Epidemiologic Reviews, 22*(1), 112–119.

Maggi, G., Aliberti, F., Petrone, G., et al. (1998). Extradural hematomas in children. *Journal of Neurosurgical Sciences, 42*(2), 95–99.

The management of spasticity. (2000). *Drug and Therapeutics Bulletin, 38*(6), 44–46.

Mansfield, R.T. (1997). Head injuries in children and adults. *Critical Care Clinics, 13,* 611–628.

Massagli, T.L., Jaffe, K.M., Fay, G.C., et al. (1996). Neurobehavioral sequelae of severe pediatric traumatic brain injury: A cohort study. *Archives of Physical Medicine and Rehabilitation, 77,* 223–231.

Massagli, T.L., Michaud, L.J., & Rivara, F.P. (1996). Association between injury indices and outcome after severe traumatic brain injury in children. *Archives of Physical Medicine and Rehabilitation, 77,* 125–132.

Max, J.E., Schachar, R.J., Levin, H.S., et al. (2005). Predictors of secondary attention-deficit/hyperactivity disorder in children and adolescents 6 to 24 months after traumatic brain injury. *Journal of the American Academy of Child and Adolescent Psychiatry, 44*(10), 1041–1049.

McCabe, C.F., & Donahue, S.P. (2000). Prognostic indicators for vision and mortality in shaken baby syndrome. *Archives of Ophthalmology, 118,* 373–377.

Meekes, J., Jennekens-Schinkel, A., & van Schooneveld, M.M. (2006). Recovery after childhood traumatic brain injury: Vulnerability and plasticity. *Pediatrics, 117*(6), 2330.

Mello, M.J., Linakis, J., Meyer, S., et al. (2005). Bicycle related traumatic brain injury at Hasbro Children's Hospital: 1997–2003. *Medicine and Health, Rhode Island, 88*(6),192–193.

Meyer, P., Legros, C., & Orliaguet, G. (1999). Critical care management of neurotrauma in children: New trends and perspectives. *Child's Nervous System, 15,* 732–739.

Meythaler, J.M., Guin-Renfroe, S., Grabb, P., et al. (1999). Long-term continuously infused intrathecal baclofen for spastic-dystonic hypertonia in traumatic brain injury: 1-year experience. *Archives of Physical Medicine and Rehabilitation, 80,* 13–19.

Michaud, L.J. (2003). Inflicted childhood neurotrauma: Outcomes and rehabilitation. In R.M. Reece & C.E.

Nicholson (Eds.), *Inflicted childhood neurotrauma* (pp. 255–264). Chicago: American Academy of Pediatrics.

Michaud, L.J., Rivara, F.P., Grady, M.S., et al. (1992). Predictors of survival and severity of disability after severe brain injury in children. *Neurosurgery, 31,* 254–264.

Michaud, L.J., Rivara, F.P., Jaffe, K.M., et al. (1993). Traumatic brain injury as a risk factor for behavioral disorders in children. *Archives of Physical Medicine and Rehabilitation, 74,* 368–375.

Miller, P.A., Binns, H.J., & Christoffel, K.K. (1996). Children's bicycle helmet attitudes and use: Association with parental rules. The Pediatric Practice Research Group. *Archives of Pediatric and Adolescent Medicine, 150,* 1259–1264.

Mittenberg, W., Wittner, M.S., & Miller, L.J. (1997). Postconcussion syndrome occurs in children. *Neuropsychology, 11*(3), 447–452.

Montgomery, V., Oliver, R., Reisner, A., et al. (2002). The effect of severe traumatic brain injury on the family. *The Journal of Trauma, 52*(6), 1121–1124.

Morgan, A., Ward, E., Murdoch, B., et al. (2003). Incidence, characteristics, and predictive factors for dysphagia after pediatric traumatic brain injury. *The Journal of Head Trauma Rehabilitation, 18*(3), 239–251.

Murgio, A., Andrade, F.A., Sanchez Munoz, M.A., et al. (1999). International multicenter study of head injury in children: ISHIP Group. *Child's Nervous System, 15,* 318–321.

Murray, J.A., Chen, D., Velmahos, G.C., et al. (2000). Pediatric falls: Is height a predictor of injury and outcome? *American Surgeon, 66*(9), 863–865.

Narayan, R.K., Michel, M.E., Ansell, B., et al. (2002). Clinical trials in head injury. *Journal of Neurotrauma, 19,* 503–557.

Natale, J.E., Joseph, J.G., Helfaer, M.A., et al. (2000). Early hyperthermia after traumatic brain injury in children: Risk factors, influence on length of stay, and effect on short term neurologic status. *Critical Care Medicine, 28,* 2608–2615.

National Institutes of Health Consensus Development Panel on Rehabilitation of Persons with Traumatic Brain Injury. (1999). Consensus conference: Rehabilitation of persons with traumatic brain injury. *Journal of the American Medical Association, 282,* 974–983.

Newgard, C.D., & Lewis, R.J. (2005). Effects of child age and body size on serious injury from passenger airbag presence in motor vehicle crashes. *Pediatrics, 115*(6), 1579–1585.

Newton, A.W., & Vandeven, A.M. (2005). Update on child maltreatment with a special focus on shaken baby syndrome. *Current Opinion in Pediatrics, 17*(2), 246–251. Review.

Nybo, T., & Koskiniemi, M. (1999). Cognitive indicators of vocational outcome after severe traumatic brain injury (TBI) in childhood. *Brain Injury, 13*(10), 759–766.

Parslow, R.C., Morris, K.P., Tasker, R.C., et al. (2005). Epidemiology of traumatic brain injury in children receiving intensive care in the UK. *Archives of Disease in Childhood, 90*(11), 1182–1187. Epub 2005 Jul 27.

Passler, M.A., & Riggs, R.V. (2001). Positive outcomes in traumatic brain injury-vegetative state: Patients treated with bromocriptine. *Archives of Physical Medicine and Rehabilitation, 82,* 311–315.

Paterakis, K., Karantanas, A.H., Komnos, A., et al. (2000). Outcome of patients with diffuse axonal injury: The significance and prognostic value of MRI in the acute phase. *The Journal of Trauma, 49,* 1071–1075.

Poirier, M.P., & Wadsworth, M.R. (2000). Sports-related concussions. *Pediatric Emergency Care, 16*(4), 278–283; quiz, 284–286.

Ponsford, J., Willmott, C., Rothwell, A., et al. (1999). Cognitive and behavioral outcome following mild traumatic head injury in children. *The Journal of Head Trauma Rehabilitation, 14*, 360–372.

Quayle, K.S. (1999). Minor head injury in the pediatric patient. *Pediatric Clinics of North America, 46*, 1189–1199, vii.

Rawlins, P.K. (2004). Intrathecal baclofen therapy over 10 years. *Journal of Neuroscience Nursing, 36*(6), 322–327.

Reece, R.M., & Sege, R. (2000). Childhood head injuries: Accidental or inflicted? *Archives of Pediatric and Adolescent Medicine, 154*, 11–15.

Rivara, J.B., Jaffe, K.M., Polissar, N.L., et al. (1994). Family functioning and children's academic performance and behavior problems in the year following traumatic brain injury. *Archives of Physical Medicine and Rehabilitation, 75*(4), 369–379.

Rocchi, G., Caroli, E., Raco, A., et al. (2005). Traumatic epidural hematoma in children. *Journal of Child Neurology, 20*(7), 569–572.

Roizen, N.J. (1999). Etiology of hearing loss in children. Nongenetic causes. *Pediatric Clinics of North America, 46*(1), 49–64, x.

Salehi-Had, H., Brandt, J.D., Rosas, A.J., et al. (2006). Findings in older children with abusive head injury: Does shaken-child syndrome exist? *Pediatrics, 117*(5), e1039–1044.

Savage, R.C., DePompei, R., Tyler, J., et al. (2005). Paediatric traumatic brain injury: A review of pertinent issues. *Pediatric Rehabilitation, 8*(2), 92–103.

Savitsky, E.A., & Votey, S.R. (2000). Current controversies in the management of minor pediatric head injuries. *American Journal of Emergency Medicine, 18*, 96–101.

Schneier, A.J., Shields, B.J., Hostetler, S.G., et al. (2006). Incidence of pediatric traumatic brain injury and associated hospital resource utilization in the United States. *Pediatrics, 118*(2), 483–492.

Schutzman, S.A., Barnes, P., Duhaime, A.-C., et al. (2001). Evaluation and management of children younger than 2 years old with apparently minor head trauma: Proposed guidelines. *Pediatrics, 107*, 983–993.

Schutzman, S.A., & Greenes, D.S. (2001). Pediatric minor head trauma. *Annals of Emergency Medicine, 37*, 65–74.

Senturia, Y.D., Christoffel, K.K., & Donovan, M. (1996). Gun storage patterns in US homes with children: A pediatric practice-based survey. *Archives of Pediatric and Adolescent Medicine, 150*, 265–269.

Senturia, Y.D., Morehead, T., LeBailly, S., et al. (1997). Bicycle-riding circumstances and injuries in school-aged children: A case-control study. *Archives of Pediatric and Adolescent Medicine, 151*, 485–489.

Sheehan, K., DiCara, J.A., LeBailly, S., et al. (1997). Children's exposure to violence in an urban setting. *Archives of Pediatric and Adolescent Medicine, 151*, 502–504.

Shields, B.J., & Smith, G.A. (2006). Success in the prevention of infant walker-related injuries: An analysis of national data, 1990–2001. *Pediatrics, 117*(3), e452–e459.

Sills, M.R., Libby, A.M., & Orton, H.D. (2005). Prehospital and in-hospital mortality: A comparison of intentional and unintentional traumatic brain injuries in Colorado children. *Archives of Pediatrics and Adolescent Medicine, 159*(7), 665–670.

Sosin, D.M., Sacks, J.J., & Webb, K.W. (1996). Pediatric head injuries and deaths from bicycling in the United States. *Pediatrics, 98*(5), 868–870.

Statler, K.D. (2006). Pediatric posttraumatic seizures: Epidemiology, putative mechanisms of epileptogenesis and promising investigational progress. *Developmental Neuroscience, 28*(4–5), 354–363.

Strauss, D.J., Shavelle, R.M., & Anderson, T.W. (1998). Long-term survival of children and adolescents after traumatic brain injury. *Archives of Physical Medicine and Rehabilitation, 79*, 1095–1100.

Tasker, R.C. (1999). Pharmacological advance in the treatment of acute brain injury. *Archives of Diseases in Childhood, 81*, 90–95.

Taylor, H.G., & Alden, J. (1997). Age-related differences in outcomes following childhood brain insults: An introduction and overview. *Journal of the International Neuropsychological Society, 3*, 555–567.

Taylor, H.G., Yeates, K.O., Wade, S.L., et al. (1999). Influences on first-year recovery from traumatic brain injury in children. *Neuropsychology, 13*(1), 76–89.

Taylor, H.G., Yeates, K.O., Wade, S.L., et al. (2003). Long-term educational interventions after traumatic brain injury in children. *Rehabilitation Psychology, 48*, 227–236.

Telzrow, C.F. (1991). The school psychologist's perspective on testing students with traumatic brain injury. *The Journal of Head Trauma Rehabilitation, 6*(1), 23–34.

Thiessen, M.L., & Woolridge, D.P. (2006). Pediatric minor closed head injury. *Pediatric Clinics of North America, 53*(1), 1–26, v.

Thompson, M.D., & Irby, J.W., Jr. (2003). Recovery from mild head injury in pediatric populations. *Seminars in Pediatric Neurology, 10*(2), 130–139.

van Rhijn, J., Molenaers, G., & Ceulemans, B. (2005). Botulinum toxin type A in the treatment of children and adolescents with an acquired brain injury. *Brain Injury, 19*(5), 331–335.

Vandeven, A.M., & Newton, A.W. (2006). Update on child physical abuse, sexual abuse, and prevention. *Current Opinion in Pediatrics, 18*(2), 201–205.

Varney, N.R., & Roberts, R.J. (Eds.). (1999). *The evaluation and treatment of mild traumatic brain injury.* Mahwah, NJ: Lawrence Erlbaum Associates.

Verger, K., Junque, C., Jurado, M.A., et al. (2000). Age effects on long-term neuropsychological outcome in paediatric traumatic brain injury. *Brain Injury, 14*, 495–503.

Wade, S.L., Taylor, H.G., Drotar, D., et al. (2004). Interpersonal stressors and resources as predictors of parental adaptation following pediatric traumatic injury. *Journal of Consulting and Clinical Psychology, 72*, 776–784.

Warschausky, S., Kewman, D., & Kay, J. (1999). Empirically supported psychological and behavioral therapies in pediatric rehabilitation of TBI. *The Journal of Head Trauma Rehabilitation, 14*, 373–383.

Watts, R., & Perlesz, A. (1999). Psychosocial outcome risk indicator: Predicting psychosocial outcome following traumatic brain injury. *Brain Injury, 13*, 113–124.

Wechsler, D. (2003). *Wechsler Intelligence Scale for Children–Fourth Edition (WISC-IV).* San Antonio, TX: Harcourt Assessment.

Wilde, E.A., Bigler, E.D., Pedroza, C., et al. (2006). Post-traumatic amnesia predicts long-term cerebral atrophy in traumatic brain injury. *Brain Injury, 20*(7), 695–699.

Wills, K.E., Christoffel, K.K., Lavigne, J.V., et al. (1997).

Patterns and correlates of supervision in child pedestrian injury: The Kids 'N' Cars Research Team. *Journal of Pediatric Psychology, 22*(1), 89–104.

Yeates, K.O., & Taylor, H.G. (2005). Neurobehavioural outcomes of mild head injury in children and adolescents. *Pediatrics Rehabilitation, 8*(1), 5–16.

Yeates, K.O., Taylor, H.G., Woodrome, S.E., et al. (2002). Race as a moderator of parent and family outcomes following pediatric traumatic brain injury. *Journal of Pediatric Psychology, 27*, 393–404.

Ylvisaker, M. (Ed.). (1985). *Head injury rehabilitation: Children and adolescents.* San Diego: College-Hill.

Ylvisaker, M., Adelson, P.D., Braga, L.W., et al. (2005). Rehabilitation and ongoing support after pediatric TBI: Twenty years of progress. *The Journal of Head Trauma Rehabilitation, 20*(1), 95–109.

Ylvisaker, M., & Feeney, T. (1998). *Collaborative brain injury intervention: Positive everyday routines.* San Diego: Singular Publishing Group.

Ylvisaker, M., Todis, B., Glang, A., et al. (2001). Educating students with TBI: Themes and recommendations. *The Journal of Head Trauma Rehabilitation, 16*(1), 76–93.

Ylvisaker, M., Turkstra, L.S., & Coelho, C. (2005). Behavioral and social interventions for individuals with traumatic brain injury: A summary of the research with clinical implications. *Seminars in Speech and Language, 26*(4), 256–267.

Zafonte, R.D., Mann, N.R., Millis, S.R., et al. (1997). Posttraumatic amnesia: Its relation to functional outcome. *Archives of Physical Medicine and Rehabilitation, 78*, 1103–1106.

Zeman, A. (1997). Persistent vegetative state. *The Lancet, 350*, 795–799.

Zuccarello, M., Facco, E., Zampieri, P., et al. (1985). Severe head injury in children: Early prognosis and outcome. *Child's Nervous System, 1*, 158–162.

Zuckerman, G.B., & Conway, E.E., Jr. (1997). Accidental head injury. *Pediatric Annals, 26*, 621–632.

IV Interventions, Families, and Outcomes

31 Feeding

Peggy S. Eicher

> Upon completion of this chapter, the reader will be able to
>
> - Describe the normal swallowing process and how it changes from infancy to adulthood
> - Understand the influence of medical, motor, and motivational problems on the process of feeding in children
> - Recognize some of the common feeding problems that occur in children with developmental disabilities
> - Identify the basic components of a treatment approach to feeding problems

Feeding problems frequently arise in children with developmental disabilities, interfering with their ability to obtain adequate nutrition (Rudolph & Link, 2002; Schwarz, Corredor, & Fisher-Medina, 2001). In fact, some reports indicate that one third of all children with a developmental disability will develop a feeding problem significant enough to interfere with their nutrition, medical well-being, or social inclusion (Sullivan et al., 2000). Feeding problems may vary in presentation from difficulty chewing, to unsafe swallowing with aspiration, to severe food selectivity, to recurrent vomiting, to total food refusal. Most of the time, a feeding problem results from a combination of several factors: anatomical abnormality, motor or sensory dysfunction, medical or psychological condition, growth abnormality, difficulty learning, or difficulty with social interactions (Rommel et al., 2003). The challenge in treating feeding problems for children with developmental disabilities is not only identifying all of the factors interfering with the child's feeding function but also understanding how they interrelate. Such an understanding enables the treating team to minimize the influence of the interaction of the active factors on the child's feeding function and thereby more effectively intervene at the level of the limiting factors themselves (Kerwin & Eicher, 2004; Miller & Willging, 2003).

This chapter first provides a brief review of the typical swallowing process and the changes in that process that normally occur with growth and development. Building from there, the chapter describes the influence of various medical and developmental conditions on the feeding process and how they result in the feeding problems frequently affecting children with developmental disabilities. A case history helps to illustrate the interaction of the different influences and their impact on feeding function. Examples of common feeding and digestive disorders are discussed, along with approaches to therapy.

HECTOR

Hector is a 15-month-old referred for evaluation because he "doesn't eat enough." Hector has the diagnosis of Sturge-Weber syndrome (see Appendix B), a genetic disorder associated with a "port wine stain" facial hemangioma (birthmark involving blood vessels), intellectual disability, and seizures. At 15 months he is healthy but mildly hypotonic (has low muscle tone). He has not had any seizure activity.

Hector was fed by bottle from birth, initially taking good volumes and gaining weight well. Spoon feeding was difficult to introduce; he finally accepted baby foods at 8 months, after 2 months of repeated attempts. Two months later, table foods were introduced and Hector stopped accepting all purées. For the past 3 months, he has eaten only Cheerios, French fries, chicken nuggets, and fish sticks. Hector eats in a highchair with an insert to help him maintain a balanced, upright sitting position. Oral-motor problems include difficulty with tongue control and chewing, use of the bottle to help transport food into the **pharynx** (throat), and oral defensiveness. Hector's weight percentile has drifted down steadily from 6 months of age.

Hector drinks 3 ounces of his formula at breakfast and 4–5 ounces every 3 hours, for a total of 25–27 ounces per day. He eats two cheese curls and half of a fish stick or chicken nugget for lunch and dinner. Breakfast is his worst meal; Hector accepts only three Cheerios. Meals end when he becomes irritable and pushes the food away. Hector's mother reports that he extends his neck during meals and frequently pulls away from the nipple while drinking. Stooling is difficult, with one hard stool produced every 2–3 days.

On physical examination, Hector's height and weight are at the 5% for age. Hector is hypotonic, with a lax jaw and open mouth posture. He can breathe through his nose if his mouth is closed. His tonsils are not enlarged. His abdomen is soft but with stool palpable through the left side. During a mealtime observation, Hector attempts to eat French fries and chicken nuggets. He demonstrates difficulty moving his tongue separately from his jaw; they move from side to side as a unit. As a result, food becomes pocketed in his cheek, and he drinks from the bottle to help clear the food. As the meal progresses, Hector becomes more irritable, turning his head away from the spoon, pushing the food away, and ending the meal.

Hector is "stuck"; he does not have the skills for the textures he accepts and cannot practice an effective pattern. Hector will not progress from his current level of functioning without some intervention. To intervene effectively, it is necessary to identify what factors are preventing him from more successful functioning. To identify those factors correctly, the normal swallowing process must first be understood.

THE FEEDING PROCESS

Swallowing

Swallowing is one of the most complex motor activities humans perform. It entails the coordinated function of striated and smooth muscles of the head and neck, respiratory and gastrointestinal tracts with input from the central, peripheral, and autonomic nervous systems (Miller, 1986). Swallowing can be divided into four phases (Figure 31.1). Phase I and II, the **oral preparatory** and **oral transport phases,** are primarily under volitional control. During these oral phases, food is broken up and collected into a bolus by the tongue, which then transports it to the back of the throat. The **pharyngeal transfer phase** (Phase III) begins when the bolus passes the faucial arches (near the tonsils) and triggers the start of the swallowing cascade. The swallowing cascade is the involuntary sequence of highly coordinated movements of the **pharyngeal** (throat) and esophageal (tube to the stomach) muscles. With each swallow, respiration ceases as the soft palate elevates to close off the nasopharynx (entrance to the nasal airway at the back of the mouth). Forward movement and elevation of the hyoid bone results in:1) tipping of the epiglottis (a projecting piece of cartilage) to cover the trachea (entrance to the lungs) so that food does not slip into the airway, and 2) opening the upper esophageal sphincter (UES, or entrance to the esophagus). A wave-like motion originating in the back wall of the throat propels the bolus past the closed airway, through the open UES, and into the esophagus, marking the start of the **esophageal transport phase** (Phase IV).

Developmental Changes in Oral Motor Skills

The process of swallowing evolves as the nervous system matures. The first phase of swallowing is most influenced by growth and development. Reflexive oral-motor patterns in the infant are integrated into more complex oral-motor patterns that are learned through practice. Cortical maturation enables more independent and finely graded tongue and jaw movements to develop under increasing volitional control (Bosma, 1986). Acquisition of oral motor skills occurs in a sequential, stepwise progression. Mastery of skills at each level provides the foundation for skills at the next level. Thus, no stage can be skipped without interfering with the foundation skills for the next stage.

Suckling Suckling is the most primitive oral pattern. The tongue moves in and out while riding up and down with the jaw, creating a wave-like motion. Suckling motions and swallowing activity have been reported in fetuses as early as 12–14 weeks' gestation (Rudolph & Link, 2002). They are gradually coupled over

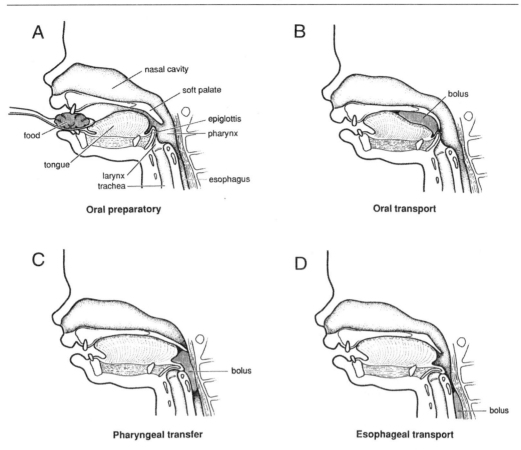

Figure 31.1. The four phases of swallowing. A) Phase I, oral preparatory: Food is taken into the mouth, processed to a manageable consistency, and then collected into a small parcel, or bolus. B) Phase II, oral transport: The bolus is then pushed backward by the tongue toward the pharynx. C) Phase III, pharyngeal transfer: As swallowing begins, the epiglottis normally folds over the opening of the trachea to direct food down the esophagus and not into the lungs. D) Phase IV, esophageal transport: The peristaltic wave moves the bolus down the esophagus toward the stomach.

the course of gestation so that the fetus can swallow half an ounce at 20 weeks' gestation and up to 15 ounces at 38–40 weeks' gestation. Only following delivery and with some practice, however, does the suck/swallow pattern become coordinated with breathing to allow functional feeding. This stepwise coupling of suck/swallow and then suck/swallow/breath is one of the reasons that even healthy premature infants usually require tube feedings during the first weeks of life (Comrie & Helm, 1997).

Initially, suckling is a reflexive activity that occurs involuntarily whenever something enters the child's mouth. With brain maturation, the reflex is integrated and the child can control initiation of the suckle pattern. The suckle pattern is normally refined with practice and increasing jaw stability to the next stage, which is sucking.

Sucking During sucking, the lips purse, the jaw opening is smaller and more controlled than in suckling, and the tongue is raised and lowered independently of the jaw. When sucking replaces the **anterior/posterior** pattern of suckling, usually around 5 months of age, the child can progress to spoon feeding. Because of the predominant up and down pattern of sucking, food can be transported to the back of the mouth without first riding out of the mouth on the tongue.

Munching and Chewing With munching, small pieces of food are broken off, flattened, and then collected for swallowing. Munching consists of a rhythmical bite-and-release pattern with a series of well-graded jaw openings and closings. More important, however, the emergence of tongue lateralization at this stage enables the child to move food from side to side and then recollect it in the mid-line. Chewing food and grinding it into smaller pieces does not occur until the child acquires a rotary component to jaw movement. This emerges around 9 months of age and is gradually modified with practice to the adult pattern by around 2 years of age (Rudolph & Link, 2002).

The Influence of Growth on Oral-Motor Structures

Typically, the attainment of new oral-motor skills is timed to integrate with the change in oral-motor structures occurring with growth. The infant, for example, is perfectly equipped for nipple feeding. The cheek fat pads confine the oral cavity while the tongue, soft palate, and epiglottis fill much of the mouth, making it easier to generate the vacuum necessary to draw fluids out of the nipple. The larynx (voice box at the entry way to the lungs) is almost tucked under the tongue, necessitating less throat control to guide the liquid passed the airway and into the esophagus (Bosma, 1986).

With growth, the jaw and palate enlarge in relation to the soft tissue structures, allowing room for teeth (Figure 31.2). The larger oral cavity is not as efficient for nipple feeding but facilitates spoon entry and lateralization. The

larynx descends and moves backward as the neck lengthens. This elongation necessitates increased postural control of the head and neck to enable safe swallowing. This is achieved as the child develops gross motor control for head righting and independent sitting. Meanwhile, the changes occurring in the child's oral-motor pattern afford the tongue increasing control of collection and propulsion of the food in the mouth and pharynx, enhancing the child's ability to guide the food safely past the airway.

The integration of growth and enlarging structures with increasing neurologic control over posture and oral motor pattern is so important that a delay in gross motor or oral-motor development can result in decreased feeding efficiency and lead to swallowing incompetency (Manno et al., 2005). Similarly, any anatomical defect involving the oral or nasal cavities, pharynx, or esophagus can adversely affect swallowing. Clefts such as those in the lip or palate interfere with sealing off the oral cavity, decreasing the child's efficiency at generating negative pressure and collecting the food in preparation for swallowing. A structural change that affects coordination can also be a significant problem; for example, enlarged tonsils and adenoids may render the child dependent on his or her mouth as an airway, influencing suck/swallow/breath timing and even coordination if

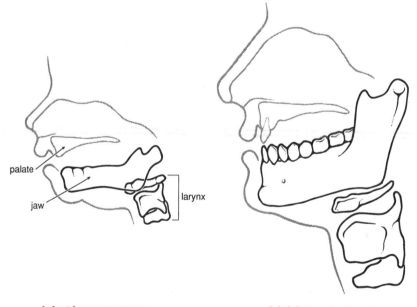

Infant bony structures   **Adult bony structures**

Figure 31.2.   The influence of growth on the bony structures of the oropharynx. The mandible (jaw) enlarges, enabling room for teeth and a larger oral cavity. The larynx descends and moves posteriorly, necessitating increased control of bolus propulsion to guide it past the airway.

the flow of the food bolus is disrupted by the tonsils. Normal esophageal peristalsis is interrupted in children with esophageal atresia or fistulae. Thus, even after repair of the anatomical defect, the child's swallow will be influenced by the degree of abnormal peristalsis remaining in the esophageal phase of the swallow.

Reference to Hector's case illustrates some of the concepts covered in this section. Munching is the level at which Hector presents with obvious problems. He has decreased and asymmetric bite strength and difficulty lateralizing the tongue to recollect the spoonful of food into the mid-line, resulting in pocketing of the food in his cheek. Despite interest in his favorite finger foods, it is very hard for Hector to successfully prepare them for swallowing, contributing to his refusal to continue eating after only a few bites. Hector's feeding history, however, suggests that he initially had difficulty advancing to spoon feeding. Thus, he did not have adequate practice with the foundation skill of sucking and its jaw stability and independent tongue movement to build on that stability for lateral movement of the tongue. The next section shows what factors could play a role in his difficulty advancing to spoon feeding.

FEEDING AND THE INFLUENCE OF MEDICAL CONDITIONS

Successful feeding is dependent not only on the anatomy and function of the oral and pharyngeal structures involved in swallowing but also on the child's medical status, especially with regard to respiration and digestion (Manno, 2005). Sensory information from the lungs, heart, and gastrointestinal (GI) tract goes directly to the swallowing center in the brain. Through this input, a child with breathing difficulty (e.g., wheezing) may start to drool because swallowing frequency slows as a result of the need for increased respiratory rate (Timms et al., 1993). Current research suggests that the feeding difficulties of preterm infants may relate more to an inappropriate swallow/respiration interface than to the suck/swallow interaction (Lau, Smith, & Schanler, 2003).

Esophagus to Stomach: Gastroesophageal Reflux

Input from the GI tract (one long tube, from mouth to anus) also has significant impact on the feeding process (Figure 31.3). The lower esophageal sphincter (LES) is a muscle at the

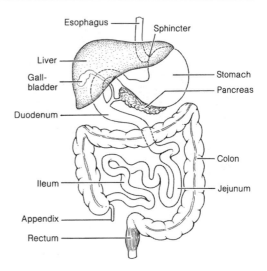

Figure 31.3. After food enters the stomach, it is mixed with acid and is partially digested. Then it passes through the three segments of the small intestine (duodenum, jejunum, and ileum). There, digestive juices are added, and nutrients are removed. The remaining water and electrolytes pass through the colon, where water is removed. Voluntary stooling is controlled by the rectal sphincter muscles.

bottom of the esophagus that functions as a one-way valve to prevent the backward flow or reflux of food up into the esophagus (termed *gastroesophageal reflux [GER]*) (Figure 31.4). GER can result in vomiting, and if the stomach contents enter the airway, the reflux can cause coughing, wheezing, and even pneumonia (Gold, 2005). In addition, the escape of stomach acid into the esophagus can cause inflammation (esophagitis) that makes eating painful. The child may respond to GER by vomiting, refusing to eat, or taking frequent breaks in the meal. GER can result from a number of abnormalities, and some forms can be inherited (Hu et al., 2004). The most common problem is transient relaxation of the LES, or lowered LES resting tone, that allows reflux of gastric contents (Gold, 2004). LES function can be influenced by meal volume and composition (Salvia et al., 2001). Reflux also can result from increased abdominal pressure caused by straining or poor posture (Kawahara et al., 2001).

Vomiting is not the only impact that GER can have on the feeding process. A child with GER who feels uncomfortable all the time may not be interested in eating or may only accept a few favorite foods (Hassall, 2005). GER can also influence the movement of the tongue, throat, and esophagus, causing the child to choose foods that are lower in texture and therefore easier to swallow. The resulting lack of practice

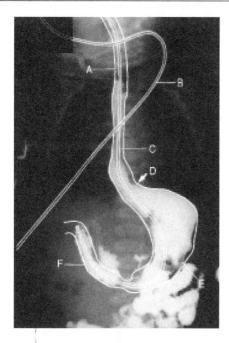

Figure 31.4. Gastroesophageal reflux (GER). Food passes down the esophagus (A), through the lower esophageal sphincter (D), and into the stomach (E) and duodenum (F). If the sphincter does not remain closed after the passage of food, reflux (C) occurs, as shown in this barium study in a child with a nasogastric tube (B) in place.

with higher textured food can lead to delayed oral-motor development. The most common conditions associated with GER are cerebral palsy and prematurity.

Vomiting, feeding problems, poor weight gain, and irritability are also characteristic of food allergy. Cow's milk allergy affects between 0.3% and 7.5% of term infants, usually within the first 4 months of life (Salvatore & Vandenplas, 2002). Symptoms of allergy to other foods may be noted as spoon feedings are introduced.

Typically, stomach wall contractions mix and push the stomach contents into the **duodenum,** the upper part of the small intestine. Delayed stomach emptying can result in stomach distension that increases the risk for reflux (Estevao-Costa et al., 2001). Delayed stomach emptying can be caused by abnormal stomach contractions, poor intestinal motility, or large amounts of fat or protein in a meal.

The Small Bowel: Lactase Deficiency

Enzymes and other substances from the pancreas and bile ducts are released into the duodenum and aid in the breakdown of food particles into sugars, fatty acids, amino acids, vitamins, and minerals. Approximately 10%–20% of African American, Asian, and Jewish children have an inherited deficiency of the enzyme **lactase,** which normally breaks down milk sugar (lactose) to allow its absorption (Rings, Grand, & Buller, 1994). With lactase deficiency, unabsorbed lactose irritates the gastrointestinal wall and causes vomiting and diarrhea after ingesting milk products. These symptoms of GI irritation can be minimized by taking lactase pills before ingesting a milk product, using lactase-containing dairy products, or using lactose-free dairy products.

The Colon: Diarrhea and Constipation

The **jejunum** and **ileum,** the middle and lower portions of the small intestine, absorb digested nutrients. The nonabsorbable nutrients, called **bulk** or fiber, pass to the large intestine or colon. Although movement from the stomach to the end of the ileum may take only 30–90 minutes, passage through the colon may require 1–7 days. Rapid movement leads to diarrhea; slower movement causes more water to be absorbed, resulting in hard stools and constipation. Proper bowel evacuation requires adequate fluid, fiber, and coordinated propulsive muscle activity (Williams, Bollella, & Wynder, 1995).

Influence of Other Medical Conditions

Any medical condition that impairs the function of the respiratory or GI tract can influence the feeding and swallowing process. For example, asthma, kidney disease, and inborn errors of metabolism (see Chapter 20) can contribute to the development of a feeding problem. Moreover, these disorders can influence one another. An increase in the work of breathing can influence GI function by changing pressure relationships between the chest and abdomen (Bibi et al., 2001). During an asthma attack, the child generates increased negative lung pressure to breathe; therefore, abdominal pressure is increased relative to chest pressure, increasing the probability of GER. Likewise, GER can contribute to reactive airway narrowing, wheezing, and increased work of breathing (Gold, 2005). Thus, a vicious cycle can start fairly easily. Unfortunately, if oral feeding is stopped for prolonged periods of time for any reason, the child may lose oral-motor skills and require gradual retraining (Monahan, Shapiro, & Fox, 1988).

FEEDING AND THE INFLUENCE OF TONE, POSTURE, AND DEVELOPMENT

The sensory and motor systems provide both the structural foundation and the sensory information that enable a child to practice and master oral-motor skills. Because the feeding process involves internal activities such as breathing, digestion, and elimination, structural alignment, control, and sensory input affect the feeding process and are affected by it. Abnormal muscle tone, whether high or low, and/or persistent primitive reflex activity (as seen in cerebral palsy; see Chapter 26) interfere with trunk support and the appropriate trunk, neck, and head alignment necessary for successful feeding. Likewise, medical conditions can have a significant influence on posture and alignment. GI discomfort, whether from irritation (as with esophagitis) or distension (as with constipation), compels the child to postures that put less pressure on the abdomen. Respiratory conditions that increase the child's work of breathing compel the child to assume postures that increase the size of the airway. These tend to be extensor positions that interfere with control and alignment through the hips, back, head, and neck. Lack of adequate trunk support

and improper alignment greatly hinder rib cage expansion, which ultimately interferes with respiration and increases pressure on the stomach and abdominal cavity. With inadequate support and restricted respiration, the shoulders typically elevate, reducing the stability of the base of support for the head and neck. Improper head and neck alignment makes guiding a bolus past the airway more difficult, increasing the risk of aspiration of food into the lungs (Larnert & Ekberg, 1995). Improper alignment also limits tongue movement and interferes with oral-motor patterns (Figure 31.5).

For all of these reasons, a child should be seated during feedings with a firm base of support to control positioning of the hips and provided with adequate trunk support to allow neutral positioning of the head and neck, with the ears and shoulders aligned in the same plane as the hips. This may require a slightly reclined position if the child has not yet accomplished independent sitting. Some children, in fact, prefer to drink while lying down. This may start as a way to stretch out and decrease the·pressure on the abdomen, if the child has gastrointestinal problems, or as a means of supporting the rib cage to facilitate breathing. However, the child then may become dependent on gravity moving the bolus rather than on active tongue transport. As a result, spoon feeding or drinking in an upright position, which requires active oral transport, is not successful.

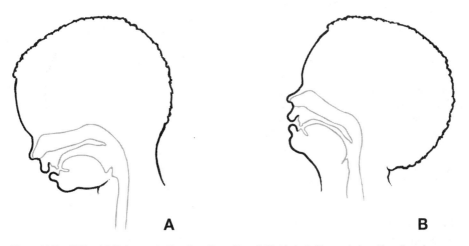

A　　　　　　　　**B**

Figure 31.5.　A) The child is in a neutral head position with a slight chin tuck. The neutral position allows for open airway while allowing the epiglottis to fall away from the tongue base, opening the vallecular space. This position gives the tongue a strong base of support off of which to move effectively with increased range and control. Widening the vallecular space acts as a "safety net" to catch any early leak of the food bolus from the oral cavity before the swallow. B) The child is in a position of head and neck extension. With neck extension, the tongue base retracts apposing the epiglottis and eliminating the vallecular space. Tongue retraction decreases control of posterior tongue transport. Moreover, by minimizing the vallecular space, this position decreases the possibility of the vallecular "safety net."

Frequently children will avoid certain sensory experiences that cause them discomfort because a sensation is associated with past painful stimuli or the sensation is currently perceived as negative. In regards to feeding, this may involve refusal of certain textures, avoidance or oral stimulation, or even a hypersensitivity to the smells or visualization of nonpreferred foods. This hypersensitivity may result from an abnormal response of the child's sensory system, but also it can be seen as part of the sensory feedback from a medical condition. For example, a child with GI discomfort may refuse new textures or feel nauseated and anxious with certain smells or at the sight of a spoon. With treatment of the medical condition, the sensory problems resolve.

The child's fine motor and adaptive skills influence the choice of utensils and level of independence at mealtime, and cognitive abilities help to shape how the child interacts with the mealtime environment. Because children are dependent on their caregivers for nutrition, effective caregiver–child communication during mealtime is crucial. An understanding of the child's cognitive level and sensitivity to nonverbal cues prepare the caregiver to effectively communicate with the child. The absence of effective communication increases the likelihood of maladaptive behaviors at mealtime, such as expelling, refusal, or tantrums. Approaching the child at his or her cognitive level also engages the child's interest and makes meals more enjoyable.

Many feeding transitions occur in the first 3 years of life, and a child with a developmental disability may have more difficulty in adjusting to changes in textures, utensils, and settings that happen during this period. This heightens the importance of a stable mealtime environment and consistent interactions between the caregiver and child (Manno et al., 2005). Consistency imparts a sense of familiarity that enables children to be comfortable and more tolerant of mealtimes.

FEEDING PROBLEMS IN CHILDREN WITH DISABILITIES

Oral motor problems in children may have a number of causes, including 1) abnormalities in muscle tone; 2) compensatory posture and breathing patterns resulting from various medical issues, especially respiratory and gastrointestinal problems; and 3) limited practice of more mature oral-motor patterns. Because children with developmental disabilities have a higher frequency of medical, motor, and learning problems, they have an increased risk for feeding problems. A feeding interruption may result from structural or neurological abnormalities that affect the mouth, nose, respiratory system, or GI tract and interfere with safe feeding. Or, a feeding problem may develop if a medical or developmental condition chronically prevents the child from having a positive feeding experience. The child then starts to associate discomfort and pain with feeding and learns to avoid feeding situations. This food avoidance or aversion can continue even after the medical condition has resolved, especially in children who have difficulty interpreting or integrating sensory input from elsewhere in the body. An explanation of some of the more common feeding problems follows.

Increased Oral Losses

Loss of food from the mouth signals oral-motor dysfunction (Chigira et al., 1994), whether related primarily to oral pharyngeal musculature or the influence of medical or postural conditions. The child may have poor lip closure or jaw instability caused by abnormal tone in the facial muscles. Once in the mouth, food may be 1) carried out on the tongue as a result of a persistent suckle pattern; 2) fall out of the mouth if the child has not practiced an active transport pattern; or 3) expelled in an attempt to control bolus size, as when there is swallowing difficulty related to GER or throat infection (Eicher et al., 2000). Sometimes food may be exhaled from the mouth if the oral cavity also serves as the primary airway.

Prolonged Feeding Time

Prolonged feeding time (greater than 30 minutes) usually results from a combination of factors. Oral transport may be slowed by difficulty in collecting food in the mouth or by weakened tongue movements. If pharyngeal transfer is weak or uncoordinated, the child may need more swallows between bites to clear the food bolus from the pharynx. The child may also slow the meal to allow more time for breathing between bites or to complete transport through the esophagus. Prolonged feeding time is a difficult problem for both the child and caregiver and signals the need for an evaluation (Kedesdy & Budd, 1998).

Food Pocketing

Food pocketing (holding food in the cheeks or the front of the mouth for prolonged periods) suggests either problematic oral transport or food refusal. Children who have difficulty moving their tongue from side to side or those who use an immature central transport pattern often have trouble bringing food back to the mid-line before a swallow. As a result, mashed food or chunks migrate toward the cheeks. Alternatively, if a child does not want to swallow the food because of its texture or taste, he or she may trap it in the cheeks like a chipmunk or under the tongue.

Coughing, Gagging, and Choking

Coughing and gagging indicate difficulty with swallowing. Both are normal defense mechanisms to prevent aspiration. The times when coughing and gagging occur during the meal may indicate which textures are troublesome. For example, if a child gags on lumpy foods but not on purées, he or she may have difficulty adequately chewing or transporting the more highly textured food. The child who coughs while drinking may have a problem controlling flow through the pharynx and past the airway. If the child coughs or gags at the end of or after a meal but not during the meal, GER should be considered. Coughing or gagging during meals that persists for several weeks is a serious warning sign and requires evaluation as soon as possible (Rudolph & Link, 2002).

Choking occurs when a piece of food becomes stuck in the pharynx or airway and the child has difficulty dislodging it. This happens most commonly when large pieces of soft solids are given to a child who has an inadequate munching pattern or suckle transport or if the child tends to stuff his or her mouth before swallowing. Cutting foods up into smaller pieces or offering only a couple of pieces at a time may decrease choking. After some practice and with positive reinforcement, the child may be able to gradually advance the size and/or number of chunks accepted. Choking can also occur when there is dysfunction in the upper esophageal sphincter, as with GER, or when the child uses his or her mouth as an airway while eating (Eicher et al., 2000). A full evaluation can help to ascertain the etiology quickly and limit anxiety.

Aspiration

Aspiration refers to the entry of food or a foreign substance into the airway (Figure 31.6). It may occur before, during, or after a swallow or as a result of reflux. Everyone aspirates small amounts of food occasionally, but our protective responses—gagging and coughing—help to clear them from the airway. Children with developmental disabilities that affect sensory or motor coordination of the oropharynx, larynx, or trachea, however, are at increased risk for recurrent aspiration (Morton et al., 2002). Furthermore, these children often have impaired protective responses that limit their ability to clear their airway once aspiration has occurred. Signs of aspiration are influenced by the age of the child. In infants, it may present as apnea and bradycardia during meals, whereas in older infants and children, it may appear as coughing, congestion, or wheezing. Some children aspirate without evoking any protective response; this is called silent aspiration and is particularly dangerous because it often goes undetected. Recurrent aspiration and resultant accumulation of foodstuffs in the airway causes irritation and inflammation that can lead to pneumonia, bronchitis, or tracheitis (Loughlin & Lefton-Greif, 1994). If there are concerns of aspiration, the child should be seen by a multidisciplinary feeding team to evaluate whether the child is aspirating and, if so, why (Fung et al., 2004).

Food Refusal

Food refusal can be total, in which case the child does not accept and swallow any food, or partial, in which the child eats some food but not enough to sustain adequate growth and nutritional health. Food refusal is most often associated with an ongoing medical problem such as asthma or GER. Because of the resulting lack of practice eating, these children also commonly show immaturity or dysfunction in their oral-motor skills that further complicates matters. Food refusal requires a coordinated approach among the child's medical provider, an oral-motor therapist, and a behavioral therapist.

Food Selectivity

Food selectivity implies that the child will accept only a small number of foods, although he or she may eat large quantities of these items. Selectivity of foods is often seen in children with autism spectrum disorders (see Chapter 23). Selectivity by texture is most commonly seen in children with cerebral palsy who have oral-motor problems. Selectivity may be associated with an underlying medical condition

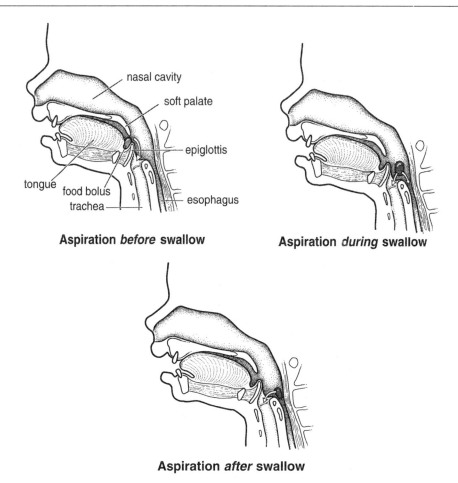

Figure 31.6. Aspiration. a) If a part of the bolus leaks past the soft palate before a swallow is triggered, it can flow past the open epiglottis and into the trachea. b) If the epiglottis is not completely closed as the bolus passes, aspiration can also occur. c) Food residua in the pharynx after a swallow can be carried into the airway with the next breath, resulting in aspiration after the swallow.

initially but then becomes a learned response perpetuated by environmental or interactional factors, even after the instigating factor has resolved (Manno et al., 2005). Food selectivity is a difficult problem that requires the coordinated efforts of a medical care provider, oral-motor specialist, and behavioral therapist.

Vomiting

GI issues including vomiting and constipation are a major problem for children with developmental disabilities (Chong, 2001). Not all vomiting is a consequence of GER. Increased intracranial pressure, obstruction of the stomach's outflow tract as with **pyloric stenosis** or intestinal malrotation, kidney disease, and food allergies are other medical conditions that produce vomiting and gastric intolerance that

mimic reflux (American Academy of Pediatrics, Committee on Nutrition, 2000). Therefore, an appropriate medical evaluation is important. Sometimes the pattern or content of emesis can suggest a cause (e.g., bilious vomiting suggests obstruction, emesis immediately after a certain food suggests an allergy).

Irregular Stooling

Constipation is a major problem for many children with developmental disabilities. It is defined as a delay or difficulty in defecation, present for 2 or more weeks and sufficient to cause significant distress to the patient (Loening-Baucke, 2005). Besides increasing abdominal pressure, and thereby the risk of reflux, constipation can be associated with cramping and discomfort that interferes with appetite, positioning, and sleep.

Overly loose stools can also be a problem. This may be caused by a lack of dietary fiber, dumping, overaggressive use of laxatives or enemas, or passage of loose stool around an impaction. Dumping, when the stomach empties too rapidly, can also compromise the function of the small intestine. Symptoms of dumping include nausea, vomiting, diarrhea, heart palpitations, and weakness. Children receiving carbohydrate-based high-caloric supplements or formulas are particularly at risk. Avoidance of dumping requires slowing the rate of stomach emptying or decreasing the concentration of food delivered to the duodenum. This can be accomplished by 1) slowing the feeding rate, using continuous feeding; 2) using fat-based instead of carbohydrate-based calorie supplements; or 3) changing to a formula with a lower caloric concentration.

Failure to Thrive

Failure to thrive is the term used to describe growth that is falling away from the normal growth curve or from the child's previously established growth curve. It can result from inadequate caloric intake, excessive caloric expenditures, or an inability to use the calories that have been ingested. Nutritionists can be very helpful in determining the caloric intake and nutritional balance of a child's diet as well as providing an estimate of the child's daily caloric and protein needs (Kovar, 1997). This information then guides further evaluation for the underlying cause of the failure to thrive. Children with developmental disabilities are at increased risk of failure to thrive for both nutritional and nonnutritional reasons (see Chapter 10).

Again, Hector's story helps illustrate topics discussed in this section. Hector's feeding problems could be described as difficulty advancing texture (food pocketed in his cheek), food selectivity by texture (in this case, refusal of purées), and partial food refusal (volume limitation) in that he stops eating after only a few bites. He uses an immature pattern with ineffective tongue lateralization. It is possible that Hector's persistent use of his stronger but more immature suckle pattern is related to his oral muscular hypotonia, which would hinder stability and development of dissociated tongue and jaw movements. Hypotonia, however, does not explain his volume limitation with liquids or his refusal of purées. Hector's neck extension with meals and frequent interruptions in nipple feeding are consistent with 1) fatigue; 2) the need for increased respiratory support, as with nasal

airway obstruction—but there is no evidence of nasal obstruction by history or physical exam; or 3) GER and resultant discomfort. Hector's difficulty with the introduction of spoon feeding is consistent with persistence of an immature suckle pattern and avoidance of spoon pressure on his tongue. Children usually avoid tongue pressure because of an increased gag response related to GI discomfort as with GER. GER, in turn, can contribute to persistence of the immature suckle pattern. Furthermore, the constipation and arching reported also suggest that Hector has GI dysmotility in the form of constipation and GER. Hector's constipation slows his GI motility and increases intra-abdominal pressure and the possibility of GER, which can make him less motivated to eat and also result in food selectivity and refusal.

Because of his hypotonia, Hector uses an adapted insert for feeding in order to maintain good head, neck, and trunk alignment in sitting. However, his constipation makes it more uncomfortable for him to sit for prolonged periods with hips flexed to 90 degrees; thus, he may try to end the meal early. Because pulling away from the nipple, neck extension, and pocketing were not recognized by his parents as subtle signs of discomfort or fatigue, Hector has escalated his behavior to include head turning, pushing food away, and refusal. However, Hector has stumbled on an effective communication strategy; when he cries and pushes food away, his mother offers him only his favorite foods. Because she is concerned about giving him adequate calories, she tries to give him something he has been more willing to take (i.e., his preferred snack foods). Hector prefers these foods not only because he likes the taste but also because he can self-feed them, which increases his independence (and, more important, keeps his mother away from his mouth) and helps him to avoid spoon placement on his tongue. Problems associated with Hector's self-feeding are that he has total control over what he accepts and where he puts it in his mouth. Thus, he can avoid any therapeutic benefit that his mother's placement of the spoon could provide him. Meal duration is limited for Hector due to the influence of constipation, fatigue, and so forth; thus, his total caloric intake remains very limited.

EVALUATION OF A FEEDING PROBLEM

Because of the complexity of the feeding process and the multiple influences on it, evaluation of a feeding problem should employ a multidisciplinary perspective (Miller & Willging, 2003). Information is needed regarding how and when the feeding problem started, how it has changed over time, and what interventions have been used. Background information regarding the child's medical, motor, and behavioral history is also important. A thorough evaluation includes the child's medical history and physical examination, neurodevelopmental assessment, oral-pharyngeal evaluation, feeding history, and mealtime observation (Miller & Willging, 2003). A nutritional analysis of a 3-day record of the child's intake can provide helpful information regarding the total calories ingested, vitamin and mineral content, and nutritional balance of the diet (Kovar, 1997). The information gleaned from the evaluation will identify the feeding problem and the medical, motor, and motivational factors contributing to it.

Diagnostic procedures may be needed to provide further information to support or clarify the clinical impression. Airway films can help to detect upper airway obstruction. If aspiration of oral feedings is suspected, a modified barium swallow with video fluoroscopy is commonly used. In this study, the child is positioned in the usual feeding position and offered foods to which barium has been added. The radiologist uses a video fluoroscope to visualize the pharynx and watch how the pharyngeal muscles guide the food bolus past the airway. The texture of the food and liquids can be varied to evaluate whether the child has more difficulty with one texture than another (Fung et al., 2004). Videofluoroscopy can also give information about airway size and the interface of the swallow with respiration.

If GI dysmotility is suspected, an upper GI series can be done to rule out anatomical problems. Barium, a milk-like substance visible on an X ray, is either ingested by the child or infused into the stomach by a **nasogastric (NG) tube.** As the fluid moves through the esophagus, stomach, and small intestine, the radiologist can identify structural abnormalities (Figure 31.4; Kramer & Eicher, 1993). A second procedure, the milk scan or gastric emptying study, provides information about height and frequency of GER episodes and assesses the rate of gastric emptying (Figure 31.7; Heyman, Eicher, & Alavi, 1995). During the milk scan, the child swallows a formula to which a small amount of a radioactive tracer has been added, enabling the radiologist to track the milk as it moves through the GI tract. In addition, if the radioactive tracer is found in the lung after several

hours, it suggests that aspiration has occurred during a reflux episode.

The final two studies, the pH probe and gastroesophageal duodenoscopy (endoscopy), are considered the gold standards in the evaluation of GER and esophagitis, respectively (Schwarz et al., 2001). For the pH probe study, an NG-like tube is inserted through the nose and passed down the esophagus to just above the junction of the stomach and esophagus. At the tip of the tube is a small sensor, which detects the pH, or acidity, above the gastroesophageal junction. If acid in the stomach refluxes into the esophagus, the sensor records a sudden drop in the pH level, signaling GER (Figure 31.8). A symptom diary of the child's activities and behaviors during the study period enhances the interpretation of the pH changes (Gold, 2004). Endoscopy entails passing a fiber-optic tube through the mouth down the esophagus and into the stomach. The child is sedated during this procedure. The gastroenterologist can then visualize the esophagus and stomach and take small biopsy specimens to look for signs of inflammation, allergy, or infection with organisms such as *Candida* or *Helicobacter pylori* (Rudolph et al., 2001).

MANAGING FEEDING PROBLEMS

Because feeding difficulties in children with developmental disabilities usually result from the interaction of multiple factors, managing them can be difficult, time consuming, and frustrating. Effective treatment usually requires intervention from more than one therapeutic discipline and a plan of intervention that can be effectively applied across the child's environments (home, school, and therapist's office). The treatment team, which should include the child's caregiver, teacher, medical care provider(s), and therapists, needs to prioritize the goals of treatment and outline an integrated plan within the context of the child's medical, nutritional, and developmental needs (Homer, 2003; Schwarz et al., 2001). The primary caregiver, with input from the team, oversees the plan and monitors progress toward the goals. Clear lines of communication among all members of the team are essential for success. Components of a successful treatment strategy include 1) minimizing negative medical influences; 2) ensuring positioning for feeding; 3) facilitating oral-motor function; 4) improving the mealtime environment; 5) promoting appetite; and 6) if needed, using alternative methods of feeding.

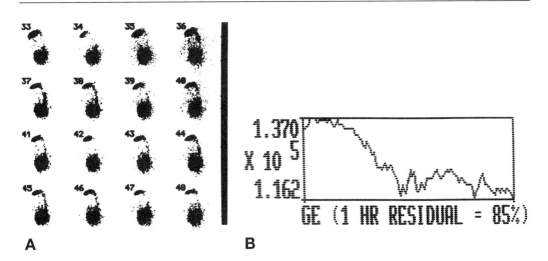

Figure 31.7. Milk scan. In this study, the child is fed a milk formula containing minute amounts of a radioactive label that can be seen on scanning. A) Shown here is a sequence of images taken after the child drinks the milk. The images are generated by a computer from information obtained by the scanner every 120 seconds. The area of radioactivity at the top of each image represents residual formula in the mouth, whereas the lower area of radioactivity is the stomach. Images 34–39 show increased activity in the mouth and esophagus, reflecting a reflux episode to the mouth and descending back to the stomach. In frames 44–48, radioactivity can be seen flowing up from the stomach into the mid-esophagus, indicating another episode of reflux. A repeat scan after the child was placed on antireflux medication would show an absence of stomach reflux. B) In addition to diagnosing reflux, the milk scan can also evaluate whether the stomach is emptying food into the small intestine at a normal rate. Delayed gastric emptying increases stomach pressure and the possibility of reflux or vomiting. In the study shown, residual gastric radioactivity decreased by 15% 1 hour after the labeled milk was ingested (decreasing from 1.370×10^5 counters per minute to 1.162×10^5). This 85% 1-hour residual is high, the normal being 67% or less. Prokinetic agents such as metoclopramide (Reglan) not only decrease gastroesophageal reflux directly but also indirectly by increasing gastric emptying. Following effective medication, the rate of gastric emptying would be expected to increase, potentially to normal levels.

All of these components should involve constant monitoring of the child's progress. Recognizing the interaction among the medical, motor, and motivational components enables the team to anticipate changes and work on several components at the same time (Manno et al., 2005). Obviously, for a feeding program to be successful, the therapists working with the child need to be consistent in and mindful of how the skills they are working on will affect the child's feeding function.

Minimize Negative Medical Influences

Because feeding is a complex skill, a child's feeding function may be very sensitive to even minor medical issues. Thus, parents' and therapists' observations of subtle changes in the child's behaviors, especially during and after feedings, are important and should be shared with medical care providers. Problems with GI irritation and dysmotility can adversely affect respiratory and GI function, as well as the child's level of comfort, and should be treated effectively. For ex-

ample, when Hector began to have daily, easily passed stools, he stopped extending his neck and pulling away from the nipple during nipple feedings. This improved his volume of intake and interest in purées and a wider variety of soft solid foods. Constipation can be remediated by 1) establishing regular toileting times to take advantage of the gastrocolic reflex that occurs after meals; 2) providing adequate fluids to minimize dry, cakey stools; and 3) encouraging active or passive physical exercise. Dietary fiber in the form of fruits, vegetables, and whole grain foods can increase movement through the GI tract (Tse et al., 2000). Fiber products (e.g., Metamucil, Benefiber) may also be helpful (Muller-Lissner et al., 2005).

When constipation is persistent, additional measures may be needed. Laxatives and suppositories can be used, including milk of magnesia, senna concentrate (Senokot), bisacodyl (Dulcolax), lactulose, polyethylene glycol, or glycerin suppositories (Fritz et al., 2005; Loening-Baucke, 2005). Enemas, such as Fleet Enema for Children, also may help, but constant use of enemas can interfere with normal rectal sphincter control and should be avoided.

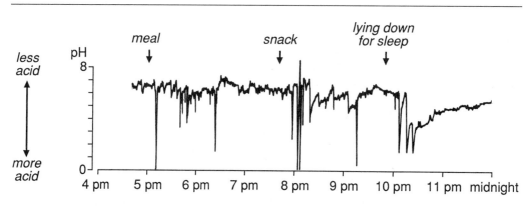

Figure 31.8. A pH probe study is done by passing a tube containing a pH electrode down the esophagus and positioning it just above the stomach. If there is reflux, the pH should drop as the acid contents of the stomach reach the lower esophagus, where the probe is placed. Shown here is an abnormal study with multiple episodes of low pH, occurring about half an hour after feeding and when the child is laid down to sleep. (From Batshaw, M.L. [1991]. *Your child has a disability: A complete sourcebook of daily and medical care* [p. 224]. Baltimore: Paul H. Brookes Publishing Co.; reprinted by permission. Copyright © 1991 Mark L. Batshaw. Illustration copyright © 1991 by Lynn Reynolds. All rights reserved.)

A combination of these approaches may be needed to establish regular bowel movements.

If GI irritation or GER is present, a number of therapeutic modalities are available, including proper positioning, meal modification, medications, and surgery (Gremse, 2004). The goal is to minimize gastric irritation and protect the esophagus from reflux of stomach acid, either by reducing the amount of gastric contents or by decreasing stomach acid production.

Small, frequent meals help to decrease the volume of food in the stomach at a time. In addition, studies have found that whey-based formulas improve stomach emptying and decrease vomiting in children with certain forms of spastic cerebral palsy (Fried et al., 1992). Similarly, a change in formula to a different protein source or predigested protein may decrease irritation in those children with milk or soy protein intolerance (Poets, 2004). Upright positioning and thickened feedings use gravity to help keep stomach contents from refluxing into the esophagus. Medications such as H2 antagonists (cimetidine [Tagamet], ranitidine [Zantac], and famotidine [Pepcid]), as well as proton pump inhibitors (omeprazole [Prilosec], lansoprazole [Prevacid], and esomeprazole [Nexium]) are used to decrease stomach acidity and thereby lower the risk of inflammation of the esophagus from reflux (Patel, Pohl, & Easley, 2003). Motility agents such as urecholine (Bethanechol), metoclopramide (Reglan), and erythromycin increase the tone or movement in the esophageal sphincter and stomach, making it harder for reflux to occur (Chicella, 2005). (See Appendix C for more information on these medications.)

When GER cannot be controlled by positioning and medication alone, surgery may be needed to prevent problems associated with prolonged reflux. These include failure to thrive, recurrent aspiration pneumonia, esophageal stricture, and recurrent apneic episodes (Hassall, 2005; Spitz & McLeod, 2003). The most common surgical procedure is **fundoplication,** in which the top of the stomach is wrapped around the opening of the esophagus (Figure 31.9). This decreases reflux while permitting continued oral feeding. An alternative to fundoplication is the surgical placement of a gastrojejunal (G-J) tube that allows access to the stomach as well as the jejunum, permitting some portion of the feeds to bypass the stomach, thereby decreasing the risk of reflux (Figure 31.10; Gilger et al., 2004).

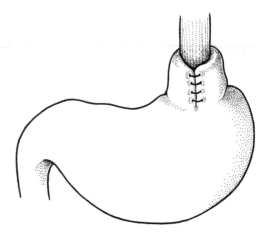

Figure 31.9. In the surgical procedure of fundoplication, the upper stomach is wrapped around the lower esophagus to create a muscular valve that prevents reflux.

Ensure Proper Positioning for Feeding

Feeding is a flexor activity that requires good breath support. Appropriate positioning maximizes the child's ability to breathe as well as providing the best alignment to optimize function of the muscles involved in the swallowing process (Larnert & Ekberg, 1995). The child should be firmly supported though the hips and trunk to provide a stable base. The head and neck should be aligned in a neutral (upright) position, which decreases extension through the oral musculature while maintaining an open airway (Figure 31.11). Such positioning allows improved coordination and more control of the steps in oral-motor preparation and transport. This, in turn, results in more positive feedback to the child and caregiver as a result of good feeding experiences (Manno et al., 2005). If the child does not appear comfortable or appropriately supported for feeding in the currently constructed chair, the child's occupational or physical therapist can make changes to improve the support and alignment.

Facilitate Oral-Motor Function

Chewing can be enhanced by placing food between the upper and lower back teeth. This encourages the child to move the jaw and use the

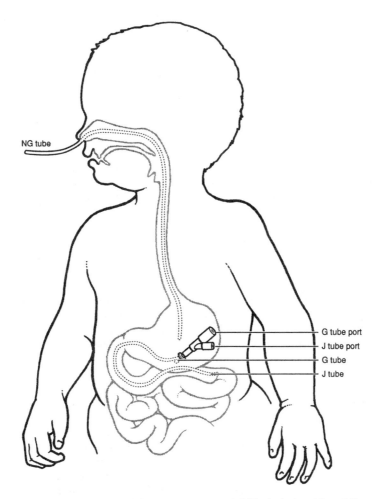

NG tube

G tube port
J tube port
G tube
J tube

Figure 31.10. Enteral feeding tubes. The nasogastric (NG) tube is placed through the nostril and into the stomach. An NG tube is helpful when problems with the child's oral function are the primary obstacle to adequate nutrition and are temporary. A gastrojejunal (G-J) tube allows access to the stomach as well as directly into the intestine. The G-J tube has 2 openings, or ports, and two parts of tubing. The G port connects with the G tube, which empties the stomach. The J port connects with the J tube, which empties into the intestine. A G-J tube can be helpful when the stomach is unable to tolerate the quantity of nutrients needed for adequate growth.

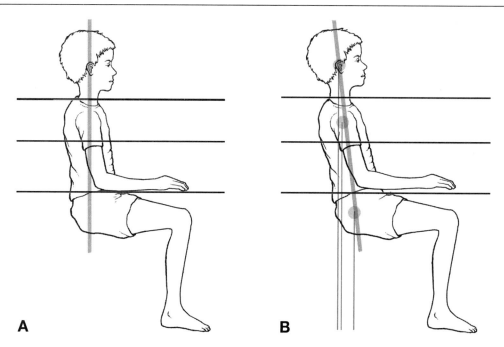

A   **B**

Figure 31.11. A) A child with a neutral pelvis and adequate trunk support to allow neutral positioning of the head and neck. Note how the ears and shoulders align in the same plane as the hips. B) A child is seated with a posterior pelvic tilt, which decreases lordosis, increases kyphosis, and throws him into a head-forward posture. Note how in this position ear, shoulder, and hip are out of alignment.

tongue in an effort to dislodge the food. Another technique is manipulating food textures to facilitate safe, controlled swallowing (Manno et al., 2005). Thickening of liquids slows their rate of flow, allowing more time for the child to organize and initiate a swallow. Thickening agents (e.g., Thick-It, instant pudding powders) can transform any thin liquid into a nectar-, honey-, or milkshake-like consistency. Almost any food can be chopped fine or puréed to a texture that the child can more competently manage.

It is important to remember that the primary goal of eating is to achieve adequate nutrition. Thus, when a child is first learning to accept a higher texture of foods, these foods should be presented during snack time, when volumes are smaller. During this transition period, easier textures should be used at mealtimes to ensure consumption of adequate calories for continued growth. A speech-language pathologist or an occupational therapist can provide information about the child's oral-motor patterns and the appropriate food textures to facilitate improvement in feeding efforts.

Improve the Mealtime Environment

Eating requires more coordination among muscle groups than any other motor activity, in-

cluding speech. Failure to perform the work competently can result in aspiration, which is unpleasant, frightening, and dangerous. Therefore, it is important to make eating as easy as possible (Kerwin et al., 1995). This can be accomplished by increasing the child's focus on the meal and including foods in each meal that are desirable and easier for the child to control. Let the child know that mealtime is coming so that he or she can prepare for the work to be done. This may entail a premeal time routine of going to a special corner of the room and putting on a bib or napkin or performing relaxation therapy followed by oral stimulation to get the needed muscles ready for eating. Children with feeding difficulties usually eat better in one-to-one situations or in small groups, because there are fewer distractions and the children are better able to focus on the eating process (Kerwin, 2003). Parental provision of undivided attention also makes mealtimes more reinforcing.

When a child is eating well and interested in self-feeding, a number of adaptive devices can promote independence in eating. These include bowls with high sides, spoons with built-up or curved handles, and cups with rocker bottoms. The satisfaction children obtain from eating can be increased by social attention during the meal or earning time for a favorite activity after the meal is completed.

Social interaction is an important part of mealtime as well, although it can be distracting. When peer interaction is the focus, it may be helpful to make the meal small (e.g., a snack) and to provide less challenging foods that do not require as much concentration for the child to be successful.

Promote Appetite

Some children have little or no appetite, regardless of whether they are receiving enough calories to progress along their growth curve. This may be caused by an underlying medical condition, such as a kidney or metabolic disorder or zinc deficiency, or it may be a sign that a chronic medical condition (e.g., diabetes) is inadequately controlled. Alternately, some children's appetite may be poor as a consequence of their schedule of tube or supplemental feedings. In Hector's case, bottle feedings of a formula were initially offered upon his awakening and then every 3 hours, leaving little time for him to become interested in spoon feedings. In consultation with his nutritionist, the spacing of bottle feedings was increased to 4-hour intervals, resulting in Hector's increased interest in spoon feeding and an increased overall nutritional intake.

There are differing opinions about whether day versus night or bolus versus continuous tube feedings are better for promoting appetite. Actually, the important thing is to look at how the child is tolerating the tube feedings. If the child retches, gags, vomits, or needs time to recover after tube feedings, he or she is not tolerating them adequately. Sometimes it takes hours for the child to feel comfortable enough to eat orally again. With this in mind, the best tube-feeding schedule to promote a child's appetite is the one that is tolerated without GI discomfort, even if this involves continuous feedings.

Use Alternative Methods of Feeding

In some cases, oral feeding may not be safe or sufficient to permit adequate nutrition (Kovar, 1997). For these children, NG tube feedings or the placement of a gastrostomy (G) or gastrojejunostomy (G-J) feeding tube is required (see Figure 31.10). A commercially prepared enteral formula (e.g., Nutren Jr., Pediasure) can be used with any of these tubes. Although puréed table food feedings can be given through an NG or a G tube, they are not appropriate for a J tube because they will obstruct it. With an NG or a G tube, feedings can be given as single large volumes (boluses) of 3–8 ounces every 3–6 hours or as a continuous drip throughout the day or overnight. J tube feedings must be given continuously, not as a bolus. The advantage of large-volume feedings is that they do not interfere with typical daily activities. The feeding itself takes about 30 minutes. As mentioned previously, however, the large volume may be difficult for the child to tolerate and may lead to vomiting or abdominal discomfort. If this happens, continuous drip feedings can be instituted. A Kangaroo or similar type of automated pump is then used to deliver the formula at a set rate. Sometimes tube feedings are used to supplement oral feedings. In this case, the tube feedings generally are used at night so that the child remains hungry for oral feedings during the day. A nutritionist can recommend the appropriate type of enteral formula as well as the amount of supplementation necessary to provide a nutritionally balanced intake that meets the child's daily caloric needs.

SUMMARY

Feeding a child with a developmental disability often requires a number of creative approaches and the involvement of a variety of health care professionals (Manno et al., 2005). When well integrated, these methods not only allow the child to have optimal oral feeding experiences with their positive social and developmental ramifications but also allow him or her to receive the necessary combination of nutrients and fluids needed to grow and remain healthy.

REFERENCES

American Academy of Pediatrics, Committee on Nutrition. (2000). Hypoallergenic infant formulas. *Pediatrics, 106*, 346–349.

Batshaw, M.L. (1991). *Your child has a disability: A complete sourcebook of daily and medical care.* Baltimore: Paul H. Brookes Publishing Co.

Bibi, H., Khvolis, E., Shoseyov, D., et al. (2001). The prevalence of gastroesophageal reflux in children with tracheomalacia and laryngomalacia. *Chest, 119*, 409–413.

Bosma, J.F. (1986). Development of feeding. *Clinical Nutrition, 5*, 210–218.

Chicella, M.F. (2005). Prokinetic drug therapy in children: a review of current options. *The Annals of Pharmacotherapy, 39*, 706–711.

Chigira, A., Omoto, K., Mukai, Y., et al. (1994). Lip closing pressure in disabled children: A comparison with normal children. *Dysphagia, 9*, 193–198.

Chong, S.K. (2001). Gastrointestinal problems in the handicapped child. *Current Opinion in Pediatrics, 13*(5), 441–446.

Comrie, J.D., & Helm, J.M. (1997). Common feeding problems in the intensive care nursery: Maturation, organization, evaluation, and management strategies. *Seminars in Speech and Language, 18,* 239–260.

Eicher, P.S., McDonald-McGinn, D.M., Fox, C.A., et al. (2000). Dysphagia in children with a 22q11.2 deletion: Unusual pattern found on modified barium swallow. *The Journal of Pediatrics, 137,* 158–164.

Estevao-Costa, J., Campos, M., Dias, J.A., et al. (2001). Delayed gastric emptying and gastroesophageal reflux: A pathophysiologic relationship. *Journal of Pediatric Gastroenterology and Nutrition, 32,* 471–474.

Fried, M.D., Khoshoo, V., Secker, D.J., et al. (1992). Decrease in gastric emptying time and episodes of regurgitation in children with spastic quadriplegia fed a whey-based formula. *The Journal of Pediatrics, 120,* 569–572.

Fritz, E., Hammer, H.F., Lipp, R.W., et al. (2005). Effects of lactulose and polyethylene glycol on colonic transit. *Alimentary Pharmacology & Therapeutics, 21,* 259–268.

Fung, C.W., Khong, P.L., To, R., et al. (2004). Videofluoroscopic study of swallowing in children with neurodevelopmental disorders. *Pediatrics International, 46,* 26–30.

Gilger, M.A., Yeh, C., Chiang, J., et al. (2004). Outcomes of surgical fundoplication in children. *Clinical Gastroenterology and Hepatology, 2*(11), 978–984.

Gold, B.D. (2004). Gastroesophageal reflux disease: could intervention in childhood reduce the risk of later complications? *American Journal of Medicine, 117,* 23S–29S.

Gold, B.D. (2005). Asthma and gastroesophageal reflux disease in children: Exploring the relationship. *The Journal of Pediatrics, 146,* S13–S20.

Gremse, D.A. (2004). GERD in the pediatric patient: Management considerations. *Medscape General Medicine 6*(2), 2004.

Hassall, E. (2005). Decisions in diagnosing and managing chronic gastroesophageal reflux disease in children. *The Journal of Pediatrics, 146,* S3–S12.

Heyman, S., Eicher, P.S., & Alavi, A. (1995). Radionuclide studies of the upper gastrointestinal tract in children with feeding disorders. *Journal of Nuclear Medicine, 36,* 351–354.

Homer, E.M. (2003). An interdisciplinary team approach to providing dysphagia treatment in the schools. *Seminars in Speech and Language, 24,* 215–234.

Hu, F.Z., Donfack, J., Ahmed, A., et al. (2004). Fine mapping a gene for pediatric gastroesophageal reflux on human chromosome 13q14. *Human Genetics, 114,* 562–572.

Kawahara, H., Dent, J., Davidson, G., et al. (2001). Relationship between straining, transient lower esophageal sphincter relaxation, and gastroesophageal reflux in children. *The American Journal of Gastroenterology, 96,* 2019–2025.

Kedesdy, J.H., & Budd, K.S. (1998). *Childhood feeding disorders: Behavioral assessment and intervention.* Baltimore: Paul H. Brookes Publishing Co.

Kerwin, M.E., Ahearn, W.H., Eicher, P.S., et al. (1995). The costs of eating: A behavioral economic analysis of food refusal. *Journal of Applied Behavior Analysis, 28,* 245–260.

Kerwin, M.L.E. (2003). Pediatric Feeding Disorders. *The Behavior Analyst Today, 4,* 160–174.

Kerwin, M.L.E., & Eicher, P.S. (2004). Behavioral intervention and prevention of feeding difficulties in infants and toddlers. *Journal of Early and Intensive Behavioral Interventions, 1,* 129–140.

Kovar, A.J. (1997). Nutrition assessment and management in pediatric dysphagia. *Seminars in Speech and Language, 18,* 5–11.

Kramer, S.S., & Eicher, P.M. (1993). The evaluation of pediatric feeding abnormalities. *Dysphagia, 8,* 215–224.

Larnert, G., & Ekberg, O. (1995). Positioning improves the oral and pharyngeal swallowing function in children with cerebral palsy. *Acta Paediatrica, 84,* 689–692.

Lau, C., Smith, E.O., & Schanler, R.J. (2003). Coordination of suck-swallow and swallow respiration in pre-term infants. *Acta Paediatrica, 92,* 721–727.

Loening-Baucke, V. (2005). Prevalence, symptoms and outcome or constipation in infants and toddlers. *The Journal of Pediatrics, 146,* 359–63.

Loughlin, G.M., & Lefton-Greif, M.A. (1994). Dysfunctional swallowing and respiratory disease in children. *Advances in Pediatrics, 41,* 135–162.

Manno, C.J., Fox, C.A., Eicher, P.S., et al. (2005). Early oral-motor interventions for pediatric feeding problems: What, when and how. *The Journal of Early and Intensive Behavior Intervention, 3,* 145–159.

Miller, A.J. (1986). Neurophysiological basis of swallowing. *Dysphagia, 1,* 91–100.

Miller, C.K., & Willging, J.P. (2003). Advances in the evaluation and management of pediatric dysphagia. *Current Opinion in Otolaryngology & Head and Neck Surgery, 11,* 442–446.

Monahan, P., Shapiro, B., & Fox, C. (1988). Effect of tube feeding on oral function. *Developmental Medicine and Child Neurology, 30,* 7.

Morton, R., Minford, J., Ellis, R., et al. (2002). Aspiration with dysphagia: The interaction between oropharyngeal and respiratory impairments. *Dysphagia, 17,* 192–196.

Muller-Lissner, S.A., Kamm, M.A., Scarpignato, C., et al. (2005). Myths and misconception about chronic constipation. *American Journal of Gastroenterology, 100,* 232–242.

Patel, A.S., Pohl, J.F., & Easley, D.J. (2003). Proton pump inhibitors and pediatrics. *Pediatrics in Review, 24,* 12–15.

Poets, C.F. (2004). Gastoresophageal reflux: A critical review of its role in preterm infants. *Pediatrics, 113,* 128–132.

Rings, E.H., Grand, R.J., & Buller, H.A. (1994). Lactose intolerance and lactase deficiency in children. *Current Opinion in Pediatrics, 6,* 562–567.

Rommel, N., DeMeyer, A., Feenstra, L., et al. (2003). The complexity of feeding problems in 700 infants and young children presenting to a tertiary care institution. *Journal of Pediatric Gastroenterology and Nutrition, 37,* 75–84.

Rudolph, C., & Link, D.T. (2002). Feeding disorders in infants and children. *Pediatric Clinics of North America: Pediatric Gastroenterology and Nutrition, 49,* 97–112.

Rudolph, D.D., Mazur, L.J., Liptak, G.S., et al. (2001). Guidelines for evaluation and treatment of gastroesophageal reflux in infants and children: Recommendations of the North American Society for Pediatric Gastroenterology and Nutrition. *Journal of Pediatric Gastroenterology and Nutrition, 32,*(Suppl. 2), S1–S31.

Salvatore, S., & Vandenplas, Y. (2002). Gastroesophageal reflux and cow milk allergy: Is there a link? *Pediatrics, 110,* 972–984.

Salvia, G., DeVizia, B., Manguso, F., et al. (2001). Effect of intragastric volume and osmolality on mechanisms of gastroesophageal reflux in children with gastroesophageal reflux disease. *American Journal of Gastroenterology, 96,* 1725–1732.

Schwarz, S.M., Corredor, J., & Fisher-Medina, J. (2001). Diagnosis and treatment of feeding disorders in children with developmental disabilities. *Pediatrics, 108,* 671–676.

Spitz, L., & McLeod, E. (2003). Gastroesophageal reflux. *Seminars in Pediatric Surgery, 12,* 237–240.

Sullivan, P.B., Lambert, B., Rose, M., et al. (2000). Prevalence and severity of feeding and nutritional problems in children with neurological impairment: Oxford Feeding Study. *Developmental Medicine and Child Neurology, 42,* 674–680.

Timms, B.J.M., Defiore, J.M., Martin, R.J., et al. (1993). Increased respiratory drive as an inhibitor of oral feeding of preterm infants. *The Journal of Pediatrics, 123,* 127–131.

Tse, P.W., Leung, S.S., Chan, T., et al. (2000). Dietary fibre intake and constipation in children with severe developmental disabilities. *Journal of Paediatric Child Health, 36,* 236–239.

Williams, C.L., Bollella, M., & Wynder, E.L. (1995). A new recommendation for dietary fiber in childhood. *Pediatrics, 96,* 985–988.

32 Dental Care

Promoting Health and Preventing Disease

George Acs, Man Wai Ng,
Mark L. Helpin, Howard M. Rosenberg, and Seth Canion

> Upon completion of this chapter, the reader will
> - Become familiar with the patterns of dental development and tooth emergence as well as potential factors affecting them
> - Understand the causes of dental decay and periodontal disease and become familiar with preventive strategies and treatment
> - Become aware of the special oral considerations for children with disabilities

Increasingly, the important association among dental disease and nutrition, growth, and development has been recognized (Acs et al., 1992; Acs et al., 1999; Beck et al., 1996; Offenbacher et al., 1996; Thomas & Primosch, 2002). Children with developmental disabilities are at a particularly high risk for dental disease that may affect their overall health and development. Yet, for many of these children, oral health is given a low priority in the presence of other major health concerns. Many families of children with disabilities also face barriers to receiving adequate dental care, including transportation difficulties, architectural and physical barriers, unwilling or unprepared dental providers, lack of awareness of available services, and inadequate financing of dental care (Mouradian, Wehr, & Crall, 2000; Newacheck et al., 2000; Schultz, Shenkin, & Horowitz, 2001; Waldman & Perlman, 2003). This chapter introduces basic concepts of dentistry for children, with a focus on children with special needs. It describes the causes, prevention, and treatment of common dental diseases and the relationship between developmental disabilities and dental problems.

CRYSTAL, ALAN, AND DOMINIQUE

Crystal is a 10-year-old with cerebral palsy. Because of feeding difficulties, all of her food must be puréed. Feeding times are prolonged because she uses her tongue to first push food against her teeth and then propel it backward for swallowing. Although Crystal has had dental checkups, it is difficult for both her parents and the dental hygienist to visualize or brush her front teeth due to her tongue thrusting. Her parents are also frustrated by the frequent wetting of her clothing and her face due to the uncontrolled drooling. Although Crystal's caregivers are dedicated to providing her needed therapy, the parents have sensed some hesitancy from these caregivers to be hands on due to the excessive drooling. Crystal's caregivers will need to devote considerable attention to maintaining her oral hygiene in order to prevent dental decay and periodontal disease. They may require special appliances, such as a nonlatex or custom-made mouth prop, to help keep Crystal's mouth open during toothbrushing.

Alan is an 8-year-old with Down syndrome. The first of his permanent teeth is only now erupting, even though his younger brother had his first permanent tooth at age 5 years. Alan's baby teeth are very crowded. His first permanent tooth, in the lower jaw, is erupting behind the baby teeth, and some teeth are malformed. As Alan gets older, he may require extraction of a number of primary (baby) teeth because they may not fall out as the permanent teeth erupt. It is interesting to note that even though Alan loves to eat sweets, he has never had a cavity. His parents do, however, complain that he has bad breath, even though he brushes his teeth daily. He also accumulates significant amounts of plaque on his crowded teeth. He will require frequent dental cleanings to prevent gingival inflammation that may contribute to periodontal disease as he gets older. In addition, Alan needs to be instructed to brush his tongue when he brushes his teeth.

Dominique is an 8-year-old who has a seizure disorder. Phenytoin (Dilantin) was prescribed to control her seizures, following unsuccessful attempts with a number of other antiepileptic drugs. Although Dominique's parents attempted toothbrushing, her clenching, tight lip musculature and head movements made it very difficult. Because of poor oral hygiene and phenytoin therapy, Dominique's gums have overgrown most of her teeth. Despite previous surgery to remove the gingival overgrowth, it has recurred.

FORMATION AND EMERGENCE OF TEETH

Human tooth formation begins when the embryo is only 4–6 weeks old. The oral ectodermal (outer) layer of tissue forms the **dental lamina,** a thickened band of cells along the future dental arches. At specific points along the dental lamina, rapid growth of cells occurs. This forms small knobs that press downward into the underlying mesodermal (middle) layer of tissue (Figure 32.1). There is one such knob (dental organ, or tooth bud) for each of the 20 primary teeth, 10 in the maxilla (upper jaw) and 10 in the **mandible** (lower jaw; Sicher, 1991) as shown in Figure 32.2. With time, permanent **incisors,** canines, and **premolars** develop from the corresponding primary tooth bud predecessors. In contrast, permanent molars develop from the dental lamina itself. Calcification of primary teeth begins at approximately 14 weeks in utero; permanent teeth begin to develop around the time of birth, and the vast majority of calcification occurs during early childhood (Avery, Dean, & McDonald, 2004).

The calcified layer of the tooth is made up of enamel, which arises from the ectoderm (Figure 32.1). The layer under the enamel, called **dentin,** arises from the mesodermal cells. The soft tissue under the dentin, called the **pulp,** also arises from the mesoderm. The pulp contains the vital parts of the tooth: its blood vessels, lymph vessels, connective tissue, and nerve fibers (Sicher, 1991).

Although it is commonly said that the first baby tooth should erupt by 6 months of age, there is actually a wide variation in the age of eruption; the first baby tooth can erupt anywhere between 4 and 17 months of age. The full complement of primary teeth takes 2–3 years to appear. The first permanent tooth typically emerges around 6 years of age, and most permanent teeth have erupted by 12–13 years of age. Although frequently congenitally absent, the third molars ("wisdom teeth") may erupt between 17 and 21 years of age, making a total of 32 permanent teeth.

When a permanent tooth emerges, a primary tooth is shed, except in the case of the first, second, and third molars, which do not have primary teeth counterparts (Avery et al., 2004). As noted previously, caution should be taken when evaluating tooth eruption in relation to tables and time schedules, especially in children with developmental disabilities, as each child has his or her own timetable. Symmetry in eruption is more important than adherence to a strict time schedule. What occurs on the right side should occur, within a few months, on the left; and what occurs in the mandible should occur in the maxilla, again within a few months.

PROBLEMS AFFECTING THE DEVELOPMENT OF TEETH

Many genetic syndromes associated with developmental disabilities have characteristic developmental dental alterations. These include the presence of extra teeth, congenital absence of multiple teeth, unusually shaped teeth, abnormalities in their mineralization, and delays in eruption. These abnormalities may contribute to orthodontic malocclusion (e.g., an overbite) and/or to an increased risk for **dental caries** (decay; Poole & Redford-Badwal, 1991). Anodontia (the absence of all teeth) is rare, but oligodontia (the absence of one or several teeth) can be seen in children with a number of genetic syndromes (see Appendix B), including Hallermann-Streiff syndrome, chondroectodermal dysplasia, Williams syndrome, Crouzon syndrome, achondroplasia, incontinentia pigmenti, ectodermal dysplasia, and cleft lip and palate. Disorders affecting development of teeth may also lead to thinly enameled and abnormally shaped teeth or contribute to eruption difficulties as seen in Cornelia de Lange syn-

8 Weeks

12 Weeks

6 Months

after birth and eruption

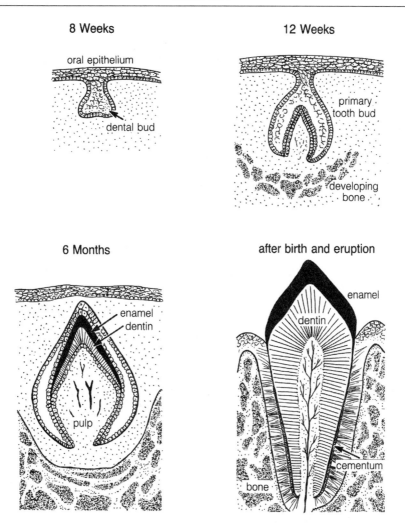

Figure 32.1. Development of teeth. By the time the fetus is 8 weeks old, the dental bud has formed, and by 12 weeks it begins to assume a tooth-like shape. At 6 months' gestation, the layers of the tooth (enamel, dentin, and pulp) are evident. About 16 months after birth, the primary cuspid, completely formed, erupts.

drome. Dentition anomalies may also be seen in children with chromosomal disorders such as Down syndrome, inborn errors of metabolism such as mucopolysaccharidoses and Lesch-Nyhan syndrome, and inherited disorders of bone formation such as osteogenesis imperfecta. Environmental influences can also affect intrauterine tooth development. For example, nutritional deficiencies—especially of calcium; phosphorus; and vitamins A, C, and D—may result in generalized enamel hypoplasia (underdevelopment), reflecting a disruption in the mineralization of the teeth during their development. Although many syndromes are characterized by specific dental alterations, each child must be individually assessed to determine the

treatment that is most appropriate. Malocclusions may be treated with a range of orthodontic approaches, whereas missing, hypoplastic, and abnormally shaped teeth may be treated with cosmetic bonding procedures. As with many elective procedures, however, the individual desires and abilities of the patient and primary caregivers to participate in treatment and to maintain treatment outcomes must be considered.

Developmental anomalies of teeth may occur as a result of childhood illness or its treatment. If a developing fetus or child between 4 months and 8 years of age is exposed to the antibiotic tetracycline, the primary or **secondary** teeth may be discolored yellow, brown, or gray

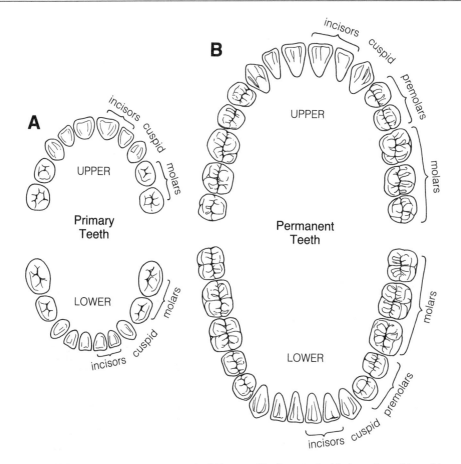

Figure 32.2. Primary and permanent teeth. A) There are 20 primary teeth: 4 incisors, 2 cuspids, and 4 molars on the top and on the bottom of the mouth. B) There are 32 permanent teeth: 4 incisors, 2 cuspids, 4 premolars, and 6 molars on the top and bottom.

when they erupt. Traumatic injury to a tooth can cause a small white or brown spot on a single tooth, whereas infectious diseases (e.g., measles, chickenpox) and chronic diseases (e.g., liver failure, congenital heart disease) can cause hypoplasia of multiple teeth (Avery et al., 2004).

ORAL DISEASES

There are two basic types of oral diseases: dental caries and periodontal diseases. Both are usually initiated by specific bacteria and, therefore, can be considered infectious in nature.

Dental Caries

Dental caries, commonly called dental decay or cavities, occur mainly in children and adolescents and are related to the presence of the bacteria *Streptococcus mutans* and *Lactobacillus acidophilus.* Decay is a multifactorial process that

involves the teeth themselves, bacteria, diet, saliva, the immune system, biochemistry, and physiology. The "chain of decay" can be seen in Figure 32.3. Bacteria adhering to the teeth break down food, creating acid as a by-product. The acid damages the integrity of the enamel, and cavity formation begins. Tooth breakdown and ultimately abscess formation can occur when caries is left untreated.

Bacteria adhere to the teeth in an organized mass called **dental plaque.** Plaque consists of bacteria, bacterial by-products, **epithelial** cells (from the linings of the lips and mouth), and food particles (Pinkham, 2005). When plaque becomes calcified, it is called **calculus,** or tartar. Plaque, as well as unremoved tartar, can cause inflammation, tenderness, and swelling of the gums. This is an early phase of periodontal, or gum, disease and can lead to loss of stability of the teeth. The process of decay is

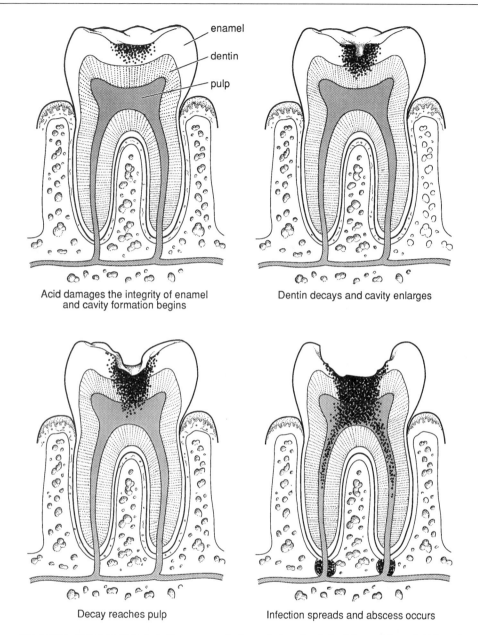

enamel
dentin
pulp

Acid damages the integrity of enamel and cavity formation begins

Dentin decays and cavity enlarges

Decay reaches pulp

Infection spreads and abscess occurs

Figure 32.3. The chain of decay. In the presence of adverse factors, the chain of decays follows: Acid formed from the action of bacteria on carbohydrates damages the enamel, leading to cavity formation. If untreated, the decay eventually affects the dentin and pulp layer of the tooth and may lead to abscess formation.

one of demineralization of enamel and dentin. The prevalence of dental caries has been cited as more than 40% in 5-year-olds and 85% in 17-year-olds (Edelstein & Douglas, 1995).

One form of caries that merits special attention is nursing or early childhood caries, caused by falling asleep while sucking on a bottle filled with milk or a sugar-containing beverage. The causative factor is prolonged contact of the fluid acids and acid breakdown products with the tooth surface, leading to demineralization. Because this starts on the tongue side of the top teeth, it is often detected late; by this time, the same process may have begun on the upper and lower back teeth. In patients with developmental abnormalities of the teeth, particularly those affecting mineralization, the ravages of nursing caries may be even more pronounced.

For young children who are receiving carbohydrate-enriched diets to treat growth failure or who require chronic liquid medications that contain sugar, rampant cavities may also occur, even in the absence of a juice-filled nighttime bottle. Evidence suggests that the impact of infant formula on the development of early childhood caries depends on the specific properties of the formula. Until more definitive information is available, children should not be allowed to fall asleep with a nursing bottle containing any liquid other than water. The same principle applies to children who are breast-fed. Prolonged breast feeding and falling asleep with the nipple in the mouth can also promote decay by acid demineralization. In addition, dipping pacifiers in sweetened solutions increases the risk of cavities.

In considering the role of bacteria in the cycle of tooth decay, it is important to note that children acquire cavity-causing bacteria during the early phases of eruption of their first few teeth. They usually contract the bacteria from their primary caregiver. If that person has a high bacterial count or possesses bacteria that are more efficient in causing cavities, the child is at increased risk for future cavities. Parents can help reduce the risk of bacterial spread by undergoing frequent dental cleanings and repairing all of their own cavities.

Periodontal Diseases

Periodontal diseases involve the gingiva (gums) and bony sockets of the teeth. Like caries, gingivitis (the most common form of periodontal disease) is associated with plaque and specific bacterial organisms (Matthewson & Primosch, 1995). The early signs of periodontal disease involve swelling and bleeding of the gums. It is often an insidious process that can go unrecognized for years. Later phases lead to loss of the alveolar bone that supports the tooth. Periodontal disease involves both local and systemic factors. Local factors include dental crowding, poor oral hygiene, overly aggressive oral hygiene, dry mouth, finger sucking, and destructive dental habits. Systemic factors include certain chronic medications, hormonal alterations, and immune deficiency states. For example, patients requiring long-term use of the drugs phenytoin (an antiepileptic drug), cyclosporine (Sandimmune; an immune suppressant agent), and nifedipine (Procardia; a blood pressure medication) are at particular risk for overgrowth of the gums. Although the exact cause of this condition is unknown, the overgrowth is generally regarded as an exaggerated response to a local irritant. Overall, gingivitis can be found in up to half of children 4–5 years of age (Pinkham, 2005).

MALOCCLUSION

Malocclusion is the improper interdigitation or relationship of the teeth or jaws. It can interfere with oral functions such as speech and chewing and increase the risk of dental caries and periodontal diseases. In addition, it can create problems with facial appearance and self-image. Although many malocclusions are minor and require attention only for cosmetic reasons, others are more severe and debilitating. The prevalence of severe malocclusion has been reported to be as high as 14%; children with certain developmental disabilities, such as cerebral palsy, have an even higher prevalence (Avery et al., 2004). In these children, the correction of this improper alignment of the teeth by orthodontic treatment to position the teeth properly also decreases the risk of dental disease by making routine oral hygiene easier.

Certain habits, including tooth grinding (**bruxism**) and pacifier/thumb sucking, may predispose to malocclusion. Bruxism is often an adaptive mechanism that allows the child to develop a comfortable occlusion or bite, but typically, the tooth grinding stops by school age when the permanent teeth erupt. In some children, however, especially those with intellectual disability, cerebral palsy, and autism spectrum disorders, bruxism becomes abnormal in intensity and persistence. Both behavior management techniques and dental appliances have been used to arrest the habit before it causes permanent dental changes. These techniques, however, only work when the child is motivated to stop the habit and is compliant in using the device.

DENTAL TRAUMA

It is estimated that half of all children experience traumatic injury to the primary or permanent teeth prior to graduation from high school. Injuries to the primary teeth are more frequent than injuries to permanent teeth. Although the incidence of primary tooth injury is approximately equal in boys and girls, males have twice as many injuries to permanent teeth (Andreasen & Andreasen, 1994). The risk of dental trauma in children with cerebral palsy and seizure disorders is increased because of their more frequent falls. The maxillary incisors, both primary and permanent, are the teeth most frequently traumatized. The presence of prominent maxillary anterior "buck" teeth, a consequence of malocclusion, is an important predisposing factor to injury of the teeth. Trauma to primary teeth generally causes tooth displacement. This is a result of the softer, spongier quality of the young bone that supports the teeth. Trauma to permanent teeth most often results in fracture of tooth structure (chipped teeth; Andreasen & Andreasen, 1994).

The management of trauma to the primary dentition is relatively straightforward. Either no treatment is necessary or the damaged tooth requires extraction. Treatment considerations of traumatized permanent teeth, however, are more complex and merit dental evaluation the same day. Although primary teeth are not re-implanted, a permanent tooth that has been knocked out should be replaced into the tooth socket by a caregiver as soon as possible after the accident. Reimplantation within 30 minutes maximizes the likelihood of successful tooth retention. If immediate reimplantation is not possible, the tooth should be kept in cold milk or in the child's saliva, as this appears to extend the time a tooth may be out of the mouth before successful reimplantation.

Because many dental injuries can be avoided, prevention is extremely important. Athletic mouth guards or helmets with protective adaptations, when they can be tolerated, significantly decrease the risk of dental injuries in children participating in contact sports and in children with developmental disabilities, who are at high risk for falls or self-injury (Andreasen & Andreasen, 1994; McDonald & Avery, 2004).

PREVENTION OF DENTAL CARIES AND PERIODONTAL DISEASE

Perhaps the most important component of preventing dental decay begins even before a child's birth. Eliminating or reducing the transmission of cavity causing bacteria from the primary caregiver to the child, particularly during the susceptible period of bacterial colonization as the first teeth are erupting, can have enormous benefits. Therefore, strategies such as frequent professional dental cleanings, rinsing with the antimicrobial chlorhexidine, or using xylitol containing chewing gum can suppress the number of cavity-forming bacteria that would ulti-

mately be transmitted to the child (Soderling et al., 2000).

Once the child's teeth have erupted, the three most important factors in protecting the teeth from dental decay are maintaining good oral hygiene, limiting ingestion of carbohydrates, and eliminating or reducing cavity-causing bacteria. Tools for preventive dentistry include brushing, flossing, and the use of fluoride and **dental sealants.**

Brushing

Children younger than 6 years generally have not developed the manual dexterity to effectively remove plaque from teeth. They should be encouraged to participate in their own oral hygiene; however, adults must take an active role and be responsible for adequately cleaning the teeth and gum regions. A soft, nylon bristle brush with polished, rounded ends works best. A scrubbing motion of the brush is a quick and easy method with which to begin. An electric toothbrush can be helpful and may be advantageous for gingival health (Barnes, Weatherford, & Menaker, 1993). When brushing, a small, pea-sized amount of toothpaste with fluoride may be used. If bubbles and foam from the paste cause a problem for the child or guardian performing the tooth brushing, an alternative to paste would be to use water or a fluoride containing mouth rinse (ACT or Fluorigard). Positioning the child in a supine (reclining) position facilitates good vision, access, and head control and will be helpful for the adult doing the brushing. The myriad successful positions are as unique as the disability with which the child presents. Successful positioning for the child must consider the following:

- Specific disability

- Comfort for the person performing the toothbrushing

- Comfort for the child having his or her teeth brushed

- Good head control and access for the child having his or her teeth brushed

- Good lighting and vision for the person performing the toothbrushing

One should allow for flexibility to find the best all-around position and time to perform these oral hygiene procedures (Avery et al., 2004; Pinkham, 2005).

Flossing

Adults should floss for a child until he or she has demonstrated facility with this procedure. Improper flossing can harm gingival tissues. Flossing should be performed wherever teeth are in contact with each other and the toothbrush cannot clean between the teeth. Unwaxed floss is preferred; however, any floss may be used. Floss-holding devices are available and can be employed by parents and/or caregivers when dexterity is a problem or when the child closes the mouth or bites (Avery et al., 2004).

Fluorides

Whether present in the municipal water supply, taken as a daily supplement found in toothpaste, contained in a mouth rinse, or professionally applied, fluoride treatment has been shown to significantly reduce the incidence of dental decay and is an integral part of a preventive program. Studies have demonstrated that fluoride in water can decrease the prevalence of tooth decay by up to 60% (Pinkham, 2005). Fluoride makes enamel more resistant to decay and remineralizes new carious lesions, making them hard again. Fluoride supplementation should be considered if fluoride is not available in the community drinking water or in the water where child care is provided. Although reverse osmosis home filtration does remove fluoride from water, other systems do not. Bottled water must disclose its fluoride content if fluoride has been added but not if it is naturally occurring. On the basis of the child's needs and abilities, specific fluoride supplements may be recommended. It should be noted that excessive systemic fluoride, however, could cause fluorosis, a condition in which permanent teeth are discolored or malformed.

Many different fluoride formulations are available, each with specifically indicated uses. For children who are capable of rinsing, low-potency over-the-counter fluoride rinses may be helpful in preventing cavities. In addition, there may be indications for the use of prescribed fluoride rinses or gels that contain higher concentrations of fluoride. Very often, these higher concentrations are provided to attempt reversal of the early stages of cavity formation. For some patients at high risk for developing cavities, and for those for whom it may be difficult to apply daily fluoride supplements, professionally applied fluoride varnishes may be of benefit. These varnish applications may provide benefits for up to 3 months.

Dental Sealants

Sealants consist of a plastic coating that is bonded to the chewing surface of molars to prevent decay. Most children have deep grooves on their permanent molars that are difficult to keep clean, but the molars can be protected by the application of sealants. Sealants are most indicated within the first 3–4 years of eruption of the permanent molars (commonly around 6–10 years of age). Studies have shown that in the absence of sealants, two thirds of children will have a cavity on at least one of their first permanent molars (Pinkham, 2005).

For sealants to be successfully applied, the tooth must be kept dry and free of moisture or salivary contamination for at least 1 minute. Otherwise, the sealant will fail or may place the child at increased risk for developing a cavity underneath the faulty sealant. If the only mechanism for ensuring a dry environment is sedation or general anesthesia, the benefit gained from applying the sealant may be outweighed by the risk of anesthesia. Thus, children with cerebral palsy may not be good candidates, and children with Down syndrome (who have few grooves in their teeth) may not need it.

Diet

Frequent feedings or snacking, as needs to occur in children with failure to thrive, increase the total amount of time that teeth are exposed to foods or liquids that facilitate the development of dental caries. For prevention of caries, these children require more frequent and intensive oral hygiene measures. Similarly, children with neuromuscular disorders that result in decreased oral-motor abilities need an extended period of time to clear food from their mouths. The increased contact time between food, especially puréed carbohydrates, and teeth places these children at greater risk for cavity development. Children with food "squirreling/pocketing" habits are also more likely to develop caries. In addition, children with chronic rumination behavior or gastroesophageal reflux (see Chapter 31) are at increased risk because of the contact of stomach acid with the enamel of teeth. Children with neurological impairments who have gastrostomy tubes often have poor oral hygiene

Table 32.1. Foods that are good to use as snacks to maintain dental health

Raw vegetables

Carrot sticks	Green pepper rings
Celery sticks	Lettuce wedges
Cauliflower bits	Radishes
Cucumber sticks	Tomatoes

Drinks

Milk	Unsweetened vegetable juices
Sugar-free carbonated beverages	

Other snacks

Nuts	Unsweetened peanut butter
Popcorn	
Unsweetened plain yogurt	Cheese
	Sugarless gum or candy

Source: American Dental Association (1983).

and low salivary flow, which may lead to a higher experience of aspiration pneumonia and significant build up of calculus (Jawadi et al., 2004). Even for typically developing children, the consistency, frequency, and timing of snacks contribute to the potential for decay. Snacks that are sticky (not just caramels but also foods such as sweet rolls, pretzels, and potato chips), eaten frequently, and eaten between meals have a high potential for causing dental decay (see Table 32.1 for a list of snacks that do not compromise dental health).

PROVIDING DENTAL AND ORTHODONTIC TREATMENT

The American Academy of Pediatric Dentistry (AAPD) recommends that all children have their first dental visit by 12 months of age. At this time, parents or primary caregivers are educated about likely events during development that affect the teeth and are taught strategies to effectively prevent dental disease. Greatest benefit is derived when a combination of preventive dentistry techniques is used. Usually, very little if any treatment is necessary at this time (AADP, 2004–2005a; Edelstein, 1994; Griffen & Goepferd, 1991; Newbrun, 1992).

In order to establish heightened interaction among the patient, parents, medical professionals, and other health care professionals, the child's global oral health needs are best served in a "dental home." The concept of a dental home is derived from the American Academy of Pediatrics' (AAP's) definition of a "medical home," which states that primary health care is best delivered when comprehen-

sive, continuously accessible, family centered, compassionate, and culturally effective care is delivered or supervised by qualified child health specialists (AAP, 2002). The AAPD supports the concept of a dental home for all infants, children, adolescents, and people with special health care needs (AAPD, 2004–2005b). Children who have a dental home are more likely to receive appropriate preventive and routine oral health care.

This first visit should be followed by check-ups at regular intervals, depending on the child's risk for oral disease. During these checkups, cleaning and topical fluoride application will be performed to help minimize the risk of caries and periodontal disease. If caries do appear despite all preventive efforts, the dentist will treat this condition by removing the decay and placing a filling material or a crown. The newest dental materials offer the advantages of good strength, aesthetics, and anticaries activity.

To minimize anxiety and help the child cope with the stress of treatment, the dentist may employ behavior management techniques or use sedation agents (e.g., nitrous oxide [laughing gas], sedative medications). Behavior management techniques focus on increasing the occurrence of desired behaviors and decreasing inappropriate behaviors (see Chapter 35). These approaches may be very effective in both improving compliance with dental health at home and in the dentist's office. For children requiring dental procedures, nitrous oxide and oxygen inhalation analgesia may be used. Onset is fast, the delivery of nitrous oxide can be controlled, and recovery is rapid and complete. Nitrous oxide analgesia may also be very effective when adjunct in providing dental treatment to young children and to those with attention-deficit/hyperactivity disorder (see Chapter 24) or with cognitive impairments that limit attention and cooperation. Inhalation sedation, however, requires a patient to voluntarily breathe the agent. If nitrous oxide, when alone, is inadequate to allow a patient to become cooperative, then conscious sedation or general anesthesia may be considered. Here, the risks and benefits must be weighed to determine if the dental needs warrant this approach. There is usually consultation with the child's primary care provider or other specialists, such as neurologist or cardiologist, to review any unique considerations or precautions required in using sedation (Pinkham, 2005).

In terms of orthodontic care, the objectives are to move the teeth into new positions using retainers and other techniques. Although mal-occlusion is the most common reason to recommend orthodontic care, there may be other aesthetic, functional, or periodontal considerations. Orthodontic care may be particularly helpful in certain genetic syndromes associated with developmental dental abnormalities. For patients with Down syndrome, cleft palate, or ectodermal dysplasia, for example, orthodontic therapy may be used to create more room for teeth, to create a more appropriate shape for the dental arches, or to align teeth to fabricate a well-fitting and functional partial denture, bridge, or implant. In patients with poor oral hygiene or who have a history of high caries activity, however, orthodontic braces should be deferred until there is an improved level of oral hygiene. This is necessary to protect against the development of new cavities or periodontal disease, both of which are more likely to occur if braces are worn for extended periods.

DENTAL CARE FOR CHILDREN WITH DEVELOPMENTAL DISABILITIES

The basic principles of pediatric dental care and oral health apply to all children. There are, however, specific issues related to several common developmental disabilities, including Down syndrome, cerebral palsy, meningomyelocele, and seizure disorders, that deserve further discussion.

Down Syndrome

In addition to having intellectual disability, children with Down syndrome have congenital anomalies and crowded dentition that place them at increased risk for oral disease. Their mid-face hypoplasia and extra, missing, or small teeth contribute to the development of malocclusion and periodontal disease by adolescence (Cooley & Sanders, 1991). Their open-mouth posture with mouth breathing can lead to dry gum tissue that bleeds easily. Excellent oral hygiene methods may delay the onset, but tight musculature and oral hypersensitivity may lead to brushing difficulties and inadequate plaque removal. An additional consideration is congenital heart disease, which places these children at increased risk for bacterial **endocarditis** (a severe infection of the inner lining of the heart chambers) and may require antibiotic prophylaxis prior to dental procedures. It is interesting to note that children with Down syndrome seem to be at less risk than usual for den-

tal caries, because their biting surfaces are smooth rather than having the typical grooving that shelters plaque formation.

Cerebral Palsy

Poor motor control and altered muscle tone may interfere with routine dental care in children with cerebral palsy (see Chapter 26). Although no specific oral problems are unique to children with cerebral palsy, several findings are more common or more severe in this population. Malocclusion is more likely to occur as a consequence of the uncoordinated movements of the muscles of the jaws, lips, and tongue. Persistent tongue thrusting or a forward positioned tongue is a particular concern. As the tongue is a powerful muscle, it can reposition the teeth, leading to an open bite and flared, widely spaced teeth. Poor motor control also results in a high incidence of uncontrolled drooling; unfortunately, there is no sure solution to the management of this problem. Surgical intervention has been proposed, along with anecdotal reports of appliance therapy to control chronic drooling (Inga et al., 2001).

The predilection for falling and the frequent prominence of the maxillary incisors also place these children at increased risk for dental trauma. In addition, mouth breathing and bruxism are often present (Avery, Dean, & McDonald, 2004; Cooley & Sanders, 1991; Nowak, 1976). Furthermore, the incidence of caries and periodontal disease is higher because of problems in the oral clearing of food; difficulty in brushing and flossing; and the soft, sticky, high-carbohydrate diet that may be needed to maintain adequate nutrition. Despite receiving limited or no nutrition by mouth, children with cerebral palsy who are fed through gastrostomy tubes (see Chapter 31) are still susceptible to reflux of stomach acid as well as plaque and calculus buildup, placing them at increased risk for dental caries and periodontal disease.

In addition, anticholinergic medications used to control drooling may cause increased susceptibility to dental caries. Psychotropic drugs may do likewise, due to an increased likelihood of xerostomia (dry mouth due to decreased production of saliva).

A number of treatment approaches can help. Providing dental care in the child's wheelchair or using positioning supports such as pillows in the dental chair adds to the comfort of the child. If toothbrushing after eating is not possible, wiping soft food debris from the mouth using a moistened face cloth or gauze pad is of benefit. In older children, an adapted toothbrush with handle modifications, an electric toothbrush, and floss holders can be of assistance in maintaining good oral hygiene.

Meningomyelocele

Individuals with meningomyelocele have a caries rate similar to that found in the general population. As a result of compromised oral hygiene, however, they have a high level of periodontal disease. Because of the spinal curvatures so often seen in these individuals and considering that many of these individuals ambulate using a wheelchair, positioning and comfort are important in dental care. The presence of hydrocephalus with a shunt may also have a bearing on the child's dental treatment; individuals with ventricular shunts may require antibiotic prophylaxis prior to dental procedures. Also, individuals with meningomyelocele have an increased risk of developing an allergic reaction to latex (Engibous, Kittle, & Jones, 1993); thus, latex gloves and other latex products should not be used.

Seizure Disorders

In children with seizure disorders, the major issues are side effects from certain antiepileptic drugs (see Chapter 29), as discussed previously, and from dental trauma. Approximately half of the children receiving the antiepileptic drug phenytoin, and occasionally those receiving phenobarbital (Luminal), develop overgrowth of the gingiva. Stopping the medication may begin to reverse the condition, but often the child will require surgical removal of the overgrown tissue. In children with poorly controlled generalized tonic-clonic seizures, the use of a helmet throughout the day to reduce risk of dental trauma from falls may be appropriate until seizure control is gained (Avery et al., 2004; Cooley & Sanders, 1991; Nowak, 1976).

Other Conditions

The range of special dental considerations in patients with chronic medical illnesses or developmental disabilities is very large. For example, although patients with sickle cell disease tend to have a very low decay rate, they may experience jaw pain that is a sign of an infarction, or sickle crisis. Children with cystic fibrosis also tend to have a low decay rate, but when dental care is needed, nitrous oxide should not be used because of its potential for adversely affecting respiration. Due to the large number of conditions that have special and ongoing dental considerations, parents should seek consultation with the pediatric dentist and create a dental home for their child that will attend to near- and long-term oral health needs and coordinate care among the child's medical specialists.

SUMMARY

Oral health is an important component of overall health (U.S. Department of Health and Human Services, National Institutes of Health, National Institute of Dental and Craniofacial Research, 2000). It contributes to wellness of the child, eliminates pain and discomfort, and enhances quality of life. Furthermore, good oral health maximizes the chances for adequate nutrition, speech, and appearance. The emphasis in oral care for the child with a developmental disability should be the same as it is for a typically developing child: prevention through home dental care and regular office checkups in the dental home.

REFERENCES

Acs, G., Lodolini, G., Kaminsky, S., et al. (1992). Effect of nursing caries on body weight in a pediatric population. *Pediatric Dentistry, 14,* 302–305.

Acs, G., Shulman, R., Ng, M.W., et al. (1999). The effect of dental rehabilitation on the body weight of children with early childhood caries. *Pediatric Dentistry, 21,* 109–113.

American Academy of Pediatric Dentistry. (2004–2005a). American Academy of Pediatric Dentistry reference manual. *Pediatric Dentistry, 26,* 67–70.

American Academy of Pediatric Dentistry. (2004–2005b). Oral health policy on the dental home. American Academy of Pediatric Dentistry reference manual. *Pediatric Dentistry, 26,* 58–59.

American Academy of Pediatrics (2002). The medical home. *Pediatrics, 100,* 184–186.

American Dental Association. (1983). *Diet and dental health.* Chicago: American Dental Association, Bureau of Health Education and Audiovisual Services.

Andreasen, J.O., & Andreasen, F.M. (1994). *Textbook and color atlas of traumatic injuries to the teeth* (3rd ed.). St. Louis: Mosby.

Avery, R.E., Dean, D.R., & McDonald, J.A. (2004). *Dentistry for the child and adolescent* (8th ed.). St. Louis: Mosby/Esevier.

Barnes, C.M., Weatherford, T.W., & Menaker, L. (1993). A comparison of the Braun Oral-B plaque remover electric and a manual toothbrush in affecting gingivitis. *Journal of Dentistry for Children, 4,* 48–51.

Beck, J., Garcia, R., Heiss, G., et al. (1996). Periodontal disease and cardiovascular disease. *Journal of Periodontology, 67*(10, Suppl.), 1123–1137.

Cooley, R.O., & Sanders, V.J. (1991). The pediatrician's involvement in prevention and treatment of oral disease in medically compromised children. *Pediatric Clinics of North America, 38,* 1265–1288.

Edelstein, B.L. (1994). Medical management of dental caries. *The Journal of the American Dental Association, 125*(Suppl.), 31S–39S.

Edelstein, B.L., & Douglas, C.W. (1995). Dispelling the myth that 50% of U.S. school children have never had a cavity. *Public Health Report, 110,* 6–13.

Engibous, P.J., Kittle, P.E., & Jones, H.L. (1993). Latex allergy in patients with spina bifida. *Pediatric Dentistry, 15,* 364–366.

Griffen, A.L., & Goepferd, S.J. (1991). Preventive oral health for the infant, child, and adolescent. *Pediatric Clinics of North America, 38,* 1209–1226.

Inga C.J., Reddy A.K., Richardson S.A., et al. (2001). Appliance for chronic drooling in cerebral palsy patients. *Pediatric Dentistry, 23,* 241–242.

Jawadi, A.H., Casamassimo, P.S., Griffen, A., et al. (2004). Comparison of oral findings in special needs children with and without gastrostomy. *Pediatric Dentistry, 26,* 283–288.

Matthewson, R.J., & Primosch, R.E. (1995). *Fundamentals of pediatric dentistry* (3rd ed.). Chicago: Quintessence Publishing.

Mouradian, W.E., Wehr, E., & Crall, J.J. (2000). Disparities in children's oral health and access to dental care. *Journal of the American Medical Association, 284,* 2625–2631.

Newacheck, P.W., McManus, M., Fox, H.B., et al. (2000). Access to health care for children with special health care needs. *Pediatrics, 105,* 760–766.

Newbrun, E. (1992). Preventing dental caries: Current and prospective strategies. *The Journal of the American Dental Association, 123,* 68–73.

Nowak, A.J. (1976). *Dentistry for the handicapped patient.* St. Louis: Mosby.

Offenbacher, S., Katz, V., Fertik, G., et al. (1996). Periodontal infection as a possible risk factor for preterm low birth weight. *Journal of Periodontology, 67*(10, Suppl.), 1103–1113.

Pinkham, J.R. (2005). *Pediatric dentistry: Infancy through adolescence* (4th ed.). Philadelphia: W.B. Saunders.

Poole, A.E., & Redford-Badwal, D.A. (1991). Structural abnormalities of the craniofacial complex and congenital malformations. *Pediatric Clinics of North America, 38,* 1089–1125.

Schultz, S.T., Shenkin, J.D., & Horowitz, A.M. (2001). Parental perceptions of unmet dental need and cost barriers to care for developmentally disabled children. *Pediatric Dentistry, 20,* 321–325.

Sicher, H. (1991). *Orban's histology and embryology* (11th ed.). St. Louis: Mosby.

Soderling, E., Isokangas, P., Pienihakkinen, K., et al. (2000). Influence of maternal xylitol consumption on acquisition of Mutans streptococci by infants. *Journal of Dental Research, 79,* 882–887.

Thomas C.W., & Primosch R.E. (2002).Changes in incremental weight and well-being of children with rampant caries following complete dental rehabilitation. *Pediatric Dentistry, 24,* 109–113.

U.S. Department of Health and Human Services, National Institutes of Health, National Institute of Dental and Craniofacial Research. (2000). *Oral health in America: A report of the Surgeon General.* Rockville, MD: U.S. Department of Health and Human Services.

Waldman H.B., & Perlman S. (2003). Why is providing dental care to people with mental retardation and other developmental disabilities such a low priority? [Monograph]. *Oral Health Care for People with Special Needs,* 12–14.

33 Early Intervention

Michael J. Guralnick and Charles J. Conlon

Upon completion of this chapter, the reader will

- Know the rationale for early intervention services
- Understand the principles of early intervention
- Be aware of the services provided

The commitment to provide early intervention services and supports for infants and toddlers with established developmental disabilities and their families is now evident in virtually every community in the United States, as well as many other parts of the world (Guralnick, 2005a). Community programs are now well organized to provide early intervention in the form of comprehensive services and supports to enhance children's development, usually provided in the context of federal early intervention legislation (initially passed as the Education of the Handicapped Act Amendments of 1986, PL 99-457) in which all states participate. Services and supports available through this legislation include various therapies, family counseling and support, and special instruction, among many others. This array of services can be provided at home, at clinics, at child care programs, or at specialized early intervention centers with numerous agencies and professional disciplines involved. As discussed shortly, this legislation defines the many structural components and principles governing state-based early intervention systems for infants and toddlers with disabilities.

CARL

Carl is a 6-month-old who was born at a gestational age of 26 weeks. After a difficult 4-month hospitalization in the neonatal intensive care unit, he was discharged home. Neurodevelopmental assessment just prior to discharge showed that he had cognitive function at a newborn level and markedly increased tone in his legs. Carl was considered to have significant developmental delays

and was referred to the local early intervention program. After a comprehensive, multidisciplinary assessment, he was found to be eligible for services, and a treatment plan (**individualized family service plan,** or IFSP) was developed. Because both of Carl's parents worked outside the home, a physical therapist and early childhood educator came to Carl's child care center once a week to provide early intervention services. Carl's parents arranged their work schedules so that at least one of them could meet with the early intervention professional every other week at the child care center. Together, Carl's parents, educators, and child care workers have come up with creative activities that encourage Carl to develop his motor skills. As a result of these interactions, both parents are feeling increasingly comfortable in caring for Carl and in playing with him at home.

DISABILITY-RELATED DEVELOPMENTAL SCIENCE

Within a larger context of support for early childhood development in general, a corresponding science of disability-related knowledge has emerged. For example, it was found that parents of children with developmental disabilities often experience difficulties in establishing developmentally enhancing interactions with their children due to their children's frequent lack of emotional expressiveness, a general inability to initiate, and an uneven and, in certain instances, highly atypical developmental pattern (Spiker, Boyce, & Boyce, 2002). Joint attention routines between parents and children, a critical activity for promoting many aspects of development, is

511

a good example of a process easily disrupted (Mundy & Stella, 2000). One consequence of this growing body of knowledge was to create a sense of urgency to apply this information and to encourage intervention approaches to center on families and to consider the value and relevance of a general developmental framework. This was underscored by related research that documented that many families of children with an established disability experienced considerable stress and even disruption during the early childhood period (Orsmond, 2005). The prospects for families becoming isolated were real, making it even more difficult to optimize their children's development. This awareness occurred in parallel with philosophical movements in the disability community intended to maximize the integration and inclusion of individuals with disabilities (Guralnick, 2001b).

AN INVESTMENT IN EFFECTIVENESS

The provision of early intervention programs also came to be seen as an "investment" in the future. The expectation was that a focus on the early years would achieve immediate and sustained child developmental benefits and that many of those benefits would be cost effective as well (Guralnick, 2004). This argument also helped establish a positive political climate for a national agenda for early intervention programs for children with established disabilities, as represented in the Education of the Handicapped Act Amendments of 1986. In point of fact, a large body of scientific knowledge, often involving highly specific forms of intervention, existed suggesting that early intervention programs had the potential to generate important benefits for young children at risk for disability as well as for those with established disabilities (Farran, 2000; Guralnick, 1997). Considerable research also was conducted focusing on intellectual development involving children from heterogeneous etiologic groups, as evidence suggested that the intellectual development of these children declines in the absence of early intervention across the first few years of life (Guralnick, 1998). Numerous studies have now revealed that this decline in development can be prevented or at least mitigated through the provision of comprehensive early intervention programs. For example, consistent evidence for children with Down syndrome from model early intervention programs in many countries demonstrated that although these children still manifested significant intellectual and related

disabilities, declines in intellectual development could be prevented (Guralnick, 2005b). It should also be pointed out that despite these positive findings for children with disabilities, considerable individual and subgroup variability in responsiveness to early intervention exists and consistent evidence for long-term effectiveness is lacking. Increasing evidence suggests, however, that the intensity of an early intervention program can substantially affect outcome effectiveness, sometimes dramatically increasing effect sizes for children and families participating in the most intensive programs (Hill, Brooks-Gunn, & Waldfogel, 2003).

STRUCTURAL COMPONENTS OF THE EARLY INTERVENTION SYSTEM

The first early intervention (previously referred to as *infant stimulation*) programs focused on improving the function of children with intellectual disability, cerebral palsy, and genetic conditions/syndromes such as Down syndrome (Denhoff, 1981). Subsequently, these programs have evolved into including not only children with established disabilities but also those at high risk for developmental disabilities because of other biological conditions (e.g., prematurity, perinatal asphyxia, certain congenital malformations, abnormal or atypical neuromuscular findings). Certain environmental risk factors, such as parental intellectual disability and psychiatric disorders, child maltreatment, and drug exposure of infants and toddlers, have also been used to define populations at risk (Meisels & Wasik, 1990).

The national agenda for an early intervention system for infants and toddlers with established disabilities culminated with the passage of the Education of the Handicapped Act Amendments of 1986, with continuing refinements over time incorporated into the Individuals with Disabilities Education Act (IDEA), which was reauthorized in 2004 (IDEA 2004, PL 108-446). Part C of that Act makes the national agenda quite clear: "to develop and implement a statewide, comprehensive, coordinated, multidisciplinary, interagency system that provides early intervention services for infants and toddlers with disabilities and their families" (§ 631, [6], [1]). Structural components of the system included establishing eligibility criteria and a process to ensure that all children meeting those criteria in a state were indeed served. To maximize participation in the program, a "Child Find" system and public awareness program were included in the required structural components designed to promote awareness of children's developmental problems by parents and professionals and to encourage early detection and identification. Once a referral was made, a timely multidisciplinary assessment component was required to evaluate the child's strengths and weaknesses in major developmental domains. A corresponding component was an assessment of needs and priorities of the family, relevant to their child's development. These are further discussed next.

Identification and Referral

Child Find efforts are most effective when coordinated with other early identification programs such as Medicaid's Early and Periodic Screening, Diagnosis, and Treatment (EPSDT) program. Primary care providers (e.g., physicians, nurses, social workers) are in a key position to identify young children who are at risk for or who have developmental delays or disabilities (American Academy of Pediatrics [AAP], Committee on Children with Disabilities, 2001; Sand et al., 2005).

Often the first step in the identification and referral of infants and toddlers who could benefit from early intervention services is developmental screening. When this occurs in the context of a well-child visit, it reinforces the concept that health and development are interrelated. An equally valid approach is to recognize parental concerns about a child's development as an effective method for early identification. Parental concern has, in fact, been shown to be as effective in identifying developmental delay as is professional opinion and/or standardized screening (Glascoe, 2000). Thus, an infant or toddler can be referred to the local early intervention program directly by anyone (including a relative or friend) who suspects that the child has a developmental delay or disability.

Developmental screening is mandated in Part C of IDEA 2004. It should involve the family and other sources of information, using a process that is culturally sensitive. It should be reliable, valid, cost effective, and time efficient. It should be seen not only as a means of early identification but also as a service that helps the family understand the child's developmental progress. Several developmental screening tests are commercially available. The following are some of the commonly used screening tools: 1) the Denver II (Frankenburg et al., 1992), 2) the Ages & Stages Questionnaires® (ASQ; Bricker & Squires, 1999), and 3) Parents' Evaluations of Developmental Status (PEDS; Glascoe, 1997).

Assessment for Early Intervention Services

Assessment is the process used to identify a child's strengths and needs. It often begins when the family first calls the infant and toddler program for assistance and is the link to develop an effective treatment plan. Once a referral is made to the local agency that coordinates early intervention services, assessment, eligibility determination, and the IFSP meeting must be completed within 45 calendar days. After a family is referred, a service coordinator is assigned to help plan and coordinate all of the steps leading to the development of a service plan (provided that the child is found to be eligible for early intervention).

Each assessment must be timely, comprehensive, and multidisciplinary. Pertinent records relating to the child's current health status as well as medical history must be reviewed. The assessment should be comprehensive and include the child's level of functioning in five development domains: physical (including vision/hearing and gross and fine motor development), cognition, communication, social-emotional, and adaptive. The multidisciplinary assessment team must include a family member and two professionals representing different disciplinary expertise (Bagnato & Neisworth, 1999). For example, the professionals might include an early childhood special educator and a speech-language pathologist or perhaps a motor therapist such as an occupational therapist or a physical therapist. The assessment must reflect the unique strengths and needs of the child. In addition, family members provide information about their circumstances, priorities, and resources that may have an impact on their child.

Development of an Individualized Family Service Plan

Following these child and family assessments, an IFSP is developed by a multidisciplinary team including the parents, ensuring that the diverse services identified are coordinated as much as possible. In fact, the array of services available in Part C is quite extraordinary, including speech, physical, and occupational therapies; psychological services; family training; counseling; home visits; medical services for diagnostic or evaluation purposes; social work services; and assistive technology devices and services. Also stipulated is that services identified in the IFSP be provided in environments that are as natural as possible for the child and family. Clearly, minimizing isolation and maximizing inclusion is important.

The importance of the IFSP can be seen in the law's detailed requirements regarding the plan's contents. These requirements are as follows (IDEA 2004; § 636 [d], [1–8]):

(1) a statement of the infant's or toddler's present levels of physical development, cognitive development, communication development, social or emotional development, and adaptive development, based on objective criteria;

(2) a statement of the family's resources, priorities, and concerns relating to enhancing the development of the family's infant or toddler with a disability;

(3) a statement of the major outcomes expected to be achieved for the infant or toddler and the family, and the criteria, procedures, and timelines used to determine the degree to which progress toward achieving the outcomes is being made and whether modifications or revisions of the outcomes or services are necessary;

(4) a statement of specific early intervention services necessary to meet the unique needs of the infant or toddler and the family, including the frequency, intensity, and method of delivering services;

(5) a statement of the natural environments in which early intervention services shall appropriately be provided, including a justification of the extent, if any, to which the services will not be provided in a natural environment;

(6) the projected dates for initiation of services and the anticipated duration of the services;

(7) the identification of the service coordinator from the professional most immediately relevant to the infant's or toddler's or family's needs (or who is otherwise qualified to carry out all applicable responsibilities under this part) who will be responsible for the implementation of the plan and coordination with other agencies and persons; and

(8) the steps to be taken to support the transition of the toddler with a disability to preschool or other appropriate services.

States also are required to ensure that those providing the services are appropriately qualified and that a central directory is available to help identify resources of all kinds relevant to early intervention. Other structural components are administrative in nature, addressing interagency cooperation, reimbursement, and procedural safeguards, among others. Taken together, Part C defines the critical structural components for an early intervention system required of each state, components that should be found in each local community as well.

Provided Services

The frequency and intensity of early intervention services continue to be controversial topics. Frequent hands-on intervention, similar to a medical rehabilitation model, is often expected by families as well as by some early intervention providers. Yet, choosing services to assist young children and families to achieve specific outcomes is a complex process. It requires that meaningful outcomes be identified and that early intervention professionals provide an array of consultative and direct services. This approach often departs from the traditional frequency and intensity model of "so many times per week." Meaningful outcomes should go beyond specific disciplinary goals (e.g., increasing the mean length of utterance, reducing limb spasticity) to effectively address the child's and family's functioning within the home and/or in a child care setting and during play or while the child is learning in any environment.

Different services as well as service levels may be needed depending on the number of caregivers and the number of locations of care. On the one hand, a biweekly visit with a parent and child who spend the day together at home may be sufficient to accomplish the desired outcome. On the other hand, a multiple caregiver situation often requires more frequent contacts to demonstrate strategies and allow for more collaboration with key adults. It should be noted that not all goals can be worked on at the same time. A flexible model might emphasize sequential rather than simultaneous services; for example, once one goal is accomplished, a new one can be introduced. Each goal should have distinct services, frequency, intensity, and location identified prior to its implementation. Frequency and intensity of services are not as important as what providers do with their time in guiding the child and family. Shifting to a flexible, outcomes-guided model that is family directed increases the likelihood that the recommendations for services will emerge from a thorough analysis of child and family priorities. This contrasts with the traditional medical model of providing a predetermined group of services by specific disciplines that are driven by a particular disability rather than by the specific goals of the family (Hanft & Feinberg, 1997).

TRANSITION FROM EARLY INTERVENTION TO PRESCHOOL SERVICES

Transition is a process that children and families go through as they move from one program or setting to another. Families of young children with developmental delays and disabilities may need to move between home and hospital or from one community-based program to another. At about 3 years of age, the child will need to make the transition from early intervention to early childhood special education services, such as an inclusive preschool or child care program or to other appropriate services. Some children may be exiting the early intervention program. Careful planning and preparation for each transition can ensure that change occurs in a timely and effective manner. Transition planning may also help to alleviate parental stress and may be an opportunity for family growth as new skills are developed that can be applied to new settings. To ensure a seamless move from early intervention to preschool services, the IFSP must include a transition plan.

STATUS OF EARLY INTERVENTION SERVICES

It has now been approximately 20 years since the establishment of a formal early intervention system in the United States. Judged by the usual standards, this program has been highly successful. All 50 states are participating in Part C, providing evidence that each of the required structural components is in place. Moreover, the number of children served continues to grow on an annual basis. Including those at risk, approximately 250,000 children received services in 2001 (U.S. Department of Education, 2002). This constitutes approximately 2% of the U.S. population in this age group. An analysis utilizing a nationally representative sample ($N = 3,338$) from the National Early Intervention Longitudinal Study (NEILS) also suggested that Part C was achieving its intended effects. Overall, approximately 62% of children became eligible because of a developmental delay, 22% as a result of a diagnosed medical condition, and 17% were enrolled due to biomedical and/or environmental risk factors (Scarborough et al., 2004). It was also clear that the early intervention system was reaching disadvantaged groups, as 26% of families served received welfare payments around the time of services, and 32% were at or below the poverty level. Given the well-established association between disadvantaged status and disability (Park, Turnbull, & Turnbull, 2002), the ability of the system to enroll large numbers of these families is consistent with a national pattern. Previous research has also suggested that service utilization patterns are generally not constrained by sociodemographic factors (Kochanek & Buka, 1998). Yet, it is reasonable to expect that, conservatively, 5% of children in this age group in the general population would experience a developmental problem that could benefit from early intervention services. Whether this discrepancy with the actual number of children receiving services (2%) is due to children receiving services outside of Part C, to parent decisions to delay services, or to difficulties in early detection and identification awaits further study.

In many respects, the early intervention system has proven to be highly responsive. In the NEILS study, for example, the average time intervals (indicated within parentheses) for critical points in the process were as follows: first concern about child's health or development (7.4 months), first diagnosis or identification (8.8 months), first looked for early intervention (11.9 months), first referred for early intervention (14.0 months), and age at which IFSP was developed (15.7 months) (Bailey, Hebbeler, Scarborough, et al., 2004). Moreover, most families found an early intervention program easily, with 79% of children receiving an IFSP within 10 weeks of referral (Bailey et al., 2004). The NEILS data also revealed that families received numerous services offered in Part C, with more than three quarters receiving two to six different services and 10% receiving eight or more services (U.S. Department of Education, 2001). Of note, the vast majority (80%) utilized the service coordination component of Part C. As might be expected, the most frequently utilized specific services were special instruction, speech and language therapy, and physical and occupational therapy (Perry, Greer, Goldhammer, et al., 2001). An interesting finding was that the array of family support services available was not usually provided to more than 20% of families. Despite these impressive service utilization rates, it is important to note that the number of actual service hours turns out to be actually quite small. Although considerable variability can be found, the average intensity of services is approximately 7 hours per month (e.g., Feinberg & Beyer, 1998; Perry et al., 2001).

From the perspective of parents, the services received have been consistently highly rated in terms of satisfaction (see Harbin, Mc-William, & Gallagher, 2000). The NEILS study addressed this issue in depth as well, finding that the overwhelming majority of families (approximately 80%) noted that their child received sufficient therapies and other early intervention services, considered them to be individualized with adequate parent input into the plan, indicated that the services were of high quality, and said that the professionals they interacted with were positively perceived (Bailey et al., 2004). Approximately 14% of families thought that additional needed services were not being provided.

Taken together, it is evident that a comprehensive early intervention system composed of well-defined structural components can be found in states and communities in the United States, providing services and supports to increasing numbers of infants and toddlers with established disabilities and their families. There is, however, also a recognition that such complex and evolving systems can be substantially improved to more effectively and efficiently meet the needs of children and families (Guralnick, 2000a). The next section discusses some directions for the future. This discussion is organized by considering each of the 10 principles that represent the Developmental Systems Model of Early Intervention (Guralnick, 2005c), an approach that integrates the developmental science of normative development, the developmental science of risk and disability, and intervention science (Guralnick, 2006).

DIRECTIONS FOR THE FUTURE: PRINCIPLES OF EARLY INTERVENTION

1. A developmental framework informs all components of the early intervention system and centers on families. Based on research from the developmental science of normative development, three family patterns of interaction have been shown to be critical for optimal child development: 1) parent–child transactions—including relationship patterns such as sensitivity, responsivity, reciprocity, scaffolding, affective warmth, and nonintrusive interactions; 2) family-orchestrated child experiences—including providing developmentally appropriate toys and materials, identifying high-quality child care, establishing family routines and related

activities involving all members, and arranging play dates; and 3) ensuring the child's health and safety—including proper nutrition, organizing the environment to protect the child from harm, and maintaining immunization schedules (see Guralnick, 1998).

Correspondingly, when a child with an established disability becomes part of a family, the developmental science of risk and disability has demonstrated how children's characteristics can perturb or exert stress on one or more of these three family patterns of interaction leading to nonoptimal child development. Stressors to these family patterns of interaction come in many forms but can be categorized into four domains. First, a child with a disability creates an extraordinary need for information. Details regarding a child's diagnosis, prognosis, responding to uneven or atypical developmental patterns, or emerging behavioral issues are among the seemingly never-ending series of issues that arise, especially over the first 3 years of the child's life (see Bailey & Powell, 2005; Guralnick, 2001a). Second, interpersonal and family distress is often created by a child with an established disability (Orsmond, 2005). Among other issues, families need to rethink their aspirations for their child and standard family routines frequently must be modified, often substantially. Social isolation can easily follow, including families feeling stigmatized by their child with a disability. Third, even with resources provided by Part C, a considerable resource burden falls to families. In particular, financial costs mount and respite care is always a concern (Shannon, Grinde, & Cox, 2003; Spiker, Hebbeler, & Mallik, 2005). Finally, optimal family patterns of interaction are frequently stressed by parents' self-doubts with respect to their ability to properly parent their child. Moreover, all of these stressors can easily be exacerbated by families who are stressed by poverty, mental health problems, a lack of social support from spouse or other family members, or the absence of helpful social networks, among others (Guralnick, 1998).

It is apparent that for early intervention programs to be consistent with this developmental framework it requires that programs center on families, seeking to strengthen them and help them address the many stressors that may be adversely affecting family patterns of interaction. Yet, available evidence suggests that a developmental approach centering on families has not yet been well integrated into the early intervention system (e.g., Bruder, 2000; Harbin et al., 2000). Even family-directed assessments, especially guided by a developmental framework, are difficult to accomplish (McWilliam, Snyder, Harbin, et al., 2000), and many intervention efforts remain in the professional comfort zone of being primarily child focused (e.g., McBride & Peterson, 1997). Clearly, encouraging the early intervention system to more fully understand and effectively implement this critical principle remains a major task for the field.

2. Integration and coordination at all levels are apparent. This includes interdisciplinary assessments, assessments for program planning, developing and implementing comprehensive intervention plans, and systems level integration. Numerous problems regarding team processes factors and collaborative problem-solving difficulties, among others, have been identified and provide clear directions for improvement (Guralnick, 2000b). From an implementation perspective, the importance of service coordination was clearly recognized in Part C, and it was identified as a separate and required service in the law. However, for this to be most effective, simply coordinating independent services, with the potential for duplication and redundancy, may not be optimal. Rather, new approaches, such as collaborative consultation models (McWilliam, 1996) that attempt to truly integrate services, will achieve outcomes that are more likely to be of functional value for the child and family (Dunst, Trivette, Humphries, et al., 2001; Hanft & Pilkington, 2000).

Moreover, similar difficulties are apparent at the systems level, where only limited leadership is being displayed by states and communities to address these issues (Spiker, Hebbeler, Wagner, et al., 2000). The leadership issue is clearly urgent in view of the increasingly diverse and complex array of services and supports required by children and families. Integrating and coordinating services from agencies not commonly part of the early intervention system, such as those related to the mental health of children and families, pose special challenges (National Research Council & Institute of Medicine, 2000).

3. The inclusion and participation of children and families in typical community programs and activities is maximized. For infants and toddlers, Part C requires that children and families receive services in "natural environments" to the extent possible. Although this has been a very difficult principle to implement due to barriers

related to financing, finding the proper service setting, definitional issues, and parent preferences, among others (see Bruder, 2001; Rabb & Dunst, 2004), much has been accomplished. Focusing intervention on activity routines in the home and plans to take advantage of natural learning activities in community environments have been important directions for early intervention, prompted in part by the principle of inclusion, and will continue as a major future direction (see Bruder, 2001; Dunst, 2001).

4. Early detection and identification procedures are in place. This principle is based on the assumption that the sooner children and families receive intervention the better. Yet, the relatively low percentage of infants and toddlers served by Part C compared with expected prevalence rates of children with disabilities, even correcting for later acquired or emerging disability, suggests that early detection and identification processes may be inadequate (see Gilliam, Meisels, & Mayes, 2005). Despite dramatic improvements in the reliability and validity of screening instruments for infants and the existence of explicit guidance from critical professional groups such as pediatricians (AAP, Committee on Children with Disabilities, 2001), a comprehensive early detection and identification system is not yet in place. Hospital personnel, primary care physicians, child care staff, and parents are all essential partners. Important technical, cost, and coordination problems remain to be addressed. Problems are further compounded by the fact that states can and do establish different eligibility requirements for services. Nevertheless, models of community-based screening are emerging, birth defect registry models can be effective (see Farel, Meyer, Hicken, et al., 2003), and the validity and reliability of instruments continues to increase, suggesting important future directions (Gilliam et al., 2005).

5. Surveillance and monitoring are integral parts of the system. This principle is intended to maximize the possibility that a child who 1) exhibits some developmental concerns but does not meet state eligibility requirements for service, 2) does not meet criteria for standard diagnostic categories, or 3) is at risk for a disability (e.g., has a sibling with an autism spectrum disorder) will receive special attention by the system. Methods of developmental surveillance can be of value (Dworkin, 2000) but require substantial, continuous, and knowledgeable participation of a pediatrician or other health professional.

6. All parts of the system are individualized. Even children sharing a similar etiology, such as Down syndrome, often vary substantially in their individual characteristics, developmental trajectories, and responsiveness to intervention (Spiker & Hopmann, 1997). The IFSP process of Part C is the major structural component of the system within which this principle is realized. Its success, however, hinges on the ability of the system to comprehensively and accurately assess stressors that can affect optimal child development, a problem noted in the previous section. Similarly, although Part C has been successful in obtaining resources for families, the NEILS data suggest that the scope of these services and supports needs to be expanded (Spiker et al., 2005).

7. A strong evaluation and feedback system is evident. Research on the effectiveness of early intervention indicates that a structured program with explicit goals and objectives and regular feedback are essential to achieve positive outcomes (Shonkoff & Houser-Cram, 1987). Consequently, careful attention to ensure that evaluation and feedback occur at every level and for every component of the system is vital. A multitiered evaluation system will likely be required. Leaders in the field have suggested such an evaluation must encompass needs assessments, monitoring and accountability of services and supports, quality reviews and program clarifications, and evaluating specific outcomes (Warfield & Hauser-Cram, 2005).

8. It is recognized that true partnerships with families cannot occur without sensitivity to cultural differences and an understanding of their developmental implications. Valuable guidelines for addressing these issues have been published (Lynch & Hanson, 2004), and professionals' ability to display cultural competence is essential to Part C. Available evidence suggests, however, that more work needs to be carried out for this principle to be fully implemented. For example, data from the NEILS analysis and related studies on parent satisfaction with early intervention services suggest that minority families are less likely to have positive experiences with the early intervention system (Bailey et al., 2004; Bailey et al., 1999).

9. Recommendations to families and practices should be evidence based. The increase in scientific knowledge based on evidence from numerous sources has been able to identify best practices and weed out those practices that have little validity. The early intervention field has been subject to many claims of dramatic success, often demanding enormous resources from families and communities, that have failed to be supported by the evidence (Nickel, 1996; Starrett, 1996). Part C notes that interventions should be based on peer-reviewed, scientifically based findings. Accomplishing this continues to remain a major challenge for the early intervention field, as the research-to-practice gap is considerable (National Research Council & Institute of Medicine, 2000; Rule et al., 1998). The recent publication of clinical guidelines and best practice manuals based on careful reviews of the available scientific literature for screening, diagnosis, and intervention in the field of early intervention has been a welcome addition (e.g., Filipek et al., 2000; Sandall, McLean, & Smith, 2000; National Research Council, 2001).

10. A systems perspective is maintained, recognizing interrelationships among all components. A major issue for the future is to determine whether the ultimate aspiration of the early intervention system should be to retain its mainly specialized focus on children with disabilities or be embedded in a larger early childhood system (Harbin et al., 2000). As Harbin (2005) pointed out, such a systems perspective is relevant to the many concerns associated with the various principles that have been previously discussed. The early intervention system must have the visionary leadership to be responsive to the changing needs of children and families and to develop strategies and organizational structures that advance the field.

SUMMARY

Infants and toddlers with disabilities and their families now have access to a well-designed early intervention system with all important structural components effectively in place. Increasing numbers of children and families continue gaining access to the system, experiencing high levels of parental satisfaction while receiving an extensive array of services and supports. Research on the effectiveness of early intervention has demonstrated the potential for achieving important benefits for children and families. Nevertheless, the full implementation of the principles that guide early intervention within a developmental systems framework that maximize intervention effectiveness has not been achieved. As noted, this circumstance is to be expected in complex, evolving systems. Fortunately, there now exists a better understanding of the meaning of those critical principles and a recognition of the interconnections among the principles, providing clear directions to ensure that the system will continue to evolve to meet the needs of young vulnerable children and their families.

REFERENCES

American Academy of Pediatrics, Committee on Children with Disabilities. (2001). Developmental surveillance and screening of infants and young children. *Pediatrics, 108*, 192–195.

Bagnato, S., & Neisworth, J. (1999). Collaboration and teamwork in assessment for early intervention. *Child and Adolescent Psychiatric Clinics of North America, 8*, 347–363.

Bailey, D.B., Jr., & Powell, T. (2005). Assessing the information needs of families in early intervention. In M.J. Guralnick (Series Ed.) & M.J. Guralnick (Vol. Ed.), *International issues in early intervention: The developmental systems approach to early intervention* (pp. 151–183). Baltimore: Paul H. Brookes Publishing Co.

Bailey, D., Hebbeler, K., Scarborough, A., et al. (2004). First experiences with early intervention: A national perspective. *Pediatrics, 113*, 887–896.

Bailey, D.B., Skinner, D., Rodriguez, P., et al. (1999). Awareness, use, and satisfaction with services for Latino parents of young children with disabilities. *Exceptional Children, 65*(3), 367–381.

Bricker, D., & Squires, J. (with Mounts, L., Potter, L., Nickel, R., et al.). (1999). *Ages & Stages Questionnaires® (ASQ): A parent-completed, child-monitoring system* (2nd ed.). Baltimore: Paul H. Brookes Publishing Co.

Bruder, M.B. (2000). Family-centered early intervention: Clarifying our values for the new millennium. *Topics in Early Childhood Special Education, 20*, 105–115.

Bruder, M.B. (2001). Inclusion of infants and toddlers: Outcomes and ecology. In M.J. Guralnick (Ed.), *Early childhood inclusion: Focus on change* (pp. 203–228). Baltimore: Paul H. Brookes Publishing Co.

Denhoff, E. (1981). Current status of infant stimulation or enrichment programs for children with developmental disabilities. *Pediatrics, 67*, 32–37.

Dunst, C.J. (2001). Participation of young children with disabilities in community learning activities. In M.J. Guralnick (Ed.), *Early childhood inclusion: Focus on change* (pp. 307–333). Baltimore: Paul H. Brookes Publishing Co.

Dunst, C.J., Trivette, C.M., Humphries, T., et al. (2001). Contrasting approaches to natural learning environment interventions. *Infants & Young Children, 14*(2), 48–63.

Dworkin, P.H. (2000). Preventive health care and anticipatory guidance. In J.P. Shonkoff & S.J. Meisels (Eds.), *Handbook of early childhood intervention* (2nd ed., pp. 327–338). New York: Cambridge University Press.

Education of the Handicapped Act Amendments of 1986, PL 99-457, 20 U.S.C. §§ 1400 *et seq.*

Farel, A.M., Meyer, R.E., Hicken, M., et al. (2003). Registry to referral: A promising means for identifying and referring infants and toddlers for early intervention services. *Infants & Young Children, 16*, 99–105.

Farran, D.C. (2000). Another decade of intervention for children who are low income or disabled: What do we know now? In J.P. Shonkoff & S.J. Meisels (Eds.), *Handbook of early childhood intervention* (2nd ed., pp. 510–548). New York: Cambridge University Press.

Feinberg, E., & Beyer, J. (1998). Creating public policy in a climate of clinical indeterminancy: Lovaas as the case example du jour. *Infants & Young Children, 10*(3), 54–66.

Filipek, P.A., Accardo, P.J., Ashwal, S., et al. (2000). Practice parameter: Screening and diagnosis of autism. *Neurology, 55*, 468–479.

Frankenburg, W.K., Dodds, J.B., Archer, P., et al. (1992). *Denver II.* Denver, CO: Denver Developmental Materials. (Available from the publisher, Post Office Box 371075, Denver, CO 80237-5075; 800-419-4729)

Gilliam, W.S., Meisels, S.J., & Mayes, L.C. (2005). Screening and surveillance in early intervention systems. In M.J. Guralnick (Ed.), *The developmental systems approach to early intervention* (pp. 73–98). Baltimore: Paul H. Brookes Publishing Co.

Glascoe, F.P. (1997). *Parents' Evaluations of Developmental Status (PEDS).* Nashville, TN: Ellsworth and Vandermeer Press.

Glascoe, F.P. (2000). Evidence-based approach to developmental and behavioural surveillance using parents' concerns. *Child: Care, Health and Development, 26*(2), 137–149.

Guralnick, M.J. (Ed.). (1997). *The effectiveness of early intervention.* Baltimore: Paul H. Brookes Publishing Co.

Guralnick, M.J. (1998). The effectiveness of early intervention for vulnerable children: A developmental perspective. *American Journal on Mental Retardation, 102*, 319–345.

Guralnick, M.J. (2000a). Early childhood intervention: Evolution of a system. In M. Wehmeyer & J.R. Patton (Eds.), *Mental retardation in the 21st century* (pp. 37–58). Austin, TX: PRO-ED.

Guralnick, M.J. (2000b). Interdisciplinary team assessment for young children: Purposes and processes. In M.J. Guralnick (Ed.), *Interdisciplinary clinical assessment for young children with developmental disabilities* (pp. 3–15). Baltimore: Paul H. Brookes Publishing Co.

Guralnick, M.J. (2001a). A developmental systems model for early intervention. *Infants & Young Children, 14*(2), 1–18.

Guralnick, M.J. (2001b). A framework for change in early childhood inclusion. In M.J. Guralnick (Ed.), *Early childhood inclusion: Focus on change* (pp. 3–35). Baltimore: Paul H. Brookes Publishing Co.

Guralnick, M.J. (2004). Family investments in response to the developmental challenges of young children with disabilities. In A. Kalil & T. Deleire (Eds.), *Family investments in children's potential: Resources and parenting behaviors that promote success* (pp. 119–137). Mahwah, NJ: Lawrence Erlbaum Associates.

Guralnick, M.J. (Ed.). (2005a). *The developmental systems approach to early intervention.* Baltimore: Paul H. Brookes Publishing Co.

Guralnick, M.J. (2005b). Early intervention for children with intellectual disabilities: Current knowledge and future prospects. *Journal of Applied Research in Intellectual Disabilities, 18*, 313–324.

Guralnick, M.J. (2005c). An overview of the developmental systems approach to early intervention. In M.J. Guralnick (Ed.), *The developmental systems approach to early intervention* (pp. 3–28). Baltimore: Paul H. Brookes Publishing Co.

Guralnick, M.J. (2006). Family influences on early development: Integrating the science of normative development, risk and disability, and intervention. In K. McCartney & D. Phillips (Eds.), *Blackwell handbook of early childhood development* (pp. 46–61). Oxford, United Kingdom: Blackwell Publishers.

Hanft, B., & Feinberg, E. (1997). Toward the development of a framework for determining the frequency and intensity of early intervention services. *Infants & Young Children, 10*(1), 27–37.

Hanft, B.E., & Pilkington, K.O. (2000). Therapy in natural environments: The means or end goal for early intervention? *Infants & Young Children, 12*(4), 1–13.

Harbin, G.L. (2005). Designing an integrated point of access in the early intervention system. In M.J. Guralnick (Ed.), *The developmental systems approach to early intervention* (pp. 99–131). Baltimore: Paul H. Brookes Publishing Co.

Harbin, G.L., McWilliam, R.C., & Gallagher, J.J. (2000). Services for young children with disabilities and their families. In J.P. Shonkoff & S.J. Meisels (Eds.), *Handbook of early childhood intervention* (2nd ed., pp. 387–415). New York: Cambridge University Press.

Hill, J.L., Brooks-Gunn, J., & Waldfogel, J. (2003). Sustained effects of high participation in an early intervention for low-birth-weight premature infants. *Developmental Psychology, 39*, 730–744.

Individuals with Disabilities Education Improvement Act of 2004, PL 108-446, 20 U.S.C. §§ 1400 *et seq.*

Kochanek, T.T., & Buka, S.L. (1998). Patterns of service utilization: Child, maternal, and service provider factors. *Journal of Early Intervention, 21*, 217–231.

Lynch, E.W., & Hanson, M.J. (Eds.). (2004). *Developing cross-cultural competence: A guide for working with children and their families* (3rd ed.). Baltimore: Paul H. Brookes Publishing Co.

McBride, S.L., & Peterson, C. (1997). Home-based early intervention with families of children with disabilities: Who is doing what? *Topics in Early Childhood Special Education, 17*, 209–233.

McWilliam, R.A. (Ed.). (1996). *Rethinking pull-out services in early intervention: A professional resource.* Baltimore: Paul H. Brookes Publishing Co.

McWilliam, R.A., Snyder, P., Harbin, G.L., et al. (2000). Professionals' and families' perceptions of family-centered practices in infant-toddler services. *Early Education and Development, 11*, 519–538.

Meisels, S.J., & Wasik, B.A. (1990). Who should be served? Identifying children in need of early intervention. In S.J. Meisels & J.P. Shonkoff (Eds.), *Handbook of early childhood intervention* (pp. 605–632). New York: Cambridge University Press.

Mundy, P., & Stella, J. (2000). Joint attention, social orienting, and communication in autism. In S.F. Warren & J. Reichle (Series Eds.) & A.M. Wetherby & B.M. Prizant (Eds.), *Communication and language intervention series: Vol. 9. Autism spectrum disorders: A transactional developmental perspective* (pp. 55–77). Baltimore: Paul H. Brookes Publishing Co.

National Research Council. (2001). *Educating children with autism.* (Committee on Educational Interventions for Children with Autism. Division of Behavioral and Social Sciences and Education.) Washington, DC: National Academies Press.

National Research Council & Institute of Medicine. (2000). *From neurons to neighborhoods: The science of early child development.* (Committee on Integrating the Science of Early Childhood Development. Jack P. Shonkoff and Deborah A. Phillips, eds. Board on Children, Youth, and Families, Commission on Behavioral and

Social Sciences and Education.) Washington, DC: National Academies Press.

Nickel, E.D. (1996). Controversial therapies for young children with developmental disabilities. *Infants & Young Children, 8*(4), 29–40.

Orsmond, G.I. (2005). Assessing interpersonal and family distress and threats to confident parenting in the context of early intervention. In M.J. Guralnick (Ed.), *The developmental systems approach to early intervention* (pp. 185–213). Baltimore: Paul H. Brookes Publishing Co.

Park, J., Turnbull, A.P., & Turnbull, H.R. (2002). Impacts of poverty on quality of life in families of children with disabilities. *Exceptional Children, 68*, 151–170.

Perry, D.F., Greer, M., Goldhammer, K., et al. (2001). Fulfilling the promise of early intervention: Rates of delivered IFSP services. *Journal of Early Intervention, 24*, 90–102.

Rabb, M., & Dunst, C.J. (2004). Early intervention practitioner approaches to natural environment interventions. *Journal of Early Intervention, 27*, 15–26.

Rule, S., Losardo, A., Dinnebeil, L.A., et al. (1998). Research challenges in naturalistic intervention. *Journal of Early Intervention, 21*, 283–293.

Sand, N., Silverstein, M., Glascoe, F.P., et al. (2005). Pediatricians' reported practices regarding developmental screening: Do guidelines work? Do they help? *Pediatrics, 116*, 174–179.

Sandall, S., McLean, M., & Smith, B. (2000). *DEC recommended practices in intervention/early childhood special education.* Longmont, CO: Sopris West.

Scarborough, A.A., Spiker, D., Mallik, S., et al. (2004). A national look at children and families entering early intervention. *Exceptional Children, 70*, 469–483.

Shannon, P., Grinde, L.R., & Cox, A.W. (2003). Families' perceptions of the ability to pay for early intervention services. *Journal of Early Intervention, 25*, 164–172.

Shonkoff, J.P., & Hauser-Cram, P. (1987). Early intervention for disabled infants and their families: A quantitative analysis. *Pediatrics, 80*, 650–658.

Spiker, D., Boyce, G.C., & Boyce, L.K. (2002). Parent-child interactions when young children have disabilities. In L.M. Glidden (Ed.), *International review of research in mental retardation* (Vol. 25, pp. 35–70). San Diego: Academic Press.

Spiker, D., Hebbeler, K., & Mallik, S. (2005). Developing and implementing early intervention programs for children with established disabilities. In M.J. Guralnick (Ed.), *The developmental systems approach to early intervention* (pp. 305–349). Baltimore: Paul H. Brookes Publishing Co.

Spiker, D., Hebbeler, K., Wagner, M., et al. (2000). A framework for describing variations in state early intervention systems. *Topics in Early Childhood Special Education, 20*, 195–207.

Spiker, D., & Hopmann, M.R. (1997). The effectiveness of early intervention for children with Down syndrome. In M.J. Guralnick (Ed.), *The effectiveness of early intervention* (pp. 271–305). Baltimore: Paul H. Brookes Publishing Co.

Starrett, A.L. (1996). Nonstandard therapies in developmental disabilities. In A.J. Capute & P.J. Accardo (Eds.), *Developmental disabilities in infancy and childhood: Vol. 1. Neurodevelopmental diagnosis and treatment* (2nd ed., pp. 593–608). Baltimore: Paul H. Brookes Publishing Co.

U.S. Department of Education. (2001). *Twenty-third an-*

nual report to Congress on the implementation of the Individuals with Disabilities Education Act. Washington, DC: U.S. Government Printing Office.

U.S. Department of Education. (2002). *Twenty-fourth annual report to Congress on the implementation of the Individuals with Disabilities Education Act.* Washington, DC: U.S. Government Printing Office.

Warfield, M.E., & Hauser-Cram, P. (2005). Monitoring and evaluation in early intervention programs. In M.J. Guralnick (Ed.), *The developmental systems approach to early intervention* (pp. 351–372). Baltimore: Paul H. Brookes Publishing Co.

34 Special Education Services

Elissa Batshaw Clair, Robin P. Church, and Mark L. Batshaw

Upon completion of this chapter, the reader will

- Be aware of the history of special education services
- Understand the components of an individualized education program
- Be familiar with the Individuals with Disabilities Education Improvement Act of 2004 and other legislation pertaining to education for children with disabilities
- Be knowledgeable about services and support available for children with disabilities

---

Special education is defined by the Individuals with Disabilities Education Improvement Act of 2004 (IDEA 2004; PL 108-446) as "specially designed instruction, at no cost to parents, to meet the unique needs of a child with a disability" (§ 602[29]). Special education includes direct educational instruction by a special education teacher, language therapy, physical therapy, paraprofessional support, or consultation from the special education professional to the general education teacher. All special education services are individualized to provide the instruction necessary to reach each child's goals. IDEA 2004 guarantees a free appropriate public education (FAPE) for all children with disabilities ages 3–21. A zero-reject provision mandates that even students who have severe and multiple impairments have the right to FAPE in the least restrictive environment (LRE).

Before the date of enactment of the Education for All Handicapped Children Act of 1975 (PL 94-142) the educational needs of millions of children with disabilities were not being fully met because they did not receive appropriate educational services, were excluded entirely from the public school system and from being educated with their peers, had undiagnosed disabilities that prevented them from having a successful educational experience, or had a lack of adequate resources within the public school system to find services outside of the public school system (PL 108-446 § [601][c][(2)]). Since the 1970s, a series of legislation has attempted to address each of these issues. Figure 34.1 summarizes the history of educational law prior to the current law, IDEA 2004. A major change in the current law is that it requires special education teachers to be highly qualified—that is, state certified in both special education and general education unless the teacher only teaches students who will take alternative assessments (Council for Exceptional Children [CEC], 2004; see Table 34.1).

JOHN

John did not walk or speak his first word until 18 months. As a toddler, John received speech therapy in his home once per week in accordance with an individualized family service plan (IFSP) provided under Part C (Infants and Toddlers with Disabilities) of IDEA. These services were designed to help John's parents facilitate their son's communication skills. When John entered kindergarten, he was soon identified as having significant delays as compared with his classmates and in need of assessment for special education services. His parents gave permission for testing, which showed him to be functioning in the range of mild intellectual disabilities and thus eligible for special education services.

An individualized educational program (IEP) was developed with input from a team consisting of a psychologist, a general education and a special education teacher, a speech-language pathologist, and John's parents. The IEP identified the goals John would work toward, the amount of time he would spend receiving special education services, and the **related services** that would be provided to support his educational progress.

The IEP team reviewed information from his most recent evaluation as well as teacher data collection, parental input, and IEP team discussion to determine the most appropriate setting for providing special education services for John. The IEP team determined that the most appropriate placement was in an inclusive environment, a class that was co-taught by a general education teacher and a special education teacher. The class contained children with and without disabilities. The two teachers worked together so that all children could have access to the same core curriculum, with differentiated instruction and **modifications** to the schoolwork. The team also decided that John would require related services from a speech-language pathologist. Sometimes this therapist would teach all or part of the class a lesson; at other times she would work with John individually.

John made good progress in this program and was reassessed on an ongoing basis so that adjustments to his IEP could be made. When John was 16 years old, he began the transition planning process mandated by IDEA. With his input during a transition-planning inventory, an **individualized transition plan (ITP)** was developed as part of his IEP. John was very interested in cooking, often preparing creative meals at home. He chose to attend prevocational food service classes in addition to his academic courses. The high school offered career cluster experiences in culinary arts, and John continued taking vocational classes, honing his skills as a chef. With the help of a job coach provided by the Bureau of Vocational Rehabilitation, John secured a summer job at a local restaurant. He continued in his school program through age 21 because special education legislation mandates services through this age for students with disabilities who 1) have not earned all of their credits toward graduation, 2) need additional transition services, or 3) are earning an alternative certificate rather than a general education diploma. Beginning in eleventh grade, when John was 19, he worked half days at the restaurant while continuing to attend school part time. At 20 years old, he enrolled in culinary classes at a community college as part of his ITP. At 21, he completed his public education, receiving a diploma, and has subsequently been hired full time as an assistant chef at the restaurant.

LEGISLATION THAT DEFINES DISABILITY

One might expect that IDEA 2004, as a special education law, contains a definition of disability. Other laws, however, also define this concept.

Individuals with Disabilities Education Improvement Act of 2004

For a child to receive special education services, he or she must have a physical, cognitive, or behavioral impairment that interferes with the ability to benefit from instruction in the general classroom curriculum. The specific disabilities recognized by IDEA 2004 legislation fall under the following categories: mental retardation (intellectual disability), hearing impairments (including deafness), speech or language impairments, visual impairments (including blindness), emotional disturbances, orthopedic impairments, autism, traumatic brain injury, other health impairments (including attention deficit/hyperactivity disorder), and specific learning disabilities (multiple disabilities and developmental delays) for children ages 3–9 (§ 602[3][a]). Among these impairments, autism is the fastest growing segment of the special education population, with an almost fifteen-fold increase (from 5,415 reported students to 78,749 reported students) between the school years 1991–1992 to 2000–2001 (U.S. Department of Education, 2002).

Other Legislation

The basic concept of IDEA is that of zero reject—in other words, that every child with disabilities should be accommodated within the public school system. If a child does not satisfy the IDEA 2004 criteria for disabilities, he or she may still receive special education services through Section 504 of the Rehabilitation Act of 1973 (PL 93-112) or through the Americans with Disabilities Act (ADA) of 1990 (PL 101-336), the objectives and language of which are very similar. These two acts are intended to establish a "level playing field" by eliminating barriers that exclude people with disabilities from participation in the community and work-

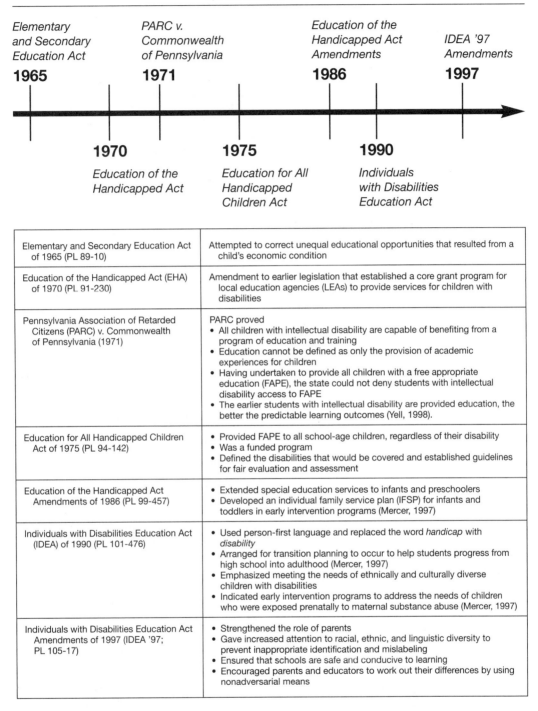

Elementary and Secondary Education Act of 1965 (PL 89-10)	Attempted to correct unequal educational opportunities that resulted from a child's economic condition
Education of the Handicapped Act (EHA) of 1970 (PL 91-230)	Amendment to earlier legislation that established a core grant program for local education agencies (LEAs) to provide services for children with disabilities
Pennsylvania Association of Retarded Citizens (PARC) v. Commonwealth of Pennsylvania (1971)	PARC proved • All children with intellectual disability are capable of benefiting from a program of education and training • Education cannot be defined as only the provision of academic experiences for children • Having undertaken to provide all children with a free appropriate education (FAPE), the state could not deny students with intellectual disability access to FAPE • The earlier students with intellectual disability are provided education, the better the predictable learning outcomes (Yell, 1998).
Education for All Handicapped Children Act of 1975 (PL 94-142)	• Provided FAPE to all school-age children, regardless of their disability • Was a funded program • Defined the disabilities that would be covered and established guidelines for fair evaluation and assessment
Education of the Handicapped Act Amendments of 1986 (PL 99-457)	• Extended special education services to infants and preschoolers • Developed an individual family service plan (IFSP) for infants and toddlers in early intervention programs (Mercer, 1997)
Individuals with Disabilities Education Act (IDEA) of 1990 (PL 101-476)	• Used person-first language and replaced the word *handicap* with *disability* • Arranged for transition planning to occur to help students progress from high school into adulthood (Mercer, 1997) • Emphasized meeting the needs of ethnically and culturally diverse children with disabilities • Indicated early intervention programs to address the needs of children who were exposed prenatally to maternal substance abuse (Mercer, 1997)
Individuals with Disabilities Education Act Amendments of 1997 (IDEA '97; PL 105-17)	• Strengthened the role of parents • Gave increased attention to racial, ethnic, and linguistic diversity to prevent inappropriate identification and mislabeling • Ensured that schools are safe and conducive to learning • Encouraged parents and educators to work out their differences by using nonadversarial means

Figure 34.1. History of educational law prior to the current law, the Individuals with Disabilities Education Improvement Act of 2004 (IDEA 2004; PL 108-446).

place. The acts try to eliminate hurdles and discrimination from participation, be they physical (e.g., steps instead of ramps) or programmatic (e.g., exclusion of a child with HIV from the classroom).

The definition of disability is broader under Section 504 than under IDEA 2004. Although Section 504 covers all students covered by IDEA 2004, the reverse is not the case. Specifically, Section 504 protects all people who

Table 34.1.　Summary of requirements to be a highly qualified special education teacher per the Individuals with Disabilities Education Improvement Act of 2004 (PL 108-446)

Category of special education teachers	Requirements
All special education teachers—general requirements	Hold at least a Bachelor of Arts degree
	Must obtain full state special education certification or equivalent licensure
	Cannot hold an emergency or temporary certificate
New or veteran elementary school teachers teaching one or more core academic subjects only to children with disabilities held to alternative academic standards (most severe cognitive disabilities)	In addition to the general requirements listed above, may demonstrate academic subject competence through a High, Objective, Uniform State Standard of Evaluation (HOUSSE) process
New or veteran middle or high school teachers teaching one or more core academic subjects only to children with disabilities held to alternative academic standards (most severe cognitive disabilities)	In addition to the general requirements, may demonstrate "subject matter knowledge appropriate to the level of instruction being provided, as determined by the State, needed to effectively teach to those standards"
New teachers of two or more academic subjects who are highly qualified in math, language arts, or science	In addition to the general requirements, has 2-year window in which to become highly qualified in the other core academic subjects and may do this through the HOUSSE process
Veteran teachers who teach two or more core academic subjects only to children with disabilities	In addition to the general requirements, may demonstrate academic subject competence through the HOUSSE process (including a single evaluation for all core academic subjects)
Consultative teachers and other special education teachers who do not teach core academic subjects	Only meet general requirements
Other special education teachers teaching core academic subjects	In addition to the general requirements, meet relevant requirements for new elementary school teachers, new middle or high school teachers, or veteran teachers

have a physical or mental impairment that substantially limits one or more major life activities, have a record of such impairment, or are regarded as having such an impairment. The following are examples of students who may be covered by Section 504 to receive special education services but are not covered by IDEA 2004: students with communicable diseases (e.g., HIV); students who are addicted to drugs, including alcohol; students with temporary disabilities resulting from accidents who may need short-term hospitalizations or homebound recovery; students with attention disorders without significant academic deficiencies; and students with Tourette syndrome.

NONDISCRIMINATORY ASSESSMENT AND ELIGIBILITY

Public schools are obligated to provide a nondiscriminatory evaluation for any child suspected of having a disability. This includes children enrolled in private schools and children ages 3–5 years who are not yet registered for school. The implementation of this requirement varies from state to state, but in addition to having access to official preschool Child Find (early intervention) programs, generally parents can bring their child to the local school district and request an evaluation. The stated purpose of the initial evaluation is to determine whether a child has a disability and, if present, to establish the educational needs of the child (PL 108-446, §§ 612 [a][10][A][ii] and § 614[a] [1][A]).

Parental consent is required prior to an evaluation. This consent, however, does not serve as consent for placement of the child in a special education program; this must be obtained separately. A child is usually evaluated by a multidisciplinary team consisting of a psychologist and one or more of the following education professionals: speech-language pathologist, occupational therapist, physical therapist, and social worker. The evaluation team should use a comprehensive assessment process to address the child's strengths, interests, goals, and needs in order to determine whether and which special education services are required. The typical evaluation may include tests of intelligence, academic skills, memory, visual-motor integration, adaptive behavior, reading, math, social-emotional skills, motor skills, sensory integration, and language. For children whose cognitive functioning is at a preschool level, testing focuses on communication, social, and adaptive skills.

The multidisciplinary team must follow specific guidelines during the evaluation of the child. These guidelines were created in response to certain faulty evaluation practices in the past, which had led to many children (especially minority children; see the Overrepresentation section) being incorrectly placed in special education. These children were often labeled "mentally retarded" on the basis of one test, typically an IQ test. With this in mind, a number of mandates for nondiscriminatory evaluation procedures were put in place as part of IDEA 2004. The key mandates are that a number of tests must be used to determine if the child has a disability and that parental input must be included. Specific guidelines include use of a variety of assessment tools and strategies, consideration of information provided by the parent, use of multiple procedures to determine whether a child has a disability, use of multiple procedures to determine an appropriate educational program for the child, use of technically sound instruments that may assess the relative contribution of cognitive and behavioral factors, in addition to physical or developmental factors, and use of the child's native language in all evaluation procedures (PL 108-466, § 614[a][2][A–C] and 614[b][3][A]).

With increasing concerns about the rising number of students classified as having a learning disability, IDEA 2004 prohibits eligibility decisions from being made based on a lack of instruction or as a result of limited English proficiency (PL 108-446, § 614 [b][5][A–C]). Reevaluation of a child with a disability is required to take place no more than once per year or less than once every 3 years unless the parent and local education agency (LEA) agree that the time lines should be altered.

Overrepresentation

One of the purposes of IDEA 2004 is to reduce the overrepresentation of minorities in special education. African Americans have the highest level of overrepresentation. This is most pronounced in the areas of intellectual disability and emotional disturbances. African American students make up 34% of the intellectual disability population in public schools, although they represent only 14% of the population (U.S. Department of Education, 2002). Two factors have been found to be the best predictors of receiving a diagnosis of intellectual disability or emotional disturbances: poverty and being African American (Hosp & Reschily, 2004). African American students are also significantly overrepresented in receiving special education services for 60% or more of the day, or 31% compared with 15% of Caucasian students (U.S. Department of Education, 2001).

SERVICES PROVIDED BY SPECIAL EDUCATION TEACHERS

Special education teachers provide the majority of services to students with disabilities. The task of the special education teacher is to provide the educational instruction and support necessary for each child to achieve his or her personal best and to prepare the child for life after school. Special education teachers collaborate with general education teachers to instruct students in a general education setting. However, a more substantial amount of time is spent directly instructing children with disabilities. Teachers develop lessons for each child that are uniquely designed to meet the student's needs.

Special education teachers give direct instruction in academic, functional, and behavioral areas. In academics, they may teach the same material that is taught in the general education setting but with an emphasis on specific areas of need. Alternately, the special education teacher may teach similar academic subject matter but using simplified materials. Special education teachers instruct in functional skills such as reading environmental signs (e.g., those that say "Stop" or "Exit"), learning their address and telephone number, or counting money to make purchases. For older students, the teacher may instruct in vocational skills such as filling out an employment application or setting tables at a restaurant. Students with disabilities often have social skill impairments and benefit from explicit social skills instruction. The special education teacher develops lessons for skills such as joining a game, resolving conflicts, or appropriately getting the teacher's attention.

One of the most beneficial outcomes from special education services comes from instruction in strategies. Students are taught tactics for learning, remembering, and responding to material that has been taught in the general education setting. They may learn how to look for key words and highlight important information (e.g., the operation in a math assignment) or to use mnemonic devices to help them remember information (e.g., for a science test). They may also be taught how to sketch out their ideas to help them organize their thoughts before answering an extended question on a test.

RELATED SERVICES

In addition to the academic services provided by the teacher, children with disabilities are eligible to receive related services. The term *related services* is defined as "transportation and such developmental, corrective, and other supportive services . . . as may be required to assist a child with a disability to benefit from special education" (PL 108-446, § 601[26]). According to IDEA 2004, these services include speech-language pathology and audiology services; psychological services; physical and occupational therapy; recreation, including therapeutic recreation; social work services; counseling services, including rehabilitation counseling; orientation and mobility services, interpreting therapeutic recreation; medical services; and nurse services (PL 108-446, § 602[26]).

These services can be provided in or outside of the classroom. Services provided in the classroom have the advantage of allowing teachers to know what is going on with their students by integrating the special education services into the general academic curriculum and preventing the children from missing material during a period outside the classroom. In recognition of these benefits, the principle of LRE requires that related services be provided in the classroom whenever appropriate.

One type of related services category that is changing significantly is medical services. As a result of the 1999 U.S. Supreme Court ruling in the case of *Cedar Rapids Community School District v. Garret F. and Charlene F.* (526 U.S.66-1999), cost cannot be a consideration in providing needed medical-related services for a child to receive FAPE. Thus, children who use technology assistance (see Chapter 36) must be provided the medical supervision necessary for their attendance in public schools. See Table 34.2 for some overall examples of related services.

THE INDIVIDUALIZED EDUCATION PROGAM

The IEP is a written plan that maps out the goals that the child is expected to achieve over the course of the school year. According to IDEA 2004, these goals must be developed based on the strengths of the child; the concerns of the parents; the results of the most recent evaluation of the child; and the academic, developmental, and functional needs of the child (§ 614[d][3][A]). A new IEP must be written at least once per year and should be modified as often as needed based on an assessment of the child's progress; however, pilot programs have been commissioned to develop an IEP that lasts up to 3 years. In addition, an IEP can now be amended when changes are necessary (as opposed to rewriting the entire IEP) if the changes are covered within the time frame of the original IEP (CEC, 2004).

A team that consists of professionals and the child's parents creates the IEP (see the Participants section). The child is also encouraged to participate in the process, when appropriate. To ensure that parents are active participants, certain arrangements may be made: parents who are not well versed in education law can bring a surrogate to the IEP planning meeting; parents whose native language is not English and who have difficulty understanding or speaking English must be provided a translator for the meeting; and parents who are unable to comprehend, for any reason, aspects of the disability or IEP must be given explanations they can understand. The following sections describe the process of developing an IEP, the provisions that must be covered, and examples of IEPs for children with varying disabilities.

Participants

Members of an IEP team include the parent(s), the child (when appropriate), the special education teacher, representatives of related services, the general education teacher (if the student is likely to participate in the general education environment), a representative of the LEA, and an individual who can interpret evaluation results (PL 108-446, § 614 [d] [1][B] [i–vii]).

Under IDEA 2004, certain changes to IEP team procedures were enacted. A parent may give written permission for a member of the IEP team to be excused from attending the IEP meeting if that individual's specific area of curriculum or related services is not being modified or discussed. In addition, a parent can con-

Table 34.2. Examples of disabilities and typical related services provided

Disability	Speech-language pathology	Audiology	Behavior support and counseling	Physical therapy	Occupational therapy	Services — Vision (orientation and mobility)	Social work	Assistive technology	Transportation	Medical services
Vision impairment	X		X	X	X	X	X	X		
Hearing impairment	X	X	X				X	X		
Intellectual disability	X		X				X			
Autism	X		X		X		X			
Attention-deficit/hyperactivity disorder			X				X			
Learning disabilities			X				X			
Cerebral palsy	X		X	X	X	X	X	X	X	X
Traumatic brain injury	X		X	X	X	X	X	X	X	X

sent to excuse a member of the IEP team, in whole or in part, even when the meeting involves a modification to or discussion of the member's area of the curriculum or related services if 1) the parent and local school system consent and 2) the member submits (in writing and to the parents and team) input into the development of the IEP prior to the meeting (§ 614[d][1][c][i–ii]). Finally, the parent and the local school district may agree not to convene an IEP meeting for the purposes of making changes to the child's IEP after the annual IEP meeting for the school year has occurred. Instead, they may develop a written document to amend or modify the child's current IEP (§ 614 [d][3][D]).

Contents

The law is very specific about what to include in an IEP. According to IDEA 2004, an IEP must contain the following items (PL 108-446, § 614 [d][1][A]):

- A statement of the child's present level of academic achievement and functional performance

- A statement of measurable annual goals, including academic and functional goals

- A description of how the child's progress toward the annual goals will be measured

- A statement of the special education and related services and supplementary aids and services, based on peer-reviewed research to the extent practicable, that will be provided to the child or on behalf of the child and a statement of modifications or supports for school personnel that will be provided for the child

- An explanation of the extent, if any, to which the child will not participate with children who do not have disabilities in the general education classroom

- A statement of any individual modifications that are needed for the child to participate in state- or districtwide assessments of student achievement

- A statement of the projected date for the beginning of the services and modifications, along with descriptions and an indication of the anticipated frequency, location, and duration of those services and modifications

- A statement for students 16 years or older of postsecondary goals based on age-appropriate transition assessments related to training, education, employment and, when appropriate, independent living skills

Development of Annual Goals and Benchmarks

IDEA 2004 requires the development of measurable annual goals to enable parents and educators to determine a student's progress. These goals should address both academic and nonacademic concerns and be based on the student's current education and behavior level. Parents of children with disabilities are to be informed of their child's progress as often as are parents of children without disabilities. Therefore, if general education report cards are distributed quarterly, reports on goal progress must also be distributed quarterly. Progress toward reaching annual goals does not necessarily require a letter grade but can be performance based or criterion referenced and can be rated on a spectrum—for example, from "no progress" to "goal met." In addition to goals, students who participate in alternative assessments require benchmarks that delineate smaller steps that are needed to meet the goal (CEC, 2004). For example, a child with a goal of writing personal information might have the benchmarks of 1) writing first and last name, 2) writing street address, and 3) writing city and state.

Individualized Transition Plan

An adolescent with a disability needs to start preparing for life in the community. According to IDEA 2004, the transition plans (ITPs) for meeting this goal may include preparing for "post-secondary education, vocational training, integrated employment (including supported employment), competitive employment, continuing and adult education, adult services, independent living, or community participation" (§ 602[30][A]). Beginning when the child is age 14, a formal ITP must be part of the IEP and should be based on the individual student's needs, interests, and choices. A transition planning inventory can be helpful in beginning this process. The inventory identifies comprehensive aspects for planning, such as the likely postschool environment, vocational interests, further training needs, daily living skills, future living arrangements, recreation and leisure interests, transportation or mobility needs, legal planning, health and medical concerns, interpersonal relationships, financial resources, existing supports and those needed for the future, and links to outside agencies. A transition plan will map out "instruction, related services, community experiences, the development of employment and other post-school adult living objectives, and, when appropriate, acquisition of daily living skills and functional vocational evaluation" (§ 602[30][C]).

The specific items to be included within the IEP relating to transition are as follows (PL 108-466, § 614[d][1][A][viii]):

- Beginning at age 16, and updated annually, a statement of the child's transition service needs (e.g., participation in advanced-placement courses or a vocational education program) that focuses on the child's course of study

- Beginning at age 16 (or younger, if determined appropriate by the IEP Team), a statement of needed transition services for the child, including, when appropriate, a statement of the interagency responsibilities or any needed linkages

- Beginning at least 1 year before the child reaches the age of majority under state law, a statement that the child has been informed of the **rights** that will transfer to him or her on reaching the age of majority

FEDERAL FUNDING OF SPECIAL EDUCATION SERVICES

Federal funding for IDEA 2004 services is received by the state education agency and then distributed to the LEA. It should be noted, however, that federal funds cover only about 10% of the total cost of special education services; the remainder is funded by the state and local school districts (Advocacy Institute, 2002). Furthermore, the federal government caps the number of students in special education in each state to 12% of the total number of school-age students. Thus, although IDEA 2004 is the law of the land, the federal government supports but a fraction of the total costs of special education and related services. This level of funding accounts to some extent for the variability of its application across states and districts. At the federal level, there are ongoing discussions and proposed plans for fully funding IDEA.

ESTABLISHMENT OF THE LEAST RESTRICTIVE ENVIRONMENT

IDEA 2004 emphasizes that the general education curriculum is presumed to be the appropriate beginning point for planning an IEP. Only when participation in the general education curriculum can be demonstrated as not beneficial to the student should an alternative curriculum be considered. There has been a great improvement in reducing the time students spend in special education environments. Between 1984–1985 and 1998–1999, the percentage of students with disabilities receiving services outside of the general education environment for less than 21% of the day almost doubled, from 24.6% to 47.4%. It should be emphasized that many variables go into making a decision about placement (e.g., what the parents want for their child, what the child wants, what cultural and ethnic issues affect the decision).

Approaches for Providing Services in the Least Restrictive Environment

If those evaluating the IEP determine that a child has a disability that interferes with his or her ability to benefit from the general education curriculum without adaptations, modifications, or support, the multidisciplinary team must determine the level and approach to providing special educational services. The principle of LRE requires that students with disabilities should be educated as much as possible with their peers who do not have disabilities. Table 34.3 summarizes the different approaches and environments for providing special education services and the distribution of students within these environments.

Although the inclusiveness of the environment is a factor in a student's academic or social success, the classroom environment and quality of instruction also are of great importance. The most effective interventions for a student with disabilities have the following components: 1) a case-by-case approach to decision making about the student's instruction and placement, 2) intensive and reasonably individualized instruction combined with close cooperation between the general and special education teachers, and 3) careful and frequent monitoring of the student's progress (Hocutt, 1996; Kauffman, 1995).

Inclusion Practices

A number of practices have been developed to accomplish the goal of inclusion. One is *coopera-*

Table 34.3. Levels of educational placement, from least to most restrictive

Environment	% of all students with disabilities	Means of service provision
0% of the day spent in a special education setting	All Disabilities 28 Learning Disabilities 20 Speech/Language Impairments 55 Emotional Disturbance 16 Intellectual Disability 7	*General education class:* The child with a disability has been determined to need no services at this time and receives no special help or materials from the teacher or any other service provider. *General education class with consulting special education teacher services and special materials:* A special education teacher assists the general education teacher in adapting the general education curriculum to best meet the needs of the child with a disability. The special education teacher or related service provider may come into the classroom to work directly with the child. The special education teacher may co-teach class with the general education teacher.
1%–21% of the day spent in a special education setting	All Disabilities 18 Learning Disabilities 25 Speech/Language Impairments 31 Emotional Disturbance 11 Intellectual Disability 6	*Modified general education class:* The child receives services from a special education teacher and/or related service provider (e.g., physical therapist, occupational therapist, speech-language pathologist) outside of the general education setting.
22%–60% of the day spent in a special education setting	All Disabilities 29.8 Learning Disabilities 40 Speech/Language Impairments 8 Emotional Disturbance 23 Intellectual Disability 29	*General education class with resource services:* The child joins a small group of students in a separate classroom (21%–60% of the school day) to work on areas of need with a special education teacher.
61%–100% of the day spent in a special education setting	All Disabilities 19.5 Learning Disabilities 14 Speech/Language Impairments 5 Emotional Disturbance 32 Intellectual Disability 51	*Self-contained environment:* The child is in a separate special education class for the majority (61%–100%) of the school day but typically has lunch and nonacademic classes with peers without disabilities.
	All Disabilities 2.9 Multiple Disabilities 26 Deaf Blind 38	*Special day school:* The child attends a school that serves only children with disabilities, and he or she spends no time during the school day with children without disabilities.
	0.7	*Residential school:* The child attends an overnight special education program.
	0.5	*Hospital or home instruction:* The child is unable to attend school and is educated in the hospital during a hospital stay or is educated at home.

Sources: Mercer (1997); U.S. Department of Education, Office of Special Education and Rehabilitative Services (2002); U.S. Department of Education, Office of Special Services (2002); Ysseldyke & Algozzine (1995).

tive learning, a term used to describe a range of team-based learning strategies (Jenkins, 2003). Students are divided into small teams with varying abilities and are assigned a task that they complete together. Team members monitor, assist, and provide feedback to each other. Methods such as direct instruction, small-group instruction, and independent practice can be combined with cooperative learning to teach skills and information. This strategy may be helpful in teaching both academic and social skills.

Another strategy is peer tutoring, in which one student acts as a teacher, providing instruction to a peer. A third strategy involves the use of instructional tools. These may include mnemonic devices, flow charts, study guides, and role-playing activities. Content enhancement routines that combine an interactive instructional sequence with instructional tools can be particularly helpful when combined with strategies of instruction that assist students in becoming self-regulated learners (Fisher, Schumaker, & Deshler, 1995).

Accommodations and Modifications to the General Curriculum

Students with disabilities can be supported within the general education curriculum in many different ways, including through the provision of accommodations, curriculum modifications, and adaptations. Accommodations are defined as changes that are made in how a student has access to the curriculum or demonstrates learning. Accommodations provide equal access to learning, do not substantially change the instructional level or content, are based on individual strengths and needs, and may vary in intensity or degree. An example of this would be reducing a spelling list that teaches the concept of the -*it* ending from 10 words to 5 words. The student with a disability is responsible for learning the same material as the students without disabilities, although with a reduced output. Modifications to curriculum provide material that substantially changes the general education curriculum. An example of this would be a student working on addition when his classmates are working on multiplication. Some examples of adaptations include reading directions to the student, providing extended time to complete assignments, providing study aids, giving frequent reminders of rules, providing taped texts, and giving note taking assistance.

In addition to supporting students through accommodations and/or modifications, instruction can be differentiated to meet the needs of high-, low-, and average-achieving students with disabilities in the classroom. As each student with a disability has individual interests and learning styles, differentiating instruction is also a way to meet the needs of a diverse class and engage everyone in the learning process (Smith et al., 2001; Tomlinson, 2000). Instructional elements that can be differentiated include content, process, product, and learning environment. Successful differentiation involves ongoing assessment that is closely tied to the curriculum, creating quality work that is interesting and appealing and using flexible groupings that give students the opportunity to work in a variety of environments and with a mix of their peers (CEC, 1993).

ROLE OF THE SPECIAL EDUCATION TEACHER IN THE GENERAL CURRICULUM

It is the responsibility of special education teachers to support students who qualify for special education services during instruction in the general education classroom. The amount of support needed depends on the individual needs of the child. The special education teacher may take on one of two roles, that of a collaborator or of a co-teacher. As a collaborator, the special education teacher must familiarize the general education teacher with the adaptations and modifications that will be necessary to enable the child to benefit from instruction in the general education classroom. The two teachers then discuss who will be responsible for which aspects of the student's instructional needs. For a student who needs only limited support, the special education teacher might create modified tests and check on the student at the end of the day to make sure that all of the homework assignments have been written down. On the advice of the special education teacher, the general education teacher might assign only even-numbered test problems or give the student extended time. For a student who needs more extensive supports, the special education teacher may supply adapted assignments that cover the same content as the general education lesson but are at the student's functional level.

As a co-teacher, the special education teacher shares the classroom with a general education teacher. The two teachers take joint responsibility for all of the students in the class, regardless of ability, and take turns teaching lessons. While one teaches the entire class, the other helps any students in need. The two teachers may divide the class into small groups for instruction, but grouping is not made according to disability. Research has found this method to be successful for students with a specific learning disability (see Chapter 25). It was found that students who participated in a co-teaching environment earned higher grades and preformed higher on nationally normed standardized tests (Rea et al., 2002).

PARTICIPATION IN STATE- AND DISTRICTWIDE ASSESSMENTS

Congress passed the No Child Left Behind Act (NCLB) of 2001 (PL 107-110) with the goal of setting standards that would improve education for all students. This legislation requires that all students in public schools take a standardized assessment annually in Grades 3–8, 10, and 11 in the areas of English language arts, mathematics, and science. IDEA 2004 requires that all students with disabilities be included in these state- and districtwide assessments. The IDEA requirement is intended to "improve opinions about people with disabilities in general, improve access to the general education curriculum for students with disabilities, and improve instruction in special education programs" (Browder & Cooper-Duffy, 2003; Browder et al., 2003). Browder noted that if students are left out of accountability systems, they also will be left out of policy decisions.

The majority of students with disabilities participate in the same assessment as their peers without disabilities. If modifications or accommodations are necessary, they are included in the IEP. The basic intention is that all students should have the opportunity to demonstrate what they have learned. Some examples of modifications or accommodations to this testing include dictation to a scribe, oral reading of assessment, use of a calculator or manipulatives, testing over multiple sessions, and taking tests in a small group.

A small percentage of students with disabilities (typically 1%–2%) participate in an alternative assessment. These include students 1) with the most severe disabilities, who cannot complete a standardized test even with assistance (e.g., a scribe or some other type of facilitator), and 2) who will earn a differentiated diploma or certificate of completion.

Alternative assessment methods vary from state to state. One common method is to collect a portfolio of student achievement and artifacts that demonstrate mastery. According to IDEA 2004, alternative assessments must be aligned with the state's challenging academic content standards and/or adopted alternated academic achievement standards (§ 612[a][16][C][ii]). For example, in Maryland, the Maryland School Assessment (MSA) program has an alternative assessment that includes goals that align to the state's regular or extended reading and mathematics content standards and measures a student's progress in five domains: 1) personal management, 2) community functioning, 3) career/vocational skills, 4) leisure/recreation skills, and 5) communication and decision-making skills. The Maryland State Department of Education (2007) provides examples of how this would be done.

Other states, such as Missouri, measure the progress of students with severe to profound intellectual disabilities using curriculum-based measurement. The teacher designs tasks that allow the student to demonstrate the application of skills aligned to state academic standards. For example, the state standard "understanding numbers, ways of representing numbers, relationships among numbers and number systems" might be fulfilled by the skill "recognize a collection of 1 to 2 items (e.g., pointing to 1 or 2 items)" (Missouri Department of Elementary and Secondary Education, 2005). Each skill is assessed a number of times over the testing period, which, in Missouri, lasts for 3 months.

The goal of alternative assessments is to ensure that the child is achieving his or her personal best and that the child continues to achieve at progressively higher levels. To accomplish this, the student's curriculum should fit his or her needs, rather than having the student fit into a particular existing curriculum. The intention of IDEA 2004 is that the child's special education and related services are in addition to and affected by the general curriculum, not separate from it.

IDEA 2004 addresses the issue of accountability by making assessment data public. States are required to report the number of children with disabilities who are participating in general assessments and in alternate assessments and their overall performance on these evaluations. States are also required to publish graduation rates, as well as postsecondary education and employment rates. These rates are to be compared with and reported in the same amount of detail as those of students without disabilities (PL 108-446, §§ 664[3][4][B] and 612[a][16][D][i], respectively). The purpose of gathering and reporting this information is to increase efforts toward attaining improved student results and has implications for funding streams at the school, district, and/or state level.

PROCEDURAL SAFEGUARDS: DUE PROCESS

Identifying a child with a disability, planning his or her program, and choosing a placement is a complicated legal process. To ensure that the rights of the students and parents are respected, IDEA 2004 regulates procedural safeguards that are to be used during all special education decision making. IDEA mandates that parents are given a copy of their procedural rights at their child's annual IEP. Parents are part of the team making IEP decisions, but they occasionally disagree with the school's decision regarding their child. When parents disagree with the school about any aspect of an IEP decision, there is a legal proceeding that allows them to challenge the decision. This is called an impartial due process hearing (PL 108-446, § 615[a] [b][c][d][e][f]).

In cases of extreme disagreement, parents may feel that the public school cannot meet their child's FAPE needs. Under these circumstances, the parents may be able to send the child to private school at the public school's expense. If the school does not agree that the student does not have access to FAPE at his or her current placement, the two parties will enter a due process hearing. The possibility of the public school paying for a private school education can only exist if three important steps are followed. First, the parents must notify the school at the most recent IEP meeting that they are rejecting the proposed placement, as it does not provide FAPE for their child. Second, the parents must notify the school in writing of their intent to send their child to a private school at least 10 business days before enrolling their child in a private school. Finally, the parents must have made the child available for any evaluations the school identified as necessary for providing FAPE.

THE SCHOOL–PARENT CONNECTION

One of the keys to positive results for students with disabilities is the teamwork between the school and family. Educators only see one facet of a child's abilities—his or her performance at school. Parents, conversely, see the whole child. For example, a parent might know of a special interest or enjoyable activity that the educator might provide as a motivator for the child's school performance. Goals and placements also need to be decided jointly by the parents and the special education team. It is encouraging to note that parent attendance at IEP meetings is strong. A federal longitudinal study (Special Education Elementary Longitudinal Study, or SEELS) found that 92% of parents of students with disabilities attended their child's IEP meeting (SRI International, 2004).

The close partnership between special educators and parents has another direct benefit: the parents understand and appreciate the efforts being made for their children. The SEELS study found that 93% of parents believed that IEP goals were challenging and appropriate, and 90% were satisfied with special education services provided. In contrast, only 75% of those parents were satisfied with the school as a whole (SRI International, 2004).

OUTCOME

In 2000, more than $77 billion was spent on students with disabilities, an average of $12,474 per student as compared with $6,556 per general education student (Advocacy Institute, 2002). With this level of expenditure, it is important to evaluate outcomes. As one marker of success, the high school graduation rate with a standard diploma for students receiving special education services increased from 51.9% in 1994 to 57.4% percent in 1999 (Advocacy Institute, 2002; U.S. Department of Education, 2002). This ranges from 75% for students with visual impairments to 42% for those with intellectual disability and emotional disturbance (U.S. Department of Education, 2002). This compares favorably with the nationwide average that shows 68% of general education students graduating (Swanson, 2004). In addition to the 57% who obtain standard diplomas, 11% of students with disabilities earn alternative credentials (Goldstein, 2003).

Although gradation rates are an important indicator of positive educational outcomes, the outcome for many students with disabilities is more adequately represented through other means. The National Longitudinal Study–2 (National Center on Secondary Education and Transition, 2003) surveyed outcomes of young adults with disabilities in many areas. As an example, 83% liked their job very much or fairly well. One of the goals of education is to provide students with the tools they need to succeed in life. Individuals who have benefited from their education should feel positively about their future. Table 34.4 represents the percent of students who feel hopeful about the future, broken down by disability. The results are quite positive, with over half of students with a wide range of disabilities indicating that they are hopeful about the future a lot or all of the time.

SUMMARY

Special education and related services are mandated by federal law to be provided to all students with defined disabilities. IDEA 2004 em-

Table 34.4. How often youth felt hopeful about the future (Item np2V2d): Overall and by primary disability category

	Total	Learning disability	Speech impairment	Mental retardation	Emotional disturbance	Hearing impairment	Visual impairment	Orthopedic impairment	Other health impairment	Autism	Traumatic brain injury	Multiple disabilities	Deaf/ blindness
(1) Rarely or never	12.3%	11.9%	11.8%	17.1%	10.4%	6.6%	8.2%	8.1%	14.5%	7.1%	12.2%	13.6%	*
(2) Some-times	24.3%	22.9%	30.2%	29.6%	22.8%	28.4%	20.2%	21.9%	27.7%	30.2%	31.1%	24.3%	*
(3) A lot of the time	22.8%	23.3%	19.9%	24.4%	19.1%	28.3%	25.4%	23.1%	21.1%	28.8%	10.0%	25.7%	20.8%
(4) Most or all of the time	40.6%	41.9%	38.2%	28.8%	47.7%	36.8%	46.2%	47.0%	36.7%	33.9%	46.8%	36.4%	56.3%
n	3,303	396	357	257	305	263	314	400	454	208	137	164	48

From National Center on Secondary Education and Transition, Institute on Community Integration. (2003). *NLTS2 Wave 2 Parent/Youth Survey Youth Report of Youth Social Involvement Table 340 Estimates*
Retrieved January 26, 2007, from http://www.nlts2.org/data_tables/tables/8/np2V2dfrm.html.

*Too few to reliably report (fewer than 10 in a cell or 20 in a column)

phasizes student participation in the general education curriculum and stresses that students with disabilities are entitled to a free and appropriate public education in the least restrictive environment to the greatest possible extent. A more collaborative relationship between general education and special education teachers is also implied by this law. The most popular approach to providing this service is by inclusion. Whether this is the best approach for all children with disabilities is still unclear, and there remains a spectrum of approaches and strategies to provide special education services. Outcome is best when support services are provided early and in the quantity and quality required for progress to be made. The IEP guides this process, and assessment of progress at regular intervals is critical for success.

REFERENCES

Advocacy Institute. (2002). *Students with learning disabilities: A national review.* Retrieved June 6, 2002, from http://www.advocacyinstitute.org/rescouces/LD_Reviews02.pdf

Americans with Disabilities Act (ADA) of 1990, PL 101-336, 42 U.S.C. §§ 12101 *et seq.*

Browder, D.M., & Cooper-Duffy, K. (2003). Evidence-based practices for students with severe disabilities and the requirement for accountability in "No Child Left Behind." *Journal of Special Education, 37,* 157-163.

Browder, D.M., Spooner, F., & Algozzine, R., et al. (2003). What we know and need to know about alternative assessment. *Exceptional Children, 70,* 45-67.

Cedar Rapids Community School Dist. v. Garret F., 526 U.S. 66 (1999).

Council for Exceptional Children. (1993). *Including students with disabilities in general education classrooms.* Reston, VA: Author. (ERIC Document Reproduction Service No. ED 434435)

Council for Exceptional Children. (2004). *The New IDEA: CEC's summary of significant issues.* Reston, VA: Author.

Council for Exceptional Children (CEC) & IDEA Partnerships. (2000). *Making assessment accommodations: A toolkit for educators.* Reston, VA: Author.

Education for All Handicapped Children Act of 1975, PL 94-142, 20 U.S.C. §§ 1400 *et seq.*

Education of the Handicapped Act Amendments of 1986, PL 99-457, 20 U.S.C. §§ 1400 *et seq.*

Education of the Handicapped Act of 1970 (EHA), PL 91-230, 84 Stat. 121-154, 20 U.S.C. §§ 1400 *et seq.*

Elementary and Secondary Education Act of 1965, PL 89-10, 20 U.S.C. §§ 241 *et seq.*

Fisher, J.B., Schumaker, J.B., & Deshler, D.D. (1995). Searching for validated inclusive practices: A review of the literature. *Focus on Exceptional Children, 28*(4), 1-20.

Goldstein, L.F. (2003). *Special education graduation rates steadily increase.* Retrieved April 2004 from http://www.ldonline.org.php?id=60&loc=49

Hocutt, A.M. (1996). Effectiveness of special education: Is placement the critical factor? *The Future of Children, 6,* 77-102.

Hosp, J.L., & Reschily, D.J. (2004). Disproportionate representation of minority students in special education: Academic, demographic, and economic predictors. *Exceptional Children, 70,* 185-199.

Individuals with Disabilities Education Act Amendments of 1997, PL 105-17, 20 U.S.C.§§ 1400 *et seq.*

Individuals with Disabilities Education Act (IDEA) of 1990, PL 101-476, 20 U.S.C. §§ 1400 *et seq.*

Individuals with Disabilities Education Improvement Act of 2004, PL 108-446, 20 U.S.C. §§ 1400 *et seq.*

Jenkins, J.R. (2003). How cooperative learning works for special education and remedial students. *Exceptional Children, 69,* 279-292.

Kauffman, J.M. (1995). Why we must celebrate a diversity of restrictive environments. *Learning Disabilities: Research & Practice, 10,* 225-232.

Maryland State Department of Education. (2007). *2007 ALT-MSA handbook.* Retrieved October 24, 2006, from http://www.marylandpublicschools.org/msde/testing/alt_msa/2007_alt-msa_handbook.htm

Mercer, C.D. (1997). *Students with learning disabilities.* Upper Saddle River, NJ: Prentice Hall.

Missouri Department of Elementary and Secondary Education, Division of Improvement. (2005). *Missouri Assessment Plan–Alternate (MAP-A): Instructor's guide and administration manual, 2005–2006.* Jefferson City, MO: Author.

National Center on Secondary Education and Transition, Institute on Community Integration. (2003). *NLTS2 Wave 2 Parent/Youth Survey Youth Report of Youth Social Involvement Table 340 Estimates* Retrieved January 26, 2007, from http://www.nlts2.org/data_tables/tables/8/np2V2dfrm.html

National Center on Secondary Education and Transition, Institute on Community Integration. (2003). Youth employment. *NCSET NLTS2 Data Brief, 2*(2). Minneapolis, MN: Author.

No Child Left Behind Act of 2001, PL 107-110, 115 Stat. 1425, 20 U.S.C. §§ 6301 et seq.

Pennsylvania Association for Retarded Citizens v. Commonwealth of Pennsylvania, 334 F. Supp. 1257 (E.D. Pa. 1971).

Praisner, C.L. (2003). Attitudes of elementary school principals toward the inclusion of students with disabilities. *Exceptional Children, 69,* 135-145.

Rea, P.T., McLaughlin, V.L., Walther-Thomas, C. (2002). Outcomes for students with disabilities in inclusive and pullout programs. *Exceptional Children, 68,* 203-222.

Rehabilitation Act of 1973, PL 93-112, 29 U.S.C. §§ 701 *et seq.*

Smith, T.E.C., Polloway, E.A., Patton, J.R., et al. (2001). *Teaching students with special needs in inclusive settings* (3rd ed.). Needham Heights, MA: Allyn & Bacon.

SRI International. (2004). *Special Education Elementary Longitudinal Study.* Retrieved October 3, 2006, from http://www.seels.net

Swanson, C.B. (2004). *Who graduates? Who doesn't? A statistical profile of public high school graduation.* Retrieved April 2004 from http://www.urban.org/url.cfm?ID=41034

Tomlinson, C.A. (2000, August). Differentiation of instruction in the elementary grades. *ERIC Digest.* (ERIC Document Reproduction Service No. ED 443572)

U.S. Department of Education, Office of Special Education and Rehabilitative Services (OSERS). (2000).

Twenty-second annual report to Congress on the implementation of the Individuals with Disabilities Education Act. Retrieved January 21, 2001, from http://www.ed.gov/about/reports/OSEPAnlRpt/ExecSumm.html?

U.S. Department of Education. (2001). *Twenty-third annual report to Congress on the implementation of the Individuals with Disabilities Education Act* (pp. III-1 to III-6). Washington, DC: U.S. Government Printing Office.

U.S Department of Education, Office of Education and Rehabilitative Services (OSERS). (2002). *Twenty-fourth annual report to Congress on the implementation of the Individuals with Disabilities Education Act.* Retrieved May 1, 2004, from http://www.ed.gov/offices/OSERS/OSEP/Products/OSEP2000AnlRpt/ExecSumm.html

Yell, M.L. (1998). *The law and special education.* Upper Saddle River, NJ: Prentice Hall.

Ysseldyke, J., & Algozzine, B. (1995). *Special education: A practical approach for teachers* (3rd ed.). Boston: Houghton Mifflin.

35 Behavioral Principles, Assessment, and Therapy

Michael F. Cataldo, SungWoo Kahng, Iser G. DeLeon,
Brian K. Martens, Patrick C. Friman, and Marilyn Cataldo

Upon completion of this chapter, the reader will

- Be familiar with the role of operant learning approaches in helping individuals with developmental disabilities

- Be acquainted with operant principles and their application to important everyday problems

- Be familiar with operant learning approaches for decreasing problematic behaviors and increasing adaptive behaviors

- Understand how operant principles can be used to treat severe behavior problems

- Have several practical techniques based on operant principles for parents and teachers to address mild behavior problems

---

Since the 1950s, a remarkable change has occurred in society's response to the needs and challenges of people with developmental disabilities. In the mid-1950s, diagnosis, treatment, and education programs were virtually nonexistent. Many people with developmental disabilities spent most of their lives in residential facilities located outside the mainstream of society. As of 2007, many of these facilities have been closed. With rare exception, children and adults with developmental disabilities now live in the community, attend school, and have jobs. This dramatic change has evolved, in a large part, because of two factors: 1) studies showing that people with developmental disabilities can learn, and 2) the civil rights movement of the 1950s and 1960s. This first factor has come about because of studies based on learning theory, particularly operant learning. The purpose of this chapter is to first briefly explain the principles of operant learning that pertain to people with developmental disabilities and then to provide examples of practical applications for both mild and severe behavioral challenges of children with developmental disabilities.

OPERANT LEARNING PRINCIPLES AND PRACTICES

Experts on the use of operant learning approaches generally have degrees in psychology or education and have several terms for what they do. These terms include *behavior modification, applied behavior analysis, behavior analysis,* and *positive behavioral support (PBS)*. The differences have mainly to do with changes in terms over the development of this field of research and practice, both with regard to preferred terminology and emphasis on specific techniques. For example, most recently, an emphasis has been placed on using only "positive" approaches to help people with developmental disabilities. This emphasis has validity because it makes less likely abuses due to inappropriate use of operant approaches and it is sufficient for the vast majority of people needing help.

In all instances, regardless of the term used, the approaches refer to behavioral challenges as "behavioral excesses and deficits" that adversely affect the lives of people with developmental disabilities. These excesses range from common problems such as bedtime difficulties to rarer but more dramatic disorders such as self-injurious behavior (SIB). Behavioral deficits include poor academic performance, inadequate social skills, and deficient communication skills, as well as an inability to independently complete activities of daily living. These behavioral excesses and deficits are often interrelated; children who engage in SIB and other severe forms of problem behavior often display skill deficits of various sorts (Baghdadli et al., 2003; Chadwick et al., 2000). Current operant-learning-based practices are grounded in a rich tradition of learning theory. Although biologic/genetic factors must be taken into account, the assumption is that typically, both appropriate and inappropriate behaviors are learned over time through their effects on the environment. Stated differently, behavior is functionally altered based on whether it results in valuable outcomes or in escaping or avoiding unpleasant ones. This simple yet powerful functional relationship between behavior and its consequences, sometimes characterized as the "Law of Effect," forms the basis for current operant learning approaches. Because behavior is considered to operate on the environment and to result in differential consequences, it is termed *operant behavior*.

Reinforcement, Extinction, and Punishment

Reinforcement is fundamental to all behavior programs. Strictly defined, it is a process in which the consequences that follow a given behavior result in an increase in the future strength of that behavior. Reinforcement can be formally divided into two subclasses: positive and negative (Figure 35.1). **Positive reinforcement** exists when the contingent delivery of an outcome produces an increase in the likelihood of the behavior(s) upon which it is contingent. Negative reinforcement is in effect when the

contingent removal of a stimulus produces an increase in the likelihood of the behavior. Both can be used in the acquisition of new behaviors as well as in the maintenance or reduction of problem behaviors. **Extinction** is the process through which reinforcement is withheld for a previously reinforced response, resulting in a decrease in the future occurrence of that response.

Punishment is technically defined as a process in which consequences delivered contingent upon a behavior result in a decrease in the future occurrence of that behavior. Thus, it produces an effect opposite to that of reinforcement. Punishment, too, can involve separate classes (Figure 35.1). Positive punishment involves the contingent delivery of a consequence (sometimes termed an aversive stimulus), whereas negative punishment involves the contingent removal of a consequence (i.e., positive **reinforcer**). Common examples of the latter include **time-out** (the individual is removed from potential sources of reinforcement) and response–cost (previously earned reinforcers, such as tokens that can be redeemed for a reward, are removed contingent on inappropriate behavior). Punitive therapeutic arrangements have become less common over the years owing to a variety of factors, including diminished social acceptability and the development of assessment methods that have improved the efficacy of reinforcement-based interventions (Pelios et al., 1999). Furthermore, the term *punishment* relates a basic learning principle to legal and negative associations. Yet, the facts are that regardless of the term employed, most learning cannot occur without feedback about incorrect responses. And, when feedback on incorrect responses occurs and enhances learning, it meets the technical definition of punishment. From a technical, operant learning perspective, grades in school can serve as reinforcement or as punishment.

It is important to note that punishing and reinforcing stimuli are not characterized by their outward appearance but by their effects on the behaviors upon which they are made contingent. The success of many behavior programs hinges upon the parent's, caregiver's, or teacher's ability to arrange or rearrange the relations between behavior and its consequences. However, knowing which stimuli can be effective as consequences to increase or decrease behavior is not always intuitively obvious. For example, normally punitive consequences, such as

		EFFECT	
		Increases likelihood of behavior	Decreases likelihood of behavior
ACTION	Stimulus presented	Positive reinforcement	Positive punishment
ACTION	Stimulus removed	Negative reinforcement	Negative punishment

Figure 35.1. Distinction between positive and negative reinforcement and punishment.

verbal reprimands (e.g., Fisher et al., 1996) and physical restraint (e.g., Magee & Ellis, 2001) under certain circumstances actually function as reinforcers for some individuals. Thus, an important part of successful behavior management is the process of identifying stimuli that are effective consequences for each individual.

Motivation

Both behavior and response–consequence interactions are dynamic. Motivation is an important concept in understanding how the effectiveness of consequences varies across time. Establishing operations (EOs) play a central role in the operant learning conceptualization of motivation (Michael, 2000). An EO produces two effects: 1) a change in the value of a consequence, and 2) a corresponding change in the strength (e.g., frequency, amount) of behavior that has historically been influenced by that consequence. For example, a lengthy period of deprivation from attention can make attention a stronger reinforcer and increase the frequency of behavior that has historically produced attention (McComas, Thompson, & Johnson, 2003; O'Reilly et al., 2006). Regarding human clinical problems (especially with people with developmental disabilities), examination of EOs has become increasingly prevalent in research and intervention programs. For example, the presence or absence of recurrent medical conditions (e.g., Kennedy & Meyer, 1996), medications (e.g., Crosland et al., 2003), and general states of alertness (e.g., O'Reilly & Lancioni, 2000) have all been shown to alter the effectiveness of certain consequences as reinforcers and, thus, alter the frequency of problem behaviors maintained by those reinforcers.

Single-Case Experimental Design and Treatment Accountability

Another distinguishing feature of operant learning approaches is the unique set of experimental arrangements that characterize research in this field. This research has historically relied on single-subject (single-case, small *n*) designs because of the ability of this approach to explore individual variation in subjects' responses to experimental conditions and because of its immediate relevance to individualized treatment. Such designs, thus, enhance treatment accountability because the specific effects on each individual participant are examined separately.

FROM BASIC PRINCIPLE TO APPLICATION

Many of the earliest studies of behavioral principles involved groups of people with developmental disabilities. Initially, this was because people with intellectual disability, in general, learn more slowly, thus making it easier to study the learning process. This had two important sequelae: 1) it led to studies of clinical problems, and 2) it provided the necessary evidence for landmark court cases on the rights of those with intellectual disability (Levy & Rubenstein, 1996).

In the late 1960s, the field of psychology dedicated to studying operant learning began to emphasize applications (Baer, Wolf, & Risley, 1968). Since then, hundreds of studies have reported the clinical utility of operant learning principles to change behavior, both excesses and deficits. Successful behavior change has been demonstrated for self-care and a variety of other skills related to activities of daily living, leisure, recreation, vocation, and the like. Studies also have shown how to improve language acquisition and various forms of communication, academic performance, community preparation, and health and safety training. In addition, this literature has analyzed and demonstrated techniques for reducing stereotypies, inappropriate sexual contact, self-injury, aggression toward others, and property destruction. Furthermore, these approaches have been shown to be successful with almost every diagnosis in the spectrum of developmental disabilities.

COMMON BEHAVIOR PROBLEMS

Research has clearly demonstrated that from these basic operant learning principles, a broad variety of applications for treatment of routine child behavior problems can be derived, a sample of which will be discussed next (see Friman, 2005, and Friman & Blum, 2003, for elaboration).

Routine Oppositional Behavior

Optimal treatment of routine oppositional behavior usually includes at least five components.

1. Establish the clarity and simplicity of the instructions or requests that are to be followed in the program.

2. Dramatically increase pleasant social and physical contact between the child and caregiver; this is sometimes called "time-

in." The more pleasant the circumstances at the time of oppositional behavior, the less intensive or intrusive an intervention has to be in order to produce a behavior changing aversive experience. Mere cessation of or removal from the pleasant circumstances is often highly aversive (an example of negative punishment).

3. Cause a temporary dramatic decrease in pleasant social and physical contact between child and caregiver, cessation of all preferred activity, and confinement to a specified location, usually a chair or a bedroom; this is usually called time-out (the obverse of the second component). The key to effectiveness is its contiguity with and contingency upon the targeted oppositional behavior and its release criteria. Generally, release requires quiet acceptance of the time-out (which can take a while to achieve, especially in the beginning stages) and verbal or gestural assent to a request by the caregiver, asking whether the child would like to leave time-out.

4. Provide an immediate and brief but intensive practice session wherein the child is instructed to complete several small tasks (e.g., put pencil on desk, place paper in wastebasket) and is praised for compliance or sent back to time-out for noncompliance.

5. Make an ardent attempt to catch the child complying with commands or following instructions in his or her everyday life and to praise (reinforce) the performance. This is sometimes called incidental teaching.

Variations on this procedure have been used successfully with oppositional behavior with more children at more developmental levels than any other documented treatment.

Toileting

Toileting accidents are common in young children and continue to be present in many typically developing children through age 6 (especially boys). When achievement of developmental milestones is slowed by developmental disability, the probability of toileting accidents increases substantially and extends well past age 6. Effective treatment of toileting accidents usually includes at least four components.

1. Detection of accidents by child and caregiver must be heightened. Market forces in the United States are actually working against this first component through the use of diapers and pull-ups in increasingly older children. Both garments inhibit detection. The polymer structure of the garments prevents urine from dampening clothing, thus interfering with visual detection by caregivers. The structure also traps urine within the garment itself and maintains its temperature at or near body levels, and so sensory detection of accidents is also delayed. Not surprisingly, the development of continence is inhibited by wearing the garments (Tarbox, Williams, & Friman, 2004). As a result, achieving the first component involves removing diapers and pull-ups when and where possible (Figure 35.2).

2. Learning trials must be increased in frequency. This can be accomplished by increasing fluid loads, usually by providing unlimited amounts of the child's favorite beverages.

3. Any movement associated with imminent urination should be quickly followed by a guided trip to the bathroom. In addition, during the training period, guided trips should be scheduled at least every 2 hours.

4. Attempts to urinate should be praised, and successes should be rewarded (positive reinforcement). If timing is critical or if the previously listed components do not yield success, a vibrating urine alarm can be added. Alarms are moisture sensitive, and they simultaneously increase detection of accidents by child and caregiver (there is a detectable sound) and supply a mildly unpleasant consequence for the accident. This increases inhibitory learning (Friman & Vollmer, 1995).

Bedtime Problems

Crying, calling, and/or coming out of the bedroom after bedtime are among the most common behavior problems for young children, and this is true whether they are typically developing or have developmental disabilities. The possibility of bedtime problems is high because faced with the prospect of being alone in the dark for hours, children often exhibit distress. Furthermore, any response from caregivers to the bedtime problem, pleasant or unpleasant, creates a reinforcing experience, because human contact is preferred to being alone (Friman & Blum, 2003).

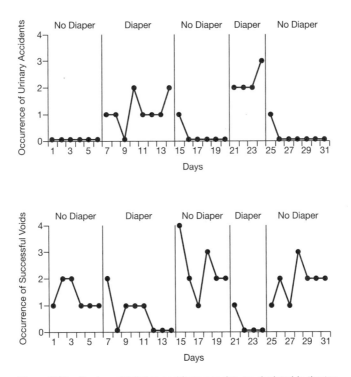

Figure 35.2. Number of toileting accidents per day are depicted in the top panel. Number of successful voids per day are depicted in the bottom panel. (From Tarbox, R., Williams, L., & Friman, P.C. [2004]. Extended diaper wearing: Effects on continence in and out of the diaper. *Journal of Applied Behavior Analysis, 37,* 99; reprinted by permission.)

Treatment involves a variation on ignoring distress calls and preventing bedroom exits, essentially an extinction procedure. The intensity and duration of the child's distress, however, frequently limits caregiver compliance with extinction. Fortunately, a method used to reduce disruptive behavior can be adapted to improve bedtime problems and increase parental compliance. This method involves providing children with a brief period of time during which their (appropriate) requests and demands are met, contingent upon their exhibiting the **target behaviors** (Bowman et al., 1997). The derived method involves giving children who appropriately prepare for bed (e.g., brushed teeth, put pajamas on) a "bedtime pass" (usually a laminated piece of cardboard) that they are allowed to use in exchange for the satisfaction of one (appropriate) request. The children are allowed to call out the request or get up and deliver it to the caregiver. Following satisfaction of the request, the pass is surrendered, the child is tucked in bed for the night, and all subsequent distress calls are ignored. The pass has successfully eliminated bedtime problems in children

between the ages of 3 and 10 years (Friman et al., 1999) and is rated as highly acceptable by parents and pediatricians. The fact that the bedtime pass program has been so successful with children as young as 3 years of age suggests it could be mastered by children with disabilities whose developmental abilities approach the 3-year level.

Common Habit Disorders

Habit disorders are highly prevalent in children, and especially in children with developmental disabilities. The likelihood of a habit increases along with the size and frequency of intervals between stimulating or nurturing events in the lives of children (e.g., contacts with people, absorbing social activities) (Friman, Byrd, & Oksal, 2001). Thus, habits are more prevalent in industrialized societies than in agrarian societies, because children in agrarian societies have abundantly more "skin-to-skin" contact with caregivers in the early periods of their lives (e.g., they sleep with parents for years, are swaddled with a parent throughout the day). Because of the abundance of highly stimulating contact and activities throughout the day, the pleasant experiential contrast provided by self-stimulatory habits is insufficient to lead to their development or maintenance.

Common habits include fingernail biting, skin picking, teeth grinding, and hair play and pulling; however, the most prevalent is probably thumb sucking and, with minor exceptions, its successful treatment is prototypical for most habits. Because all of these behaviors, like other pediatric presenting problems, can be signs of underlying medical or psychiatric problems, a proper evaluation is a prerequisite for behavioral treatment. If warranted, however, a behavioral approach would proceed as follows.

1. A version of time-in (as previously described) is used. To the extent possible, the frequency and length of intervals associated with limited external stimulation is reduced by increasing the delivery of pleasant social and physical contact.

2. Detection of the habit is increased through intensive monitoring.

3. The child's awareness of the habit is raised through methods that increase its recognition. With thumb sucking, this is achieved by applying edible but bitter-tasting substances to the thumbnail.

4. All public exhibitions of the habit result in a brief time-out, but private practice of the habit is allowed. The logic behind allowing private practice is that unless a child spends an inordinate amount of time alone, the likelihood that a private habit will cause social or physical problems is minimal.

5. An incentive system is employed to reward the child when the habit is not exhibited during an established number of defined intervals.

Variations on this form of treatment for thumb sucking have been shown to be highly successful in research studies (e.g., Friman & Leibowitz, 1990), even when the sucking is part of a cluster of self-stimulatory behaviors (e.g., see Friman, 1990). Other variations have been used to treat a broad range of behavior problems including fingernail biting and chronic hair pulling (Woods & Miltenberger, 2001).

Obviously, the previously mentioned problems form a much abbreviated sample of common behavior problems, but it is representative of the kind of problems for which operant–learning-based strategies have been proven effective. Thus, these techniques are evidence based and can easily be disseminated to parents through brief well-child visits.

SEVERE PROBLEM BEHAVIORS

Problem behaviors such as SIB, aggression, and property destruction cannot be dealt with in the same practical manner described in the preceding section. Although there is compelling evidence that problem behaviors (e.g., SIB) involve neurobiological mechanisms (e.g., Nyhan, 2002), medical approaches, such as the use of atypical antipsychotics (i.e., risperidone), are only partially successful. Research shows that these problem behaviors also have a learned component (which influences frequency and long-term disability) and can be reduced by applying operant–learning-based approaches (Iwata, Pace, Dorsey, et al., 1994; National Institutes of Health, 1991).

For example, SIB has been shown to be maintained by environmental contingencies such as negative reinforcement (escape) and positive reinforcement (attention) (Carr, Newsom, & Binkoff, 1976; Lovaas et al., 1965). Numerous studies have demonstrated that other problem behaviors such as aggression and property destruction can be maintained through similar environmental contingencies (e.g., Carr & Durand, 1985; Marcus et al., 2001). Therefore, children with severe behavior problems (e.g., SIB, aggression, property destruction) should be referred to properly trained and credentialed behavior analysts[1], psychologists, or educators.

The environmental contingencies that maintain problem behavior can be categorized into three groups: social-positive reinforcement, social-negative reinforcement, and automatic reinforcement (Iwata et al., 2000). These are described next.

Social-Positive Reinforcement

Events or stimuli that follow the occurrence of a behavior may function to strengthen that be-

---

[1]One type of professional that is well-trained in operant learning approaches is termed a behavior analyst. Recently, rigorous credentialing processes have been put into place for these individuals and have been recognized by some states as being on a par with the process of licensing psychologists and certifying special educators. The credentialing is conducted by the Behavior Analyst Certification Board (http://www.bacb.com).

havior. Oftentimes, these consequences are socially mediated (i.e., delivered by other individuals) and take the form of attention or items (e.g., toys, food). For example, a common response by parents when their child engages in less intensive forms of SIB (or stereotypic behavior) may be to provide a verbal reprimand (e.g., saying "Don't do that") or physical comfort (e.g., hugging the child). Although these consequences may lead to a temporary decrease in the problem behavior, repeated pairing of either consequence with the problem behavior may inadvertently result in a future increase in both the frequency and intensity of this problem behavior.

Social-Negative Reinforcement

The removal of some unwanted or aversive event contingent on a behavior may also result in strengthening of that behavior and may take the form of escape or avoidance from the unwanted event. For example, a teacher may present a student with a challenging task (e.g., answering a difficult question), which may result in the child becoming aggressive. This aggressive behavior may eventually lead the teacher to terminate the task and provide the student a break so that he or she will calm down. In this situation, the escape may lead to a temporary reduction of aggression. However, the inadvertent pairing of the escape with the aggression may lead to future increases in aggression by the student when he or she is presented with similarly challenging tasks.

Automatic Reinforcement

Some forms of SIB occur independent of environmental or socially mediated consequences (Vollmer, 1994). These behaviors are oftentimes said to be self-stimulatory, and a variety of biological explanations have been suggested. These include biochemical deficiencies, insensitivity to pain, and the body's response to opiate-like substances (Cataldo & Harris, 1982). These nonsocially mediated contingencies have collectively become referred to as automatic reinforcement (Vaughan & Michael, 1982).

BEHAVIORAL ASSESSMENT OF PROBLEM BEHAVIORS

Since the early 1990s, the dominant approach to severe problem behaviors initially involves a category of assessments collectively referred to as functional assessment. The basic goal is to identify the antecedent events and consequences that serve as motivational variables for problem behavior. There are three types of functional assessment: indirect assessment, descriptive analysis, and functional (experimental) analysis (Iwata et al., 2000).

Indirect assessment is the simplest method of gathering information about behavioral function. Indirect assessments consist of questionnaires and rating scales (e.g., Matson et al., 1999) that are completed by caregivers (e.g., parents, teachers, school staff, child care staff). The caregivers are asked a series of questions about the problem behavior and related events (i.e., antecedent events and consequences). Typically, a score is derived from this assessment that may be suggestive of behavioral function. Indirect assessments are quick and efficient means of gathering preliminary information about the problem behaviors. However, it is not generally recommended that these assessments be the sole source of information about behavior because of their questionable reliability and validity.

Descriptive analyses involve the quantitative, direct observation of the individual's behaviors as well as antecedent events and consequences under naturalistic conditions (e.g., Bijou, Peterson, & Ault, 1968; Lerman & Iwata, 1993). Conditional probability of occurrence between the behavior and the antecedents/consequences can then be determined. This can help identify a relationship between the problem behavior and environmental events. Descriptive analyses are objective means of gathering more information about variables that may be maintaining a problem behavior. They permit determination of the degree of correspondence between a behavior and environmental events. However, descriptive analyses tend to be time consuming, and because they are correlational, they may not identify the variables that are maintaining the problem behavior.

The most powerful demonstration of the relationship between antecedent and consequent events on problem behaviors consists of the controlled manipulation of these events, typically called a functional analysis (Iwata et al., 1982/1994).

FUNCTIONAL ASSESSMENT AND TREATMENT DEVELOPMENT

Interest in functional assessments as a treatment development tool has increased since the early 1980s (Kahng, Iwata, & Lewin, 2002;

Iwata et al., 1982/1994). This interest and a corresponding body of research has resulted in providing mandates in the Individuals with Disabilities Education Act Amendments of 1997 (IDEA '97; PL 105-17) and the law's 2004 reauthorization (IDEA 2004; PL 108-446) and in being specifically addressed in the No Child Left Behind (NCLB) Act of 2001 (PL 107-110). Using a functional assessment, the antecedent conditions that influence a problem behavior can be identified and changed to reduce the likelihood of the problem behavior. Once identified, the source of reinforcement for the problem behavior can be minimized or eliminated. Then, the reinforcer that maintains the behavior can be used in the behavioral intervention to reduce it. Finally, identification of a behavioral function may permit one to eliminate unnecessary or irrelevant components of a treatment.

The adoption of functional assessments has changed the manner in which behavioral interventions are developed (Mace, 1994). Prior to the advent of functional assessment, individuals attempted to change problem behaviors without consideration of the likely cause. In most cases, this resulted in a standard selection of treatment components. Functional assessment technology has led to hypothesis-based (i.e., function-based) treatment development, which has resulted in an increase in the number of treatment options and the individualization of treatments. When behavioral treatment fails to produce a positive outcome, functional assessment has provided information on factors responsible for the failure. Once the likely maintaining contingencies for problem behavior have been identified, a hypothesis-driven approach to treatment development is possible. Some examples using the previously described types of reinforcement are described next.

Social-Positive Reinforcement

The most basic reinforcement-based intervention for problem behaviors that are maintained by social-positive reinforcement is the termination of the reinforcer, such as attention or access to **tangibles.** This extinction approach typically involves ignoring the problem behavior (e.g., Hagopian, Toole, Long, Bowman, & Lieving, 2004). However, extinction is sometimes associated with initial bursts in the problem behavior, followed by a gradual decrease, and increases in other nontargeted behaviors (Lerman & Iwata, 1996). In most instances, extinction is combined with differential reinforcement procedures, such as differential reinforcement of

other behaviors (DRO) or differential reinforcement of alternative behaviors (DRA). DRO consists of the delivery of reinforcers (e.g., attention) contingent on the absence of problem behaviors. Reinforcers are typically provided after prespecified intervals of time in which the problem behavior has not occurred (e.g., Conyers et al., 2004). DRA is the delivery of the reinforcer contingent on the performance of alternative, more appropriate behaviors. Oftentimes this alternative response takes the form of appropriate communicative responses, such as requesting attention or access to the tangible item (e.g., functional communication training [FCT]; Lerman et al., 2002).

Social-Negative Reinforcement

Procedurally, extinction of problem behaviors that are maintained by social-negative reinforcement is different from extinction of problem behaviors maintained by social-positive reinforcement. Whereas the latter involves terminating (i.e., ignoring) the problem behaviors, extinction of escape-maintained problem behaviors involves preventing escape; that is, the aversive event (e.g., demand) is continued and NOT terminated (Iwata, Pace, Cowdery, et al., 1994). Hypothesis-based differential reinforcement procedures have also been effective in reducing escape-maintained problem behaviors. As with attention-maintained problem behaviors, DRO consists of the delivery of a brief period of escape that is contingent on the absence of problem behavior (Kodak, Miltenberger, & Romaniuk, 2003). DRA typically consists of the delivery of brief escape that is contingent on the performance of alternative behaviors, such as appropriate communication or compliance (Johnson, McComas, Thompson, & Symons, 2004).

Automatic Reinforcement

Although it is difficult to identify the specific source of stimulation for problem behaviors that are maintained by automatic reinforcement, the fact that responding occurs regardless of social stimulation provides useful information for treatment development. Extinction of problem behaviors maintained by automatic reinforcement requires the attenuation or elimination of the source of reinforcement. This typically involves the use of protective equipment, such as mitts or helmets, that permit the occurrence of the behavior, but it minimizes the amount of reinforcement produced by that behavior (Moore, Fisher, & Pennington, 2004).

Another type of treatment focuses on providing stimuli that compete with problem behaviors. These procedures are sometimes referred to as "enriched environments" or "competing stimuli" and consist of the presentation of stimuli that are incompatible with the problem behavior (Piazza et al., 2000). Finally, some studies have attempted to replace the hypothesized source of sensory stimulation produced by the behavior. Although difficult to determine, researchers have provided alterative sources of stimulation based on the appearance of the behavior. For example, studies have provided alternative sources of visual stimulation for individuals who demonstrate self-injury to their eyes (Kennedy, & Souza, 1995), and others have provided alternative, safe items to ingest to eliminate pica, which is the eating of nonfood items (Piazza et al., 2000).

PRACTICAL STRATEGIES FOR THE CLASSROOM

For children and youth with developmental disabilities, the primary venues for operant–learning-based approaches are the home and school. For children older than 5–6 years, in terms of hours per day, the school becomes as important as the home. Teachers should create and design a learning environment that will maximize student performance and minimize the occurrence of maladaptive behaviors. This can be aided by principles of operant learning as described in previous sections. Once assessments have been conducted and the functions of those behaviors considered, the following practical strategies will give teachers some tools to create, improve, and maintain an organized and predictable classroom environment. For the previously described operant learning principles and approaches to be employed effectively, a few organizational matters should be addressed.

Establishing Routines and Schedules

To reduce behavior problems and create an organized, predictable classroom, it is key to establish individual student and classroom schedules. Using schedules in a classroom provides students with predictability and can teach them to tolerate waiting and transitions between activities.

Several types of schedules that can be used, such as picture schedules, word schedules, and checklists. Choosing the appropriate schedule and its design should be influenced by each student's cognitive level, adaptive skills, and motor abilities. For example, a student with minimal reading or word identification skills may benefit most from a picture schedule (McClannahan & Krantz, 1999), with each picture corresponding to an activity or step within an activity (e.g., see Figure 35.3). During a morning routine, a child may be required to remove his or her jacket and bag, place them in a locker, collect materials for an independent activity, and then sit at a desk. Each step would be depicted by a picture that appears on a board or folder and is removed as the step is completed.

Arranging the Classroom for Maximum Impact

The concept of space management and positioning of staff and students can have a powerful effect on behavior, and it is one of the easiest variables to manipulate (e.g., see Figure 35.4). First, it may be necessary to assess the level of supervision each student requires. Some students may need to sit close to the teacher or

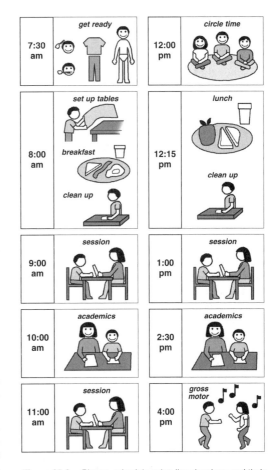

Figure 35.3. Picture schedule using line drawings and their corresponding words.

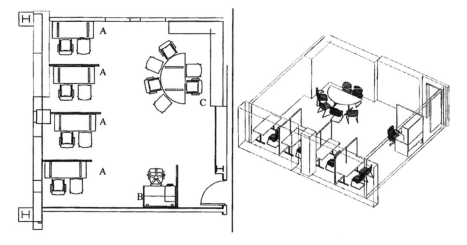

Figure 35.4. Schematic of classroom. (A) Carrels to help decrease visual distraction. This design is used for one-to-one instruction or independent work. (B) A computer workstation, separate from the rest of the stations with a divider to minimize distraction. (C) Table for small group instruction.

might benefit from working one to one with a support staff person, either periodically or for extended periods. Second, the use of individual carrels, and the proper location of them in the room, can reduce distractibility in students with attention problems. If carrels are located in high-traffic areas, it should be determined whether they can be relocated to a quieter or less traveled section of the room. In addition, the location of group activities and lessons should be considered, and if possible, moved away from individual work stations into an area where group work will not be distracting to other students. It is critical to frequently assess auditory and visual stimulation during the day and make modifications as needed for students who are easily distracted.

Providing Instruction

First and foremost, readiness skills such as remaining seated, attending to materials, and listening to instructions are extremely important. If a child is unable to sit in a chair or make eye contact with an instructor, he or she will be more likely to become distracted or focused on irrelevant stimuli. A good strategy for addressing attention problems is to teach students to ready themselves. Each student can be taught a "ready position." For example, before any instruction begins, the students can be prompted to "get ready to learn," meaning that they should sit quietly in their chairs with their feet on the floor and hands on their desk, looking at the instructor, and listening for instructions.

For children who are very distractible, it may be necessary to teach these attending skills one at a time (e.g., sitting, then keeping feet on floor, then keeping hands still, then looking at instructor, and so forth) before beginning to address other educational objectives.

Where and how instructions are given also play an important role in providing an optimal learning environment. For some activities and students, written instructions on the board may be most effective in conjunction with verbal instructions, whereas for other activities and students, tape-recorded instructions may be necessary so that students can replay them as needed. Regardless of the activity, instructions should be determined by student ability and modified based on performance progress.

Just as instructions should be individualized based on activity and ability, the types of instructional materials chosen for each student should to be individualized. These materials may need to address a number of variables including motor abilities, sight limitations, hearing deficits, attention deficits, and student interests. For instance, if a student has a hearing impairment, materials should be visually stimulating. By choosing materials based on these criteria, a teacher is less likely to encounter problem behaviors that arise out of boredom or frustration.

Another important variable is the appropriate arrangement of educational materials. Although material choice that is based on cognitive and motor abilities is important, the presentation of these materials is equally important. The use of easily destroyed or thrown materials with a child who has disruptive behavior will only contribute to these problems. Conversely, the use of Velcro to attach materials to a table could serve to decrease the opportunity for problem behaviors to occur, therefore maximizing the student's opportunity to learn. In addition, it is always a good idea to keep any excess materials out of reach or sight of the student. This will also help in reducing distractions and self-stimulatory or disruptive behaviors.

Finally, prompting procedures (both verbal and nonverbal) are critical tools for improving skill acquisition and minimizing the occurrence of maladaptive behaviors. Prompting procedures should be selected according to the students' abilities, as some students learn best from models whereas others learn best from more restrictive guidance. Severe aggression might warrant use of limited physical prompting, focusing mainly on verbal and gestural models, and extremely disruptive behavior, such as ripping and throwing materials, may require more intrusive physical guidance, at least initially.

These recommendations use arrangements of space, materials, routines, and the like to reduce the probability of problem behavior and increase the occurrence of behavior that is appropriate and necessary for learning skills and academics. This attention to setting events or EOs, as discussed previously, decreases reliance on staff intensive behavioral programs that employ positive and negative social contingencies. These approaches stem from operant learning principles and are just good common sense. Suc-

cessful, experienced teachers have used these techniques for decades.

Reinforcement

Every classroom should have a system of reinforcement. Ideally, this system would include reinforcement programs for both individuals and the group as a whole. However, it is important to remember that individual students have specific preferences and that what works to reinforce appropriate behavior for one student may not work for another. In addition, a student's preferences can change, either gradually or frequently. Therefore, students should be assessed regularly and reinforcement systems changed accordingly. This may seem excessive, but in the end it will save teachers time and energy in dealing with maladaptive behaviors and noncompliance (DeLeon et al., 2001; Hanley, Iwata, & Roscoe, 2006).

Some examples of reinforcement systems that are commonly used in the classroom are token boards and economies, sticker charts, edible and tangible reinforcers (including access to self-stimulatory behaviors), classroom "stores," and earning participation in preferred or extracurricular activities (e.g., see Figure 35.5). In addition, reinforcement may be provided for a variety of contingencies. Students may earn tokens, for instance, for the absence of a problem behavior, the completion of some specified task, or the appropriate communication of a want or need. Furthermore, the frequency at which

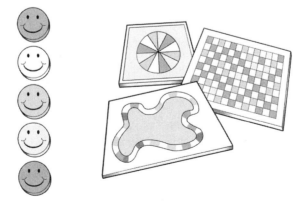

5 tokens = 5 minutes of playing a board game of Michael's choice

Figure 35.5. Example of a token board. The icon on the right is the reinforcer for which the child is working.

these reinforcers should be delivered is determined by a number of factors, including the student's skill level, compliance, and motivation. It is common practice to deliver reinforcement more frequently when a system is first initiated and then gradually thin the schedule of reinforcement as student compliance and behavior problems improve. As the frequency of reinforcement is decreased, it may be beneficial to provide visual cues (e.g., tokens, pieces of a puzzle) that indicate progress toward receipt of a reinforcer (McClannahan & Krantz, 1999).

BEHAVIORAL TEACHING STRATEGIES

Goals of Effective Teaching

Teachers are rarely satisfied if their students can perform a new skill or behavior accurately but only with considerable assistance and under simplified conditions. Rather, instruction is considered effective when learners can perform the skills taught accurately, independently, and in situations outside of training, or what is termed generalization (Alberto & Troutman, 2006; Stokes & Baer, 1977). Common forms of generalization include performing the same skill when the stimuli that signal it differ in some way (e.g., saying "cat" when the letters of the word are typed in different fonts), performing the same skill when the stimuli that signal it are presented in different contexts (e.g., saying "cat" when the word appears in different sentences), and combining different skills in ways that were not trained (e.g., pointing to a picture of a cat when shown the word).

A prerequisite to all forms of generalization is the development of stimulus control, or bringing the learner's response under the control of certain key stimuli. Stimulus control does not happen all at once but accumulates gradually over time as learners are given multiple opportunities to practice skills with feedback and reinforcement. Notice that as practice progresses, two types of learning take place: *how* to perform the behavior correctly (e.g., tearing lettuce into bite-sized pieces) and *when* performance of the behavior will be reinforced (e.g., in response to the instruction, "Let's make a salad"). Key factors in the development of stimulus control are the ability to perform the behavior, differential reinforcement of correct responding, and attention to the relevant situational cues that signal that the behavior will be reinforced. Early in training, a learner's response becomes more accurate and eventually efficient as a result of feedback and reinforcement. At the same time, the key features of stimuli that control responding become more evident, making them easier to detect across learning trials. Later in training, when nonessential features of the controlling stimuli are varied (e.g., font of text, person giving the command) or their context changes, stimulus control enables the learner to continue responding correctly. Stimulus control and generalization, therefore, can be viewed as two ends of a skill-training continuum that are linked in the middle by repeated practice opportunities together with feedback and reinforcement.

Tailoring Instruction to Student Performance Levels

Whether learning to read, prepare meals, or engage in leisure or sporting activities, mastery of a skill is attained through a sequence of stages referred to as the instructional hierarchy (Martens & Witt, 2004). This describes behaviors to be learned, not by their form (e.g., single-digit addition, sums to 18), but by the level of proficiency with which they are performed (e.g., at least 90% of problems correct with assistance, at least 20 digits correct per minute in the face of distraction). Each stage of the instructional hierarchy (i.e., acquisition, fluency and maintenance, and generalization) can be described by a different training goal, performance measure, and associated set of teaching strategies. Once the training goal at each stage is reached, opportunities for learning are maximized by then "shifting" instruction to the next stage. The instructional hierarchy is an important teaching tool for several reasons. First, it offers a practical description of how performance improves over time that can be applied to a wide range of behaviors and skills. Second, because learning at each stage of the instructional hierarchy is promoted in different ways, knowing how well a learner performs a skill enables one to select the most effective teaching strategy for that student's proficiency level (Daly, Lentz, & Boyer, 1996). Third, frequent performance monitoring allows one to change teaching procedures as needed in order to maximize practice opportunities, minimize errors, and avoid escape-motivated problem behavior. In this respect, behavioral approaches to effective teaching require educators to be active and responsive in changing their instructional activities as a learner's skills improve.

Acquisition   The goal of training at the first stage, acquisition, is for learners to perform a new skill or behavior accurately on repeated occasions without assistance. Performance measures during acquisition typically include number or percent correct attempts, number or percent errors, and type of assistance provided. Because acquisition-level training involves first attempts at new skills and behaviors, some learners have difficulty acquiring the skill in its natural context. For these students, teaching the skill in isolation first can be effective. This requires teachers to guide students through a number of discrete practice opportunities with assistance (prompting), feedback, and reinforcement, or what are termed learning trials (Alberto & Troutman, 2006). A complete learning trial refers to an opportunity to practice a skill that is controlled by the trainer. Complete learning trials include several components as illustrated in the following example: 1) a task direction that includes key stimuli (saying, "Pick up the *fork*"), 2) a controlling prompt (picking up another fork as a model), 3) an opportunity to respond (waiting 10 seconds), 4) corrective feedback for incorrect responses (providing hand-over-hand guidance), and 5) reinforcement for correct responding (the child's taking a bite of a preferred food item). Although prompts may take a variety of forms (i.e., gesturing, verbal instructions, modeling, pictures, partial physical guidance, full physical guidance), controlling prompts consistently produce the correct response.

Once a learner can perform a skill accurately with a certain amount of assistance, the assistance is withdrawn or gradually faded until the skill can be performed accurately and independently. Numerous procedures for systematically **fading** prompts have been reported in the literature and include the following (Alberto & Troutman, 2006):

1. *Prompt and test,* in which a set number of prompted trials are followed by unprompted test trials to assess learning

2. *Prompt and fade,* in which the prompt presented on initial trials is gradually withdrawn on later trials

3. *Most-to-least prompting,* in which successively less intrusive prompts from a hierarchy are presented after learners meet a performance criterion at each level

4. *Least-to-most prompting,* in which successively more intrusive prompts from a hier-

archy are presented if needed after a delay on each trial

5. ***Graduated guidance,*** in which prompts are provided as needed

6. *Time delay* (constant or progressive), in which the trainer delays presenting the controlling prompt after the key stimulus is presented

The careful use and gradual withdrawal of prompts during acquisition enables accuracy goals to be reached with few or no errors, promotes positive interactions between teachers and learners as well as high rates of reinforcement, reduces problem behavior that is motivated by escape or avoidance, and decreases the chances of practicing errors.

Fluency and Maintenance   During fluency building, the goal is to perform an already acquired skill accurately but at higher rates as indexed by the frequency of correct responses during brief timings (e.g., the number of letter sounds read correctly in 1 minute; McDowell & Keenan, 2001). In order for practice time to be productive, it should include 1) tasks and/or materials that the learner can respond to with high accuracy and minimal assistance (i.e., instructionally matched materials); 2) brief, repeated practice opportunities with feedback and reinforcement; 3) monitoring and charting of performance; and 4) performance criteria for changing to more difficult material (Chard, Vaughn, & Tyler, 2002; Martens & Witt, 2004). Implicit in these requirements is the need to assemble a large enough pool of materials, sequenced by difficulty and of sufficient variety, in order to allow for repeated practice opportunities over time. Students are initially assigned material to which they can respond with high accuracy but minimum fluency (e.g., at least 90% accuracy and between 50 and 70 words correct per minute in reading). When students reach the performance goal on material at this level (e.g., 100 words correct per minute on grade-one passages), practice begins again using more difficult material (e.g., grade-two passages), and the sequence is repeated. Two aspects of this sequence are noteworthy. First, fluency building is a dynamic process that requires periodic changes in practice material to ensure that it is matched to the student's proficiency level. Second, when using instructionally matched material, students require less assistance to respond correctly. This means that practice can still be productive in the absence of direct teacher involvement.

Because fluency building occurs gradually and involves a variety of tasks and materials, students are inevitably exposed to both programmed variations (e.g., different types of clothing and fasteners when learning to dress) and naturally occurring variation (e.g., interruptions by staff, dropped clothing items) in the stimulus conditions surrounding performance. Under such conditions, practice to high levels of fluency promotes the generalization of responding in two ways. First, as performance becomes more efficient and even automatic, it becomes easier to execute at different times and in different contexts (Goldstein & Martens, 2000). Second, when correct performance is reinforced under different practice conditions and with different materials, relevant dimensions of the key stimuli that control behavior become more easily recognized. From this perspective, the benefits of fluency building result, not only from increases in response rate per se (Doughty, Chase, & O'Shields, 2004) but also from the stimulus control and stimulus generalization of prolonged practice under varying conditions.

In order to prepare both typically developing children and children with disabilities for testing that is mandated by NCLB, public educators emphasize the training of complex composite skills (e.g., reading a word problem in math, executing the relevant computations, graphing or writing a narrative of the answer) instead of basic component skills (e.g., fluency with multiplication facts). Fluency researchers advocate the opposite approach and have found an interesting, albeit counterintuitive, benefit of devoting time to basic skill practice. As learners develop basic component skills to higher levels of fluency, less instruction and assistance is needed to perform more difficult tasks (Johnson & Layng, 1996).

Generalization The goal of generalization training is to achieve accurate and rapid performance of behavior in the natural environment or in situations that differ from previous training levels. Generalization is best promoted by reinforcing the correct use and application of skills with diverse materials, people, or contexts (Alberto & Troutman, 2006). By varying practice conditions, learners gain experience in responding to key stimuli in different contexts (e.g., identifying the symbol for *men* on bathroom doors in different public locations) and responding to key stimuli that differ in non-

essential ways (e.g., identifying different symbols for *men* on bathroom doors).

Based on the principle of stimulus control, a rule of thumb for promoting generalization is that skills trained in one condition will transfer to another condition to the extent that the two conditions are identical (i.e., contain the same key stimuli or reinforce the same behaviors in the same way). In order to promote generalization, training can occur in the natural environment or training conditions can be made to resemble the natural environment in terms of stimuli, behaviors, or reinforcers. Focusing on stimuli has involved using common people or objects as props, training in multiple and varied settings, using multiple trainers, or using a range of stimulus examples (Lumley et al., 1998). Focusing on behaviors has included training to high levels of fluency, as discussed previously (Johnson & Layng, 1996); training behaviors that are useful in a variety of settings (e.g., functional communication training; Charlop-Christy et al., 2002), or training behaviors that remind the child of what to do (e.g., self-instruction training; Mithaug & Mithaug, 2003). Finally, focusing on reinforcers has involved using reinforcers from the natural environment during training trials, providing reinforcement on an irregular schedule and thereby encouraging persistence, and teaching children to recruit reinforcement (Craft, Alber, & Heward, 1998).

BEHAVIORAL INSTRUCTION PROGRAMS

Direct instruction (DI) is a behavioral instruction program based on the instructional hierarchy that uses scripted routines to promote the development of student skills (Adams & Engelmann, 1996; Carnine, Silbert, & Kameenui, 1997). DI lessons are characterized by clear instructions and materials, frequent opportunities to respond to both examples and nonexamples, and consistent consequences for correct responding (Daly et al., 1996). Research suggests that students receiving DI outperform those receiving all other instructional programs on basic skill, comprehension, and affective measures (Adams & Engelmann, 1996; Watkins, 1997). Nevertheless, DI was never promoted or disseminated on a large scale, and the majority of preservice special education teachers continue to receive little or no training in the DI model (Begeny & Martens, 2006).

Precision teaching (PT) is a behavioral instruction and monitoring program, also based on the instructional hierarchy, that emphasizes practicing skills to high levels of fluency and performance charting (Binder, 1996). PT involves daily, timed practices of basic skills (e.g., writing answers to math problems or reading aloud for 1 minute) until learners reach fluency levels high enough to promote maintenance and application (i.e., Retention, Endurance, Stability, Application, and Adduction [RESAA] fluency aims). Frequencies of performance during these brief, timed practices (e.g., 50 words correct per minute) are displayed on charts that make it easy for teachers to see changes in learning rate. The charts, in turn, are used to evaluate the effectiveness of instruction and to make changes as needed. Students in PT classroom have been shown to gain between two and three grade levels per year on group-administered achievement tests (Johnson & Layng, 1992).

SUMMARY

The decades since the 1950s have proven to be a dynamic period of advancement in the support provided by society to individuals with developmental disabilities. Behavioral research, based on operant learning theory, has resulted in innovative and effective approaches that have led to significant improvements in the lives of individuals with developmental disabilities. Much of this research has focused on making socially significant changes to harmful behaviors, as well as improvements in skills necessary for success in everyday community living.

REFERENCES

Adams, G.L., & Engelmann, S. (1996). *Research on Direct instruction: 25 years beyond DISTAR*. Seattle: Educational Achievement systems.

Alberto, P.A., & Troutman, A.C. (2006). *Applied behavior analysis for teachers* (7th ed.). Upper Saddle River, NJ: Prentice Hall.

Ayllon, T., & Michael, J. (1959). The psychiatric nurse as a behavioral engineer. *Journal of the Experimental Analysis of Behavior, 2*, 323–334.

Baer, D.M., Wolf, M.M., & Risley, T.R. (1968). Some current dimensions of applied behavior analysis. *Journal of Applied Behavior Analysis, 1*, 91–97.

Baghdadli, A., Pascal, C., Grisi, S., et al. (2003). Risk factors for self-injurious behaviours among 222 young children with autistic disorders. *Journal of Intellectual Disability Research, 47*, 622.

Begeny, J.C., & Martens, B.K. (2006). Assessing pre-service teachers' training in empirically-validated behavioral instruction practices. *School Psychology Quarterly, 21*, 262–285.

Bijou, S.W., Peterson, R.F., & Ault, M.H. (1968). A method to integrate descriptive and experimental field studies at the level of data and empirical concepts. *Journal of Applied Behavior Analysis, 1*, 175–191.

Binder, C. (1996). Behavioral fluency: Evolution of a new paradigm. *The Behavior Analyst, 19*, 163–197.

Bowman, L.G., Fisher, W.W., Thompson, R.H., et al. (1997). On the relation of mands and the function of destructive behavior. *Journal of Applied Behavior Analysis, 30*, 251–266.

Carnine, D., Silbert, J., & Kameenui, E. (1997). *Direct instruction reading* (3rd ed.). Upper Saddle River, NJ: Prentice Hall.

Carr, E.G., & Durand, V.M. (1985). Reducing behavior problems through functional communication training. *Journal of Applied Behavior Analysis, 18*, 111–126.

Carr, E.G., Newsom, C.D., & Binkoff, J.A. (1976). Stimulus control of self-destructive behavior in a psychotic child. *Journal of Abnormal Child Psychology, 4*, 139–153.

Cataldo, M.F., & Harris, J. (1982). The biological basis for self-injury in the mentally retarded. *Analysis and Intervention in Developmental Disabilities, 2*, 21–39.

Chadwick, O., Piroth, N., Walker, J., et al. (2000). Factors affecting the risk of behavior problems in children with severe intellectual disability. *Journal of Intellectual Disability Research, 44*, 108–123.

Chard, D.J., Vaughn, S., & Tyler, B.J. (2002). A synthesis of research on effective interventions for building reading fluency with elementary students with learning disabilities. *Journal of Learning Disabilities, 35*, 386–406.

Charlop-Christy, M.H., Carpenter, M., Le, L., et al. (2002). Using the Picture Exchange Communication System (PECS) with children with autism: Assessment of PECS acquisition, speech, social-communicative behavior, and problem behavior. *Journal of Applied Behavior Analysis, 35*, 213–231.

Conyers, C., Miltenberger, R., Maki, A., et al. (2004). A comparison of response cost and differential reinforcement of other behavior to reduce disruptive behavior in a preschool classroom. *Journal of Applied Behavior Analysis, 37*, 411–415.

Craft, M.A., Alber, S.R., & Heward, W.L. (1998). Teaching elementary students with developmental disabilities to recruit teacher attention in a general education classroom: Effects on teacher praise and academic productivity. *Journal of Applied Behavior Analysis, 31*, 399–415.

Crosland, K.A., Zarcone, J.R., Lindauer, S.E., et al. (2003). Use of functional analysis methodology in the evaluation of medication effects. *Journal of Autism and Developmental Disorders, 33*, 271–279.

Daly, E.J., III, Lentz, F.E., & Boyer, J. (1996). The instructional hierarchy: A conceptual model for understanding the effective components of reading interventions. *School Psychology Quarterly, 11*, 369–386.

DeLeon, I.G., Fisher, W.W., Rodriguez-Catter, V., et al. (2001). Examination of relative reinforcement effects of stimuli identified through pretreatment and daily brief preference assessments. *Journal of Applied Behavior Analysis, 34*, 463–473.

Doughty, S.S., Chase, P.N., & O'Shields, E.M. (2004). Effects of rate building on fluent performance: A review and commentary. *The Behavior Analyst, 27*, 7–23.

Durand, V.M., & Crimmins, D.B. (1988). Identifying the variables maintaining self-injurious behavior. *Journal of Autism and Developmental Disorders, 18*, 99–117.

Fisher, W.W., Ninness, H.A.C., Piazza, C.C., et al. (1996). On the reinforcing effects of the content of verbal attention. *Journal of Applied Behavior Analysis, 29*, 235–238.

Friman, P.C. (1990). Concurrent habits: What would Linus do with his blanket if his thumb sucking were treated? *American Journal of Diseases of Children, 144*, 1316–1318.

Friman, P.C. (2005). Behavioral pediatrics. In M. Hersen (Ed.), *Encyclopedia of behavior modification and therapy Vol. II* (pp. 731–739). Thousand Oaks, CA: Sage Publications.

Friman, P.C., Barone, V.J., & Christophersen, E.R. (1986). Aversive taste treatment of finger and thumb sucking. *Pediatrics, 78*, 174–176.

Friman, P.C., & Blum, N.J. (2003). Primary care behavioral pediatrics. M. Hersen & W. Sledge (Eds.), *Encyclopedia of psychotherapy* (pp. 379–399). San Diego: Academic Press.

Friman, P.C., Byrd, M.R., & Oksol, E.M. (2001). Oral digital habits: Demographics, phenomenology, causes, functions, and clinical associations. In D.W. Woods & R. Miltenberger (Eds.), *Tic disorders, trichotillomania, and other repetitive behavior disorders: Behavioral approaches to analysis and treatment* (pp. 197–222). New York: Kluwer Academic/Plenum Publishers.

Friman, P.C., Hoff, K.E., Schnoes, C., et al. (1999). The bedtime pass: An approach to bedtime crying and leaving the room. *Archives of Pediatrics and Adolescent Medicine, 153*, 1027–1029.

Friman, P.C., & Leibowitz, J.M. (1990). An effective and acceptable treatment alternative for chronic thumb and finger sucking. *The Journal of Pediatric Psychology, 15*, 57–65.

Friman, P.C., & Vollmer, D. (1995). Successful use of the nocturnal urine alarm for diurnal enuresis. *Journal of Applied Behavior Analysis, 28*, 89–91.

Goldstein, A.P., & Martens, B.K. (2000). *Lasting change: Methods for enhancing generalization of gain.* Champaign, IL: Research Press.

Hagopian, L.P., Toole, L.M., Long, E.S., et al. (2004). A comparison of dense-to-lean and fixed lean schedules of alternative reinforcement and extinction. *Journal of Applied Behavior Analysis, 37*, 323–337.

Hanley, G.P., Iwata, B.A., & Roscoe, E.M. (2006). Some determinants of changes in preference over time. *Journal of Applied Behavior Analysis, 39*, 189–202.

Individuals with Disabilities Education Act Amendments of 1997, PL 105-17, 20 U.S.C. §§ 1400 *et seq.*

Individuals with Disabilities Education Improvement Act of 2004, PL 108-446, 20 U.S.C. §§ 1400 *et seq.*

Iwata, B.A., Dorsey, M.F., Slifer, K.J., et al. (1994). Toward a functional analysis of self-injury. *Journal of Applied Behavior Analysis, 27*, 197–209. (Reprinted from *Analysis and Intervention in Developmental Disabilities, 2*, 3–20, 1982)

Iwata, B.A., Pace, G.M., Cowdery, G.E., et al. (1994). What makes extinction work: An analysis of procedural form and function. *Journal of Applied Behavior Analysis, 27*, 131–144.

Iwata, B.A., Pace, G.M., Dorsey, M.F., et al. (1994). The functions of self-injurious behavior: An experimental-epidemiological analysis. *Journal of Applied Behavior Analysis, 27*, 215–240.

Iwata, B.A., Kahng, S., Wallace, M.D., et al. (2000). Functional analysis of behavior disorders. In J. Austin & J.E. Carr (Eds.), *Handbook of applied behavior analysis* (pp. 61–89). Reno, NV: Context Press.

Johnson, K.R., & Layng, T.V.J. (1992). Breaking the structuralist barrier: Literacy and numeracy with fluency. *American Psychologist, 47*, 1475–1490.

Johnson, K.R., & Layng, T.V.J. (1996). On terms and procedures: Fluency. *The Behavior Analyst, 19*, 281–288.

Johnson, L., McComas, J., Thompson, A., et al. (2004). Obtained versus programmed reinforcement: Practical considerations in the treatment of escape-reinforced aggression. *Journal of Applied Behavior Analysis, 37*, 239–242.

Kahng, S., Iwata, B.A., & Lewin, A. (2002). The impact of functional assessment on the treatment of self-injurious behavior. In S. Schroeder, M.L. Oster-Granite, & T. Thompson (Eds.), *Self-injurious behavior: Gene-brain-behavior relationships* (pp. 119–131). Washington, DC: American Psychological Association.

Kennedy, C.H., & Meyer, K.A. (1996). Sleep deprivation, allergy symptoms, and negatively reinforced problem behavior. *Journal of Applied Behavior Analysis, 29*, 133–135.

Kennedy, C.H., & Souza, G. (1995). Functional analysis and treatment of eye poking. *Journal of Applied Behavior Analysis, 28*, 27–37.

Kodak, T., Miltenberger, R.G., & Romaniuk, C. (2003). A comparison of differential reinforcement and noncontingent reinforcement for the treatment of a child's multiply controlled problem behavior. *Behavioral Interventions, 18*, 267–278.

Lerman, D.C., & Iwata, B.A. (1993). Descriptive and experimental analyses of variables maintaining self-injurious behavior. *Journal of Applied Behavior Analysis, 26*, 293–319.

Lerman, D.C., & Iwata, B.A. (1996). Developing a technology for the use of operant extinction in clinical settings: An examination of basic and applied research. *Journal of Applied Behavior Analysis, 29*, 345–382.

Lerman, D.C., Kelley, M.E., Vorndran, C.M., et al. (2002). Reinforcement magnitude and responding during treatment with differential reinforcement. *Journal of Applied Behavior Analysis, 35*, 29–48.

Levy, R.M., & Rubenstein, L.S. (1996). *The rights of people with mental disabilities: The authoritative ACLU guide to the rights of people with mental illness and intellectual disability.* Carbondale: Southern Illinois University.

Lovaas, O.I., Freitag, G., Gold, V.J., et al. (1965). Experimental studies in childhood schizophrenia: Analysis of self-destructive behavior. *Journal of Experimental Child Psychology, 2*, 67–84.

Lumley, V.A., Miltenberger, R.G., Long, E.S., et al. (1998). Evaluation of sexual abuse prevention program for adults with intellectual disability. *Journal of Applied Behavior Analysis, 31*, 91–101.

Mace, F.C. (1994). The significance and future of functional analysis methodologies. *Journal of Applied Behavior Analysis, 27*, 385–384.

Magee, S.K., & Ellis, J. (2001). The detrimental effects of physical restraint as a consequence for inappropriate classroom behavior. *Journal of Applied Behavior Analysis, 34*, 501–504.

Marcus, B.A., & Vollmer, T.R. (1995). Effects of differential negative reinforcement on disruption and compliance. *Journal of Applied Behavior Analysis, 28*, 229–230.

Marcus, B.A., Vollmer, T.R., Swanson, V., et al. (2001). An experimental analysis of aggression. *Behavior Modification, 25*, 189–213.

Martens, B.K., & Witt, J.C. (2004). Competence, persistence, and success: The positive psychology of behavioral skill instruction. *Psychology in the Schools, 41*, 19–30.

Matson, J.L., Bamburg, J.W., Cherry, K.E., et al. (1999). A validity study on the Questions About Behavioral Function (QABF) scale: Predicting treatment success for self-injury, aggression, and stereotypies. *Research in Developmental Disabilities, 20*, 163–176.

McClannahan, L.E, & Krantz, P.J. (1999). *Activity schedules for children with autism: Teaching independent behavior.* Bethesda, MD: Woodbine House.

McComas, J.J., Thompson, A., & Johnson, L. (2003). The effects of presession attention on problem behavior maintained by different reinforcers. *Journal of Applied Behavior Analysis, 36*, 297–307.

McDowell, C., & Keenan, M. (2001). Developing fluency and endurance in a child diagnosed with attention deficit hyperactivity disorder. *Journal of Applied Behavior Analysis, 34*, 345–348.

Michael, J. (2000). Implications and refinements of the establishing operation concept. *Journal of Applied Behavior Analysis, 33*, 401–410

Mithaug, D.K., & Mithaug, D.E. (2003). Effects of teacher-directed versus student-directed instruction on self-management of young children with disabilities. *Journal of Applied Behavior Analysis, 36*, 133–136.

Moore, J.W., Fisher, W.W., & Pennington, A. (2004). Systematic application and removal of protective equipment in the assessment of multiple topographies of self-injury. *Journal of Applied Behavior Analysis*(37), 73–77.

National Institutes of Health. (1991). *Treatment of destructive behaviors in persons with developmental disabilities.* Washington, DC: U.S. Department of Health and Human Services.

No Child Left Behind Act of 2001, PL 107-110, 115 Stat. 1425, 20 U.S.C. §§ 6301 *et seq.*

Nyhan, W.L. (2002). Lessons from Lesch-Nyhan Syndrome. In S. Schroeder, M.L. Oster-Granite, & T. Thompson (Eds.), *Self-injurious behavior: Gene-brain-behavior relationships* (pp. 251–267). Washington, DC: American Psychological Association.

O'Reilly, M.F., & Lancioni, G. (2000). Response covariation of escape-maintained aberrant behavior correlated with sleep deprivation. *Research in Developmental Disabilities, 21*, 125–136.

O'Reilly, M., Sigafoos, J., Edrisinha, C., et al. (2006). A preliminary examination of the evocative effects of the establishing operation. *Journal of Applied Behavior Analysis, 39*, 239–242.

Pelios, L., Morren, J., Tesch, D., et al. (1999). The impact of functional analysis methodology on treatment choice for self-injurious and aggressive behavior. *Journal of Applied Behavior Analysis, 32*, 185–195.

Piazza, C.C., Adelinis, J.D., Hanley, G.P., et al. (2000). An evaluation of the effects of matched stimuli on behaviors maintained by automatic reinforcement. *Journal of Applied Behavior Analysis, 33*, 13–27.

Stokes, T.F., & Baer, D.M. (1977). An implicit technology of generalization. *Journal of Applied Behavior Analysis, 10*, 349–367.

Tarbox, R., Williams, L., & Friman, P.C. (2004). Extended diaper wearing: Effects on continence in and out of the diaper. *Journal of Applied Behavior Analysis, 37*, 97–101.

Vaughan, M.E., & Michael, J. (1982). Automatic reinforcement: An important but ignored concept. *Behaviorism, 10*, 217–227.

Vollmer, T.R. (1994). The concept of automatic reinforcement: Implications for behavioral research in developmental disabilities. *Research in Developmental Disabilities, 15*, 187–207.

Watkins, C.L. (1997). *Project Follow Through: A case study of contingencies influencing instructional practices of the educational establishment.* Concord, MA: Cambridge Center for Behavioral Studies.

Woods, D.W., & Miltenberger, R. (2001). *Tic disorders, trichotillomania, and other repetitive behavior disorders: Behavioral approaches to analysis and treatment.* New York: Kluwer Academic/Plenum Publishers.

36 Technological Assistance

Larry W. Desch

Upon completion of this chapter, the reader will

- Know the definitions of *assistive technology* and *medical assistive technology*
- Be aware of the types of both rehabilitative and medical assistive technology and examples of each
- Understand conditions leading to a need for assistive technology
- Understand the basics of assessment and funding for assistive technology

The goal of this chapter is to provide information about the categories of currently available rehabilitative and medical technology assistance and the process for evaluating their use and effectiveness. This chapter does not address complementary, or alternative, therapies—for example, devices using unproven or disproven methodologies, such as colored lenses for treatment of dyslexia (Committee on Children with Disabilities, 1998). The devices discussed in this chapter have at least some basic empirical or scientific evidence to document their effectiveness. The chapter also focuses on "mid-tech" and "high-tech" devices, as "low-tech" devices are discussed in Chapter 37.

Many children with disabilities are able to have more independent function through the use of assistive, adaptive, or augmentative devices. Although definitions for these devices vary, there seems to be some consensus emerging. Assistive devices are those that help alleviate the impact of a disability, thus reducing the functional limitations (e.g., tape-recorded lessons for students with a specific reading disability). Adaptive technology substitutes or makes up for the loss of function brought on by a disability (e.g., a sophisticated robotic feeding device provides independence for people with spastic quadriplegia). Augmentative devices increase an area of functioning that is deficient, sometimes severely, but for which there are some residual abilities (e.g., a microchip-powered voice output augmentative device for a person with dysarthria). The term *augmentative devices*

currently only refers to devices used to improve communication. In this chapter, the term *assistive* is used to encompass all of these terms. The chapter uses this general term for medical devices as well. *Medical assistive technology refers* to that subset of assistive technology that is used for primarily medical or life-sustaining reasons (e.g., ventilators, feeding pumps). These devices also improve functioning, but perhaps in more basic ways.

For many years, assistive technology (sometimes called "AT") has been thought of as referring only to devices containing microcomputers or other electronics. Although such complicated devices may be the only answer for a particular disability-related problem, they represent the higher end of the spectrum of assistive technology that includes low-tech, mid-tech, and high-tech (and everything in between) (Desch, 1986). Many people, even professionals working in the field, do not realize that they may themselves be using assistive technology on a daily basis. For example, a foam or rubber cushion placed over a pencil or pen to help with one's grip and prevent writer's cramp is a low-tech assistive device. However, the use of assistive technology is usually reserved for people with considerably more loss of function due to disability.

Table 36.1 provides examples of assistive devices. Some items on the table are low-tech assistive technology—that is, those using low-cost materials and not requiring batteries or other electric sources to operate. Examples include wheelchair ramps, gastrostomy feeding tubes, and printed picture communication boards.

Table 36.1.　Examples of available assistive devices

Area of disability	Type of technology		
	Low-tech	Mid-tech	High-tech
Physical	Swivel spoon (and other feeding aids)	Reciprocating gait orthosis	Electronically controlled/ adapted wheelchairs
	Wheelchair ramps	Lightweight wheelchairs	Environmental control units
	Adapted playgrounds	Adapted toys	Robotic devices
	Most orthotics		Functional electric stimulation
	Grips for pencils		Voice input and eye gaze input devices
Communication	Simple picture/word boards	On/off light for yes/no responses	Adapted laptops
	Eye gaze picture boards	Digital voice recorder	Commercially available computerized devices (e.g., TouchTalker)
	Visual schedule/planner	Scanning light board	
Sensory	Magnifying lenses	Alerting systems (to movement/sound)	Digital hearing aids
	Large-print books	Braille typewriters	Cochlear implants
	Books on tape	FM transmitting	Kurzweil 1000 voice output computer
Learning	Color-coded notebooks	Talking calculators	Kurzweil 3000 reading software
	Post-it notes	Electronic spelling/ dictionary	Hypertext learning programs
	Flash-cards	Tape recorders	Software for cognitive/attention rehabilitation
	Visual schedule/planner	Books on tape	
Medical assistance	Nasogastric tubes	Oxygen systems	Home ventilators
	Bladder catheters	Gastrostomy tubes	Oxygen monitors
		Indwelling intravenous (IV) tubes	Apnea monitors
			Dialysis machines

Mid-tech devices generally require battery/ electrical power or are more complex in their use—for example, teletypewriter (TTY) devices for those who are deaf, home-infusion pumps, suction machines, and sophisticated manual wheelchairs. Finally, high-tech devices are those that are complicated and often expensive to own and maintain. Examples include microcomputer-enabled voice output devices, home ventilators, cochlear implants, and electronic wheelchairs.

Assistive devices, across the spectrum, are acquired in one of three ways: 1) direct purchase from a commercial supplier; 2) development of a custom-made device (these can be simple, handmade devices or complex, one-of-a-kind devices made by an engineer or technician for use by one person); or 3) modification of an existing device such as a desktop computer, laptop computer, or telephone (these modifications can also be commercially available items). Some of these modified devices are constructed at rehabilitation centers at a high cost. However, the

availability of microprocessing technology has increased such that the purchase of commercial devices or commercial modifications to devices is becoming the most common way to acquire even the most complex, high-tech assistive devices. Where assistive devices can be obtained also varies, from public schools and therapy providers to large university or private rehabilitation centers. Most assistive devices, excluding the medical assistive devices, can be obtained without prescriptions from physicians.

BRIAN

Brian is a 10-year-old who, according to his mother, is doing "just wonderful," but this was not always so. Brian was born 8 weeks premature and had severe hyperbilirubinemia (jaundice) due to blood group incompatibility and neonatal sepsis (a blood infection). He spent more than a month in the neonatal intensive care unit. Initially, he was placed on a ventilator for help with breathing. Brian also had occasional episodes of apnea and bradycardia (periodic breathing arrests accompanied by low heart rate) and was sent home on a cardiorespiratory monitor. At 6 months of age, he had severe oral-motor feeding problems and gastroesophageal reflux (GER) that led to placement of a gastrojejunal tube. This required Brian's parents to learn how to use a feeding pump that would give him formula over several hours. At 18 months of age, Brian was diagnosed with severe dyskinetic cerebral palsy and his mother was told that he would never walk. His mother, however, always had high hopes for Brian, and at the age of 3 years, Brian obtained a power wheelchair that he began using both at home and school. He also used a special spoon so that he could better control getting food to his mouth. Brian became quite a good artist by using low-tech splints to help him hold paint brushes and crayons. Although Brian's family usually comprehended his speech, his peers at school had trouble understanding him, and at age 5 years Brian obtained a computerized voice output device. He has not stopped "talking" since.

TECHNOLOGY FOR MEDICAL ASSISTANCE

The Office of Technology Assessment (OTA) defines a child who receives medical technology assistance as one "who requires a mechanical device and substantial daily skilled nursing care to avert death or further disability" (OTA, 1987). These medical devices replace or augment a vital body function and include respiratory technology assistance (e.g., nasal cannulae for oxygen supplementation, mechanical ventilators, positive airway pressure devices, artificial airways such as tracheotomy tubes), surveillance devices (e.g., cardiorespiratory monitors, pulse oximeters), nutritive assistive devices (e.g., nasogastric or gastrostomy feeding tubes), equipment for **intravenous (IV)** therapy (e.g., parenteral nutrition, medication infusion), devices to augment or protect kidney function (e.g., dialysis, urethral catheterization), and ostomies (e.g., gastrostomy, colostomy). The use of medical technology assistance by children is uncommon—occurring in only 1 per 1,000 children—and most of these uses are temporary (e.g., following premature birth, injury, or surgery) (Storgion, 1996). The incidence does appear to be increasing, however, in children younger than

1 year of age, primarily as a result of improved survival of very low birth weight infants. In a 1987–1990 survey of children in Massachusetts who are dependent on technology, more than half (57%) had neurological involvement, and 13% had multisystem involvement (Palfrey et al., 1994). The types of medical assistive devices that are required in a number of these are described next (see also Table 36.1 for a summary).

Respiratory Support

Infants and children who require respiratory support most often fall into one of two categories: 1) those with problems with their lungs and/or hearts, and 2) those with problems with neurological control of breathing and/or weakness of the muscles used to control breathing. As an example of the first category, severe damage to the lungs related to prematurity, called bronchopulmonary dysplasia, can lead to the prolonged need for supplemental oxygen (Bass et al., 2004; see Chapter 9). Another example is the child with spastic quadriplegic cerebral palsy who may develop a severe scoliosis (curvature of the spine), leading to rib cage distortion and stiffness (see Chapter 26). This chest wall abnormality can cause a decrease in respiratory muscle power and lung function necessitating supplemental oxygen. An example of the second category is neuromuscular disorders, including Duchenne muscular dystrophy and spinal muscular atrophy (Bush et al., 2005; Gilgoff et al., 2003; see Chapter 14).

Children who have chronic respiratory failure require medical technology assistance to maintain normal oxygen levels in the blood, prevent additional lung injury from recurrent infections, and promote optimal growth and development. These goals usually can be accomplished via a combination of oxygen supplementation, continuous positive airway pressure (CPAP), chest physiotherapy (CPT), suctioning, and medications (e.g., bronchodilators). When these treatments are ineffective or insufficient, however, mechanical ventilation and tracheostomy tube placement are considered. Equipment that is used to monitor the child's cardiorespiratory status may also be required (e.g., heart rate and blood oxygen monitors).

Oxygen is the single most effective agent in treating the infant or child with chronic lung disease, and supplemental oxygen may be required for months or even years. Oxygen can be administered by nasal cannulae (plastic prongs placed in the nose and connected to a tube that delivers an oxygen/air mixture), facemask, oxygen tent or hood, or an artificial airway (e.g., tracheostomy).

For the child with mild respiratory failure or obstructive sleep apnea, CPAP may be employed (Downey, Perkin, & MacQuarrie, 2000). CPAP can be applied to the child's natural airway (via a tight-fitting mask or nasal pillows); more commonly, it is given chronically through a tracheostomy tube (Lemrye, Davis, & de Paoli, 2002). If a child is on a mechanical ventilator, positive pressure can be administered between mechanical breaths, in which case the technique is referred to as positive end expiratory pressure (PEEP).

Children with respiratory or oral-motor problems also may produce excessive secretions (e.g., saliva) and/or be unable to cough effectively. CPT and suctioning, which can be taught to all caregivers, help clear pulmonary secretions (Krause & Hoehn, 2000). CPT involves the repetitive manual percussion of the chest wall. For infants, this often involves using a vibrator. Secretions are loosened and can then be cleared by coughing or, in children with tracheostomies, by suctioning. Typically, supplemental oxygen is administered before and after suctioning to prevent hypoxia from occurring during the procedure (Flenady & Gray, 2000). Suctioning and CPT are done as often as necessary, usually several times a day. The newest modality for CPT is the use of an automatic device, the high-frequency chest compression vest. A number of recent studies attest to its effectiveness, especially in people who have cystic fibrosis (Davidson, 2002; Dosman & Jones, 2005).

A tracheostomy involves the insertion of a plastic tube through a surgically created incision in the cartilage of the trachea, just below the Adam's apple. It is secured around the neck with foam-padded strings. This open airway can then be attached to a mechanical ventilator or to a CPAP device with tubing that provides humidified air or an air/oxygen mixture. If ventilatory support or oxygen is not needed, then a humidifying device (an "artificial nose") is attached to the tracheostomy tube. A **speaking valve** (e.g., Passey-Muir valve) often is used with the tracheostomy tube to allow more air to go through the vocal cords to allow phonation. The tracheostomy tube also allows the caregiver to have direct access to the airway, permitting suctioning of secretions or removal of other blockages. Children who have tracheostomies may spend part or all of their day connected to a mechanical ventilator that augments or replaces the their own respiratory efforts (Edwards, O'Toole, & Wallis, 2004).

Monitoring and Surveillance Devices

Children with disorders that affect the heart or lungs are likely to require the use of monitoring or surveillance devices. Although these instruments provide no direct therapeutic benefit, they give early warning of problems and thereby improve care indirectly. The two most common types of electronic surveillance devices are pulse oximeters and cardiorespiratory monitors. They can be used individually or in combination in the hospital and at home.

To avoid giving too much or too little oxygen, oxygen saturation (the oxygen-carrying capacity of red blood cells) can be monitored using a device called a **pulse oximeter.** The pulse oximeter measures oxygen saturation in the arterial blood, using a probe that is attached with a special tape to one of the child's fingers or toes (Nadkarni, Shah, & Deshmukh, 2000). An alarm can be set to sound below a certain oxygen saturation level. This most commonly occurs when there is low oxygen delivery (e.g., kinked tubing, low oxygen level in the oxygen tank) or a change in the child's condition (e.g., an increased need for supplemental oxygen because of a respiratory infection). Because this device reflects how well oxygen is being delivered to vital organs, it is an important monitor; unfortunately, it is quite susceptible to false alarms resulting from probe displacement, movement of the extremity, or electrical interference.

A cardiorespiratory monitor has electrodes that are pasted to the child's chest to record heart and respiratory rate (Silvestri et al., 2005). An alarm is part of the system and is set off by rates that are either too high or too low. If the alarm sounds, the caregiver should examine the child's respiratory, cardiovascular, and neurological status. Like the oximeter, the cardiorespiratory monitor can produce false alarms, most commonly resulting from the inadvertent detachment of the chest leads. In the very rare event that the alarm sounds because of a cardiorespiratory arrest (i.e., slowing or stopping of breathing and/or heart rate), cardiopulmonary resuscitation (CPR) and possibly the use of an automated external defibrillator (AED) must be instituted immediately.

Nutritional (Gastrointestinal) Fluid Assistance

Children with cerebral palsy and other chronic neurological conditions are often limited in their ability to take in nutrition by mouth. Despite often needing an increased food intake as a result of their motor-control problems (e.g., dyskinesia), these children may be unable to ingest even a normal intake because of oral-motor impairments, GER, or food refusal. In these instances, nutritional assistance devices may prove helpful. Tube feedings can be provided in a number of ways. The tube can be temporarily inserted into one nostril and passed into the stomach (nasogastric tube) or the second part of the intestine (nasojejunal tube). When long-term feedings are required, a permanent tube can be placed directly through the skin and into the stomach (gastrostomy tube, or G tube) or intestine (jejunostomy tube, or J tube) A G-J tube combines a G tube and a J tube. The J tube portion travels through the stomach, the duodenum, and into the jejunum to prevent reflux of nutrients. If the child has GER, the intervention of choice may be the combination of a surgical antireflux procedure (e.g., fundoplication by open or laparoscopic route; see Chapter 31) and insertion of a G tube or G-J tube. Once the feeding tube is inserted, nutrition can be provided by using a commercially available formula, such as Jevity or Ensure or foods from the family's meals that have been puréed.

Intravenous Fluid Assistive Devices

Long-term IV therapy, generally provided through a central venous line, is most often used to provide nutrition and/or to administer medication (McInally, 2005). Total parenteral nutrition involves the provision of a high-calorie, high-protein solution directly into the bloodstream by intravenous administration. Prolonged intravenous access may also be needed to provide antibiotics (e.g., when a child has osteomyelitis, a deep bone infection) or for cancer chemotherapy. In these situations, a catheter (often called a central line or Broviac line) may be placed into a vein under radiological guidance and advanced to a more central position, near the heart. This type of catheter averts the need for repeated placement of peripheral venous lines. In addition, a central venous catheter allows the child to receive medication and/or nutrition at home rather than having to remain in the hospital. Central lines are more stable than peripheral lines and can be maintained for months or years, provided that there is strict adherence to sterile techniques and proper care.

TECHNOLOGY FOR PHYSICAL DISABILITIES

Children with cerebral palsy or neuromuscular disorders commonly use assistive technology, especially low-tech devices such as ankle-foot orthoses, hand splints, and spinal braces (see Chapter 26 and 37). Mid-tech devices include functional electrical stimulators (FES), which provide neural stimulation to increase mobility); treadmills with support frames to increase strength even in nonambulatory people; and dynamic braces for treatment of a hemiplegic arm. Personal computers, with the appropriate adaptations, can be very useful high-tech tools for people with physical disabilities. Transparent modifications to a computer can be made using add-on equipment and/or specialized software programs. These modifications permit most commercially available software programs (including computer games, word-processing programs, and instructional programs) to be used. Transparent modifications do not modify or interfere with either the computer or the standard software program. An example is the keyboard emulator, which a device such as a joystick that replaces the keyboard (Keates & Robinson, 1999). Keyboard emulators are electronic circuits that function by taking the output from a special keyboard or input device, altering it, and then transmitting a standard signal format by wires to the appropriate connectors in the computer. The emulator translates the original signal into a different format that the computer interprets as coming from its own keyboard.

In addition to multiple-use devices, such as computers, many single-application devices have been designed or adapted for people with physical disabilities. Examples range from relatively simple mid-tech feeding devices to elaborate high-tech environmental control units that can turn lights and appliances on and off and can dial a telephone.

TECHNOLOGY FOR SENSORY IMPAIRMENTS

People with sensory impairments have been helped in many ways by assistive devices. For people with visual impairments there are low-tech magnification devices; mid-tech aids such as alerting systems, laser canes, and taped books or digital recorded systems; and high-tech systems such as personal computers with extra-large type on video screens. Various devices using electronic technology have also been developed for people who are blind. These include the Kurzweil1000 reading machine that translates the written word to voice-synthesized output and refreshable braille displays (e.g., ALVA Satellite) that provide an alternative access in the form of braille to the text or content displayed on a computer monitor. See Chapter 11 for more information on assistive technology for people with visual impairments.

Since the mid-1980s, there has been an explosion in the complexity and efficacy of hearing aids for people with hearing impairment. Digital programmable hearing aids have become more available, allowing improved customization for an individual's specific degree and range of hearing loss. Many mid-tech solutions are also available—for example, assistive listening devices (infrared or FM transmitters) in movie theaters and classrooms and palm-sized telecommunication devices for use with telephones.

For the child or adult with a severe hearing impairment, as well as for their families and others, there have been advances in methods to learn lip-reading and sign language by computer modeling programs. In addition, versions of the electronic cochlear implant have been gradually improving; for some individuals, this device can restore a type of hearing or at least an improved awareness of sounds (Stern et al., 2005; Zwolan et al., 2004; see Chapter 12). See Chapter 12 for more information on assistive technology for people with hearing impairments.

TECHNOLOGY FOR COMMUNICATION DISABILITIES

Many types of augmentative and alternative communication (AAC) devices exist to assist a person who is unable to use speech for communication (see Table 36.1). Low-tech devices include various lists of words or pictures mounted on durable material. These communication boards are used in face-to-face communication; the user points to the selected word or picture to communicate a specific message. A battery-operated scanning communication device is an example of a mid-tech AAC device. Other mid-

tech AAC devices include portable voice output storage units that require direct selection and hold only a few minutes of prerecorded sentences or phrases.

High-tech electronic communication aids, often incorporating single symbols to substitute for groups of words, are becoming more commercially available. Various companies have started using laptop computers as the core part of a communication system, increasing the versatility of these communication aids. Rather than being used only for person-to-person communication, these adapted laptops can be used for all types of communication—letter writing, telecommunications, and e-mail. These computers also can be the foundation for environmental controls, safety systems, and recreation (e.g., Internet, virtual-reality computer games; Sigafoos et al., 2004; Weiss, Bialik, & Kizony, 2003).

When compared with high-tech computerized AAC technology, there are significant problems with low-tech and mid-tech devices: 1) they are slow in getting the message across, 2) they provide limited messages (i.e., usually only those about basic needs), and 3) they require face-to-face interaction. Spoken communication among typical individuals is normally performed at such high speed that patience is needed for conversations between typically communicating people and those using a communication system (especially low-tech systems involving symbols, letters, or word boards). Although these methods are extremely slow, such boards should not be abandoned. They often are just as effective, if not more so, than high-tech devices in face-to-face communication. Electronic devices are often limited by their need for a power source, and most are not suitable for outdoor activities such as going to the beach or walking in the rain. Thus, low-tech solutions such as word and picture boards should always be part of an overall communication system and should be available as a backup to electronic devices.

TECHNOLOGY FOR COGNITIVE AND LEARNING DISABILITIES

Children who have learning differences have been helped by various assistive technology devices and strategies (Behrmann & Schaff, 2001; Hetzroni & Shrieber, 2004). Many software programs have been developed since the late 1980s that use computers to assist in reading, math, and other types of special education instruction. These programs range widely in price and utility, and only recently has enough research been performed to begin to determine their effectiveness and generalizability, especially over the long term (Lahm et al., 2001). Computer-based instruction, however, has several unique advantages, perhaps the most important of which is the ease of individualization. It is possible to build on children's strengths and talents and develop alternative ways of learning. Very few children in special education have their own personal teacher on a full-time basis, so the use of a computer can allow these children to begin to develop independent learning skills. It is crucial to first fully evaluate the educational strengths and needs of a student who has learning difficulties and then apply the assistive technology where it can best alleviate problems. Most of the time, however, low-tech and mid-tech solutions should be considered initially. A high-tech solution is often not the best answer for a specific problem that a child is having in school.

ASSESSMENT FOR ASSISTIVE TECHNOLOGY

It is important that the assessment process and the prescribing of any assistive device be done by a knowledgeable team of individuals. Depending on the type of assistive device to be prescribed, this interdisciplinary team may include a speech-language therapist, a physical therapist, an occupational therapist, a rehabilitation engineer, a neurodevelopmental pediatrician, a neurologist, a physiatrist or other physician, a special educator, a social worker, and a computer specialist. Also included in the team are the child who will be using the device(s) and his or her family members, who can offer advice that is critical in making final device recommendations. This team approach is needed to properly evaluate the child's motor and intellectual capabilities and to narrow down the devices that may fit within the child's abilities and needs (e.g., educational plans).

Figure 36.1 summarizes the assessment process. (See the Functional Evaluation of the Individual section for more information on the assessment tools mentioned in this figure.) An important aspect of assessment is the consideration of the range of assistive technology that may be useful. The best approach is to begin with the low-tech devices and to move on to mid-tech or high-tech devices only if needed. For example, to get around the home, a child with a severe physical disability may benefit more from ramps and wider doors than from a

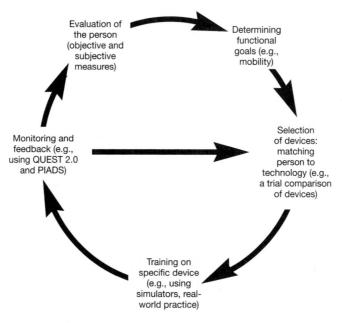

Figure 36.1. The assistive device assessment cycle. (*Key:* QUEST 2.0, Quebec User Evaluation of Satisfaction with Assistive Technology, Version 2.0 [Demers, Weiss-Lambrou, & Ska, 2000]; PIADS, Psychosocial Impact of Assistive Devices Scale [Day, Jutai, & Campbell, 2002; Routhier et al., 2001].)

power wheelchair. The assessment process often involves making educated guesses (based on prior experiences with other people with similar disabilities) and then having the individual try out the devices chosen. The most complete evaluation possible should be undertaken prior to purchasing the equipment, including testing the device in ALL settings where it will be used. This avoids buying a device that is unusable or inappropriate.

Functional Evaluation of the Individual

The ultimate goal for a person using an assistive device is to achieve the highest possible level of functioning. The World Health Organization (WHO) introduced the International Classification of Functioning, Disability and Health (ICF), a system that produces an overall picture of the capabilities of an individual, rather than solely focusing on the disability (WHO, 2001). A number of other standardized instruments have been developed that can be used to evaluate the current functioning and impact of treatment or intervention, including assistive technology, on children with various types of disabilities. These include the children's version of the Functional Independence Measure (Wee-FIM; Wong et al., 2005; Wong et al., 2004) and the Pediatric Disability Inventory (PEDI; Ostensjo et al., 2006; Msall et al., 1997).

A number of studies have shown that between one third and three quarters of assistive devices are abandoned shortly after they are obtained (Galvin & Scherer, 2004; Phillips & Zhao, 1993). To improve utilization, techniques have been developed to predict the successful use of assistive devices. One approach is the Matching Persons and Technology (MPT) model (Scherer, 1998a) that stresses the importance of addressing environmental, personal, and technology related issues. Environmental issues include the family structure and the work or school settings. The personal area includes recognition of functional limitations, motivation, coping skills, and personality traits (e.g., optimism). The technology area includes the characteristics of the assistive device: reliability, ease of use, adaptability, and whether any discomfort or stress is caused by its use. Scherer and colleagues developed an assessment tool, the Assistive Technology Device Predisposition Assessment, which uses the MPT model to facilitate a match between the device and the per-

Table 36.2. Factors associated with abandonment of an assistive device (from the Matching Persons and Technology model).

Improper or ineffective training on the use of a device (e.g., single-session training without follow-up and feedback)

Problems or obstacles in the environment preventing use of a device (e.g., second-floor rooms inaccessible to a power wheelchair user)

Faults or failures in performance of the device (e.g., AAC device that is too sensitive to movement)

Device size, weight, or appearance (e.g., AAC device decorated with pink roses given to a boy)

Motivational factors in the user and/or family members (e.g., depression occurring after traumatic injuries)

Perceived lack of or minimal need for the device (e.g., decision made not to leave the house rather than to use a wheelchair)

Functional abilities that worsen or improve (e.g., progressive disorder or recovery)

Source: Scherer (1998a).

son to ensure a good long-term result (Scherer, 1998a, 1998b). Table 36.2 lists factors that relate to this model. There are also assessment tools that determine the efficacy and satisfaction of the device once in place: the Quebec User Evaluation of Satisfaction with Assistive Technology (QUEST), now called QUEST 2.0 (Demers et al., 1996; Demers, Weiss-Lambrou, & Ska, 2000), and the Psychosocial Impact of Assistive Devices Scale (PIADS; Day, Jutai, & Campbell, 2002; Routhier et al., 2001).

Training in the Use of the Device

The physicians, therapists, or educators who prescribe or recommend electronic assistive devices or assistive devices in general must also ensure that the child receives proper training and monitoring for using the device. For some devices and software, demos and simulators are available (e.g., power wheelchair controls, AAC devices), which can help with training before the actual device is ordered (Harrison et al., 2002). Simulators are especially helpful in evaluating reaction time, speed, and accuracy.

EFFECTS OF ASSISTIVE TECHNOLOGY ON THE FAMILY AND COMMUNITY

Assistive technology compensates for or builds on the individual skills that each person already possesses. It can lead to increased feelings of success and self-worth and, it is hoped, improved functioning (Kirk & Glendinning, 2004; Wang & Barnard, 2004). For example, several studies have provided evidence for the positive effects of adapted toys on intellectual development (Besio, 2002; Brodin, 1999). Although much uncertainty remains about the earliest age at which a child can successfully use an assistive device, some pilot studies suggest children younger than 5 years of age can benefit. For example, studies of power wheelchair use demonstrated that children as young as 2 years old can be quite successful and reap considerable social benefits as well (Bottos et al., 2001). One study suggests that for children with communicative disabilities, if AAC devices are not being successfully used by first grade, the child will not be an active participant in the classroom setting (Buekelman & Mirenda, 2005).

Although assistive devices can markedly improve function, medical technology especially can promote social isolation. In school, the child is likely to be treated differently because of the accompanying equipment and medical/nursing needs. The presence of a tracheostomy and ventilator can be particularly intimidating. This can be partially offset by educating classmates and teachers and providing psychological counseling for the child. The child and family must also learn to deal with the underlying medical problem that led to the technology dependence. It is generally easier for a child and family to cope with medical technology assistance on a short-term basis, such as when intravenous antibiotics are necessary to treat a severe infection or when a temporary ostomy is required following abdominal surgery. If the child has a severe chronic disease, however, adaptation to assistive technology is only one issue that the child and family must face. Studies have suggested that families fare better if the more significant type of technological assistance, such as mechanical ventilation, lasts less than 2 years. More prolonged periods are associated with an increased risk of parental stress and depression (Montagnino & Mauricio, 2004). The provision of in-home respite care and family-to-family support systems can be extremely helpful in these situations.

Despite financial and psychosocial difficulties, children who require chronic and substantial medical technology assistance are being included in the community (Feudtner et al., 2005; O'Brien & Wegner, 2002; Rehm & Rohr, 2002). Home care, especially when ventilator assistance is required, becomes a viable option only after a number of requirements have been met (Carnevale et al., 2006; Heaton et al., 2005; Parker et al., 2006):

1. The family must master the child's medical and nursing care.

2. The family needs to select a nursing agency if home nursing services are required and a durable medical equipment supplier for equipment, disposable supplies, and in-home support (e.g., equipment maintenance and monitoring).

3. The funds to pay for all of these services also must be arranged.

4. Modifications to the family's home may be needed, such as changing existing electrical systems and adding ramps for wheelchair or adapted stroller accessibility.

5. If mechanical ventilation is required, local electric, ambulance, and telephone companies must be notified that a person dependent on life-support technology will be living in the family's home so that the household can be placed on a priority list in the event of a power failure or a medical emergency.

Medical, educational, and therapy (e.g., occupational therapy, physical therapy) services also need to be arranged before discharge from the hospital. A pediatrician or family physician in the community should be identified to provide general medical care. The discharging team should contact this physician prior to the child's hospital discharge to introduce the child and encourage the community physician's active participation in the child's care. If the child requires special rehabilitation therapies after discharge, either center- or home-based providers should be arranged. Educational services also need to be identified, and the child's health care and rehabilitative plans should be written into an individualized family service plan (IFSP) for early intervention services if the child is younger than age 3 or into an individualized education program (IEP) if the child is preschool or school age (Committee on Children with Disabilities, 1999, 2000; Palfrey et al., 1994). In addition, the school nurse needs to develop an individualized health care plan as well as emergency plans for the child. A center- or school-based educational program offers the child the opportunity to interact with other children in a stimulating environment. These out-of-home experiences should be encouraged if the child's physical condition permits and if appropriate medical or nursing supports are available.

FUNDING ISSUES

Assistive technology can be very expensive, depending on the type of equipment required and the extent of the disability and the professional staffing needs of the child (Miller et al., 1998; Smith, 1998). For medical assistive technology, the two major issues are payment for nursing care and durable medical equipment/supplies (including technological assistance). It is sometimes easier to obtain funding for the former than for the latter. The primary source of funding of both is insurance, private and public, and each has restrictions that may affect the provision of medical assistive technology (see Chapter 42).

For assistive technology that can be used in schools, the Individuals with Disabilities Education Improvement Act of 2004 (PL 108-446) as well as other laws (e.g., the Technology-Related Assistance for Individuals with Disabilities Act of 1988 [PL 100-407], or "Tech Act") and legal opinions specifically indicate that funding should be provided for "technological" devices (including software) that are part of a student's IEP. Yet, there are difficulties in actually finding funds to support this, and cooperative efforts among insurance companies, philanthropic agencies, school systems, and parents are often required. Another concern is that usually schools will restrict the use of the software or device to the school program (and the student is not able to take it for use at home).

For some devices, such as home ventilators, suctioning, or specialized feeding equipment, insurance companies universally recognize that these are medically necessary and will pay for them. There continues to be controversy, however, as to whether other assistive devices are medically necessary or whether they are educationally necessary. For example, AAC devices, wheelchairs, or standing frames for children who have cerebral palsy could be used both at home and at school. If a device is shown to be primarily medically necessary, it may be possible to obtain funding from medical insurance companies. If they are educationally necessary, the school system should purchase the needed devices. The Tech Act has tried to solve this problem of discriminating between medical and educational use by legally allowing Medicaid funding to be used by the school to purchase the assistive device. The Tech Act further requires letting the child take home such devices for educationally related purposes. This sets a precedent for medical funding to be at least considered for the purchase of essentially all assistive devices.

For years, most forms of private and government medical insurance have been willing to pay for the purchase of wheelchairs, and they gradually are beginning to fund other types of assistive devices. Fortunately, AAC devices are increasingly being seen as medically necessary in much the same way as wheelchairs are. Physicians are often called upon to send medical necessity letters and prescriptions to funding sources for assistive technology (Committee on Children with Disabilities, 1999, 2000; Sneed, May, & Stencel, 2004). This can best be done after the physician consults with the child's therapists and then summarizes current abilities and expected outcomes from using the assistive device. Many assistive devices and their related professional services are relatively new and specialized, and they usually are not included on lists of approved products that are eligible for funding. As a result, many funding agencies need to be properly educated about the potential of these devices to improve functioning and independence for individuals with disabilities. Patience and perseverance are frequently necessary for funding to be secured. Initial denials of payment are almost automatic for some funding sources; however, these denials are usually subject to appeal and reversal.

ADVOCACY INFORMATION

Fortunately, increasingly accessible sources of information about assistive technology have developed. Statewide Technological Assistance Services (Tech Act sites) are now available in all states, and information from them is becoming more widely accessible. ABLEDATA, which is funded by the National Institute for Disability and Rehabilitation Research, is an example of a large database that holds continuously updated information about assistive technology pertinent to many disabilities. Various organizations dealing with children who have disabilities, such as the Council for Exceptional Children (http://www.cec.sped.org) and *Exceptional Parent* magazine (http://www.eparent.com), have developed services that can be used to obtain references and abstracts about many facets of assistive technology, especially in regard to school-related services. On the Internet, there is an increasing number of sites offering resources for people interested in assistive technology, although many of these are thinly veiled advertisements from companies or sites that propose "alternative therapies." Therefore, all web sites must be evaluated critically.

SUMMARY

Most children with disabilities who use rehabilitative assistive technology employ it to make their day-to-day living easier or to improve functioning. However, some children use a medical assistive device that replaces or augments a vital bodily function, such as breathing. For the group using rehabilitative assistive technology (e.g., power wheelchairs, AAC, hearing and vision aids), perhaps the best way to ensure the availability of future vocational opportunities is to provide access to appropriate assistive devices at an early age—thereby allowing the children to become proficient in use of the devices by the time they are young adults. Improved access to these devices also has social implications. As children with disabilities become better able to use their assistive devices or communication devices, they likely will be less isolated and have more contact with the community.

For children who require medical assistive technology (e.g., respiratory technology devices, surveillance devices, nutritive assistive devices, ostomies, dialysis), the requirement for prolonged medical technology assistance places both financial and emotional stresses on the family. It also leads to considerable challenges for health care professionals and other caregivers. Knowledge about the correct use of medical devices and confidence in dealing with potential emergencies is important for parents, educators, and other caregivers. Training of caregivers and others in the use of medical technology assistance is best done while the child is hospitalized. Arrangement for financial, nursing, and equipment support is essential before the child goes home. Ultimately, the outcome for the child who depends on assistive technology appears to be more a function of the underlying disorder than the type or extent of technology, but the role of the family cannot be overemphasized (Fuhrer et al., 2003).

REFERENCES

Bass, J.L., Corwin, M., Gozal, D., et al. (2004). The effect of chronic or intermittent hypoxia on cognition in childhood: A review of the evidence. *Pediatrics, 114*(3), 805–816.

Behrmann, M., & Schaff, J. (2001). Assisting educators with assistive technology: Enabling children to achieve independence in living and learning. *Children and Families, 42*(3), 24–28.

Besio, S. (2002). An Italian research project to study the play of children with motor disabilities: The first year of activity. *Disability and Rehabilitation, 24,* 72–79.

Bottos, M., Bolcati, C., Scuito, L., et al. (2001). Powered wheelchairs and independence in young children with tetraplegia. *Developmental Medicine and Child Neurology, 43,* 769–777.

Brodin, J. (1999). Play in children with severe multiple disabilities: Play with toys—a review. *International Journal of Disability, Development and Education, 46,* 25–34.

Buekelman, D.R., & Mirenda, P. (2005). *Augmentative and alternative communication: Supporting children and adults with complex communication needs* (3rd ed.). Baltimore: Paul H. Brookes Publishing Co.

Bush, A., Fraser, J., Jardine, E., et al. (2005). Respiratory management of the infant with type 1 spinal muscular atrophy. *Archives of Disease in Childhood, 90*(7), 709–711.

Carnevale, F.A., Alexander, E., Davis, M., et al. (2006). Daily living with distress and enrichment: The moral experience of families with ventilator-assisted children at home. *Pediatrics, 117*(1), e48–e60.

Committee on Children with Disabilities. (1998). Learning disabilities, dyslexia and vision: A subject review. *Pediatrics, 102*(5), 1217–1219.

Committee on Children with Disabilities. (1999). The pediatrician's role in development and implementation of an individual education plan (IEP) and/or an individual family service plan (IFSP). *Pediatrics, 104* (1), 124–127

Committee on Children with Disabilities. (2000). Provision of educationally-related services for children and adolescents with chronic diseases and disabling conditions. *Pediatrics, 105*(2), 448–451.

Davidson, K.L. (2002). Airway clearance strategies for the pediatric patient. *Respiratory Care, 47*(7), 823–828.

Day, H., Jutai, J. & Campbell, K.A. (2002). Development of a scale to measure the psychosocial impact of assistive devices: Lessons learned and the road ahead. *Disability and Rehabilitation, 24,* 31–37.

Demers, L., Weiss-Lambrou, R., & Ska, B. (1996). Development of the Quebec User Evaluation of Satisfaction with Assistive Technology (QUEST). *Assistive Technology, 8,* 3–13.

Demers, L., Weiss-Lambrou, R., & Ska, B. (2000). *Quebec User Evaluation of Satisfaction with Assistive Technology (QUEST) Version 2.0: An outcome measure for assistive technology devices.* Webster, NY: Institute for Matching Person and Technology.

Desch, L.W. (1986). High technology for handicapped children. *Pediatrics, 77,* 71–85.

Dosman C.F., & Jones R.L. (2005). High-frequency chest compression: A summary of the literature. *Canadian Respiratory Journal, 12*(1), 37–41.

Downey, R., III, Perkin, R.M., & MacQuarrie, J. (2000). Nasal continuous positive airway pressure use in children with obstructive sleep apnea younger than 2 years of age. *Chest, 117,* 1608–1612.

Edwards, E.A., O'Toole, M., & Wallis, C. (2004). Sending children home on tracheostomy dependent ventilation: Pitfalls and outcomes. *Archives of Disease in Childhood, 89*(3), 251–255.

Feudtner, C., Villareale, N.L., Morray, B., et al. (2005). Technology-dependency among patients discharged from a children's hospital: A retrospective cohort study. *BioMedCentral Pediatrics, 5*(1), 8.

Flenady, V.J., & Gray, P.H. (2000). Chest physiotherapy for preventing morbidity in babies being extubated from mechanical ventilation. *Cochrane Database of Systemic Reviews, 2,* CD000283.

Fuhrer, M.J., Jutai, J.W., Scherer, et al. (2003). A framework for the conceptual modeling of assistive device outcomes. *Disability and Rehabilitation, 25,* 1243–1251.

Galvin, J.C., & Scherer, M.J. (Eds.) (2004). *Evaluating, selecting and using appropriate assistive technology.* Austin, TX: PRO-ED.

Gilgoff, R.L., & Gilgoff, I.S. (2003). Long-term follow-up of home mechanical ventilation in young children with spinal cord injury and neuromuscular conditions. *The Journal of Pediatrics, 142*(5), 476–480.

Harrison, A., Derwent G., Enticknap, et al. (2002). The role of virtual reality technology in the assessment and training of inexperienced powered wheelchair users. *Disability and Rehabilitation, 24,* 599–607.

Heaton, J., Noyes, J., Sloper, P., et al. (2005). Families' experiences of caring for technology-dependent children: A temporal perspective. *Health and Social Care in the Community, 13*(5), 441–450.

Hetzroni, O.E., & Shrieber, B. (2004). Word processing as an assistive technology tool for enhancing academic outcomes of students with writing disabilities in the general classroom. *Journal of Learning Disabilities, 37* (2), 143–154.

Individuals with Disabilities Education Improvement Act of 2004, PL 108-446, 20 U.S.C. §§ 1400 *et seq.*

Keates, S., & Robinson, P. (1999). Gestures and multimodal input. *Behavior and Information Technology, 18* (1), 36–44.

Kirk, S., & Glendinning, C. (2004). Developing services to support parents caring for a technology-dependent child at home. *Child: Care, Health and Development, 30*(3), 209–218; discussion, 219.

Krause, M.F., & Hoehn, T. (2000). Chest physiotherapy in mechanically ventilated children: A review. *Critical Care Medicine, 28,* 1648–1651.

Lahm, E.A., Bausch, M.E., Hasselbring, T.S., et al. (2001). National assistive technology research institute. *Journal of Special Education Technology, 16,* 19–26.

Lemyre, B., Davis, P.G., & de Paoli, A.G. (2002). Nasal intermittent positive pressure ventilation (NIPPV) versus nasal continuous positive airway pressure (NCPAP) for apnea of prematurity. *Cochrane Database of Systematic Reviews, 1,* CD002272.

McInally, W. (2005). Whose line is it anyway? Management of central venous catheters in children. *Paediatric Nursing, 17*(5), 14–18.

Miller, V.L., Rice, J.C., DeVoe, M., et al. (1998). An analysis of program and family costs of case managed care in technology-dependent infants with bronchopulmonary dysplasia. *Journal of Pediatric Nursing, 13,* 244–251.

Montagnino, B.A., & Mauricio, R.V. (2004). The child with a tracheostomy and gastrostomy: Parental stress and coping in the home—a pilot study. *Pediatric Nursing, 30*(5), 373–380, 401.

Msall, M.K., Rogers, B.T., Ripstein, H., et al. (1997). Measurements of functional outcomes in children with cerebral palsy. *Mental Retardation and Developmental Disabilities Research Reviews, 3*(2), 194–204.

Nadkarni, U.B., Shah, A.M., & Deshmukh, C.T. (2000). Non-invasive respiratory monitoring in paediatric intensive care. *Journal of Postgraduate Medicine, 46,* 149–152.

No Child Left Behind Act of 2001, PL 107-110, 115 Stat 1425, 20 U.S.C. §§ 6301 *et seq.*

O'Brien, M.E., & Wegner, C.B. (2002). Rearing the child who is technology dependent: Perceptions of parents and home care nurses. *Journal for Specialists in Pediatric Nursing, 7*(1), 7–15.

Office of Technology Assessment. (1987). *Technology-dependent children: Hospital versus home care: A technical memorandum* (DHHS Publication No. TM-H-38). Washington, DC: U.S. Government Printing Office.

Ostensjo, S., Bjorbaekmo, W., Carlberg, E.B., et al. (2006). Assessment of everyday functioning in young children with disabilities: An ICF-based analysis of concepts and content of the Pediatric Evaluation of Disability Inventory (PEDI). *Disability and Rehabilitation, 28*(8), 489–504.

Palfrey, J.S., Haynie, M., Porter, S., et al. (1994). Prevalence of medical technology assistance among children in Massachusetts in 1987 and 1990. *Public Health Reports, 109,* 226–233.

Parker, G., Bhakta, P., Lovett, C., et al. (2006). Paediatric home care: A systematic review of randomized trials on costs and effectiveness. *Journal of Health Services Research and Policy, 11*(2), 110–119.

Phillips, B., & Zhao, H. (1993) Predictors of assistive technology abandonment. *Assistive Technology, 5,* 36–45.

Rehm, R.S., & Rohr, J.A. (2002). Parents', nurses', and educators' perceptions of risks and benefits of school attendance by children who are medically fragile/technology-dependent. *Journal of Pediatric Nursing, 17*(5), 345–353.

Routhier, F., Vincent, C., Morrissette, M.J. et al. (2001). Clinical results of an investigation of paediatric upper limb myoelectric prosthesis fitting at the Quebec Rehabilitation Institute. *Prosthetics and Orthotics International, 25,* 119–131.

Scherer, M.J. (1998a). *Matching person and technology model and accompanying assessment forms* (3rd ed.). Webster, NY: Institute for Matching Person and Technology.

Scherer, M.J. (1998b). The impact of assistive technology on the lives of people with disabilities. In D.B. Gray, L.A. Quatrano, & M.L. Lieberman (Eds.), *Designing and using assistive technology: The human perspective* (pp. 99–115). Baltimore: Paul H. Brookes Publishing Co.

Sigafoos, J., O'Reilly, M.F., Seely-York, S., et al. (2004). Transferring AAC intervention to the home. *Disability and Rehabilitation, 26*(21–22), 1330–1334.

Silvestri, J.M., Lister, G., Corwin, M.J., et al. (2005). Collaborative Home Infant Monitoring Evaluation Study Group—Factors that influence use of a home cardiorespiratory monitor for infants: The collaborative home infant monitoring evaluation. *Archives of Pediatrics and Adolescent Medicine, 159*(1), 18–24.

Smith, D.C. (1998). Assistive technology: Funding options and strategies. *Mental and Physical Disability Law Reports, 22,* 115–123.

Sneed, R.C., May, W.L., & Stencel, C. (2004). Policy versus practice: Comparison of prescribing therapy and durable medical equipment in medical and educational settings. *Pediatrics, 114*(5), e612–e625

Stern, R.E., Yueh, B., Lewis, C., et al. (2005). Recent epidemiology of pediatric cochlear implantation in the United States: Disparity among children of different ethnicity and socioeconomic status. *Laryngoscope, 115,* 125–131.

Storgion, S.A. (1996). Care of the technology-dependent child. *Pediatric Annals, 25,* 677–684.

Technology-Related Assistance for Individuals with Disabilities Act of 1988, PL 100–407, 29 U.S.C. §§ 2201 *et seq.*

Wang, K.W., & Barnard, A. (2004). Technology-dependent children and their families: A review. *Journal of Advanced Nursing, 45*(1), 36–46.

Weiss, P.L., Bialik, P., & Kizony, R. (2003). Virtual reality provides leisure time opportunities for young adults with physical and intellectual disabilities. *CyberPsychology and Behavior, 6,* 335–343.

Wong, V., Au-Yeung, Y.C., & Law, P.K. (2005). Correlation of Functional Independence Measure for Children (WeeFIM) with developmental language tests in children with developmental delay. *Journal of Child Neurology, 20*(7), 613–616.

Wong, V., Chung, B., & Hui, S., et al. (2004). Cerebral palsy: Correlation of risk factors and functional performance using the Functional Independence Measure for Children (WeeFIM). *Journal of Child Neurology, 19*(11), 887–893.

World Health Organization. (2001). *International Classification of Functioning, Disability and Health (ICF).* Geneva: Author.

Zhan, S., & Ottenbacher, K.J. (2001). Single subject research designs for disability research. *Disability and Rehabilitation, 23,* 1–9.

Zwolan, T.A., Ashbaugh, C.M., Alarfaj, A., et al. (2004). Pediatric cochlear implant patient performance as a function of age at implantation. *Otology and Neurotology, 25,* 112–120.

37

Physical Therapy and Occupational Therapy

Lisa A. Kurtz

Upon completion of this chapter, the reader will

- Appreciate the contribution made by occupational therapists and physical therapists in helping children with disabilities to achieve their potential

- Recognize when and how to recommend therapy services

- Become familiar with some common approaches to intervention, including motor learning theory, sensory integration therapy, orthotics, and nonmedical assistive technology

---

Children with disabilities may experience a wide range of impairments in body structure and function, limitations in their ability to participate meaningfully in activities of daily life, and restrictions in their ability to be an active part of their community (World Health Organization [WHO], 2001). Occupational therapy and physical therapy are commonly recommended to address these issues.

Physical therapists focus on evaluating the influence of motor development, along with the child's physical capacities and limitations, on the child's potential for functional mobility within the environment. Occupational therapists focus on evaluating the cognitive, motor, and sensory processing skills needed for independence in self-care, play, and school performance, which are the primary "occupations" of childhood. Although play is the medium of choice for most young children, therapy incorporates a variety of interventions including exercise, sensory stimulation, physical agents, splinting or casting, adaptive aids and equipment, and behavioral training, depending upon the needs of the individual child (American Occupational Therapy Association [AOTA], 2002; American Physical Therapy Association [APTA], 2001). Overlap in the roles of physical and occupational therapists exists for several reasons. Both professions require similar educational backgrounds in human development, anatomy and physiology, the scope and nature of disabil-

ities, and a general approach to habilitation (teaching skills that have not yet been learned) and rehabilitation (teaching skills that have been lost through illness or injury). Postgraduate continuing education allows therapists from both disciplines to develop advanced skills in selected interventions, such as splinting, application of assistive technology, and other specialized therapy approaches. The interests and talents of individual therapists, along with the philosophy and needs of the workplace, often dictate the exact nature of a therapist's role in that setting. Table 37.1 reviews some of the ways that occupational therapists and physical therapists might approach similar goals from different perspectives.

KIA: A CHILD WITH CEREBRAL PALSY

Kia was born prematurely and was diagnosed with periventricular leukomalacia (a cause of cerebral palsy; see Chapter 9) shortly after birth. Physical therapy intervention began in the neonatal intensive care unit in the form of consultation with parents and unit staff regarding positioning and handling techniques designed to help her develop postural control and the ability to maintain a quiet, alert state during her waking hours. By 6 months of age, Kia was actively engaged in her environment, playing with toys and interacting with people. However, the muscle tone in her legs

571

was increased compared with the tone in her arms, and she was unable to sit unsupported. A diagnosis of spastic diplegic cerebral palsy was made, and she was referred for early intervention services. Outpatient physical therapy focused on a home management program, bilateral foot orthoses, adaptive seating, and helping Kia learn to sit and crawl. By 3 years of age, Kia was able to walk with canes, and was enrolled in a preschool program where she began occupational therapy with an emphasis on learning dressing and other self-care skills. Although she had typical intellectual development and was not a candidate for special education services upon entering kindergarten, Kia was eligible to continue receiving consultative physical therapy and occupational therapy services under the provisions of Section 504 of the Rehabilitation Act of 1973 (PL 93-112).

At age 6, Kia underwent orthopedic surgery to lengthen her lower extremity muscles, followed by a period of intensive physical therapy to improve her hip and knee control. This allowed her to continue to be a community ambulator with the use of canes, although Kia preferred a manual wheelchair for extended trips. By third grade, Kia was falling behind in schoolwork due to handwriting difficulties, and the occupational therapist recommended classroom modifications that included instruction in word processing that allowed Kia to complete classroom assignments more efficiently.

Kia has continued her schooling, attending general education classes, receiving good grades, and participating fully in extracurricular activities that she enjoys. As she enters high school, she is considering a power scooter to improve speed and freedom of mobility in her expanded school environment and in the community with her peers. She continues to be monitored by a physical therapist to address current or potential activity limitations.

CONTEMPORARY ISSUES IN PHYSICAL THERAPY AND OCCUPATIONAL THERAPY

Therapists practicing in the 21st century have witnessed many changes in the way that their services are conceptualized and delivered. In the past, the focus was on identifying and treating the deficits that limited a child's participation in activities. Using a bottom-up problem solving approach, goals and interventions were selected according to professional judgment as to the child's potential for remediation of these underlying deficits. Therapy most commonly occurred in a clinical setting where therapists could create a controlled environment for producing change. Current practice supports ability-based models of service delivery, in which goals and interventions are determined based on the priorities of the child and family, as well as on the environmental and cultural context of the child's participation in daily activities. Therapy frequently takes place in natural environmental settings, recognizing that this will likely result in increased caregiver carryover of therapy goals and increased generalization of learning. Official practice guidelines for both occupational therapists and physical therapists have recently undergone revision, using language and terminology consistent with WHO's International Classification of Functioning, Disability and

Table 37.1. Comparison of occupational therapy (OT) and physical therapy (PT)

Desired outcome	Typical OT emphasis	Typical PT emphasis
Promote developmental skills	Fine motor, adaptive, and personal-social domains	Gross motor domain
Teach functional skills needed for daily living	Dressing, eating, toileting, personal hygiene, and household chores	Ambulation, transfers, and other mobility demands
Maintain or increase strength and range of motion	Upper body	Lower body
Promote environmental accessibility	Organizing work and play areas for efficiency	Reducing architectural barriers to mobility
	Modifying the environment to promote attention and information processing	Providing adapted car seats or transportation devices
Provide assistive technology	Adapted toys, school materials, computers, self-care aids, and environmental controls	Wheelchairs, ambulation aids, transfer equipment, and positioning devices for bath and toilet

Health (ICF) (AOTA 2002; APTA, 2001; WHO, 2001). This is recognition that the ultimate goal of intervention is to prevent or ameliorate social disadvantages that may develop as consequences of the underlying impairment (Christiansen, 1993). In addition, there is increasing emphasis on interventions for health promotion and the prevention of secondary complications, such as obesity, social isolation, and depression (Kniepmann, 1997; Rimmer, 1999).

Specific models of service delivery are often influenced by factors outside the control of the individual therapist, for example: 1) federal and state legislation imposes strict guidelines for service delivery within early intervention and school settings, 2) managed care approaches to cost containment and outcomes-based intervention limit the length and scope of treatment in hospital or rehabilitation settings, and 3) rising health care costs and varying reimbursement practices of insurance companies limit access to outpatient services (Effgen, 2005; Rice et al., 2004). Therapy may be provided on an individual, group, or consultative basis and in varying levels of intensity. It may be delivered in a variety of settings, including hospitals, rehabilitation settings, schools, and naturalistic community environments. Therapists are required to be creative and flexible in adapting to continually changing demands of the workplace.

GUIDELINES FOR REFERRAL

Referral to physical therapy should be considered whenever a child exhibits a physical impairment, a delay in motor development, or a qualitative impairment in postural or movement skills that causes limitations in activity participation. Referral to occupational therapy should be considered whenever there is delay or qualitative impairment in the performance of daily tasks and routines, including self-care, play, social participation, or the performance of school-related tasks (Michaud & Committee on Children with Disabilities, 2004). Referral is recommended as soon as a problem is identified in order to help family members and other caregivers learn about the diagnosis, identify additional supportive services, and undertake intervention practices that will promote development and prevent further complications.

ASSESSMENT AND PLANNING FOR INTERVENTION

Initial assessment should include 1) a review of background information from records and dis-

cussion with other professionals involved with the child; 2) an interview with family or other caregivers to determine their needs, concerns, and priorities for the child; and 3) observation of the child at play or when performing functional activities within his or her natural environment. Therapists then clinically assess the child for muscle tone and strength, joint range of motion, sensory responses and perception, neurological maturation and organization, and social and behavioral responses. Standardized tests of motor, perceptual, and functional development are usually administered to confirm impressions gained from the clinical assessment.

A treatment plan is then developed based on the results of the assessment, the priorities of the child and family, and the coordinated recommendations of other professionals involved with the child. It is extremely important that the referring physician, the family, and other team members are in agreement with the plan so that there will be a coordinated approach to intervention. The plan should address the model of intervention that is recommended (e.g., individual, group, consultative), the optimal frequency of therapy sessions, recommendations for special equipment or environmental adaptations, and the plan for instruction to family members and others. Goals are developed for a specific time period, with objective and measurable objectives delineated. Periodically, the plan is reevaluated and revised as necessary.

THERAPY IN EARLY INTERVENTION PROGRAMS

Therapy services in early intervention programs may include screening for motor or perceptual problems, monitoring the development of the child over time, consulting with families and other members of the team, and providing direct therapy. Often, the emphasis is more on helping the family to adjust to the developmental delay or disability than on correcting specific problems. Attention is given to encouraging parents to develop a satisfying and nurturing relationship with their child and to learn practical methods for supporting their child's development in the natural environments of the home and community. Through the process of developing an individualized family service plan (IFSP), therapy goals are organized around helping the family engage in daily routines and meaningful rituals that are unique to the child's family unit (DeGrace, 2003).

THERAPY IN EDUCATIONAL SETTINGS

Since the passage of the Education for All Handicapped Children Act of 1975 (PL 94-142), occupational therapists and physical therapists have worked with students with disabilities in public school settings as a "related service" to help the student benefit from special education or gain access to the general education program. Other legislation, including the Individuals with Disabilities Education Act (IDEA) of 1990 (PL 101-476) and its reauthorizations in 1997 (PL 105-17) and 2004 (PL 108-446) have further clarified the model of service delivery in this setting. Even children with disabilities who do not require special education services (e.g., those with congenital amputations or a medical condition such as juvenile rheumatoid arthritis) may be eligible for services and accommodations under other entitlements, including the Americans with Disabilities Act (ADA) of 1990 (PL 101-336), Section 504 of the Rehabilitation Act of 1973 (PL 93-112), or state regulations governing education.

Therapists may fulfill multiple roles in support of a student's educational objectives. These may include 1) promoting safe and efficient mobility, 2) recommending classroom positioning that supports optimal postural control, 3) modifying materials and routines to improve attention and organization, 4) treating perceptual and motor impairments and functional limitations to assist the student from benefiting from special education, 5) promoting independence in self-care, and 6) planning for transitions and contributing to prevocational training. Because federal legislation is designed to support the student's performance only in the school environment, some children with disabilities may require additional therapy in a clinical setting for their functional needs to be fully addressed.

A variety of service models are used for implementing school-based therapy (Case-Smith, Rogers & Johnson, 2001; Effgen, 2005). Direct service means that the therapist has frequent contact with the student, either individually or in a group, to provide selected interventions. This service model is often used for students with severe or newly acquired disabilities that limit performance or for those who require consistent, hands-on therapy to meet educational objectives. Monitoring involves the development of an intervention plan that can be effectively carried out by the teacher or other school personnel. Infrequent direct contact by the therapist is required to establish the effectiveness of the intervention and to update and revise the plan based on the student's progress. Consultation refers to the sharing of specialized knowledge with other education team members to support the overall goals of the educational program. Consultation may be oriented toward 1) the student (e.g., recommending adapted sports equipment to allow a student to participate with peers during gym class, 2) colleagues (e.g., providing in-service education to teachers regarding strategies to promote good handwriting habits), or 3) the educational system (e.g., recommending environmental adaptations that allow all students with mobility limitations to participate in extracurricular activities). Therapists may also be involved in prereferral assessments and interventions for students who are struggling in school but have not yet been identified as having a specific disability. Current practice supports the concept of inclusion so that interventions are often carried out in the student's natural environment, in the presence of peers, and with the typical tasks and materials that are expected of other students (Case-Smith & Cable, 1996).

SELECTED APPROACHES TO INTERVENTION

Many frames of reference exist to guide a therapist's selection of specific interventions. They are based on theories that reflect the philosophical beliefs of the profession and include an organized scheme for methods of treatment and for evaluation of the expected outcome of intervention. The following sections describe several popular approaches to intervention for children with developmental disabilities.

Motor Learning

Theories underlying how children with neuromuscular disorders, such as cerebral palsy, learn to move are in continual evolution. In the past, most physical therapists and occupational therapists approached treatment using one of several developmental frames of reference with the belief that motor development progressed according to a hierarchy of predictable, sequential steps and that progression of these steps was dependent on maturation of the central nervous system. Neurodevelopmental therapy (NDT), based on the work of Drs. Karel and Berta Bobath, has been one of the most widely used developmental approaches to motor learning

(Bigsby, 2003; Bobath & Bobath, 1984; Howle, 2002). Historically, treatment using this approach focused on individualized handling techniques designed to control abnormal patterns of movement while facilitating more normal patterns, thus promoting motor learning through the sensory feedback associated with active movement. Research on the efficacy of NDT poses many challenges, as treatment is not delivered in a standardized manner because there are considerable differences in the skill level of individual therapists and in the family's participation in daily therapy routines (Law & King, 1993). Nevertheless, current evidence suggests that although there may be some improvement in range of motion and quality of movement during treatment using an NDT approach, there is no evidence of long-term changes that produce normal movement patterns or increase functional movement (Butler & Darrah, 2001).

Newer theories of motor learning suggest that a systems approach to motor development is more efficacious than a purely developmental approach (Duff & Quinn, 2002; Larin, 2000). Some of the specific positioning and handling techniques used in NDT remain popular. However, the central nervous system is no longer believed to be the primary structure involved in learning to move. Therapists now recognize that multiple variables—including underlying impairments of the musculoskeletal system, cognitive ability to solve a motor dilemma, motivation to learn, task requirements, and practice effect—must be manipulated in varying combinations to cause lasting changes in motor behavior (Westcott & Goulet, 2005). Rigorous study of the effects of these combined approaches to therapy has yet to occur.

Sensory Integration Therapy

Sensory integration (SI) refers both to a theory and a model for therapy that has evolved since its introduction by A. Jean Ayres in the 1960s (Ayres, 1972; Bundy et al., 2002; Schaaf & Miller, 2005). It was originally developed to address the sensory processing, perceptual, and motor impairments of children with learning disabilities or other forms of developmental disability, but is now applied to children with a wide range of disabilities (Roley, Blanche, & Schaaf, 2001). Ayres defined sensory integration as a normal developmental process involving the ability of the child's central nervous system to organize sensory feedback from the body and the environment in order to make

successful adaptive responses. Children who have impairments in processing and integrating sensory inputs may exhibit problems with motor planning and execution and behavioral organization, which can have a significant impact on their learning and emotional well-being. Therapy is individually planned and focuses on providing the child with controlled sensory input to create a milieu that promotes the child's success in making adaptive responses to environmental challenges. Proponents of SI contend that therapy enhances neural organization, leading to more mature learning and behavior patterns. Thus, rather than teach specific skills, the goal of intervention is to enhance the brain's ability to learn. As with other developmental approaches to intervention, there is limited evidence to support its efficacy as a primary intervention (Holm, 2000; Mulligan, 2002; Vargas & Camilli, 1999).

As with NDT, current application of SI may be best viewed as a systems approach to manipulating multiple variables in an effort to help the child achieve progressively more mature adaptive responses. Modification of classroom materials and routines to reduce motor challenges can help the child focus attention more effectively on the cognitive aspects of learning. Examples include providing a chair with armrests and a nonslip seat for the child who fidgets in class, using an adapted pencil grip for the child with immature grasp who fatigues during writing, or placing color-coded page separators for the child who is slow to locate assignments in a workbook. Cognitive and behavioral strategies may be effective in helping children learn specific functional motor behaviors that limit their successful participation in sports or recreational activities (Mandich et al., 2001; Polatajko et al., 2001). Group therapy organized around a common recreational interest may focus on preventing or minimizing the negative social consequences associated with learning differences, including problems with peer social interaction and self-esteem (Williamson, 1993).

Constraint-Induced Movement Therapy

Constraint-induced (CI) movement therapy is a promising new treatment approach for improving upper-limb function in children with hemiplegia resulting from cerebral palsy or acquired neurological injury (Gordon, 2005; Plummer, 2003). In hemiplegia, the sensory and motor impairments that compromise unilateral movement efficiency cause many children to avoid using the affected extremity. Over time, this can result in a learned pattern of nonuse that can further exacerbate the impairments. The methodology used in CI therapy involves several components. First, the unaffected extremity is gently restrained, often using a removable cast or sling. Next, the child is engaged in unilateral exercises, games, and other motivating activities that demand forced use of the affected extremity. The choice of activities is based on specific movement goals that are selected by the therapist and are then broken down into small steps to be accomplished in a process known as shaping. Intensive practice in movement activities combined with positive reinforcement for each small success are critical components of the approach. Studies suggest that CI therapy may improve both motor function and quality of life for children with hemiplegia and that gains appear to be sustainable over time (Bonnier, Eliasson, & Krumlinde-Sundholm, 2006; Gordon & Wolf, 2006; Taub et al., 2004).

Orthotics

Orthotic management refers to the use of splints or braces to improve or maintain motor function. It may be used as an isolated intervention or as an adjunct to therapy. Splints may be either static (rigid) or dynamic (with moveable parts). They may serve a variety of purposes: 1) to support weak muscles, 2) to increase or maintain muscle length needed for mobility, 3) to control involuntary movement, 4) to immo-

bilize a body part, and 5) to serve as a base of support for the attachment of toys or self-care devices (Blanchet & McGee, 1996).

Lower extremity orthotics, such as molded ankle-foot orthoses (MAFOs), are worn inside the shoes. For example, they are commonly used to enhance ambulatory function in children who have neuromuscular problems, like Kia. Children with significant lower extremity weakness may require more extensive orthoses that support the knees and/or hips to achieve ambulation.

Static resting hand splints are often used to maintain muscle length and prevent the development of secondary musculoskeletal deformity in children with increased muscle tone. Their use during periods of inactivity, such as sleep, may promote increased flexibility and improved hand function when they are removed. Other splints support the hand in positions that improve function during purposeful activity. For example, a splint that supports the wrist in slight extension may make it easier for the child to oppose the thumb to other fingers, allowing a more functional grasp of objects. **Dynamic** hand splints may be designed to selectively increase muscle strength or to control abnormal patterns of movement. Figure 37.1 presents two examples of static splints commonly used by physical and occupational therapists.

Assistive Technology and Assistive Technology Services

The broad term *assistive technology*, sometimes called "AT," is used to describe a variety of de-

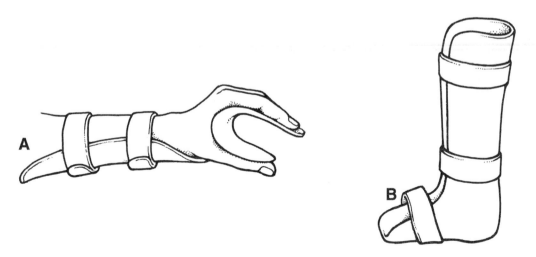

Figure 37.1.   A) Resting hand splint prevents deformity by maintaining a flaccid or spastic hand in a functional position; B) molded ankle-foot orthosis (MAFO) maintains the ankle in a desired position and prevents unwanted motion during gait.

vices and services that help children with disabilities to be included in a full range of social experiences and to function more independently, thus improving their quality of life (see Chapter 36). Assistive technology may be as simple as an enlarged spoon handle to compensate for a weak grasp, as commonplace as a wheelchair to promote mobility within the environment, or as sophisticated as individually designed computerized systems for augmentative communication using synthesized speech. Assistive technology devices include products that are purchased commercially, modified, or custom designed according to the specific needs of the user. Occupational therapists and physical therapists work with other team members to select or design appropriate assistive technology intervention, to secure funding, and to provide training to the child and other caregivers.

Even very young children may benefit from early training in the use of technology (Ostensjo, Carlberg, & Vollestad, 2005). For example, typically developing infants as young as 6 months are capable of understanding the cause-and-effect relationships necessary to operate a single-switch computer program. Early intervention programs teach young children how to use devices that promote their independence, because children who are able to enter school with these technologies in place may be better prepared to meet with success in the general education classroom.

A number of laws—including the Technology-Related Assistance for Individuals with Disabilities Act of 1988 (PL 100-407) and its recent amendments, the Assistive Technology Act of 2004 (PL 108-364), the ADA, the Rehabilitation Act of 1973, and IDEA 2004—have improved access to assistive technology devices and services for children. These laws have provided funding not only for the purchase or lease of equipment but also for services to ensure success with their use. Services supported under IDEA 2004 include 1) evaluation of the child's technological needs; 2) obtaining the needed equipment; 3) modifying, maintaining, and repairing equipment; 4) coordination of technology with other therapy services; 5) training the child and family; and 6) training for school personnel (Jones & Gray, 2005). If an evaluation indicates that a student requires assistive technology in order to benefit from special education, it must be provided as an integral element of the student's IEP. This means that public schools hold the legal responsibility for evaluation, device selection and acquisition, and train-

ing in the use of educationally relevant assistive devices. When assistive devices are recommended for purposes that are not related to educational objectives, creative strategies for funding equipment must be identified. Examples of potential funding sources include Medical Assistance, Supplemental Security Income (SSI), private foundations or donors, and durable medical equipment riders on private insurance policies.

OUTCOMES OF THERAPY

Therapists are increasingly challenged to demonstrate that the interventions they select are supported by scientific evidence and focus on relevant outcomes. They use a variety of sources of evidence to support their treatment decisions, including review of published research, personal experience and tradition, textbooks and manuals, the values and beliefs of the client, and the opinions of others who are considered to be expert (Lee & Miller, 2003; Maher et al., 2004; O'Donnell & Roxborough, 2002). Although research is an important component of evidence-based practice, the nature of therapy does not easily lend itself to the randomized controlled trials (RCT) traditionally accepted by the medical community. Methodological issues exist, including those in the measurement of treatment-related change in the presence of developmental maturation and the heterogeneity of populations. In addition, physical therapy and occupational therapy differ from most medical interventions in that they are more aptly described as dynamic processes that involve active participation by the child and family, as opposed to standardized procedures in which the child assumes a more passive role (Lee & Miller, 2003; Michaud & Committee on Children with Disabilities, 2004).

Tools used to measure the effectiveness of intervention need to demonstrate not only that gains made during therapy can be sustained over time and in the child's natural environment but also that they result in an improved quality of life for the child and family (Chen et al., 2004; Law, 2003). For example, children like Kia with cerebral palsy frequently receive physical therapy to improve mobility skills. One typical outcome measure, easy to obtain during therapy, is increased joint range of motion as measured by goniometry. The real value of this outcome must be questioned, however, unless mobility gains can 1) be easily maintained by parents or other caregivers at home; 2) prevent the need for more invasive orthopedic or other medical intervention; 3) reduce the costs for special education and related services; or 4) promote access to social, educational, or recreational experiences that are important to the child and family. Therapists must be prepared to justify that recommended interventions are appropriate (i.e., address the needs as stated by the consumer), effective (i.e., achieve targeted outcomes), and efficient (i.e., are available at the lowest cost possible). Examples of pediatric functional assessment tools in common use include the Pediatric Evaluation of Disability Inventory (PEDI; Coster & Haley, 1992; Ostensjo et al., 2006), the Uniform Data Set for Medical Rehabilitation for Children (WeeFIM; Msall, DiGaudio, & Duffy, 1993), and the School Function Assessment (SFA; Coster et al., 1998).

SUMMARY

Pediatric occupational therapy and physical therapy strive to minimize the effects of impairment, to promote full inclusion into society, and to enhance the overall quality of life for children with disabilities and their families. Although the two disciplines may overlap in certain knowledge and skills, there are important differences in their primary focus for intervention. Although therapists use a variety of sources of evidence to support their methodology, further research is needed to support the clinical efficacy of certain interventions commonly used in practice.

REFERENCES

American Occupational Therapy Association. (2002). Occupational therapy practice framework: Domain and process. *American Journal of Occupational Therapy, 56*, 609–639.

American Physical Therapy Association. (2001). Guide to physical therapy practice (2nd ed.). *Physical Therapy, 81*, 9–744.

Americans with Disabilities Act (ADA) of 1990, PL 101-336, 42 U.S.C. §§ 12101 *et seq.*

Assistive Technology Act of 2004, PL 108-364, 29 U.S.C. §§ 3001 *et seq.*

Ayres, A.J. (1972). *Sensory integration and learning disorders.* Los Angeles: Western Psychological Services.

Bigsby, R. (2003). Developmental and neurological perspectives. In E.B. Crepeau, E.S. Cohn, & B.A.B. Schell (Eds.), *Willard and Spackman's occupational therapy* (10th ed., pp. 243–252). Philadelphia: Lippincott, Williams & Wilkins.

Blanchet, D., & McGee, S.M. (1996). Principles of splint design and use. In L.A. Kurtz, P.W. Dowrick, S.E. Levy, et al. (Eds.), *Handbook on developmental disabilities: Resources for interdisciplinary care* (pp. 465–480). Gaithersburg, MD: Aspen Publishers.

Bobath, K., & Bobath, B. (1984). Neuro-developmental treatment. In D. Scrutton (Ed.), *Clinics in developmental medicine: No.90. Management of the motor disorders of children with cerebral palsy* (pp. 6–18). New York: Cambridge University Press.

Bonnier, B., Eliasson, A.C., & Krumlinde-Sundholm, L. (2006). Effects of constraint-induced movement therapy in adolescents with hemiplegic cerebral palsy: A day camp model. *Scandinavian Journal of Occupational Therapy, 13*(1) 13–22.

Bundy, A.C., Lane, S., Murray, E.A., et al. (2002). *Sensory integration: Theory and practice* (2nd ed.). Philadelphia: F.A. Davis.

Butler, C., & Darrah, J. (2001). Effects of neurodevelopmental treatment (NDT) for cerebral palsy: An AACPDM evidence report. *Developmental Medicine and Child Neurology, 43*, 778–790.

Case-Smith, J., & Cable, J. (1996). Perceptions of occupational therapists regarding service delivery models in school-based practice. *The Occupational Therapy Journal of Research, 16*(1), 23–44.

Case-Smith, J., Rogers, J., & Johnson, J.H. (2001). School-based occupational therapy. In J. Case-Smith (Ed.), *Occupational therapy for children* (4th ed., pp. 757–779). St. Louis: Mosby.

Chen, C.C., Heinemann, A.W., Bode, R.K., et al. (2004). Impact of pediatric rehabilitation services on children's functional outcomes. *American Journal of Occupational Therapy, 58*(1), 44–53.

Christiansen, C. (1993). Continued challenges of functional assessment in rehabilitation: Recommended changes. *American Journal of Occupational Therapy, 47*, 258–259.

Coster, W., Deeney, T., Haltiwanger, J, et al. (1998). *School Function Assessment.* San Antonio, TX: Harcourt Assessment.

Coster, W.J., & Haley, S.M. (1992). Conceptualization and measurement of disablement in infants and young children. *Infants and Young Children, 4*(4), 11–22.

DeGrace, B.W. (2003). Occupation-based and family-centered care: A challenge for current practice. *American Journal of Occupational Therapy, 57*(3), 347–350.

Duff, S., & Quinn, L. (2002). Motor learning and motor control. In D. Cech & S. Martin (Eds.), *Functional movement development across the life span* (2nd ed., pp. 86–117). Philadelphia: W.B. Saunders.

Education for All Handicapped Children Act of 1975, PL 94-142, 20 U.S.C. §§ 1400 *et seq.*

Effgen, S.K. (Ed.). (2005). *Meeting the physical therapy needs of children.* Philadelphia: F.A. Davis.

Gordon, C.J. (2005). A critical review of constraint-induced movement therapy and forced use in children with hemiplegia. *Neural Plasticity 12*(2–3), 245–61.

Gordon, C.J., & Wolf, S.L. (2006). Efficacy of constraint-induced movement therapy on involved upper-extremity use in children with hemiplegic cerebral palsy is not age-dependent. *Pediatrics, 117*(3), 363–373.

Holm, M.B. (2000). Our mandate for the new millennium: Evidence-based practice [Eleanor Clark Slagle Lecture]. *American Journal of Occupational Therapy, 54*(6), 575–585.

Howle, J.M. (Ed.). (2002). *Neuro-developmental treatment approach: Theoretical foundations and principles of clinical practice.* Laguna Beach, CA: NDTA Treatment Association.

Individuals with Disabilities Education Act Amendments of 1997, PL 105-17, 20 U.S.C. §§ 1400 *et seq.*

Individuals with Disabilities Education Act (IDEA) of 1990, PL 101-476, 20 U.S.C. §§ 1400 *et seq.*

Individuals with Disabilities Education Improvement Act of 2004, PL 108-446, 20 U.S.C. §§ 1400 *et seq.*

Jones, M., & Gray, S. (2005). Assistive technology: Positioning and mobility. In S.K. Effgen (Ed.), *Meeting the physical therapy needs of children* (pp. 455–474). Philadelphia: F.A. Davis.

Kniepmann, K. (1997). Prevention of disability and maintenance of health. In C. Christiansen & C. Baum (Eds.), *Occupational therapy: Enabling function and well-being* (pp. 530–555). Thorofare, NJ: Slack.

Larin, H. (2000). Motor learning: Theories and strategies for the practitioner. In S.K. Campbell, D.W. Vander Linden, & R.J. Palisano (Eds.), *Physical therapy for children* (2nd ed., pp. 170–195). Philadelphia: W.B. Saunders.

Law, M. (2003). Outcome measurement in pediatric rehabilitation. *Physical and Occupational Therapy in Pediatrics, 23*(2), 1–4.

Law, M., & King, G. (1993). Parent compliance with therapeutic interventions for children with cerebral palsy. *Developmental Medicine and Child Neurology, 35*, 983–990.

Lee, C.J., & Miller, L.T. (2003). The process of evidence-based clinical decision making in occupational therapy. *American Journal of Occupational Therapy, 57*(4), 473–477.

Maher, C.G., Sherrington, C., Elkins, M., et al. (2004). Challenges for evidence-based physical therapy: Accessing and interpreting high-quality evidence on therapy. *Physical Therapy, 84*(7), 644–654.

Mandich, A.D., Polatajko, H.J., Missiuna, C., et al. (2001). Cognitive strategies and motor performance in children with developmental coordination disorder. *Physical and Occupational Therapy in Pediatrics, 20*(2/3), 125–143.

Michaud, L.A., & Committee on Children with Disabilities. (2004). Prescribing therapy services for children with motor disabilities. *Pediatrics, 113*(6), 1836–1838.

Mulligan, S. (2002). Advances in sensory integration research. In A.C. Bundy, S.J. Lane, & E.A. Murray (Eds.), *Sensory integration: Theory and practice* (2nd ed., pp. 397–411). Philadelphia: F.A. Davis.

Msall, M.E., DiGaudio, K.M., & Duffy, L.C. (1993). Use of functional assessment on children with developmental disabilities. *Physical Medicine and Rehabilitation Clinics of North America, 4*, 517–527.

O'Donnell, M.E., & Roxborough, L. (2002). Evidence-based practice in pediatric rehabilitation. *Physical Medicine and Rehabilitation Clinics of North America, 13*(4), 991–1005.

Ostensjo, S., Bjorbackmo, W., Carlberg, E.G., et al. (2006). Assessment of everyday functioning in young children with disabilities: An ICF-based analysis of concepts and content of the Pediatric Evaluation of Disability Inventory (PEDI). *Disability and Rehabilitation, 28*(8), 489–504.

Ostensjo, S., Carlberg, E.B., & Vollestad, N.K. (2005). The use and impact of assistive devices and other environmental modifications on everyday activities and care in young children with cerebral palsy. *Disability and Rehabilitation, 27*(14), 849–861.

Plummer, A.C. (2003). Constraint-induced therapy and the motor learning literature that underpins its application. *Physical Therapy Reviews, 8*(3), 143–149.

Polatajko, H.J., Mandich, A.D., Miller, L.T., et al. (2001). Cognitive orientation to daily occupational performance: Part II. The evidence. *Physical and Occupational Therapy in Pediatrics, 20*(2/3), 125–143.

Rehabilitation Act of 1973, PL 93-112, 29, U.S.C. §§ 701 *et seq.*

Rice, S.A., Allaire, J., Elgin, K., et al. (2004). Effect of shortened length of stay on functional and educational outcome after pediatric rehabilitation. *American Journal of Physical Medicine and Rehabilitation, 83*(1) 27–32.

Rimmer, J.M. (1999). Health promotion for people with disabilities: The emerging paradigm shift from disability prevention to prevention of secondary conditions. *Physical Therapy, 79*, 495–502.

Roley, S., Blanche, E.I., & Schaaf, R.C. (2001). *Understanding the nature of sensory integration with diverse populations.* San Antonio, TX: Therapy Skill Builders.

Schaaf, R.C., & Miller, L.J. (2005). Occupational therapy using a sensory integrative approach for children with developmental disabilities. *Mental Retardation and Developmental Disabilities Research Reviews, 11*(2), 143–148.

Taub, E., Ramsey, S.L., DeLuca, S., et al. (2004). Efficacy of constraint-induced movement therapy for children with cerebral palsy with asymmetric motor impairment. *Pediatrics, 113*(2), 305–312.

Technology-Related Assistance for Individuals with Disabilities Act of 1988, PL 100-407, 29 U.S.C. §§ 2201 *et seq.*

Vargas, S., & Camilli, G. (1999). A meta-analysis of research on sensory integration treatment. *American Journal of Occupational Therapy, 53*(2), 189–198.

Westcott, S.L., & Goulet, C. (2005). Neuromuscular system: Structures, function, diagnoses, and evaluation. In S.K. Effgen (Ed.), *Meeting the physical therapy needs of children* (pp. 185–244). Philadelphia: F.A. Davis.

Williamson, G.G. (1993). Enhancing the social competence of children with learning disabilities. *Sensory Integration Special Interest Section Newsletter, 16*(1), 1–2.

World Health Organization. (2001). *International Classification of Functioning, Disability and Health (ICF).* Geneva: Author.

38 Exercise, Sports, and Recreation

Sarah Helen Evans and Terry Adirim

Upon completion of this chapter, the reader will

- Be familiar with the specific benefits of exercise for the child with special needs
- Be aware of the laws regarding the inclusion of children with physical and cognitive disabilities in physical education and community programs
- Understand how to incorporate physical education adaptations into a child's individualized education program based on his or her abilities
- Be aware of community sports and recreation programs available to children with special needs
- Know about the preparticipation evaluation for children and adolescents with disabilities
- Have knowledge of the types of injuries encountered in athletes with disabilities

---

One of the goals of the U.S. government's Healthy People 2010 initiative (a statement of national health objectives) is to have 85% of adolescents participate in vigorous physical activity for more than 20 minutes, three times per week (U.S. Public Health Service, 2000). It is recommended that children younger than the age of 12 accumulate 60 minutes of physical activity per day, with 10–15 minutes of that time devoted to moderate-vigorous activity. Despite this recommendation, it has been noted that people with disabilities tend to engage in very low rates of physical activity. Wilson (2002) reported that only 39% of children with disabilities were physically active, compared to the 64% of their peers without disabilities. As a result of this finding, there has been increased interest in incorporating exercise, sports, and recreation into the lives of children with disabilities. In addition to the improved health that results from increased fitness, this impetus reflects a commitment to full inclusion of children with disabilities in all aspects of life.

Ideally, all children should have the opportunity to participate in recreational activities and sports that capitalize on their abilities and teach new skills. For any child, free play and sporting activities promote fitness, endurance, coordination, and self-esteem. Physical activity has also been credited with maximizing muscle and bone growth and strength, increasing lean muscle mass, reducing body fat, and preventing or reducing symptoms of depression and anxiety (Chang, 2000). In addition, sports provide children with achievable goals that promote a sense of accomplishment and increase self-esteem. Recreational activities also provide the opportunity for children with developmental disabilities to be included in their broader community. This is beneficial to both children with and without disabilities. Children with disabilities develop important social skills, and typically developing children learn sensitivity to others who are different. Very few conditions preclude children from participating in exercise and sports, and almost none preclude participation in more sedentary recreational activities.

581

Thus, professionals working with children with disabilities should actively promote their participation in sport and recreation activities.

JAMIE

Jamie is a 14-year-old with Down syndrome who is interested in playing on a Special Olympics basketball team. He became interested in the Special Olympics because one of his classmates plays in a local league. In preparation for his participation, Jamie visited his pediatrician, who noted that Jamie has not had many of the medical complications associated with Down syndrome. Jamie's pediatrician first asked about symptoms suggestive of atlantoaxial subluxation, including neck pain, stiff neck, torticollis (wry neck), progressive loss of bowel or bladder control, change in strength or sensation in any of his limbs, or change in gait pattern. Jamie's mother indicated that her son had not had any of these symptoms. The pediatrician then examined Jamie and concluded that he was mildly overweight and had mild to moderate ligamentous laxity (hyperflexible, flat feet) but had no neurologic signs or symptoms suggestive of atlantoaxial subluxation.

After discussing the findings with Jamie's family, the pediatrician decided to obtain special cervical spine (neck) X rays to screen for atlantoaxial subluxation; these were found to be normal. As a result of the examination, the pediatrician signed the form permitting Jamie's participation in sports activities without specific limitations. She also told the family that this physical activity could be helpful to Jamie in a number of ways. It could aid in weight control, which is often an issue for people with Down syndrome. It could also support Jamie's emerging social skills and self-esteem. The pediatrician, however, counseled the family about certain injuries that Jamie was at higher risk to sustain as a result of his generalized ligamentous laxity. To avoid these, she suggested that he perform particular warm-up exercises and avoid certain sustained activities that would predispose him to injury. She also recommended a generalized strengthening program, explaining that stronger muscles around the joints would help stabilize and protect them.

MARISOL AND CARLY

Marisol and Carly are third-graders who are enrolled in general education classes. Although neither has cognitive limitations, Marisol has spina bifida and Carly has cerebral palsy. Both girls can walk but require the use of crutches to maintain balance and keep up with their peers. The girls know each other from playing soccer in a community league. In kindergarten and first grade, they played on teams with other children in their classes and easily used their crutches to run around on the field with their peers who did not have disabilities. Last year, in the second grade, the games became more competitive and the other children ran too fast for Marisol and Carly to keep up. In addition, as play became more aggressive, it was difficult for the girls to avoid having their crutches kicked out from under them. Both girls' parents were unwilling to allow their daughters to continue to play in the soccer league. Their parents tried interesting the girls in Special Olympic events, but Marisol and Carly were looking for the level of competition at which their peers were playing.

Through the adaptive physical education (PE) teacher in the school, Marisol and Carly's parents learned that BlazeSports sponsored a basketball team for children with disabilities in the next town. Following the preparticipation medical evaluation with their pediatricians, the designated specialist for the team assessed the girls. Marisol and Carly each underwent an evaluation via the functional classification system prior to inclusion in the program. Although neither of the girls owned wheelchairs or required them for household or community ambulation, the girls were taught to use them to play basketball. Doing so allowed the girls to have increased balance while playing the sport, as well as a significant increase in the use of their hands for ball handling.

PHYSICAL ACTIVITY IN CHILDREN WITH DISABILITIES

Developmental disabilities carry varying challenges for participation in physical activities. For example, cerebral palsy is associated with significantly impaired movements (see Chapter 26), and neuromuscular disorders such as muscular dystrophy (see Chapter 14) may be associated with decreased levels of cardiorespiratory fitness and muscular endurance. Yet, the lack of participation in physical activity by affected individuals predisposes them to more health problems, including osteoporosis and obesity, than does involvement (Dykens, Rosner, & Butterbaugh, 1998; Takeuchi, 1994). Rates of obesity are especially high in people with Down syndrome, muscular dystrophy, and spina bifida (see Chapters 18 and 28; Fernhall et al., 1996; Prasher, 1995).

Exercise, particularly aerobic activity, has been shown to aid in weight control and to be feasible in most children (Rimmer, 1992). In addition, it can improve self-confidence and offer opportunities for social interactions. Studies have shown that low self-esteem is a particular concern in children with intellectual disability (Bybee, Ennis, & Zigler, 1990; Widaman et al., 1992) and that participants in Special Olympics have greater self-esteem and confidence as compared with nonparticipating individuals (Edmiston, 1990; Klein, Gilman, & Zigler, 1993).

People with intellectual disability are also at increased risk for maladaptive behaviors including aggression, impulsivity, stereotypies, and self-injurious behaviors (Dykens et al., 1998; see Chapter 17). Studies have shown that exercise is beneficial in reducing some of these behaviors, especially in individuals with autism spectrum disorders (Celiberti et al., 1997; see Chapter 23).

Another area that is being actively investigated is the effect of sports on improving social competence in individuals with intellectual disability. In one study, participants in Special Olympics programs were shown to be more involved in extracurricular activities, hobbies, and friendships than nonparticipants (Dykens & Cohen, 1996). Other studies have demonstrated that sports activities improve social adjustment in children with learning disabilities (Rosenthal-Malek & Mitchell, 1997). A few studies have explored the effects of exercise on learning, but no significant change has been noted. Despite the paucity of data, taken as a whole, these studies suggest that children with developmental disabilities should be encouraged to participate in some form of exercise or sport activity on an ongoing basis. In support of such a conclusion, the American Academy of Orthopaedic Surgeons (1985/1992) issued a report strongly endorsing the participation of people with physical disabilities in sports and recreational activities. These activities include both regular sports (e.g., track and field, martial arts, swimming) and adapted sports (e.g., horseback riding to improve balance in the child with cerebral palsy, wheelchair races for individuals with spina bifida).

Individual sports may be more fulfilling than team sports for children who are focused on personal achievement or personal best. In contrast to team sports that tend to be organized for the youth population (e.g., Little League Baseball, soccer), individual sports (e.g., swimming) allow participation throughout a person's life span. Individual sports also allow the individual with a disability to improve at his or her own pace, without being compared with other children. As a result, even small improvement can lead to a sense of accomplishment. It should be emphasized that although individual activities may not be conducted with a team of other athletes, they can be performed in the company of other children. In this inclusive setting, the child with a disability can benefit from learning to cooperate with other children and to engage in socially appropriate behavior. The participation of a child with a disability in community recreation programs should be presented in a positive manner to the other participating children. Children without disabilities may benefit from liberal inclusion policies by becoming more accepting of individuals with disabilities not only in sporting activities but also in other aspects of life.

INCLUSION OF THE CHILD WITH DISABILITIES IN EXERCISE AND SPORTS PROGRAMS IN SCHOOL

The school curriculum should provide the time, the instruction, and the role models for all children to exercise. In fact, the Individuals with Disabilities Education Improvement Act of 2004 (IDEA 2004; PL 108-446) includes a provision that PE be part of a free appropriate public education and should be incorporated into educational curriculum for a student with disabilities as part of his or her individualized education program (IEP; see Chapter 34).

Despite these goals and the IDEA legislation, children with disabilities continue to be excluded from many general PE programs. In order to prevent this exclusion, specific goals and objectives for PE should be included in each IEP. These should be developmentally appropriate for the child and include the provision of adaptive techniques and technology when needed. Developmentally, children ages 3–5 are learning fundamental motor skills beyond walking, such as throwing, running, and using a wheelchair independently. Children ages 6–9 are finalizing development of upper-level balance skills and can successfully participate in recreational sports. Children with physical disabilities begin to develop more complex motor skills as well and are primed to learn to participate in different sports and recreational activities. Preteens (10- to 12-year-olds) are ready for more complex motor and cognitive activities and can compete in entry-level team sports (Block, 2007). Children with developmental disabilities, especially those associated with cognitive impairment, may be better suited to participate in age-normed activities when they are slightly older, as readiness is determined by developmental rather than chronological age.

Adapted PE programs are those that have the same objectives as general PE but involve adjustments in the regular program to meet the needs and abilities of students with disabilities (Dunn, 1997). In many special education departments, there are teachers specially trained in adapted PE. In the event that such a specialist is not available, adaptations can be made to the general PE program within the school to allow the student to participate. Often, these adaptations are made with the input and recommendations of the treating pediatricians and/or physical and occupational therapists. Some examples include modifying equipment, changing the rules of the game, having a student participate in alternate activities, and providing peer assistance. The purpose of these adaptations is to allow the child to be included in the general PE class with peers who do not have disabilities to the greatest extent possible.

Accommodations to team and individual sports also can be made for children with physical and sensory disabilities. For example, ball sports can be adapted by using larger or smaller balls, varying the distance required to travel while dribbling in basketball or soccer, using textured balls that facilitate catching, using brightly colored balls for a child with a visual impairment, or using softer balls for safety. A student who has a wheelchair can play these sports by holding the ball on his or her lap while moving the chair to the basket or goal or by being permitted to push the wheelchair a few times, bounce the ball, and then move the wheelchair again. Students in power wheelchairs can play field sports, especially soccer, by moving their chairs to the ball and using the power of the chair to propel or kick the ball. A student who uses a wheelchair should be encouraged to pass the ball by throwing overhead instead of from the chest. In softball, an athlete can hit the ball off a tee use larger balls or be given extra strikes before he or she is called out. In addition, an athlete with visual impairments can receive verbal cues when the ball is pitched.

During a game, a peer without a disability can be paired with the athlete with a disability to provide assistance (Block, 2007).

COMMUNITY SPORTS PROGRAMS

It was not until 1948 that the first organized sporting event for people with disabilities occurred. At that time Dr. Ludwig Guttman incorporated wheelchair sports into the rehabilitation of war veterans who were paralyzed. In the United States, federal legislation has been instrumental in both the creation of special/adapted community recreation programs for children with disabilities and in the inclusion of these children in general community recreation programs. This movement started with the Rehabilitation Act of 1973 (PL 93-112), which prohibited discrimination in recreation programs on the basis of disability. The Americans with Disabilities Act (ADA) of 1990 (PL 101-336) opened doors for the nondiscriminatory participation of individuals with disabilities in all aspects of public life, including recreational activities (Paciorek & Jones, 2001).

Still, there remain barriers to participation in both special/adapted and inclusive recreational programs. For example, in any one school or community there may not be a sufficient number of children with a particular disability to form a special team, or the special program that is available may be too far away. Barriers to inclusion also involve reluctance on the part of athletes without disabilities and their families, coaches, and teachers to allow children with disabilities to participate. Families may face a difficult decision, especially in the younger age groups, as to whether to focus participation on inclusion with peers who do not have disabilities (with or without modifications to the sport) or on more specialized sports programs for children with disabilities.

There are clearly effective ways to include individuals with disabilities in existing recreation/sports programs as well as to develop special programs (Schleien, Ray, & Green, 1997). Many of the more innovative programs are taking place in community centers and in parks and recreation programs that are supported by federal funds and, therefore, must be responsive to federal mandates. These include swimming, adapted sports, and camp programs geared to the child with physical or cognitive impairments (Chang, 1994).

As communities are becoming aware of the barriers to participation in recreational activities for children with disabilities, new opportunities and ideas for inclusion are being tested. One example is the construction of adapted playgrounds that have ramps and wheelchair-accessible equipment; another example is ball ramps in bowling alleys that allow people in wheelchairs to bowl, albeit currently from a stationary position in the chair.

A number of national organizations (with local affiliates) provide an infrastructure for programs involving athletes with disabilities; many are under the direction of the United States Olympic Committee. Certain organizations address specific disabilities; others are sports-specific organizations (see Appendix D). As an example, the United States Tennis Association and U.S. Disabled Athletes Fund have entered a partnership to jointly develop a wheelchair tennis instruction and competition program that is implemented at the community and national level. These organizations not only provide the opportunity for children with disabilities to play specific sports but also allow these children to partner with peers without disabilities.

Each of these organizations has criteria for determining how athletes are grouped according to abilities. Originally, the criteria were unique to each organization and were anatomically determined. Now athletes with disabilities are grouped according to functional skills rather than to specific medical diagnosis. The International Paralympic Committee (2000) criteria state that a person is eligible to participate in the Paralympic Games if he or she cannot participate on reasonably equal terms in a sport for people without disabilities because of a functional disadvantage due to a permanent disability. The functional classification system requires that an athlete be evaluated both by a bench examination and a sports specific examination. These examinations are technical and can be done only by designated physicians, and they do not replace the need for preparticipation medical evaluations (Wind, Schwend, & Larson, 2004).

Since the inception of the function oriented grouping in sports classification, individuals with a range of diagnoses have been able to compete against each other. A wide range of sports are available, including archery, track and field, cycling, equestrian activities, fencing, judo, powerlifting, sailing, soccer, swimming, table tennis, wheelchair basketball, wheelchair rugby, wheelchair tennis, volleyball, alpine and cross-country skiing, ice-sledge hockey, and wheelchair dance sport. The number of competitive events continues to grow each year.

The Special Olympics is probably the best known of the private agencies promoting sports programs for individuals with developmental disabilities. Its mission is stated as follows:

> Providing year-round sports training and athletic competition in a variety of Olympic-type sports for all children and adults with intellectual disability, giving them continuing opportunities to develop physical fitness, demonstrate courage, experience joy, participate in the sharing of gifts, skills and friendship with their families, other Special Olympic athletes and the community. (Special Olympics, n.d.)

At the opposite end of the disability spectrum, and new since the 1996 Paralympic Games, is the U.S. Disabled Athletes Fund and its offshoot, the BlazeSports Program, organized specifically for children with physical disabilities. This program supports numerous basketball and tennis teams around the country. Equally devoted to increasing self-esteem and providing sports and recreation to its members, the BlazeSports program is closer to traditional community-based organizations for children without disabilities in that the level of competition increases as children grow and their skills increase and the activities can help identify elite athletes among the participants.

THE PREPARTICIPATION EXAMINATION

The preparticipation examination is an essential component of injury and illness prevention in athletes. Every athlete with a disability should have this exam performed at least once per year by a physician knowledgeable about sports medicine issues (American Academy of Pediatrics, Committee on Sports Medicine and Committee on Children with Disabilities, 1987). The purpose is not to determine whether a child should be excluded from participation but rather to provide an opportunity for the physician to recommend prevention measures and/or adapted activities based on development skills and physical challenges. This evaluation may include special tests to uncover conditions problematic or hazardous to the athlete. In addition, it can provide advice in choosing an appropriate sport and/or the adaptive equipment needed for that sport. The general approach to the preparticipation examination for the athlete with disabilities should be similar to that of the approach to the preparticipation examination for the athlete without disabilities. In this way, the focus is directed away from the primary disabling condition so that the examiner will not overlook common medical issues apart from the primary disability.

Following completion of the regular exam, attention should be turned to any unique aspects or concerns arising from or secondary to the primary disabling condition. When considering Jamie's request to participate in the Special Olympics, Jamie's doctor was aware that individuals with Down syndrome have physical differences that may affect their ability to participate in contact sports or those requiring vigorous effort. Approximately 15% of people with Down syndrome have atlantoaxial subluxation (see Chapter 18), a condition caused by laxity of the ligament that holds the first neck vertebra (C1) in place. Excessive motion at this level has the potential to cause permanent damage to the spinal cord, potentially leading to quadraplegia with ventilator dependency and/or death (Sullivan & Anderson, 2000). As a result, screening for this problem is mandated by the Special Olympics prior to an individual's participating in certain sports: butterfly stroke and diving starts in swimming (as well as individual medley events), pentathlon, high jump, squat lifts, equestrian sports, artistic gymnastics, football (soccer), alpine skiing, snowboarding, and any warm-up exercises placing undue stress on the head and neck (Special Olympics, 2007). Children with significant atlantoaxial subluxation are encouraged to take part in lower impact sports and to be followed closely for any signs of spinal cord impingement.

A physician who is familiar with the child's needs should perform the annual preparticipation examination. Each year, the physician should identify new physical/developmental accomplishments and challenges as well as address ongoing issues. Topics to review should include the use of adaptive equipment (e.g., a wheelchair); presence of allergies; special dietary needs; risk of exercise-induced wheezing; emotional, psychiatric, or behavioral problems that could interfere with participation in sports; bone or joint disorders; hearing impairment and hearing aid use; contact lens or eyeglasses use; use of dentures; immunization record (especially tetanus); and long-term medications that could enhance performance (e.g., steroids) or interfere with it (e.g., sedating medication). The physician should also ask about past medical problems that may place the child at in-

creased risk for sports injury. These include exercise-induced fainting or seizures, past heat or cold injuries, prior fractures or dislocations, a history of menstrual problems, prior medical disqualification, and the level of previous sports participation.

The physical examination should include all organ systems, with a special focus on those areas affected by the child's disability. Finally, athletes who use wheelchairs, prosthetics, or other medical assistive devices (e.g., ostomies) should have this equipment checked periodically for fit and wear.

Some sports are clearly inappropriate for children with certain disabilities. For example, contact sports are contraindicated in a child with brittle bones due to osteogenesis imperfecta (see Chapter 14) or for the child with Down syndrome who has atlantoaxial subluxation. Similarly, children with neuromuscular diseases such as Duchenne muscular dystrophy cannot safely participate in strength training or in activities that require excessive eccentric contraction of the muscles. In the past, however, children with disabilities were often excluded from sports unnecessarily. Take the example of swimming and diving for children with seizure disorders (see Chapter 29). Previously, neither swimming nor diving was permitted; now it is clear that provided that there is adequate supervision and the child's seizures are under good control, these activities carry little risk of injury.

The Committee on Sports Medicine and Fitness of the American Academy of Pediatrics (2001) devised a classification system for sports. Sports are classified as either contact or noncontact and then are further subclassified into strenuous, moderately strenuous, and nonstrenuous activities. The committee also set forth recommendations for participation by children with various medical conditions on the basis of this classification system. In this system, very few conditions exclude a child from playing all sport activities. Even children with Down syndrome who have complex congenital cardiac malformations may be able to participate in some sporting activities, depending on the severity of the condition and following consultation with the child's cardiologist. Some children are excluded from contact sports but are cleared for participation in nonstrenuous, noncontact activities. These individuals should consult with their physician before deciding on a sport.

SPORT INJURIES IN THE ATHLETE WITH DISABILITIES

The types of sport injuries sustained by children with disabilities are usually the same as those in typically developing children, and injury should be assessed in a similar manner. If the child is unable to describe what happened, obtaining a history of the injury from witnesses or parents is helpful. In a child with no history of acute trauma, overuse injuries ranging from muscle strains to stress fractures should be considered. After the history is taken, a thorough physical examination is performed, including a careful evaluation of the affected extremity and related body regions. For example, the hips should be examined in a child with knee pain because hip pain often is perceived to be coming from the knee. In some children, a more comprehensive examination is indicated to uncover unappreciated injuries. Finally, tests may be taken, including blood work, bone density measurements, X rays of the injured extremity, or more advanced imaging techniques (e.g., computed tomography, magnetic resonance imaging).

Children with certain developmental disabilities and associated physical impairments are at greater risk for specific injuries resulting from exercise or sports. The child with spina bifida or a spinal cord injury may not be able to perceive pain in an injured area. As a result, he or she is at risk for undetected soft-tissue damage from contusions, abrasions, lacerations, or crush injuries. In addition, many of these individuals will be participating in sports using their wheelchairs. This shifts the site of the most common injuries from the lower extremities to the upper extremities; wrist and shoulder sprains and pain are common. Athletes with spinal cord lesions at or above the sixth thoracic vertebra (T6) may also have problems with autonomic dysreflexia, potentially resulting in poor thermoregulation and altered blood pressure control. Therefore careful attention to appropriate dress and hydration is essential.

For children with cerebral palsy, there is an increased risk for ligament sprains and muscle strains because of tone abnormalities and inadequate muscle control resulting in muscle imbalance around the joints. The presence of contractures is more likely to place stress on affected joints, leading to a higher risk of injury with exercise. Attention to using appropriately sized adaptive equipment (e.g., braces, wheelchairs) and padding of the equipment, in addition to the use of otherwise required safety equipment, is essential in preventing injury.

Individuals with Down syndrome have other specific physical concerns with regard to sports and recreation, especially involving the cervical spine. These children should be screened for an abnormality prior to participating in exercises or sports that place the neck at risk for injury (e.g., gymnastics, contact sports, diving). If a child is found to have a cervical spine abnormality, alternative sports activities should be chosen. Another medical concern for some children with Down syndrome is congenital heart disease that may decrease endurance or predispose the individual to arrhythmias during intense exercise. In this case, consultation with a pediatric cardiologist should be sought. Children with Down syndrome also have a higher incidence of orthopedic issues resulting from hypotonia and ligamentous laxity. This can lead to flat feet, scoliosis, a slipped capital femoral epiphysis, and patellar instability (see Chapter 18). These conditions can be caused or exacerbated by physical activity. Awareness that the child with Down syndrome is at risk for these problems can help anticipate and prevent these complications. For example, orthotic shoe inserts can be used to treat flat feet, and orthoses may help patellar instability.

Wheelchair athletes are particularly susceptible to injuries related to the extensive use of their upper extremities in sports such as road racing, basketball, track, and tennis. Injuries most commonly involve sprains and strains of the wrists and shoulders. To avoid these problems, it is important that athletes use appropriate equipment and that they stretch, train, and rest properly. Very aggressive or very young athletes should pay particular attention to the availability of new or evolving equipment or modifications designed to minimize repetitive use injuries. Healing of skin lesions may also be an issue for these athletes, especially among those who have insensate areas, so careful attention to skin care of blisters and lacerations is important. Proper attire, including helmets for high-speed activities, is also important in wheelchair athletes. For children who are in wheelchairs both inside and outside the sports arena, osteopenia is common in the lower extremities. This leads to an increased risk of fractures in the legs in situations where the force involved might not otherwise cause a problem (Wilson, 2002).

NONPHYSICAL RECREATION

WordNet (http://www.wordnet.com) defines recreation as "an activity that diverts, amuses or stimulates, that refreshes and renews health and spirits by enjoyment and relaxation." Children would likely define recreation as play. Play can take forms both physically active and sedentary. Either can be challenging for a child with a disability. To assist with sedentary recreation such as games or art, multiple adapted toys with various switches and modifications exist, allowing children with disabilities to play more independently. Initially such toys could only be found in specialized catalogues. Now, stores as common as Toys-R-Us carry an extensive line of adapted toys, and many toys manufactured for children without disabilities have switches that make the toys fun for everyone.

In this millennium, play for all children has been affected by technological development that has resulted in a significant increase in video entertainment. Many types of electronic game controls are easily accessible to children with disabilities and in some cases result in a more evenly matched opportunity for competition with children who do not have disabilities. The dexterity required to use video game controls adeptly is significantly less than that required to write, type, or fasten buttons. This also means that remote television controls are often mastered at an early age. As with all children, although speed and dexterity increase with adroitness at video games, generalized learning is not as great as with reading and mathematic games. The American Academy of Pediatrics recommends a limit of 2 hours of screen time per day for children.

Other recreational activities include trips to restaurants and attractions and participation in art and music classes. Most commercial movie theaters are wheelchair accessible, and spectator sports arenas and concert halls have wheelchair-accessible seating. Many amusement parks have rides that can accommodate wheelchairs or transfers from wheelchairs to allow children with disabilities to enjoy the rides. Disneyland Resorts list its rides according to wheelchair accessibility on its web site; information is categorized for guests with hearing impairments as well. Although most places have wheelchairs available on site for use by their patrons, children should take their own chairs with them whenever possible. A rental chair is never as light or as supportive, nor can it position the child as well as a chair custom made for the child. Careful attention should be paid to the details of such customized chairs, keeping recreation in mind, so that children may participate in outings easily. For example, a child who goes to restaurants regularly should have a chair that fits easily under a commercial dinner table.

Art and music classes can be easily adapted for children with disabilities and, although these activities are therapeutic, they are very different from art and/or music therapy. Sometimes, changes in media or the way in which media are worked is necessary in the art class. Adaptive equipment is also available to help the individual hold writing, drawing, or painting utensils. Similar adaptations are available for some musical instruments, especially percussion instruments (e.g., drums). Music volume and bass level can be adjusted for children who are deaf to allow the children to interact with the music via vibratory input.

SUMMARY

Sports and recreational activities are important to promote the physical and emotional health of all children, including children with disabilities. Virtually all children can participate in these activities, although some modification or use of adaptive equipment may be required. An effective exercise/sports program can improve weight control, socialization, self-esteem, and acceptance of the child into the community. The mission of many organizations is to assist the family of a child with disabilities in identifying appropriate sport and recreational opportunities. Medical assessment prior to participation in sports is important, especially for individuals with disorders that carry enhanced risks of injury.

REFERENCES

American Academy of Orthopaedic Surgeons. (1992). *Support of sports and recreational programs for physically disabled people* (Document No. 1123). Rosemont, IL: Author. (Original work published 1985)

American Academy of Pediatrics, Committee on Sports Medicine and Committee on Children with Disabilities. (1987). Exercise for children who are mentally retarded. *Pediatrics, 80,* 447–448.

American Academy of Pediatrics, Committee on Sports Medicine and Fitness. (2001). Medical conditions affecting sports participation. *Pediatrics, 107,* 1205–1209.

Americans with Disabilities Act (ADA) of 1990, PL 101-336, 42 U.S.C. §§ 12101 *et seq.*

Block, M.B. (2007). *A teacher's guide to including students with disabilities in general physical education* (3rd ed.). Baltimore: Paul H. Brookes Publishing Co.

Bybee, J., Ennis, P., & Zigler, B. (1990). Effects of institutionalization on the self-concept and outerdirectedness of adolescents with intellectual disability. *Exceptionality*, *1*, 215–216.

Celiberti, D.A., Bobo, H.E., Kelly, K.S., et al. (1997). The differential and temporal effects of antecedent exercise on the self-stimulatory behavior of a child with autism. *Research in Developmental Disabilities, 18*, 139–150.

Chang, F.M. (1994). The child athlete with chronic disease. In C.L. Stanitski, J.C. De Lee, & D. Drez, Jr. (Eds.), *Pediatric and adolescent sports medicine* (Vol. 3, pp. 34–43). Philadelphia: W.B. Saunders.

Chang, F.M. (2000). Physically challenged athletes. In J.A. Sullivan & S.J. Anderson (Eds.), *Care of the young athlete*. Rosemont, IL: American Academy of Orthopaedic Surgeons.

Dunn, J.M. (1997). *Special physical education*. Salem, OR: Bookbyte/Norwest Textbooks.

Dykens, E.M., & Cohen, D.J. (1996). Effects of Special Olympics International on social competence in persons with intellectual disability. *Journal of American Academy of Child and Adolescent Psychiatry, 35*, 223–229.

Dykens, E.M., Rosner, B.A., & Butterbaugh, G. (1998). Exercise and sports in children and adolescents with developmental disabilities: Positive physical and psychosocial effects. *Child and Adolescent Psychiatric Clinics of North America, 7*, 757–771.

Edmiston, P.A. (1990). *The influence of participation in a sports training program on the self concepts of the educable mentally retarded attending a one-week Special Olympics sports camp* (Special Olympics International, Inc., research monograph). Washington, DC: Joseph P. Kennedy, Jr. Foundation.

Fernhall, B., Pitetti, K.H., Rimmer, J.H., et al. (1996). Cardiorespiratory capacity of individuals with intellectual disability including Down syndrome. *Medicine and Science in Sports and Exercise, 28*, 366–371.

Individuals with Disabilities Education Improvement Act of 2004, PL 108-446, 20 U.S.C. §§ 1400 *et seq.*

International Paralympic Committee. (2000, January). Sports: Classifications. Section IT: Eligibility of competitors. Retrieved January 14, 2002, from http://www.paralympic.org

Klein, T., Gilman, E., & Zigler, E. (1993). Special Olympics: An evaluation by parents and professionals. *Mental Retardation, 31*, 15–23.

Paciorek, M.J., & Jones, J.A. (2001). *Disability, sport and recreation resources*. Traverse City: Cooper Publishing Group.

Prasher, V.P. (1995). Overweight and obesity amongst Down syndrome adults. *Journal of Intellectual Disability Research, 39*, 437–441.

Rehabilitation Act of 1973, PL 93-112, 29 U.S.C. §§ 701 *et seq.*

Rimmer, J.R. (1992). Cardiovascular fitness programming for adults with intellectual disability: Translating research into practice. *Adapted Physical Activity Quarterly, 9*, 237–248.

Rosenthal-Malek, A., & Mitchell, S. (1997). Brief report: The effects of exercise on the self-stimulatory behaviors and positive responding of adolescents with autism. *Journal of Autism and Developmental Disorders, 27*, 193–202.

Schleien, S.J., Ray, M.T., & Green, F.P. (1997). *Community recreation and people with disabilities: Strategies for inclusion* (2nd ed.). Baltimore: Paul H. Brookes Publishing Co.

Special Olympics. (n.d.). *Special Olympics: About us.* Retrieved October 4, 2006, from http://www.specialolympics.org / Special + Olympics + Public + Website/ English/About_Us/default.htm

Special Olympics. (2007). *Special Olympics sports rules: Summer sports.* Retrieved February 13, 2007, from http://www.specialolympics.org/special+olympics+public+website/english/coach/sports_rules/summer+sports.htm

Sullivan, J.A., & Anderson, S.J. (Eds.). (2000). *Care of the young athlete*. Rosemont, IL: American Academy of Orthopaedic Surgeons.

Takeuchi, E. (1994). Incidence of obesity among school children with intellectual disability in Japan. *American Journal of Intellectual disability, 99*, 283–288.

U.S. Public Health Service. (2000). *Healthy People 2010: National health promotion and disease prevention objectives.* Washington, DC: U.S. Department of Health and Human Services.

Widaman, K.F., MacMillan, D.L., Hemsley, R.R., et al. (1992). Differences in adolescents' self-concept as a function of academic level, ethnicity, and gender. *American Journal on Intellectual Disability, 96*, 387–404.

Wilson, P. (2002). Exercise and sports for children who have disabilities. *Physical Medicine and Rehabilitation Clinics of North America, 13*, 907–923.

Wind, W.M., Schwend, M.D., & Larson, J. (2004). Sports for the physically challenged child. *The Journal of the American Academy of Orthopaedic Surgeons, 12*, 126–137.

39   Ethical Dilemmas

Tomas Jose Silber

Upon completion of this chapter, the reader will

- Become familiar with medical ethical issues concerning children with disabilities, such as informed consent and assent, medical rights of minors, prenatal diagnosis, genetic testing and screening, withholding of treatment, advanced directives, sexual and reproductive rights, and human subject research

- Learn the vocabulary of ethics, including language related to parental rights, the best interest of the child, and the mature minor doctrine

- Review moral reasoning and understand how it involves the balancing of competing ethical theories, principles, and casuistry to resolve ethical dilemmas

- Understand the differences and similarities between ethical decision making and legal requirements

- Be cognizant of ethics committees and the availability of ethics consultations

---

Moral issues are interwoven with professional practice, and it is the duty of every educator and health care professional to recognize, reflect on, and process ethical dilemmas. This obligation of being available to patients and families when they are making morally charged decisions is no different, and the responsibility is no less than that involved in aiding them with educational and clinical decisions. Yet, although most professionals are well prepared for the latter, they are often intimidated by the former.

The purpose of this chapter is to empower those who take care of children with disabilities for the "daily practice" of clinical ethics. To begin, it must be recognized that we do not come to ethical deliberations in a naïve state. Our membership in a culture, religion, gender, and so on has immersed us in the world of ethics since childhood. People come to their profession with certain core beliefs and biases, and they must be careful to "disarm" or at least acknowledge these in all clinical, educational, and ethical considerations (Engelhardt, 2003). This awareness is particularly important in the traditional hospital environment, where there is the potential for a power differential between professionals and the families they serve. This disparity, fortunately, is changing.

In the old prototype, parents came as supplicants to receive care for their child; professionals were the ones with all the knowledge. In the new prototype of family-centered care, recognition is given to the role of parents who, through time spent caring for their child, have become "experts" in the disease and intricate care issues, including the availability or lack of availability of appropriate services. These families also think about ethical dilemmas involving the care of their child. Therefore, clinicians and educators need to consider the experiential expertise of patients and families and acknowledge their own values and abilities for ethical decision making (American Academy of Pediatrics, Committee on Hospital Care, 2003).

In addition to the general ethical issues relating to the medical care of children, there are some that are specific to children with disabilities. Advances in reproductive, genetic, and life-support technology continue to raise a number of unique ethical questions in the care of these children. Are there instances in which medical care can be ethically withheld? Should all technologically feasible genetic screening be done? Is it ethical to offer risky research procedures to children who may not have the capacity to provide **assent?**

The sheer complexity of the ethical dilemmas that relate to children with disabilities, the magnitude of the various possible outcomes, and the strongly held opposing viewpoints encountered all call for careful and deliberate reflection. For example, there may be tension between adhering to the precepts of disability rights and proposing options of care, such as palliative care only. Indeed, respect for the rights of individuals with disabilities and willingness to advocate for them at times may contrast with (but should not prevent or inhibit discussions about) limiting aggressive life-sustaining therapy. This style of thoughtful balancing of competing values, referred to as *moral reasoning*, is the function of clinical ethics. This can be best exemplified with a case.

SIDNEY

Sidney was a child noted to have marked hypotonia in infancy. Sidney developed a disability over time and was discovered to suffer from an inherited and ultimately fatal mitochondrial disease. Sidney's abnormal swallowing function led to a progressive worsening of the nutritional status, accompanied by occasional bouts of respiratory distress. Sidney's mother, a physician, was increasingly concerned that her child was faced with a diminished quality of life and one filled with pain, discomfort, and similar to that of many patients for whom she had cared. She and Sidney's father had, over the years, worked intensely with their child's pediatrician and genetics team, as well as a child neurologist, a developmental psychologist, and professionals in the respiratory, physical, and occupational therapy fields. When Sidney's pediatrician proposed placing a tracheostomy to facilitate airway suctioning and in preparation for a respirator, as well as inserting a gastrostomy feeding tube to improve his nutrition, the parents refused to give consent. A number of members of the multidisciplinary rehabilitation team became very upset with this decision and requested a consultation from the medical ethics consult service.

During the consultation, it became clear that the parents were very caring and loving of Sidney, their only child. They considered quality of life, however, to be a paramount issue, and they wanted to protect their child from further suffering with this potentially painful proposed medical/surgical intervention. Sidney's parents noted that they had thought through this decision with the help of their extended family. They felt comfortable with their decision and believed that it was justified. An "ethics conversation" was held with both parents, and a case conference was conducted with the medical multidisciplinary team. After considering the issues, the medical ethics consultation team recommended that because of the serious nature and grim prognosis of the condition, and because the parents' decision was congruent with their value system, the parents were entitled to exercise their parental right of surrogate decision making. Following the communication of this ethics consult, the parents formally refused any further intervention. Sidney died peacefully at home a few months later.

This painful story raises many issues: Was this decision right? Who has the right to make a decision? What are legitimate considerations on which to base a decision? What should be done regarding dissent? The sheer number of ethical dilemmas that relate to the treatment of children with disabilities and the importance of the various possible outcomes call for careful and deliberate reflection. To complicate matters, there is no consensus among ethicists about many ethical issues. Moreover, there is no accepted methodology to verify if a right moral decision has been made (Society for Health and Human Values-Society for Bioethics Consultation, 1998). This places a lot of responsibility on all professionals dealing with children with disabilities. To get acquainted with the field of clinical ethics, there is a need to familiarize oneself with the vocabulary of ethics and ethical theory.

THE VOCABULARY OF ETHICS

Understanding ethical terms and their various applications may facilitate thinking through ethical dilemmas. Students and professionals should also become familiar with ethical principles, ethical theory, casuistry, and the basic knowledge of regulations and legal requirements.

Ethical Principles

Ethical principles are general statements about what types of actions are right and wrong. Proposed principles include autonomy (the right to self-determination), beneficence (an obligation to act to benefit an individual), nonmaleficence ("first, do no harm"), and justice (fairness in the distribution of resources) (Beauchamp & Childress, 1994).

Ethical Theories

Ethical theories are attempts to construct a "master approach" to evaluate moral issues (Mappes & Degrazia, 2000). They involve systematic connections among moral principles. The main difference among competing ethical theories is the criteria utilized to decide what is "right." Theories differ in their account of what makes something good. Some theories focus on the consequence of a behavior (consequentialist ethics). Within this group, some see pleasure (or the avoidance of suffering) as the deciding criterion (hedonism). Others still look at the consequences of an act and embrace the greatest happiness for the greatest number (utilitarianism). The "formalists" appeal to the concept of deontological ethics (from the Greek word for "duty"). They postulate that the rightness of an act does not flow from the goodness of the outcome but rather from the kind of act it is. Usually this is specified in terms of universal principles of moral duty (Kantian moral imperatives). Often, distinctions are not that clear. The ethics of caring, which focuses on ethical decisions as embedded in the context of relationships, combines elements of consequentialism and deontology.

A different viewpoint altogether has originated in virtue ethics, in which the right behavior is the one that comes from a virtuous person. This follows the Aristotelian view that it is the moral person who will make moral decisions out of the strength of his or her character. Finally, in the last decades of the 20th century, new thoughts enriched the field of bioethics, ranging from feminist philosophy to multicultural and international perspectives. Most recently, the theory of urban ethics has emerged, addressing issues of discrimination and disparity in health care (Cesire, Blustein, & Fleischman, 2000).

Ethical theories do not give a concrete answer to specific problems, but they may serve as guides for looking for an answer and deciding which factors are relevant. A theory of morality aspires to explain decisions, to illuminate conclusions, and to test for consistency. Criticism of both principled ethics and ethical theory frequently includes the potential for getting lost in abstractions and separating theory from practice.

Casuistry is the fine tuning of ethical choices based on previous resolutions of similar dilemmas. It emphasizes the point that theory finds its meaning mostly in the context of practice.

Many classic terms, originating from both casuistry and jurisprudence, have been added to the ethics vocabulary, such as the *doctrine of double effect, ordinary versus extraordinary means, substituted judgment* (a concept that entails representing what a person would have desired for him- or herself if able to express his or her wishes), and *surrogate decision making* (see the Pediatric Ethics section). The doctrine of double effect makes it permissible ethically to have a bad outcome (e.g., death) if the intention was to pursue a benefit and not to inflict harm (e.g., to alleviate respiratory distress with morphine in a terminal patient with cystic fibrosis). The concept of ordinary versus extraordinary treatment is understood to apply not to the treatment technology itself (e.g., tracheostomy and gastrostomy tube placement are now "ordinary" procedures) but to how a procedure relates to a patient's situation (i.e., these procedures may be considered an extraordinary intervention for a child with a very severe acquired cognitive impairment).

ETHICS AND THE LAW

Ethics has been referred to as moral reflection with all things considered. Some acquaintance with the law is, therefore, a necessary part of this equation, especially when considering specific decisions such as reporting child abuse, child neglect, or sterilization of adolescents with severe intellectual disability. Knowledge of the law is also needed for practical implementations, such as the use of courts to intervene in health care decisions, appointment of guardians, and interpretation of statutes. Although the law is also informed by ethical principles, legal dispositions per se do not necessarily imply right ethical conclusions and on occasion it may be necessary to challenge a law on moral grounds.

PEDIATRIC ETHICS

A number of ethical concepts are associated specifically with children. These include child assent, **informed consent** (parental permission), surrogate decision making, parental rights, medical rights of minors, and the best interest of the child (Cassidy & Fleischman, 1996). Moreover, some ethical dilemmas present themselves repeatedly, such as decisions to forgo treatments, genetic testing, fetal therapy, sexual and reproductive rights of individuals with disabilities, organ donation, and rationing of care.

Informed Consent and Assent

Informed consent means that any person who will be affected by a proposed treatment has the right to learn about the proposed treatment, alternative treatments (or nontreatment), and the possible outcomes (American Academy of Pediatrics, Committee on Bioethics, 1995). Although studies have shown that older children and adolescents have the capacity to understand and make medical decisions, from a legal perspective, it is the parents who make binding decisions for the child. Parents therefore exercise a right of surrogate decision making by giving permission for the treatment of their children (Bartholome, 1995). These parental rights are seldom questioned unless unusual circumstances occur (e.g., cases of parental abuse or neglect). Despite their inability to give consent, children should receive explanations about any proposed evaluations or treatments, as discussed in the next section.

Medical Rights of Minors

Special ethical issues arise during adolescence, when risky behaviors and budding autonomy challenge the need for parental consent for treatment. Under certain circumstances, minors may have the legal authority to give consent and make medical decisions (Ford, English & Sigman, 2004; Sigman & O'Connor, 1991). Responding to the concern that many adolescents would remain untreated if parental consent were required, certain statutes developed since the 1960s came to be known as the medical rights of minors. The statutes' most important outcome is allowing mature adolescents to consent to treatment under some circumstances (e.g., reproductive health care, mental health care) (Ford et al., 2004). It is the treating clinician who decides if a particular adolescent qualifies as a mature minor (Sigman & O'Connor, 1991). This pivotal concept has been expressed long ago in the legal literature as follows: "A 'mature minor' makes his or her decisions on daily affairs, is mobile, independent, and can

manage financial affairs; can initiate own appointments, understands risks, benefits, and informed consent" (Brown & Truitt, 1979).

Indeed, an adolescent who has lived with his or her disability for 15 years certainly would have some valuable insight into his situation and therefore the right to participate in decisions regarding medical treatments. The medical rights of minors therefore need to be taken into consideration in determining the degree of participation in decisions by older children and teenagers with disabilities. Although it is true that, legally, consent belongs to the parents (with exceptions allowed for statutes and state laws), it makes sense for **mature minors** to have varying degrees of participation. Reluctance to allow this participation or conflicts among parents, adolescents, and professionals can lead to ethical dilemmas, especially when dealing with end-of-life issues.

Forgoing Treatment

Some children with severe developmental disabilities are born with medical conditions that are life shortening. Decisions about whether and/or how to treat these conditions require thoughtful weighing of risks and benefits (American Academy of Pediatrics, Committee on Bioethics, 1994, 1996; Street et al., 2000). To give informed consent for treatment, parents must receive information about the risks of the procedure, the possible benefits, and the long-term prognosis. In providing this information, physicians and other health care professionals may be influenced by their own personal or professional experiences and biases concerning a particular infant's disability. Research has shown that physicians and nurses are often disinclined to treat infants with severe disabilities based on issues of quality of life, effect on the family, and cost of care. They are also less optimistic about achieving a "satisfactory outcome" than are occupational and physical therapists, social workers, teachers, and parents—a strong argument in favor of bringing these other professionals into the ethical decision-making process (Lee, Penner, & Cox, 1991).

As a result of bias, clinicians may consciously or unconsciously accentuate certain risks, underestimate the quality of life of people with disabilities, and unduly influence the parents' treatment decisions (Bach & Campagnolo, 1992; Gerhart et al., 1994). From the perspective of medical ethics, professionals should be aware of their own biases and attempt to suppress or acknowledge them when providing information about the risks and benefits of a procedure or treatment (Engelhardt, 2003).

Even if parents can receive and process information, some clinicians maintain that parents still are not in a position to give informed consent. They argue that parents faced with a child with severe disabilities are in such a state of shock and so overwhelmed by fear, guilt, and horror that they are not capable of making an informed decision. Others argue with equal conviction that even though parents have these feelings, they still retain their right to decide and their wishes should not be overridden. Generally, it has been noted that parents' decisions in these situations are thoughtful and responsible, especially if they are given sufficient time to consider their choices (Carter & Levetown, 2004). In most instances, delays of a few days will not adversely affect an infant's outcome, may lead to more informed decision making, and help preserve the parents' right to make decisions about their child's care. Most important, parents need to be reassured that they are "good parents" no matter what decision they make (Carter & Levetown, 2004). A special commission acknowledged the importance of parental involvement: "In nearly all cases, parents are best suited to collaborate with practitioners in making decisions about an infant's care, and the range of choices practitioners offer should typically reflect the parents' preferences regarding treatment" (President's Commission, 1983).

Current mores propose that when treatment of an ill infant has a reasonable chance of being successful and the infant is likely to survive and be able to interact with his or her environment, even with a serious disability, the best interests of that infant are served by treatment. When treatment is likely to be futile, however, it need not be instituted (Carter & Levetown, 2004; Loewy, 1994).

Advance Directives

The term *advance directive* originated in the world of adult medicine and refers to instructions a patient leaves about the medical care he or she desires in advance of a time when incompetence or loss of consciousness prevents that person from giving directives. More loosely, advance directives refer to a physician's order, in a patient's medical chart, to prospectively limit the amount of intervention that should occur in the event of a medical emergency (Walsh-Kelly et al., 1999). Such an order might indicate that in the event of a cardiopulmonary arrest, no resuscitative actions should be taken. Alternatively, it might limit, rather than exclude, intervention in such an emergency.

These advance directives have also been used for children with disabilities, most often for those who are neurologically devastated and have no hope of improvement. In such cases, parents often stipulate that normal care be provided but extraordinary measures not be taken simply to prolong life. Under such circumstances, a **do not resuscitate (DNR)** order is written by an attending physician after discussion with and consent by the parents. This order can be rescinded at any time at the parents' request. The DNR terminology is imbedded in the medical culture, yet can at times be misinterpreted as abandonment of the patient, a sense that nothing can be done. This should never be the case, as palliative and comfort care are important treatment modalities. Many clinicians are now proposing that a DNR would benefit families more if formulated and understood as an allowing for natural death (AND) order.

Genetic Testing and Screening Programs

Tests for genetic conditions such as fragile X syndrome can provide information not only about the child who is being tested but also about his or her family (Ross & Moon, 2000). This is a potential ethical problem; people who do not want to know this information about themselves may have their autonomy violated as a consequence of another person's test. Furthermore, genetic tests may be used to predict the development of a currently asymptomatic disease in the future (e.g., Huntington disease, breast cancer), rather than to diagnose a current illness (Terrenoire, 1992). If test results become part of a medical record, insurance companies could gain access to them and could use them as a basis for denying health care, disability, or life insurance coverage for the tested individual or other family members (Miller, 1998).

As new genetic tests become available, society will need to consider whether the benefit to the person being tested outweighs the possible harm not only to that person but also others in the family. Several issues need to be contemplated for ethical decision making. Is there a treatment for the condition being detected by the test? How accurate is the test? What are the consequences of false positives and false negatives? Will the parents or other family members be at risk of losing their health or life insurance as a consequence of a test result (Ross, 2004)?

Advances in genetic research promise great advances in the diagnosis and treatment of many childhood diseases. Yet, although emerging genetic technology may facilitate testing and screening, this often takes place before prevention or treatment can be established. It is therefore crucial to consider each discovery, whether it involves newborn screening, carrier testing, or testing for susceptibility to late-onset conditions, from the perspective of what is in the best interest of the child. The American Academy of Pediatrics recently tackled the issue and made a series of recommendations. Among them are periodic review and evaluation of established newborn screening, informed parental consent and older child/adolescent assent, deferral of genetic testing for adult-onset conditions whenever this does not reduce morbidity or mortality, and need for counseling about the limits of genetic knowledge (American Academy of Pediatrics, Committee on Bioethics, 2001a).

Screening programs differ from genetic testing because they are performed on large populations that consist mostly of individuals who are at low risk of having the condition. The purpose of screening usually is to identify those at high risk for a condition before it becomes clinically apparent. This is beneficial if it permits early institution of therapy to prevent or lessen the impact of the disease. Common examples are blood pressure and cholesterol screening programs. If a person is identified as having an abnormal screen, after further testing to confirm the risk, he or she may receive medications or be placed on a special diet to control the blood pressure or reduce the cholesterol level. This, in turn, may decrease the risk of stroke or heart attack.

Most people agree that these screening programs are in the best interest of the person being tested and do not represent ethical dilemmas. However, if the benefits are not substantial, screening programs can be at odds with the principles of voluntary participation, privacy, confidentiality, and informed consent. For example, if screening tests were required prior to being hired for a job, problems could arise if abnormal test results were used to prevent an individual from obtaining the job or health insurance (Ad Hoc Committee on Genetic Testing/Insurance Issues, 1995).

Health Insurance Portability and Accountability (HIPPA) Act and Genetics

Genetic information and material is covered by the Privacy Rule, a portion of the Health Insurance Portability and Accountability (HIPPA) Act of 1996 (PL 104-191). The full text of the Privacy Rule, also known as the Standards for Privacy of Individually Identifiable Health Information, can be found on the web site of the Office for Civil Rights (http://www.hhs.gov/ocr/hipaa/).

There are two aspects of genetics covered by the rule:

1. *Genetic material* is considered private health information (PHI), even when "deidentified" (e.g., stripping labels from specimens), because ultimately genetic material is always identifiable.

2. The *findings of genetic testing* also have special protections—for example, when parents sign an authorization for disclosure and there is genetic information within the record to be disclosed, additional warnings should be given to alert the parents that they are releasing genetic information.

Unauthorized sharing of PHI can be prosecuted, and both civil and criminal penalties may apply. The Federal HIPAA legislation preempts weaker state law and serves as the standard. However if a state law has stronger protections regarding genetic information, the state law trumps the federal dispositions.

Prenatal Diagnosis and Selective Abortion

Closely linked to the question of genetic screening are the issues surrounding prenatal diagnosis and abortion (Silber, 1981). The ethics of abortion is one of the most difficult questions to resolve, as discussion is often complicated by religious, legal, and political arguments. The main ethical questions revolve around the issues of the personhood of the fetus in conflict with the autonomy of the woman. The possibility of fetal therapy has added a new dimension to the prenatal diagnosis and termination of pregnancy (Yang, 1999).

Some view prenatal diagnosis as a threat to individuals with disabilities (Glover & Glover, 1996). They state that if the human variances that are reflected in disabilities are devalued, then the person with the disability also is devalued. Others argue that it is a family's right to be given information about an identified genetic disorder, because this can provide a wider range of choices about the decision they wish to make. Consensus is building that if this knowledge is available, families should not be deprived of it; rather, they should be taught how to use this knowledge in an effective and ethical manner.

The potential conflict between the disability rights movement and the feminist movement was addressed as follows:

> How is it possible to contest the eugenic and stigmatizing definition of disabilities, which seems to underlie prenatal diagnosis, while still upholding the rights of the individual women to determine what kind of medical care and what sort of pregnancy decisions are in their own best interest? (Rapp, 1999)

Dr. Rapp's answer was that it is possible to complement both views by supporting reproductive rights *and* optimal services for children with disabilities. Finally, a strong argument can be made that prevention of the gestation of an infant with a severe disability does not equate with unwillingness to provide comprehensive care and support of the child and family who decide in favor of the birth of a child with the same disability.

Preimplantation Diagnosis

A recent ethical/genetic issue is preimplantation diagnosis using in vitro fertilization (IVF) (Fost, 1999). This technique holds the possibility of choosing the genetic makeup of our children in ways that were not previously possible, of creating "designer babies." By removing a single cell from an early embryo prior to implanting it, one can now test for sex, certain genetic diseases, and chromosomal abnormalities. With the availability of gene chip technology, thousands of potential mutations could be screened in this manner. This raises obvious ethical dilemmas: whether it is permissible to use IVF to choose gender, whether all embryos carrying genetic disorders should be discarded, and whether IVF should be used to create babies who have a genetic makeup that will help another family member. The last of these questions is already becoming a reality (Fost, 2004).

Organ Donation and Rationing of Care

There is a significant need for hearts, livers, and kidneys to be transplanted in children who have been born with or developed life-threatening malformations of these organs. However, few infant organ donors are available. Research is now focusing on the use of partial transplants of organs from adults, organs from nonhuman primates, and artificial organs.

An ethical issue regarding transplantation is whether individuals with disabilities should have equal access to organ transplants. Traditionally, organ transplantation was reserved for typically developing individuals. Since the 1990s, however, access has increased for people with disabilities, although they still remain at a disadvantage and prone to discrimination in organ transplantation. Quality of life and ability to comply with posttransplant drug regimens are among the reasons given for assigning a low priority to individuals with disabilities.

The basic issue of rationing of care is likely to become more, rather than less, pervasive in this era of managed care and concern over health care costs. It will be important to be vigilant to ensure that individuals with disabilities are not discriminated against when these decisions are being made (Woodstock Theological Center, 1999).

Sexual and Reproductive Rights

Progress in medicine has allowed most people with disabilities to reach reproductive age, in turn leading to new concerns. What are the rights of people with intellectual disability to have sexual relations, marry, and procreate? Sexual drive is presumed to be as strong in individuals with intellectual disability as it is in the general population, although it may be somewhat delayed and may be less evident in individuals with intellectual disability requiring extensive aid and supervision (Monat-Haller, 1992). Nevertheless, the attitude that previously ignored sexual drive and the right to sexual activity in individuals with intellectual disability can be questioned.

In the past, a paternalistic attitude toward sex in people with intellectual disability resulted in institutional policies of separation by gender and punishment of sexual "acting out" behavior. This policy is now considered ethically suspect, as it denies individual autonomy to engage in activities that are pleasurable and, under protected circumstances, not necessarily harmful to anyone (Crichton, 1998). Obviously, there are appropriate and inappropriate times and places to engage in sexual behavior, and those guidelines should be taught. For example, people with intellectual disability can learn that masturbation is an acceptable but private expression of sexuality. Similarly, most individuals with intellectual disability can learn how to use contraception, take precautions against sexually transmitted diseases (STDs), and decline sexual opportunities.

Although in some states laws remain that deny marriage and sexual relations to people with intellectual disability, these regulations have not been enforced; furthermore, they may be unconstitutional. The rights to marry and bear children are protected under the Fourteenth Amendment to the Constitution. The right to procreate, however, is not absolute; it is accompanied by responsibility for the new human being that is created. Therefore, decisions about marriage and procreation in individuals with disabilities may involve not only the couple but also the broader family unit and should benefit from professional guidance.

Sterilization of Adolescents with Intellectual Disabilities

From an ethical perspective, it is problematic to consider sterilization for a person with intellectual disability because of concerns for his or her capacity to care for children. Some traditions (e.g., Catholic teachings) consider this procedure to be an inadmissible practice or mutilation, considering that the reproductive organs exist to benefit the species and cannot be subordinated to benefit an individual. Others oppose sterilization for different reasons; they fear potential abuse of the technology by the power of the state and the proponents of eugenics. Finally, others invoke the right of persons with intellectual disability not to be invaded by a surgical procedure they cannot understand and maintain that rather than sterilization, they require more parental and societal support, protection, and supervision.

Despite these objections, there is a place for sterilization whenever ethical considerations point toward making the procedure morally permissible. The principle of beneficence—for example, calling for protection of vulnerable individuals from a pregnancy they could not possibly handle—can justify sterilization, as sterilization is the most effective contraception with the least side effects. Such measures, though, should require that the decision be transparent, be made publicly, be made with a multidisciplinary assessment, and be clearly documented (American Academy of Pediatrics, Committee on Bioethics, 1990).

ETHICS CONSULTATION AND ETHICS COMMITTEES

Most clinical and ethical decisions are resolved between professionals and families following the process of moral reflection, or the give and take outlined previously. On occasion, however, this process does not work and more questions are raised than answered. In this case, an ethics consultation can be of help. Professionals and families may not be knowledgeable about when an ethics consult is needed, who should have access to the case, and how an ethics consultant or the ethics committee can be reached. The following discussion addresses these issues.

Ethics consultations for patients with disabilities can be requested when there is concern about the moral appropriateness of a decision, when there is disagreement among members of the health care team or between the professionals and the family, or when members of the family have diverging views. The issues involved may cover a wide spectrum, ranging from informed consent to withdrawal of treatment. Ethics committees are usually located in hospitals. Access to the ethics consult should be available to patients, families, surrogates, health care providers, and other involved parties because open access is a way of ensuring that the rights and values of all involved parties are respected. Although institutions may differ, the current recommendation is to proceed with open consultation—that is, the request for a consultation can come from sources other than the attending physician, such as the patient, family, and other professionals (American Academy of Pediatrics, Committee on Bioethics, 2001b). To get the most out of an ethics consultation, it is useful to be familiar with the role of the ethics consultant, the types of consultations, and the functions of ethics committees (see American Academy of Pediatrics, Committee on Bioethics, 2001b; Society for Health and Human Values–Society for Bioethics Consultation, 1998).

RESEARCH INVOLVING CHILDREN WITH DISABILITIES

Many of the guidelines for medical research with children were developed in response to abuse in research studies that took advantage of the vulnerable nature of children, people with disabilities, and people in institutions (Dresser, 1996). One of the most controversial examples occurred in the early 1950s, when research was conducted on healthy children with intellectual disability in a state institution in New York. Researchers infected the children with a hepatitis virus to study the efficacy of a new vaccine. Some parents were not able to admit their child to the institution unless they permitted the researchers to enroll the child in the study (Kodish, 2005; Levine, 1988). When this information became public, there was a great uproar, eventually leading to guidelines for research on children and other vulnerable individuals (American Academy of Pediatrics, 1995; Field & Behrman, 2004). These were subsequently codified as federal regulations (Code of Federal Regulations, 2001). Parents can receive guidance about pediatric research from professionals and web sites (Hoehn & Nelson, 2004).

SOCIAL JUSTICE

Children with disabilities have to face life issues that go beyond health care (Savage, 1998). Minorities and the poor are overrepresented in this group, often as a consequence of their limited socioeconomic circumstances (e.g., lack of or late prenatal care). There is also a gender component, as single mothers are at higher risk for poverty. Moreover, these mothers and many of the allied health workers aiding in the care of children with disabilities are chronically overworked, underpaid, and ignored. Inquiry on the sociopolitical implications of this situation raises the question of what political equality means for those who perform the "labor of dependency" (MacIntyre, 1999). Insufficient attention has been paid to society's unfairness toward those who provide most of the care—mothers and low-paid women. At issue is how dependency workers, overwhelmingly female, will have the time, energy, or resources to represent their personal interest in a public sphere designed for autonomous people. It has been proposed that justice and equality cannot be obtained without alterations in the way society meets the needs of the dependent (MacIntyre, 1999). An additional disturbing fact is the existence of health disparities, as "not all Americans are benefiting equally from advances in health prevention and technology" (Fedder Kitay, 1998). Indeed, there is compelling evidence that gender, race, ethnicity, and disability correlate with persistent health inequalities in the burden of both chronic illness and death, and this calls for rectification (Cesire et al., 2000).

SUMMARY

Issues relating to the treatment of children with disabilities, such as withholding treatment, organ donation, research, genetic screening, and prenatal diagnosis all can entail ethical dilemmas. Ethical problems most often arise in the medical treatment of children with severe disabilities because they may not be able to make autonomous choices. They often cannot participate voluntarily in medical care, nor can they usually give informed consent. Parents or guardians become the substitute decision makers who ideally make choices in the best interests of the child. In situations in which treatment decisions are made by proxy, professionals must try to ensure a higher benefit-to-risk ratio than what people are making decisions on their own behalf would make. It is generally assumed that parents can make the best decisions about their children's care; parental authority, however, is not absolute. Ethical concerns need to be discussed in an open and frank manner. By identifying relevant principles, one can reflect on which take precedence and what is ethically permissible. As with so many other medical responsibilities, this can be consulted, learned, practiced, and improved upon. Professionals caring for children with disabilities can study and enhance their capacity for ethical reflection so as to participate fully in these important decision-making processes (Silber & Batshaw, 2004).

REFERENCES

Ad Hoc Committee on Genetic Testing/Insurance Issues. (1995). Genetic testing and insurance. *American Journal of Human Genetics, 56,* 327–331.

American Academy of Pediatrics, Committee on Bioethics. (1990). Sterilization of women who are mentally handicapped. *Pediatrics, 85,* 868–871.

American Academy of Pediatrics, Committee on Bioethics. (1994). Guidelines on forgoing life-sustaining medical treatment. *Pediatrics, 93,* 532–536.

American Academy of Pediatrics, Committee on Bioethics. (1995). Informed consent, parental permission, and assent I pediatric practice. *Pediatrics, 95*(2), 314–317.

American Academy of Pediatrics, Committee on Bioethics. (1996). Ethics and the care of critically ill infants and children. *Pediatrics, 98*(1), 149–152.

American Academy of Pediatrics, Committee on Bioethics. (2001a). Ethical issues with genetic testing in pediatrics. *Pediatrics, 107,* 1451–1453.

American Academy of Pediatrics, Committee on Bioethics. (2001b). Institutional ethic committees. *Pediatrics, 107,* 205–209.

American Academy of Pediatrics, Committee on Drugs. (1995). Guidelines for the ethical conduct of studies to evaluate drugs in pediatric populations. *Pediatrics, 95*, 286–294.

American Academy of Pediatrics, Committee on Hospital Care. (2003). Family centered care and the pediatrician's role. *Pediatrics, 112*, 691–697.

Bach, J.R., & Campagnolo, D.I. (1992). Psychosocial adjustment of post-poliomyelitis ventilator assisted individuals. *Archives of Physical Medicine and Rehabilitation, 73*, 934–939.

Bartholome, W.G. (1995). Informed consent, parental permission, and assent in pediatric practice. *Pediatrics, 96*(5, Pt. 1), 981–982.

Beauchamp, T.L., & Childress, J.F. (1994). *Principles of biomedical ethics* (4th ed.). New York: Oxford University Press.

Brown, R.H., & Truitt, R.B. (1979). Rights of minors to Medicaid treatment. *De Paul Law Review, 28*, 290–295.

Carter, B.S., & Levetown, M. (Eds.). (2004). *Palliative care for infants, children and adolescents: A practical handbook.* Baltimore: The Johns Hopkins University Press.

Cassidy, R.C., & Fleischman, A.R. (1996). *Pediatric ethics: From principles to practice.* Amsterdam, The Netherlands: Harwood Academic Publishers.

Cesire, V.R., Blustein, J., & Fleischman, A.R. (2000). Urban bioethics. *Kennedy Institute of Ethics Journal, 10*, 1–21.

Code of Federal Regulations. (2001). 45 CFG 46; 21 CFR 50,56.66 FR 20598, April 24, 2001.

Crichton, J. (1998). Balancing restriction and freedom in the care of people with intellectual disability. *Journal of Intellectual Disability Research, 42*(Pt. 2), 189–95.

Dresser, R. (1996). Mentally disabled research subjects: The enduring policy issues. *Journal of the American Medical Association, 276*, 67–72.

Engelhardt, Jr., H.T. (2003). The bioethics consultant: Giving moral advice in the midst of moral controversy. *HEC Forum, 15*, 362–382.

Fedder Kitay, E. (1998). *Love's labor: Essay on women, equality and dependency.* New York: Rutledge.

Field, M., & Behrman, R. (Eds.). (2004). *Ethical conduct of clinical research involving children.* Washington, DC: National Academies Press.

Ford, C., English, A., & Sigman G. (2004). Confidential health care for adolescents: Position paper for the Society for Adolescent Medicine. *Journal of Adolescent Health, 35*, 160–167.

Fost, N. (1999). Access to IVF. *Pediatrics in Review, 20*(8), e36–e37; discussion e38–e39.

Fost, N.C. (2004). Conception for donation. *Journal of the American Medical Association, 291*, 2125–2126.

Gerhart, K.A., Koziol-McLain, J., Lowenstein, S.R., et al. (1994). Quality of life following spinal cord injury: Knowledge and attitude of emergency care providers. *Annals of Emergency Medicine, 23*, 807–812.

Glover, N.M., & Glover, S.J. (1996). Ethical and legal issues regarding selective abortion of fetuses with Down syndrome. *Mental Retardation, 34*(4), 207–214.

Health Insurance Portability and Accountability Act (HIPAA) of 1996, PL 104-191, 42 U.S.C. §§ 201 *et seq.*

Hoehn, K.S., & Nelson, R.M. (2004). Advising parents about children's participation in clinical research. *Pediatric Annals, 33*(11), 778–781.

Kodish E. (Ed). (2005). *Ethics and research with children.* Oxford, England: Oxford University Press.

Lee, S.K., Penner, P.L., & Cox, M. (1991). Comparison of the attitudes of health care professionals and parents toward active treatment of very low birth weight infants. *Pediatrics, 88*, 110–114.

Levine, R.J. (1988). *Ethics and regulation of clinical research* (2nd ed.). New Haven, CT; Yale University Press.

Loewy, E.H. (1994). Limiting but not abandoning treatment in severely mentally impaired patients: A troubling issue for ethics consultants and ethics committees. *Cambridge Quarterly of Healthcare Ethics, 3*, 216–225.

MacIntyre, A. (1999). *Dependent rational animals: Why human beings need virtues.* New York: Open Court.

Mappes, T., & Degrazia, D. (Eds.). (2000). *Biomedical ethics* (5th ed.). New York: McGraw Hill Higher Education.

Miller, P.S. (1998). Genetic discrimination in the workplace. *Journal of Law and Medical Ethics, 26*(3), 178, 189–197.

Monat-Haller, R.K. (1992). *Understanding and expressing sexuality: Responsible choices for individuals with developmental disabilities.* Baltimore: Paul H. Brookes Publishing Co.

President's Commission for the Study of Ethical Problems in Medicine and Biomedical and Behavioral Research. (1983). *Seriously ill newborns: Deciding to forgo life-sustaining treatment* (pp. 197–229). Washington, DC: U.S. Government Printing Office.

Rapp, R. (1999). *Testing women, testing the fetus: The social impact of amniocentesis in America.* New York: Routledge.

Ross, L.F. (2004). Should children and adolescents undergo genetic testing? *Pediatric Annals, 33*(11), 762–769.

Ross, L.F., & Moon, M.R. (2000). Ethical issues in genetic testing of children. *Archives of Pediatrics & Adolescent Medicine, 154*(9), 873–879.

Savage, T.A. (1998). Children with severe and profound disabilities and the issue of social justice. *Advanced Practice Nursing Quarterly, 4*(2), 53–58.

Sigman, A.S., & O'Connor, C. (1991). Exploration for physicians the mature minor doctrine. *Journal of Pediatrics, 119*, 520–525.

Silber, T.J. (1981). Amniocentesis and selective abortion. *Pediatric Annals, 1981*, 31–34.

Silber, T.J., & Batshaw, M.L. (2004). Ethical dilemmas in the treatment of children with disabilities. *Pediatric Annals, 33*(11), 752–761.

Society for Health and Human Values–Society for Bioethics Consultation. (1998). *Task force on Standards for Bioethics consultation, Core competencies for Health Care Ethics Consultation: The report of the American Society for Bioethics and Humanities.* Glenview, IL: American Society for Bioethics and Humanities.

Street, K., Ashcroft, R., Henderson, J., et al. (2000). The decision making process regarding the withdrawal or withholding of potential life-saving treatments in a children's hospital. *Journal of Medical Ethics, 26*(5), 346–352.

Terrenoire, G. (1992). Huntington's disease and the ethics of genetic prediction. *Journal of Medical Ethics, 18*, 79–85.

Walsh-Kelly, C.M., Lang, K.R., Chevako, J., et al. (1999). Advance directives in a pediatric emergency department. *Pediatrics, 103*(4, Pt. 1), 826–830.

Woodstock Theological Center. (1999). *Ethical issues in managed health care organizations.* Washington, DC: Georgetown University Press.

Yang, E.Y., Flake, A.W., & Adzick, N.S. (1999). Prospects for fetal gene therapy. *Seminars in Perinatology, 23*(6), 524–534.

40 Caring and Coping

Helping the Family of a Child with a Disability

Symme Wilson Trachtenberg, Karen Batshaw, and Michael Batshaw

---

Upon completion of this chapter, the reader will

- Understand the impact of having a child with a disability on family development during the life cycle of the child

- Learn the principles of family-centered care

- Be knowledgeable about strategies and resources to help families cope with a disability

- Recognize the influence of societal attitudes on the outcome of children with disabilities

---

The preceding chapters have focused on the medical, rehabilitative, and educational supports for various developmental disabilities. Equally important is the impact of these disabilities on the function of the child–family unit. How the family handles the day-to-day stresses, concerns, and needs of its members influences to a great extent the outcome of the child with disabilities (Green et al., 2005). Traditionally, professionals offered only those resources they believed were "appropriate" or "best" for the child and family, and they focused exclusively on their area of perceived responsibility. It is now recognized that to be effective in working with these families, professionals must take a holistic, family-centered care approach. This chapter focuses on the issues that families face through the life of a child with a disability and the approaches professionals can take to help them. For the purposes of this chapter, the term *family* is used to refer to children and their parent(s) or family member(s) who are primary caregivers. Families today have many different structures: traditional two-parent families, single-parent families, adoptive families, stepfamilies, gay and lesbian families, foster families, and intergenerational families (Farber & Maharaj, 2005; Hanson & Lynch, 2004). Each family is a culture unto itself (Arrango, 1999). The family unit, regardless of its composition, transmits traditions, values, ethnic heritage, religious beliefs, and personal spirituality. The family's traditions provide members with stability, support, comfort, strength, guidance, and strategies for coping with the difficulties of daily life (Harry, 2002; Ochieng, 2003). These family cultures and belief systems must be respected and incorporated into the care plan.

SAMANTHA

Samantha (Sam) is an 8-year-old with Down syndrome and the daughter of Monica and Sean. When Sam was born, her parents were excited by the arrival of their first child, a healthy and active baby. Shortly after birth, however, they were told that Sam had Down syndrome. They were devastated. Khandra, the social worker from the Down syndrome clinic, met with Monica and Sean as well as Sam's grandparents. They were all distressed by this diagnosis that was so unexpected, especially as Monica was just 25 years old. The grandparents had visions of Sam needing to be institutionalized, while Monica and Sean were overwhelmed with sadness. Khandra answered questions about what they could do to help Sam. She was very encouraging, noting that most children with Down syndrome have a long and productive life. She supplied information about Down syndrome and resources available to support the family. She also helped the family contact the early intervention program in order for Sam to begin receiving weekly home visits from the early intervention specialist. Khandra continued to meet with the family each time they came for follow-up to the Down syndrome clinic. She noted that Monica was very loving and appropriate in her care for Sam and that her sorrow had been replaced by commitment. Khandra helped Monica become involved with the local Down syndrome support group, where Monica eventually became an officer. Sean became involved in the Special Olympics, where Sam excelled in track and field. The grandparents, however, have had a hard time accepting Sam, and this has created tension. Monica would call Khandra when she needed advice or just when she needed to talk a bit. When interviewed by a local newspaper, Monica said "Khandra is like part of the family. We feel blessed to have her."

HOW FAMILIES COPE WITH THE DIAGNOSIS

Individuals and families differ widely in their initial responses to being told they have a child with a disability. Their responses may depend on the severity of the disability and the health care professional's manner of delivery of the news. Oftentimes it is the timing, the words used, the time spent, and the emotional support provided by the professional that has a great deal of influence. The impact on the family also depends on past life experiences, religious and cultural backgrounds, and age of the child at diagnosis (Leiter et al., 2004). Other factors that may influence familial reactions include their attitudes about individuals with disabilities; knowledge about health care practitioners; and receptiveness to accepting help from professionals, friends, and other family members (Sullivan-Bolyai et al., 2003). Some individuals with a strong religious faith may believe that God has chosen them to care for a child with a disability. Others may be able to adjust more easily because of previous experience with a family member with a disability. If the diagnosis has been delayed, parents may be relieved to finally receive answers and help for their child. Yet, they also may be angry with health care professionals, friends, or family members who previously reassured them that their child would "grow out of it." It is difficult to predict how a particular family member will react to the news that a child has a disability. Furthermore, what one family considers a mild disability may be a major disability to another family.

The most common initial response of parents who are told that their child has a severe disability is some combination of shock, denial, disbelief, guilt, and an overwhelming sense of loss. Some parents initially deny their child's diagnosis and visit various professionals looking for a more optimistic diagnosis or prognosis (Ho & Keiley, 2003; Sullivan-Bolyai et al., 2003).

Families with a child who initially developed typically but later acquired a disability as a result of an illness or an injury have some additional challenges. They often have a difficult time accepting that aspirations for their child must be adjusted and that family relationships may be altered. After the initial period of shock and denial, some family members experience depression (Rolland, 2003). This can result from emotional stress combined with the physical strain of following through on the many appointments, procedures, recommendations, and care required for their child (Ello & Donovan, 2005). Other factors contributing to depression may be spousal disagreement over acceptance of the diagnosis, assignment of blame, choice of treatment options, and/or responsibility in caring for the child (Singer & Powers, 1993). The mother, usually the primary caregiver, is more often affected. Symptoms of depression include extreme fatigue, restlessness or irritability, insomnia, changes in appetite, and/or loss of sex drive. Professionals should screen for depression and refer the family member for further evaluation and treatment if concerned.

Depression may be accompanied or followed by anger, which may be directed at a person, an event, God, or life in general. If directed at a person, it may be the doctor, other professionals caring for the child, the other parent, one of the other children in the family, or even the child with the disability (Tunali & Power, 1992). Alternately, the anger may be self-directed. A parent may ask, "What did I do or not do that contributed to or caused the disability?" Regardless of where the anger is directed, it is important to recognize that such expressions are part of a coping strategy. Anger may well be an appropriate expression of frustration when parents feel their opinions are not being heard or respected. However, it may be inappropriately directed at a "safe" target (i.e., the spouse) rather than at the person for whom it is felt (i.e., the professional who communicated the diagnosis). Counseling and advocacy training can help parents or other family members channel their anger into productive interactions, so they can learn how to obtain the resources they need for their child and find ways to express their feelings more effectively (Banks, 2003). Support from family members and friends is critical. Families who have strong relationships are better able to meet the challenges they encounter. However, at a time when the parent(s) are most in need of support, family and friends may be unable to provide it. The extended family may not accept the diagnosis or may assign blame to one of the parents, most commonly to the one unrelated to them. Friends may feel uncomfortable in the presence of the child with a severe disability or not know what to say in consolation; as a result, they often stay away. In addition, parents may be embarrassed by their child's disability or behavior and rarely venture into the community with the child. Parents may find it difficult to see their friends' typically developing children, knowing their own child will follow a different trajectory. All of these factors can lead to social isolation. Even if parents want to maintain social contacts, their child's physical, behavioral, and medical challenges may be so complex that simply going shopping and/or finding a skilled baby sitter becomes a major production.

Finances also play a role. Families come from a wide range of educational and socioeconomic circumstances. Some families are very knowledgeable about their choices and can afford to obtain multiple expert opinions and services. Other families have neither a good understanding of the health care and educational systems nor the means to obtain private fee-for service programs. These disparities can directly affect the outcome of the child. Family-centered care involves educating all parents about their child's condition, resources, and entitlements. Parents who learn advocacy skills in the individualized education program (IEP) process (see Chapter 34) are better able to meet their child's needs.

Most parents are eventually able to cope with their child's disability and recognize positive outcomes from the experience. This leads to improved family cohesion and hardiness, increased understanding and compassion among

family members, and, for some, a more enriched and meaningful life (Ho & Keiley, 2003). Parents become experts in meeting their children's needs. They learn to ask for and obtain what is needed. This strength and ability in many cases benefits the child, who may achieve more than what was originally expected at the time of diagnosis. For example, in some communities, families who receive a prenatal diagnosis of Down syndrome are immediately connected with the Down syndrome parent group in their area. Positive experiences are shared and families immediately begin to receive the help they need. After birth, the child and family are welcomed into the community of Down syndrome families, which creates a supportive environment of hope and positive expectation throughout the life span (Bittles & Glasson, 2004).

For most families, the sadness lessens as members develop a routine of care, gain access to early intervention and respite care services, and begin seeing progress in the child's development (Turnbull et al., 1993). The need for support and/or therapy, however, may recur at various developmental stages. Support from friends, extended family, and other parents of children with disabilities also can be (re)established over time. Parenting networks, in which parents educate and support one another, are often very powerful and may be even more effective than professional information and support (see Appendix D for examples of such resources).

LONG-TERM EFFECTS ON THE PARENTS

The problems engendered by having a child with a disability may include physical and time demands for in-home care that interfere with employment; requirements for medical, educational, and therapy appointments; financial burdens; added stress level; and specialized needs for recreational programs, legal services, and transportation (Trachtenberg & Lewis, 1996). Parents or partners often react differently to these problems, perhaps as a result of their separate roles within the family unit or gender-specific issues.

In most families, women continue to carry most child care responsibilities, although men often are participating more than in the past. This responsibility carries both potential risks and benefits. A mother caring for a child who will remain dependent in daily living skills throughout life is at high risk for developing stress, depression, and burnout over time (Johnson et al., 2005). If the mother can efficiently and effectively master the child's care, however, she may feel a sense of accomplishment and competency that is positively reinforcing (Leiter et al., 2004). Meanwhile, the traditional father who focuses on financial issues and long-term planning rather than taking part in the child's daily living activities may be avoiding having to deal with the reality of the child or the disability (Green et al., 2005). In contrast, he may find that by participating actively in the child's care, he not only provides relief for the mother but also experiences pleasure from an enhanced role in daily family life (Willoughby & Glidden, 1995).

Gender-specific differences also are found in communication styles. Although men tend to talk in order to impart information, women talk to communicate feelings as well. This can lead to miscommunication. The husband may think his wife is complaining when she is actually just sharing her feelings and experiences of the day. The wife may think her husband is insensitive when he imparts information without emotional content. This difference in communication styles is not unique to families of children with disabilities, but it is often accentuated in an environment of increased stress and inadequate financial and emotional resources. Fathers may also feel that they must keep their emotions internalized and be the strong partner.

Given these stresses, it has been found that strong marital relationships, good parenting and problem-solving skills, financial stability, and supportive social networks are predictors of a good outcome for parents who have a child with a disability (Power, 2004; Rolland, 2003). For families who lack these supports, professionals need to be available to provide advice and support to ensure the child's optimal growth, development, and safety. Although some marriages are strengthened by the challenge, others deteriorate, especially if the relationship had previous troubles (Banks, 2003). Strong religious and community affiliation and effective behavioral interventions in the home are also associated with an increased likelihood of effective family functioning (Hanson & Lynch, 2004; Power, 2004; Rolland, 2003). Related life experiences may have sometimes unpredictable effects. For example, a parent who has dealt with a chronic illness or disability in another family member may feel more competent in handling this new disability. Alternatively, a previous difficult caregiving experience may

leave the parent burned out and unable to cope with this new responsibility.

Parents may also fear for the safety of their child, especially as the child attends preschool or school outside of the home environment. An ever-present concern is that their child will be injured, teased, or bullied by other children or physically/sexually assaulted by other children or by adults. For children who are violent, with or without intent, the concern is that they may injure themselves, other children, or staff. This fear is heightened when a child has a disability that interferes with communication skills. The parents may also face increasing behavior problems, new health care and physical needs, mounting financial concerns, or feelings of inadequacy in meeting the needs of other family members. Parents of children with the most severe developmental disabilities and/or medical fragility—for example, requiring prolonged technology assistance such as a ventilator—are at greatest risk for caregiver burnout and decreased family functioning (Ello & Donovan, 2005; Trachtenberg & Trachtenberg, 1996). Many families, however, do well and thrive at home with children who have technology dependence (O'Brien, 2001). Some parents have difficulty finding or accepting respite care or other assistance for their child. As a result, they continue to experience chronic stress, which can lead to depression or physical illness and ultimately render them incapable of continuing to meet the demands of care. Parents whose children have mild disabilities may also experience recurrent episodes of sadness and feelings of despair, which, in some instances, become a condition called chronic sorrow (Wickler, Wasow, Hatfield, 1981). When the feelings of sadness and grief become chronic and interfere with the parent's ability to function, psychological intervention is indicated.

EFFECTS ON SIBLINGS

The siblings of a child with a disability have special needs and concerns that vary with gender, age, birth order, and temperament (Burke, 2004; Stalker & Connors, 2004). Coleby (1995) found that older male siblings had an increased appreciation for children with disabilities, whereas older female siblings showed increased behavior problems (perhaps because of being overburdened with child care responsibilities). The same study showed that near-age siblings had less contact with peers, and younger siblings showed increased anxiety. Sibling concerns also appeared to reflect such situational variables as whether their own needs were being met, how the parents were handling the diagnosis emotionally, what the children were being told, and how much they understood.

In addition to recognizing age and gender differences, it is important to acknowledge that children, in general, have mixed feelings about their siblings with or without disabilities. They may be glad that they do not have a disability yet feel guilty about this fact as well. They may worry that they will "catch" the disability or fantasize that they actually caused it by having bad thoughts about their sibling. Adolescents may question whether they will pass a similar disability on to their future children. Furthermore, because of the extra care and time required by the child with a disability, the typically developing children may think that their parents love their brother or sister more than them. As a consequence, they may act out in order to get attention, or they may withdraw, not wanting to ask for attention from their overly burdened parents (Williams, Williams, & Graff, 2003). Care must be taken to balance the parenting efforts so that the typically developing sibling(s) continue to feel appropriately supported. When the siblings reach adolescence, it may be the appropriate time for a family discussion of planning for the future. This discussion should include the eventuality of the parents' death and/or the parents being unable to continue providing care for the child with a severe disability. The discussion should include the participation of the affected child to whatever extent possible. Getting assistance from professionals who have training in self-determination or person-centered planning may be useful for some individuals (DePoy & Gilson, 2004). There may also be a need for an attorney to set up an estate plan and a special needs trust and guardianship, as well as an evaluation to determine the person's competence to make financial and/or medical decisions for him- or herself (see Chapter 41).

Despite these concerns, having a child with a disability in a family does not necessarily adversely affect the typically developing siblings. In fact, there is some evidence that these children demonstrate increased maturity, a sense of responsibility, a tolerance for being different, a feeling of closeness to the family, and enhanced self-confidence and independence. In one study, siblings ages 3–6 years showed more involvement in social play and nurturing activities than children in a control group (Lobato, Miller, Barbour, et al., 1991). Many siblings of individuals with disabilities ultimately enter helping professions (Lobato, 1990).

Siblings fare best psychologically when 1) their parents' marriage is stable and supportive, 2) feelings are discussed openly, 3) the disability is explained completely, and 4) they are not overburdened with child care responsibilities (Lobato, 1990; Pilowsky et al., 2004; Williams et al., 2003). Parents must remember that children take their lead. If the parents are upset, so too will be the children, even if they do not understand why. In contrast, parents who acknowledge their pain while being proud of the accomplishments of all their children show their ability to adapt to the increased emotional and physical demands of having a child with special needs. This sets the tone for the entire family. Parents also should avoid burdening siblings with caregiving responsibilities. It has been shown that mothers of children with disabilities are more likely to put child care demands on the siblings and reprimand them more (Lobato et al., 1991).

Parents must recognize that their other children often feel torn between protecting and caring for their brother or sister with a disability and being accepted by children outside the family who may tease them and their sibling. Siblings should be informed at an early age about their brother or sister's disability so their knowledge is based on fact, not misconception. This must be done in an age-appropriate fashion, with the siblings feeling free to ask questions. These sessions will need to be repeated as the children grow older and require more information. By the time siblings have reached adolescence, the parents may be ready to share with them information about genetics, estate planning, guardianship arrangements, and wills. It is helpful for siblings to know what resources and options are available. Some siblings will choose to have their sibling with a disability live with them in the future or they may promote their sibling's independence by finding living arrangements and/or the available systems of care in their community (Rivers & Stoneman, 2003). The family should stay current with services offered in their community as well as be aware of any waiting lists for those services.

EFFECTS ON THE EXTENDED FAMILY

Having grandchildren creates strong feelings in most people. These include feelings of satisfaction, connectedness, fulfillment of life's purpose, joy, and comfort. Learning that a grandchild has a disability leads to more mixed feelings. To the extent that the grandparents have or do not have a quality relationship with their own children further affects their own coping with the disability and with their support of the child. Typically, when a grandchild is born with a disability, grandparents grieve for their own loss as well as for their child's loss. They may experience denial more strongly than do the parents of the child with the disability, and this can interfere with the family's adaptation to the disability. Yet, grandparents can be extremely helpful to the family as a strong source of emotional support. They also may provide respite care and financial assistance that may be crucial for having a child with a severe disability live at home (Sandler, Warren, & Raver, 1995). Counseling, support groups for grandparents, and/or information given via the parents can help them deal with the reality of the child's disability and lead them to become more involved in supporting the family.

Other extended family members and friends also can help or hinder the parents' ability to cope. Some family members may have their own issues that will interfere with their ability to be supportive. For example, parents' siblings may be concerned about their own risk for having a child with a genetically based condition, in addition to experiencing sadness or discomfort with the diagnosis. Professionals can suggest ways to discuss these issues with family and friends and should encourage parents to utilize support groups and community service agencies that fully include people with disabilities.

EFFECTS ON THE CHILD WITH A DISABILITY

Some effects on the child with a disability vary across the life span. Issues common at particular ages are discussed next.

Preschool Age

Prior to school age, the child with a disability may not recognize that he or she is different from other children. During this period parent–child interactions and child–peer interactions are crucial to prepare for future school-age interactions. Referral to early intervention and special preschool services is very important at this stage (see Chapter 34). This will lead to interactions between parents and professionals to set up the individualized family service plan (IFSP), setting the tone for dealing with the disability.

School Age

By school age, most children with disabilities are aware of their abilities and challenges and may need help in dealing with feelings of being different. If the child is given proper supports, he or she can learn to cope with the disability effectively. Full acceptance must first come from the home. If the child is seen as being worthwhile by parents and siblings, the child's self-image is usually good. This acceptance includes being part of family activities (e.g., attending religious services, taking part in recreational programs, going on vacations), participating as much as possible in developmentally appropriate family responsibilities, and being permitted to discuss the disability openly.

Discussing and modeling how to handle different situations at home improves the child's ability to cope with social situations in the community as well. This is very important because acceptance outside of the home can be difficult to achieve. Classmates may tease the child, and schoolwork may prove difficult in an inclusive setting. Furthermore, if the child's communication or social skills are limited, this may interfere with interpersonal interactions. If others do not accept the child, he or she may develop a poor self-image and exhibit behavior problems. In order for inclusion to work, teachers and school personnel must be adequately informed and trained about the specific physical and cognitive needs of the child (Ross-Watt, 2005).

Planning for the child's entry into school should begin while the child is in preschool and with the help of professionals. The transition to school also can be eased by preparing the class for the child's entrance (Cutler, 1993). The child's parents must be included in this planning. They can help explain the child's disorder and the necessary adaptations to both the teacher and students. They also can share with the school staff their hopes and fears for their child's education and future during the IEP meeting (see Chapter 34). It should be noted that in the case of a recent disability (e.g., a traumatic brain injury [TBI], Chapter 30), as opposed to a congenital disorder (e.g., meningomyelocele; see Chapter 28), the parents may be less able to take such a proactive role, because they may be coping with their own adjustment to the disability. Professionals from the treating hospital can assist in school reentry.

The child with disabilities gains self-confidence through participation in activities in which he or she can be successful. These can be either general or special activities. The philosophy of inclusion is that children who are differently challenged are accepted in general activities with appropriate adaptations or assistance. This, however, should not preclude either participation in segregated programs, such as the Special Olympics, or development of friendships with children who have similar disabilities.

Some children with disabilities will need encouragement and assistance in socializing and developing friendships. Summer camps (be they inclusive or special) that welcome children with special needs provide an avenue for children to develop important socialization skills and experience independence from parents. This not only encourages personal growth for the child but also for his or her parents and camp mates as well. In camps with inclusive programs, the typically developing children learn to appreciate people with differences. This will prepare them for a future where they will live, work, and befriend people with disabilities (Davern & Schnorr, 1991).

Adolescence

Adolescence is one of the most difficult periods for both children and their families, not only because of the many biological and social changes taking place but also because society does not have a well-developed support system for adults with disabilities in education, employment, and socialization (Kim & Turnbull, 2004). For parents, adolescence signals their child's proximity to adulthood and adult responsibilities. It quite naturally elicits anxieties and fears about independence, self-sufficiency, and maturity. Adolescents may become preoccupied with comparing themselves with their peers (Orsmond, Krauss, & Seltzer, 2004). Yet, the desire for sameness and peer approval in areas of physical and intellectual development may be unattainable because of the developmental disability. This will be less of an issue if the adolescent with a disability has a strong peer group or has already come to terms with being "different." If the adolescent has just acquired a disability (e.g., from TBI) or is having emotional or behavior difficulties, counseling may be helpful in working through his or her concerns and learning effective behavioral strategies. There are specific interventions that are effective to assist adolescents as they move to-

ward becoming productive adults (White et al., 2002).

It is important to use this time to start developing a reasonable plan for enhancing the adolescents' capacity for independent behavior and self-sufficiency as they make the transition to young adulthood. As an example, they should be acknowledged as sexual beings. They should be given appropriate material about intimate relationships and "safe sex" and encouraged to discuss issues of sexuality with parents, peers, and professionals in a way and at a level they feel comfortable with and can understand. Although promiscuity or sexual exploitation is sometimes an issue, social isolation is a far more common problem during adolescence. This can result either from limitations imposed on the child by the disability or by attitudes and reactions of peers and family (Hill, 1993). For some developmental disabilities (e.g., autism spectrum disorder), social skills impairments are an integral part of the disability. These adolescents may act in an odd manner in social interactions, often making peers feel uncomfortable in their presence. They may benefit from social skills training that entails modeling appropriate social interactions and learning to participate successfully in group activities. They also can learn to enjoy individual recreational activities, such as listening to music, watching movies, and participating in sports activities (e.g., swimming, horseback riding) (Orsmond et al., 2004).

Adolescence is a critical time for predicting future independence; individuals who remain dependent through adolescence tend not to move from this stage in later life (Powers, Singer, & Sowers, 1996). Adolescents who have the potential for independence but face difficulties with issues of separation and individuation need assistance with these developmental tasks. Parents should be encouraged to give them the necessary freedom to become independent. At times, this requires taking certain reasonable risks and providing psychosocial intervention. If parents persist in managing their child's life and the disability, however, they are giving the adolescent the message that he or she is not competent to manage independently. This can have long-term adverse consequences.

Young Adulthood

The transition to adulthood is both important and difficult for parents and children with disabilities (see Chapter 41). It must be viewed as a dynamic lifelong process that meets individual needs by providing developmentally appropriate services that continue uninterrupted as the individual moves from adolescence to adulthood (White et al., 2002).

The young adult's ability to cope and become as independent as possible depends on the degree of the disability and the effectiveness of the family in planning and managing this transition emotionally and financially (Hallum, 1995). The individual may be ready to move out of the family home and into an independent living arrangement. If he or she is affiliated with an agency focused on the needs of young adults with disabilities, the support offered can provide important socialization opportunities within the community, contributing to personal development, competency, maturity, and adaptive functioning. It also can be a very difficult time, however, disrupting the established family structure. The family may need assistance in successfully supporting the young adult at this point.

PRINCIPLES OF FAMILY-CENTERED CARE: ROLE OF THE PROFESSIONAL

Table 40.1 lists principles of family-centered care. The goal of family-centered care is to facilitate the best possible outcome for a child with a developmental disability. To achieve this goal, the professional must establish a relationship with the family based on mutual respect and open communication. This means that the family sees the professional as someone who is nonjudgmental, open to constructive feedback, respectful of cultural diversity, and able to listen empathically (Arrango, 1999; Johnson, 2000; see also http://www.familycenteredcare.org). Once this relationship has been established, both parties will be in a strong position to receive and appreciate the unique expertise that each contributes.

Families of children with disabilities come into contact with a bevy of professionals (e.g., physicians, nurses, teachers, physical and occupational therapists, psychologists, social workers). Individually and as a group, they are responsible for explaining the results of the initial evaluation and testing, presenting various treatment options, and teaching intervention and advocacy strategies. The initial contact the family has with professionals generally sets the tone for future interactions (Miceli & Clark, 2005).

Professionals need to be flexible and responsive while recognizing the importance of coordinating efforts with the family and other professionals. As a result of their training, experience, and expertise, professionals often have strong opinions about what is best for the child and family. However, people with disabilities and their families have the right to choose their own path. If a family encounters difficulties along the way, it can always turn to a professional for further assistance to accomplish its goals. It is important to remember that families who make their own choices are empowered to continue making decisions that best meet their needs (Miceli & Clark, 2005).

The overall approach of the professional toward the family should be one of respect and support, promoting decision making and mastery of care by the family. This family-centered practice leads to a true partnership between parents and professionals (Cavet & Sloper, 2004; Singer & Powers, 1993). Families who find programs consistent with their personal needs and cultural values are much more likely to follow through, to their child's advantage (Banks, 2003; Hanson & Lynch, 2004; Harry, 2002; Ochieng, 2003). Professionals should pro-

Table 40.1.   Principles of family-centered care

1. Respecting each child and his or her family
2. Honoring racial, ethnic, cultural, and socioeconomic diversity and its effect on the family's experience and perception of care
3. Recognizing and building on strengths of each child and family, even in difficult and challenging situations
4. Supporting and facilitating choice for the child and family about care and support
5. Ensuring flexibility in organizational policies and procedures, and providers practices so services can be tailored to the needs, beliefs, and cultural values of each child and family
6. Sharing honest and unbiased information with families on an on-going basis and in ways they find useful and affirming
7. Providing and/or ensuring formal and informal support (e.g., family-to-family support) for the child and parent(s) and/or guardian(s) during pregnancy, childbirth, infancy, childhood, adolescence , and young adulthood
8. Collaborating with families at all levels of healthcare, in the care of the individual child and in professional education, policy making and program development
9. Empowering each child and family to discover their own strengths, build confidence, and make choices and decisions about their health

From Johnson, B.H. & Eichner, J.M. (2003). Family-centered care and the pediatrician's role. *Pediatrics, 112*(3), 692; reprinted by permission.

mote self-determination by encouraging families to become actively involved in understanding the disability, setting goals, and making decisions. Families often use the Internet for information and guidance, and professionals need to understand that it contains a wealth of both information and misinformation. Therefore, they need to be proactive in helping families evaluate the quality of the information and its appropriateness for their child.

A consequence of feeling empowered is that families are more likely to make decisions on their own and challenge the advice of professionals (Sullivan-Bolyai et al., 2004). A family may request additional information or referral for a second opinion. Families may not follow advice because of specific child-rearing and medical care practices advanced by ethnic and religious affiliations, specific cultural values, family authority figures and communication patterns, or decision-making practices (Trachtenberg & Hale Sills, 1996). Professionals should work within the family's system of beliefs, if at all possible. Collaboration with another colleague, often a social worker or psychologist, may clarify the family's perspective, and compromises may be reached that provide good care for the child and are acceptable to both family and professionals. If the professional is persistent and uncompromising in pushing his or her approach, the likely result is that the prescription will not be filled, the therapeutic intervention will not be followed, and the family will not return to the professional for further care.

The professional must take action, however, if the choices the individual or family makes are perceived as inappropriate. For example, a family may decide to pursue treatment that has not been proven scientifically valid, is potentially harmful, and/or costs the family a great deal of time and money. It is the professional's responsibility to inform the family of the risks of nonvalidated interventions while respecting the family's autonomy. This action should not be performed in a demeaning or controlling manner. The decision must always remain in the family's hands. The one exception is if it is believed that the family's actions may be harmful to the child. The professional must then contact the local child welfare agency (or other authority) to report suspected child abuse or neglect.

Sometimes isolation and depression are experienced by one family member or the entire family. In these situations, the professional can suggest several proven methods of psychotherapy to assist the family. At the present time, the two most validated time limited therapies are cognitive-behavioral therapy (CBT) and interpersonal psychotherapy (IPT). CBT uses cognitive approaches to problem solving (Dobson, 2002). Professionals can help families deal with isolation, depression, and discord, especially if these feelings are interfering with the parents' ability to care for their child. These cognitive therapies provide family members with an opportunity to examine feelings and develop solutions. IPT is helpful in identifying the places of interpersonal discord in the family that have led to the depressive symptoms. This therapy helps individuals understand and change interactions that cause strife in the family. The therapy usually lasts for 4 months at the most and has been shown to be effective in treating a variety of interpersonal issues (Blanco, Lipsitz, & Caligor, 2001; Stuart, 1999; Weissman, Markowitz, & Klerman, 2000). Although CBT and IPT are the most rigorously proven psychological therapies, there are other modalities that can be helpful to a family. These include supportive therapies and family therapy (Carr, 2000; Serketich & Dumas, 1996).

THE ROLE OF SOCIETY AND COMMUNITY

The family's social context plays an important role in determining the outcome of its members. Fortunately, in today's society there is greater appreciation for people with disabilities. There are more educational, vocational, and housing services, as well as entitlements, available. Federal funding provides for a protection and advocacy system for people with disabilities in each state.

Federal legislation also guarantees equal opportunities for all members of society. The Individuals with Disabilities Education Improvement Act of 2004 (IDEA 2004; PL 108-446) mandates free educational and rehabilitative services for school-age children (see Chapter 34). Reaching citizens of all ages with disabilities, the Americans with Disabilities Act (ADA) of 1990 (PL 101-336) focuses on the establishment of rights regarding access to employment, transportation, telecommunications, and public accommodations. The effects of the ADA are increasingly visible. City sidewalks now have direct curb access so that wheelchairs can be used, and buses are equipped with wheelchair lifts. Buildings have wheelchair access ramps, and theater and sporting events are able to accommodate individuals with disabilities. Public telephones have adjustable speaker volumes, and many offices have teletypewriter (TTY) capability. More, however, needs to be done.

As a result of these and other laws, people with disabilities and their families and friends are guaranteed the same civil rights as people without disabilities. Parent advocates have paved the way for the current focus on family-centered care, with parents acting as true partners with professionals to enable the child to function at the highest possible level.

Although laws are important, they need to be accompanied by a change in the public's perception and attitudes toward individuals with disabilities. This too seems to be happening, perhaps as a consequence of "mainstreaming" that began in the mid-1970s. Young adults who have grown up in schools with children with disabilities are more sensitive to their needs and more cognizant of their abilities. Individuals with disabilities are in the workforce and are productive members of society. They are seen in movies, on television shows, in television commercials, and in magazine advertisements. Although society has made itself more accessible to and supportive of individuals with disabilities, the future remains challenging.

Supplemental Security Income, medical assistance, and food stamps all currently provide financial support for parents and eventually for children with disabilities when they turn 18. Many of these entitlement programs are being challenged, however, and may not exist in their current form in the future (Chapter 42). For example, managed care plans may not cover all long-term medications, rehabilitation therapies, and technologies that are presently funded by mandated programs (Giardino et al., 2002). New cost-effective care models must be developed to promote quality and outcome-oriented services that build on the strengths of the children, their families, and the professionals who serve them.

SUMMARY

As a family journeys through its life cycle, its members face many challenges and changes. This trip is particularly challenging for the family of a child with a disability. The child, parents, siblings, extended family members, and friends are all affected and may initially undergo a period of grieving for their loss of a "normal child." Over time, the family's coping strategies generally improve. Parents learn to master the child's care and to advocate effectively for necessary medical, educational, and other services. The child learns to cope with the disability at school and in the community and to become a self-advocate. Working closely with the parents and child in a family-centered approach, the social worker, therapists, teachers, and physicians can play a crucial role in promoting these adjustments and may be instrumental in determining the prognosis of the child and the outcome of the entire family.

REFERENCES

Americans with Disabilities Act (ADA) of 1990, PL 101-336, 42 U.S.C. §§ 12101 *et seq.*

Arango, P. (1999). A parent's perspective on family-centered care. *Journal of Developmental and Behavioral Pediatrics, 20*(2), 123–123.

Banks, M.E. (2003). Disability in the family: A life span perspective. *Ethnic Minority Psychology, 9*(4), 367–384.

Bittles, A.H., & Glasson, E.J. (2004). Clinical, social, and ethical implications of changing life expectancy in Down syndrome. *Developmental Medicine and Child Neurology, 46,* 282–286.

Blanco, C., Lipsitz, J., & Caligor, E. (2001). Treatment of chronic depression with a 12-week program of interpersonal psychotherapy. *American Journal of Psychiatry, 158,* 371–375.

Burke, P. (2004). *Brothers and sisters of disabled children.* Philadelphia: Jessica Kingsley Publishers.

Carr, A. (2000). Evidence-based practice in family therapy and systemic consultation I. *Journal of Family Therapy, 22,* 29–60.

Cavet, J., & Sloper, P. (2004). Disabled children's participation in decision-making. *Children and Society, 18,* 278–290.

Coleby, M. (1995). The school-aged siblings of children with disabilities. *Developmental Medicine and Child Neurology, 37,* 415–426.

Cutler, B.C. (1993). *You, your child, and "special" education: A guide to making the system work.* Baltimore: Paul H. Brookes Publishing Co.

Davern, L., & Schnorr, R. (1991). Public schools welcome students with disabilities as full members. *Children Today, 20*(2), 21–25.

DePoy, E., & Gilson, S.F. (2004). *Rethinking disability: Principles for professional and social change.* Belmont, CA: Brooks/Cole.

Dobson, K.S. (Ed.). (2002). *Handbook of cognitive-behavioral therapies* (2nd ed.). New York: The Guilford Press.

Ello, L.M., & Donovan, S.J. (2005). Assessment of the relationship between parenting stress and a child's ability to functionally communicate. *Research on Social Work Practice, 15*(6), 531–544.

Farber, M., & Maharaj, R. (2005). Empowering high-risk families of children with disabilities. *Research on Social Work Practice, 15*(6), 501–515.

Giardino, A.P., Kohrt, A.E., Arye, L., et al. (2002). Health care delivery systems and financing issues. In

M.L. Batshaw (Ed.), *Children with disabilities* (5th ed., 707–724). Baltimore: Paul H. Brookes Publishing Co.

Green, S., Davis, C., Karshmer, E., et al. (2005). Living stigma: The impact of labeling, stereotyping, separation, status loss and discrimination in the lives of individuals with disabilities and their families. *Sociological Inquiry, 75*(2), 197–215.

Hallum, A. (1995). Disability and the transition to adulthood: Issues for the disabled child, the family, and the pediatrician. *Current Problems in Pediatrics, 25*(1), 12–50.

Hanson, M.J., & Lynch, E.W. (2004). *Understanding families: Approaches to diversity, disability, and risk.* Baltimore: Paul H. Brookes Publishing Co.

Harry, B. (2002). Trends and issues serving culturally diverse families of children with disabilities. *Journal of Special Education, 36*(3), 131–138.

Hill, A.E., (1993). Problems in relation to independent living: A retrospective study of physically disabled school leavers. *Developmental Medicine and Child Neurology, 35*(12), 1111–1115.

Ho, K.M., & Keiley, M.K. (2003). Dealing with denial: A systems approach for family professionals working with parents of individuals with multiple disabilities. *The Family Journal: Counseling and Therapy for Couples and Families, 11*(3), 239–247.

Individuals with Disabilities Education Improvement Act of 2004, PL 108-446, 20 U.S.C. §§ 1400 *et seq.*

Johnson, B. (2000). Family-centered care: Four decades of progress. *Families, Systems & Health. Special issue on consumers and collaborative care, 18*(2), 137–156.

Johnson, C.P., Kastner, T.A., & Committee/Section on Children with Disabilities. (2005). Helping families raise children with special health care needs at home. *Pediatrics, 115*(2), 507–511.

Kim, K., & Turnbull, A. (2004). Transition to adulthood for students with severe intellectual disabilities: Shifting toward person-family interdependent planning. *Research and Practice for Persons with Severe Disabilities, 29*(1), 111–124.

Leiter, V., Krauss, M.W., Anderson, B., et al. (2004). The consequences of caring: Effects of mothering a child with special needs. *Journal of Family Issues, 25*(3), 379–403.

Lobato, D.J. (1990). *Brothers, sisters, and special needs: Information and activities for helping young siblings of children with chronic illnesses and developmental disabilities.* Baltimore: Paul H. Brookes Publishing Co.

Lobato, D.J., Miller, C.T., Barbour, L., et al. (1991). Preschool siblings of handicapped children: Interactions with mothers, brothers and sisters. *Research in Developmental Disabilities, 12*(4), 387–399.

Miceli, P.J., & Clark, P.A. (2005). Your patient–my child: Seven priorities for improving pediatric care from the parent's perspective. *Journal of Nursing Care Quality, 20*(1), 43–53.

O'Brien, M.E. (2001). Living in a house of cards: Family experiences with long-term childhood technology dependence. *Journal of Pediatric Nursing, 16,* 13–22.

Ochieng, B.M. (2003). Minority ethnic families and family-centered care. *Journal of Child Health Care, 7*(2), 123–132.

Orsmond, G., Krauss, M., & Seltzer, M. (2004). Peer relationships and social and recreational activities among adolescents and adults with autism. *Journal of Autism and Developmental Disorders, 34*(3), 245–256.

Pilowsky, T., Yirmiya, N., Doppelt, O., et al. (2004). Social and emotional adjustment of siblings of children with autism. *Journal of Child Psychology and Psychiatry, 45*(4), 855–865.

Power, P.W. (2004). *Families living with chronic illness and disability: Interventions, challenges, and opportunities.* New York: Springer Publishing Co.

Powers, L.E., Singer, G.H.S., & Sowers, J-A. (Eds.). (1996). *On the road to autonomy: Promoting self-competence in children and youth with disabilities.* Baltimore: Paul H. Brookes Publishing Co.

Rivers, J., & Stoneman, Z. (2003). Sibling relationships when a child has autism: Marital stress and support coping. *Journal of Autism and Developmental Disorders, 33*(4), 383–394.

Rolland, J.S. (2003). Mastering family challenges in illness and disability. In F. Walsh (Ed.), *Normal family processes: Growing diversity and complexity* (3rd ed.). New York: The Guilford Press.

Ross-Watt, F. (2005). Inclusion in the early years: From rhetoric to reality. *Child Care in Practice, 11*(2), 103–118.

Sandler, A.G., Warren, S.H., & Raver, S.A. (1995). Grandparents as a source of support for parents of children with disabilities: A brief report. *Mental Retardation, 33,* 248–250.

Serketich, W., & Dumas, J.E. (1996). The effectiveness of behavioural parent training to modify antisocial behaviour in children: A meta-analysis. *Behaviour Therapy, 27,* 171–186.

Singer, G.H.S., & Powers, L.E. (Eds.). (1993). *Families, disability, and empowerment: Active coping skills and strategies for family interventions.* Baltimore: Paul H. Brookes Publishing Co.

Stalker, K., & Connors, C. (2004). Children's perceptions of their disabled siblings: 'She's different but it's normal for us.' *Children and Society, 18,* 218–230.

Stuart, S. (1999). Interpersonal psychotherapy for postpartum depression. In L. Miller (Ed.), *Postpartum psychiatric disorders* (pp. 143–162). Washington, DC: American Psychiatric Press.

Sullivan-Bolyai, S., Sadler, L., Knafl, K.A., et al. (2003). Great expectations: A position description for parents as caregivers: Part I. *Pediatric Nursing, 29*(6), 457–461.

Sullivan-Bolyai, S., Sadler, L., Knafl, K.A., et al. (2004). Great expectations: A position description for parents as caregivers: Part II. *Pediatric Nursing, 30*(1), 52–56.

Trachtenberg, S.W., & Hale Sills, N. (1996). Collaboration with parent and child. In L. Kurtz, P.W. Dowrick, S.E. Levy, et al. (Eds.), *Children's Seashore House handbook of developmental disabilities: Resources for interdisciplinary care* (pp. 526–533). Gaithersburg, MD: Aspen Publishers.

Trachtenberg, S.W., & Lewis, D.F. (1996). Case management. In L. Kurtz, P.W. Dowrick, S.E. Levy, et al. (Eds.), *Children's Seashore House handbook of developmental disabilities: Resources for interdisciplinary care* (pp. 203–208). Gaithersburg, MD: Aspen Publishers.

Trachtenberg, S.W., & Trachtenberg, J.I. (1996). Prevention of burnout for parents and professionals. In L. Kurtz, P.W. Dowrick, S.E. Levy, et al. (Eds.), *Children's Seashore House handbook of developmental disabilities: Resources for interdisciplinary care* (pp. 593–596). Gaithersburg, MD: Aspen Publishers.

Tunali, B., & Power, T.G. (1992). Creating satisfaction: A psychological perspective on stress and coping in families of handicapped children. *Journal of Child Psychology and Psychiatry, 34*(6), 945–957.

Turnbull, A.P., Patterson, J.M., Behr, S.K., et al. (Eds.). (1993). *Cognitive coping, families, and disability.* Baltimore: Paul H. Brookes Publishing Co.

Weissman, M.M., Markowitz, J.C., & Klerman, G.L. (2000). *Comprehensive guide to interpersonal psychotherapy*. New York: Basic Books.

White, P.H., Schuyler, V., Edelman, A., et al. (2002). Future expectations: Transition from adolescence to adulthood. In M.L. Batshaw (Ed.), *Children with disabilities* (5th ed., 693–705). Baltimore: Paul H. Brookes Publishing Co.

Wickler, L., Wasow, M., & Hatfield, E. (1981). Chronic sorrow revisited: Parent vs. professional depiction of the adjustment of parents of mentally retarded children. *American Journal of Orthopsychiatry, 51*, 63–70.

Williams, P.D., Williams, A.R., & Graff, J.C. (2003). A community-based intervention for siblings and parents of children with chronic illness or disability: The ISEE study. *The Journal of Pediatrics, 143*(3), 386–393.

Willoughby, J.C., & Glidden, L.M. (1995). Fathers helping out: Shared child care and marital satisfaction of parents of children with disabilities. *American Journal on Mental Retardation, 99*, 399–406.

41 Future Expectations

Transition from Adolescence to Adulthood

Nienke P. Dosa, Patience H. White, and Vincent Schuyler

Upon completion of this chapter, the reader will

- Be aware of the importance of planning for the transition to adulthood for youth with disabilities
- Understand the relationship between self-determination and health outcomes and social participation
- Understand the resources and mandated laws available to assist youth with disabilities
- Know the role of employment and postsecondary education in the transition process
- Understand the role health care providers play in promoting successful transition to adulthood of youth with disabilities

---

Individuals with developmental disabilities encounter the same life transitions as typically developing people do. Perhaps the most challenging of these is the transition to adulthood, a period of complex biological, social, and emotional change. This transition involves learning to move from 1) school to work, 2) home to community, and 3) pediatric- to adult-oriented health care. This chapter focuses on the steps involved in the successful transition of an individual with developmental disabilities from adolescence to adulthood.

BRYAN

Bryan is a 23-year-old former premature infant who has cerebral palsy and intellectual disability. Since he completed his public school education 2 years ago, Bryan has worked in a supported employment position at a local supermarket. He receives support and guidance from co-workers who were trained by a local job placement program to provide natural supports in the workplace. After work he participates in many recreational and leisure activities with friends. With his increasing job satisfaction and financial independence, this past year Bryan expressed a desire to live on his own. He and his parents contacted the local United Cerebral Palsy Association chapter and with assistance from the staff found an apartment and a live-in personal care attendant. Bryan still goes to his parent's house for family dinners and events at least once per week and spends additional time with his two younger siblings, ages 16 and 18, who come to visit him frequently in his apartment. Bryan has recently started dating a young woman he met at his job.

GENERAL PRINCIPLES OF TRANSITION

There are three basic tenets of successful transition. First, transition is a process, not an event. Planning should begin as early as possible on a flexible schedule that recognizes the young person's increasing autonomy and capacity for making choices. Transition to adult services should occur prospectively rather than during a crisis

(American Academy of Pediatrics, American Academy of Family Physicians, & American College of Physicians–American Society of Internal Medicine, 2002). Second, coordination among health care, educational, vocational, and social service systems is essential. It is particularly important to recognize the complex interplay between health and social outcomes as youth with developmental disabilities age into an employment-based health insurance system. Third, self-determination skills should be fostered throughout the transition process. Practice standards for transition services call for a youth-centered and asset-oriented approach that involves youth as decision makers during the entire transition process (Rosen et al., 2003).

MOVING TOWARD INDEPENDENCE: SELF-DETERMINATION

Self-determination is a combination of attitudes and abilities that lead people to set goals for themselves and to take the initiative to reach these goals (Ryan & Deci, 2000). The capabilities needed to become self-determined are learned through real-world experience (including mistakes) and an open, supportive acknowledgement of disability (Bremer, Kachgal, & Schoeller, 2003). Too often families, teachers, and other well-intentioned people protect youth with disabilities from making mistakes and avoid discussing the ramifications of a child's disability. This approach can set the child up for failure or can result in learned helplessness. Teachers and other individuals providing assistance to families can and should begin preparing children with developmental disabilities for independence as early as possible. For example, young children between 3 and 5 years of age can begin to incorporate chores into their daily routine. Families that give children opportunities to demonstrate competence through developmentally appropriate household chores send a clear message of support and capability. By the developmental age of 6–11 years, children should begin to assume responsibility for their self-care. During adolescence, self-determination skills can next be focused on identifying and meeting educational and vocational goals (Malian & Nevin, 2002; Wehmeyer et al., 2000). In early adulthood, these skills can then be used to identify and meet goals related to independent living. Curricula, tools, and policies have been developed to enhance self-determination for students with disabilities (Wood et al., 2000).

MOVING FROM SCHOOL TO WORK

The concept of transition planning originated with schools, and education policies are the driving force for almost all aspects of transition. Four pieces of legislation—the Individuals with Disabilities Education Improvement Act of 2004 (PL 108-446; IDEA 2004), the School-to-Work Opportunities Act of 1994 (PL 103-239), the Workforce Investment Act (WIA) of 1998 (PL105-220), and the Americans with Disabilities Act (ADA) of 1990 (PL 101-336)—outline important educational practices that lead to successful adult outcomes for students with disabilities. (See Chapter 34 for a discussion of the transition plan and how it affects an individualized education program [IEP].) Certain aspects of these laws are discussed in the following sections.

Vocational Rehabilitation

Linking schools with systems of care that serve adults with disabilities, including vocational rehabilitation (VR) agencies, strengthens the transition process. The School-to-Work Opportunities Act of 1994 provides workplace mentoring and skills certificates for youth with developmental disabilities. The WIA links education, employment, and training services to a network of resources in local areas called One-Stop Career Centers (Barnow & King, 2005). Transition planning as mandated by IDEA 2004 stipulates that VR counselors must participate in transition planning before the student exits the school system. It is important to note that VR counselors are typically assigned to students only during their last 2 years of school but that parents and students can request their participation as early as age 14 via One-Stop Career Centers (U.S. Department of Labor, 2005) or through the school.

Unlike the entitlement based system for K–12 education, all adult services and systems are eligibility based and require that individuals meet the established requirements, including financial eligibility criteria, to receive services. Once individuals are determined to be eligible, the VR agency can provide or arrange for a host of training, educational, medical, and other services designed to help these individuals acquire and maintain gainful employment. Similar to the IEP in the school system, all services are guided by the development of an individualized plan for employment (IPE) (previously called an individualized written rehabilitation program [IWRP]), which is individualized to meet the needs of the young person. Although VR counselors can provide direct services to the young adult, they more often refer the individual to appropriate community-based agencies. Services covered by VR may include self-advocacy training, the development of employment readiness skills, adaptive driving evaluation and instruction, identification and procurement of assistive technology, job coaching, and so forth.

Moving Toward Postsecondary Education

Postsecondary education can take many forms. Although traditionally thought of as college, it may be any form of education or training that takes place after a young adult leaves high school, including on-the-job training, specialized coursework, or even courses through postgraduate study. Most colleges and universities have an office designated as a Disability Support Services (DSS) or, at a minimum, an individual designated to assist students with disabilities. To receive assistance or request accommodations for disability-related needs, a student must take the lead in disclosing his or her disability, providing current documentation of the disability and identifying needed accommodations. Accommodations are established on a case-by-case basis and do not necessarily replicate those provided in the K–12 setting. Examples of accommodations that can be requested of DSS include extra time in test taking, a sign language interpreter, a note taker, recorded books, and coordination with other services. Postsecondary education facilities that receive federal funding are required to provide reasonable accommodations to qualified individuals with disabilities under Section 504 of the Rehabilitation Act of 1973 (PL 93-112) and under Titles II and/or III of the ADA. A number of organizations can give students and parents information about laws that have an impact on the education of individuals with disabilities (see also Appendix D).

Entering the Workforce

Work experience is a prerequisite for many jobs. Unfortunately, most youth with developmental disabilities enter the workforce later than their peers who do not have disabilities. Nationwide, 41% of high school freshman and 85% of high school seniors hold down regular jobs either during the school year or during summer months (U.S. Department of Labor, 2005). In contrast, only 54% of adolescents with developmental disabilities are wage earners prior to high school graduation (Cameto et al., 2003). Those with learning disabilities, emotional disturbances, other health impairments, or speech impairments are most likely to be employed. Only 15% of youth with autism spectrum disorders; approximately one fourth of youth with multiple disabilities, deaf-blindness, or orthopedic impairments; and about one third of youth with intellectual disability or visual impairments are employed during high school. The implications of limited early job experience on workforce readiness, long-term employment, economic status, and social functioning in adulthood are profound. In 2004, employment rates for the 14 million U.S. adults who have a disability (7.9% of adults ages 18–64 years) were substantially lower than for adults who do not have a disability (19% versus 77%). The correlate to this is a poverty rate for adults who have a disability that is substantially higher than that of the population without disabilities (28% versus 9.2%) (Houtenville, 2005).

Paid work experiences should be written into a student's transition plan starting no later than age 16 years. Job choice should be based on individual interests, abilities, and postsecondary goals. For example if a student has set a goal to work as a computer operator, it would not be appropriate to place that student in a job reshelving books in the school library. The appropriate placement would be one that allows the student to work with a computer in some fashion—for example, doing basic data entry.

Work Options

Individuals with disabilities, like those without disabilities, have the option of participating in competitive employment, but they also have a range of other work alternatives (Wittenburg, Fishman, & Golden, 2002). Competitive employment and alternatives are described next.

Competitive Employment An individual engaged in competitive employment is working in a job in which he or she is expected to perform the essential functions of a job at the same level as other employees without disabilities. Individuals with disabilities may request an accommodation under the protections of the ADA that enable them to perform these functions as long as the accommodation does not fundamentally alter the nature of the job. This could include adaptive seating, computer input devices, large-print text, and so forth. To succeed in a competitive employment setting, individuals with disabilities must have the same skills requisite for any employee to succeed in the workplace: appropriate social skills, effective communication skills, and motivation. Individuals with disabilities also must have appropriate independent living skills and the skills and abilities to manage their disability related needs, such as hiring and managing personal care attendants and transportation services. Individuals with an intellectual disability can be successful in competitive employment settings given the appropriate level of support.

Work-Study Employment Work-study employment is part-time work for students, on or off the school campus, that is sanctioned by the school. Youth should be cautioned to avoid vocational counseling that purveys cultural stereotypes. For example, the number of individuals with developmental disabilities employed in food service (19% of work-study jobs and 16% of regular jobs) and maintenance (16% of work-study jobs and 24% of regular jobs) far exceeds what one would expect to be representative of the interest level for these jobs among youth with developmental disabilities (Cameto et al., 2003).

Supported Employment Supported employment is defined by the Rehabilitation Act Amendments of 1986 (PL 99-506) and 1992 (PL 102-569) as employment in an inclusive setting with ongoing support services for an individual with a disability. Supported employment programs are generally administered through the state-level Bureaus of Vocational Rehabilitation and state developmental disability agencies. These agencies help people with disabilities to obtain employment by identifying supports through supervisor or co-worker assistance (natural supports) or job coaches. A job coach or employment consultant is a person who is hired by the individual or the placement agency to provide specialized on-site training to assist the employee with a disability in learning and performing his or her job and adjusting to the work environment. It should be recognized, however, that a job coach sometimes interferes with worksite inclusion (Degeneffe, 2000).

Customized Employment Customized employment is a blend of services designed to increase employment options for individuals with significant disabilities such as self-employment, entrepreneurship, job carving and restructuring, personal agents and customized training (Martin-Luecking & Luecking, 2004).

Enclaves Enclaves were once considered a viable employment option for individuals with severe disabilities. The enclave structure groups of individuals with disabilities together at one site with a common job coach engaged around a work task. Enclaves are seen as a cost-saving model for agencies but are controversial because individuals often are paid subwages and the model does not promote worksite inclusion. Placement of individuals in enclave settings is not recommended.

Volunteering In today's competitive job market, volunteering is an opportunity for adolescents to gain valuable insight into the world of work, develop skills, and build work related experience. However, volunteer experiences should not take the place of paid work experiences. Doing so may inadvertently promote cultural stereotypes about the employability of individuals with developmental disabilities.

Other Options Some youth with intellectual disabilities may not be ready to make the transition into a work-related setting immediately after exiting the school system. For these individuals, other more supportive options are available, such as day treatment/habilitation or work-readiness programs. These programs provide a more intensive level of support and focus on the development of daily living skills rather than job skills. The ultimate goal for any of these programs should remain moving the individual toward employment.

MOVING FROM HOME INTO THE COMMUNITY

It is important to address several key financial and legal issues prior to age 18 to avoid loss of income and/or services, to protect family assets, and to ensure that youth with developmental disabilities have suitable independent living options as they move from home to the community. Financial barriers are the most common reason youth with developmental disabilities fail to make the transition to independent living in the community (McPherson et al., 2004). It is essential that families be proactive about legal and financial matters as youth with developmental disabilities make the transition to adulthood. Key issues are summarized next.

Financial Independence

Supplemental Security Income (SSI) is a monthly payment for individuals with disabilities. To qualify for SSI, individuals must meet both disability and financial eligibility requirements. SSI eligibility is generally determined again using adult criteria when adolescents turn 18 years old, with the exception being youth enrolled in a Social Security Administration (SSA) work incentive program. Young people with developmental disabilities may lose their SSI at this time if they fail to meet the adult disability criteria. Conversely, some individuals with disabilities may now qualify for SSI when they had previously been ineligible because individual income, rather than household income, is used to determine income eligibility at age 18. Generally speaking, adults who receive SSI cannot have assets greater than $1,500 and still remain eligible. The SSA, however, does allow several important exceptions to this rule, which are referred to as work incentives (see http://www.SSA.gov/work).

Despite these incentive programs, a significant number of youth with developmental disabilities lose SSI benefits when they become adults. In 2002, SSI recipients in the 13–17 year age bracket numbered 321,114, compared with 243,689 recipients in the 18–21 year age bracket (Nadel, Wamhoff, & Wiseman, 2003). Youth who lose SSI benefits when eligibility is determined at age 18 should request a second review because nearly one third of such requests result in the reinstatement of SSI benefits (Schulzinger, 2000). Some individuals who are found ineligible can continue to receive SSI benefits as long as they participate in approved VR programs. In most states, people who receive SSI automatically also qualify for Medicaid.

Social Security Disability Insurance (SSDI) is a monthly payment for individuals with disabilities. There are two ways to qualify for SSDI benefits. Workers (including those in sheltered or supported work settings) who have paid into the Social Security system are eligible for SSDI if they are no longer able to work. Monthly SSDI benefits are also paid to an adult with developmental disabilities when a parent or guardian meets disability criteria and cannot work. It is important to know that beneficiaries who receive SSDI for more than 2 years are eligible for health care coverage under Medicare.

Legal Status/Guardianship

In most states, the natural guardianship of parents ends when children reach age 18 years. At that point, parents no longer have the legal ability to make decisions and sign consent forms for their child unless they submit an application for guardianship at their local probate court. Two prerequisites should exist before a court appoints a guardian: 1) the child must show incompetence in at least one important area of life, such as health care decisions or financial matters, and 2) there must be a present need for the guardianship. In accord with the principles of self-determination, it is important to evaluate the extent to which an individual can participate in decisions that affect his or her own life. This allows probate courts to appoint someone as a guardian only over the portion of a person's life where he or she both shows incompetence and has a need (e.g., health care guardianship). There are several alternatives to guardianship that may be preferable because they avoid legal "red tape" and are more specific to the needs and rights of an individual. A representative payeeship can be useful when the only income an individual receives is his or her monthly SSI check and there are no major financial decisions. A special needs trust permits adults with developmental disabilities to inherit money, which can be used for services not covered by Medicaid or Medicare without interrupting these government benefits. A conservatorship is established when an individual is mentally competent but has a physical disability that limits his or her ability to participate in the decision-making process. Adult protective services can be ordered by a court if abuse or neglect of an adult with developmental disabilities is suspected. A circle of support is an informal group of volunteer advocates who make sure that an individual with developmental disabilities has a support system that meets all of his or her needs. A microboard is a circle of support that is incorporated to include the individual with developmental disabilities as the chairperson.

Although informal alternatives to guardianship are gaining acceptance, it should be noted that a legal guardian or a representative payee is often required by programs and services in order to disburse funds to an individual with developmental disabilities. The paperwork for this should be completed before age 18 to avoid interruption in benefits.

Housing

Approximately 35% of adults with developmental disabilities live in their own homes, 60% live with their families, and 15% reside in publicly funded residential settings (Braddock et al., 2001; Seltzer & Krauss, 2001). Community living programs for young adults with developmental disabilities are in high demand, and waiting lists are the norm (Larson, Lakin, & Huang, 2003; Prouty, Smith, & Lakin, 2004).

Services and programs that assist individuals with community living have increased dramatically since the 1990s as a result of the New Freedom Initiative (Executive Order No. 13217), the ADA, and the Olmstead decision. The Olmstead decision interpreted Title II of the ADA to require states to administer their services, programs, and activities "in the most integrated setting appropriate to the needs of qualified individuals with disabilities." State-funded programs as well as private nonprofit agencies—such as The Arc of the United States, Easter Seals, and United Cerebral Palsy (UCP) —provide service coordination and access to a wide array of independent living options. Independent living centers foster networking among people with disabilities and offer assistance in four key areas: information and referral, independent living skills and training, peer counseling, and advocacy (Seekins, Enders, & Innes, 1999). Various housing options are discussed next.

Family Home Many families whose grown children have developmental disabilities will choose for the individual to continue to live at home. The aging of these families is an emerging concern. Approximately 25% of home-based adults with developmental disabilities live in homes headed by elderly parents. Support systems for aging parents of adults with developmental disabilities are lacking (Fujiura, 2003).

Group Home The most common form of assisted living program (outside of the family home) is the group home. The trend is toward smaller group homes of one to three residents (Prouty et al., 2004). Most group homes have on-site counselors who provide supervision and support in daily living skills, employment, and recreation.

Supported Living Services (SLS) Supported living services (SLS) provide services to adults with developmental disabilities who live in homes that they own or lease in the community. SLS may include assistance with 1) selecting and moving into a home, 2) choosing personal attendants and housemates, 3) acquiring household furnishings, 4) addressing common daily living activities and emergencies, 5) becoming a participating member in community life, and 6) managing personal financial affairs.

MOVING FROM PEDIATRIC- TO ADULT-ORIENTED HEALTH CARE

As a result of advances in medical technology and dramatic improvements in the delivery of acute health care, the vast majority of children with developmental disabilities can now expect to survive to adulthood (Glasson et al., 2002; Hunt & Oakeshott, 2003). As life expectancy for individuals with developmental disabilities approaches that of the general population, socioeconomic factors are increasingly being recognized as important determinants of health (Newachek & Kim, 2005), and quality of life and social inclusion are being recognized as meaningful health outcomes (Anderson, Krajci, & Vogel, 2003; Liptak & Accardo, 2003; Turk et al., 2001). The International Classification of Functioning, Disability and Health (ICF) provides a framework for understanding the impact of the social and physical environment on health for individuals with developmental disabilities (World Health Organization, 2001). This framework broadens the array of interventions to be considered as strategies for improving health and social outcomes. For example, identifying accessible recreation opportunities in the community may be one of the most effective ways to "treat" obesity individuals with spina bifida. Coincidental with the ICF reconceptualization of functioning, disability, and health is a paradigm shift in the way health care is delivered to people with developmental disabilities. Institutions and hospital-based programs are rapidly being replaced by home and community-based supports and services. This trend is reflected by the federal health care goal (in *Healthy People 2010*) that young people with developmental disabilities receive services needed to make necessary transitions to *all* aspects of adult life, including health care, work, and independent living (U.S. Department of Health and Human Services, 2000).

A major obstacle with transition to adult-oriented care is that youth have "nowhere to go" (Reiss & Gibson, 2002). Many adult health care providers lack training in the care of individuals with developmental disabilities. Low patient satisfaction with adult providers has been reported in terms of availability, thoroughness, respect, and privacy (Larson et al., 2003). Pediatric providers, in turn, are inadequately mobilized to "let go" of their adolescent patients (Reiss, Gibson, & Walker, 2005). Studies have documented that only one out of six pediatricians routinely discuss health care transition with young adult patients who have developmental disabilities (Scal & Ireland, 2005). Lack of insurance and underinsurance are also major barriers to health care transition (see chapter 42). In the United States, nearly one in three young adults with developmental disabilities ages 18–24 years is uninsured (Callahan & Cooper, 2006).

A professional consensus statement put forth in 2002 established several first steps to ensuring a successful transition to adult-oriented health care for youth with developmental disabilities (American Academy of Pediatrics, American Academy of Family Physicians, & American College of Physicians–American Society of Internal Medicine, 2002). These recommendations include 1) identifying a health care professional who acts as a transition coordinator in partnership with the youth and his or her family; 2) educating health care professionals to provide developmentally appropriate transition services; 3) preparing and maintaining an up-to-date medical summary that is portable and accessible; 4) creating a written health care transition by age 14 together with the youth and his or her family; 5) applying same guidelines for primary and preventive care; and 6) ensuring affordable, continuous health insurance coverage that includes compensation for transition planning and care coordination.

Health care transition involves not only the transfer of medical information from pediatric to adult providers but also the transition of responsibility for health-related issues from the parent to the individual with developmental disabilities (Betz, 2004). In addition to the previously mentioned systems-level issues, several clinical topics generic to adolescent health care have unique applications for youth with developmental disabilities during the transition to adulthood.

Adherence and Health Literacy

To be ready to move to the adult system, the adolescent needs to be responsible for taking medications (with supervision when necessary); to develop the ability to understand and discuss his or her disability; and to use required adaptive equipment or appliances. During this process, health care professionals should consider when to start seeing the individual alone and when to develop a confidential relationship with him or her. For many adolescents this is appropriately at age 12–13 years. Health care autonomy checklists are available to help youth with developmental disabilities and their health care providers to assess health related skills and learn what is needed to navigate the adult oriented health care system (University of Washington, n.d.). Checklists are also available at the Healthy & Ready to Work national resource center (http//www.HRTW.org). Some youth with developmental disabilities may qualify for state-funded medical service coordination and assistance with developing self care skills.

Health Promotion

Good nutrition and regular exercise are the basis of health. Adults with developmental disabilities have similar rates of obesity and risky behaviors (e.g., tobacco use) as people without disabilities but are less likely to participate in prevention programs or to receive periodic cancer screening (Havercamp, Scandlin, & Roth, 2004). Adults with developmental disabilities are also at risk for preventable "secondary conditions" such as osteoporosis and decubitus ulcers. Early and sustained participation in community-based programs is essential for adolescents to maintain healthy lifestyles beyond the school years (Liptak & Accardo, 2004; Turk et al. 2001). Leisure activities are particularly important for young adults with developmental disabilities, who tend to become socially isolated. People with developmental disabilities requiring extensive to pervasive support are less likely to participate in leisure activities (Felce & Emerson, 2001). Therapeutic recreation programs that incorporate social skills training can help individuals with developmental disabilities to develop conversation skills, maintain eye contact, use appropriate body language, or recover from rejection. Examples of therapeutic recreation programs include Special Olympics for individuals with cognitive impairments and Games for the Physically Challenged for individuals with physical disabilities. The National Center on Physical Activity and Disability (http://www.ncpad.org) is a clearinghouse for information to promote physical activity among individuals with disabilities.

Sexuality

Sexuality is a natural aspect of human development and important to all individuals regardless of age, gender, orientation, or developmental level (Ailey et al., 2003). Adolescents with developmental disabilities often do not receive information about sexuality and reproductive health. Professionals and parents either lack the awareness to consider sexuality as part of the adolescent's normal growth and development or are fearful of discussing sensitive issues and acknowledging vulnerability (Shapland, 1999). This results in an information void that may increase the chances of sexual exploitation and unintended pregnancy. Youth with developmental disabilities are four times more likely to be sexually abused or exploited than their typical counterparts. Lack of knowledge of sexuality, lack of information on exploitation, cognitive difficulties, poor social skills, poor self-esteem, and poor body image are just some of the factors that place adolescents with developmental disabilities at risk (Schwier & Hingsberger, 2000).

Mental Health

Individuals with developmental disabilities are at high risk for developing mental health problems. Among adults with developmental disabilities, the prevalence of mental illness is approximately four times higher than that found in the general population (Rush et al., 2004). Furthermore, adults with developmental disabilities are seven times more likely to report inadequate emotional support, compared with adults who do not have disabilities (Havercamp et. al., 2004; see also Chapter 21). Behavioral concerns should be investigated rather than being ascribed to the individual's developmental disability. It is important to question adolescents and their families about physical symptoms of anxiety and depression, such as altered sleep and appetite. Excessive school absence is also a red flag. Environmental factors should also be considered when adolescents with developmental disabilities present with challenging behaviors. For example, it is not unusual for an adolescent with developmental disabilities to experience anxiety when a long-time aide is no longer available at school or when opportunities to socialize diminish with high school graduation. Surgery, prolonged hospitalization, or medical setbacks can also precipitate depressive episodes. Behaviors that occur across all settings are more likely to be due to organic causes. Treatments can include psychological, behavioral, and/or environmental interventions along with pharmacotherapy, if needed. Community-based models of support with neuropsychiatric intervention can be a potent therapeutic combination in the management of challenging behaviors in individuals with developmental disabilities (Ferrell et al., 2004; see also Chapter 35).

SUMMARY

Health care providers, educators, other professionals, and families must foster the expectation that youth with developmental disabilities will become healthy, happy, active, and productive members of their community. Youth should be provided with opportunities to learn about their strengths, abilities, skills, needs, and interests. They should also be allowed to take risks and to learn from failure. They should assume responsibility for themselves and understand the difference between the protected worlds of school and home and the worlds of work and adult life. Most of all, they must believe they are capable of success. These goals can be accomplished through comprehensive transition planning and advocacy, including self-advocacy, to promote full participation in society.

REFERENCES

Ailey, S.H., Marks, B.A., Crisp, C., et al. (2003). Promoting sexuality across the life span for individuals with intellectual and developmental disabilities. *Nursing Clinics of North America, 38*(2), 229–352.

American Academy of Pediatrics, American Academy of Family Physicians, & American College of Physicians–American Society of Internal Medicine. (2002). A consensus statement on health care transitions for young adults with special health care needs. *Pediatrics, 110*(6, Pt. 2), 1304–1306.

Americans with Disabilities Act (ADA) of 1990, PL 101-336, 42 U.S.C. §§ 12101 *et seq.*

Anderson, C.J., Krajci, K.A., & Vogel, L.C. (2003). Community integration among adults with spinal cord injuries sustained as children or adolescents. *Developmental Medicine & Child Neurology, 45*(2), 129–134.

Barnow, B.S., & King, C.T. (2005). *Workforce Investment Act in eight states* (U.S. Department of Labor Employment and Training Administration Occasional Reports 2005-1 [AK-12224-01-60].) Retrieved February 10, 2007 from http://rockinst.org/publications/federalism/wia/Rockefeller_Institute_WIA%20_Final_Report2-17-05.pdf

Betz, C.L. (2004). Transition of adolescents with special health care needs: Review and analysis of the literature. *Issues in Comprehensive Pediatric Nursing, 27*(3), 179–241.

Braddock, D., Emerson, E., Felce, D., et al. (2001). Living circumstances of children and adults with mental retardation or developmental disabilities in the United States, Canada, England and Wales, and Australia. *Mental Retardation and Developmental Disabilities Research Reviews, 7,* 115–121.

Bremer C.D., Kachgal M., & Schoeller K. (2003). Self-determination: Supporting successful transition. *Research to Practice Brief: Improving Secondary Education and Transition Services Through Research, 2*(1). Retrieved June 16, 2005, from http://ncset.org/publications/viewdesc.asp?id=962

Callahan, S.T., & Cooper, W.O. (2006). Access to health care for young adults with disabling chronic conditions. *Archives of Pediatrics & Adolescent Medicine, 160*(2), 178–182.

Cameto, R., Marder, C., Wagner, M., et al. (2003). Youth employment. *NLTS2 Data Brief, 2*(2). Retrieved June 16, 2005, from http://www.ncset.org/publications/viewdesc.asp?id=1310

Casey Family Programs. (2004). *Adolescent Autonomy Checklists.* Seattle, WA: Author.

Degeneffe, C.E. (2000). Supported employment services for persons with developmental disabilities: Unmet promises and future challenges for rehabilitation counselors. *Journal of Applied Rehabilitation Counseling, 31*(2), 41–47.

Edelman, A., Schuyler, V.E., & White, P.H. (1998). *Maximizing success for young adults with chronic health-related illnesses: Transition planning for education after high school.* Washington, DC: HEATH Resource Center.

Executive Order No. 13217, 66 Federal Register 33155 (21 June 2001).

Felce, D., & Emerson, E. (2001). Living with support in a home in the community: Predictors of behavioral development and household and community activity. *Mental Retardation and Developmental Disabilities Research Reviews, 7,* 75–83.

Ferrell R.B., Wolinsky E.J., Kauffman C.I., et al. (2004). Neuropsychiatric syndromes in adults with mental retardation: Issues in assessment and treatment. *Current Psychiatry Reports, 6*(5), 380–390.

Fujiura, G.T. (2003). Continuum of mental retardation: Demographic evidence for the "forgotten generation." *Intellectual Disability, 41*(6), 420–429.

Glasson, E.J., Sullivan, S.G., Hussain, R., et al. (2002). The changing survival profile of people with Down's syndrome: Implications for genetic counselling. *Clinical Genetics, 62*(5), 390–393.

Havercamp, S.M., Scandlin, D., & Roth, M. (2004). Health disparities among adults with developmental disabilities, adults with other disabilities, and adults not reporting disability in North Carolina. *Public Health Reports, 119*(4), 418–426.

Houtenville, A.J. (2005). *Disability statistics in the United States.* Ithaca, NY: Cornell University Rehabilitation Research and Training Center on Disability Demographics and Statistics (StatsRRTC).

Hunt, G.M., & Oakeshott, P. (2003). Outcome in people with open spina bifida at age 35: Prospective community based cohort study. *British Medical Journal, 326*(7403), 1365–1366.

Individuals with Disabilities Education Improvement Act of 2004, PL 108-446, 20 U.S.C. §§ 1400 *et seq.*

Larson, S., Lakin, C., & Huang, J. (2003). Service Use by and needs of adults with functional limitations or ID/DD in the NHIS-D: Difference by age, gender, and disability. *DD Data Brief, 5*(2), 10.

Levey, E.B., & Murphy, N.A. (2005). Addressing transition to adulthood with special needs patients. *AAP News, 26*(2), 19.

Liptak, G.S., & Accardo, P.J. (2004). Health and social outcomes of children with cerebral palsy. *Journal of Pediatrics, 145*(2, Suppl.), S36–S41.

Malian, I., & Nevin, A. (2002). A review of self-determination literature: Implications for practitioners. *Remedial and Special Education, 23*(2), 68–74.

Martin-Luecking, D., & Luecking, R.G. (2004). Organization change: Building employer-friendly services. In R.G. Luecking, E.S. Fabian, & G. P. Tilson (Eds.), *Working relationships: Creating career opportunities for job seekers with disabilities through employer partnerships* (pp. 217–233). Baltimore: Paul H. Brookes Publishing Co.

McPherson, M., Weissman, G., Strickland, B.B., et al. (2004). Implementing community-based systems of services for children and youths with special health care needs: how well are we doing? *Pediatrics, 113*(5, Suppl.), 1538–1544.

Nadel, M., Wamhoff, S., & Wiseman, M. (2003). Disability, welfare reform and supplemental security income. *Social Security Bulletin, 65,* 14–30.

Newacheck, P.W., & Kim, S.E. (2005). A national profile of health care utilization and expenditures for children with special health care needs. *Archives of Pediatrics & Adolescent Medicine, 159*(1), 10–17. [erratum in *Archives of Pediatrics & Adolescent Medicine, 159*(4), 318].

Olmstead v. L.C., 527 U.S. 581 (1999).

Olsen, D.G., & Swigonski, N.L. (2004). Transition to adulthood: The important role of the pediatrician. *Pediatrics, 113,* e159–e162.

Prouty, R., Smith, G., & Lakin, K.C. (Eds.). (2004). *Residential services for persons with developmental disabilities: Status and trends through 2003.* Minneapolis: University of Minnesota, Research and Training Center on Community Living.

Rehabilitation Act Amendments of 1986, PL 99-506, 29 U.S.C. §§ 701 *et seq.*

Rehabilitation Act Amendments of 1992, PL 102-569, 29 U.S.C. §§ 701 *et seq.*

Rehabilitation Act of 1973, PL 93-112, 29 U.S.C. §§ 701 *et seq.*

Reiss, J., & Gibson, R. (2002). Health care transition: Destinations unknown. *Pediatrics, 110*(6, Pt. 2), 1307–1314.

Reiss, J.G., Gibson, R.W., & Walker, L.R. (2005). Health care transition: Youth, family, and provider perspectives. *Pediatrics, 115*(1), 112–120.

Rosen, D.S., Blum, R.W., Britto, M., et al. (2003). Transition to adult health care for adolescents and young adults with chronic conditions: Position paper of the Society for Adolescent Medicine. *Journal of Adolescent Health, 33*(4), 309–311.

Rush, K.S., Bowman, L.G., Eidman, S.L., et al. (2004). Assessing psychopathology in individuals with developmental disabilities. *Behavior Modification, 28*(5), 621–637.

Ryan, R.M., & Deci, E.L. (2000). Self-determination theory and the facilitation of intrinsic motivation, social development, and well-being. *American Psychologist, 55*(1), 68–78.

Scal, P., & Ireland, M. (2005). Addressing transition to adult health care for adolescents with special health care needs. *Pediatrics, 115,* 1607–1612.

Schwier, K.M., & Hingsburger, D. (2000). *Sexuality: Your sons and daughters with intellectual disabilities.* Baltimore: Paul H. Brookes Publishing Co.

School-to-Work Opportunities Act of 1994, PL 103-239, 20 U.S.C. 6101 *et seq.*

Schulzinger, R. (2000). *Youth with disabilities in transition: Health insurance options and obstacles. An occasional policy brief of the Institute for Child Health Policy.* Gainesville, FL: Institute for Child Health Policy.

Section 504 of the Rehabilitation Act, 29 U.S.C. § 794d.

Seekins, T., Enders, A., & Innes, B. (1999). *Ruralfacts: Centers for independent living, rural and urban distribution.* Missoula: The University of Montana, The Research and Training Center on Rural Rehabilitation Services. Retrieved October 4, 2006, fromhttp://rtc.ruralinstitute.umt.edu/IL/Ruralfacts/RuCILfacts.htm

Seltzer, M.M., & Krauss, M.W. (2001). Quality of life of adults with mental retardation/developmental disabilities who live with family. *Mental Retardation and Developmental Disabilities Research Reviews, 7,* 105–114.

Shapland, C. (1999). *Sexuality issues for youth with disabilities and chronic conditions* (An occasional policy brief of the Institute of Child Health Policy). Gainesville, FL: Institute of Child Health Policy.

Turk, M.A., Scandale, J., Rosenbaum, P.F., et al. (2001). The health of women with cerebral palsy. *Physical Medicine and Rehabilitation Clinics of North America, 12* (1), 153–168.

University of Washington, Center on Human Development and Disability, Adolescent Health Transition Project. (n.d.). *Transition timeline for children and adolescents with special health care needs: Developmental disabilities/delays.* Retrieved February 10, 2007, from http://depts.washington.edu/healthtr/Timeline/DDD_timeline_Eng.PPT

U.S. Department of Health and Human Services. (2000). *Healthy People 2010:Understanding and improving health* (2nd ed.). Washington, DC: U.S. Government Printing Office.

U.S. Department of Labor. (2005). *Work activity of high school students: Data from the National Longitudinal Survey of Youth 1997* (USDL reports: 05-732). Retrieved June 16, 2005, from http://www.bls.gov/nls/nlsy97r6.pdf

U.S. Department of Labor, Employment and Training Administration. (2005). *Map of state One-Stop web sites.* Retrieved June 16, 2005, from http://www.doleta.gov/usworkforce/onestop/onestopmap.cfm

Wehmeyer, M.L., Palmer, S.B., Agran, M., et al. (2000). Promoting causal agency: The self-determined learning model of instruction. *Exceptional Children, 66*(4), 439–453.

Wittenburg, D., Fishman, M., & Golden, T. (2002). Transition options for youth with disabilities: An overview of the programs and policies that affect the transition from school. *Journal of Vocational Rehabilitation, 17,* 195–206.

Wood, W.M., Test, D.W., Browder, D.M., et al. (2000). *Self-Determination Synthesis Project.* Retrieved October 4, 2006, from http://www.uncc.edu/sdsp/home.asp

Workforce Investment Act (WIA) of 1998, PL 105-220, 29 U.S.C. §§ 2801 *et seq.*

World Health Organization. (2001). *International Classification of Functioning, Disability and Health (ICF).* Geneva: Author.

42 Health Care Delivery Systems and Financing Issues

Angelo P. Giardino, Renee M. Turchi, and Alan E. Kohrt

Upon completion of this chapter, the reader will

- Understand the definition of the term *children with special health care needs* and see how such a definition affects health care delivery and financing issues
- Appreciate the complexity involved in developing a system that adequately coordinates various services and supports
- Be aware of insurance coverage issues that affect the provision of health care to these children
- Recognize the various public health care programs and benefits that may be of value to these children and their families

The federal Maternal and Child Health Bureau (MCHB) defines children and youth with special health care needs (CYSHCN) as "those who have or are at increased risk for a chronic physical, developmental, behavioral or emotional condition and who also require health and related services of a type or amount beyond that required by children generally" (McPherson et al., 1998, p. 138). Approximately 13%–18% of children in the United States who are younger than 18 years (9–12.5 million children) satisfy these criteria (Newacheck, McManus, et al., 2000; Strickland et al., 2004). Not all children with developmental disabilities have special health care needs, and not all CYSHCN have developmental disabilities, however. For example, children with learning disabilities do not generally have special medical needs, and children with asthma, who do have special medical needs, do not generally have developmental disabilities. Therefore, the term CYSHCN includes both a subgroup of children with developmental disabilities (e.g., cerebral palsy, meningomyelocele) and a group of typically developing children with complex medical problems (e.g., hemophilia, diabetes) (Newacheck et al., 1998). The National Survey of Children with Special Health Care Needs estimated that 12.8% of U.S. children have special health care needs (van Dyck et al., 2004).

Developing an effective health care system for CYSHCN is the focus of this chapter. Several of the core features of this system, however, are important for all children. CYSHCN may require an array of services beyond the primary care doctor, including those provided by specialists, therapists, pharmacists, educators, mental health providers, and home health providers (Wells et al., 2000). The Institute of Medicine (2001) suggested the fragmentation of health care in the United States jeopardizes quality of care. Thus, the most important principles are that children should be provided comprehensive health care, that all care is coordinated, and that all children should have a "medical home."

PROBLEMS IN ARRANGING COORDINATION OF CARE

Given the many services that may be needed and the number of providers and professionals potentially involved in coordinating the various health care services required by a CYSHCN,

623

there are many challenges for the child's family and health care providers. The child's needs are complex, and a great deal of time, energy, and skill are needed to ensure the efforts of different agencies, institutions, and professionals work effectively together in developing a comprehensive plan of care (American Academy of Pediatrics [AAP], 1998, 1999). Required services may include some not traditionally seen as health related, such as education and housing. When provided, care coordination services are readily accepted by families and minimize the burden of the child's condition (Palfry et al., 2004). However, recent estimates suggest that less than half of families received effective care coordination when it was needed (McPherson et al., 2004). Care coordination can result in cost savings and decrease hospital stays. (Liptak et al., 1998; Palfrey et al., 2004). In fact, more than half of the time that a health care provider spends with CYSHCN may involve care coordination without reimbursement (Antonelli & Antonelli, 2004). Even when obtained, many services are not available in convenient, community-based settings, thus further depleting the families' energy and resources.

In an attempt to deal with these issues, insurers, hospitals, and public and private agencies have developed case management programs. The purpose and scope of these programs vary with the type of agency and often are not focused on the overall coordination of care. Hospitals use case management to provide information to payers and assist with discharge planning. Case management done for insurers and managed care organizations (MCOs) focuses more on benefits management and resource utilization and less on care coordination, although some Medicaid MCOs do organize and coordinate a broader package of benefits (Abt Associates, 2000). Many social agencies and public programs provide case management services because these are often mandated by public policy. Title V programs, which are state programs for CYSHCN that are funded via block grants from the MCHB, have a special mandate to monitor and provide care coordination, but programs vary from state to state. Although Medicaid payment for case management may be allocated for a child, families may find their case manager lacks the necessary medical information or adequate communication with clinicians. Many specialty programs in children's hospitals have nurse specialists who help coordinate the medical care. These specialty-based care coordinators may have the most informa-

tion about the particular specialty (e.g., diabetes) but may lack knowledge of resources and other aspects of comprehensive medical care at the community or primary care level. One of the few estimates of the cost of providing care coordination services in a community-based practice suggested that although substantial, it is not cost prohibitive (Antonelli & Antonelli, 2004). This rather disjointed system often results in 1) the community-based primary care practice team and the primary care physicians saying that they want to be the care coordinators; 2) the specialty clinicians and their team providing some coordination; 3) the insurers, including Medicaid MCOs, providing benefits management; 4) early intervention, mental health, and Title V programs paying for and delivering different aspects of case management; and 5) families valuing whatever help with coordination they receive but often doing most of the coordination themselves and asking for more organized and consistent help (Wells et al., 2000).

THE CONCEPT OF A MEDICAL HOME

To help families with care coordination and to improve care, the AAP called for all children to have "a medical home that provides accessible, continuous, comprehensive, family centered, coordinated, and compassionate health care in an atmosphere of mutual responsibility and trust among clinician, child, and caregiver(s)" (1992, p. 774; see also Johnson & Kastner, 2005). The MCHB strongly supports these concepts and also emphasized the importance of culturally competent and community-based care. Table 42.1 describes the ideal medical home.

Prior to the emergence of managed care as a dominant force in health care delivery, primary care was beginning to be recognized as a valuable component in the highly specialized, technology dependent, tertiary care–based health care delivery system in the United States. Starfield (1992) defined primary care as health care that is first contact (involving an initial physician to whom the family goes to for routine and nonroutine care), community based (accessible), longitudinal (continuous), coordinated, and comprehensive. In addition, primary care clinicians for children (e.g., community pediatricians, family physicians, nurse practitioners) provide preventive care such as well-child examinations; immunizations; and vision, hearing, developmental, and medical screenings. Pri-

Table 42.1. Attributes of the ideal medical home

Attributes	Description
A medical home provides care that is accessible.	The family can obtain care in the community, and there are no barriers to receiving care based on race, ethnic, or cultural background; based on type of health insurance, including Medicaid and the Children's Health Insurance Program (CHIP); or based on lack of insurance coverage. When families are forced to change insurance because of employer decisions, the health care practice makes an effort to accommodate the change and maintain continuity of care.
The medical home is family centered.	Family members are recognized by the clinicians and staff as the principal caregivers and partners in caring for the child. Information is shared with parents in an unbiased, ongoing, and complete manner. All care plans reinforce the family as the center of support and decision makers for the child.
Care from a medical home is continuous.	Families and children value the ongoing relationship with primary care providers, subspecialty clinicians, and staff. The medical home provides continuity of care as the child and family make the transition from the hospital to the community and to child care, to school, or to home-based care. The continuity of care from infancy through young adulthood is the foundation of the medical home; it allows the clinician to know the family and patient and permits the family to trust the physician and his or her staff. This continuity shapes clinical judgment so that unnecessary tests are avoided and psychosocial factors can be weighed in decision making. The long-term relationship finally fosters the young adult and family to make a smooth transition to adult-based care with a new provider with support and information from the pediatrician or pediatric nurse practitioner.
Primary care medical homes provide care that is comprehensive.	Families can receive health care or advice 24 hours per day, 7 days per week. The child can receive preventive, acute, or chronic care within the scope and knowledge of the clinician. Because of the complexity of medical conditions today, many children require appropriate referral to subspecialists for management of acute and chronic conditions.
Medical homes coordinate care.	Not only are families assisted in contacting and utilizing appropriate support, educational services, and community-based services, but also the care provided in hospital, ambulatory, and community settings is planned and coordinated to the benefit of the family and child. Medical records, care plans, and other information are shared between providers and across systems avoiding duplication and fragmentation.
Medical homes are characterized by compassion.	The clinic- and office-based teams in the medical home demonstrate concern for the well-being of the child and family. This compassion is communicated by every member of the staff and felt by the family.
Care in the medical home also must be culturally competent.	The medical home must be able to deliver care in cross-cultural situations; therefore, the staff members must value diversity, be aware of how their own culture affects their thoughts and actions, understand the dynamics when cultures interact, and have a practice-wide cultural education program that helps ensure culturally competent clinical care and service delivery.
Care delivered by the medical home is community based.	Primary care is community based. Although children and families with special health care needs often require care by subspecialists who may not be available in their own community, the medical home should be in the community where the family lives whenever possible. The staff and clinicians of the medical home coordinate and communicate with the subspecialists. In addition, other providers—including pediatric physical, occupational, speech, and feeding therapists; home nursing staff; and providers of other important services—should be available in the community or as close to home as possible.

Source: American Academy of Pediatrics (1992).

mary care also includes personalized care that demonstrates the clinician's knowledge of the patient and family environment, including work; personal; emotional; and, at times, financial concerns. For the child and family, often the primary care team's medical home coordinates care with the pediatric subspecialist(s), staff, school system, and community providers to ensure comprehensive care. In a few instances, the subspecialist assumes the majority of the responsibilities for the medical home; in some albeit unusual cases, the specialist may even provide well-child care (e.g., for a child with cystic fibrosis).

THE HEALTH CARE ENVIRONMENT AND FINANCING

For most of its history, the health care system in the United States utilized a fee-for-service model in which the health care provider received a payment for each unit of service rendered (MacLeod, 2001). The typical was based on a "usual and customary" charge for the service. This system was a **retrospective** payment system; payment was made after the service was rendered. This approach was criticized because of its potential to encourage health care professionals to provide too many services (i.e., overutilization). In response to skyrocketing costs, the U.S. health care system experienced a revolution in the later years of the 20th century, and it continues to evolve toward a **prospective,** or prepayment, approach which, if structured correctly, would encourage "appropriate" utilization and avoid the potential for underutilization of necessary services (Deal, Shiono, & Behrman, 1998; Wagner, 2001). This is a particular issue for CYSHCN, whose health care costs are three times that of other children (Newacheck & Kim, 2005). In addition, providing comprehensive ambulatory services to children with chronic conditions demonstrated reduced cost, admissions, lengths of stays, with subsequent savings for insurers (Liptak, et al., 1998). Table 42.2 compares expenditures and utilization for health care services for CYSHCN with those for typically developing children.

Managed Care

The notion of prepayment is a defining feature of what has become known as managed care. In its purest form, the provider is paid a set fee based solely on the number of individuals to be served, in an arrangement referred to as capitation. No additional payment is made when services are provided. This approach is expected to result in the provision of only appropriate services because providers are not compensated for "doing more." A criticism of managed care is that such a system has the potential to encourage providers to do less than is optimal (i.e., underutilization). In looking at how financial aspects of the health care environment relate to CYSHCN, it is important to consider managed care as an approach; to review types of insurance coverage, including private and public programs; and to weigh the overall importance of Medicaid (also referred to as Medical Assistance, or MA) to these children and their families.

Managed care is defined by five key elements: 1) prospective payment, 2) networks of selected providers, 3) credentialing of providers using explicit standards, 4) quality and utilization management programs, and 5) incentives for use of network providers (Freund & Lewit, 1993). Using these components, managed care organizations (MCOs) in theory develop a more comprehensive range of health care services with incentives and oversight devices intended to maximize health benefits while limiting unnecessary utilization and expenditures. In their purest form, MCOs operating as health maintenance organizations (HMOs) usually reimburse providers on a capitated basis, providing a set payment each month for each individual covered regardless of the amount of services that the individual uses (typically referred to as the per-member-per-month rate, or the PMPM)

Table 42.2. Comparison of health care expenditures and utilization between children and youth with special health care needs and children without disabilities

Category	Children and youth with special health care needs	Children without disabilities	Comparison
Hospital days	464 days/1,000	55 days/1,000	8 times higher
Physician visits	4.6 visits/year	1.9 visits/year	2 times more visits
Nonphysician professional visits	3 visits/year	0.6 visits/year	5 times more visits
Prescriptions	6.2 medications/year	1.8 medications/year	3 times the number of prescriptions
Home health provider days	3.8 days/year	0.04 days/year	95 times more days
Health care expenditures	$2669/year	$676/year	4 times the cost
Out-of-pocket expenditures	$297/year	$189/year	1.5 times the cost

Source: Newacheck, Inkelas, and Kim (2004).

Secondary data analysis of 1999 and 2000 Medical Expenditure Panel Survey, with total sample of 13,792 children younger than 18 years of age and overall response rate of 65.5%. All comparisons are statistically significant.

(Fox & Fama, 1996). If the individuals, on average, use fewer services than expected that month, the providers may realize a financial gain; if the individuals use more services than expected, the providers may face a financial loss (Kongstvedt, 2001). Thus, the MCOs seek to keep health care expenditures at or below monthly or annual expectations to maximize potential financial gain. It is thought that the financial incentive structure discourages overuse of services and should lead to appropriate service delivery.

Increasingly, MCOs are adopting the less restrictive preferred provider organization (PPO) structure, which pays providers on a discounted fee for service model rather than the HMOs' capitation approach, and avoiding the hassle attributed to needing to get a referral for specialty care from one's primary care provider. PPOs do not always have all the specialists needed by CYSHCN, however, and parents sometimes have to go out of the plan network and pay out of pocket until they reach a deductible. They also have much higher copays than if they use PPO-contracted providers alone.

The Kaiser Family Foundation (KFF; 2005) reported all forms of managed care demonstrate continue growth, rising from 27% of workers covered by employer plans in 1988 to 97% in 2005. PPO enrollment increased from 11% in 1988 to 61% in 2005, compared with an HMO enrollment increase from 16% in 1988 to 21% in 2005.

Insurance Coverage: Public and Private

Access and use of health care services is affected by insurance coverage, family income, and sociodemographics (Newacheck, McManus, et al., 2000). The principal form of health insurance for all Americans younger than age 65 is private or commercial insurance provided by employers. The number of workers receiving employer-provided insurance continues to decline, with a subsequent reduction in the number of children covered under such plans (Children's Defense Fund, 2004). As employer-based insurance coverage for children declines, coverage from public forms of insurance tends to increase. If this increase occurs at a slower rate than the decrease in private insurance, it results in an expanding number of uninsured children.

To avoid the problem of uninsured children, the federal government has developed several publicly funded insurance programs that provide avenues for children to receive health care coverage. Table 42.3 lists each program. In 1965, Medicaid was launched. Medicaid is a jointly funded federal/state program that serves as a societal safety net for children who are inadequately covered by private insurance, who do not have private insurance, or who meet other eligibility criteria. It should be noted that coverage under Medicare, the other kind of public insurance, is uncommon in children except for those with end-stage kidney disease. In addition, Congress created the Children's Health Insurance Program (CHIP) in 1997, which provides states with an incentive to extend health care coverage to uninsured children who do not qualify for traditional Medicaid (Deal & Shiono, 1998). Many states have CHIP programs (called SCHIP) with coverage that deviates from that of Medicaid. One study concluded that CHIP coverage may not be sufficient to care for CYSHCN, suggesting that care coordination and reviewing of insurer's coverage decisions should be integral parts of CHIP program design (Markus et al., 2006). Despite the availability of public coverage via Medicaid and CHIP, there remain children who do not have adequate health insurance coverage (Brodsky & Somers, 1997; Children's Defense Fund, 2004; Newacheck, Halfon, & Inkelas, 2000).

The federal and state governments provide several other avenues for CYSHCN and their families to gain access to a range of health care services and funding for these services. These include 1) the Social Security Administration's Supplemental Security Income (SSI) program, which provides income support and/or access to Medicaid; 2) the MCHB's Title V programs, which provide enhanced services (e.g., case management) above the covered Medicaid services; 3) and the Individuals with Disabilities Education Improvement Act of 2004 (IDEA 2004; PL 108-446), which may link educational and health care needs with Medicaid funding. In practical terms, these programs may demonstrate considerable state-to-state variability in eligibility criteria, types of services covered or offered, and amount of care provided.

Private–public insurance coverage issues and programmatic variability further complicate the task of fashioning care plans for CYSHCN. Children and families experience this variability most acutely when navigating through a number of agencies, institutions, and providers, each with its own set of eligibility requirements, regulations, and service provisions that may or may not meet the child's needs. In

Table 42.3. Overview of assistance programs for children with special health care needs

Program	Description	Web resources
Supplemental Security Income (SSI)	SSI provides benefits to low-income people who meet financial and other eligibility requirements. SSI qualifies children and adults (including those with disabilities) for Medicaid health care services in many states	http://www.ssa.gov/notices/supplemental-security-income http://www.ssa.gov/notices/supplemental-security-income/text-understanding-ssi.htm http://www.ssa.gov/notices/supplemental-security-income/text-child-ussi.htm
Medicaid (MA)	Medicaid provides low-income individuals access to health coverage. States are mandated to cover a core set of benefits (e.g., hospital; outpatient physician services; laboratory and X ray; basic home health services; and early and periodic screening, diagnosis, and treatment [EPSDT]). EPSDT requires states to cover all medically necessary services for children, even those optional for adults.	http://www.cms.hhs.gov/medicaid http://www.cms.hhs.gov/medicaid/consumer.asp http://www.cms.hhs.gov/medicaid/whoiseligible.asp#children
Children's Health Insurance Program (CHIP)	CHIP funds states to insure children from working families with incomes too high to qualify for Medicaid but too low to afford private health insurance	http://www.cms.hhs.gov/schip
Title V	Provides children with special health care needs and their families with family-centered, coordinated, and community-based services, such as case management or care coordination, transportation, home visiting, and health education. Also, Title V helps to provide wraparound services (individualized direct services designed to support a child in his or her home, school, and community) and provides rehabilitation services for individuals younger than 16 who are blind or who have disabilities and who receive SSI. Title V may also provide partial funding for categorical programs (e.g., for children with spina bifida, cerebral palsy, sickle cell disease, and hemophilia).	https://performance.hrsa.gov/mchb/mchreports/tvisreports.asp ftp://ftp.hrsa.gov/mchb/titlevtoday/UnderstandingTitleV.pdf
Individuals with Disabilities Education Improvement Act of 2004 (IDEA 2004; PL 108-446)	IDEA guarantees all students with disabilities ages 3–21 the right to a free appropriate public education in the least restrictive environment. It also provides federal funds to states and local school districts to help pay the costs of special education, including related services such as speech-language and physical therapy.	http://www.ed.gov/policy/speced/guid/idea/idea2004.html http://thomas.loc.gov/cgi-bin/query/z?c108:h.r.1350.enr:

addition, publicly funded programs are coming under increased scrutiny as legislative and budgetary debates focus on cost cutting (National Research Council & Institute of Medicine, 1996; Smith, 2004; White et al., 2005).

Managed Care and Children and Youth with Special Health Care Needs

CYSHCN could potentially experience benefits from managed care, especially as compared with the parameters of the traditional fee-for-service plans (Mitchell & Gaskin, 2004). In the best-case scenario, MCOs provide the following: 1) increased flexibility to design programs that will meet the children's special needs; 2) coverage of well-child care, routine immunizations, and other preventive care that are often excluded in traditional plans; 3) protection of families from excessive medical costs;

and 4) point-of-service (POS) plans that provide families with the benefits of managed care while retaining the choice of physicians even if they are not in the standard network of providers (Smith & Ashbaugh, 1995). Managed care systems, in the worst case scenario, could also work to the disadvantage of these children, especially because more than 90% of child health care expenditures are consumed by approximately 15% of children who have disabilities or chronic illnesses (Deal et al., 1998; Kuhithau et al., 1998; Smith & Ashbaugh, 1995). CYSHCN, therefore, represent a group of high service utilizers, which makes them ready cost-reduction targets in a system that is essentially designed to manage routine populations and that usually limits access to specialists and reduces utilization of high-cost services. Taking this into account, potential downsides identified for CYSHCN include 1) a lack of choice; 2) decreased access to specialty providers; 3) availability of specialized

Table 42.4. Components of an optimal care system for children with special health care needs

- Integration of primary and specialty care in a way that combines the expertise of the specialists with the breadth of perspective provided by a generalist
- Integration of medical care with home- and community-based services, effectively linking the person with visiting nurses, Meals on Wheels, transportation, respite care, housekeeping, educational, and housing services
- Integration of patient and family perspectives into the care process and planning, using patient-centered communication and a consumer-oriented focus to service delivery
- Emphasis on functional status and quality of life so systems are tracked to be accountable for their effectiveness
- Improved screening and risk assessment to identify children early, when specialized services developmentally have the most effect
- Individual and group health education targeted to improve self-care skills and appropriate use of health care services
- Flexible gatekeeping that allows children and families access to a variety of services on a limited basis without prior authorization
- Comprehensive case management moving beyond benefit management and achieving real case coordination
- Coordination with public health, education, and social services, including collaborative arrangements, to organize and provide services
- An understanding of the differences between adult and childhood disability and the need for managed care models to be flexible in meeting pediatric needs
- Access to a medical home
- Fair reimbursement that compensates physicians for the increased time and complexity associated with care coordination (sometimes referred to as risk-adjusted rates in capitated systems)
- Viable systems of monitoring the care delivered

Sources: American Academy of Pediatrics (1998); McManus & Fox (1996a, 1996b); Sandy & Gibson (1996).

services only when significant improvement is expected over a short period; 4) high co-payments, especially for out-of-network providers; and 5) lack of information about the needs of these children. Decreased access is a particular concern in the care of such children, who often require the services of pediatric specialists. In addition, limiting therapy services to those resulting in immediate improvement would exclude treatment for children who require ongoing treatment to improve age-appropriate function (e.g., physical therapy for children with cerebral palsy or meningomyelocele).

The findings in the literature regarding the impact of managed care on children in general and those with special health care needs in particular are equivocal (Mitchell & Gaskin, 2004; Szilagyi, 1998). What is clear is that some plans can successfully implement strategies that reduce 1) inpatient hospital bed days (which account for between 40% and 50% of total health care expenditures) and 2) emergency department usage by enrollees. The impact on primary care in the outpatient setting and access to specialists is less clear. A trend is emerging, however, showing that MCOs may reduce the use of specialty services, especially of high-cost procedures (Szilagyi, 1998).

Recognizing the potential disadvantages of a managed care approach for these children and realizing that a significant number of these chil-dren receive some or all of their overall health care coverage under state-run Medicaid pro-grams, the Centers for Medicare & Medicaid Services (CMS; formerly called the Health Care Financing Administration), which has federal oversight responsibility for Medicaid, has established a set of safeguards promoting attention to the unique aspects of caring for CYSHCN in a managed care environment. These safeguards provide protection for children and families involved in Medicaid programs and outline some of the potentially problematic areas that CYSHCN may face in managed care. To deal with this issue, some states have conceived "carve-outs" for these children in which the child is handled separately from the general population. In addition, CYSHCN may be eligible for Medicaid waivers, including the 1915(c) or Katie Beckett waiver (home and community-based services waiver program). The 1915(c) waiver waives (or permits exceptions to) certain federal requirements to provide home and community based services as an alternative to institutionalization or continued hospitalization. Such a waiver, for example, may permit a family with a CYSHCN to receive Medicaid in order to have health care services and support for keeping that child at home rather than in a hospital or institution. One advantage of the 1915(c) waiver is that the family income is not considered in determining eligibility for Medicaid. The

Table 42.5 Quality indicators in health care and the questions they address

Dimension	Indicators examined	Examples of questions
Structure	Facilities Equipment Conformance to standards Staffing patterns Personnel qualifications and experience Organizational structure descriptions Financing patterns	Are primary care and specialty care clinics and hospitals accessible? How is the service delivery system structured? Do clinicians providing care communicate with each other? Are the health care professionals well educated, well trained, and board certified? Are medical records well maintained?
Process	Technical and professional skill Documentation of care Safety practices Monitoring assessment tools	Was the blood test for lead done for a child at risk for lead poisoning? Was the child with asthma treated in the most up-to-date manner?
Outcome	Health status Health-related knowledge Health-related behavior Satisfaction with care	Did the patient get better? Was the impact of the disability reduced? Does a child with special health care needs have the highest level of functioning possible given what is known to be possible? If not, why not?

Source: Monahan & Sykora (1999).

Note: Not all outcomes are the result of purely clinical decision making. Clinicians need to acknowledge that parents of children with special health care needs and other consumers of health care also consider personal preferences and experience when making health care plan choices.

waivers are state-run programs and thus each state has different approaches to waivers with different eligibility requirements or services.

There are several perspectives on what constitutes an optimal care system for CYSHCN. These are listed in Table 42.4.

LOOKING TOWARD THE FUTURE

Measuring outcomes and demonstrating high quality (e.g., pay for performance models) will become increasingly necessary in order to justify the enhanced service delivery and higher costs for CYSHCN in what is increasingly a market-based system (Palfry et al., 2004). This will require rigorous collection of data on the health care services delivered and analysis of the data using increasingly sophisticated health services techniques. The success that various HIV/AIDS programs have had in achieving adequately funded comprehensive sets of service for affected patients serves as a model for what can be done with rigorously collected data that supports the care delivered (Havens et al., 1997).

Classically, the measurable dimensions of health care quality are the structure, the process, and the actual outcomes (Donabedian, 1980). Structure, from a quality and health services perspective, describes aspects of the health care system such as facilities, staffing patterns, and qualifications. Process in this context deals with the policies and procedures that govern aspects of care such as technical and professional skills, documentation of care, safety practices,

and the use of assessment tools. Finally, outcomes deal with the health status of the people served, their health-related knowledge and behavior, and their satisfaction with care (Monahan & Sykora, 1999). Table 42.5 lists the types of quality questions that can be answered when looking at structure, process, and outcomes, and Table 42.6 outlines potential problems with assessing outcomes.

SUMMARY

Given the many services needed and the number of providers and professionals involved, coordinating health care services for CYSHCN presents a unique challenge to the child's family and health care providers. The complexity of the child's needs necessitate a great deal of time, energy, and skill to coordinate the efforts of different agencies, institutions, and professionals so that they work effectively together in a comprehensive plan of care. This coordination is particularly complex both because of the relative lack of comprehensive case management and care coordination services and because the child's needs may span a range of services, including some that are not traditionally seen as health related. Further complicating matters are the many federal and state agencies and programs involved in providing and funding services and the revolutionary changes in the heath care marketplace. Managed care may prove to be a combination of a blessing and a curse for CYSHCN. All of this points to the importance of each child having a medical home and effective case management to assist the family in navigating this system.

Table 42.6.   Potential problems with assessing outcomes

Self-limited conditions may improve or resolve on their own/even without therapy over time, so attributing the improvement to the treatment may be difficult.

Treatment of some chronic conditions is only partially effective and is not expected to be curative, so the presence of the condition cannot be used as a measure because the diagnosis does not change even though the treatment makes an improvement.

Lack of understanding of the natural history of some chronic conditions leads some authorities to disagree on what is expected and what the result of therapy should be.

External factors that may be involved in improvement, such as supportive family involvement and the responsiveness of community supports, are not easily measured but surely can have an impact on outcome.

Source: Monahan & Sykora (1999).

REFERENCES

Abt Associates, Inc. (2000, June). *Evaluation of the District of Columbia's demonstration program, "Managed Care System for Disabled and Special Needs Children": Final report summary.* Retrieved November 20, 2001, from http://aspe.hhs.gov/daltcp/reports/dc-frs.htm

American Academy of Pediatrics. (1992). American Academy of Pediatrics Ad Hoc Task Force on Definition of the Medical Home: The medical home (RE9262). *Pediatrics, 90,* 774.

American Academy of Pediatrics. (1998). Managed care and children with special health care needs: A subject review (RE9814). *Pediatrics, 102,* 657–660.

American Academy of Pediatrics. (1999). Care coordination: Integrating health and related systems of care for children with special health care needs (RE9902). *Pediatrics, 104,* 978–981.

Americans with Disabilities Act (ADA) of 1990, PL 101-336, 42 U.S.C. §§ 12101 *et seq.*

Antonelli, R.C., & Antonelli, D.M. (2004). Providing a

medical home: The cost of care coordination services in a community-based general pediatric practice. *Pediatrics, 113*(5), 1522–1528.

Balanced Budget Act of 1997, PL 105-33, 111 Stat. 251.

Beers, N.S., Kemeny, A., Sherritt, L., et al. (2003). Variations in state-level definitions: Children with special health care needs. *Public Health Reports, 118*(95), 434–447.

Bethell, C.D., Read, D., Stein, R.E., et al. (2002). Identifying children with special health care needs: Development and evaluation of a short screening tool. *Ambulatory Pediatrics, 2*, 38–48.

Bodenheimer, T., Lo, B., & Casalino, L. (1999). Primary care physicians should be coordinators, not gatekeepers. *Journal of the American Medical Association, 282*, 2045–2049.

Brodsky, K.L., & Somers, S.A. (1997). Medicaid managed care for special needs population: Making it work. *Health Strategies Quarterly, 1*(2), 1–2.

Chen, A., Brown, R., Archibald, N., et al. (2000). *Best practices in coordinated care* (Contract No. HCFA 500-95-0048 [04]; MPR Reference No. 8534-004). Baltimore: Health Care Financing Administration.

Children's Defense Fund. (2004). CDF calls on country to insure all children during "cover the uninsured week." Washington, DC: Children's Defense Fund.

CHIP and seamless health care: New programs expand both coverage and confusion. (1999, March). *State Initiatives in Health Care Reform*(30), 7–10.

Deal, L.W., & Shiono, P.H. (1998). Medicaid managed care and children: An overview. *The Future of Children, 8*(2), 93–104.

Deal, L.W., Shiono, P.H., & Behrman, R.E. (1998). Children and managed health care: Analysis and recommendations. *The Future of Children, 8*(2), 4–24.

Donabedian, A. (1980). *The definition of quality and approaches to its assessment.* Ann Arbor, MI: Health Administration Press.

Education for All Handicapped Children Act of 1975, PL 94-142, 20 U.S.C. §§ 1400 *et seq.*

Fox, P.D., & Fama, T. (Eds.). (1996). *Managed care and chronic illness: Challenges and opportunities.* Gaithersburg, MD: Aspen Publishers.

Freund, D.A., & Lewit, E.M. (1993). Managed care for children and pregnant women: Promises and pitfalls. *The Future of Children, 3*(2), 92–122.

Gupta, V.B., O'Connor, K.G., & Quezada-Gomez, C. (2004). Care coordination services in pediatric practices. *Pediatrics, 113*(5), 1517–1528.

Havens, P.L., Cuene, B.E., Waters, D., et al. (1997). Structure of a primary care support system to coordinate comprehensive care for children and families infected/affected by human immunodeficiency virus in a managed care environment. *The Pediatric Infectious Disease Journal, 16*, 211–216.

Health Care Financing Administration. (2001). *State Children's Health Insurance Program (SCHIP): Aggregate enrollment statistics for the 50 states and the District of Columbia for federal fiscal years (FFY) 2000 and 1999.* Retrieved from http://www.hcfa.gov/init/fy99-00.pdf

Hughes, D.C., & Luft, H.S. (1998). Managed care and children: An overview. *The Future of Children, 8*(2), 25–38.

Implementing Title XXI: States face choices. (1997). *Health Policy and Child Health, 4*(4), 1–4.

Individuals with Disabilities Education Act Amendments of 1997, PL 105-17, 20 U.S.C. §§ 1400 *et seq.*

Individuals with Disabilities Education Act (IDEA) of 1990, PL 101-476, 20 U.S.C. §§ 1400 *et seq.*

Individuals with Disabilities Education Improvement Act of 2004, PL 108-446, 20 U.S.C. §§ 1400 *et seq.*

Institute of Medicine. (2001). *Crossing the quality chasm: A new health system for the 21rst century.* Washington DC: National Academies Press.

Institute of Medicine. (2003). *Priority areas for national action: Transforming healthcare quality.* Washington DC: National Academies Press.

Ireys, H.T., Grason, H.A., & Guyer, B. (1996). Assuring quality care for children with special needs in managed care organizations: Roles for pediatricians. *Pediatrics, 98*, 178–185.

Johnson, C.P., & Kastner, T.A. (2005). Helping families raise children with special health care needs at home. *Pediatrics, 115*(2), 507–511.

Kaiser Family Foundation. (2005). Trends and indicators in the changing health care marketplace. In *2005 Annual Survey of Employer Health Benefits.* Retrieved July 24, 2006, from http://www.kff.org/insurance/7031/print-sec2.cfm

Kastner, T.A. (2004). Managed care and children with special health care needs. *Pediatrics, 114*(6), 1693–1698.

Kongstvedt, P.R. (Ed.). (2001). *The managed health care handbook* (4th ed.). Gaithersburg, MD: Aspen Publishers.

Kuhithau, K., Perrin, J.M., Ettner, S.L., et al. (1998). High-expenditure children with Supplemental Security Income. *Pediatrics, 102*, 610–615.

Lewit, E.M., & Baker, L.S. (1996). Children in special education: The future of children. *Special Education for Students with Disabilities, 6*(1), 139–151.

Liptak, G.S., Burns, C.M., Davidson, P.W., et al. (1998). Effects of providing comprehensive ambulatory services to children with chronic conditions. *Archives Pediatrics and Adolescent Medicine, 152*, 1003–1008.

Liptak, G.S., & Revell, G.M. (1989). Community physician's role in case management of children with chronic illnesses. *Pediatrics, 84*, 465–471.

MacLeod, G.K. (2001). An overview of managed health care. In P.R. Kongstvedt (Ed.), *The managed health care handbook* (4th ed., pp. 3–16). Gaithersburg, MD: Aspen Publishers.

Markus, A., Rosenbaum, S., Stein, R.E., et al. (2006). *From SCHIP benefit design to individual coverage decisions* (Policy brief #6). Washington, DC: The George Washington University Department of Health Policy.

McManus, M.A., & Fox, H.B. (1996a). Enhancing preventive and primary care. *Managed Care Quarterly, 4* (3), 19–29.

McManus, M.A., & Fox, H.B. (1996b). Enhancing preventive and primary care for children with chronic or disabling conditions served in health maintenance organizations. In P.D. Fox & T. Fama (Eds.), *Managed care and chronic illness: Challenges and opportunities* (pp. 197–112). Gaithersburg, MD: Aspen Publishers.

McNeil, J.M. (1993). *Americans with disabilities, 1991–1992* (Current Population Reports; series P70, no.–33). Washington, DC: U.S. Department of Commerce, Bureau of Census.

McPherson, M., Arango, P., Fox, H., et al. (1998). A new definition of children with special needs. *Pediatrics, 102*, 137–140.

McPherson, M., Weissman, G., Strickland, B.B., et al. (2004). Implementing community-based systems of services for children with special health care needs: How well are we doing? *Pediatrics, 113*(5), 1538–1544.

Milligan, M. (2003). *Center for Health Care Strategies, Inc. A model for integrating children with special health care needs into Medicaid-managed care*. Retrieved February 6, 2007, from http://www.chcs.org/usr_doc/texas-childrenpdf.pdf

Mitchell, J.M., & Gaskin, D.J. (2004). Do children receiving Supplemental Security Income who are enrolled in Medicaid fare better under fee-for-service or comprehensive capitation model? *Pediatrics, 114(1),* 196–204.

Monahan, C.A., & Sykora, J. (1999). *Developing and analyzing performance measures: A guide for assessing quality care for children with special health care needs*. Vienna, VA: National Maternal and Child Health Clearinghouse.

National Research Council & Institute of Medicine. (1996). *Paying attention to children in a changing health care system: Summaries of workshops*. Washington, DC: National Academies Press.

Newacheck, P.W., Halfon, N., & Inkelas, M. (2000). Commentary: Monitoring expanded health insurance for children. Challenges and opportunities. *Pediatrics, 105,* 1004–1005.

Newacheck, P.W., Inkelas, M., & Kim, S.E. (2004). Health services use and health care expenditures for children with disabilities. *Pediatrics, 114*(1), 79–85.

Newacheck, P.W., McManus, M., Fox, H.B., et al. (2000). Access to health care for children with special health care needs. *Pediatrics, 105,* 760–766.

Newacheck, P.W., Strickland, B., Shonkoff, J.P., et al. (1998). An epidemiologic profile of children with special health care needs. *Pediatrics, 102,* 117–122.

Newacheck, P.W., & Kim, S.E. (2005). A national profile of health care utilization and expenditures for children with special health care needs. *Pediatrics, 159*(1), 10–17.

Omnibus Budget Reconciliation Act (OBRA) of 1981, PL 97-35, 95 Stat. 357.

Palfry, J.S., Sofis, L.A., Davidson, E.J., et al. (2004). The pediatric alliance for coordinated care: Evaluation of a medical home model. *Pediatrics, 113*(5), 1507–1516.

Personal Responsibility and Work Opportunity Reconciliation Act of 1996, PL 104-193, 42 U.S.C. §§ 211 *et seq.*

Sandy, L.G., & Gibson, R. (1996). Managed care and chronic care: Challenges and opportunities. In P.D. Fox & T. Fama (Eds.), *Managed care and chronic illness: Challenges and opportunities* (pp. 8–17). Gaithersburg, MD: Aspen Publishers.

Shaller, D. (2004). Implementing and using quality measures for children's health care: Perspectives on the state of the practice. *Pediatrics, 113,* 217–27.

Silva, T.J., Sofis, L.A., & Palfrey, J.S. (2000). *Practicing comprehensive care: A physician's operations manual for implementing a medical home for children with special health care needs*. Boston: Institute for Community Inclusion/UAP.

Smith, G., & Ashbaugh, J. (1995). *Managed care and people with developmental disabilities: A guidebook*. Alexandria, VA: National Association of State Directors of Developmental Disabilities Services.

Smith V. (2004, October). *The continuing Medicaid budget challenge: State Medicaid spending growth and cost containment in fiscal years 2004 and 2005*. Washington, DC: Kaiser Commission on Medicaid and the Uninsured.

Starfield, B. (1992). *Primary care: Concept, evaluation and policy*. New York: Oxford University Press.

Strickland, B.B., McPherson, M., Weissman, G., et al. (2004). Access to the medical home: Results of the National Survey of Children with Special Health Care Needs. *Pediatrics, 113*(5), 1485–1492.

State legislative agendas focus on managed care and CHIP: Potential and value of further state reform debated. (1999, March). *State Initiatives in Health Care Reform (No. 30),* 1–3, 10.

Stroul, B.A., Pires, S.A., Armstrong, M.I., et al. (1998). The impact of managed care on mental health services for children and their families. *The Future of Children, 8*(2), 119–133.

Szilagyi, P.G. (1998). Managed care for children: Effect on access to care and utilization of health services. *The Future of Children, 8*(2), 39–59.

U.S. General Accounting Office. (2000, March). *Medicaid managed care: Challenges in implementing safeguards for children with special needs* (Report No. GAO/HEHS-00-37). Washington, DC: Author.

van Dyck, P.C., Kogan, M.D., McPherson, M.G., et al. (2004). Prevalence and characteristics of children with special health care needs. *Archives of Pediatrics and Adolescent Medicine, 158,* 884–890.

Wagner, E.R. (2001). Types of managed care organizations. In P.R. Kongstvedt (Ed.), *The managed health care handbook* (4th ed., pp. 28–41). Gaithersburg, MD: Aspen Publishers.

Wells, N., Knauss, M.W., Anderson, B., et al. (2000). *What do families say about health care for children with special health care needs? Your voice counts!! The Family Partners Project report to families* Unpublished manuscript, Family at the Federation for Children with Special Needs, Boston.

White, C., Fisher, C., Mendelson, D., et al. (2005). *State Medicaid disease management: Lessons learned from Florida*. Lambertville, NJ: The Health Strategies Consultancy LLC, in collaboration with Duke University.

World Health Organization. (1980). *International Classification of Impairments, Disabilities, and Handicaps: A manual of classification relating to the consequences of disease*. Geneva: Author.

World Health Organization. (2001). *International classification of Functioning, Disability and Health (ICF)*. Geneva: Author.

A Glossary

Gaetano R. Lotrecchiano

abduction Moving part of the body away from one's mid-line.

ABR *See* auditory brainstem response.

abruptio placenta Premature detachment of a normally situated placenta; *also called* placental abruption.

abscesses Localized collections of pus in cavities caused by the disintegration of tissue, usually the consequence of bacterial infections.

accommodation 1) In special education, a change in how a student gains access to the curriculum or demonstrates his or her learning that does not substantially alter the content or level of instruction (e.g., allowing a student to record test answers in the test booklet instead of on a separate bubble sheet); 2) the change in the shape of the lens of the eye that allows it to focus on objects at varying distances.

acetabulum The cup-shaped cavity of the hip bone that holds the head of the femur in place, creating a joint.

acetylcholine A neurotransmitter for cholinergic neurons that innervate many tissues, including smooth muscle and skeletal muscle.

acid–base balance In metabolism, the ratio of acidic to basic compounds (or pH).

acidosis Too much acid in the bloodstream. The normal pH is 7.42; acidosis is generally less than 7.30.

acquired immunodeficiency syndrome (AIDS) Severe immune deficiency disease caused by human immunodeficiency virus (HIV; *see Chapter 6*).

actin Protein involved in muscle contraction.

acute inflammatory peripheral neuropathy Ascending paralysis following a viral infection; *also called* Guillain-Barré syndrome (*see Chapter 14*).

adduction Moving a body part, usually a limb, toward the mid-line.

adenine One of the four nucleotides (chemicals) that comprise DNA.

adenoid Lymphatic tissue located behind the nasal passages.

adenoidectomy The surgical removal of the adenoids.

adenoma sebaceum Benign cutaneous growths, usually seen around the nose, that resemble acne; these occur in individuals with tuberous sclerosis (*see Appendix B*).

adjustment disorders A group of psychiatric disorders, usually of childhood, associated with difficulty adjusting to life changes.

adrenaline A potent stimulant of the autonomic nervous system. It increases blood pressure and heart rate and stimulates other physiological changes needed for a "fight or flight" response.

advance directives In children with severe disabilities, the term is used to define the level of intervention a parent wants provided in the event of life-threatening emergency or illness in the child.

afferent Pertaining to the neural signals sent from the peripheral nervous system to the central nervous system (CNS).

AFP *See* alpha-fetoprotein.

afterbirth *See* placenta.

agenesis of the corpus callosum Absence of the band of white matter that normally connects the two hemispheres of the brain.

agonist 1) A medication that enhances certain neural activity; 2) a muscle that works in concert with another muscle to produce movement.

agyria Absence of normal convolutions on the surface of the brain.

AIDS *See* acquired immunodeficiency syndrome.

alcohol-related neurodevelopmental disorder (ARND) *Previously called* fetal alcohol effects (FAE), refers to the range of neurological and developmental impairments that can affect a child who has been exposed in utero to alcohol.

alleles Alternate forms of a gene that may exist at the same site on the chromosome.

alopecia Hair loss.

alpha-fetoprotein (AFP) Fetal protein found in amniotic fluid and serum of pregnant women. Its measurement is used to test for meningomyelocele and Down syndrome in the fetus.

alveoli Small air sacs in the lungs. Carbon dioxide and oxygen are exchanged through their walls.

amalgam An alloy of mercury and silver used in dental fillings.

amaurosis Blindness.

amblyopia Partial loss of sight resulting from disuse atrophy of neural circuitry during a critical period of development, most often associated with untreated strabismus in children.

amino acid Building block of protein needed for normal growth.

amino acid disorders Inborn errors of metabolism resulting from an enzyme deficiency involving amino acids, the building blocks of protein.

amniocentesis A prenatal diagnostic procedure performed in the second trimester in which amniotic fluid is removed by a needle inserted through the abdominal wall and into the uterine cavity.

amniotic fluid Clear fluid that surrounds the fetus during pregnancy, acting as a physical buffer for fetal movements and physical development. It is formed by fetal urine production and lung fluid secretion during fetal respirations.

anaphase The stage in cell division (mitosis and meiosis) when the chromosomes move from the center of the nucleus toward the poles of the cell.

anaphylaxis A life-threatening hypersensitivity response to a medication or food, marked by breathing difficulty, hives, and shock.

anemia Disorder in which the blood has either too few red blood cells or too little hemoglobin.

anencephaly Neural tube defect (NTD) in which either the entire brain or all but the most primitive regions of the brain are missing.

anophthalmia Congenital absence of the eyes.

anorexia A severe loss of appetite.

antagonists Working at cross-purposes (e.g., the adductor and abductor muscles of the hip oppose each others' actions).

antecedents Events or contextual factors that precede or coincide with a behavior.

anterior The front part of a structure.

anterior fontanelle The membrane-covered area on the top of the head; *also called* the soft spot. It generally closes by 18 months of age.

anterior horn cells Cells in the spinal column that transmit impulses from the pyramidal tract to the peripheral nervous system.

anthropometrics Measurements of the body and its parts.

antibody A protein formed in the bloodstream to fight infection.

anticholingeric medications A group of medications that acts by antagonizing the effects of the neurotransmitter acetycholine.

anticipation A term used in genetics to denote an expansion in triplet repeats from one generation to the next, leading to a more severe manifestation of the disease (e.g., in fragile X syndrome).

anticonvulsants Medications (e.g., phenobarbital, dilantin) used for control of seizures.

antidepressants Medications used to control major depression.

antihistamine A drug that counteracts the effects of histamines, substances involved in allergic reactions.

antipsychotic medications Medications used to treat psychosis.

antiretroviral agents (ARVs) A category of medications used to treat retroviral infections (i.e., HIV/AIDS).

anxiety disorders Psychiatric disorders characterized by feelings of anxiety. The disorders include panic attacks, separation anxiety, obsessive-compulsive disorder (OCD), and posttraumatic stress disorder (PTSD).

aorta The major artery of the body. It originates in the left ventricle of the heart and carries oxygenated blood to the rest of the body.

Apgar scoring system Scoring system developed by Virginia Apgar to assess neurological status in the newborn infant. Scores range from 0 to 10.

apical At the tip of a structure.

apnea A lack of spontaneous breathing effort.

apneic Pertaining to an episodic arrest of breathing.

apraxia The loss of the ability to perform coordinated movements or manipulate objects in the absence of a motor or sensory impairment.

aqueous humor The fluid in the eyeball that fills the space between the lens and the cornea.

architectonic dysplasias Developmental malformations affecting the neuronal architecture of the brain.

arterial blood gas A laboratory profile test of sampled arterial blood, including pH, PaO_2, and $PaCO_2$.

arterial-venous malformation (AVM) Birth

defect of blood vessels, often associated with a disastrous postthrombotic hemorrhage.

arthritis   An inflammatory disease of joints.

articular   Referring to the surface of a bone at a joint space.

articulation   1) The formulation of individual speech sounds; 2) the connection at a joint.

asphyxia   Interference with oxygenation of the blood that leads to loss of consciousness and possible brain damage.

aspiration   Inhalation of a foreign body, usually a food particle, into the lungs.

aspiration pneumonia   Inflammation of the lung(s) caused by inhaling a foreign body, such as food, into the lungs.

assent   Agreement to research or treatment, given by a child or minor who is too young to give legally valid informed consent.

assistive devices   Any device used to assist in a body function (e.g., a wheelchair).

astigmatism   A condition of unequal curvature of the cornea that leads to blurred vision.

astrocytes   Support cells in the central nervous system (CNS) that help form the white matter.

asymmetrical tonic neck reflex (ATNR)   A primitive reflex, *also called* fencer's response, found in infants; usually is no longer evident by 3 months of age. When the neck is turned in one direction, the arm shoots out on the same side and flexes on the opposite side; similar changes occur in the legs.

ataxia   An unbalanced gait caused by a disturbance of cerebellar control.

ataxic cerebral palsy   A form of dyskinetic cerebral palsy in which the prominent feature is ataxia.

athetoid cerebral palsy   A form of dyskinetic cerebral palsy associated with athetosis.

athetosis   Constant random, writhing involuntary movements of the limbs.

atonic   Pertaining to the absence of normal muscle tone.

atopic dermatitis   Eczema.

atresia   Congenital absence of a normal body opening; *adjective:* atretic.

atria   The two upper chambers of the heart.

atrial septal defect   A congenital heart defect in which where there is lack of closure of the wall separating the two upper chambers of the heart.

attention-deficit / hyperactivity disorder (ADHD)   A developmental disorder characterized by impulsivity, hyperactivity, and inattention to a degree that leads to impairment in functioning.

audiometry   A hearing test using a device called an audiometer that yields results in the form of a graph showing hearing levels in sound intensity at various wavelengths of sound presented through earphones.

auditory brainstem response (ABR)   A test of central nervous system (CNS) hearing pathways.

augmentative and alternative communication (AAC)   Devices that assist individuals in communicating with others.

aura   A sensation, usually visual and/or olfactory, marking the onset of a seizure.

auricle   The outer ear.

autism/autism spectrum disorders (ASDs)   Autistic Disorder (or autism), Asperger syndrome, and pervasive developmental disorder–not otherwise specified.

autoimmune   Pertaining to a reaction in which one's immune system attacks other parts of the body.

automatic movement reactions   *See* postural reactions.

automatisms   Automatic fine motor movements (e.g., unbuttoning one's clothing) that are part of a seizure.

autonomic   Describing the part of the nervous system that regulates certain automatic functions of the body (i.e., heart rate, sweating, and bowel movement).

autonomy   The ability and/or right to be self-determining; to be able to choose for oneself.

autosomal dominant   Mendelian inheritance pattern in which a single copy of a gene leads to expression of the trait.

autosomal recessive   Mendelian inheritance pattern in which two carrier parents have a 25% chance of passing the trait to each child.

autosomes   The first 22 pairs of chromosomes. All chromosomes are autosomes except for the two sex chromosomes.

aversive   Pertaining to a stimulus, often unpleasant that decreases the likelihood a particular response will subsequently occur.

AVM   *See* arterial-venous malformation.

backward chaining   Method of teaching a task in which the instructor begins by teaching the last step in a sequence because this step is most likely to be associated with a potent positive reinforcer.

bacteremia   Spread of a bacterial organism throughout the bloodstream.

banding   In genetics, pertaining to a series of dark and light bars that appear on chromosomes after they are stained. Each chromosome has a distinct banding pattern.

barotrauma Injury related to excess pressure, especially to the lungs or ears.

basal 1) Near the base; 2) relating to a standard or reference point (e.g., basal metabolic rate).

basal ganglia Brain structure at the base of the cerebral hemispheres involved in motor control, cognition, emotions, and learning.

baseline In behavior management, the frequency, duration, and intensity of a behavior prior to intervention.

beriberi Disease caused by a deficiency of the vitamin B_1 (thiamin) and manifested as edema, heart problems, and peripheral neuropathy.

beta-blockers Medications (e.g., propranolol [Inderal]) that were initially used to control high blood pressure and have subsequently been found to be useful in treating tremor and migraine headache.

binocular vision The focusing of both eyes on an object to provide a stereoscopic image.

biotin One of the B-complex vitamins needed to activate a number of important enzymatic reactions in the body.

biotinidase deficiency An inborn error of metabolism involving an enzyme deficiency leading to the accumulation of toxic organic acids.

bipolar disorder A psychiatric disorder manifested by cycles of mania and depression; *previously called* manic depression.

blastocyst The embryonic group of cells that exists at the time of implantation.

blood PaO$_2$ A measurement of the partial pressure of arterial oxygen (i.e., the amount of oxygen in the blood).

blood pH Blood acidity normally 7.25–7.40.

blood poisoning *See* sepsis.

body mass index (BMI) A measurement of the relative percentages of fat and muscle mass in the human body, in which weight in kilograms is divided by height in meters and the result used as an index of obesity.

bolus 1) A small rounded mass of food made ready by tongue and jaw movement for swallowing; 2) a single dose of a large amount of medication given to rapidly attain a therapeutic drug level.

botulism Poisoning by botulin toxin and manifested as muscle weakness or paralysis.

BPD *See* bronchopulmonary dysplasia.

brachialis A muscle in the upper arm.

brachycephaly Tall head shape with flat back part of the skull.

bradycardia Abnormal slowing of the heart rate, usually to fewer than 60 beats per minute.

braille A system of writing and printing for people who are blind or visually impaired.

brainstem The primitive portion of the brain that lies between the cerebrum and the spinal cord.

branchial arches A series of archlike thickenings of the body wall in the pharyngeal region of the embryo.

bronchopulmonary dysplasia (BPD) A chronic lung disorder that occurs in a minority of premature infants who previously had respiratory distress syndrome. It is associated with "stiff" lungs that do not permit adequate exchange of oxygen and carbon dioxide, frequently leads to dependence on ventilator assistance for extended periods, and markedly increases the risk for the child developing asthma in the future.

bronchospasm Acute constriction of the bronchial tube, most commonly associated with asthma.

bruxism Repetitive grinding of the teeth.

bulk Foodstuffs that increase the quantity of intestinal contents and stimulate regular bowel movements. Fruits, vegetables, and other foods containing fiber provide bulk in the diet.

caffeine A central nervous system (CNS) stimulant found in coffee, tea, and cola.

calcify To become hardened through the laying down of calcium salts.

calculus An abnormal collection of mineral salts on the tooth, predisposing it to decay; *also called* tartar.

callus A disorganized network of bone tissue that forms around the edges of a fracture during the healing process.

camptodactyly Deformity of fingers or toes in which they are permanently flexed.

cancellous Referring to the lattice-like structure in long bones (e.g., the femur).

cardiorespiratory monitor A device used to monitor heart and respiratory rate.

case control study An observational epidemiologic study of people with a specific disease (or other outcome) of interest and a suitable control (e.g., comparison, reference) group of people without the disease.

catalyze To stimulate a chemical reaction via a compound that is not used up.

cataracts Clouding of the lenses of the eyes.

catheterization Use of a tube to infuse or remove fluids.

CBF *See* cerebral blood flow.

cecostomy Surgical formation of a permanent artificial opening into the cecum, the end of the colon.

celiac disease Congenital malabsorption syndrome that leads to the inability to gain weight and the passage of loose, foul-smelling stools. It is caused by intolerance of cereal products that contain gluten (e.g., wheat).

central nervous system (CNS) The portion of the nervous system that consists of the brain and spinal cord. It is primarily involved in voluntary movement and thought processes.

central venous line A catheter that is advanced through a peripheral vein to a position directly above the opening to the right atrium of the heart. It is used to infuse long-term medication and/or nutrition.

centrioles Tiny organelles that migrate to the opposite poles of a cell during cell division and align the spindles.

centromere The constricted area of the chromosome that usually marks the point of attachment of the sister chromatids to the spindle during cell division.

cephalocaudal From head to tail; refers to neurological development that proceeds from the head downward.

cephalohematoma A swelling of the head resulting from bleeding of scalp veins. Often found in newborn infants, it is usually not harmful.

cerebellum A cauliflower-shaped brain structure located just above the brainstem beneath the occipital lobes at the base of the skull that is principally involved in muscle tone and coordination of movement.

cerebral blood flow (CBF) Poorly autoregulated blood flow within the early developing brain, making the newborn particularly vulnerable to any changes in blood pressure.

cerebral contusion A bruise on the cerebrum.

cerebral hemisphere Either of the two halves of brain substance.

cerebral palsy A disorder of movement and posture due to a nonprogressive defect of the immature brain (*see Chapter 26*).

cerebral vascular accident (CVA) A thrombotic (clot) or hemorrhagic (bleed) stroke that can damage large regions of the brain in the location of a particular blood vessel (artery or vein).

cerebrospinal fluid (CSF) Clear, watery fluid that fills the ventricular cavities within the brain and circulates around the brain and spinal cord.

cerumen Ear wax.

cervical Pertaining 1) to the cervix, or 2) to the neck.

cesarean section (C-section) A surgical operation for delivering a baby through incising the uterus rather than via the vagina.

cheilitis An inflammation of the lips.

chemotherapy Drugs used to treat cancer.

choanal atresia Congenital closure of the nasal passage; part of the CHARGE association.

cholesteatoma A complication of otitis media in which skin cells from the ear canal migrate through the perforated eardrum into the middle ear, or mastoid region, forming a mass that must be removed surgically.

chorea A disorder marked by involuntary jerky movements of the extremities.

choreoathetosis Movement disorder, characteristic of dyskinetic cerebral palsy, involving frequent involuntary spasms of the limbs.

chorioamnionitis An infection of the amniotic sac that surrounds and contains the fetus and amniotic fluid.

chorion The outermost covering of the membrane surrounding the fetus.

chorionic villus sampling (CVS) A prenatal diagnostic procedure done in the first trimester of pregnancy to obtain fetal cells for genetic analysis.

chorioretinitis An inflammation of the retina and choroid that produces severe visual loss.

choroid The middle layer of the eyeball between the sclera and the retina.

choroid plexus Cells that line the walls of the ventricles of the brain and produce cerebrospinal fluid.

chromatids Term given to chromosomes during cell division.

chromosomes Thread-like strands of DNA and associated proteins in the nucleus of cells that carry the genes transmitting hereditary information.

ciliary muscles Small muscles that affect the shape of the lens of the eye, permitting accommodation.

CK *See* creatine kinase.

clonus Alternate muscle contraction and relaxation in rapid succession.

clubfoot A congenital foot deformity; *also called* talipes equinovarus.

CMV *See* cytomegalovirus.

CNS *See* central nervous system.

coagulation Blood clotting.

coarctation A congenital narrowing, such as of a blood vessel, most commonly of the aorta.

cochlea The snail-shaped structure in the inner ear containing the hearing organ.

cochlear implant A device surgically implanted in the cochlear of the ear that permits a form of hearing in individuals with deafness.

codons Triplets of nucleotides that form the DNA code for specific amino acids.

cohort study An epidemiologic study of subgroups of a population identified with some common characteristic (e.g., an exposure, an ethnic background) that are followed or traced over a period of time for the occurrence of disease.

colic A condition in infancy marked by uncontrollable crying usually caused by abdominal discomfort and often the result of gastroesophageal reflux (GER).

coloboma Congenital cleft in the retina, iris, or other ocular structure.

comorbid A coexisting condition that worsens an underlying disorder.

competent Legally recognized to be able to make decisions for oneself. Minors are presumed to be incompetent, except under certain specified conditions that may vary from state to state.

compliance training An important prerequisite to instructional training. The instructor orients the child to attend to the instructor and then issues a developmentally appropriate "do" request.

computed tomography (CT) An imaging technique in which X-ray "slices" of a structure are viewed and synthesized by a computer, forming an image. It is most commonly used to visualize the brain. CT scans are less clear than magnetic resonance imaging (MRI) scans but are better at localizing certain tumors and areas of calcification.

concave Having a curved, indented surface.

concussion A clinical syndrome caused by a blow to the head, characterized by transient loss of consciousness.

cones Photoreceptor cells of the eye associated with color vision.

congenital Originating prior to birth.

congenital myopathies A group of inherited muscle disorders often associated with mitochondrial dysfunction.

conjunctiva The mucous membrane that lines the inner surface of the eyelid and the exposed surface of the eyeball.

consanguinity Relationship by blood.

conscience A personal sense, generally intuitive and urgent, of the way one should respond under specific circumstances; often described, as by Socrates, an inner voice that forbids certain actions.

consequences Events or contextual factors that occur subsequent to a behavior and may or may not be causally related to it.

conservatorship A circumstance in which the court declares an individual unable to take care of legal matters and appoints another individual (a conservator) to handle these matters on the individual's behalf.

contiguous gene syndrome A genetic syndrome resulting from defects in a number of adjacent genes.

contingent stimulation Applying punishment following the occurrence of a misbehavior.

contingent withdrawal The removal of access to positive reinforcement following a misbehavior.

contracture A shortening of muscle fibers that causes decreased joint mobility and is almost always irreversible.

contusion (of brain) Structural damage limited to the surface layer of the brain caused by a blow to the head.

convex Having a curved, elevated/protruding surface, such as a dome.

cordocentesis See percutaneous umbilical blood sampling (PUBS).

cornea The transparent, dome-like covering of the iris.

corpus callosotomy Surgical procedure in which the corpus callosum is cut to prevent the generalized spread of seizures from one hemisphere to another.

corpus callosum The bridge of white matter connecting the two cerebral hemispheres.

cortical Pertaining to the cortex or gray matter of the brain.

corticospinal pathways White matter pathways leading from the brain through the spinal corticospinal tract; see pyramidal tract.

cortisol A steroid.

craniofacial Relating to the skull and bones of the face.

craniosynostosis Premature closure of cranial bones.

creatine kinase (CK) An enzyme released by damaged muscle cells. Its level is elevated in muscular dystrophy.

crib death See sudden infant death syndrome (SIDS).

Crohn's disease An inflammatory bowel disorder.

crossover The exchange of genetic material between two closely aligned chromosomes during the first meiotic division.

cryotherapy The use of freezing temperatures to destroy tissue. A cryotherapy probe has been used to treat retinoblastoma and retinopathy of prematurity.

cryptorchidism Undescended testicles.

C-section *See* cesarean section.

CSF *See* cerebrospinal fluid.

CT *See* computed tomography.

CVA *See* cerebral vascular accident.

CVS *See* chorionic villus sampling.

cystic fibrosis An autosomal recessively inherited disorder of the secretory glands leading to malabsorption and lung disease.

cytomegalovirus (CMV) A virus that may be asymptomatic or cause symptoms in adults that may resemble mononucleosis. In the fetus, it can lead to severe malformations similar to congenital rubella.

cytoplasm The contents of the cell outside the nucleus.

cytosine One of the four nucleotides (chemicals) that comprise DNA.

DAIs *See* diffuse axonal injuries.

dB *See* decibel.

DDH *See* developmental dislocation of the hip.

debridement The removal of dead tissue (e.g., after a burn or an infection).

decibel (dB) A measure of loudness used in hearing testing.

decubitus ulcers Bed sores.

deletion Loss of genetic material from a chromosome.

delirium An organically based psychosis characterized by impaired attention, disorganized thinking, altered and fluctuating levels of consciousness, and memory impairment. It may be caused by encephalitis, diabetes, or intoxication and is usually reversed by treating the underlying medical problem.

delusions False beliefs, often quite bizarre, that are symptoms of psychosis or drug intoxication.

dementia A progressive neurological disorder marked by the loss of memory, decreased speech, impairment in abstract thinking and judgment, other disturbances of higher cortical function, and personality change (e.g., Alzheimer's disease).

dental caries Tooth decay.

dental lamina A thickened band of tissue along the future dental arches in the human embryo.

dental organ The embryonic tissue that is the precursor of the tooth; *also called* tooth bud.

dental plaque Patches of bacteria, bacterial by-products, and food particles on teeth that predispose them to decay.

dental sealant Plastic substance administered to teeth, most commonly the molars, to increase their resistance to decay.

dentin The principal substance of the tooth surrounding the tooth pulp and covered by the enamel.

deoxyribonucleic acid (DNA) The fundamental component of living tissue. It contains an organism's genetic code.

depolarization The eliminating of the electrical charge of a cell.

depressed fracture Fracture of bone, usually the skull, that results in an inward displacement of the bone at the point of impact. It requires surgical intervention to prevent damage to underlying tissue.

deprivation In behavior management, denial of access to a reinforcing item or event.

dermal sinus A cavity lined extending from the skin surface to a deeper structure, most notably the spinal cord.

descriptive and functional analysis Observation period in behavior management that precedes treatment.

detoxification The conversion of a toxic compound to a nontoxic product.

developmental disabilities A group of chronic conditions that are attributable to an impairment in physical, cognitive, speech or language, psychological, or self-care areas and that are manifested during the developmental period (younger than 21 years of age).

developmental dislocation of the hip (DDH) A congenital hip dislocation, usually evident at birth, occurring more commonly in girls.

dextrose A simple sugar similar to glucose and used to medically correct or to prevent low blood sugar.

diagnostic test A test used to confirm a medical diagnosis.

dialysis A detoxification procedure of the blood (hemodialysis) or across the peritoneum (peritoneal dialysis) used to treat kidney failure.

diaphysis The shaft of a long bone lying under the epiphysis.

diastematomyelia A congenital defect in which the spinal cord is divided into halves by a bony or cartilaginous divider, often seen in spina bifida.

differential reinforcement A behavior management technique in which a preferred alternate behavior is positively reinforced while a less preferred behavior is ignored.

diffuse axonal injuries (DAIs) Diffuse injuries to nerve cell components, usually resulting from shearing forces. This type of traumatic brain injury is commonly associated with motor vehicle accidents.

diffusion-weighted imaging (DWI) A new form of magnetic resonance imaging (MRI) scanning that can identify with great sensitivity areas of brain that have suffered an acute injury.

diopters Units of refractive power of a lens.

diploid Having paired chromosomes in nondividing cells (i.e., 46 chromosomes in 23 pairs).

dislocation The displacement of a bone out of a joint space.

disorders of carbohydrate metabolism Inborn errors of metabolism involving enzyme deficiencies in the breakdown of sugars.

distal Pertaining to the part farthest from the mid-line or trunk.

diuretics Medications used to reduce intercellular fluid buildup in the body (edema), especially in the lungs.

diving reflex Named for its presence in diving seals, this also occurs in infants during hypoxic ischemic encepolopathy (HIE) and results in the redistribution of blood away from "nonvital organs" (e.g., kidneys, liver, lungs, intestines, and skeletal muscles) to preserve the perfusion of the "vital organs" (i.e., heart, brain, and adrenal glands). This reflex if prolonged may result in insufficient blood supply and damage to the nonvital organs.

DMD *See* Duchenne muscular dystrophy; *see Chapter 14 and Appendix B.*

DNA *See* deoxyribonucleic acid.

DNR *See* do not resuscitate.

dominant In genetics, referring to a trait that only requires one copy of a gene to be expressed phenotypically. For example, having brown eyes is a dominant trait, so a child receiving a gene for brown eyes from his or her mother or father (or from both parents) will have brown eyes.

do not resuscitate (DNR) Medical orders that, should a patient develop a cardiopulmonary arrest, no attempts at resuscitation should be undertaken (i.e., "No Code" orders).

dopamine A neurotransmitter involved in attention deficits (i.e., attention-deficit/hyper-activity disorder [ADHD]) and motor function (i.e., Parkinson's disease).

double effect Principle of a moral argument used to defend certain actions that can be anticipated to have both good and bad outcomes.

double helix The coiled structure of DNA.

dual diagnosis Intellectual disability and psychiatric disorder.

Duchenne muscular dystrophy (DMD) *See Chapter 14 and Appendix B.*

ductus arteriosus An arterial connection open during fetal life that diverts the blood flow from the pulmonary artery into the aorta, thereby bypassing the not yet functional lungs.

ductus venosus Open during fetal life, it is a shunt that allows oxygenated blood from the placenta to bypass the liver and return to the systemic circulation for distribution to the rest of the body.

duodenal atresia Congenital absence of a portion of the first section of the small intestine; often seen in individuals with Down syndrome.

duodenum The first part of the small intestine.

DWI scan *See* diffusion-weighted imaging.

dynamic In the context of orthotics, capable of active movement.

dysarthria Difficulty with speech due to impairment of oral motor structures or musculature.

dyscalculia Learning disability affecting skills in mathematics.

dysgraphia Learning disability in areas of processing and reporting information in written form.

dyskinesia An impairment in the ability to control movements characterized by spasmodic or repetitive motions.

dyskinetic cerebral palsy Type of "extrapyramidal" cerebral palsy often involving abnormalities of the basal ganglia and manifesting as rigidity, dystonia, or choreoathetosis.

dyslexia Learning disability affecting reading skills.

dysmorphic Unusual facial appearance as a result of a genetic disorder.

dysmotility Abnormal motility of the gut.

dysostosis An abnormal bony formation.

dysphagia Difficulty in swallowing function.

dysphasia Impairment of speech consisting of a lack of coordination and failure to arrange words in proper order due to a central brain lesion.

dysplasia Abnormal tissue development.

dyspraxia Inability to perform coordinated movements despite normal function of the central and peripheral nervous systems and muscles.

dysthymia A mild form of depression characterized by a mood disturbance that is present most of the time and is associated with feelings of low self-esteem, hopelessness, poor concentration, low energy, and changes in sleep and appetite; often seen in depressed adolescents.

dystocia Structural abnormalities of the uterus that cause a difficult labor or childbirth.

dystonia A disorder of the basal ganglia associated with altered muscle tone leading to contorted body positioning.

dystonic cerebral palsy A form of dyskinetic cerebral palsy, the prominent feature of which is dystonia.

E. coli *See Escherichia coli.*

ECG *See* electrocardiogram.

echocardiography An ultrasonic method of imaging the heart. It can be used to detect congenital heart defects.

echolalic Pertaining to immediate or delayed repetition of a word or phrase said by others; often evident in children with certain autism spectrum disorders (ASDs).

ECMO *See* extracorporeal membrane oxygenation.

ectoderm Outer cell layer in the embryo.

ectodermal dysplasia Abnormal skin development.

ectopias Congenital displacement of a body organ or tissue.

ectopic pregnancy Embryo implanted outside the uterus.

ectrodactyly Congenital absence of all or parts of digits.

eczema A common skin problem, often occurring in childhood, marked by an itchy inflammatory reaction manifested by tiny blisters with reddening, swelling, bumps, and crusting.

EDC *See* estimated date of confinement.

EDD Estimated due date; *also called* estimated date of confinement.

edema An abnormal accumulation of fluid in the tissues of the body.

EEG *See* electroencephalogram.

efferent Pertaining to the impulses that go to a nerve or muscle from the central nervous system (CNS).

effusion Fluid escaping from blood vessels or lymphatics that collects in body cavities (e.g., a pleural, or lung, effusion).

EKG *See* electrocardiogram.

ELBW *See* extremely low birth weight.

electrocardiogram (EKG, ECG) The graphic record of an electronic recording of heart rate and rhythm.

electroencephalogram (EEG) A recording of the electrical activity in the brain that is often used in the evaluation of seizures.

electrolytes Minerals contained in solution (e.g., in the blood).

electromyography A technique for measuring muscle activity and function.

electroretinogram (ERG) A graphic record of the electrical activity of the retina.

eloquent cortex The area of the cortex involved in the production of speech.

emancipated minor A teenage minor who is free of parental control for giving informed consent to any medical treatment. Status is based on legal statutes that vary among states but use relatively objective criteria (e.g., marriage, pregnancy, parenthood, independent living, military service, high school graduation, parents have surrendered their parental rights).

embryo The earliest stage of conceptional development after fertilization and during the first 8 weeks of pregnancy. The placenta and most of the primitive organs are formed into the major systems during this time.

embryogenesis Up until full term at 37–40 weeks' human gestation. The major organs become larger and more complex as they begin to differentiate and establish physiologic function.

embryotic period The first 8 weeks of pregnancy.

enamel The calcified outer layer of the tooth.

encephalitis Inflammation of the brain, generally from a viral infection.

encephalocele Congenital cystic malformation of the brain associated with severe disabilities.

encephalopathy Disorder or disease of the brain.

endocardial cushion defect A congenital heart defect found often in Down syndrome where there is a lack of closure of the wall separating the two sides of the heart.

endocarditis Inflammation of the inner lining of the heart.

endochondral ossification Formation of bone from cartilage.

endoderm The inner cell layer in the embryo.

enteral nutrition Feeding directly into the stomach through the nose or mouth to ensure that nutrition requirements are met.

epicanthal folds Crescent-shaped fold of skin on either side of the nose, commonly associated with Down syndrome.

epidemiology The study of the distribution and determinants of disease frequency in specific populations.

epidural anesthesia Pain relief by infusing an anesthetic agent into the epidural space of the spine.

epidural hematoma Localized collection of clotted blood lying between the skull and the outer (dural) membrane of the brain, resulting from the hemorrhage of a blood vessel resting in the dura. This most often results from traumatic head injury.

epiglottis A lid-like structure that hangs over the entrance to the windpipe and prevents aspiration of food or liquid into the lungs during swallowing.

epilepsy A disorder of the brain characterized by an enduring predisposition to generate epileptic seizures and by the neurobiologic, cognitive, psychological, and social consequences of this condition.

epiphyses The end plates of long bones where linear growth occurs.

epithelial Pertaining to cells that are found on exposed surfaces of the body, (e.g., skin, mucous membranes, intestinal walls).

equinus Involuntary extension (plantar flexion) of the foot (like a horse); this position is often found in spastic cerebral palsy.

ERG *See* electroretinogram.

erythrocytosis An abnormal increase in the number of circulating red blood cells.

Escherichia coli (E. coli) Bacteria that can cause infections ranging from diarrhea to urinary tract infection to sepsis.

esophageal atresia A congenital defect in which there is a stricture in the esophagus preventing food from entering the stomach.

esophageal transport phase Phase of swallowing in which the rhythmic contraction of esophageal muscles transports food from the pharynx to the stomach.

esophagus Tube through which food passes from the pharynx to the stomach.

esotropia A form of strabismus in which one or both eyes turn in; "cross-eyed."

estimated date of confinement (EDC) Expected date of delivery; *also called* estimated due date (EDD).

estrogen Female sex hormone.

etiology Cause.

eustachian tube Connection between oral cavity and middle ear, allowing equilibration of pressure and drainage of fluid.

everted Turned outward.

excitotoxic Pertaining to excitotoxins, neurochemicals that can cause neuronal cell death and have been implicated in hypoxic brain damage and acquired immunodeficiency syndrome (AIDS) encephalopathy.

executive function Brain processing involved in planning; it is thought to be deficient in individuals with learning disabilities, attention-deficit/hyperactivity disorder (ADHD), and autism spectrum disorders (ASDs).

exotropia A form of strabismus in which one or both eyes turn out; "wall-eyed."

expressive language Communication by spoken language, gesture, signing, or body language.

extension Movement of a limb at a joint to bring the joint into a more straightened position.

extinction *See* planned ignoring.

extinction burst A transient increase in the frequency and intensity of a challenging behavior before a subsequent reduction occurs.

extracorporeal membrane oxygenation (ECMO) An extreme and invasive life support technique that involves putting a patient onto a heart–lung bypass machine.

extract In the context of medication, a concentrated preparation.

extrapyramidal system Areas of the brain involved in subconscious, automatic aspects of motor coordination.

extremely low birth weight (ELBW) Term often used to describe an infant with a birth weight less than 1,000 grams (2¼ pounds).

fading Behavioral instruction process by which prompts are withdrawn gradually.

failure to thrive (FTT) Inadequate growth of both weight and height in infancy or early childhood caused by malnutrition, chronic disease, or a congenital anomaly.

fatty acid oxidation disorders Inborn errors of metabolism involving enzyme deficiencies in the breakdown of fatty acids.

febrile Having an elevated body temperature. A child is considered febrile when registering a fever above 100.4 degrees Fahrenheit (38 degrees Celsius).

femur Long bone in the thigh connecting the hip to the knee.

fencer's response *See* asymmetrical tonic neck reflex (ATNR).

fertilization The entrance of a sperm into the egg resulting in a conception.

fetal alcohol effects (FAE) Former term for alcohol-related neurodevelopmental disorder (ARND; *see Chapter 5*).

fetal heart rate (FHR) Normally 120–140 beats per minute and routinely monitored by ultrasound throughout labor to indicate fetal well-being versus fetal distress (FHR < 100).

fetal period The period of pregnancy following the eighth week of gestation.

fetus Refers to the stages of development during pregnancy after the first eight weeks.

FHR *See* fetal heart rate.

FISH *See* fluorescent *in situ* hybridization.

flexion Movement of a limb to bend at a joint.

flexor A muscle with the primary function of flexion or bending at a joint.

flora In medicine, bacteria normally residing within a body organ and not causing disease, such as *E. coli* in the intestine.

fluency Aspect of speech production; producing speech in a fluid manner.

fluorescent *in situ* hybridizationa (FISH) A technique to identify small chromosomal defects such as those found in Prader-Willi Syndrome.

fMRI *See* functional magnetic resonance imaging.

focal Localized.

focal neurological changes Findings on neurological exams that are abnormal and indicative of a lesion in a particular part of the brain; *also called* focal neurological impairments.

folic acid A vitamin, a deficiency of which during early pregnancy has been linked to neural tube defects.

patent foramen ovale (PFO) A tiny open window in the atrial wall of the heart passing oxygenated blood from the right atrium into the left atrium, thus bypassing circulation to the fetal lungs in utero.

forebrain The front portion of the brain during fetal development; *also called* the prosencephalon.

forward chaining A behavior management technique in which the first skill in a sequence is taught first and the last skill is taught last.

fovea centralis The small pit in the center of the macula; the area of clearest vision, containing only cones.

frame shift A type of gene mutation in which the insertion or deletion of a single nucleotide leads to the misreading of all subsequent codons.

free level In pharmacotherapy, the amount of active drug that is able to produce an effect on the body.

free radicals Chemical compounds, the abnormal accumulation of which has been linked to cancer and neurotoxicity.

frequency Cycles per second, or hertz (Hz), a measure of sound.

FTT *See* failure to thrive.

functional magnetic resonance imaging (fMRI) A neuroimaging procedure that permits evaluation of the effects of activities, such as reading, on brain function.

fundoplication An operation in which the top of the stomach is wrapped around the opening of the esophagus to prevent gastroesophageal reflux (GER).

FXS Fragile X syndrome; *see* Chapter 19.

galactosemia An inborn error of metabolism involving an enzyme deficiency that prevents the breakdown of the sugar galactose, a component of many foods.

gamma-aminobutyric acid (GABA) An amino acid that acts as an inhibitory neurotransmitter.

gastroenteritis An acute illness marked by vomiting and diarrhea usually associated with a viral infection (e.g., rotavirus in infants) that generally lasts a few days; *also called* stomach flu.

gastroesophageal reflux (GER) The backward flow of food into the esophagus after it has entered the stomach.

gastroschisis Congenital malformation of the abdominal wall resulting in the protrusion of abdominal contents.

gastrostomy An operation in which an artificial opening is made into the stomach through the wall of the abdomen. This is usually done in order to place a feeding tube into the stomach.

GBS *See* group B *streptococcus.*

gene A unit of genetic material (DNA) that encodes a single protein.

genome The complete set of hereditary factors (genes) in an organism.

genomic imprinting A condition manifested differently depending on whether the trait is inherited from the mother or father; *also called* uniparental disomy. An example is a deletion in chromosome 15q11–q13, which when inherited from the mother results in Angelman syndrome and when inherited from the father results in Prader-Willi syndrome (*see Appendix B*).

genotype The genetic composition of an individual.

GER *See* gastroesophageal reflux.

germ cells The cells involved in reproduction (i.e., sperm, eggs).

German measles *See* rubella.

glaucoma Increased pressure within the anterior chamber of the eye, which can cause blindness.

glial cells Cells that compose the white matter and provide a support function for neurons.

glossoptosis Protruding tongue.

glucose A sugar; *also called* sucrose; contained in fruits and other carbohydrates.

glutaminergic neurons Brain cells that release the chemical glutamate, an exactatory neurotransmitter.

glycine An amino acid that can serve as an excitotoxin, causing seizures.

glycogen The chief carbohydrate stored in the body, primarily in the liver and muscles.

Gogli apparatus The intracellular organelle that packages proteins in a form that can be released through the cell membrane and carried throughout the body.

goiter Enlargement of the thyroid gland.

goniometry Use of a hinged measuring tool to determine joint range of motion.

graduated guidance A behavior management technique in which only the level of assistance (guidance) necessary for the child to complete the task is provided.

graft versus host disease A mechanism of the body's immune system that destroys foreign proteins. It can be life-threatening when it occurs in a child who has received a bone marrow or organ transplant and has a suppressed immune system. Symptoms include diarrhea, skin breakdown, and shock.

grammar The system of and rules for using units of meaning (morphemes) and syntax in language.

grapheme A unit, such as a letter, of a writing system.

gravida/para The number of times a woman has been pregnant (gravid) and has delivered (parous) a living infant.

group B *streptococcus* Bacteria, causing one of the most common and severe neonatal infections.

guanine One of the four nucleotides (chemicals) that comprise DNA.

guided compliance A behavior management technique involving the use of graduated guidance to teach functional tasks.

Guillain-Barré syndrome An acute neuropathy (*see Appendix B*).

gynecomastia Excessive breast growth in males.

gyri Convolutions of the surface of the brain; *singular:* gyrus.

habilitation The teaching of new skills to children with developmental disabilities. It is called habilitation rather than rehabilitation

because these children did not possess these skills previously.

hallucinations Sensory perceptions without a source in the external world. These most commonly occur as symptoms of psychosis, drug intoxication, or seizures.

haploid Having a single set of human chromosomes, 23, as in the sperm or egg.

hCG *See* human chorionic gonadotropin.

hearing loss A condition characterized by a decrease in the ability to hear based on decreased intensity, loudness as measured in decibels (dB), or frequency of sound.

hemangiomas Congenital masses of blood vessels.

hematocrit Percentage of red blood cells in whole blood, normally about 35%–40%.

hematologic Relating to the blood system.

hematopoietic Relating to the formation of red blood cells.

hemihypertrophy Asymmetric hypertrophy of face or limbs.

hemiplegia Paralysis of one side of the body.

hemodialysis A detoxification procedure in which an individual's blood is gradually removed through an artery, passed through an artificial kidney machine, and then returned cleansed. It is used most commonly to treat chronic renal (kidney) failure.

hemoglobin Blood protein capable of carrying oxygen to body tissues.

hemostat A small surgical clamp used to constrict a tube or blood vessel.

hepatosplenomegaly Enlargement of the liver and spleen.

herpes simplex virus (HSV) A virus leading to symptoms that range from cold sores to genital lesions to encephalitis; also a cause of fetal malformations and sepsis in early infancy.

hertz (Hz) Cycles per second; a measure of the frequency of sound.

heterotopia Migration and development of normal neural tissue in an abnormal location in the brain.

heterozygous Carrying genes dissimilar for one trait.

hexosaminidase An enzyme, a deficiency of which leads to Tay-Sachs disease.

HIE *See* hypoxic ischemic encephalopathy.

hippocampus A region of the brain in the floor of each lateral ventricle that has a central role in the formation of memory and emotion.

hippotherapy The therapeutic use of horseback riding.

HIV *See* human immunodeficiency virus.

homeobox (HOX) A group of genes involved in early embryonic development.

homeostasis Equilibrium of fluid, chemical, and temperature regulation in the body.

homozygous Carrying identical genes for any given trait.

HSV *See* herpes simplex virus.

human chorionic gonadotropin (hCG) The hormone secreted by the embryo that prevents its expulsion from the uterus. A pregnancy test measures the presence of this hormone in the blood or urine.

human immunodeficiency virus (HIV) *See Chapter 6.*

hybrid Offspring of parents of dissimilar species.

hydrocephalus A condition characterized by the abnormal accumulation of cerebrospinal fluid within the ventricles of the brain. In infants, this leads to enlargement of the head.

hyperalimentation *See* parenteral feeding.

hyperbilirubinemia Excess accumulation of bilirubin in the blood, which can result in jaundice, a yellowing of the complexion and/or the whites of the eyes, or kernicterus, the yellow staining of certain central parts of the brain.

hyperglycemia High blood sugar level as seen in diabetes.

hyperimmune globulin Blood that is especially rich in antibodies against a virus.

hyperopia Farsightedness.

hyperparathyroidism High level of blood parathyroid hormone, which causes abnormalities in calcium and phosphorous metabolism.

hypersynchronous In the context of the central nervous system (CNS), pertaining to the discharge of many neurons at the same time that leads to a seizure.

hypertelorism Widely spaced eyes.

hypertension High blood pressure.

hyperthyroidism Condition resulting from excessive production of thyroid hormone.

hypertrichosis Excessive hair growth.

hypertrophy Overgrowth of a body part or organ.

hypocalcemia Low blood calcium level.

hypogenitalism Having small genitalia.

hypoglycemia Low blood sugar level usually below a concentration of 40–50 milligrams of glucose per 100 milliliters of blood for a period of time.

hypogonadism Decreased function of sex glands with resultant retarded growth and sexual development.

hypoplasia Defective formation of a tissue or body organ.

hypoplastic lungs Small lungs that are not fully developed; associated with oligohydramnios and lack of fetal breathing efforts.

hypospadias Abnormal urethral opening in penis.

hypotension Low blood pressure.

hypothermia Excessively low body temperature.

hypothyroidism Condition resulting from deficient production of thyroid hormone.

hypotonia Decreased muscle tone.

hypoxemia Seriously low blood oxygen supply to the entire body.

hypoxic Having reduced oxygen content in body tissues.

hypoxic ischemic encephalopathy (HIE) An acute brain malfunction often resulting in coma caused by acute reduction in the blood flow and the oxygen supply to the brain.

hypsarrhythmia Electroencephalographic (EEG) abnormality seen in infants with infantile spasms; marked by chaotic spike–wave activity.

ictal Pertaining to a seizure event.

IDDM *See* insulin-dependent diabetes mellitus.

IEP *See* individualized education program.

IFSP *See* individualized family service plan.

ileostomy A surgically placed opening from the small intestine through the abdominal wall to divert bowel or bladder contents after an operation.

ileum Lower portion of the small intestine.

imitation training A behavior management technique in which the teacher demonstrates the desired behavior, asks the child to complete the action, and provides positive reinforcement when the task is completed.

immunoglobulin An antibody produced by the body after exposure to a foreign agent, such as a virus.

impact In reference to traumatic head injury, the forcible striking of the head against an object.

imperforate Lacking a normal opening in a body organ. The most common example in childhood is an absent or closed anus.

implantation An attachment and imbedding of the fertilized egg (blastocyst) into the mucous lining of the uterus.

in utero Occurring during fetal development.

inborn error of metabolism An inherited enzyme deficiency leading to the disruption of normal bodily metabolism (e.g., phenylketonuria [PKU]).

incidence The rate of occurrence of new cases of a disorder in a population.

incidence rate The rate at which new events occur in the population expressed as a function of time.

incisors Front teeth used for cutting.

incus One of the three small bones in the middle ear that help amplify sound.

individualized education program (IEP) A written plan, mandated by federal law, that maps out the objectives and goals that a child receiving special education services is expected to achieve over the course of the school year.

individualized family service plan (IFSP) A written plan detailing early intervention and related services to be provided to an infant or toddler with disabilities in accordance with federal law.

individualized transition plan (ITP) A written plan for an adolescent receiving special education services that maps out his or her postschool education, services, and employment and adult living goals; required by federal law to be part of the student's individualized education program (IEP) starting at age 14.

inertial Pertaining to inertia, which is the tendency to keep moving in the same direction as the force that produced a movement.

infantile spasms A seizure type in infancy marked by brief flexor spasms, usually lasting 1–3 seconds.

inferior In anatomy, below.

influenza An acute illness caused by a virus that attacks respiratory and gastrointestinal tracts.

informed consent The written consent of a person to undergo a procedure or treatment after its risks and benefits have been explained in easily understood language.

inhaled nitric oxide (iNO) A new therapeutic gas for treating persistent pulmony hypertension of the neonate (PPHN). It is mixed with the baby's oxygen supply in miniscule amounts and directly stimulates pulmonary function.

instructional training A behavior management technique in which the teacher describes the desired behavior, asks the child to perform it, and provides positive reinforcement upon completion of the task.

insulin-dependent diabetes mellitus (IDDM) A disorder in which blood sugar level is high enough to require treatment with insulin.

insult An attack on a body organ that causes damage to it. This may be physical, metabolic, immunological, or infectious.

intellectual disability Significantly subaverage general intellectual functioning accompanied by significant limitations in adaptive functioning; *previously called* mental retardation.

intensity Strength.

interictal In an individual with a seizure disorder, pertaining to the periods when seizures are not occurring.

interphase The period in the cell life cycle when the cell is not dividing.

interval schedules Provision of reinforcement based on the passage of a certain amount of time relative to the child's performance of a behavior or task.

intrathecal The infusion of medication into the spinal space.

intrauterine growth restriction (IUGR) Restricted growth in the fetus, producing a small for gestational age at-birth baby, often resulting from abnormal placental development.

intravenous Infusion into a vein.

intraventricular hemorrhage (IVH) A hemorrhage into the cerebral ventricles.

intubation Insertion of a tube through the nose or mouth into the trachea to permit mechanical ventilation.

inversion The result of two breaks on a chromosome followed by the reinsertion of the missing fragment at its original site but in the inverted order.

inverted 1) Reversed; 2) in anatomy, turned inward.

ionic Pertaining to mineral ions, a group of atoms carrying a charge of electricity.

iris The circular, colored membrane behind the cornea that surrounds the pupil.

ischemia A decreased blood flow to an area of the body that leads to tissue death.

isochromosome A chromosome with two copies of one arm and no copy of the other.

ITP *See* individualized transition plan.

IUGR *See* intrauterine growth restriction.

IVH *See* intraventricular hemorrhage.

J tube *See* jejunostomy tube.

jaundice A yellowing of the complexion and the whites of the eyes resulting from hyperbilirubinemia.

jejunostomy (J) tube A tube placed through the skin of the abdomen and directly into the jejunum to provide nutrition.

jejunum The second portion of the small intestine.

karyotyping Photographing the chromosomal makeup of a cell. In a human, there are 23 pairs of chromosomes in a normal karyotype.

ketogenic diet Special diet high in fat used to promote the use of ketones as an energy source.

ketosis The buildup of acid in the body, most often associated with starvation, inborn errors of metabolism, or diabetes.

kyphoscoliosis A combination of humping and curvature of the spine.

kyphosis Humping deformity of the spine; "hunchback."

labyrinth One of the major components of the inner ear, the other being the cochlea.

lactase Enzyme necessary to digest the milk sugar lactose.

lactic acid Chemical produced in muscles as a result of anaerobic glucose metabolism.

lactose Milk sugar composed of glucose and galactose.

lag of mineralization of bone *See* spondyloepiphyseal dysplasia.

lanugo Fine body hair.

large for gestational age (LGA) Weighing more than 4 kilograms, about 9 or more pounds at birth, which makes vaginal delivery mechanically difficult through the normal pelvic birth canal. This typically occurs in infants of mothers with diabetes.

lateral To the side; away from the mid-line.

lateral ventricles Cavities in the interior of the cerebral hemisphere containing cerebrospinal fluid. They are enlarged with hydrocephalus or with brain atrophy.

LBW *See* low birth weight.

lens The biconvex, translucent body that rests in front of the vitreous humor of the eye and refracts light.

lesions Injuries or loss of function.

LGA *See* large for gestational age.

ligament A sheet or band of tough, fibrous tissue connecting bones or cartilage at a joint.

linear fracture Break of a bone in a straight line; refers to a type of skull fracture or fracture of a long bone (arm or leg).

lipoma A benign, fatty tissue tumor.

lissencephaly A smooth brain due to incomplete neuronal proliferation and migration.

locus Focus or location.

low birth weight (LBW) Term often used to describe an infant with a birth weight less than 2,500 grams (5½ pounds).

lower esophageal sphincter The muscular valve connecting the esophagus and stomach and normally preventing reflux.

lumbar Pertaining to the lower back.

lumbar puncture The tapping of the subarachnoid space to obtain cerebrospinal fluid from the lower back region. This procedure is used to diagnose meningitis and to measure chemicals in the spinal fluid; *also called* a spinal tap.

lymphadenopathy An enlargement of lymph nodes.

lymphocyte A type of white blood cell.

lymphoma A cancerous growth of lymphoid tissue.

lyonization The genetic principle discovered by Mary Lyon that there is X-chromosome inactivation in females.

lysosome Minute organelle in a cell that contains enzymes used to digest potentially toxic material.

macrocephaly Large head size.

macroorchidism Having abnormally large testicles; found in fragile X syndrome.

macrosomia Large body size.

macrostomia Large mouth.

macula The area of the retina that contains the greatest concentration of cones and the fovea centralis.

magnetic resonance imaging (MRI) Imaging procedure that uses the magnetic resonance of atoms to provide clear images of interior parts of the body. It is particularly useful in diagnosing structural abnormalities of the brain.

magnetic resonance spectroscopy (MRS) A study that can be done as part of a regular MRI scan. Rather than provide a picture of the brain, it analyzes the presence and amount of certain metabolic components in various brain regions. It is particularly helpful in diagnosing certain inborn errors of metabolism, such as mitochondrial disorders (*see Appendix B*).

major depression A prolonged period of depressed mood.

malleus One of the three small bones in the middle ear that help amplify sound.

malnutrition Inadequate nutrition for typical growth and development to occur.

malocclusion The improper fitting together of the upper and lower teeth.

mandible Lower jaw bone.

mania A distinct period of abnormally and persistently elevated, expansive, or irritable mood. This mood disturbance is sufficiently severe to cause impairment in function.

manic depression *See* bipolar disorder.

mass spectrometry A technique used for identifying chemical, drug, or metabolic abnormalities in the blood or urine.

mastoiditis   Infection of the mastoid air cells that rest in the temporal bone behind the ear. This is an infrequent complication of chronic middle-ear infection.

mature minor   A teenage minor who may give consent because the physician judges that he or she understands the nature, purpose, and risks of the proposed treatment; generally limited to minors at least 15 years old where the treatment is for the patient's own benefit and is judged necessary by conservative medical opinion (compare with *emancipated minor*).

maxilla   The bony region of the upper jaw.

maxillary hypoplasia   Incomplete development of the upper jaw.

meconium   The thick and tarry stool that is formed during fetal life consisting of swallowed amniotic fluid debris, gastrointestinal mucous and green bile secretions from the liver, and sloughed off gastrointestinal epithelial cells; is not normally passed until after birth.

medial   Toward the center or mid-line.

median plane   The mid-line plane of the body. It runs vertically and separates the left and right halves of the body.

medium chain fatty acids   Fatty acids that can bypass the normal uptake process and go directly to the liver.

megavitamin therapy   The use of at least 10 times the required amount of vitamins; *also called* orthomolecular therapy.

meiosis   Reductive cell division occurring only in eggs and sperm in which the daughter cells receive half (23) the number of chromosomes of the parent cells (46).

Mendelian traits   Dominant and recessive traits inherited according to the genetic principles put forward by Gregor Mendel.

meningeal   Related to the meninges, the three membranes enveloping the brain and spinal cord.

meningitis   Infection of the meninges or sac that surround the brain, often bacterial.

meningocele   Protrusion of the meninges through a defect in the skull or vertebral column.

meningomyelocele   Protrusion of meninges and malformed spinal cord through a defect in the vertebral column; *also called* myelomeningocele.

menses   Menstrual flow.

mental retardation   *See* intellectual disability.

mesencephalon   Midbrain region.

mesoderm   Middle cell layer in the embryo.

messenger ribonucleic acid (mRNA)   RNA involved in the translation of genetic information.

metaphase   The stage in cell division in which each chromosome doubles.

metaphyses   The ends of the shaft of long bones connected to the epiphyses.

methionine   An amino acid.

methylation   The attachment of methyl groups to DNA at the cytosine base that turns gene function off.

microdeletion   A microscopic deletion in a chromosome associated with a contiguous gene syndrome.

microdeletion syndromes   Genetic disorders caused by mutations in a small number of contiguous genes, an example being velocardiofacial syndrome.

micrognathia   Receding chin.

microphthalmia   Small eye.

micropreemie   Term often used to describe an infant born weighing less than 800 grams (1.75 pounds).

microswitches   Switches used to control computers, environmental control systems, or power wheelchairs that have been adapted so that less pressure than normal is required for activation.

microtia   Small ear.

milligram   One thousandth of a gram.

milliliter   One thousandth of a liter; equal to about 15 drops.

missense mutation   Gene error resulting from the replacement of a single nucleic acid for another, resulting in a misreading of the DNA code.

mitochondrial myopathy   Congenital muscle disorder caused by a mutation in the mitochondrial DNA.

mitosis   Cell division in which two daughter cells of identical chromosomal composition to the parent cell are formed. Each contains 46 chromosomes.

mixed cerebral palsy   A form of cerebral palsy with spastic and dyskinetic components.

modification   In special education, a substantial change in the method or scoring scale used to assess a student's academic performance or knowledge (e.g., using a portfolio of work to demonstrate a student's learning).

monosomy   Chromosome disorder in which one chromosome is absent. The most common example is Turner syndrome, XO (*see Appendix B*).

monosomy X   Turner syndrome (*see Appendix B.*)

morbidity Medical complication of an illness, procedure, or operation.

moro reflex Primitive reflex present in the newborn in which the infant throws the arms out as if to give an embrace; *also called* startle reflex when a newborn infant experiences a sudden drop of the head and neck or a loud noise and responds with sudden flexion of the neck, arms, and legs, and then cries irritably; reflex becomes hyperactive in babies with hypoxic ischemic encephalopathy (HIE).

morphemes The smallest linguistic units of meaning.

morula The group of cells formed by the first divisions of a fertilized egg.

mosaicism The presence of two genetically distinct types of cells in one individual (e.g., in a child with Down syndrome who has some cells containing 46 chromosomes and some cells containing 47 chromosomes).

MOSF *See* multi-organ system failure.

motor point block The injection of a denaturing agent into the nerve supply of a spastic muscle.

MRI *See* magnetic resonance imaging.

mRNA *See* messenger ribonucleic acid.

MRS *See* magnetic resonance spectroscopy.

mucopolysaccharides Product of metabolism that may accumulate in cells and cause a progressive neurological disorder (e.g., Hurler syndrome, *see Appendix B*).

multifactorial Describing an inheritance pattern in which environment and heredity interact.

multi-organ system failure (MOSF) Results from the diving reflex during severe hypoxic ischemic encephalopathy (HIE).

muscle spindles Muscle fibers that are part of the reflex arc that controls muscle contraction.

muscular dystrophy *See Chapter 14 and Appendix B.*

musculoskeletal Referring to the muscle and bone support system of the body.

mutation A change in a gene that occurs by chance.

myasthenia gravis *See Chapter 14.*

myelination The production of a coating called myelin around an axon, which quickens neurotransmission.

myelomeningocele *See* meningomyelocele.

myoclonus Irregular, involuntary contraction of a muscle.

myopia Nearsightedness.

myosin Protein necessary for muscle contraction.

myotonia Abnormal rigidity of muscles when voluntary movement is attempted.

myringotomy The surgical incision of the eardrum, usually accompanied by the placement of pressure-equalization tubes to drain fluid from the middle ear.

nasal cannula Plastic prong placed in the nostrils to deliver oxygen: *plural*, cannulae.

nasal pillows A prop attached to an oxygen line to permit the flow of oxygen directly into the nose.

nasogastric (NG) tube A plastic feeding tube placed in the nose and extended into the stomach.

nasopharynx Posterior portion of the oral cavity above the palate.

NDT *See* neurodevelopmental therapy.

NEC *See* necrotizing enterocolitis.

necrosis Death of tissue.

necrotizing enterocolitis (NEC) Severe inflammation of the small intestine and colon, most common in premature infants.

negative reinforcement Behavioral phenomenon in which an individual's behavior permits an unpleasant event to be avoided or escaped, with a resultant increase in this behavior in the future.

neonatal intensive care unit (NICU) Hospital unit specializing in providing newborn life support treatments.

neonatal seizure A seizure that manifests as arm and/or leg tonic/clonic movements seeming like bicycling or rowing movements of the arms and/or legs. Movements may also be more subtle (e.g., orolingual movements such as spasmodic lip smacking or tongue thrusting, ocular movements such as excessive blinking or prolonged eye opening/staring, apnea, bradycardia [stopping breathing with a resultant slowing of the heart rate]).

nerve blocks Direct injection of denaturing agents into motor nerves.

nerve conduction velocity Measure of nerve function.

neural fold During embryonic life, the fold created when the neural plate expands and rises; later it becomes the spinal column.

neural network A network involving many brain regions working in concert to store and use information obtained from the environment.

neural plate Earliest fetal brain mass development derived from the ectodermal germ layer of the embryo in the first 7 weeks of gestation.

neural tube The stage of central nervous system (CNS) development that follows neural plate formation, which subsequently gives rise to the various parts of the brain (i.e., the forebrain folding into the cerebrum and the hindbrain into the cerebellum, brainstem, and spinal cord).

neural tube defects (NTDs) *See Chapter 28.*

neurodevelopmental therapy (NDT) Therapy that includes an understanding and utilization of typical developmental stages in working with children; commonly used theory underlying physical and occupational therapy.

neuroleptic malignant syndrome A rare toxic reaction to a medication in which there is a potentially life-threatening high fever.

neuromuscular Affecting both muscles and nerves.

neurotoxicant A chemical compound that can damage neurons; *also called* neurotoxin.

neurotransmitter A chemical released at the synapse that permits transmission of an impulse from one nerve to another.

neurulation Sequential central nervous system (CNS) developmental processes of neuron cell proliferation and migration of nascent neurons outward from the center of the developing brain to the outer cortex.

neutropenia Low white blood cell count.

NG tube *See* nasogastric tube.

NICU *See* neonatal intensive care unit.

nondisjunction Failure of a pair of chromosomes to separate during mitosis or meiosis, resulting in an unequal number of chromosomes in the daughter cells.

nonsense mutation Gene defect in which a single base pair substitution results in the premature termination of a message and the resultant production of an incomplete and inactive protein.

norepinephrine A neurotransmitter.

NTDs *See* neural tube defects; *see Chapter 28.*

nucleotide bases The nucleic acids that form DNA—adenine, guanine, cytosine, and thymine.

nystagmus Involuntary rapid movements of the eyes.

obsessive-compulsive disorder (OCD) A psychiatric disorder in which recurrent and persistent thoughts and ideas that cannot be suppressed (obsessions) are associated with repetitive behaviors (compulsions), such as excessive handwashing.

ocular Pertaining to the eye.

oligohydramnios The presence of too little amniotic fluid, which may result in fetal deformities, including clubfoot and hypoplastic lungs.

omphalocele Congenital herniation of abdominal organs through the navel.

onychomycosis A fungal infection of the nails.

operant control Control established and maintained by operant contingencies (i.e., the relationships in effect between the behavior and its consequences).

ophthalmologist Physician specializing in treatment of diseases of the eye.

ophthalmoscope An instrument containing a mirror and a series of magnifying lenses used to examine the interior of the eye.

opiate antagonists A category of medications that block endorphin receptors of the brain.

opisthotonos Positioning of the body in which the back is arched while the head and feet touch the bed.

optokinetic Pertaining to movement of the eyes.

oral preparatory phase The step preceding swallowing in which food is formed into a bolus in the mouth.

oral transport phase The transport of a bolus of food to the back of the mouth so that it can be swallowed.

organ of Corti A series of hair cells in the cochlea that form the beginning of the auditory nerve.

organic acidemias Inborn errors of metabolism involving enzyme deficiencies in the breakdown of organic acids (e.g., methylmalonic aciduria; *see Appendix B*).

ornithine transcarbamylase (OTC) An enzyme in the urea cycle, a deficiency of which leads to an inborn error of metabolism characterized by episodes of encephalopathy.

orthomolecular therapy *See* megavitamin therapy.

orthopedic Relating to bones or joints.

orthosis Orthopedic device (e.g., a splint or brace) used to support, align, or correct deformities or to improve the function of limbs; *plural:* orthoses; *also called* orthotic.

orthotic Device that supports or corrects the function of a limb or the torso; *also called* orthosis.

orthotist Professional trained in the fitting and construction of splints, braces, and artificial limbs.

ossicles The three small bones in the middle ear—the stapes, incus, and malleus.

ossicular chain Three small bones in the middle ear that amplify sound.

osteoarthritis Degenerative joint disease.

osteoblasts Cells that produce bony tissue.

osteoclast Cell that absorbs and removes bone.

osteoid   The substrate of bone.

osteopenia   The loss of bony tissue.

osteopetrosis   A genetic disorder marked by deficient osteoclastic activity. A buildup of bone encroaches on the eye, brain, and other body organs, leading to early death.

ostomy   An artificial opening in the abdominal region, for example, for discharge of stool or urine.

OTC   *See* ornithine transcarbamylase.

otitis media   Middle-ear infection.

otoacoustic emissions   Low-intensity sound energy emitted by the cochlea subsequent to sound stimulation as measured by a microphone coupled to the external ear canal.

ototoxic   Toxic to the auditory nerve, leading to hearing impairment.

oval window   Connects the middle to the inner ear.

oxidative phosphorylation   A chemical reaction occurring in the mitochondrion, resulting in energy production.

oxygenation   The provision of sufficient oxygen for bodily needs.

pachygyria   Abnormal convolutions on the surface of brain.

palatal   Relating to the palate, the back portion of the roof of the mouth.

palate   The roof of the mouth.

pancreatitis   An inflammation of the pancreas.

panic disorder   A psychiatric disorder in which the patient has episodes of sudden and irrational fears associated with hyperventilation and palpitations.

parasomnia   Sleep disturbances (i.e., night terrors, sleep walking).

parenteral feeding   Intravenous provision of high-quality nutrition (i.e., carbohydrates, protein, fat) used in children with malabsorption, malnutrition, and short bowel syndrome; *also called* hyperalimentation.

parietal lobe   Brain region involved in integrating sensory information and in visual-spatial processing.

Parkinson's disease   A progressive neurological disease usually occurring in older people; associated with tremor, slowed movements, and muscular rigidity.

paroxysmal   Intermittent.

partial graduated guidance   Instructor uses minimal physical contact but much praise in helping the child learn a desired task.

parvovirus   A group of extremely small DNA viruses. Intrauterine infection with one type of parvovirus increases the risk of miscarriage but has not been shown to result in fetal malformations.

patent ductus arteriosus (PDA)   The persistence of a fetal passage permitting blood to bypass the lungs.

patent foramen ovale (PFO)   A tiny open window in the atrial wall of the heart passing oxygenated blood from the right atrium into the left atrium, thus bypassing circulation to the fetal lungs in utero.

paternalism   Imposing a decision on another person for that person's welfare (e.g., the theory that "doctor knows best").

PCB   *See* polychlorinated biphenyl.

PDA   *See* patent ductus arteriosus.

PDD   Pervasive developmental disorder; *see* Chapter 23.

penetrance   The percentage of people with a particular genetic mutation who express symptoms of the disorder. A disorder shows reduced penetrance when some people with the genetic defect are completely without symptoms.

percutaneous umbilical blood sampling (PUBS)   A prenatal diagnostic procedure for obtaining fetal blood for genetic testing; *also called* cordocentesis.

percutaneously   Through the skin.

perfusion   The passage of blood through the arteries to an organ or tissue.

periodontal disease   Disease of the gums and bony structures that surround the teeth.

periosteum   Fibrous tissue covering and protecting all bones.

peripheral nervous system   The parts of the nervous system other than the brain and spinal cord.

peripheral venous lines   Catheters that are placed in a superficial vein of the arm or leg to provide medication.

peritoneal   Referring to the membrane surrounding the abdominal organs.

periventricular leukomalacia (PVL)   Injury to part of the brain near the ventricles; caused by lack of oxygen; occurs principally in premature infants.

peroxisome   A cellular organelle involved in processing fatty acids.

persistent pulmonary hypertension of the newborn/persistent fetal circulation (PPHN/PFC)   Persistent high pulmonary blood pressure in the newborn period due to vasoconstriction of the pulmonary arterial blood vessels and resulting in severe hypoxia.

pervasive developmental disorder (PDD)   One of the autism spectrum disorders; *see* Chapter 23.

pes cavus   High-arched foot.

pesticide   A chemical used to kill insects.

PET scan *See* positron emission tomography.

petechiae A small purplish spot, usually on the skin, caused by a minute hemorrhage.

PFO *See* patent foramen ovale.

phalanges Bones of the fingers and toes.

pharyngeal Pertaining to the pharynx.

pharyngeal transfer phase The transfer of a food bolus from the mouth to the pharynx on its way to being swallowed.

pharynx The back of the throat.

phenothiazines Antipsychotic medications that affect neurochemicals in the brain and are used to control aggressive behavior and psychotic symptoms.

phenotype The physical appearance of a genetic trait.

phenylalanine An amino acid, the elevation of which causes phenylketonuria (PKU).

phenylketonuria (PKU) *See Chapter 20.*

philtrum Groove between nose and mouth.

phobias Irrational fears.

phocomelia Congenitally foreshortened limbs.

phoneme The smallest unit of sound in speech.

phonetic Pertaining to the sounding out of words.

phonology The set of sounds in a language and the rules for using them.

photoreceptors Receptors for light stimuli; the rods and cones in the retina.

physes Growth plates of a developing long bone.

physiotherapy Physical therapy.

pica The hunger for or ingestion of nonfood items.

pitch The frequency of sounds, measured in cycles per second, or hertz (Hz). Low-pitched sounds have a frequency less than 500 Hz and a bass quality. High-pitched sounds have a frequency greater than 2,000 Hz and a tenor quality.

PKU *See* Phenylketonuria; *see Chapter 20 and Appendix B.*

placebo An inactive substance used as a control in a study to determine the effectiveness of a drug.

placenta The organ of nutritional exchange between the mother and the embryo. It has both maternal and embryonic portions, is disc-shaped, and is about 7 inches in diameter. The umbilical cord attaches in the center of the placenta. *Also called* the afterbirth; *adjective:* placental.

placenta accreta Abnormal adherence of the chorionic villi to the uterus.

placenta previa Condition in which the placenta is implanted in the lower segment of the uterus, extending over the cervical opening. This often leads to bleeding during labor.

placental abruption *See* abruptio placenta.

planned ignoring A behavior management technique based on withholding positive reinforcement following an occurrence of a nondangerous, nondestructive challenging behavior; *also called* extinction.

plasma The noncellular content of blood; *also called* serum.

plasmapheresis The removal of blood followed by filtering the plasma and reinfusing the blood products. This procedure is done to remove toxins and antibodies as in Guillain-Barré syndrome.

plasticity The ability of an organ or part of an organ to take over the function of another damaged organ.

***pneumocystis carinii* pneumonia** Lung infection often seen in immunocompromised individuals, such as those with acquired immunodeficiency syndrome (AIDS).

point mutation A mutation in a single nucleotide (DNA) base leading to a genetic syndrome (i.e., sickle cell disease).

polio Viral infection of the spinal cord causing an asymmetrical ascending paralysis, now prevented by vaccination.

polychlorinated biphenyl (PCB) One of a group of organic compounds originally used in industry and now recognized as an environmental pollutant.

polydactyly Extra fingers or toes.

polyhydramnios The presence of excessive amniotic fluid; often associated with certain fetal anomalies such as esophageal atresia.

polymicrogyria A brain with too many convoluted gyri that are smaller than normal, due to abnormal neuronal migration during embryogenesis of the central nervous system (CNS).

polysomnogram Procedure performed during sleep that involves monitoring electroencephalogram (EEG), electrocardiogram (EKG), and respiratory efforts. It is used to investigate individuals with sleep disorders, including sleep apnea.

POR *See* prevalence odds ratio.

positive pressure ventilation (PPV) Assistance provided during newborn resuscitation.

positive reinforcement A method of increasing desired behaviors by rewarding them.

positive reinforcers Any tangible (e.g., food, toy) or action (e.g., hug) that is reinforcing to an individual and will lead to a subsequent increase in the behavior that preceded it.

positive support reflex (PSR) Primitive reflex present in an infant, in which the child reflexively accepts weight on the feet when bounced, appearing to stand briefly.

positron emission tomography (PET) Imaging study utilizing radioactive labeled chemical compounds to study the metabolism of an organ, most commonly the brain.

posterior In back of or the back part of a structure.

postictal Immediately following a seizure episode.

postterm birth Birth after the 42nd week of gestation.

posttraumatic stress disorder (PTSD) Psychiatric disorder in which a previously experienced stressful event is reexperienced psychologically many times and associated with anxiety and fear.

postural reactions Normal reflex-like protective responses of an infant to changes in position; *also called* automatic movement reactions.

PPHN/PFC *See* persistent pulmonary hypertension of the newborn/persistent fetal circulation.

PPV *See* positive pressure ventilation.

pragmatics The study of language as it is used in a social context (e.g., conversation).

precocious puberty A condition in which the changes associated with puberty begin at an unexpectedly early age.

preeclampsia Illness of late pregnancy characterized by high blood pressure with swelling and/or protein in the mother's urine, seen especially in teenagers and women older than 35 years; *also called* toxemia of pregnancy.

premolar Teeth in the back of the mouth used for grinding.

prenatal screening Noninvasive (usually blood) tests used to screen for genetic disorders in pregnant women.

presbyopia A decrease in the accommodation of the lens of the eye that occurs with aging.

preterm birth Birth prior to the 37th week of gestation; prematurity.

prevalence odds ratio (POR) The burden or status of a disease in a defined population at a specified time, including all cases of disease in the population whether they are newly diagnosed or previously recognized.

primitive reflexes Infantile reflexes that tend to fade in the first year of life (i.e., the suck, startle, and root).

prompts Cues (e.g., verbal, visual) that direct the child to participate in a targeted activity.

prone Face down.

prophase The initial stage in cell division when the chromosomes thicken and shorten to look like separate strands.

prophylaxis Use of a preventive agent.

proptosis Appearance of protruding eyes.

prosencephalon *See* forebrain.

prosocial Socially acceptable.

prosody The intonation and rhythm of speech.

prospective Pertaining to 1) treatment in anticipation of the development of a disorder or 2) a managed health care model based on payment (e.g., of insurance premiums) before services are rendered.

proximal Describing the part nearest the midline or trunk.

proxy consent Consent for treatment or research given by a parent or guardian for a child or an incompetent adult.

pseudohypertrophy Enlarged but weak muscle, as found in muscular dystrophy.

PSR *See* positive support reflex.

psychoeducational Pertaining to the testing of intelligence, academic achievement, and other types of psychological and educational processes.

psychosis A psychiatric disorder characterized by hallucinations, delusions, loss of contact with reality, and unclear thinking; *adjective:* psychotic.

psychotherapy Nonpharmacological treatment for an individual with an emotional disorder. Various types of psychotherapy range from supportive counseling to psychoanalysis with services usually provided by a psychologist, psychiatrist, or social worker.

ptosis Drooping of eyelid.

PTSD *See* posttraumatic stress disorder.

PUBS *See* percutaneous umbilical blood sampling.

pulmonary Pertaining to the lungs.

pulmonary hypertension Increased back pressure in the pulmonary artery leading to decreased oxygenation and right heart failure.

pulmonary vascular resistance Vasoconstriction of the pulmonary blood vessels normally high during fetal life, which should relax immediately upon birth with the first breaths of life.

pulmonary vasodilation Relaxation of the lung's blood vessels soon after birth to establish lung circulation and extinguish fetal circulation.

pulp The soft tissue under the dentin layer in teeth containing blood vessels, lymphatics (lymph vessels), connective tissue, and nerve fibers.

pulse oximeter A device that measures oxygen tension noninvasively.

punishment In behavior management, a procedure or consequence that decreases the frequency of a behavior through the use of a negative stimulus or withdrawal of a preferred activity/object.

pupil The aperture in the center of the iris.

purine A type of organic molecule found in RNA and DNA.

PVL *See* periventricular leukomalacia.

PVR *See* pulmonary vascular resistance.

pyloric stenosis A congenital narrowing of the opening from the stomach to the small bowel.

pyramidal tract A nerve tract; *also called* the corticospinal tract, leading from the cortex into the spinal column and involved in the control of voluntary motor movement. Damage to this tract results in spasticity, commonly seen in cerebral palsy.

pyridoxine Vitamin B_6.

quickening The first signs of life felt by the mother as a result of fetal movements in the fourth or fifth month of pregnancy.

rad A measure of radioactivity.

radiograph A medical X ray.

ratio schedules Provision of reinforcement following a set number of correct responses.

real-time ultrasonography The use of sound waves to provide a moving (real-time) image used in fetal monitoring.

rebound A phenomenon in which as a medication dose wears off, a person's behavior or symptoms become worse than when completely off medication.

receptive aphasia Impairment of receptive language due to a disorder of the central nervous system (CNS).

receptive language The understanding of language.

recessive Pertaining to a trait that is expressed only if the child inherits two copies of the gene.

refracted Deflected through a substance (e.g., a lens).

reinforcer A response to a behavior that in-

creases the likelihood that the behavior will occur again.

related services Services (e.g., transportation, occupational and physical therapy) that supplement the special education services provided to a child with a disability.

resonance In linguistics and speech-language pathology, the balance of air flow between the nose and the mouth.

retina The photosensitive nerve layer of the eye.

retinoscope An instrument used to detect errors of refraction in the eye.

retrospective 1) Looking backward; 2) pertaining to a fee-for-service health care model in which payment occurs after services are rendered.

retrovirus 1) A type of DNA virus that is involved in gene therapy; 2) the class of viruses that includes human immunodeficiency virus (HIV), the causative agent of acquired immunodeficiency syndrome (AIDS).

Rh incompatibility Condition occurring when an Rh⁺ baby is born to an Rh⁻ mother. This leads to breakdown of red blood cells in the baby and the excessive release of bilirubin, predisposing the Rh⁺ baby to kernicterus. This condition is prevented by the use of the drug RhoGAM in the Rh⁻ mother who is carrying an Rh⁺ fetus.

rhombencephalon The hindbrain region of the embryo.

ribonucleic acid (RNA) A molecule essential for protein synthesis within the cell.

ribosome Intracellular structure concerned with protein synthesis.

rickets Bone disease resulting from nutritional deficiency of vitamin D.

rights Moral or legal claims by one party against another.

rigid Pertaining to increased tone marked by stiffness; seen in dyskinetic cerebral palsy.

ring chromosome A ring-shaped chromosome formed when deletions occur at both tips of a normal chromosome with subsequent fusion of the tips, forming a ring.

RNA *See* ribonucleic acid.

rods Photoreceptor cells of the eye associated with low-light vision.

rolandic epilepsy An inherited benign form of epilepsy occurring in children and characterized by arrested speech and muscular contractions of the side of the face.

rootlets Small branches of nerve roots.

rubella A viral infection. Generally causes a

mild elevation of temperature and skin rash and resolves in a few days. However, when it occurs in a pregnant woman during the first trimester, it can lead to intrauterine infection and severe birth defects; *also called* German measles.

SAH *See* subarachnoid hemorrhage.

salicylates Chemicals found in many food substances and in aspirin.

sarcomeres The contractile units of the muscle fiber.

Sarnat neurological score The most popular system for grading the severity of hypoxic ischemic encephalopathy (HIE); it ranges from 1 (*mild*) to 3 (*severe*) in neonates.

satiation Having had enough or too much of something.

saturated fatty acid A type of fatty acid in the diet that has been linked to heart disease more frequently than unsaturated fatty acids have been.

scala media Fluid-filled cavity within the cochlea of the ear.

schizencephaly A severely malformed brain with clefts formed because of a neuronal migrational defect during early embryogenesis.

schizophrenia A psychiatric disorder with characteristic psychotic symptoms (i.e., prominent delusions, hallucinations, catatonic behavior, and/or flat affect).

sclera The white, outer covering of the eyeball.

scoliosis Lateral curvature of the spine.

SDH *See* subdural hemorrhage.

seborrheic dermatitis Dandruff.

secondary 1) Occurring as a consequence of a primary disorder; 2) pertaining to the permanent teeth.

secretin Hormone produced in the duodenum that stimulates secretion of pancreatic enzymes.

seizure threshold Tolerance level of the brain for electrical activity. If level of tolerance is exceeded, a seizure occurs.

semantics The study of and conventions governing meanings of words.

sensory integration (SI) therapy Therapy that uses controlled sensory stimulation combined with a meaningful adaptive response to achieve changes in learning and behavior. A common method used in occupational therapy.

separation anxiety Excessive concern about separation, usually of mother from child (e.g., school phobia).

sepsis Infection that has spread throughout the bloodstream and can be life threatening; *also called* blood poisoning.

sequential modification If desired changes in behavior are not observed to occur across settings and behaviors, concrete steps are taken to introduce the effective intervention (e.g., positive reinforcement) to each of the behaviors or settings to which transfer of effects is inadequate.

serotonin reuptake inhibitors A group of psychoactive drugs, an example being fluoxetine (Prozac) used to treat depression.

serum *See* plasma.

sex chromosomes The X and Y chromosomes that determine gender.

sex-linked trait *See* X-linked trait.

shadowing Technique in which the instructor keeps his or her hands within an inch of the child's hands as the child proceeds to complete the task.

shared decision making Patient or proxy and physician participate together in committing to a treatment decision.

SI therapy *See* sensory integration therapy.

SIDS *See* sudden infant death syndrome.

single nucleotide polymorphisms (SNPs) DNA sequence variations.

single photon emission computed tomography (SPECT) An imaging technique that permits the study of the metabolism of a body organ, most commonly the brain.

sleep apnea Brief periods of arrested breathing during sleep, most commonly found in premature infants and in older children and adults with morbid obesity.

sleep myoclonus Sudden jerking movements of the body associated with various sleep stages that may be confused with a seizure.

small for gestational age (SGA) Refers to a newborn whose weight is below the third percentile for gestational age.

SNPs *See* single nucleotide polymorphisms.

soft neurological signs A group of neurological findings that are normal in young children, but when found in older children suggest immaturities in central nervous system (CNS) development (i.e., difficulty performing sequential finger–thumb opposition, rapid alternating movements).

soft spot *See* anterior fontanelle.

somatic Relating to the body.

spastic Pertaining to increased muscle tone

in which muscles are stiff and movements are difficult; caused by damage to the pyramidal tract in the brain.

spastic diplegia A form of cerebral palsy primarily seen in former premature infants that is manifested as spasticity of both lower extremities with only mild involvement of upper extremities.

spastic hemiplegia A form of cerebral palsy in which one side of the body demonstrates spasticity and the other side is unaffected.

spastic quadriplegia A form of cerebral palsy in which all four limbs are affected. Increased muscle tone (i.e., spasticity) is caused by damage to the pyramidal tract in the brain.

spasticity Abnormally increased muscle tone.

speaking valve A valve that can be used by children who have tracheostomy tubes to permit vocalizations.

specific language impairment A significant deficit in linguistic functioning that does not appear to be accompanied by deficits in hearing, intelligence, or motor functioning.

SPECT *See* single photon emission computed tomography.

spectral karyotyping An advanced form of chromosome analysis that can identify small alternations than cannot be seen by normal karyotype analysis.

speech and language disorders Problems in communication and related areas such as oral-motor function.

spermatocytes Sperm.

spina bifida A developmental defect of the spine; *also called* spinal dysraphism.

spina bifida occulta Generally benign congenital defect of the spinal column not associated with protrusion of the spinal cord or meninges.

spinal cord The thick, whitish cord of nerve tissue that extends from the base of the brain down through the spinal column.

spinal dysraphism *See* spina bifida.

spinal muscular atrophy Congenital neuromuscular disorder of childhood associated with progressive muscle weakness.

spinal tap *See* lumbar puncture.

spindle In mitosis and meiosis, a web-like figure along which the chromosomes are distributed; not to be confused with muscle spindle.

spondyloepipheseal dysplasia Congenital structural abnormality of vertebral column caused by a lack of mineralization of bone; *also called* lag of mineralization of bone.

spontaneous recovery In behavior management, the recurrence of an undesirable behavior after it has been extinguished.

sporadic In genetics, describing a disease that occurs by chance and carries little risk of recurrence.

standardized rating scales Questionnaires concerning specific behaviors that have been completed for large samples of children so that norms and normal degrees of variation are known.

stapes One of the three small bones in the middle ear that help amplify sound.

static Unchanging.

stenosis A narrowing.

stereotypic movement disorder Disorder characterized by recurring purposeless but voluntary movements (e.g., hand flapping in children with autism); *also called* stereotypies.

stereotypies *See* stereotypic movement disorder.

steroids 1) Medications used to treat severe inflammatory diseases and infantile spasms; 2) certain natural hormones in the body.

stimulant Medication used to treat attention-deficit/hyperactivity disorder (e.g., methylphenidate [Ritalin]).

stomach flu *See* gastroenteritis.

strabismus Deviation of one or both eyes during forward gaze.

subarachnoid Beneath the arachnoid membrane, or middle layer, of the meninges.

subarachnoid hemorrhage (SAH) Hemorrhage into the fluid-filled space between the arachnoid membrane and the underlying brain that can compress or contuse the underlying brain and often may follow a particularly difficult labor and delivery that sometimes requires metal forceps or vacuum assistance to the head to get the baby out.

subdural Resting between the outer (dural) and middle (arachnoid) layers of the meninges.

subdural hematoma Localized collection of clotted blood lying in the space between the dural and arachnoid membranes that surround the brain. This results from bleeding of the cerebral blood vessels that rest between these two membranes.

subdural hemorrhage (SDH) Hemorrhage between the tough outer membrane (dura) and the meninges surrounding the brain and spinal cord that can compress or contuse the underlying brain.

subluxation Partial dislocation.

substrate A compound acted upon by an enzyme in a chemical reaction.

sucrose *See* glucose.

sudden infant death syndrome (SIDS) Diagnosis given to a previously well infant (often a former premature baby) who is found lifeless in bed without apparent cause; *also called* crib death (*see Chapter 9*).

sulci Furrows of the brain; *singular:* sulcus.

superior In anatomy, above.

supine Lying on the back, face upward.

surfactant A lipoprotein normally secreted into the alveoli with the first breaths of life that acts like a soap bubble and allows for a significant decrease in the alveolar membrane's surface tension, thus making breathing much easier and the lungs much more flexible immediately after birth.

surveillance The ongoing monitoring of disease in the population.

sutures In anatomy, the fibrous joints between certain bones (e.g., skull bones).

synapses The minute spaces separating one neuron from another. Neurochemicals breach this gap.

syncopal episode Fainting spell.

syndactyly Webbed hands or feet.

synophrys Confluent eyebrow.

syntax Word order.

syphilis A sexually transmitted disease that can cause an intrauterine infection in pregnant women and result in severe birth defects.

syringomas Benign sweat glad tumors.

syringomyelia A chronic disease of the spinal cord characterized by the presence of fluid.

systemic Involving the whole body.

tachycardia Rapid heart rate.

talipes equinovarus *See* clubfoot.

tandem mass spectrometer (MS/MS) The machine used in newborn screening to detect certain inborn errors of metabolism.

tandem mass spectroscopy The method used in newborn screening to detect certain inborn errors of metabolism.

tangibles Rewards given in positive reinforcement procedures (e.g., food, toys).

tardive dyskinesia A potentially severe movement disorder resulting from the long-term use of phenothiazines or other antipsychotic medication.

target behavior Behavior selected for assessment and management.

tartar *See* calculus.

telangiectasia Abnormal cluster of small blood vessels.

teletypewriter (TTY) An electronic device for text communication via a telephone line used when one or more of the parties has hearing or speech difficulties.

telophase The final phase in cell division in which the daughter chromosomes are at the opposite poles of the cell and new nuclear membranes form.

temporal lobe Brain region involved in visual and auditory processing.

tendons Fibrous cords by which muscles are attached to bone or to one another.

teratogens Agents that can cause malformations in a developing embryo.

testosterone Male sex hormone.

tetraploid Having four copies of each chromosome (i.e., 92 chromosomes). This is incompatible with life.

thalamus Region of the brain situated in the posterior part of the forebrain that relays sensory impulses to the cerebral cortex.

thimerosal A mercury-containing organic compound that was used as a preservative in vaccines.

thrombocytopenia Low platelet count.

thrombophilia A genetic tendency for one's blood to clot more than normal (thrombus formation).

thrush Monilial (fungal) yeast infection of the oral cavity sometimes seen in infants.

thymine One of the four nucleotides (chemicals) that comprise DNA.

thyrotoxicosis A form of hyperthyroidism leading to severe symptoms.

tics Brief repetitive movements or vocalizations that occur in a stereotyped manner and do not appear to be under voluntary control.

time-out A procedure whereby the possibility of positive reinforcement is withdrawn for a predetermined brief amount of time following the occurrence of a targeted challenging behavior.

TLR *See* tonic labyrinthine reflex.

tocolysis Use of medications to stop premature labor.

tonic labyrinthine reflex (TLR) Primitive reflex in which the infant retracts the arms and extends the legs when the neck is tilted backwards, stimulating the labyrinth.

tonic-clonic Spasmodic alteration of muscle contraction and relaxation.

tonotopically Arranged spatially by tone as found in the cochlea or inner ear.

tooth bud *See* dental organ.

torticollis Wry neck in which the neck is painfully tilted to one side; a form of dystonia.

toxemia *See* preeclampsia.

toxoplasma gondii Microorganism causing toxoplasmosis.

toxoplasmosis An infectious disease caused by a microorganism, which may be asymptomatic in adults but can lead to severe fetal malformations.

trachea Windpipe.

tracheoesophageal fistula A congenital connection between the trachea and esophagus leading to aspiration of food and requiring surgical correction.

tracheomalacia Softening of the cartilage of the trachea.

tracheostomy 1) The surgical creation of an opening into the trachea to permit insertion of a tube to facilitate mechanical ventilation; 2) the tube itself.

trachoma A bacterial infection causing blindness in developing countries.

transcription The process in which mRNA is formed from a DNA template.

transitional (fetal) circulation Circulatory changes occurring at birth in the lungs and around the heart, resulting from pulmonary vasodilation and closure of the ductus arteriosus and the foramen ovale (the two fetal by-passes around the lungs during fetal life).

translation The process in which an amino acid sequence is assembled according to the pattern specified by mRNA.

translocation The transfer of a fragment of one chromosome to another chromosome.

tremor A trembling motion.

Treponema pallium Microorganism causing syphilis.

triplet repeat expansion Abnormal number of copies of identical triplet nucleotides (as occurs in fragile X syndrome; *see Chapter 19*).

triploid Having three copies of each chromosome (i.e., 69 chromosomes), which is generally incompatible with life.

trisomy A condition is which there are three copies of one chromosome rather than two (e.g., trisomy 21, Down syndrome).

trophoblast The outermost layer of cells that attaches the fertilized egg to the uterine wall.

TTY *See* teletypewriter.

tubers Benign congenital tumors found in the brain of an individual with tuberous sclerosis (*see Appendix B*).

twinning The production of twins.

tympanometry The measurement of flexibility of the tympanic membrane as an indicator

of a middle-ear infection or fluid in the middle ear.

tyrosine An amino acid.

umbilical cord prolapse The umbilical cord being born before rather than after the baby, thereby becoming compressed by the fetus during the delivery process and interfering with oxygen flow to the fetus during labor; typically occurs with polyhydramnios.

undernutrition Inadequate nutrition to sustain normal growth.

uniparental disomy *See* genomic imprinting.

unsaturated fatty acid A type of dietary fat, certain kinds of which have been linked to heart disease.

urea End product of protein metabolism.

ureterostomy Surgical procedure creating an outlet for the ureters through the abdominal wall.

urethra Canal through which urine passes from the bladder.

valgus Condition in which the distal body part is angled away from the mid-line.

varicella The virus that causes chickenpox and shingles.

varus Condition in which the distal body part is angled toward the mid-line.

vasoconstriction A decrease in the diameter of blood vessels.

ventilator A machine that provides a mixture of air and oxygen to an individual in respiratory failure. The oxygen content, pressure, volume, and frequency of respirators can be adjusted.

ventricles Fluid filled cavities, especially in the heart or brain.

ventricular septal defect A congenital heart disease in which the wall separating the two lower chambers of the heart does not close.

ventricular system Interconnecting cavities of the brain containing cerebrospinal fluid. Blockage leads to hydrocephalus.

ventriculoperitoneal shunt (VP shunt) Tube connecting a cerebral ventricle with the abdominal cavity used to treat hydrocephalus.

vertebral arches The bony arches projecting from the body of the vertebra.

vertex presentation Downward position of infant's head during vaginal delivery.

very low birth weight (VLBW) Term often used to describe an infant with a birth weight less than 1,500 grams (3⅓ pounds).

vesicles Small, fluid-containing elevations in the upper layer of skin, as seen in chickenpox.

vesicostomy The surgical creation of an opening for the bladder to empty its contents through the abdominal wall.

vestibular system Three ring-shaped bodies located in the labyrinth of the ear that are involved in maintenance of balance and sensation of the body's movement through space.

villi Vascular projections, such as those coming from the embryo that become part of the placenta; *singular:* villus.

vision impairment A condition characterized by a loss of visual acuity, where the eye does not see objects as clearly as usual, or a loss of visual field, where the eye cannot see as wide an area as usual without moving the eyes or turning the head.

vitiligo A skin disease marked by patches of lack of pigment.

vitreous humor The gelatinous content of the eye located between the lens and retina.

VLBW *See* very low birth weight.

VP shunt *See* ventriculoperitoneal shunt.

watershed area Area of tissue lying between two major arteries and thus poorly supplied by blood.

watershed infarct Injury to brain due to lack of blood flow in the brain tissues between interfacing blood vessels.

xerosis Dry skin.

X-linked trait A trait transmitted by a gene located on the X chromosome; *previously called* sex-linked.

zygote Fertilized egg.

B Syndromes and Inborn Errors of Metabolism

Erynn S. Gordon

The underlying cause of a developmental disability can be explained in some children by a single genetic or teratogenic mechanism. An understanding of the etiology can shed light on the reason for clinical features such as physical malformations, cognitive impairments, and behavior problems. Making a diagnosis in such cases may be important for physicians to implement appropriate medical management or to provide genetic or prenatal counseling. Other professionals may also find that a diagnosis assists them in the development of more global aspects of the child's care, including educational, physical, occupational, and speech-language therapy. The direct benefit to families includes the ability to gather information specific to their child's condition and to seek out support from other parents and/or affected individuals through support groups, conferences, and the Internet. Finally, attaining a specific diagnosis can lead patients, families, and health care professionals to the appropriate disease-oriented organization, which is often a great source of information and support (emotional and sometimes financial). For all of these reasons, the search for an etiology of a child's developmental disability may focus on syndrome identification.

By definition, a syndrome is a collection of two or more features with a single origin. Syndromes may have a genetic basis (see Chapter 1) or can be caused by teratogens (see Chapter 5). Genetic syndromes affect multiple organ systems because the genetic defect is usually contained in every cell of the body. This abnormality may interfere with typical development or cause abnormal differentiation of more than one tissue of the body. Most genetic and teratologic syndromes are of prenatal onset and are evident at birth, usually because of an unusual appearance (i.e., dysmorphic features) or multiple congenital abnormalities. Syndromes are usually stable conditions, and neurological regression is uncommon. An association, or a sequence, is a single localized anomaly and its secondary defects.

Unlike most syndromes, inborn errors of metabolism are usually not evident at birth. During pregnancy, the mother's normal metabolism protects the fetus. After delivery, however, there may be an accumulation of toxic metabolites as a result of an enzyme deficiency. The presentation of inborn errors varies from metabolic crisis and death within days of birth to occasional episodes in response to external factors later in childhood. Some metabolic disorders are treatable, and many in this category of genetic conditions are detectable with newborn screening through biochemical or molecular testing (see Chapters 7 and 8).

Although the clinical features associated with certain syndromes and inborn errors of metabolism have been known for centuries (e.g., Down syndrome, congenital hypothyroidism), the chromosomal and molecular bases of the disorders have only been characterized since the 1960s. An increasing number of genetic and biochemical tests can now be utilized to confirm a clinically suspected diagnosis. This is of particular importance because different therapeutic options (or the opportunity to participate in clinical research trials) may be available to individuals on the basis of a genetic diagnosis, particularly in the cases of molecularly based therapies. In addition, a genetic diagnosis allows for accurate recurrence risk estimates and appropriate genetic counseling for other family members.

Research on the cognitive abilities of individuals with genetic syndromes is uncovering specific learning and behavior patterns for many syndromes. These are called behavioral phenotypes, and they can be used to establish rational and attainable educational goals to promote the child's reaching his or her full cognitive and functional potential (see Finegan, J.A. [1998]. Study of behavioral phenotypes: Goals and methodological considerations. *American Journal of Medical Genetics, 81*, 148–155). Insight into an individual's specific condition, the behavioral phenotype, cognitive abilities, and learning strengths and weakness can be of particular importance in the classroom. References addressing the cognitive and behavioral abilities of individuals with specific genetic conditions are included in this appendix.

Many excellent resources concerning genetic conditions exist for families and health care professionals caring for children with disabilities. These include the Genetic Alliance, which has a directory of support groups, foundations, research organizations, patient advocacy groups, and tissue registries. The Genetic Alliance is based in Washington, D.C. (202-966-5557; http://www.geneticalliance.org; e-mail: info@geneticalliance.org). Two other excellent resources are GeneTests and GeneReviews (http://www.genetests.org), both administered by the University of Washington and funded by the National Institutes of Health (NIH), the Health Resources and Services Administration (HRSA), and the U.S. Department of Energy (DOE). GeneTests has a directory of clinics and laboratories that provide genetic testing. In addition, some educational tools for professionals are available. GeneReviews provides peer-reviewed articles on genetic conditions that include information on diagnosis, management, and genetic counseling of individuals with specific inherited disorders and their families. The National Organization for Rare Disorders (NORD; 203-746-6518; http://www.rarediseases.org) is a patient advocacy organization dedicated to orphan diseases (disorders occurring in less than 200,000 individuals in the United States). This organization's rare disease database, newsletter, and directory of participating organizations (including support groups and foundations) are useful to families and clinicians alike. NORD also offers research grants and fellowships to physician-scientists. The Online Mendelian Inheritance in Man (OMIM; http://www.ncbi.nlm.nih.gov/omim) catalog describes all known Mendelian disorders, providing clinical, biochemical, genetic, and therapeutic information. The National Coalition for Health Professionals Education in Genetics (NCHPEG) (http://www.nchpeg.org) is dedicated to promoting genetic knowledge among health care professionals. The NCHPEG web site offers specific web-based educational programs in a variety of areas, including dentistry, counseling, family history taking, and general core competencies in genetics. The Genetics Home Reference, sponsored by the National Library of Medicine (http://www.ghr.nlm.nih.gov/ghr), is an excellent resource for health care professionals, teachers, and families, providing basic information about genetics and searchable disease-specific data.

This appendix lists a number of syndromes and inborn errors of metabolism that are often associated with developmental disabilities. Included in each listing are the principal characteristics, pattern of inheritance, frequency of occurrence (prevalence or incidence), treatment options when available, and recent references that further define the syndrome. Cognitive and behavioral changes are noted for disorders in which common developmental abnormalities are widely accepted as being part of the syndrome or inborn error. When known, the causative gene or chromosome location is listed. In describing the chromosomal location, the first number or letter indicates the chromosome on which there is a genetic change (mutation), and the subsequent letter (p or q) indicates the short or long arm of the chromosome, respectively. The term *ter* is used when the site is at the terminal end of one arm of the chromosome, and *cen* is used when the site is near the **centromere**. The numbers following the p or q specify the location on the chromosome. For example, Aarskog-Scott syndrome is located on the short arm of the X chromosome at position 11.21, designated as Xp11.21. The inheritance patterns of genetic traits are listed as autosomal recessive (AR), autosomal dominant (AD), X-linked recessive (XLR), X-linked dominant (XLD), mitochondrial (M), new mutation (NM) (i.e., diseases caused by new mutations that arise in the sperm or the egg), or sporadic (SP) (i.e., noninherited). In the rare syndromes for which a treatment is available, a description of that treatment is included in the description. Treatment is more often available for inborn errors of metabolism. Although this appendix lists a number of the more commonly recognized syndromes associated with developmental disabilities, it is not intended to be all-inclusive. Specific medical terminology is defined in the glossary (see Appendix A); glossary terms that appear here for the first time are presented in boldface type.

Aarskog-Scott syndrome (faciodigitogenital dysplasia [FGDY]) *Clinical features:* Short stature, brachydactyly (short fingers and toes), widow's peak, broad nasal bridge with small nose, hypertelorism, shawl scrotum, **cryptorchidism** (undescended testes); learning disabilities and behavioral problems are present in a subset of patients. *Associated complications:* Ptosis, eye movement problems, strabismus, orthodontic problems, occasional cleft lip/palate. *Cause:* Mutations in the FGD1 gene at Xp11.21. *Inheritance:* XLR with partial expression in some females; rare AD cases reported. *Prevalence:* Unknown, phenotypic overlap with other conditions.

References: Logie, L.J., & Porteous, M.E.M. (1998). Intelligence and development in Aarskog syndrome. *Archives of Disease in Childhood, 79*, 359–360.

Orrico, A., Galli, L., Cavaliere M.L., et al. (2004). Phenotypic and molecular characterisation of the Aarskog-Scott syndrome: A survey of the clinical variability in light of FGD1 mutation analysis in 46 patients. *European Journal of Human Genetics, 12*(1), 16–23.

Teebi, A.S., Rucquoi, J.K., & Meyn, M.S. (1993). Aarskog syndrome: Report of a family with review and discussion of nosology. *American Journal of Medical Genetics, 46*, 501–509.

achondroplasia *Clinical features:* The most common form of short stature, associated with disproportionately shortened limbs. Narrowing of the foramen magnum may lead to apneic episodes, hydrocephalus, hypotonia, hyperreflexia, or clonus. In addition, cervical spinal cord compression may occur as a result of a narrowing of the spinal canal, which requires decompression surgery. Children with achondroplasia should be monitored for changes in their neurological status, particularly if there are concerns about delayed motor development. Cognitive development is usually typical. *Incidence:* 1 of every 15,000–25,000 live births. *Cause:* Point mutation in the gene coding for fibroblast growth factor receptor 3 or FGFR3. *Inheritance:* 80% of cases caused by NM with AD inheritance when passed from an affected individual.

References: Ho, N.C., Guarnieri, M., Brant L.J., et al. (2004). Living with achondroplasia: Quality of life evaluation following cervico-medullary decompression. *Ameri-*can *Journal of Medical Genetics Part A, 131* (2), 163–167.

Savarirayan, R., Rimoin, & D.L. (2002). The skeletal dysplasias. *Best Practice and Research in Clinical Endocrinology and Metabolism, 16*(3), 547–560.

acrocephalosyndactyly, type I *See* Apert syndrome.

acrocephalosyndactyly, type II *See* Carpenter syndrome.

acrocephalosyndactyly, type V *See* Pfeiffer syndrome.

acrofacial dysostosis (Nager syndrome) *Clinical features:* **Micrognathia** (small jaw), malar hypoplasia (underdeveloped cheeks), downward slant of eyelids, high nasal bridge, external ear defects, occasional cleft lip/palate, asymmetric limb anomalies (hypoplastic thumb or radius [a bone in the lower arm]). *Associated complications:* Scoliosis, severe conductive hearing loss, occasional heart or kidney defects, intellectual disability present in 16%. *Cause:* Proposed causative gene is CFP37 linked to chromosome 9q32. *Inheritance:* Most cases NM with evidence of AD inheritance, rare reports of AR. *Prevalence:* Rare.

References: Dreyer S.D., Zhou L, Machado M.A., et al. (1998). Cloning, characterization, and chromosomal assignment of the human ortholog of murine Zfp-37, a candidate gene for Nager syndrome. *Mammalian Genome, 9*, 458–462.

Hunt J.A., & Hobar, P.C. (2002). Common craniofacial anomalies: The facial dysostoses. *Plastic and Reconstructive Surgery, 110*, 1714–1726.

McDonald, J.T., & Gorski, J.L. (1993). Nager acrofacial dysostosis. *Journal of Medical Genetics, 30*, 779–782.

adrenoleukodystrophy (X-linked ALD) *(For neonatal form, see* adrenoleukodystrophy, neonatal form.) *Clinical features:* Progressive neurological disorder of white matter resulting from accumulation of very long chain fatty acids; both childhood and adult onset forms occur. Adult onset form is characterized mainly be adrenal insufficiency and usually presents with peripheral neuropathy (disturbance of the peripheral nerves) and causes slowly progressive paraparesis (partial paralysis) and impotence. Only 20% of adult onset cases experience brain involvement. Boys with the childhood onset form are symptom free at birth and develop typically until the end of the first decade. Symptoms often begin with behavioral problems and progress to include spasticity, ataxia, peripheral neuropathy, and speech disturbance. *Associated complications:* Progressive intellectual deterioration, seizures, endocrine abnormalities, conductive hearing loss. *Cause:* Mutations in ABCD1 gene at Xq28. The ALD protein product is localized to the peroxisomal membrane. *Inheritance:* XLR, with intrafamilial variability ranging from classical childhood onset ALD to adult onset ALD to Addison disease. *Incidence:* 1/100,000 males in the United States. *Treatment:* Adrenal hormone therapy for adrenal insufficiency (will not alter neurologic symptoms). Bone marrow transplant can provide long-term stability and may reverse some neurologic complications in the early stages. Dietary modifications including "Lorenzo's oil" (oleic acid and erucic acid) have been shown to have some benefit for presymptomatic patients but not in symptomatic patients.

References: Moser, H., Dubey, P., & Faemi, A. (2004). Progress in X-linked adrenoleukodystrophy. *Current Opinion in Neurology, 7,* 263–269.

van Geel, B.M., Assies, J., Haverkort, E.B., et al. (1999). Progression of abnormalities in adrenomyeloneuropathy and neurologically asymptomatic X-linked adrenoleukodystrophy despite treatment with "Lorenzo's oil." *Journal of Neurology, Neurosurgery, and Psychiatry, 67,* 290–299.

adrenoleukodystrophy, neonatal form *(For childhood form, see* adrenoleukodystrophy [X-linked ALD].) *Clinical features:* A disorder of peroxisomes (minute organelles in certain cells that are involved in the processing of long chain fatty acids) characterized by congenital hypotonia (low muscle tone), onset in early infancy of seizures, hypotonia, and adrenal insufficiency; mild dysmorphic facial features include high forehead, epicanthal folds (vertical fold of skin on either side of the nose), broad nasal bridge, and anteverted (forward-tipping) nostrils. Developmental progress is achieved during the first year of life followed by regression. Death in early childhood is usual, but there are known cases of affected individuals surviving until the second or third decade of life. *Associated complications:* Intellectual disability, cataracts, visual and auditory impairment. *Cause:* Absence of peroxisomes, resulting from mutations in a

number of autosomal peroxin (PEX) genes. *Inheritance:* AR. *Prevalence:* Rare.

References: Moser, A.B., Rasmussen, M., Naidu, S., et al. (1995). Phenotype of patients with peroxisomal disorders subdivided into sixteen complementation groups. *Journal of Pediatrics, 127,* 13–22.

Percey A.K., & Rutledge S.L. (2001). Adrenoleukodystrophy and related disorders. *Mental Retardation and Developmental Disabilities Research Reviews, 7,* 179–189.

Aicardi syndrome *Clinical features:* Infantile spasms beginning between three and four months of age, absence or hypoplasia of the corpus callosum, spastic hemiplegia, abnormalities of eyes (including the retina), vertebral or rib anomalies, evidence of neuronal migration disorder, severe intellectual disability. *Associated complications:* Poorly controlled seizures, visual impairment. *Cause:* Gene linked to Xp22. *Inheritance:* XLD/NM; it is presumed that mutations in this gene are lethal in males; only one familial case has been reported. *Prevalence:* Rare.

Reference: Aicardi, J. (2005). Aicardi syndrome. *Brain and Development, 27,* 164–171.

alcohol-related neurodevelopmental defects (ARND) *Previously called* fetal alcohol effects (FAE); *see Chapter 5.*

Alexander disease *Clinical features:* Progressive neurological disorder characterized by macrocephaly, exaggerated startle response, optic atrophy, intellectual decline, seizures, early death. *Associated complications:* Hydrocephalus, demyelination, progressive spasticity, visual impairment; bulbar signs are present in some patients. Infantile (diagnosed at less than 2 years old), juvenile (diagnosed between 2 to 12 years old), and adult onset forms (diagnosed beyond age 13 years) have been described. *Cause:* Mutations in the GFAP gene are known to be causative, (coding for glial fibrillary acidic protein at 17q21). *Inheritance:* Majority of cases caused by a NM with AD inheritance when passed from an affected individual; rare AD families have been reported. *Prevalence:* Rare.

References: Johnson, A.B. (2002). Alexander disease: A review and the gene. *International Journal of Developmental Neuroscience, 20,* 391–394.

Rong L., Johnson, A.B., & Salomons, G. (2005). Glial fibrillary acidic protein mutations in infantile, juvenile, and adult forms of Alexander disease. *Annals of Neurology, 57,* 310–326.

Angelman syndrome *Clinical features:* "Puppet-like" gait, large mouth, small head with bra-chycephaly (short head), prominent jaw, ataxia, sudden bursts of inappropriate laugh-ter, generalized depigmentation of hair. *Asso-ciated complications:* Seizures, severe intellec-tual disability, paucity of speech. Behavioral features include hyperactivity, chewing or mouthing of objects, fascination with water, hand flapping, sleep disturbance, and gorging food. *Cause:* Deletion of 15q11–q13 on the maternally inherited chromosome or pater-nal inheritance of both copies of chromosome 15 (uniparental disomy, or UPD) or a point mutation in the maternal copy of the UBE3A gene. *Inheritance:* All three causes arise as a re-sult of NM; mutations in the UBE3A gene may be passed in an AD fashion. *Prevalence:* 1/10,000–1/20,000.

References: Berry, R.J., Leitner, R.P., Clarke, A.R., & Einfeld, S.L. (2005). Behavioral as-pects of Angelman syndrome: A case con-trol study. *American Journal of Medical Ge-netics, 132,* 8–12.

Varela, M.C., Kok, R., Otto, P.A., & Koiff-mann, C.P. (2004). Phenotypic variability in Angelman syndrome: Comparison among different deletion cases and between dele-tion and UPD subjects. *European Journal of Human Genetics, 12,* 987–992.

Apert syndrome (acrocephalosyndactyly, type I) *Clinical features:* (craniosynostosis) pre-mature fusion of the cranial sutures with mis-shapen head, high forehead, and flat occiput (back part of head); hypertelorism with down-ward slant; flat mid-face and nasal bridge; se-vere syndactyly (webbing of fingers or toes); limb anomalies; cleft palate. *Associated compli-cations:* Hydrocephalus, varying degrees of intellectual disability, hearing loss, teeth ab-normalities, occasional heart and kidney anomalies. *Cause:* Mutations in the fibroblast growth factor receptor-2 (FGFR2) gene on chromosome 10q26. *Inheritance:* Majority of cases are caused by a NM, with AD inheri-tance when passed from an affected individ-ual. *Prevalence:* 1.5/100,000. *Treatment:* Early neurosurgical correction of fused sutures im-proves appearance and may reduce risk of in-tellectual disability; plastic/orthopedic sur-gery for limb anomalies.

References: Lajeunie, E., Cameron, R., El Ghouzzi, V., et al. (1999). Clinical variabil-ity in patients with Apert's syndrome. *Jour-nal of Neurosurgery, 90,* 443–447.

Yacubian-Fernandes A., Palhares A., Gilgio

A., et al. (2004). Apert syndrome: Analysis of associated brain malformations and con-formational changes determined by surgi-cal treatment. *Journal of Neuroradiology, 31,* 116–122.

ARND Alcohol-related neurodevelopmental disorder; *see Chapter 5.*

arthrogryposis multiplex congenita *Clinical features:* Nonprogressive joint contractures that begin prenatally; flexion contractures at the fingers, knees, and elbows, with muscle weakness around involved joints. *Associated complications:* Occasional kidney and eye anomalies, cleft palate, defects of abdominal wall, scoliosis. *Cause:* Multiple; most fre-quently related to an underlying neuropathy, myopathy (muscle weakness), or in utero crowding; may be associated with maternal myasthenia gravis; nerve conduction stud-ies/EMG and muscle biopsy may be benefi-cial in determining the basis of the condition (myopathic versus neurogenic). *Inheritance:* Usually SP and may be caused by teratogenic exposure; however both AD or AR inheri-tance also have been reported. *Incidence:* Ranges from 1/3,000 to 1/12,000. *Treatment:* Casting of affected joints or surgery, if indi-cated.

References: Gordon, N. (1998). Arthrogrypo-sis multiplex congenita. *Brain Development, 20,* 507–511.

Kang, P.B., Lidov, H.G., David, W.S., et al. (2003). Diagnostic value of electromyog-raphy and muscle biopsy in arthrogryposis multiplex congenital. *Annals of Neurology, 54,* 790–795.

ataxia telangiectasia *Clinical features:* Slowly progressive ataxia, telangiectasias (dilation of capillaries, especially in the sclera [whites of eye] and behind the earlobe), immune de-fects, elevated alpha-fetoprotein in blood. *Associated complications:* Dystonia or choreo-athetosis, dysarthric speech (imperfect artic-ulation due to decreased motor control), in-creased sensitivity to radiation, increased risk of malignancy (often lymphoma), eye move-ment abnormalities, finger contractures, in-creased risk of sinus and pulmonary infec-tions; intelligence is typically unaffected, but may decline with disease progression. *Cause:* Mutation in the ATM gene on chromosome 11q22.3. *Inheritance:* AR. *Prevalence:* 1/40,000 in the United States.

References: Chun, H.H., & Gatti, R.A. (2004). Ataxia-telangectasia: An evolving pheno-type. *DNA Repair, 3,* 1187–1196.

Crawford, T.O., Mandir, A.S., Lefton-Greif, M.A., et al. (2000). Quantitative neurologic assessment of ataxia-telangiectasia. *Neurology, 54,* 1505–1509.

Bardet-Biedl syndrome *Clinical features:* Obesity, genital anomalies, polydactyly (extra fingers or toes), retinal anomalies. *Associated complications:* Intellectual disability or learning disabilities, speech disorder, abnormal liver function, cataracts, occasional cardiac and renal (kidney) anomalies, diabetes, delayed puberty, ataxia, spasticity, night blindness. (Bardet-Biedl syndrome and Laurence-Moon syndrome were previously called Laurence-Moon-Bardet-Biedl syndrome but are now known to be separate disorders.) *Cause:* Linked to six distinct chromosomal loci: 2q31, 3p12–p13, 11q13, 15q22.3–q23, 16q21, 20p12. *Inheritance:* Unusual inheritance similar to AR. *Prevalence:* Rare in most populations; increased frequency in Newfoundland as well as in Arab population in Kuwait and in Bedouin population. It is suggested that mutations in more than one locus may be necessary for the onset of symptoms. *References:* Beales, P.L., Elcioglu, N., Woolf, A.S., et al. (1999). New criteria for improved diagnosis of Bardet-Biedl syndrome: Results of a population survey. *Journal of Medical Genetics, 36,* 437–446.

Katsanis, N., Lupski, J.R., & Beales, P.L. (2001). Exploring the molecular basis of Bardet-Biedl syndrome. *Human Molecular Genetics, 10,* 2293–2299.

Sheffield, V.C. (2004). Use of isolated populations in the study of a human obesity syndrome: The Bardet-Biedl syndrome. *Pediatric Research, 55,* 908–911.

Batten disease (neuronal ceroid lipofuscinosis, juvenile) *Clinical features:* Typical development for first 2 to 4 years of life; rapid vision loss between 4 and 7 years; gradual onset of ataxia, myoclonic or major motor seizures, and retinal degeneration; typically no survival beyond adolescence. *Associated complications:* Gradual intellectual decline, spasticity, psychosis, kyphoscoliosis, decline in speech, behavioral problems, sleep disturbance. *Cause:* CLN3 gene mapped to chromosome 16p12.1, with the common cause being a large deletion in the gene. *Inheritance:* AR. *Incidence:* 7/100,000 live births in Iceland; 0.71/100,000 live births in Germany; rarer elsewhere. Many other forms of neuronal ceroid lipofuscinosis exist including infantile, late infantile, juvenile, and adult forms. Mu-

tations in 8 CLN genes cause various forms of neuronal ceroid lipofuscinosis. *References:* Goebel, H.H., & Wisniewski, K.E. (2004). Current state of clinical and morphological features in human NCL. *Brain Pathology, 14,* 61–69.

Rider, J.A., & Rider, D.L. (1999). Thirty years of Batten disease research: Present status and future goals. *Molecular Genetics and Metabolism, 66,* 231–233.

Becker muscular dystrophy (BMD) *See* muscular dystrophy.

Beckwith-Wiedemann syndrome *Clinical features:* Omphalocele (congenital defect in abdominal wall containing the intestine); macrosomia (large body size); large organs, especially the tongue; neonatal hypoglycemia (low blood sugar). *Associated complications:* Advanced growth for the first 6 years, with advanced bone age, occasional **hemihypertrophy** (enlargement of one side of the body), kidney or adrenal anomalies, increased risk of malignancy (liver, kidney, muscle), occasional intellectual disability (may be due to hypoglycemia). *Cause:* Presumed failure to suppress gene for insulin-like growth factor, type 2 (IGF2), caused by a duplication (including uniparental disomy) of paternal chromosome 11p15.5, maternal chromosomal rearrangements involving chromosome 11p15.5, or mutations in one or more critical genes in this region. *Inheritance:* Majority of cases are caused by a NM with AD inheritance with variable penetrance when passed from an affected individual. *Prevalence:* 0.07/1,000. *Treatment:* Early treatment of hypoglycemia is critical; surgical repair of omphalocele. *References:* Bliek, J., Gicquel, C., Maas, S., et al. (2004). Epigenotyping as a tool for the prediction of tumor risk and tumor type in patients with Beckwith-Wiedemann syndrome. *Journal of Pediatrics, 145,* 796–799.

Nicholls, R.D. (2000). The impact of genomic imprinting for neurobehavioral and developmental disorders. *Journal of Clinical Investigation, 105,* 413–418.

biotinidase deficiency *See* multiple carboxylase deficiency, late onset, juvenile form.

Bloom syndrome *Clinical features:* Pre- and postnatal growth retardation, dolichocephaly (long head), microcephaly, narrow face with prominent ears and nose, genital anomalies, syndactyly and/or polydactyl, skin abnormalities (café au lait spots, hyperpigmentation, hypopigmentation, facial telangectasia, hypertrichosis), mild intellectual disability or learning disabilities. *Associated complications:* Chronic lung disease, infertility in males, reduced fertility in females, non–insulin dependant diabetes, immunoglobulin deficiency, predisposition to neoplasm (lymphoma, leukemia, adenocarcinoma, squamous cell carcinoma *Cause:* mutations in the BLM gene which encodes the BLM RecQ protein on chromosome 15q26.1. *Inheritance:* AR. *Prevalence:* Overall prevalence is rare, although it is seen more commonly in the Ashkenazi Jewish population.

Reference: Kaneko, H., & Kondo, N. (2004). Clinical features of Bloom syndrome and function of the causative gene: BLM helicase. *Expert Review of Molecular Diagnostics, 4,* 393–401.

BMD muscular dystrophy, Becker type   *See* muscular dystrophy, Duchenne and Becker types.

Börjeson-Forssman-Lehmann   syndrome *Clinical features:* Obesity; short stature; postpubertal gynecomastia (breast enlargement in males); long, thick ears; coarse facial appearance; protruding tongue; hypogonadism (small testes), cataracts or other eye anomalies; tapering fingers; varying degrees of intellectual disability. *Associated complications:* Seizures, microcephaly, hypotonia. *Cause:* Causative gene *PHF6* linked to chromosome Xq26.3. *Inheritance:* XLR, with females less severely affected than males. *Prevalence:* Rare.

References: Turner, G., Gedeon, A., Mulley, J., et al. (1989). Borjeson-Forssman-Lehmann: Clinical manifestations and gene localization to Xq26–q27. *American Journal of Medical Genetics, 34,* 463–469.

Visootsak, J., Rosner, B., Dykens, E., et al. (2004). Clinical and behavioral features of patients with Borjeson-Forssman-Lehmann syndrome with mutations in PHF6. *Journal of Pediatrics, 145,* 819–825.

Brachmann de Lange syndrome   *See* de Lange syndrome.

Canavan disease (spongy degeneration of central nervous system)   *Clinical features:* Progressive neurological disorder consisting of macrocephaly, hypotonia progressing to spasticity with age, visual impairment, and early death. Symptoms begin at 3–6 months of age; children do not develop ability to sit, walk, or talk. Despite limitations, children are interactive. *Associated complications:* Feeding difficulties with progressive swallowing problems, gastroesophageal reflux, severe in-

tellectual disability, head lag. *Cause:* Deficiency in the enzyme aspartoacylase caused by a mutation in the ASPA gene on chromosome 17pter–p13. *Inheritance:* AR. *Prevalence:* Rare in most populations; about 1/5,500 in Ashkenazi Jewish population.

References: Matalon, R.M., & Michals-Matalon, K. (2000). Spongy degeneration of the brain, Canavan disease: Biochemical and molecular findings. *Frontiers in Bioscience, 5,* D307–D311.

Surendran, S., Michals-Matalon, K., Quast. M.J., et al. (2003). Canavan disease: A monogenic trait with complex genomic interaction. *Molecular Genetics and Metabolism, 80,* 74–80.

Carpenter syndrome (acrocephalosyndactyly, type II)   *Clinical features:* Craniosynostosis, flat nasal bridge, malformed and low-set ears, short digits, syndactyly and/or polydactyly, obesity, **hypogenitalism** and/or cryptorchidism. *Associated complications:* congenital heart defects, hearing loss; 75% have mild intellectual disability. *Cause:* Unknown. *Inheritance:* Presumed AR. *Prevalence:* Rare.

References: Robinson, L.K., James, H.E., Mubarak, S.J., et al. (1985). Carpenter syndrome: Natural history and clinical spectrum. *American Journal of Medical Genetics, 20,* 461–469.

Katzen, J.T., & McCarthy, J.G. (2000). Syndromes involving craniosynostosis and midface hypoplasia. *Otolaryngology Clinics of North America, 33,* 1257–1284.

cerebrohepatorenal   syndrome   *See* Zellweger syndrome.

CHARGE syndrome   *Clinical features:* **C**oloboma (defect in iris or retina), **h**eart defect, choanal **a**tresia (congenital blockage of the nasal passages), **r**etarded growth and development, **g**enital anomalies, and **e**ar anomalies with or without hearing loss. *Associated complications:* Hypogenitalism, cryptorchidism, occasional cleft lip/palate, varying degrees of intellectual disability, potentially severe visual and hearing impairments. *Cause:* Mutations in the chromodomain helicase DNA-binding protein-7 (CHD7) and semaphorin-3E gene (SEMA3E) have been shown to cause CHARGE. *Inheritance:* Majority of cases are caused by a NM, with evidence of AD inheritance when passed from an affected individual; associated with increased paternal age. Usually SP; approximately 8% of cases are familial. *Prevalence:* 1/10,000; more common in females than males.

References: Brock, K.E., Mathiason, M.A., Rooney B.L., & Williams, M.S. (2003). Quantitative analysis of limb anomalies in CHARGE syndrome: Correlation with diagnosis and characteristic CHARGE anomalies. *American Journal of Medical Genetics, 123,* 111–121.

Verloes, A. (2005). Updated diagnostic criteria for CHARGE syndrome: A proposal. *American Journal of Medical Genetics, 133,* 306–308.

chondroectodermal dysplasia *See* Ellis-van Creveld syndrome.

chromosome 22q11 microdeletion syndromes (i.e., DiGeorge syndrome, velocardiofacial syndrome [VCFS]) *Clinical features:* Microdeletions within the long arm of chromosome 22 have varying presentations, including DiGeorge syndrome, VCFS, and isolated outflow tract defects of the heart. Characteristic facial appearance that includes a small, open mouth; short palpebral fissures (eyelid openings); flat nasal bridge; bulbous nasal tip; protuberant, low-set ears; varying degrees of palatal abnormalities ranging from cleft to velopharyngeal insufficiency; classic DiGeorge syndrome is associated with hypoplastic thymus, hypoparathyroidism, hypotonia and congenital heart defect. *Associated complications:* Feeding problems in infancy, rare seizures, hypernasal speech, developmental disabilities ranging from learning disability to more significant cognitive delays, gross and fine motor delays expressive language is delayed more significantly than receptive language. *Cause:* Deletion on chromosome 22q11.2. *Inheritance:* Usually NM, with AD inheritance when passed from an affected individual; one parent occasionally has a chromosomal rearrangement involving 22q, which increases the risk for recurrence; risk to offspring of affected individuals is 50%. *Prevalence:* Unknown.

References: Gerdes, M., Solot, C., & Wang, P.P. (1999). Cognitive and behavioral profile of preschool children with chromosome 22q11.2 deletion. *American Journal of Medical Genetics, 85,* 127–133.

Perez, E., & Sullivan, K.E. (2002). Chromosome 22q11.2 deletion syndrome (DiGeorge and velocardiofacial syndromes). *Current Opinion in Pediatrics, 14,* 678–683.

Yamagishi, H., & Srivastava, D. (2003). Unraveling the genetic and developmental mysteries of 22q11 deletion syndrome. *Trends in Molecular Medicine, 9,* 383–389.

Cohen syndrome *Clinical features:* Obesity; microcephaly; short stature; long hands with tapering fingers; characteristic facial features, including micrognathia, short philtrum, prominent incisors; varying degrees of developmental delay/intellectual disability. *Associated complications:* Hypotonia, joint laxity, ocular abnormalities, occasional heart defect. *Cause:* Mutations in the COH1 gene linked to chromosome 8q21–q22. *Inheritance:* AR. *Prevalence:* Unknown.

References: Kivitie-Kallio, S., & Norio, R. (2001). Cohen syndrome: Essential features, natural history, and heterogeneity. *American Journal of Medical Genetics, 102,* 125–135.

Kolehmainen, J., Wilkinson, R., Lehesjoki, A-E., et al. (2004). Delineation of Cohen syndrome following a large-scale genotype-phenotype screen. *American Journal of Human Genetics, 75,* 122–127.

congenital facial diplegia *See* Moebius sequence.

Cornelia de Lange syndrome *See* de Lange syndrome.

craniofacial dysostosis *See* Crouzon syndrome.

cri-du-chat syndrome (chromosome 5p–syndrome) *Clinical features:* Pre- and postnatal growth retardation, cat-like cry in infancy, hypertelorism with downward slant, microcephaly, low-set ears, micrognathia, single palmar crease, cognitive deficits ranging from learning difficulties in some patients to moderate or severe intellectual disability in others. Receptive language skills are better then expressive language. *Associated complications:* Severe respiratory and feeding difficulties in infancy, hypotonia, inguinal (groin) hernias, occasional congenital heart defects, sleep disturbance, hyperactivity. *Cause:* Partial deletion of chromosome 5p15.2. *Inheritance:* Usually NM; in 12% of cases, a parent carries a balanced translocation. *Prevalence:* 1/20,000–1/50,000.

References: Cornish, K. (2002). Cri du chat syndrome: Genotype–phenotype correlations and recommendations for clinical management. *Developmental Medicine and Child Neurology, 44,* 494–497.

Cornish, K.M., Bramble, D., Munir, F., et al. (1999). Cognitive functioning in children with typical cri du chat (5p–) syndrome. *Developmental Medicine and Child Neurology, 41,* 263–266.

Crouzon syndrome (craniofacial dysostosis) *Clinical features:* Craniosynostosis, shallow orbits with proptosis (protuberant eyeballs), hypertelorism, strabismus, parrot-beaked nose, short upper lip, maxillary hypoplasia (small upper jaw), conductive hearing loss. *Associated complications:* Increased intracranial pressure, intellectual disability, seizures, visual impairment, agenesis of corpus callosum, occasional cleft lip or palate, obstructive airway problems. *Cause:* Mutations in fibroblast growth factor receptor-2 (FGFR2) gene on chromosome 10q25.3–q26. *Inheritance:* AD with variable expression; up to 25% may represent new mutations. *Prevalence:* Unknown.

References: Hoefkens, M.F., Vermeij-Keers, C., & Vaandrager, J.M., (2004). Crouzon syndrome: Phenotypic signs and symptoms of the postnally expressed subtype. *Journal of Craniofacial Surgery, 15*, 233–240.

Proudman, T.W., Moore, M.H., Abbott, A.H., et al. (1994). Noncraniofacial manifestations of Crouzon's disease. *Journal of Craniofacial Surgery, 5*, 218–222.

de Lange syndrome (Brachmann de Lange syndrome, Cornelia de Lange syndrome) *Clinical features:* Prenatal growth retardation, postnatal short stature, hypertrichosis (excessive body hair), synophrys (confluent eyebrows), anteverted nostrils, depressed nasal bridge, long philtrum, thin upper lip, microcephaly, low-set ears, limb and digital anomalies, eye problems (myopia, ptosis, or nystagmus). *Associated complications:* Severe intellectual disability, occasional heart defect, gastrointestinal problems, features of autism, self-injurious behavior, occasional hearing loss. *Cause:* Mutation in the Nipped-B-like gene (NIPBL) Gene, which is linked to chromosome 3q26.3. *Inheritance:* Majority of cases are caused by a NM with AD inheritance when passed from an affected individual. *Prevalence:* 1/50,000.

References: Berney, T.P., Ireland, M., & Burn, J. (1999). Behavioural phenotype of Cornelia de Lange syndrome. *Archives of Disease in Childhood, 81*, 333–336.

Goodban, M.T. (1993). Survey of speech and language skills with prognostic indicators in 116 patients with Cornelia de Lange syndrome. *American Journal of Medical Genetics, 47*, 1059–1063.

Tonkin E.T., Wang T.J., & Lisgo, S. (2004). NIPBL, encoding a homolog of fungal Scc2-type sister chromatid cohesion proteins and fly Nipped-B, is mutated in Cornelia de Lange syndrome. *Nature Genetics, 36*, 636–641.

DiGeorge syndrome *See* chromosome 22q11 microdeletion syndromes.

DMD muscular dystrophy, Duchenne type *See* muscular dystrophy, Duchenne and Becker types.

Down syndrome *Clinical features:* Hypotonia, flat facial profile, upward-slanting palpebral fissures, small ears, small nose with low nasal bridge, single palmar crease, short stature, intellectual disability, congenital heart disease. *Associated complications:* Atlantoaxial (upper cervical spine) instability; hyperextensible large joints; strabismus; thyroid dysfunction; predisposition toward immune disorders and leukemia; eye abnormalities, including strabismus, nystagmus, cataracts, or glaucoma; narrow ear canals and high incidence of middle-ear infections with potential hearing loss; neurological abnormalities include risk of seizures and early-onset Alzheimer's disease. *Cause:* Extra chromosome 21 caused by trisomy, mosaicism, or translocation. *Inheritance:* NM; usually nondisjunction chromosomal abnormality. Recurrence risk in the absence of translocation is 1%–2% in women younger than 35 years and the same as the typical maternal age-related risk in women over 35 years old at delivery. If translocation is present in parent, recurrence risk is higher and is dependent on sex of carrier parent. *Prevalence:* 1/100,000–1.5/100,000. *Incidence:* 1/800 births. *See also Chapter 16.*

References: Chapman, R.S., & Hesketh, L.J. (2000). Behavioral phenotype of individuals with Down syndrome. *Mental Retardation and Developmental Disabilities Research Reviews, 6*, 84–95.

Merrick J., Kandel, I., & Vardi, G. (2004). Adolescents with Down syndrome. *International Journal of Adolescent Medical Health, 16*, 13–9.

Dubowitz syndrome *Clinical features:* Prenatal onset of growth deficiency; postnatal short stature; eczema; sparse hair; mild microcephaly; cleft palate; dysmorphic facial features, including high forehead, broad nasal bridge, ptosis, epicanthal folds. *Associated complications:* Intellectual disability, behavioral disturbances, recurrent infections, increased frequency of malignancy, occasional hypospadias (abnormality in the location of the male urethra) or cryptorchidism, hypoparathyroidism. *Cause:* Unknown. *Inheritance:* AR. *Prevalence:* Rare.

References: Swartz, K.R., Resnick, D.K., Iskandar, B.J., et al. (2003). Craniocervical anomalies in Dubowitz syndrome: Three cases and a literature review. *Pediatric Neurosurgery, 38,* 238–243.

Tsukahara, M., & Opitz, J.M. (1996). Dubowitz syndrome: Review of 141 cases, including 36 previously unreported patients. *American Journal of Medical Genetics, 63,* 277–289.

Duchenne muscular dystrophy (DMD) *See* muscular dystrophy, Duchenne and Becker types.

ectrodactyly–ectodermal dysplasia–clefting (EEC) syndrome *Clinical features:* Ectrodactyly (split hands or feet), ectodermal dysplasia (abnormal skin development), sparse hair, cleft lip and palate, lacrimal (tear) duct abnormalities; intelligence is not usually affected. *Associated complications:* Occasional renal (kidney) or genital anomalies, hearing impairment, hypodontia (underdeveloped teeth), lymphoma associated with EEC3 only. *Cause:* Mutations in p63 gene at 3q27 cause EEC type 3; EEC type 1 have been linked to chromosome 7q21–q22. *Inheritance:* AD with variable penetrance and expressivity. *Prevalence:* Unknown.

References: Akahoshi, K., Sakazume, S., Kosaki, K., et al. (2003). EEC syndrome type 3 with a heterozygous germline mutation in the P63 gene and B cell lymphoma. *American Journal of Medical Genetics, 120,* 370–373.

Roelfsema, N.M., & Cobben, J.M. (1996). The EEC syndrome: A literature study. *Clinical Dysmorphology, 5,* 115–127.

Edwards syndrome *See* trisomy 18 syndrome.

EEC syndrome *See* ectrodactyly–ectodermal dysplasia–clefting syndrome.

Ehlers-Danlos syndrome *Clinical features:* At least 10 distinct forms have been described. All include aspects of skin fragility, easy bruisability, joint hyperextensibility, and hyperelastic skin. Types I and III are most commonly described and have similar clinical presentations with the previously mentioned features; type IV is characterized by severe blood vessel involvement with risk of spontaneous arterial rupture; type VI is characterized by eye involvement, including corneal fragility; type VIII includes periodontal disease; type IX has bladder diverticula (pouches or sacs in the bladder wall), and chronic diarrhea. *Associated complications:* Occasional intellectual disability, premature loss of teeth, mitral valve prolapse, intestinal hernias, premature delivery from premature rupture of membranes, scoliosis, abnormalities of thymus. *Cause:* Each form is associated with an abnormality in the formation of collagen. Types I and II are caused by mutations in the COL5A1 and A2 genes; type III is caused by mutations in the COL3A1 gene as well as the tenascin XB gene (TNXB); type IV is caused by mutations in the COL3A1 gene; mutations in the lysyl hydroxylase gene (PLOD) cause some cases of EDS VI; EDS VII may be caused by mutations in the COL1A1 and COL1A2 ADAMTS2 gene. The genes for types V, VIII, IX, or X are yet to be identified. *Inheritance:* Types I, II, III, IV, VII, and VIII are AD with variable expression; types VI and X are AR; types V, VII, and IX are XLR. *Prevalence:* Approximately 1 in 5,000.

References: Burrows, N.P. (1999). The molecular genetics of the Ehlers-Danlos syndrome. *Clinical and Experimental Dermatology, 24,* 99–106.

Whitelaw, S.E. (2003). Ehlers-Danlos syndrome, classical type: Case management. *Pediatric Nursing, 29,* 423–426.

Ellis-van Creveld syndrome (chondroectodermal dysplasia) *Clinical features:* Short-limbed dwarfism (final height 43 to 60 inches), polydactyly, nail abnormalities, neonatal teeth, underdeveloped and premature loss of teeth, congenital heart defect in 50%; intelligence is usually not affected. *Associated complications:* Severe cardiorespiratory problems in infancy specifically atrial sepation (producing a common atrium in the heart), hydrocephalus, severe leg deformities. *Cause:* Mutations in the EVC and EVC 2 genes located on chromosome 4p16. *Inheritance:* AR. *Prevalence:* Rare, increased in Amish.

References: Avolio, A., Jr., Berman, A.T., & Israelite, C.L. (1994). Ellis-van Creveld syndrome (chondroectodermal dysplasia). *Orthopedics, 17,* 735–737.

Galdzicka, M., Patnala, S., Hirshman, M.G., et al (2002). A new gene, EVC2, is mutated in Ellis-van Creveld syndrome. *Molecular Genetics and Metabolism, 77,* 291–295.

facio-auriculo-vertebral spectrum *See* oculoauriculovertebral spectrum.

faciodigitogenital dysplasia (FGDY) *See* Aarskog-Scott syndrome.

FAE *See* fetal alcohol effects.

familial dysautonomia (Riley-Day syndrome) *Clinical features:* Absent or sparse tears, absence of fungiform papillae (knoblike projections) on tongue, diminished pain and temperature sensation, postural hypotension, abnormal sweating, episodic vomiting, swallowing disorder, ataxia, decreased reflexes. *Associated complications:* Feeding difficulties, scoliosis, joint abnormalities, hypertension, aseptic necrosis of bones (damage to bony tissue unassociated with infection or injury). *Cause:* Mutation of IKBKAP gene (stands for inhibitor of kappa light polypeptide gene enhancer in B-cells, kinase complex associated protein) localized to chromosome 9q31–q33. *Inheritance:* AR. *Prevalence:* Rare; 3% carrier frequency in Ashkenazi Jewish population.

References: Axelrod, F.B. (1998). Familial dysautonomia: A 47-year perspective. How technology confirms clinical acumen. *Journal of Pediatrics, 132,* S2–S5.

Hilz, M.J., Axelrod, F.B., Bickel, A., et al. (2004). Assessing function and pathology in familial dysautonomia: Assessing of temperature perception, sweating and cutaneous innervation. *Brain, 127,* 2090–2098.

FAS *See* fetal alcohol syndrome.

fetal alcohol effects (FAE) Former term for alcohol-related neurodevelopmental effects (ARND); *see Chapter 5.*

fetal alcohol syndrome (FAS) *See Chapter 5.*

fetal face syndrome *See* Robinow syndrome.

fetal hydantoin syndrome Phenytoin syndrome; *see Chapter 2.*

FGDY faciogenital dysplasia *See* Aarskog-Scott syndrome.

5p– syndrome *See* cri-du-chat syndrome.

45,X *See* Turner syndrome.

47,X *See* XXX, XXXX, and XXXXX syndromes.

fragile X syndrome *Clinical features:* Prominent jaw, macroorchidism (large testes), large ears, attention-deficit/hyperactivity disorder, autism spectrum disorder; affected males (full mutation) often have moderate to severe intellectual disability. Of females with a full mutation, 33% have average intelligence; 33% have average intelligence with significant learning disabilities; and 33% have intellectual disability, occasional autism spectrum disorder, or psychiatric disorders. *Associated complications:* Abnormalities of connective tissue with finger joint hypermobility or joint instability, mitral valve prolapse. *Cause:* Mutation in FMR1 gene on Xq27–q28; molecular analysis reveals an increase in cytosine-guanine-guanine (CGG) trinucleotide repeats in the coding sequence of the FMR1 gene. Normal allele sizes vary from 6 to 50 CGG

repeats. Phenotypically unaffected individuals have premutations, with allele size ranging from 50 to 200. Allele sizes of greater than 230 CGG repeats generally indicate a full mutation with phenotypic expression of the syndrome. *Inheritance:* X-linked with genetic imprinting (full mutations are not inherited from the father) and anticipation (number of repeats may increase in subsequent generations). *Prevalence:* 1/2,000 males; 1/4,000 females. *See also Chapter 19.*

References: Cornish, K., Sudhalter, V., & Turk, J. (2004). Attention and language in fragile X. *Mental Retardation and Developmental Disabilities Research Reviews, 10,* 11–16.

Fisch, G.S., Carpenter, N.J., Holden, J.J., et al. (1999). Longitudinal assessment of adaptive and maladaptive behaviors in fragile X males: Growth, development, and profiles. *American Journal of Medical Genetics, 83,* 257–263.

Maes, B., Fryns, J.P., Ghesquiere, P., et al. (2000). Phenotypic checklist to screen for fragile X syndrome in people with intellectual disability. *Mental Retardation, 38,* 207–215.

Friedreich ataxia *Clinical features:* Slowly progressive neurological disorder characterized by limb and gait ataxia, dysarthria, nystagmus, pes cavus (high-arched feet), hearing loss, kyphoscoliosis (backward curve of the spine). In rare cases, progression is rapid. Onset is before adolescence. *Associated complications:* Delayed motor milestones, cardiomyopathy (heart muscle weakness), and/or congestive heart failure; increased risk of insulin-dependent diabetes mellitus; impaired color vision. *Cause:* Usually homozygous guanine-adenosine-adenosine (GAA) expansions in the frataxin gene on chromosome 9q13; point mutations in the frataxin gene have also been identified. *Inheritance:* AR. *Prevalence:* Approximately 1/29,000–1/50,000. *Treatment:* Supportive care includes physical therapy, orthopedic surgery to correct progressive scoliosis, and close cardiology follow-up. Antioxidants such as Idebenone have been used with intial success. Additional studies must be done to confirm these results and monitor long term effects.

References: Alper, G., & Narayanan, V. (2003). Friedreich's Ataxia. *Pediatric Neurology, 28,* 335–341.

Wood, N.W. (1998). Diagnosing Friedreich's ataxia. *Archives of Disease in Childhood, 78,* 204–207.

G syndrome *See* Opitz syndrome.

galactosemia *Clinical features:* Jaundice, lethargy, hypotonia in the newborn period; failure to thrive with vomiting and diarrhea; cataracts; liver dysfunction; varying degrees of intellectual impairment (severe if untreated). In 70% of treated children, IQ score is less than 90; 50% have significant visual-perceptual impairments. Verbal dyspraxia is also seen in 62% of treated infants. *Associated complications:* Ovarian failure, hemolytic anemia, increased risk of sepsis (particularly E. coli in neonate), cerebellar ataxia, tremors, choreoathetosis. *Cause:* Onset of clinical features is in part dependant on the ingestion of dietary galactose; individuals diagnosed by newborn screening in whom galactose has been withheld still experience some cognitive deficits and ovarian failure (females). *Cause:* A deficiency of the enzyme galactose-1-phosphate uridyltransferase or (GACT), less commonly, galactokinase (both are enzymes required for digestion of galactose, a natural sugar found in milk). The GALT gene is on chromosome 9p13. *Inheritance:* AR. *Prevalence:* 1/50,000–1/70,000 in the United States. *Treatment:* Galactose-free diet.

References: Hansen, T.W., Henrichsen, B., Rasmussen, R.K., et al. (1996). Neuropsychological and linguistic follow-up studies of children with galactosaemia from an unscreened population. *Acta Paediatrica, 85,* 1197–1201.

Leslie N.D. (2003). Insights into the pathogenesis of Galactosemia. *Annual Review of Nutrition, 23,* 59–80.

Schweitzer, S., Shin, Y., Jakobs, C., et al. (1993). Long-term outcome in 134 patients with galactosemia. *European Journal of Pediatrics, 152,* 36–43.

Gaucher disease *Clinical features:* Three clinically distinct forms, the most common of which (type I) has onset in adulthood including enlarged spleen and liver, anemia, thrombocytopenia, and bone involvement; no nervous system involvement has been noted. Most individuals with type I go undiagnosed. Type II presents in infancy with an enlarged spleen, hematological abnormalities, bony lesions, abnormalities of skin pigmentation, and varying degrees of intellectual disability. Most children will die within the first 2 years of life. Type III is more variable with ataxia, seizures, eye movement disorder, and dementia. *Associated complications:* Rare associated features such as cardiac valvular involvement and Parkinsonian features have been associated with specific genotypes. *Cause:* Accumulation of glucosylceramide due to deficiency of the enzyme beta-glucosidase on chromosome 1q21. *Inheritance:* AR. *Prevalence:* Rare in general population; prevalence of type I estimated to be approximately 1/1,000 in the Ashkenazi Jewish population. *Treatment:* Enzyme replacement therapy, bone marrow transplantation.

References: Elstein, D., Abrahamov, A., Hadas-Halpern, I., et al. (1999). Recommendations for diagnosis, evaluation, and monitoring of patients with Gaucher disease. *Archives of Internal Medicine, 159,* 1254–1255.

Sidransky, E. (2004). Gaucher disease: Complexity in a "simple" disorder. *Molecular Genetics and Metabolism, 83,* 6–15.

globoid cell leukodystrophy *See* Krabbe disease.

glutaric acidemia, type I (a disorder of organic acid metabolism) *Clinical features:* Macrocephaly, hypotonia, movement disorder (dystonia), and seizures present between 6 and 18 months, interrupting otherwise typical development. This disorder may mimic dyskinetic cerebral palsy. *Associated complications:* Episodic acidosis, vomiting, lethargy, and coma. Intellectual disability is usual, although intellectual functioning may remain intact. *Cause:* Mutations in the glutaryl-CoA dehydrogenase gene on chromosome 19p13.2 result in accumulation of glutaric acid and to a lesser degree of 3-hydroxyglutaric and glutaconic acids. *Inheritance:* AR. *Prevalence:* Rare; 1/30,000 in Sweden and more common in North American aboriginals of Manitoba and Ontario as well as in the Amish population. *Treatment:* Diet low in lysine and supplemental oral carnitine.

References: Baric, I., Zschocke, J., Christensen, E., et al. (1998). Diagnosis and management of glutaric aciduria type I. *Journal of Inherited Metabolic Disease, 21,* 326–340.

Funk, C.B.R., Prasad, A.N., & Frosk, P. (2005). Neuropatholgoical, biochemical, and molecular findings in a glutaric academia type 1 cohort. *Brain, 128,* 711–722.

Hoffmann, G.F., & Zschocke, J. (1999). Glutaric aciduria type I: From clinical, biochemical, and molecular diversity to successful therapy. *Journal of Inherited Metabolic Disease, 22,* 381–391.

glutaric acidemia, type II (multiple acyl-CoA dehydrogenase deficiency) *Clinical* *features:* An inborn error of metabolism that may present in infancy with severe metabolic acidosis, hypoglycemia, and cardiomyopathy. The urine has a characteristic odor of sweaty feet, similar to that present in isovaleric acidemia. Dysmorphic facial features (macrocephaly, large anterior fontanelle [soft spot], high forehead, flat nasal bridge, and malformed ears) are seen in one half of cases. This condition also can present later in life with episodic vomiting, acidosis, and hypoglycemia. *Associated complications:* Muscle weakness, liver disease, cataracts, respiratory distress, renal (kidney) cysts. *Cause:* Mutations in at least three different genes—ETFA, ETFB, and ETFDH—have been identified. No clinical differences with respect to causative gene have been identified. *Inheritance:* AR. *Prevalence:* Rare. *Treatment:* Diet with supplemental riboflavin and carnitine.

References: al-Essa, M.A., Rashed, M.S., Bakheet, S.M., et al. (2000). Glutaric aciduria type II: Observations in seven patients with neonatal- and late-onset disease. *Journal of Perinatology, 20,* 120–128.

Frerman, F.E., & Goodman, S.I. (1995). Glutaric acidemia type II. In C.R. Scriver, A.L. Beaudet, W.S. Sly, et al. (Eds.), *The metabolic and molecular bases of inherited disease* (pp. 1619–1623). New York: McGraw-Hill.

Olsen, R.K., Andresen, B.S., & Christensen, E. (2003). Clear relationship between ETF/ETFDH genotype and phenotype in patients with multiple acyl-CoA dehydrogenation deficiency. *Human Mutation, 22,* 12–23.

glycogen storage diseases (glycogenoses) *Clinical features:* More than 12 forms of glycogen storage diseases are currently known, all caused by defects in the production or breakdown of glycogen and resulting in a wide spectrum of clinical features. They share varying degrees of liver and muscle abnormalities and can be broken down by whether they primarily affect the muscle (and therefore present with muscle cramps, easy fatigability, and progressive muscle weakness) or the liver (where an enlarged liver and decreased blood sugar are the initial symptoms). In all disease forms, patient organs have excessive glycogen accumulation. Types I (glucose-6-phosphate deficiency), II (Pompe disease, acid alpha-glucosidase deficiency), III (amylo-1, 6-glycosidase deficiency), and VI (hepatic phosphorylase deficiency) are the most common and represent almost 95% of cases. Common clinical features include hypoglycemia, short stature, enlarged spleen, and muscle weakness. *Associated complications:* Hypotonia, renal (kidney) abnormalities, gouty arthritis, bleeding abnormalities, hypertension, respiratory distress; type II disease characteristically has severe cardiac, muscle, and neurological involvement. *Cause:* Deficiencies in the various enzymes involved in the synthesis and degradation of glycogen. There are many genes and chromosome locations associated with glycogenoses. *Inheritance:* All except type VIII are inherited as AR; type VIII is XLR. *Prevalence:* Combined incidence of 1/20,000–1/25,000. *Treatment:* Increased protein intake and overnight tube feeding of starch to maintain normoglycemia have been shown to be useful for supportive care. This treatment also prevents growth and developmental problems, and can mollify the biochemical abnormalities. No more specific treatment, however, is yet available for any of the glycogenoses. Liver transplantation has been attempted in types I, III, and IV, with correction of the biochemical abnormalities but not all sequelae.

References: Chen, Y.T. (2001). Glycogen storage diseases. In C.R. Scriver, A.L. Beaudet, W.S. Sly, et al. (Eds.), *The metabolic and molecular bases of inherited disease* (pp. 1521–1551). New York: McGraw-Hill.

Wolfsdorf, J.I., & Weinstein, D.A. (2003). Glycogen storage diseases. *Reviews in Endocrine and Metabolic Disorders, 4,* 95–102.

GM2 gangliosidosis, type I *See* Tay-Sachs disease.

Goldenhar syndrome *See* oculoauriculovertebral spectrum.

Guillain-Barré Syndrome (GBS) *Clinical features:* Pain and the development over one to several days of muscle weakness, with the inability to walk and a loss of deep tendon reflexes. The weakness affects both sides of the body symmetrically, usually starting in the lower extremities. The arms are involved later, with maximum weakness occurring by 3 weeks. Most children with GBS begin to recover 2–3 weeks after the symptoms began. About 85% of affected children are able to walk within 6 months; however, some have residual weakness. The mortality rate is 3%, and the chance of relapse has been reported as 7% in children. *Cause:* It can follow an upper respiratory or gastrointestinal (GI) viral infection. A specific type of GI infection produced by the bacteria *campylobacter jejuni* has been particularly associated with GBS. GBS is considered an autoimmune disease. *Incidence*: 0.4–1.7 cases per 100,000 people each year. *Diagnosis*: Spinal fluid analysis and electromyographic evaluation. *Treatment*: Treatment is mostly supportive. About 10%–20% need to be placed on a ventilator. Medical treatment includes the use of intravenous immune globulin (IVIG) and/or plasmapheresis. *Reference*: Hughes, R.A., & Cornblath, D.R. (2005). Guillain-Barré syndrome. *The Lancet* (9497), 1653–1666.

Hallermann-Streiff syndrome (oculomandibulodyscephaly with hypotrichosis) *Clinical features:* Proportionate short stature; characteristic facial appearance, including small eyes, small, pinched nose, and small mouth; sparse, thin hair; frontal bossing (prominent central forehead). *Associated complications:* Various eye abnormalities, including nystagmus, strabismus, cataracts, and/or decreased visual acuity; neonatal teeth and other dental abnormalities; narrow upper airway or tracheomalacia (softening of the tracheal cartilages), with related respiratory difficulty; frequent respiratory infections, snoring, and feeding difficulties; clinical overlap with oculodentodigital dysplasia (ODDD) has been suggested. *Cause:* Unknown, believed to be genetic; one patient has been identified with a homozygous mutation in the GJA1 gene known to be causative in ODDD. *Inheritance:* Most reported cases are not inherited from an affected parent and are assumed to be caused by a NM. *Prevalence:* 150 cases known to exist. *References:* David, L.R., Finlon, M., Genecov, D., et al. (1999). Hallermann-Streiff syndrome: Experience with 15 patients and review of the literature. *Journal of Craniofacial Surgery, 10*, 160–168.

Pizzuti, A., Flex, E., Mingarelli, R., et al. (2004). A homozygous GJA1 gene mutation causes a Hallermann-Streiff/ODDD spectrum phenotype. *Human Mutation, 23*, 286.

hemifacial microsomia *See* oculoauriculovertebral spectrum.

hereditary progressive arthroophthalmopathy *See* Stickler syndrome.

holocarboxylase synthetase deficiency *See* multiple carboxylase deficiency, infantile or early form.

holoprosencephaly *Clinical features:* This classification encompasses a spectrum of midline defects of the brain and face. The most severe are incompatible with life. Individuals who survive have varying degrees of disability ranging from typical development with hypotelorism (widely spaced eyes) to alobar holoprosencephaly (brain without segmentation into hemispheres) and cyclopia (single central eye). *Associated complications:* Seizures, endocrine abnormalities, micropenis and other genital anomalies, cleft of retinae, and intellectual disability. Facial anomalies are seen in 80% of cases. *Cause:* Genetically heterogeneous; sonic hedgehog (SHH) gene on chromosome 7q36 implicated in some cases; many cases have involved mutations in different genes, such as those located at 2p21 (SIX3 gene), 13q32 (ZIC2 gene), or 18p11.3 (TGIF gene); cases may be caused by a single gene or a larger chromosomal abnormality. *Inheritance:* May be part of a syndrome or caused by teratogenic exposure; as an isolated birth defect may be AD or AR. *Prevalence:* 1/16,000.
References: Barr, M., Jr., & Cohen, M.M., Jr. (1999). Holoprosencephaly survival and performance. *American Journal of Medical Genetics, 89*, 116–120.

Lazaro, L., Dubourg, C., Pasquier, L., et al. (2004). Phenotypic and molecular variability of the holoprosencephalic spectrum. *American Journal of Medical Genetics, 129*, 21–24.

Holt-Oram syndrome *Clinical features:* Upper-limb defect ranging from hypoplastic (incompletely formed), abnormally placed or absent thumbs to hypoplasia of radius, ulna, or humerus (arm bones) to complete phocomelia (foreshortened limbs); 85%–95% of affected individuals also have congenital heart defect (atrial septal defect and ventricular septal defect are most common). *Associated complications:* Occasional abnormalities of chest muscles and vertebral anomalies. *Cause:* Mutations in the TBX5 gene on chromosome 12q2. *Inheritance:* AD with variable expression; may increase in severity with each generation. *Prevalence:* Approximately 1/100,000.
References: Basson, C.T., Cowley, G.S., Solomon, S.D., et al. (1994). The clinical and genetic spectrum of Holt-Oram syndrome (heart–hand syndrome). *The New England Journal of Medicine, 330*, 885–891.

Huang, T. (2002). Current advances in Holt-Oram syndrome. *Current Opinion in Pediatrics, 14*, 691–695.

Newbury-Ecob, R.A., Leanage, R., Raeburn, J.A., et al. (1996). Holt-Oram syndrome: A clinical genetic study. *Journal of Medical Genetics, 33*, 300–307.

homocystinuria *Clinical features:* Downward dislocation of lens of the eye (with myopia); tall, slim physique; hypopigmentation (fair skin); and sparse, thin hair. Two forms have been described, differing in their responsiveness to pyridoxine (vitamin B_6). *Associated complications:* Mild to moderate intellectual disability in one half to three fourths of untreated individuals; a vascular event such as myocardial infarction and stroke occurs in 50% of affected individuals by age 30 due to increased risk for blood clots; behavioral disorders, cataracts, or glaucoma; scoliosis; osteoporosis. *Cause:* Inherited defect in the enzyme cystathionine beta-synthetase caused by mutations in a gene on chromosome 21q22. *Inheritance:* AR with variable expressivity. *Incidence:* Ranges from 1/65,000 in Ireland to 1/344,000 worldwide. *Treatment:* Folic acid supplementation, use of betaine hydrochloride, and dietary restriction of methionine have shown promise; pyridoxine is used in the rare individuals who have the pyridoxine-responsive form of the disease. Early treatment with pyridoxine in responsive cases may allow typical intelligence. Treatment with above agents significantly reduces risk of vascular events.

References: Kraus, J.P. (1994). Molecular basis of phenotype expression in homocystinuria. *Journal of Inherited Metabolic Disease, 17,* 383–390.

Yap, S. (2003). Classical homocystinuria: Vascular risk and its prevention. *Journal of Inherited Metabolic Disorders, 26,* 259–265.

Yap, S., & Naughten, E. (1998). Homocystinuria due to cystathionine beta-synthase deficiency in Ireland: 25 years' experience of a newborn screened and treated population with reference to clinical outcome and biochemical control. *Journal of Inherited Metabolic Disease, 21,* 738–747.

Hunter syndrome (MPS II) *See* mucopolysaccharidoses (MPS).

Huntington disease (HD) (*previously called* Huntington chorea), juvenile *Clinical features:* Juvenile onset progressive neurological disorder. For cases to be considered juvenile HD onset must occur by 20 years of age. Children present with dysarthria, clumsiness, hyperreflexia, rigidity, and oculomotor disturbances. *Associated complications:* Joint contractures, swallowing dysfunction, seizures. *Cause:* Expansion of CAG (cytosine-adenine-guanine) trinucleotide repeat in *huntingtin* gene on chromosome 4p16.3 (normal number of CAG repeats is 11–34; individuals affected with juvenile HD have greater than 60 CAG repeats). *Inheritance:* AD with anticipation (earlier onset with each generation, especially when paternally inherited). Progression in children with paternally inherited disease is more rapid than in children with maternally inherited disease. *Prevalence:* 4/100,000–7/100,000; juvenile onset disease accounts for 5% to 10% of all cases of HD.

References: Gomez-Tortosa, E., del Barrio, A., Garcia Ruiz, P.J., et al. (1998). Severity of cognitive impairment in juvenile and late-onset Huntington disease. *Archives of Neurology, 55,* 835–843.

Seneca, S., Fagnart, D., Keymolen, K., et al. (2004). Early onset Huntington disease: A neuronal degeneration syndrome. *European Journal of Pediatrics, 163,* 717–721.

Hurler syndrome (MPS IH) *See* mucopolysaccharidoses (MPS).

hypophosphatasia *Clinical features:* A disorder of calcium and phosphate metabolism with symptoms ranging from a severe infantile form (which can be rapidly fatal) to a relatively mild childhood form. A total of 6 forms of the disease have been described (perinatal severe, perinatal moderate, infantile, childhood, adult, and odontohypophosphatasia [dental only]). Features include short stature, bowed long bones, craniosynostosis, hypocalcemia. *Associated complications:* Seizures, multiple fractures, premature loss of teeth. The neonatal form presents as short limbs and poor ossification of the skeleton. The childhood form presents with an early loss of secondary teeth, short stature, and delayed walking with a waddling gait. Joint pain and nonprogressive muscle weakness may also be present. *Cause:* Mutations in the "tissue non-specific" alkaline phosphatase gene (ALPL) on chromosome 1p36. *Inheritance:* AR (severe forms), AR/AD (milder forms). *Incidence:* 1/100,000; incidence of severe infantile form is 1/250 in Mennonite families from Manitoba, Canada.

References: Spentchian, M., Merrienl, Y., Herasse, M., et al. (2003). Severe Hypophasphatasia: Characterization of fifteen novel mutations in the ALPL gene. *Human Mutation, 22,* 105–106.

Whyte, M.P. (2001). Hypophosphatasia. In C.R. Scriver, A.L. Beaudet, W.S. Sly, et al. (Eds.), *The metabolic and molecular bases of inherited disease* (pp. 5313–5329). New York: McGraw-Hill.

incontinentia pigmenti *Clinical features:* Swirling patterns of hyperpigmented skin lesions; tooth abnormalities; microcephaly; ocular abnormalities; thin, wiry hair; hairless lesions, intellectual disability in approximately one third of cases. *Associated complications:* Spasticity, seizures, vertebral or rib abnormalities; strabismus, hydrocephalus, history of male miscarriages. *Cause:* Mutations in NEMO gene on chromosome Xq28, skewed X-inactivation. *Inheritance:* XLD with lethality in males. *Prevalence:* Rare.

References: Hadj-Rabia, S., Froidevaux, D., Bodak, N., et al. (2003). Clinical study of 40 cases of incontinentia pigmenti. *Archives of Dermatology, 139,* 1163–1170.

Landy, S.J., & Donnai, D. (1993). Incontinentia pigmenti (Bloch-Sulzberger syndrome). *Journal of Medical Genetics, 30,* 53–59.

Smahi, A., Courtois, G., Vabres, P., et al. (2000). Genomic rearrangement in NEMO impairs NF-kappa-B activation and is a cause of incontinentia pigmenti. *Nature, 405,* 466–472.

infantile Refsum disease *See* Refsum disease, infantile.

isovaleric acidemia *Clinical features:* A disorder of organic acid metabolism; an acute, often fatal neonatal form is characterized by acidosis and coma; a chronic form presents with recurrent attacks of ataxia, vomiting, lethargy, and ketoacidosis. Attacks are generally triggered by infection or increased protein load. Urine smell of sweaty feet is characteristic. *Associated complications:* Seizures, intellectual disability if untreated, enlarged liver, vomiting, hematologic abnormalities. *Cause:* Deficiency of the enzyme isovaleryl-CoA dehydrogenase; gene linked to chromosome 15q14–q15. *Inheritance:* AR. *Prevalence:* Rare. *Treatment:* Treatment consisting of a low-protein diet with supplemental oral glycine and carnitine has resulted in a relatively good cognitive outcome.

References: Berry, G.T., Yudkoff, M., & Segal, S. (1988). Isovaleric acidemia: Medical and neurodevelopmental effects of long-term therapy. *Journal of Pediatrics, 113,* 58–64.

Mehta, K.C., Zsolway, K., Osterhoudt, K.C., et al. (1996). Lessons from the late diagnosis of isovaleric acidemia in a five-year-old boy. *Journal of Pediatrics, 129,* 309–310.

Joubert syndrome *Clinical features:* Structural cerebellar abnormalities, abnormal eye movements, retinal dysplasia or coloboma, episodic hyperventilation; characteristic facial appearance including large head, prominent forehead, ptosis, epicanthal folds, upturned nose, tongue protrusion. *Associated complications:* Hypoplasia of corpus callosum, encephalocele (hernia of part of the brain and meninges through a skull defect), kidney cysts, microcephaly, abnormalities of the tongue, hypotonia, developmental delay/intellectual disability and behavioral problems; age at diagnosis ranges from the neonatal period through the first decade of life. *Cause:* Gene linked to 9q34.3 in some families. Additional genes and chromosomal regions yet to be identified are also thought to be causative. *Inheritance:* AR. *Prevalence:* Rare.

References: Fennell, E.B., Gitten, J.C., Dede, D.E., et al. (1999). Cognition, behavior, and development in Joubert syndrome. *Journal of Child Neurology, 14,* 592–596.

Kumandas, S., Akcakus, M., Coskun, A., & Gumus, H. (2004). Joubert syndrome: Review and report of seven new cases. *European Journal of Neurology, 11,* 505–510.

juvenile neuronal ceroid lipofuscinosis *See* Batten disease.

Kabuki syndrome *Clinical features:* Microcephaly, trapezoid philtrum (area between base of nose and upper lip), prominent posteriorly rotated ears, preauricular pit (small hole/indentation on the ear), long palpebral fissures, thick eyelashes, ptosis, sparse broad arched eyebrows, congenital heart defect, hirsutism (excessive hair), café au lait spots, cryptorchidism, small penis, hypotonia, joint hyperextensibility. *Associated complications:* Cleft palate, recurrent ear infections, hearing loss, aspiration pneumonia, feeding difficulties, malabsorption, anal stenosis, imperforate anus, scoliosis, congenital hip dislocation, increased susceptibility to infections, seizures, intellectual disability, premature thearche (breast development), hemolytic anemia, congenital hypothyroidism. *Cause:* Unknown. *Inheritance:* NM with AD inheritance when passed on from an affected individual. *Prevalence:* Rare.

Reference: Armstrong, L., Abd El Moneim, A., Aleck, K., et al. (2005). Further delineation of Kabuki syndrome in 48 well defined new individuals. *American Journal of Medical Genetics, 132,* 265–272.

Kearns-Sayre syndrome *See* mitochondrial disorders.

kinky hair syndrome *See* Menkes syndrome.

Klinefelter syndrome (XXY syndrome) *Clinical features:* Occurring only in males; tall, slim stature; long limbs; relatively small penis and testes; gynecomastia (breast enlargement) in 40%. *Associated complications:* Intention tremor (involuntary trembling arising when attempting a voluntary, coordinated movement) in 20%–50%, low to average intelligence, infertility, behavioral disorders, scoliosis, osteoporosis and reduced muscle strength, vascular problems; 8% have diabetes mellitus as adults, risk of extragonadal mid-line germ cell tumors. Patients may appear to have no physical changes prior to puberty with the exception of long legs. *Cause:* Chromosomal nondisjunction resulting in 47,XXY karyotype. *Inheritance:* NM caused by the presence of an additional X chromosome; about 50% of cases caused by maternal non-disjunction (error in the separation of chromosomes), while 50% are caused by paternal nondisjunction. *Prevalence:* 1/500 males. *Treatment:* Hormone treatment is needed in adolescence for the development of secondary sex characteristics.

References: Geschwind, D.H., Boone, K.B., Miller, B.L., et al. (2000). Neurobehavioral phenotype of Klinefelter syndrome. *Mental Retardation and Developmental Disabilities Research Reviews, 6,* 107–116.

Lanfranco, F., Kamischke, A., Zitmann, M., & Nieschlag, E. (2004). Klinefelter's syndrome. *The Lancet, 364,* 273–283.

Klippel-Feil syndrome *Clinical features:* Cervical vertebral fusion, hemivertebrae (incomplete development of one side of one or more vertebrae). *Associated complications:* Congenital scoliosis, torticollis (wry neck); low hairline; sacral agenesis (absence of tailbone); hearing loss; occasional congenital heart defect; extra, fused, or missing ribs; middle-ear abnormalities, genitourinary abnormalities, pain. *Cause:* Subgroup has been linked to the SGM1 gene on chromosome 8q22.2. *Inheritance:* AD with variable expressivity and reduced penetrance most common; AR and nongenetic causes have been reported. *Incidence:* Approximately 1/40,000, with a slight female predominance.

References: Clarke, R.A., Catalan, G., Diwan, A.D., et al. (1998). Heterogeneity in Klippel-Feil syndrome: A new classification. *Pediatric Radiology, 28,* 967–974.

Tracy, M.R., Dormans J.P., & Kusumi, K. (2004). Flippel-Feil syndrome: Clinical features and current understanding of etiology. *Clinical Orthopaedics and Related Research, 424,* 183–190.

Klippel-Trenauny-Weber syndrome *Clinical features:* Asymmetric hypertrophy of limb, face (lips, cheeks, tongue, teeth) or other body parts, hemangiomas (benign congenital tumors made up of newly formed blood vessels); hypertrophy and hemangiomas arise independently and are not always on the same side of the body. *Associated complications:* Dependent on the area of hypertrophy; complications may affect any organ/body part including spinal cord (resulting in weakness or paralysis), kidneys (renal obstruction), brain (intracranial hypertension). *Cause:* Linked to the VG5Q gene at 5q13.3. *Inheritance:* Believed to passed as an AD trait, where individuals are not affected unless a second, somatic (mutation arising after fertilization) occurs. *Prevalence:* Unknown.

References: Berry, S.A., Peterson, C., Mize, W., et al. (1998). Biometric and magnetic resonance imaging assessment of dento-facial abnormalities in a case of Klippel-Trenauny syndrome. *American Journal of Medical Genetics, 79,* 319–326.

Defraia, E., Baccetti, T., Marinelli, A., & Tollaro, I. (2004). Biometric and magnetic resonance imaging assessment of dento-facial abnormalities in a case of Klippel-Trenauny-Weber syndrome. *Oral Surgery, Oral Medicine, Oral Pathology, Oral Radiology, and Endodontology, 97,* 127–132.

Krabbe disease (globoid cell leukodystrophy) *Clinical features:* In the classic form of this progressive neurological disorder, symptoms begin at 4–6 months of age with irritability, progressive stiffness, optic atrophy, cognitive deterioration, and early death. Approximately 10%–15% of cases have onset of symptoms between 15 months and 17 years of age, and have slower disease progression. *Associated complications:* Hypertonicity, opisthotonos (back arching), visual and hearing impairment, episodic unexplained fevers, seizures; peripheral neuropathy. *Cause:* Accumulation of psychosine galactosylceramide caused by a galactocerebrosidase enzyme deficiency resulting from a mutation in the GALC gene on chromosome 14q24.3–q32.1. *Inheritance:* AR. *Incidence:* 0.5/100,000–1/100,000; may be increased in specific populations including Swedish populations (estimated incidence is 1/50,000) and Druze kindred in Israel (1/130). *Treatment:* Hematopoietic stem cell transplantation has been performed in a small number of patients, success is unclear.

References: Korn-Lubetzki, I., & Nevo, Y. (2003). Infantile Krabbe disease. *Archives of Neurology, 60*, 1643–1644.

Wenger, D.A., Rafi, M.A., Luzi, P., et al. (2000). Krabbe disease: Genetic aspects and progress toward therapy. *Molecular Genetics and Metabolism, 70*, 1–9.

Landau-Kleffner syndrome (LKS) *Clinical features:* Selective aphasia (loss of speech), regression in receptive and/or expressive language ability, with some recovery in older children; seizures (80% of patients); paroxysmal electroencephalogram; electrical status epilepticus in slow wave sleep with or without clinical seizures. *Associated complications:* Behavioral disturbances similar to those in autism *(see Chapter 23). Cause:* Unknown. *Inheritance:* Possibly AR. *Prevalence:* Unknown; at least 170 children have been reported in the medical literature with approximately 1/440 children with epilepsy being diagnosed with LKS; predominance of affected males. *Treatment:* Treatment of seizures with antiepileptic medications. *See also Chapter 29.*

References: Gordon, N. (1997). The Landau-Kleffner syndrome: Increased understanding. *Brain Development, 19*, 311–316.

McVicar, K.A., & Shinnar, S. (2004). Landau-Kleffner syndrome, electrical status epilepticus in slow wave sleep, and language regression in children. *Mental Retardation and Developmental Disabilities Research Reviews, 10*, 144–149.

Laurence-Moon-Bardet-Biedl syndrome *See* Bardet-Biedl syndrome.

Leber hereditary optic neuropathy *See* mitochondrial disorders.

Leber's congenital amaurosis *See* mitochondrial disorders.

Leigh syndrome *See* mitochondrial disorders.

Lennox-Gastaut syndrome *See Chapter 29.*

Lesch-Nyhan syndrome *Clinical features:* An inborn error of purine metabolism associated with elevated levels of uric acid in blood and urine. Affected males appear symptom free at birth, but dyskinetic (incomplete or fragmented) movements and spasticity develop, accompanied by severe involuntary self-injurious behavior, including biting of fingers, arms, and lips. *Associated complications:* Cognitive impairment, seizures in 50%, hematuria (blood in urine), kidney stones, and ultimate kidney failure. *Cause:* Defect in enzyme hypoxanthine-guanine phosphoribosyl transferase caused by a mutation in the HPRT gene on Xq26–q27.2. *Inheritance:* XLR. *Prevalence:* Rare. *Treatment:* Allopurinol is useful in preventing kidney and joint deposition of uric acid. Numerous medications have been used in management of self-injurious behavior without much success.

References: Olson, L., & Houlihan, D. (2000). A review of behavioral treatments used for Lesch-Nyhan syndrome. *Behavior Modification, 24*, 202–222.

Robey, K.L., Reck, J.F., Giacomini, K.D., et al. (2003). Modes and patterns of self-mutilation in persons with Lesch-Nyhan disease. *Developmental Medicine and Child Neurology, 45*, 167–171.

lissencephaly syndromes (e.g., Miller-Dieker syndrome) *Clinical features:* A group of disorders characterized by lissencephaly (smooth brain) in which Miller-Dieker syndrome is the prototype; lissencephaly syndromes can be divided into subgroups based on features. Classical lissencephaly (formerly lissencephaly type I), the most common form, is defined by the presence of a very thick cortex and subcortical band heterotopia, whereas other types of lissencephaly present with other brain malformations, including agenesis of the corpus callosum and severe cerebellar hypoplasia. Features include agyria or **pachygyria** (absent or decreased cerebral convolutions, respectively); progressive spasticity; microcephaly; characteristic facial appearance with short nose, broad nasal bridge, upturned nose, hypertelorism, prominent upper lip, malformed or malpositioned ears. *Associated complications:* Intellectual disability, infantile spasms, late tooth eruption, failure to thrive, **dysphagia** (swallowing difficulty), congenital heart defect, intestinal atresia (congenital closure). *Cause:* Five genes have been defined to date that cause lissencephaly: LIS1 (on chromosome 17p13.3), 14-3-3 epsilon (on chromosome 17p13.3), DCX (on chromosome Xq22.3), RELN (on chromosome 7q22), and ARX (on chromosome Xp22.13); a deletion of one copy (haploinsufficiency) of any of the above genes is sufficient to cause one of the lissencephaly syndromes. *Inheritance:* NM with AD inheritance when passed from an affected individual; possibly increased recurrence risk if one parent has a balanced chromosomal translocation of chromosome 17p. *Prevalence:* Rare.

References: Kato, M., & Dobyns, W.B. (2003). Lissencephaly and the molecular basis of neuronal migration. *Human Molecular Genetics, 12*, R89–R96.

Leventer, R.J., Pilz, D.T., Matsumoto, N., et al. (2000). Lissencephaly and subcortical band heterotopia: Molecular basis and diagnosis. *Molecular Medicine Today, 6*, 277–284.

Lowe syndrome (oculocerebrorenal syndrome) *Clinical features:* Bilateral cataracts at birth, hypotonia, absent deep tendon reflexes, kidney dysfunction, dysmorphic facies. *Associated complications:* Failure to thrive, vitamin D-resistant rickets, seizures, visual impairment, glaucoma, intellectual disability in 75%, behavioral problems, intention tremor, craniosynostosis, peripheral neuropathy (damage to nerves). *Cause:* Abnormal inositol phosphate metabolism caused by mutations in the OCRL1 gene on chromosome Xq26.1. *Inheritance:* XLR with one third of cases being NM. *Prevalence:* Rare.

References: Addis, M., Loi, M., & Lepiani, C. (2004). OCRL mutation analysis in Italian patients with Lowe syndrome. *Human Mutation, 23*, 524–525.

Laube, G.F., Russell-Eggitt, I.M., & van't Hoff, W.G. (2004). Early proximal tubular dysfunction in Lowe's syndrome. *Archives of Disease in Childhood, 89*, 479–480.

mandibulofacial dysostosis *See* Treacher Collins syndrome.

maple syrup urine disease (MSUD) *Clinical features:* A disorder of branched chain amino acid metabolism with four identified clinical variants (classic, intermittent, intermediate, and thiamine-responsive); the classic form comprises 75% of cases and is characterized by severe opisthotonos (spasm with body in a bowed position and head and heels bent backward), hypertonia, hypoglycemia, lethargy, and respiratory difficulties. Symptoms appear within the first 48 hours of life; if untreated, it is most often fatal within 1 month. Untreated survivors have severe intellectual disability and spasticity. The intermittent form presents with periods of ataxia, behavior disturbances, drowsiness, and seizures. Attacks are triggered by infections, excessive protein intake, or other physiological stresses. Individuals with the intermediate form usually demonstrate mild to moderate intellectual disability. *Associated complications:* Acidosis, hypoglycemia, growth retardation, feeding problems; acute episodes are characterized by muscle fatigue, vomiting, impaired cognitive ability, hyperactivity, sleep disturbance, hallucinations, dystonia, and ataxia. *Cause:* Deficiency in branched chain alpha-ketoacid dehydrogenase caused by mutations in the genes (at chromosomal locations 1p31, 6p22–p21, and 19q13.1–q13.2) making up this enzyme complex. *Prevalence:* 1/220,000; increased prevalence in Mennonite population with an incidence of 1/200. *Inheritance:* AR. *Treatment:* High-calorie diet with restriction of branched chain amino acids. If instituted early (within 2 weeks of birth), the prognosis is good for typical intelligence. Thiamine is used in the thiamine-responsive form.

References: Chuang, D.T., & Shih, V.E. (2001). Maple syrup urine disease (branched-chain ketoaciduria). In C.R. Scriver, A.L. Beaudet, W.S. Sly, et al. (Eds.), *Metabolic and molecular bases of inherited disease* (pp. 1971–2006). New York: McGraw-Hill.

Holmes, M.D., Srauss, K.A., Robinson, D.L., et al. (2002). Diagnosis and treatment of maple syrup disease: A study of 36 patients. *Pediatrics, 109*, 999–1008.

Marfan syndrome *Clinical features:* Tall, thin body; upward dislocation of ocular lens; myopia; spider-like limbs; hypermobile joints. Average intelligence expected, although learning disabilities have been reported in up to 50% of children. *Associated complications:* Aortic dilatation or dissection, congestive heart failure, mitral valve prolapse, emphysema, sleep apnea, and scoliosis. *Cause:* Mutation in the fibrillin (FBN-1) gene located on chromosome 15q15–q21.3. *Inheritance:* AD with wide clinical variability. *Prevalence:* Estimated to be about 1/5,000.

References: Nollen, G.J., & Mulder, B.M.J. (2004). What is new in the Marfan syndrome? *International Journal of Cardiology, 97*, 103–108.

Ryan-Krause, P. (2002). Identify and manage Marfan syndrome in children. *Nurse Practitioner, 27*, 26–36.

Maroteaux-Lamy syndrome (MPS VI) *See* mucopolysaccharidoses (MPS).

McCune-Albright syndrome (polyostotic fibrous dysplasia) *Clinical features:* Large café-au-lait spots with irregular borders; fibrous dysplasia of bones (thinning of the bone with replacement of bone marrow with fibrous tissue, producing pain and increasing deformity); bowing of long bones; premature onset of puberty; advanced bone age. *Associated complications:* Hearing or visual impairment, hyperthyroidism, hyperparathyroidism (increased activity of the parathyroid gland, which controls calcium metabolism), abnormal adrenal function, increased risk of malignancy, occasional spinal cord anomalies. *Cause:* Post mitotic mutation in the GNAS1 gene (causing a defect in the enzyme adenyl cyclase) localized to 20q13. *Inheritance:* NM arising after fertilization (somatic mosaic) will be passed in an AD fashion if reproductive organs involved; theoretically lethal unless present in the mosaic form. *Testing:* Mutations in the GNAS1 gene were only present in 46% of patients presenting with the classic triad. Other tissue types may need to be tested to confirm the presence of the common mutation. *Prevalence:* Unknown.

References: de Sanctis, C., Lala, R., Matarazzo, P., et al. (1999). McCune-Albright syndrome: A longitudinal clinical study of 32 patients. *Journal of Pediatric Endocrinology and Metabolism, 12,* 817–826.

Lumbroso, S., Paris, F., Sultan, C., et al. (2004). Activating Gsalpha mutations: Analysis of 113 patients with signs of McCune Albright syndrome: A European collaborative study. *Journal of Clinical Endocrinology and Metabolism, 89,* 2107–2113.

MELAS (*m*itochondrial myopathy, *e*ncephalopathy, *l*actic *a*cidosis, and *s*troke-like episodes) *See* mitochondrial disorders.

Menkes syndrome (kinky hair syndrome) *Clinical features:* An inborn error of copper metabolism presenting at age 1–2 months with "steely" texture of hair and characteristic face with pudgy cheeks. *Associated complications:* Seizures, feeding difficulties, severe intellectual disability, recurrent infections, visual loss, bony abnormalities with tendency toward easy fracture, thrombosis, early death. *Cause:* Copper deficiency from decreased absorption and/or missing enzymes caused by mutations in the adenosine triphosphatase ATP7A gene at Xq13. *Inheritance:* XLR. *Prevalence:* 1/100,000 to 1/250,000. *Treatment:* Treatment with copper-histidine has been found to prevent neurological deterioration when provided before the age of 2 months. Treatment provided after two months of age cannot prevent neurologic, connective tissue, or bone complications.

References: Kirodian, B.G., Gogtay, N.J., Udani, V.P., & Kshirsagar, N.A. (2002). Treatment of Menkes disease with parenteral copper histidine. *Indian Pediatrics, 39,* 183–185.

Menkes, J.H. (1999). Menkes disease and Wilson disease: Two sides of the same copper coin. Part I: Menkes disease. *European Journal of Paediatric Neurology, 3,* 147–158.

MERRF (*m*yoclonic *e*pilepsy with *r*agged *r*ed *f*ibers) *See* mitochondrial disorders.

metachromatic leukodystrophy (sulfatide lipidosis) *Clinical features:* One of a group of lysosomal storage disorders in which lysosomes, the cell structures that digest toxic materials, are missing a necessary enzyme; the resulting accumulation of toxins leads to varying degrees of progressive neurological impairment, ranging from unsteady gait to severe rigidity and choreoathetosis. Muscle weakness and ataxia are common. Onset of the infantile form is by age 2 years and usually results in death by age 5. The juvenile form generally begins between 4 and 10 years of age, is rarer, and progresses more slowly. Two distinct adult onset forms exist, one presenting with neurologic/motor involvement and the other with behavioral abnormalities. *Associated complications:* Seizures, abdominal distension, mental deterioration. *Cause:* Mutations in the arylsulfatase A (ASA) gene on chromosome 22q cause ASA enzyme deficiency and result in the accumulation of sphingolipid sulfatide. *Inheritance:* AR. *Prevalence:* 1/40,000 in Sweden; rarer elsewhere. *Treatment:* Bone marrow transplantation may have beneficial effects on some tissues types but does not affect lipid storage in the brain.

References: Baumann, N., Turpin, J.-C., Lefevre, M., & Colsch, B. (2002). Motor and psycho-cognitive clinical types in adult metachromatic leukodystrophy: Genotype/phenotype relationships. *Journal of Physiology—Paris, 96,* 301–306.

Gieselmann, V. (2003). Metachromatic leukodystrophy: Recent research developments. *Journal of Child Neurology, 18,* 591–594.

methylmalonic aciduria *Clinical features:* In symptomatic cases, this disorder of organic acid metabolism is characterized by repeated episodes of vomiting, lethargy, and coma resulting from acidosis due to a high intake of protein or minor infection. On newborn screening analyses, some individuals with this metabolic abnormality may remain asymptomatic. *Associated complications:* Seizures, neutropenia (decreased white blood count), osteoporosis, infections, feeding abnormalities, intellectual disability, renal failure. *Cause:* Deficiency of enzyme methylmalonyl-CoA mutase (caused by mutation in the MUT gene at 6p21). *Inheritance:* AR. *Prevalence:* 1/20,000. *Treatment:* Treatment consists of a low-protein diet and supplemental vitamin B_{12} in those who have a B_{12}-responsive form; supplementation with carnitine is also used.

References: Horster, F., & Hoffmann, G.F. (2004). Pathophysiology, diagnosis, and treatment of methylmalonic aciduria: Recent advances and new challenges. *Pediatric Nephrology, 19,* 1071–1074.

van der Meer, S.B., Poggi, F., Spada, M., et al. (1994). Clinical outcome of long-term management of patients with vitamin B_{12}-unresponsive methylmalonic acidemia. *Journal of Pediatrics, 125,* 903–908.

Miller-Dieker syndrome *See* lissencephaly syndromes.

mitochondrial disorders (mitochondrial encephalopathies and myopathies) *Clinical features:* This diverse group of disorders is linked by a common etiology: abnormal function of the mitochondria (energy-producing intracellular structures) or mitochondrial metabolism. Mitochondrial disorders can affect every organ system. Common features include ptosis, external ophthalmoplegia (paralysis of the external eye muscles), myopathy, cardiomyopathy, short stature, and hypoparathyroidism. *Associated complications:* Seizures, sensorineural hearing loss, optic atrophy, retinitis pigmentosa (pigmentary changes in retina causing loss of peripheral vision and clumping of pigment), cataracts, diabetes, migraine, intestinal pseudo-obstruction, reflux, renal problems, exercise intolerance. *Cause:* Genes encoding nuclear DNA and mitochondrial DNA (mtDNA) are known to cause mitochondrial disorders. Mutations in different genes may cause the same symptoms. *Inheritance:* AR, AD, NM, or may be inherited from the mother through mtDNA. *Prevalence:* 1/8,500 for all mitochondrial disorders combined. *Treatment:* Early diagnosis and treatment of diabetes, eye abnormalities, and cardiac disease. Coenzyme Q10 and riboflavin have been used with some reported benefit. Six mitochondrial disorders are discussed next.

References: DiMauro, S. (2004). Mitochondrial diseases. *Biochemica et Biophysica Acta, 1658,* 80–88.

Thornburn, D.R. (2004). Mitochondrial disorders: Prevalence, myths, and advances. *Journal of Inherited Metabolic Disease, 27,* 349–362.

Kearns-Sayre syndrome *Clinical features:* Short stature, progressive external ophthalmoplegia, cardiomyopathy, retinitis pigmentosa. *Associated complications:* Visual impairment, hearing loss, myopathy, ataxia, endocrine abnormalities, diabetes mellitus, dementia. *Cause:* Rearrangements in mtDNA. *Inheritance:* Maternal, through mtDNA.

Leber hereditary optic neuropathy (Leber's congenital amaurosis, LHON) *Clinical features:* Bilateral central vision loss. *Associated complications:* Occasionally seen with multiple sclerosis, dystonia, or movement disorder. *Cause:* Primarily associated with point mutations in mtDNA. *Inheritance:* Maternal, through mtDNA. Males are more commonly affected.

Leigh syndrome (subacute necrotizing encephalomyopathy) *Clinical features:* Encephalopathy, ophthalmoplegia, optic atrophy, myopathy. *Associated complications:* Developmental delay and regression, ataxia, spasticity, early death. *Cause:* Deficiency of cytochrome *c* oxidase (COX) or another enzyme involved in energy metabolism. *Inheritance:* Maternal, AR, XLR.

MELAS (*m*itochondrial myopathy, *en*cephalopathy, *l*actic *a*cidosis, and *s*troke-like episodes) *Clinical features:* Migraine headaches, seizures, stroke-like episodes, encephalopathy (degenerative disease of the brain), myopathy. *Associated complications:* Progressive hearing loss, cortical blindness, ataxia, dementia, and lactic acidosis, recurrent vomiting, hemiparesis. *Cause:* A mutation in mtDNA encoding transfer RNA causes reduced mitochondrial protein synthesis. *Inheritance:* Maternal, through mtDNA.

MERRF (*m*yoclonic *e*pilepsy with *r*agged *r*ed *f*ibers) *Clinical features:* Myoclonic epilepsy, ataxia, spasticity, myopathy. *Associated complications:* Optic atrophy, sensorineural hearing loss, peripheral neuropathy, diabetes, cardiomyopathy, dementia, lipomas (fatty tumors); characteristic ragged red muscle fibers are seen on muscle biopsy examination. *Cause:* Mutations in mtDNA encoding transfer RNA. *Inheritance:* Maternal, through mtDNA.

NARP (*n*europathy, *a*taxia, *r*etinitis *p*igmentosa) *Clinical features:* Retinitis pigmentosa, sensory neuropathy. *Associated complications:* Seizures, dementia, ataxia, proximal weakness. *Cause:* Mutation in the ATP synthase 6 gene. *Inheritance:* Maternal, through mtDNA.

Moebius sequence (congenital facial diplegia) *Clinical features:* Expressionless face and facial weakness (bilateral in 92% of cases and unilateral in 8%) due to palsies of the 6th, 7th, and occasionally 12th cranial nerves; occasional abnormalities of fingers and legs; micrognathia; eye abnormalities including esotropia ("cross-eyed") and vision problems including myopia, astigmatism, and amblyopia; craniofacial malformations. *Associated complications:* Feeding difficulties, oral motor dysfunction, articulation disorder, occasional tracheal or laryngeal anomalies, gross and fine motor delay and dysfunction. Intellectual disability in 10%–50%. *Cause:* Linked to chromosomes 13q12–q13 and 1p34. *Inheritance:* Not well characterized, most reported cases are SP, possibly due to a NM; rare reports of AR, AD and X linked cases with variable expressivity. *Prevalence:* 1/50,000.

References: Johansson, M., Wentz, E., Fernell, E., et al. (2001). Autistic spectrum disorders in Mobius sequence: A comprehensive study of 25 individuals. *Developmental Medicine and Child Neurology, 43,* 338–345.

Verzijl, H.T., van der Zwaag, B., Cruysberg, J.R., & Padberg, G.W. (2003). Mobius syndrome redefined: A syndrome of rhombencephalic maldevelopment. *Neurology, 61,* 327–333.

monosomy X *See* Turner syndrome.

Morquio syndrome (MPS IV) *See* mucopolysaccharidoses (MPS).

MSUD *See* maple syrup urine disease.

mucopolysaccharidoses (MPS) *Clinical features:* A group of lysosomal storage disorders (defined in the entry about metachromatic leukodystrophy) in which glycosaminoglycans accumulate within the lysosomes; there are seven distinguishable forms of the disorder, each with two or more subgroups. Features shared by most include coarse facial features, thick skin, hirsutism (excessive hair), corneal clouding, and organomegaly (enlargement of spleen and liver). Growth deficiency, intellectual disability, cardiomyopathy, and skeletal dysplasia are also seen. *Inheritance:* All are AR except MPS II, Hunter syndrome. The various MPS disorders are differentiated by their clinical features, enzymatic defects, genetic transmission, and urinary mucopolysaccharide pattern. *Prevalence:* Overall estimated to be 1/22,500. MPS I (Hurler, Scheie, and Hurler-Scheie), MPS II (Hunter), and MPS III (Sanfilippo) syndromes are discussed next. Others include MPS IV (Morquio), MPS VI (Maroteaux-Lamy), and MPS VII (Sly) syndromes.

References: Muenzer, J. (2004). The mucopolysaccharidoses: a heterogeneous group of disorders with variable pediatric presentations. *Journal of Pediatrics, 144,* S27–S34.

Neufeld, E.F., & Muenzer, J. (2001). The mucopolysaccharidoses. In C.R. Scriver, A.L. Beaudet, W.S. Sly, et al. (Eds.), *The metabolic and molecular bases of inherited disease* (pp. 3421–3452). New York: McGraw-Hill.

MPS I (Hurler syndrome, Scheie syndrome, Hurler-Scheie syndrome) Due to the wide spectrum of clinical variability seen in patients with MPS I, patients with the mild form were originally thought to have a distinct disorder from those with severe symptoms. The mild condition was called Scheie syndrome (*previously called* MPS V), and the severe form of the disorder was *previously called* Hurler syndrome. Determination of a common enzyme deficiency in both conditions led to the realization that these conditions represented the variable presentation of a single disease. They are now denoted as IH and IS. *Clinical features:* Patients with the severe form of the disease (Hurler) have short stature; gradual coarsening of facial features in early childhood, including hypertrichosis (excessive hair); large skull; organomegaly; prominent lips; corneal clouding; dysostosis (malformed bones); stiffening of joints. There is progressive intellectual deterioration and spasticity. The milder (Scheie) form is characterized by typical stature, typical intelligence, and survival into adulthood. *Associated complications:* Chronic ear infections, hearing loss, occasional hernia and cardiac valve changes, visual impairment, brain cysts, airway obstruction. *Cause:* Deficiency of enzyme alpha-L-iduronidase caused by mutations in the iduronidase gene on chromosome 4p16.3. *Inheritance:* AR. *Incidence:* 1/144,000–1/1,000,000. *Treatment:* Bone marrow transplantation has shown some success in early treated cases.

MPS II (Hunter syndrome) *Clinical features:* Type IIA is severe; type IIB is mild. Features include short stature; enlarged liver and spleen; coarsening of facial features, with hypertrichosis beginning in early childhood; presence of pebbly ivory colored skin lesion on the back, upper arms, and thighs. Intellectual disability is mild or absent in type IIB; this subtype is compatible with survival to adulthood. Type IIA is highlighted by progressive intellectual deterioration first noted between 2 and 3 years of age; death occurs before age 15 in most cases and is similar to MPS IH, but with clear corneas. *Associated com-*

plications: Sensorineural hearing loss; retinitis pigmentosa with visual loss; macrocephaly; stiffening of joints, particularly those in the hands; cardiac valve disease in 90%; hernia; respiratory insufficiency; chronic diarrhea in 65%; seizures in 66%. *Cause:* Deficiency of enzyme iduronate 2-sulfatase caused by mutations in this gene on chromosome Xq28. *Inheritance:* XLR. *Incidence:* 1/34,000–1/132,000. *Treatment:* Minimal success has been reported with bone marrow transplantation.

MPS III (Sanfilippo syndrome) *Clinical features:* Four distinct types representing four different enzyme defects with similar clinical features; clinical features present between 2 and 6 years in children who otherwise appear typical. There is mild coarsening of facial features, coarse hair and hirsutism, absence of corneal clouding, mild enlargement of liver, joint stiffness, sleep disorders and progressive mental deterioration. Deterioration is most rapid in type IIIA; death occurs by 10–20 years in most cases. *Associated complications:* Severe behavioral disturbances by age 4 to 6 years, dysostosis, diarrhea in 50%, progressive spasticity and ataxia, precocious puberty, central breathing problems with advancing disease. *Cause:* Type IIIA: Deficiency of enzyme heparan sulfatase caused by mutations in sulfamidase gene on 17q25.3. Type IIIB: Deficiency of enzyme alpha-N-acetylglucosaminidase caused by mutations in the NAGLU gene on 17q21. Type IIIC: Deficiency of enzyme acetyl-CoA: alpha-glucosaminide N-acetyltransferase caused by mutations in a gene linked to chromosome 14. Type IIID: Deficiency of enzyme N-acetyl-alpha-glucosaminine-6-sulfatase caused by mutations in the G6S gene linked to chromosome 12q14. *Inheritance:* AR. *Incidence:* 1/73,000–1/280,000. *Treatment:* Treatment is supportive only. Bone marrow transplantation has not been successful.

multiple acyl-CoA dehydrogenase deficiency *See* glutaric acidemia, type II.

multiple carboxylase deficiency, infantile or early form (holocarboxylase synthetase deficiency) *Clinical features:* Disorder of organic acid metabolism characterized by seizures, hypotonia, lethargy, coma, skin rash, alopecia (loss of hair from skin areas where it is normally present), and acidosis. Often, the presenting feature is feeding difficulty or respiratory distress. *Associated complications:* Intellectual disability, hearing impairment, optic atrophy with visual impairment, recurrent infections, vomiting. *Cause:* Mutations causing enzyme deficiencies of holocarboxylase synthetase, or 3-methylcrotonyl-CoA carboxylase. *Inheritance:* AR. *Prevalence:* Rare. *Treatment:* Oral biotin supplementation. Prenatal treatment with oral biotin corrects lethargy, hypotonia, and vomiting.

References: Morrone, A., Malvagia, S., Donati, M.A., et al. (2002). Clinical findings and biochemical and molecular analysis of four patients with holocarboxylase synthetase deficiency. *American Journal of Medical Genetics, 111,* 1–18.

Wolf, B. (2001). Disorders of biotin metabolism. In C.R. Scriver, A.L. Beaudet, W.S. Sly, et al. (Eds.), *The metabolic and molecular bases of inherited disease* (pp. 3935–3964). New York: McGraw-Hill.

multiple carboxylase deficiency, late onset, juvenile form (biotinidase deficiency) *Clinical features:* A disorder characterized by varying degrees of intellectual disability, hypotonia, seizures (often infantile spasms), alopecia, skin rash, delayed myelination and lactic acidosis; the onset of symptoms usually occurs between 2 weeks and 2 years of age. *Associated complications:* Hearing and visual impairment, respiratory difficulties and apnea, recurrent infections. *Cause:* Defects in various enzymes for biotin transport or metabolism; genetic mutations have been identified in the biotinidase gene on chromosome 3p25 and the holocarboxylase synthetase gene on chromosome 21q22.1. *Inheritance:* AR. *Incidence:* 1/80,000–1/100,000. *Treatment:* Supplementation with oral biotin; response is better if used early in the course of the disease.

References: Grunwald, S., Champion, M.P., Leonard, J.V., et al. (2004). Biotinidase deficiency: A treatable leukoencephalopathy. *Neuropediatrics, 35,* 211–216.

Wolf, B. (2001). Disorders of biotin metabolism. In C.R. Scriver, A.L. Beaudet, W.S. Sly, et al. (Eds.), *The metabolic and molecular bases of inherited disease* (pp. 3935–3964). New York: McGraw-Hill.

muscular dystrophy, Duchenne (DMD) and Becker (BMD) types *Clinical features:* Progressive proximal muscular degeneration, muscle wasting, hypertrophy (enlargement) of calves, cardiomyopathy; onset of symptoms in DMD occurs before 3 years. Loss of ability to walk independently occurs by adolescence in DMD. The onset in BMD is later, and the progression is slower. *Associated complications:* Congestive heart failure, scoliosis, flexion contractures, respiratory compromise, and intestinal motility dysfunction (causing constipation); approximately 1/3 of boys with DMD have learning or intellectual disabilities. *Cause:* Mutations in the gene that encodes dystrophin localized to Xp21.1. *Inheritance:* XLR with 1/3 of cases due to a NM. *Incidence:* DMD 1/3,500 male births; BMD 1/20,000 males. *Treatment:* Glucocorticosteroids have been shown to prolong ambulation. *See also Chapter 14.*

References: Muntoni, F., Torelli, S., & Ferlini, A. (2003). Dystrophin and mutations: One gene, several proteins, multiple phenotypes. *The Lancet Neurology, 2,* 731–740.

Tidball, J.G., & Wehling-Henricks, M. (2004). Evolving therapeutic strategies for Duchenne muscular dystrophy: Targeting downstream events. *Pediatric Research, 56,* 831–841.

myasthenia gravis *Clinical features:* The most common symptoms are fatigability after repetitive movements and fluctuation of the symptoms throughout the day. *Cause:* Impairment in formation, binding or use of acetylcholine at the neuromuscular junction. Although in rare instances genetic in origin, it is most often acquired as an autoimmune disorder. *Treatment:* Directed at removing the offending antibody and increasing the level of acetylcholine in the synaptic cleft; the immunological approach has employed corticosteroid medication, immunoglobulin, plasmapheresis, and the surgical removal of the thymus gland. Transient symptom improvement due to increased neurotransmitter levels in the synaptic cleft is achieved with pyridostigmine (Mestinon). Using these various treatment approaches, individuals with myasthenia can lead quite typical lives.

References: Andrews, P.I. (2004). Autoimmune myasthenia gravis in childhood. *Seminars in Neurology, 24*(1), 101–10.

Tsao, C.Y., Mendell, J.R., Lo, W.D., Luquette, M., & Rennebohm, R. (2000). Myasthenia gravis and associated autoimmune diseases in children. *Journal of Child Neurology, 15*(11), 767–769.

myotonic dystrophy (Steinert's disease) *Clinical features:* The most prominent feature is myotonia, a form of dystonia involving increased muscular contractility combined with decreased power to release (e.g., a strong handshake with the inability to release it). Other features include myopathy, dysarthria, ptosis, and frontal balding. The age of onset varies from childhood to adulthood. The congenital form is severe, with neonatal hypotonia, motor delay, intellectual disability, and facial muscle palsy. In the congenital form, feeding difficulties and severe respiratory problems are common. Classic myotonia does not begin until around 10 years of age. *Associated complications:* Cataracts, cardiac conduction abnormalities, diabetes, and hypogonadism. *Cause:* Cytosine-thymine-guanine (CTG) expansion mutations in the muscle protein kinase gene on chromosome 19q13. Severity varies with the number of CTG repeats. Unaffected people have 5–30 repeat copies. Those with the classical adult form have more than 80 copies, and individuals with the childhood onset form usually have more than 500 copies. The correlation between the number of repeats, severity and age of onset, however, is not always consistent. *Inheritance:* AD with genetic anticipation (repeat expands in subsequent generations and the onset of symptoms becomes earlier); with rare exception, it is the mother who transmits mutations, causing the congenital form. *Prevalence:* 1/10,000–1/25,000; increased prevalence in certain areas of Quebec.

References: de Swart, B.J.M., van Engelen, B.G.M., van de Kerkhof, J.P.B.M., & Maassen B.A.M. (2004). Myotonia and flaccid dysarthria in patients with adult onset myotonic dystrophy. *Journal of Neurology, Neurosurgery, and Psychiatry, 75,* 1480–482.

Perini, G.I., Menegazzo, E., Ermani, M., et al. (1999). Cognitive impairment and (CTG)n expansion in myotonic dystrophy patients. *Biological Psychiatry, 46,* 425–431.

Nager syndrome   *See* acrofacial dysostosis.

NARP (neuropathy, ataxia, retinitis, pigmentosa)   *See* mitochondrial disorders.

neonatal adrenoleukodystrophy   *See* adrenoleukodystrophy, neonatal form.

neurofibromatosis, type I (von Recklinghausen disease)   *Clinical features:* Multiple café-au-lait spots, axillary (armpit) and inguinal (groin) freckling, nerve tumors (fibromas) in body and on skin, Lisch nodules (brown bumps on the iris of the eye). *Associated complications:* Glaucoma, scoliosis, hypertension, attention-deficit/hyperactivity disorder (ADHD), macrocephaly or hydrocephalus, visual impairments (secondary to optic gliomas), increased risk of numerous malignant and benign tumors in the nervous system (malignant peripheral nerve sheath tumors in 8%–13% of patients), verbal and non-verbal learning disabilities occur in 30%–65% of patients. *Cause:* Mutation in NF1 gene, which codes for neurofibromin protein, on chromosome 17q11.2. *Inheritance:* AD with variable expression. Approximately 50% represent NM. *Prevalence:* 1/3,500.

References: Arun, D., & Gutmann, D.H. (2004). Recent advances in neurofibromatosis type 1. *Current Opinion in Neurology, 17,* 101–105.

Rosser, T.L., & Packer, R.J. (2003). Neurocognitive dysfunction in children with neurofibromatosis type 1. *Current Neurology and Neuroscience Reports, 3,* 129–136.

neurofibromatosis, type II *Clinical features:* Bilateral vestibular schwannomas (benign tumors of auditory nerve), cranial and spinal tumors, neuropathy, café-au-lait spots (usually fewer than six); in contrast to type I, no Lisch nodules or axillary freckling are seen. *Associated complications:* Deafness (average age of onset is 20 years), cataracts or other ocular abnormalities, meningiomas (tumor of the meninges); tumor growth rates are variable within the same patients and between patients. *Cause:* Mutation in tumor-suppressor (NF2) gene encoding merlin protein on chromosome 22q12.2; genotype/phenotype studies show that nonsense mutations (mutations that create a stop codon) are associated with more severe disease presentation than other type of genetic mutations. *Inheritance:* AD with significant variability between patients; up to 50% may represent NM. *Prevalence:* 1/210,000. *Incidence:* 1/33,000–1/40,000. *Treatment:* Mortality is lower for patients treated in specialty centers. Microsurgery and radiation therapy are both commonly used.

References: Baser, M.E., Evans, D.G.R., & Gutmann, D.H. (2003). Neurofibromatosis 2. *Current Opinion in Neurology, 16,* 27–33.

MacCollin, M., & Mautner, V.F. (1998). The diagnosis and management of neurofibromatosis 2 in childhood. *Seminars in Pediatric Neurology, 5,* 243–252.

neuronal ceroid lipofuscinosis, juvenile *See* Batten disease.

Niemann-Pick disease, types A and B *Clinical features:* Lysosomal storage disorder; type A presents in infancy with failure to thrive, enlarged liver and spleen, rapidly progressive neurological decline. Death occurs by age 2–3 years. *Associated complications:* Intellectual disability, ataxia, myoclonus, eye abnormalities, coronary artery disease, lung disease; type B is variable but compatible with survival to adulthood and may cause few or no neurological abnormalities. Main clinical features of type B are enlargement of the spleen and liver resulting in liver dysfunction, as well as cardiac disease, lipid abnormalities, pulmonary involvement, and growth retardation. *Cause:* Sphingomyelinase enzyme deficiency caused by mutations in the sphingomyelinase (SMPD) gene on chromosome 11p15.4. *Inheritance:* AR. *Prevalence:* Rare; incidence of type A is increased in Ashkenazi Jewish population, type B is seen equally in all ethnic groups.

References: Schuchman, E.H., & Desnick, R.J. (2001). Niemann-Pick disease types A and B: Acid sphingomyelinase deficiencies. In C.R. Scriver, A.L. Beaudet, W.S. Sly, et al. (Eds.), *The metabolic and molecular bases of inherited disease* (pp. 3589–3610). New York: McGraw-Hill.

Wasserstein, M.P., Desnick, R.J., Schuchman, E.H., et al. (2004). The natural history of type B Niemann Pick disease: Results from a 10 year longitudinal study. *Pediatrics, 114,* 672–677.

Noonan syndrome *Clinical features:* Short stature; characteristic facial features, including triangular shape, deep philtrum, downslanting palpebral fissures, ptosis; low-set ears; low posterior hair line; short or webbed neck; congenital heart defects (usually pulmonary valve stenosis); shield-shaped chest; mean IQ score of 85–90. *Associated complications:* Sensorineural deafness, malocclusion of teeth, learning disabilities with deficits in verbal learning, ADHD, poor motor coordination, bleeding abnormalities. *Cause:* Mutations in the PTPN11 gene cause approximately half of cases; additional patients have been found to have mutations in the KRAS gene. *Inheritance:* Majority of cases are due to NM with AD inheritance when passed from an affected individual. *Prevalence:* 1/1,000–1/2,500. *Treatment:* Human growth hormone has been used to treat short stature in some patients with Noonan syndrome.

References: Lee, D.A., Portnoy, S., Hill, P., et al. (2005). Psychological profile of children with Noonan syndrome. *Developmental Medicine and Child Neurology, 47,* 35–38.

van der Burgt, I., Thoonen, G., Roosenboom, N., et al. (1999). Patterns of cognitive functioning in school-aged children with Noonan syndrome associated with variability in phenotypic expression. *Journal of Pediatrics, 135,* 707–713.

oculoauriculovertebral spectrum (facio-auriculo-vertebral spectrum; Goldenhar syndrome; hemifacial microsomia) *Clinical features:* Unilateral external ear deformity ranging from absence of an ear to microtia (tiny ear), preauricular (earlobe) tags or pits, middle-ear abnormality with variable hearing loss, facial asymmetry with small size unilaterally, macrostomia (large mouth), occasional cleft palate, microphthalmia or eyelid coloboma. *Associated complications:* Vertebral anomalies, occasional heart and renal (kidney) defects, intellectual disability in 10%. *Cause:* Unknown. *Inheritance:* Genetically heterogeneous; may be SP in some cases resulting from gestational maternal diabetes; additionally cases with clear AR and AD inheritance have been reported. *Prevalence:* 1/45,000 in Northern Ireland, presumably less common in other populations. *Incidence:* 1/3,000 to 1/5,000.

References: Healey, D., Letts, M., & Jarvis, J.G. (2002). Cervical spine instability in children with Goldenhar's syndrome. *Canadian Journal of Surgery, 45,* 341–344.

Poon, C.C., Meara, J.G., & Heggie, A.A. (2003). Hemifacial microsomia: Use of the OMENS-plus classification at the Royal Children's Hospital of Melbourne. *Plastic and Reconstructive Surgery, 111,* 1011–1018.

oculocerebrorenal syndrome *See* Lowe syndrome.

oculomandibulodyscephaly with hypotrichosis *See* Hallermann-Streiff syndrome.

Optiz syndrome (Opitz-Frias syndrome; Opitz oculogenitolaryngeal syndrome; previously called G syndrome) (G refers to surname of original patient described.) *Clinical features:* Hypertelorism (wide-spaced eyes), hypospadias, imperforate anus (without an opening), dysphagia, bifurcated (divided) nasal tip, broad nasal bridge, widow's peak, occasional cleft lip/palate, mild to moderate intellectual disability in two thirds of affected individuals. *Associated complications:* Gastroesophageal reflux; esophageal dysmotility (poor movement of food through the esophagus); hoarse cry; occasional congenital heart defect; agenesis of corpus callosum; platelet abnormalities; structural cerebellar anomalies, including Dandy-Walker malformation. *Cause:* MID1 gene on Xp22.3 is known

to cause the X linked form. The gene believed to cause the AD form has been linked to 22q11.2. *Inheritance:* AD and XLR. In both the AD and XLR forms symptoms are more severe in males than in females. *Prevalence:* Unknown.

References: De Falco, F., Cainarca, S., Andolfi, G., et al. (2003). X-linked Opitz syndrome: Novel mutations in the MID1 gene and redefinition of the clinical spectrum. *American Journal of Medical Genetics, 120,* 222–228.

So, J., Suckow, V., Kijas, Z., et al. (2004). Mild phenotypes in a series of patients with Opitz GBBB syndrome with MID1 mutations. *American Journal of Medical Genetics, 132,* 1–7.

osteogenesis imperfecta *Clinical features:* Seven clinically distinct forms of this metabolic disease of bone have been described. Type I is characterized by typical height or mild short stature, bone fragility, and blue sclera. Type II usually presents with severe bone deformity and death in the newborn period. Type III is characterized by progressive bone deformity, short stature, triangular face, severe scoliosis, and dental abnormalities. Type IV is clinically similar to type I, but presents with normal sclerae, milder bone deformity, variable short stature, and dental abnormalities. Type V is associated with mild to moderate short stature, bone deformity, and other bone abnormalities. Type VI is characterized by severe bone deformity with moderate short stature and a fish scale pattern of bone deposition. Type VII causes moderate bone deformations, mild short stature, with a shortening of the long bones (humerus and femur). *Associated complications:* Increased prevalence of fractures (may be confused with physical abuse) that decreases after puberty; scoliosis; mitral valve prolapse; occasionally progressive adolescent-onset hearing loss. *Cause:* Mutations in one of the genes regulating collagen formation. Type 1 maps to 17q21–q22 (COLA1). Types II through IV map to both the COLA1 gene and 7q21–q22 (COLA2). The genetic cause of types V, VI, and VII are yet to be determined. *Inheritance:* Type I, IV, V, VI: AD; type II: AD (all type II cases are NM; recurrence risk is 6% due to gonadal mosaicism); type III is occasionally AR, type VII is AR (only seen in Indigenous Peoples in Northern Quebec). *Prevalence:* 1/30,000. *Treatment:* Cyclic intravenous pamidronate therapy to increase bone mineral density. *(See Chapter 14.)*

References: Rauch, F., & Glorieux, F.H. (2004). Osteogenesis Imperfecta. *The Lancet, 363,* 1377–1385.

Zeitlin, L., Fassier, F., & Glorieux, F.H. (2003). Modern approach to children with osteogenesis imperfecta. *Journal of Pediatric Orthopedics. Part B, 12,* 77–87.

pentasomy X   *See* XXX, XXXX, and XXXXX syndromes.

Pfeiffer syndrome (acrocephalosyndactyly, type V)   Three subtypes of Pfeiffer syndrome have been described with a range of clinical severity. *Clinical features:* Mild craniosynostosis with brachycephaly, flat mid-face, broad thumbs and toes, hypertelorism, and partial syndactyly. *Associated complications:* Hydrocephalus, airway obstruction due to mid-face hypoplasia, hearing impairment, seizures, occasional intellectual disability. *Cause:* Mutations in the genes that code for fibroblast growth factor receptors 1 and 2 (FGFR1 and FGFR2) on chromosomes 8p11.2–p11.1 and 10q26, respectively. *Inheritance:* AD with many cases due to NM. *Prevalence:* Unknown. *References:* Hockstein, N.G., McDonald-McGinn, D., Zackai, E., et al. (2004). Tracheal anomalies in Pfeiffer syndrome. *Archives of Otolaryngology, Head, and Neck Surgery, 130,* 1298–1302.

Plomp, A.S., Robin, N.H., Scott, J.A., Arnold, J.E., et al. (1998). Favorable prognosis for children with Pfeiffer syndrome types 2 and 3: Implications for classification. *American Journal of Medical Genetics, 75,* 240–244.

phenylketonuria (PKU)   *Clinical features:* Inborn error of amino acid metabolism without acute clinical symptoms; intellectual disability, microcephaly, abnormal gait, and seizures may develop in untreated individuals. Treated individuals have still been found to have mild cognitive deficits especially in executive function. Pale skin and blond hair are common features. *Associated complications:* Behavioral disturbances, cataracts, skin disorders, movement disorders. *Cause:* Classically caused by a deficiency of the enzyme phenylalanine hydroxylase, which is associated with a mutation in the PAH gene on chromosome 12q24.1. *Inheritance:* AR. *Prevalence:* 1/10,000 among Caucasians in the United States. *Treatment:* Early identification is available through newborn screening. A phenylalanine-restricted, low-protein diet should be continued at least until adulthood and in females during childbearing years. Specialized formulas are available for individuals who need to be on the restricted diet. *See also Chapter 20.*
References: Leuzzi, V., Pansini, M., Sechi, E., et al. (2004). Executive function impairment in early treated PKU subjects with normal mental development. *Journal of Inherited Metabolic Disease, 27,* 115–125.

Sullivan, J.E., & Chang, P. (1999). Review: Emotional and behavioral functioning in phenylketonuria. *Journal of Pediatric Psychology, 24,* 281–299.

phenytoin syndrome (fetal hydantoin syndrome)   *See Chapter 2.*

Pierre-Robin sequence   *Clinical features:* Micrognathia, cleft palate, glossoptosis (downward displacement of tongue). *Associated complications:* Neonatal feeding problems, apnea or respiratory distress, upper airway obstruction, GI reflux. *Cause:* Impaired closure of the posterior palatal shelves early in development; this defect can be an isolated finding or can be associated with trisomy 18 or other syndromes. *Inheritance:* AR; a rare X-linked form also exists. *Prevalence:* Unknown. *Treatment:* Surgical procedure (mandibular distraction osteogenesis) can be used to correct micrognathia, which alleviates many of the feeding and respiratory problems.
References: Kapp-Simon, K.A., & Krueckeberg, S. (2000). Mental development in infants with cleft lip and/or palate. *Cleft Palate-Craniofacial Journal, 37,* 65–70.

Monasterio, F.O., Molina, F., Berlanga, F., et al. (2004). Swallowing disorders in Pierre Robin sequence: Its correction by distraction. *Journal of Craniofacial Surgery, 15,* 934–941.

PKU   *See* phenylketonuria.

polyostotic fibrous dysplasia   *See* McCune-Albright syndrome.

Prader-Willi syndrome   *Clinical features:* Short stature; failure to thrive in infancy; hyperphagia (abnormally increased appetite); almond-shaped eyes; viscous (thick) saliva; hypotonia, particularly in neck region; hypogonadism with cryptorchidism; small hands and feet; hypopigmentation. *Associated complications:* Mild to moderate intellectual disability, behavior problems (tantrums, obsessive compulsive disorder, rigidity, food stealing, skin picking), obstructive sleep apnea, high pain threshold, osteoporosis, neonatal temperature instability, type 2 diabetes. *Cause:* Approximately 75% have a microdeletion on the long arm of the paternally inherited chromosome 15 (15q11–q13); 25% have maternal uniparental disomy. *Inheritance:* NM with AD inheritance when passed from an affected individual. *Incidence:* 1/25,000. *Prevalence:* 1/50,000.

References: Einfeld, S.L., Smith, A., Durvasula, S., et al. (1999). Behavior and emotional disturbance in Prader-Willi syndrome. *American Journal of Medical Genetics, 82,* 123–127.

Goldstone A.P. (2004). Prader-Willi syndrome: Advances in genetics, pathophysiology and treatment. *Trends in Endocrinology and Metabolism, 15,* 12–20.

propionic acidemia   *Clinical features:* A disorder of organic acid metabolism characterized by episodes of vomiting, lethargy, and coma; hypotonia; bone marrow suppression; enlarged liver (hepatomegaly), characteristic facies with puffy cheeks and exaggerated Cupid's bow upper lip. *Associated complications:* Impaired antibody production, intellectual disability, seizures in half, abnormalities of muscle tone, lack of appetite, prolonged drowsiness, rapid difficult breathing; a late-onset form of proprionic acidemia has been described with average onset at 16 months. *Cause:* Deficiency of enzyme propionyl-CoA carboxylase (PCC) caused by mutations in the PCCA gene on chromosome 13q32 and the PCCB gene on chromosome 3q21–q22. *Inheritance:* AR. Prevalence: 1/2,000–1/5,000 in Saudi Arabia; rare elsewhere. *Treatment:* Treatment consists of a diet low in valine, isoleucine, threonine, and methionine with supplement of carnitine. A commercial formula is available. Hemofiltration and peritoneal dialysis have been used with some success in patients in metabolic crisis.

References: North, K.N., Korson, M.S., Gopal, Y.R., et al. (1995). Neonatal-onset propionic acidemia: Neurologic and developmental profiles, and implications for management. *Journal of Pediatrics, 126,* 916–922.

Sass, J.O., Hofmann, M., Skladal, D., et al. (2004). Propionic academia revisited: A workshop report. *Clinical Pediatrics, 43,* 837–843.

Refsum disease, infantile   *Clinical features:* Failure to thrive, absent or tiny ear lobes, high forehead, single palmar crease, flat facial profile and nasal bridge, retinal degeneration, hypotonia, liver enlargement and dysfunction. *Associated complications:* Sensorineural hearing impairment, intellectual disability, peripheral neuropathy, hypercholesterolemia

(elevated blood cholesterol level); there is also a late-onset form of this disease. *Cause:* Accumulation of phytanic acid, very long chain fatty acids, di- and trihydroxycholestanoic acids, and pipecolic acid due to defect in peroxisomal function. *Inheritance:* AR. *Prevalence:* Rare.

References: Poll-The, B.T., Gootjes, J., & Duran, M. (2004). Peroxisome biogenesis disorders with prolonged survival: Phenotype expression in a cohort of 31 patients. *American Journal of Medical Genetics, 126,* 333–338.

Weinstein, R. (1999). Phytanic acid storage disease (Refsum's disease): Clinical characteristics, pathophysiology, and the role of the therapeutic apheresis in its management. *Journal of Clinical Apheresis, 14,* 181–184.

retinitis pigmentosa   *Clinical features:* A group of diseases associated with retinal degeneration, constricted visual fields, and progressive blindness; initial symptom is night blindness occurring in adolescence or adult life and loss of peripheral vision. *Associated complications:* May occur as an isolated condition or as part of over 30 syndromes (e.g., Usher syndrome, mitochondrial disorders). *Cause:* More than 32 different genes have been identified to date. Additional causative genes are anticipated. *Inheritance:* AD in 15%–20% of cases, AR in 20%–25%, and XLR in 10%–15%. A genetic cause is yet to be identified in the remaining 40%–55%. Recurrence risk depends on cause and family history. *Incidence:* 1/3,500.

References: Sharma, R.K., & Ehinger, B. (1999). Management of hereditary retinal degenerations: Present status and future directions. *Survey of Ophthalmology, 43,* 427–444.

Wang, D.Y., Chan, W.M., Tam, P.O., et al. (2005). Gene mutations in retinitis pigmentosa and their clinical implications. *Clinica Chemica Acta, 351,* 5–16.

Rett syndrome (Rett's Disorder)   *Clinical features:* Typical development for 6–9 months, followed by progressive encephalopathy. Features of autism, loss of purposeful hand use with characteristic ringing of hands, hyperventilation, ataxia, spasticity. *Associated complications:* Postnatal onset of microcephaly, seizures. *Cause:* Mutations in the methyl-CpG binding protein 2 (MeCP2) gene at Xq28. *Inheritance:* XLD with severe, neonatal encephalopathy or lethality in males. *Preva-*

lence: 1/10,000–1/15,000 among females. *See also Chapter 23.*

References: Hoffbuhr, K., Devaney, J., LaFleur, B., et al. (2001). MeCP2 mutations in children with and without the phenotype of Rett syndrome. *Neurology, 56,* 1486–1495.

Naidu, S., Bibat, G., Kratz, L., et al. (2003). Clinical variability in Rett syndrome. *Journal of Child Neurology, 18,* 662–668.

Riley-Day syndrome *See* familial dysautonomia.

Robinow syndrome (fetal face syndrome) *Clinical features:* Slight to moderate short stature; short forearms; macrocephaly with frontal bossing (prominent central forehead); flat facial profile with apparent hypertelorism; small, upturned nose; hypogenitalism; micrognathia; small face; tented upper lip with occasional clefting of the lower lip; hypertrophy of the gums; deficiency of the lower eyelid giving the appearance of protruding eyes (exophthalmos); congenital heart defects. *Associated complications:* Vertebral or rib anomalies, dental malocclusion, genital hypoplasia, inguinal (groin) hernia, enlarged liver and spleen, developmental delay in 15% of cases. *Cause:* Mutations in the ROR2 gene on 9q22. *Inheritance:* Rarely AD; AR form is most common, is clinically more severe, and is often accompanied by rib anomalies. *Prevalence:* Rare.

References: Patton, M.A., Afzal, A.R. (2002). Robinow syndrome. *Journal of Medical Genetics, 39,* 305–310.

Van Steensel, M. (1998). Robinow syndrome. *Journal of Medical Genetics, 35,* 349–350.

Rubinstein-Taybi syndrome *Clinical features:* Growth retardation, broad thumbs and toes, maxillary hypoplasia (small upper jaw), high arched palate, down slanted palpebral fissures, prominent nose, pouting lower lip, short upper lip, occasional agenesis of corpus callosum. *Associated complications:* Apnea, constipation, reflux, feeding difficulties, hypotonia, cardiac defects, renal anomalies, ophthalmologic problems, keloid (scar) formation, glaucoma, intellectual disability. *Cause:* Mutations of the CREB binding protein (CBP) gene on chromosome 16p13.3, most often an interstitial microdeletion of this chromosome locus. *Inheritance:* Most cases are due to a NM in the CBP gene with AD inheritance when passed from an affected individual. *Prevalence:* 1/125,000.

References: Hennekam, R.C. (1993). Rubinstein-Taybi syndrome: A history in pictures. *Clinical Dysmorphology, 2,* 87–92.

Wiley, S., Swayne, S., Rubinstein, J.H., et al. (2003). Rubinstein-Taybi syndrome medical guidelines. *American Journal of Medical Genetics, 119,* 101–110.

Russell-Silver syndrome (Silver-Russell syndrome) *Clinical features:* Short stature of prenatal onset; skeletal asymmetry with hemihypertrophy (enlargement of one side of the body) in 60%; triangular facies; beaked nose; thin upper lip; narrow, high-arched palate; blue sclerae; occasional café-au-lait spots; fifth finger clinodactyly; genital anomalies in males. *Associated complications:* Delayed fontanelle (soft spot) closure, hypocalcemia in neonatal period with sweating and rapid breathing, increased risk of fasting hypoglycemia as toddler, feeding difficulties, precocious sexual development, vertebral anomalies. *Cause:* Duplications or maternal uniparental disomy at 7p12–p11.2; some evidence that chromosome 17q25 may be a cause in a subset of cases. *Inheritance:* NM with AD inheritance when passed from an affected individual; maternal uniparental disomy in 10%; AR in rare cases. *Prevalence:* Unknown.

References: Hitchins, M.P., Stanier, P., Preece, M.A., et al. (2001). Silver-Russell syndrome: A dissection of the genetic aetiology and candidate chromosomal regions. *Journal of Medical Genetics, 38,* 810–819.

Price, S.M., Stanhope, R., Garrett, C., et al. (1999). The spectrum of Silver-Russell syndrome: A clinical and molecular genetic study and new diagnostic criteria. *Journal of Medical Genetics, 36,* 837–842.

Saethre-Chotzen syndrome *Clinical features:* Short stature, brachycephaly (forshortened skull), acrocephaly, radioulnar synostosis (fusion of lower arm bones), syndactyly of the second and third fingers and third and fourth toes, fifth finger clinodactyly, craniosynostosis, small ears, flat facies with long pointed nose and low hairline and facial asymmetry, shallow asymmetric eye orbits with hypertelorism. *Associated complications:* Late closing fontenelles (soft spot of forehead), deafness, strabismus, proptosis, lacrimal (tear) duct abnormalities. *Cause:* Mutations in the TWIST transcription factor gene on chromosome 7p21. *Inheritance:* AD. *Prevalence:* Rare.

References: Chun, K., Teebi, A.S., Jung, J.H., et al. (2002). Genetic analysis of patients with the Saethre-Chotzen phenotype. *American Journal of Medical Genetics, 110,* 136–143.

Flores-Sanart, L. (2002). New insights into craniosynostosis. *Seminar in Pediatric Neurology, 9*, 274–291.

Sanfilippo syndrome (MPS III) *See* mucopolysaccharidoses (MPS).

Scheie syndrome (MPS V) *See* mucopolysaccharidoses (MPS).

Silver-Russell syndrome *See* Russell-Silver syndrome.

Sly syndrome (MPS VII) *See* mucopolysaccharidoses (MPS).

Smith-Lemli-Opitz syndrome *Clinical features:* Microcephaly, short nose with upturned nostrils, low serum cholesterol, syndactyly of second and third toes, genitourinary abnormalities, renal anomalies, and lung malformations. *Associated complications:* Intrauterine growth restriction, hypotonia, moderate to severe intellectual disability, motor and language delay, seizures, feeding difficulties and vomiting, photosensitivity, occasional heart defect. Specific behavioral features include: irritability, sleep disturbance, self-injurious behavior. *Cause:* Defect in cholesterol metabolism (conversion of 7-DHC to cholesterol) caused by mutations in the sterol delta-7-reductase gene on chromosome 11q12–q13. Clinical features result from deficiency of cholesterol as well as toxic accumulation of 7-DHC. *Inheritance:* AR. *Prevalence:* 1/20,000–1/40,000. *Treatment:* Dietary modifications, including increased cholesterol ingestion.

References: Jira, P.E., Waterham, H.R., Wanders, R.J., et al. (2003). Smith-Lemli-Opitz syndrome and the DHCR7 gene. *Annals of Human Genetics, 67*, 26–9-280.

Sikora, D.M., Ruggiero, M., Petit-Kekel, K., et al. (2004). Cholesterol supplementation does not improve developmental progress in Smith-Lemli-Opitz syndrome. *Journal of Pediatrics, 144*, 783–791.

Smith-Magenis syndrome *Clinical features:* Short stature, brachycephaly, cleft palate, congenital heart defect, myopia, mid-face hypoplasia, prominent chin, varying degrees of intellectual disability. *Associated complications:* Genital or vertebral anomalies, scoliosis, hearing impairment, self-injurious behavior, other behavior problems. *Cause:* Microdeletion at chromosome 17p11.2. *Inheritance:* Most cases represent new mutations with AD inheritance when passed from an affected individual. *Prevalence:* 1/25,000.

References: Sarimski, K. (2004). Communicative competence and behavioral phenotype in children with Smith-Magenis syndrome. *Genetic Counseling, 15*, 347–355.

Shelley, B.P., Robertson, M.M. (2005). The neuropsychiatry and multisystem features of the Smith-Magenis syndrome: A review. *Journal of Neuropsychiatry and Clinical Neuroscience, 17*, 91–97.

Sotos syndrome *Clinical features:* An overgrowth syndrome characterized by a distinctive head shape, macrocephaly, downslanting eyes, flat nasal bridge, accelerated growth with advanced bone age, high forehead, hypertelorism, and prominent jaw. *Associated complications:* Increased risk of abdominal tumors, hypotonia, marked speech delay, congenital heart defects, varying degrees of cognitive impairment. *Cause:* Mutations in the NSD1 gene have been found to be causative; in addition, submicroscopic deletions have been identified at chromosome 5q35. *Inheritance:* AD with the majority of cases due to a NM. *Prevalence:* At least 112 cases have been reported in the medical literature.

References: Kurotaki, N., Harada, N., Shimokawa, O., et al. (2003). Fifty microdeletions among 112 cases of Sotos syndrome: Low copy repeats possibly mediate the common deletion. *Human Mutation, 22*, 378–387.

Tatton-Brown, K., & Rahman, N. (2004). Clinical features of NSD1-positive Sotos syndrome. *Clinical Dysmorphology, 13*, 199–204.

spongy degeneration of central nervous system *See* Canavan disease.

Stickler syndrome (hereditary progressive arthroophthalmopathy) *Clinical features:* Flat facies, myopia, cleft of hard or soft palate, spondyloepiphyseal dysplasia (lag of mineralization of bone). *Associated complications:* Hypotonia, hyperextensible joints, occasional scoliosis, risk of retinal detachment, cataracts, arthropathy in late childhood or adulthood, occasional hearing loss or cognitive impairment. *Cause:* Mutations in type 2 and type 11 procollagen genes (COL2A1, COL 11A1, COL11A2), which have been linked to chromosomes 12q13.11–q13.2, 1p21, and 6p 21.3, respectively. *Inheritance:* AD with variable expression. *Prevalence:* 1/20,000.

References: Donoso, L.A., Edwards, A.O., Frost, A.T., et al. (2003). Clinical variability of Stickler syndrome: Role of exon 2 of the collagen COL2A1 gene. *Survey of Ophthalmology, 48*, 191–203.

Snead, M.P., & Yates, J.R. (1999). Clinical and molecular genetics of Stickler syndrome. *Journal of Medical Genetics, 36*, 353–359.

Sturge-Weber syndrome *Clinical features:* Flat facial "port wine stains," seizures, glaucoma, intracranial vascular abnormality. *Associated complications:* Hemangiomas (benign congenital tumors made up of newly formed blood vessels) of meninges; may be progressive in some cases, with gradual visual or cognitive impairment and recurrent stroke-like episodes, hemiparesis, hemiatrophy, and hemianopia (decreased vision in one eye). *Cause:* Unknown. *Inheritance:* Usually SP, possibly due to somatic mosaicism; AD in a few reported cases. *Incidence:* 1/50,000. *Treatment:* Pharmacologic therapies can be used to treat seizures, surgical intervention can be used for glaucoma and laser therapy can be used to remove vascular facial features.

References: Powell, J. (1999). Update on hemangiomas and vascular malformations. *Current Opinion in Pediatrics, 11*, 457–463.

Thomas-Sohl, K.A., Vaslow, D.F., & Maria, B.L. (2004). Sturge-Weber syndrome: A review. *Pediatric Neurology, 30*, 303–310.

subacute necrotizing encephalomyopathy Leigh syndrome; *See* mitochondrial disorders.

sulfatide lipidosis *See* metachromatic leukodystrophy.

TAR syndrome *See* thrombocytopenia-absent radius syndrome.

Tay-Sachs disease (GM2 gangliosidosis, type I) *Clinical features:* A lysosomal storage disorder leading to a progressive neurological condition characterized by deafness, blindness, and seizures; development is typical for the first several months of life. Subsequently, there is an increased startle response, hypotonia followed by hypertonia, cherry-red spot in maculae, optic nerve atrophy. There is rapid decline and fatality by age 5 years. An adult form of this enzyme deficiency presents with ataxia. *Associated complications:* Feeding abnormalities, aspiration. *Cause:* Deficiency of the enzyme hexosaminidase A caused by mutation in the gene at chromosome 15q23–q24. *Inheritance:* AR. *Prevalence:* 1/112,000; 1/3,800 in Ashkenazi Jewish population; increased frequency in the Cajun and French Canadian populations..

References: Fernandes Filho, J.A., & Shapiro, B.E. (2004). Tay Sachs disease. *Archives of Neurology, 61*, 1466–1468.

Gravel, R.A., Kaback, M.M, Proia, R.L., et al. (2001). The GM2 gangliosidoses. In C.R. Scriver, A.L. Beaudet, W.S. Sly, et al. (Eds.), *The metabolic and molecular bases of inherited disease* (pp. 3827–3876). New York: McGraw-Hill.

tetrasomy X *See* XXX, XXXX, and XXXXX syndromes.

thrombocytopenia-absent radius syndrome (TAR syndrome) *Clinical features:* Radial aplasia (absence of one of the lower arm bones) with normal thumbs; thrombocytopenia (platelet deficiency) is present in all cases and symptomatic in 90% of cases; 50% of patients have dysmorphic features including micrognathia (small jaw) and low posteriorly rotated ears. *Associated complications:* Knee joint abnormalities, neonatal foot swelling, occasional congenital heart or renal (kidney) defect, gastrointestinal bleeding, and occasional intracerebral bleeding. *Cause:* Unknown. *Inheritance:* AR, possibly AD with variable penetrance. *Prevalence:* Unknown. *Treatment:* Platelet infusions.

References: Greenhalgh, K.L., Howell, R.T., Bottani, A., et al. (2002). Thrombocytopenia—absent radius syndrome: A clinical genetic study. *Journal of Medical Genetics, 39*, 876–881.

McLaurin, T.M., Bukrey, C.D., Lovett, R.J., et al. (1999). Management of thrombocytopenia-absent radius (TAR) syndrome. *Journal of Pediatric Orthopedics, 19*, 289–296.

Treacher Collins syndrome (mandibulofacial dysostosis) *Clinical features:* Characteristic facial appearance with malformation of external ears, small chin, flattened midface, cleft palate. *Associated complications:* Conductive or mixed (conductive and sensorineural) hearing loss; defects of middle and inner ear; respiratory and feeding problems, apnea; intelligence is average in 95% of cases. *Cause:* Mutations in TCOFI gene on chromosome 5q32–q33. *Inheritance:* AD. *Incidence:* 1/25,000–1/50,000. *Treatment:* Surgical repair of most malformations.

References: Beaune, L., Forrest, C.R., Keith, T. (2004). Adolescents' perspectives on living and growing up with Treacher Collins syndrome: A qualitative study. *Cleft Palate–Craniofacial Journal, 41*, 343–50.

Posnick, J.C. (2000). Treacher Collins syndrome: Current evaluation, treatment, and future directions. *Cleft Palate–Craniofacial Journal, 37*, 434–456.

Winter, R.M. (1996). What's in a face? *Nature Genetics, 12*, 124–129.

trisomy 13 syndrome *Clinical features:* Microphthalmia, coloboma, corneal opacity, cleft lip and palate, polydactyly, scalp defects, dysmorphic features, low-set ears, flexion deformity of fingers. *Associated complications:* Cardiac defects, kidney and gastrointestinal tract anomalies, eye abnormalities, visual impairment, sensorineural hearing loss, profound intellectual disability, cerebral palsy. *Cause:* Nondisjunction resulting in extra chromosome 13; rarely parental translocation. *Inheritance:* NM; usually nondisjunction chromosomal abnormality; may recur in families in presence of parental translocation. *Incidence:* 1/8,000 births.

References: Graham, E.M., Bradley, S.M., Shirali, G.S., et al. (2004). Effectiveness of cardiac surgery in trisomies 13 and 18 (from the Pediatric Cardiac Care Consortium). *American Journal of Cardiology, 93,* 801–803.

Matthews, A.L. (1999). Chromosomal abnormalities: Trisomy 18, trisomy 13, deletions, and microdeletions. *Journal of Perinatal and Neonatal Nursing, 13,* 59–75.

trisomy 18 syndrome (Edwards syndrome) *Clinical features:* Prenatal onset of growth retardation, low-set ears, clenched fists, congenital heart defects, microphthalmia, coloboma, corneal opacity; 30% die within first month of life, 50% by second month, and only 10% survive their first year. *Associated complications:* Feeding problems, aspiration, conductive hearing loss, profound intellectual disability. *Cause:* Nondisjunction resulting in extra chromosome 18. *Inheritance:* NM; usually nondisjunction chromosomal abnormality, may recur in families in presence of parental translocation. *Incidence:* 1/6,600 births.

References: Graham, E.M., Bradley, S.M., Shirali, G.S., et al. (2004). Effectiveness of cardiac surgery in trisomies 13 and 18 (from the Pediatric Cardiac Care Consortium). *American Journal of Cardiology, 93,* 801–803.

Matthews, A.L. (1999). Chromosomal abnormalities: Trisomy 18, trisomy 13, deletions, and microdeletions. *Journal of Perinatal and Neonatal Nursing, 13,* 59–75.

trisomy 21 *See* Down syndrome; *see also* Chapter 18.

trisomy X *See* XXX, XXXX, and XXXXX syndromes.

tuberous sclerosis *Clinical features:* Hypopigmented areas on skin, adenoma sebaceum (acne-like facial lesions), infantile spasms, iris depigmentation, retinal defects, calcium deposits in brain, benign tumor of the kidneys, pulmonary lesions. *Associated complications:* Seizures, mild to moderate intellectual disability, tumors of the heart, increased risk of malignancy, hypoplastic tooth enamel and dental pits, renal (kidney) cysts, hypertension. *Cause:* Mutations in the TSC1 and TSC2 genes on chromosomes 16p13 and 9q34, respectively. *Inheritance:* AD with variable expressivity. *Incidence:* 1/10,000.

References: Curatolo, P., Verdecchia, M., & Bombardieri, R. (2002). Tuberous sclerosis complex: A review of neurologic aspects. *European Journal of Pediatric Neurology, 6,* 15–23.

Lendvay, T.S., & Marshall, F.F. (2003). The tuberous sclerosis complex and its highly variable manifestations. *Journal of Urology, 169,* 1635–1642.

Turner syndrome (45,X; monosomy X) *Clinical features:* Affecting females only, the physical features include short stature, broad chest with widely spaced nipples, short neck with low hairline and extra skin at nape ("webbed" appearance), "puffy" hands and feet. *Associated complications:* "Streak" ovaries causing infertility and delayed puberty, congenital heart defect (often coarctation of aorta), small ear canals, eye involvement (strabismus, ptosis, nystagmus, cataracts), chronic otitis media in 90% with frequent hearing loss, hypothyroidism, renal (kidney) disease; intelligence is usually average, but prevalence of learning disabilities is high. *Cause:* Nondisjunction chromosome abnormality resulting in one copy of sex chromosome. *Inheritance:* NM; usually nondisjunction chromosomal abnormality. *Prevalence:* 1/5,000. *Incidence:* 1/2,000 *Treatment:* Growth hormone has been used successfully to increase eventual adult height. Hormone replacement therapy is needed to initiate puberty *(see also Chapter 1).*

References: Gravholt, C.H. (2004). Epidemiological, endocrine, and metabolic features in Turner syndrome. *European Journal of Endocrinology, 151,* 657–687.

Sybert, V.P., & McCauley, E. (2004). Turner's syndrome. *The New England Journal of Medicine, 351,* 1227–1238.

Usher syndromes *Clinical features:* Approximately 10 subtypes exist; all have progressive sensorineural deafness, nystagmus, retinitis pigmentosa, central nervous system defects (e.g., loss of sense of smell, vertigo, epilepsy).

Type 1 is characterized by profound hearing loss, absent vestibular function, and retinitis pigmentosa in childhood. Individuals with type 2 have normal vestibular function and less severe hearing loss with onset of retinitis pigmentosa in the second decade. Type 3 can be differentiated by the presence of a progressive loss of hearing. *Associated complications:* Ataxia, psychosis, cataracts, occasional cognitive impairment; more than 50% of adults with a combination of congenital blindness and deafness have Usher syndrome. *Cause:* Seven chromosome loci (5 genes) have been identified for type 1 alone (MYO7A, USH1C, CDH23, PCDH15, SANS). Three loci have been identified for type 2, although only one gene has been identified USH2A. One loci has been identified for type 3. *Inheritance:* AR. *Prevalence:* 2/100,000–6/100,000. *Treatment:* Cochlear implants may be beneficial for some individuals with type 1, while hearing aids are effective for individuals with type 2.

References: Keats, B.J., & Corey, D.P. (1999). The Usher syndromes. *American Journal of Medical Genetics, 89,* 158–166.

Keats, B.J., & Savas, S. (2004). Genetic heterogeneity in Usher syndrome. *American Journal of Medical Genetics, 130,* 13–16.

VATER/VACTERL association *Clinical features:* Vertebral defects, ear anomalies, facial clefting, anal atresia (imperforate anus), genitourinary anomalies, **tracheoesophageal fistula** (problem with connection between trachea and esophagus), esophageal anomalies, radial (lower arm) and other limb defects, renal (kidney) anomalies. *Associated complications:* Respiratory, cardiac, and renal (kidney) abnormalities that can be severe. Intelligence is usually not affected. *Cause:* Unknown. *Inheritance:* Usually SP, no recognized genetic or teratogenic cause; rare families with AR pattern. *Prevalence:* Unknown.

References: Bergmann, C., Zerres, K., Peschgens, T., et al. (2003). Overlap between VACTERL and hemifacial micosomia illustrating a spectrum of malformations seen in axial mesodermal dysplasia complex (AMDC). *American Journal of Medical Genetics, 121A,* 151–155.

Botto, L.D., Khoury, M.J., Mastroiacovo, P., et al. (1997). The spectrum of congenital anomalies of the VATER association: An international study. *American Journal of Medical Genetics, 71,* 8–15.

velocardiofacial syndrome (VCFS) *See* chromosome 22q11 microdeletion syndromes.

von Recklinghausen disease *See* neurofibromatosis, type I.

Waardenburg syndrome. Four clinical subtypes exist with types I and II accounting for the majority of cases. *Clinical features:* Widely spaced eyes (type I), heterochromia (irises of different colors), white hair forelock, nonprogressive sensorineural hearing loss, musculoskeletal abnormalities (type III). Types I and II have virtually identical clinical features with the only distinguishing characteristic being telecanthus (abnormally long distance from the inside corner of the eye to the nose) which is found in type I. *Associated complications:* Impaired vestibular function leading to ataxia, premature graying, vitiligo (patches of skin depigmentation), occasional glaucoma. *Cause:* Types I and III: Mutations in PAX3 gene on chromosome 2q35; type II: Mutations in various genes, including the microphthalmia-associated transcription factor (MITF) gene on chromosome 3p14.1–p12.3. *Inheritance:* AD. *Prevalence:* 1/20,000–1/40,000.

References: Black, F.O., Pesznecker, S.C., Allen, K., & Gianna C. (2001). A vestibular phenotype for Waardenburg syndrome? *Otology and Neurotology, 22,* 188–194.

Pardono, E., van Bever, Y., van den Ende, J., et al. (2003). *American Journal of Medical Genetics, 117,* 223–235.

Weaver syndrome *Clinical features:* Micrognathia; distinctive chin with dimple; hypertelorism; macrocephaly; downslanting palpebral fissures; long philtrum; depressed nasal bridge; hoarse, low-pitched cry; deep set nails. *Associated complications:* Accelerated growth with advanced bone age, hypertonia, camptodactyly (permanently flexed fingers), intellectual disability. *Cause:* Mutations have been identified in the NSD1 gene on chromosome 5q35. *Inheritance:* Select case reports suggest AD inheritance, but most cases are isolated, suggesting NM. *Prevalence:* Unknown.

References: Rio, M., Clech, L., Amiel, J., et al. (2003). Spectrum of NSD1 mutations in Sotos and Weaver syndromes. *Journal of Medical Genetics, 40,* 436–440.

Voorhoeve, P.G., van Gils, J.F., & Jansen, M. (2002). The difficulty of height prediction in Weaver syndrome. *Clinical Dysmorphology, 11,* 49–52.

Williams syndrome *Clinical features:* Characteristic "elfin" facies (full lips and cheeks, fullness of area around the eyes); short stature; star-like pattern to iris; hoarse voice;

communication delay in early childhood, followed by increasing verbal abilities later in life; characteristic friendly, talkative, extroverted personality; congenital heart defect, often supravalvular aortic stenosis. *Associated complications:* Hypercalcemia (increased blood calcium level), stenosis (stricture) of blood vessels, kidney anomalies, hypertension, joint contractures, mild to moderate intellectual disability (but with characteristic strength in verbal abilities). *Cause:* Microdeletion of a segment of chromosome 7q11.23 consisting of approximately 25 genes. *Inheritance:* AD; all cases are the result of NM (sporadic deletions). *Prevalence:* 1/10,000.

References: Carrasco, X., Castillo, S., Aravena, T. et al. (2005). Williams syndrome: pediatric, neurologic, and cognitive development. *Pediatric Neurology, 32,* 166–172.

Vicari, S., Bates, E., Caselli, M.C., et al. (2004). Neuropsychological profile of Italians with Williams syndrome: An example of a dissociation between language and cognition. *International Journal of Neuropsychology and Sociology, 10,* 862–876.

Wilson disease *Clinical features:* Liver dysfunction, jaundice, Kayser-Fleischer ring in cornea, low serum ceruloplasmin (enzyme important in regulation of copper in body). *Associated complications:* Movement disorders, dysphagia (difficulty swallowing) or other oral-motor dysfunction, behavioral disturbances; if left untreated, death from liver failure within 1–3 years of onset. *Cause:* Mutations in the copper metabolism gene, ATP7B, on chromosome 13q14.3–q21.1 lead to intracellular accumulation of copper in liver. *Inheritance:* AR. *Prevalence:* 1/50,000. *Treatment:* Administration of copper-chelating agents in conjunction with a low copper diet.

References: Ferenci, P., Caca, K., Loudianos, G., et al. (2003). Diagnosis and phenotypic classification of Wilson disease. *Liver International, 23,* 139–142.

Shimizu, N., Yamaguchi, Y., Aoki, T. (1999). Treatment and management of Wilson's disease. *Pediatrics International, 41,* 419–422.

Wolf-Hirschhorn syndrome *Clinical features:* Hypertelorism; characteristic broad, beaked nose; microcephaly; marked intrauterine growth retardation and premature birth; ear anomalies; severe intellectual disability with reductions in receptive and expressive language. *Associated complications:* Hypotonia, psychomotor delays, growth delay, renal anomalies, hypodontia (decreased number of teeth) resulting in feeding problems, seizures, occasional heart defect or cleft palate. *Cause:* Partial deletion of short arm of chromosome 4; some research shows that the HOX7 gene may be responsible as well as the Wolf-Hirschhorn syndrome candidate-1 gene (WHSC1). *Inheritance:* Occurs as a result of a NM; recurrence risk is greater if parent has a balanced translocation. *Prevalence:* 1/50,000.

References: Battaglia, A., Carey, J.C., Cederholm, P., et al. (1999). Natural history of Wolf-Hirschhorn syndrome: Experience with 15 cases. *Pediatrics, 103,* 830–836.

Sabbadini, M., Bombardi, P., Carlesimo, G.A., et al. (2002). Evaluation of communicative and functional abilities in Wolf-Hirschorn syndrome. *Journal of Intellectual Disability Research, 46,* 575–582.

X-linked ALD *See* adrenoleukodystrophy.

XXX (trisomy X; 47,XXX); XXXX (tetrasomy X); and XXXXX (pentasomy X) syndromes *Clinical features:* Females with XXX syndrome generally have above-average stature but otherwise typical physical appearance; 70% have significant learning disabilities; language delay/problems are also present in some girls. Significant malformations have been described in some patients including gonadal dysgenesis (nonfunctional ovaries), dysmorphic facial appearance, atrophic or dysplastic (absent or shrunken) kidneys, and vaginal and uterine malformations. XXXX syndrome is associated with a mildly unusual facial appearance, behavioral problems, and moderate intellectual disability. XXXXX syndrome presents with severe intellectual disability and multiple physical defects. *Associated complications:* Infertility, delayed pubertal development. *Cause:* Nondisjunction during meiosis. *Inheritance:* NM; usually nondisjunction chromosomal abnormality, may recur in families in presence of parental translocation. *Incidence:* 1/800 liveborn females.

References: Haverty, C.E., Lin, A.E., Simpson, E., et al. (2004). 47, XXX association with malformations. *American Journal of Medical Genetics, 125A,* 108–111.

Linden, M.G., Bender, M.G. (2002). Fifty-one prenatally diagnosed children and adolescents with sex chromosome abnormalities. *American Journal of Medical Genetics, 110,* 11–18.

XXY syndrome *See* Klinefelter syndrome.

XYY syndrome   *Clinical features:* Subtle findings, including tall stature, severe acne, large teeth. *Associated complications:* Poor fine motor coordination; learning disabilities; language delay; varying degrees of behavioral disturbances, including tantrums and aggression; increased risk for autism. *Cause:* Extra Y chromosome resulting from nondisjunction. *Inheritance:* NM; usually nondisjunction chromosomal abnormality, may recur in families in presence of parental translocation. *Prevalence:* 1/1,000.

References: Fryns, J.P. (1998). Mental status and psychosocial functioning in XYY males. *Prenatal Diagnosis, 18,* 303–304.

Geerts, M., Steyaert, J., & Fryns, J.P. (2003). The XYY syndrome: A follow up study on 38 boys. *Genetic Counseling, 14,* 267–279.

Zellweger syndrome (cerebrohepatorenal syndrome)   *Clinical features:* The most severe of the known peroxisomal disorders; affected infants have intrauterine growth retardation, characteristic facies (high forehead, upslanting palpebral fissures, hypoplastic supraorbital ridges, and epicanthal folds), hypotonia, eye abnormalities (cataracts, glaucoma, corneal clouding, retinitis pigmentosa), early onset of seizures. Death occurs by 1 year of age in most cases. *Associated complications:* Severe feeding difficulties with failure to thrive, liver disease, occasional cardiac disease, extremity contractures, kidney cysts. *Cause:* Impaired peroxisome synthesis caused by mutations in a number of genes, including peroxin-1 (PEX1) at chromosome 7q21–q22, peroxin-5 (PEX5) at chromosome 12, peroxin-2 (PEX2) at chromosome 8, peroxin-6 (PEX6) at chromosome 6, and peroxin-12 (PEX12). (The peroxisome is a cellular organelle involved in processing fatty acids.) *Inheritance:* AR. *Prevalence:* 1/100,000. *Treatment:* Docosahexaenoic acid (DHA) ethyl ester was shown to be helpful in a small group of patients.

References: Martinez, H., & Korman, S.H. (2003). Phenotypic variability (heterogeneity) of peroxisomal disorders. *Advances in Experimental Medicine and Biology, 544,* 9–30.

Martinez, M. (2001). Restoring the DHA levels in the brains of Zellweger patients. *Journal of Molecular Neuroscience, 16,* 309–316.

C Commonly Used Medications

Karl F. Gumpper

This appendix contains information about commonly used medications but is not meant to be used to prescribe medication. The generic name of each drug is in capital letters. The trade name is in parentheses; not all preparations are included. The drug categories, uses, standard applications, and side effects are listed. It should be noted that uses and standard applications may change during the life of this edition and that additional side effects may be discovered. Drug interactions and contraindications such as hepatic or renal insufficiency are not included; use of any medication should be discussed with a health care provider familiar with the individual's medical background.

REFERENCES

Children's National Medical Center. (2006). *CNMC Hospital Formulary (Intranet version)*. Washington, DC: Author.

MICROMEDEX Thomson Healthcare. (1974–2006). *MICROMEDEX Healthcare Series: Vol. 125*. Greenwood Village, Co: Author.

Taketomo, C.K., Hodding, J.H., & Kraus, D.M. (Eds.). (2004–2005). *Pediatric dosage handbook* (11th ed.). Cleveland, OH: Lexicomp.

Medication	Category	Use(s)	Standard application[a]	Side effects
ACYCLOVIR (Zovirax)	Antiviral agent	Used primarily in children who are immunocompromised to treat or protect against herpes simplex and varicella (chickenpox) infections	**C, L, O, T, and injection:** Depending on clinical situation	Renal impairment, headache, gastrointestinal irritation, vertigo, insomnia, rash, elevated liver function tests, adverse hematologic effects
ALPRAZOLAM (Xanax)	Psychopharmacological agent	Anxiety, aggression, panic attacks	**T:** Titrate starting at minimal doses of 0.125 mg three times daily; safety and efficacy in children younger than 18 years is not known	Drowsiness, insomnia, decreased salivation, dysarthria, ataxia, addictive potential; abrupt withdrawal can cause seizures
AMITRIPTYLINE (Elavil)	Psychopharmacological agent	Attention-deficit/hyperactivity disorder, depression, migraine prophylaxis	**T, injection:** 1–1.5 mg/kg/day, given in three doses; not recommended for children younger than 12 years	Sedation, dry mouth, blurred vision, dizziness; very rarely, sudden death from cardiac arrhythmia
AMOXICILLIN (Amoxil)	Antibiotic	First-line drug for otitis media	**C, T, L, chewables:** 20–90 mg/kg/day, given in two to three doses	Diarrhea, rash
AMOXICILLIN AND CLAVULANIC ACID (Augmentin)	Antibiotic	Otitis media	**T, L, chewables:** 50 mg/kg/day, given in two doses	Diarrhea (worse than with amoxicillin alone), rash
AMPHETAMINE/DEXTROAMPHETAMINE (Adderall and Adderall XR)	Psychopharmacological agent	Attention-deficit/hyperactivity disorder, obesity	**C, T:** One to three doses daily; not recommended for children younger than 3 years; 3- to 5-year-olds: 2.5 mg/day initially, with an increase of 2.5 mg/week until optimal response; children older than 6 years: 5 mg once or twice daily initially, with an increase of 5 mg/week until optimal response; extended release is dosed once daily	Insomnia, loss of appetite, emotional lability, addictive potential, arrhythmia; not recommended for children younger than 3 years of age.

ATOMOXETINE (Strattera)	Psychopharmacological agent	Attention-deficit/hyperactivity disorder	**C:** Initial: 0.5 mg/kg/day, increase after minimum of 3 days to ~1.2 mg/kg/day; may administer as either a single daily dose or 2 evenly divided doses in morning and late afternoon/early evening; maximum daily dose: 1.4 mg/kg or 100 mg, whichever is less	Headache, palpitations, decreased appetite, abdominal pain, nausea, vomiting, weight loss; FDA warning letter cautions about severe liver injury
BACLOFEN	Antispasticity agent	Spasticity of cerebral or spinal origin	**T:** 5 mg, two or three times daily initially; increase by 5 mg every 4–7 days to a maximum of 30–80 mg/day; *Intrathecal:* 50–600 mcg/day delivered by implantable pump	Drowsiness, muscle weakness; rarely nausea, dizziness, paresthesia (numbness and tingling); abrupt withdrawal can cause hallucinations and seizures
BENZTROPINE (Cogentin)	Anticholinergic	Movement disorders associated with antipsychotics such as haloperidol	**T, injection:** Initiate therapy with low dosage; gradually increase in increments of 0.5 mg twice daily; maximum daily dosage: 6 mg/day	Gastrointestinal upset, drowsiness, dizziness or blurred vision, dry mouth, difficult urination, constipation
BOTULINUM TOXIN A (Botox)	Antispasticity agent	Spasticity in cerebral palsy and spinal cord injury	Injections are administered by a qualified practitioner; based on review of clinical trials, dosage use in management of cerebral palsy should not exceed 4 units/kg total body weight per 2 months	Diffuse skin rash, paralysis with overdose

a*Key:* C, capsules; T, tablets; L, liquid suspension or elixir; O, ointment; P, powder; S, suppositories.

Medication	Category	Use(s)	Standard application[a]	Side effects
BUDESONIDE (Pulmicort)	Respiratory agent	Maintenance and prophylactic treatment of asthma; may be used for other reactive airway diseases	**Inhaler:** Children 12 months to 8 years: Pulmicort Respules: Titrate to lowest effective dose once patient is stable; start at 0.25 mg/day or use as follows: • Previous therapy of bronchodilators alone: 0.5 mg/day administered as a single dose or divided twice daily (maximum daily dose: 0.5 mg) • Previous therapy of inhaled corticosteroids: 0.5 mg/day administered as a single dose or divided twice daily (maximum daily dose: 1 mg) • Previous therapy of oral corticosteroids: 1 mg/day administered as a single dose or divided twice daily (maximum daily dose: 1 mg)	Runny nose, hoarseness, dry mouth epistaxis (bloody nose)
BUPROPRION (Wellbutrin)	Psychopharmacological agent	Depression, attention-deficit/hyperactivity disorder	**T:** Safety and efficacy in children younger than 18 years has not been established	Decreased seizure threshold, nausea, agitation, anxiety, insomnia, decreased appetite; FDA warns of possible increased suicidal risks in children and adolescents
BUSPIRONE (BuSpar)	Psychopharmacological agent	Attention-deficit/hyperactivity disorder, anxiety, aggression	**T:** safety and efficacy in children younger than 18 years has not been established	Chest pain, ringing in the ears, sore throat, nasal congestion, restlessness

702

Drug	Classification	Use	Dosage	Side Effects
CAFFEINE CITRATE (Cafcit)	Respiratory agent	Apnea of prematurity	**L, injection:** Loading dose: 10–20 mg/kg as caffeine citrate (5–10 mg/kg as caffeine base); maintenance dose: 5–10 mg/kg/day as caffeine citrate (2.5-5 mg/kg/day as caffeine base) once daily starting 24 hours after the loading dose; therapeutic drug level: 8–30 microgram/mL	Increased heart rate, insomnia, restlessness, agitation, irritability, hyperactivity, jitteriness, headache, nausea, vomiting, and muscle tremors or twitches; avoid in symptomatic arrhythmias
CALCIUM UNDECYLENATE (10%) (Caldesene powder)	Skin agent	Diaper rash	**O, P:** Apply three or four times daily after bath or changing	Irritation, allergic reaction
CARBAMAZEPINE (Carbatrol; Tegretol, Tegretol XR)	Antiepileptic	Generalized tonic-clonic, complex partial, and simple partial seizures; also used to treat aggression	**C, T, L:** 5–20 mg/kg/day; blood level should be maintained at 4–14 mcg/ml	Unsteady gait, double vision, drowsiness, slurred speech, dizziness, tremor, headache, nausea, abnormalities in liver function; FDA warning of reported aplastic anemia and agranulocytosis
CARNITINE (also called L-CARNITINE) (Carnitor)	Nutritional supplement	Primary and secondary carnitine deficiency, especially in inborn errors of metabolism; valproic acid–induced deficiency	**T, L, injection:** 50–100 mg/kg/day divided into doses given every 6 hours; give higher dosages with caution; start dosage at 50 mg/kg/day, and increase slowly to a maximum of 3 g/day while assessing tolerance and therapeutic response	Nausea, vomiting, abdominal cramps, diarrhea
CEPHALEXIN (Keflex, Biocef)	Antibiotic	Used to treat susceptible infections of the respiratory tract, skin, and urinary tract	**C, T, L:** 25–100mg/kg/day divided every 6–8 hours; maximum dose: 4,000 mg/day	Headache, rash, nausea, vomiting, diarrhea
CHLORAL HYDRATE (Aquachloral [supplement], Noctec)	Psychopharmacological agent	Sedation	**S, syrup:** 5–15 mg/kg every 8 hours to a maximum dosage of 2 g/day	Mucous membrane and gastro-intestinal irritation, paradoxical excitement, hypotension, myocardial/respiratory depression

[a]*Key:* C, capsules; T, tablets; L, liquid suspension or elixir; O, ointment; P, powder; S, suppositories.

Medication	Category	Use(s)	Standard application[a]	Side effects
CHLORPROMAZINE (Thorazine)	Psychopharmacological agent, antiemetic	Psychosis, anxiety, aggression, severe hyperactivity in individuals with intellectual disability (rarely used now because of newer drugs with fewer side effects)	*T, S, C, injection, syrup, L:* 2.5–6 mg/kg/day to a maximum of 40 mg in children younger than 5 years or 75 mg in children 5–12 years old	Drowsiness, tardive dyskinesia (involuntary movements of face and tongue), hypotensive, weight gain, lower seizure threshold, electrocardiogram changes, agranulocytosis (depletion of white blood cells), rash, hyperpigmentation of skin
CIMETIDINE (Tagamet)	Gastrointestinal agent	Gastroesophageal reflux, gastric/duodenal ulcers; inhibits gastric acid secretion	*T, L:* 10–40 mg/kg/day, given 4 times daily	Rarely diarrhea, headache, decreased white blood count, liver toxicity
CISAPRIDE (Propulsid)	Gastrointestinal agent	Gastroesophageal reflux; increases gastric emptying	*T, L:* 0.7–1 mg/kg/day, given three or four times daily (*Note:* Cisapride was removed from the U.S. market in July 2000 because of serious adverse events; limited-access program is available through Janssen Pharmaceutica)	Abdominal pain, diarrhea, cardiac arrhythmias
CITALOPRAM (Celexa)	Psychopharmacological agent	Treatment of depression, panic disorder, obsessive-compulsive disorder, separation anxiety	*T, L*	Somnolence, insomnia, nausea, dry mouth, increased sweating, agitation, restlessness; FDA warns of possible increased suicidal risks in children and adolescents
CLARITHROMYCIN (Biaxin)	Antibiotic	Wide-spectrum drug used against staph, strep, and mycoplasma ("walking pneumonia") infections	*T, L:* 15 mg/kg/day, given twice daily for 10 days	Stomach upset, diarrhea, nausea, cardiac arrhythmias, but tolerated better than erythromycin
CLOMIPRAMINE (Anafranil)	Psychopharmacological agent	Obsessive-compulsive disorder, trichotillomania	*C:* Initiate at 25 mg/day; gradually increase during the first 2 weeks, as tolerated, to a daily maximum of 3 mg/kg or 100–200 mg, whichever is smaller	Drowsiness, dry mouth, blurred vision

Drug	Classification	Use	Dosage	Side Effects
CLONAZEPAM (Klonopin)	Antiepileptic	Lennox-Gastaut syndrome; absence, atonic, myoclonic, and partial seizures; infantile spasms; anxiety	**T:** 0.01–0.2 mg/kg/day (usual maintenance dosage is 0.5–2 mg/day, given twice daily)	Sedation, hyperactivity, confusion, depression—especially if withdrawn quickly; do not stop abruptly; tolerance to the drug can develop
CLONIDINE (Catapres)	Psychopharmacological agent, antihypertensive agent	Hypertension, attention-deficit/hyperactivity disorder, Tourette syndrome	**T:** 0.005–0.025 mg/kg/day, four times daily; increase every 5–7 days as needed; sustained-release patch also available	Dry mouth, sedation, hypotension, headache, nausea
CLORAZEPATE (Tranxene)	Antiepileptic, psychopharmacological agent	Adjunctive therapy for partial seizures, anxiety	**T:** 3.75–7.5 mg/dose twice daily; increase dosage by 3.75 mg at weekly intervals, not to exceed 60 mg/day in two to three divided doses	Hypotension, drowsiness, dizziness (see also side effects of DIAZEPAM)
CLOTRIMAZOLE (Lotrimin, Mycelex)	Skin treatment	Antifungal, Candida albicans (yeast) infections	**Cream:** Apply twice daily for 2–4 weeks	Skin irritation, peeling
CLOZAPINE (Clozaril)	Psychopharmacological agent	Schizophrenia in which standard antipsychotic drug treatment has not worked	**T:** 25 mg once or twice daily, then continued with daily dosage increments of 25–50 mg/day, if well tolerated, to a target dosage of 300 to 450 mg/day by the end of 2 weeks (**Note:** All patients must be registered in Novartis' distribution system prior to starting the medication)	Hypotension, seizure, weight gain, sedation; FDA warning for seizures, agranulocytosis (i.e., low white blood cell count leading to infection), myocarditis (i.e., inflammation of the heart), and other cardiovascular and respiratory effects
COLLOIDAL OATMEAL (e.g., Aveeno)	Skin treatment	Dry skin, itching	**Oil, cleansing bar, cream, lotion:** Add to bath or apply as needed	Allergic reaction

aKey: C, capsules; T, tablets; L, liquid suspension or elixir; O, ointment; P, powder; S, suppositories.

Medication	Category	Use(s)	Standard application[a]	Side effects
CORTICOTROPIN (Acthar, ACTH)	Antiepileptic	Infantile spasms and Lennox-Gastaut syndrome	***Intramuscular injection:*** 20–40 units/day; many regimens exist, but ACTH is generally used for weeks to months and then tapered off slowly	Glucose in urine, hypertension, cataracts, brittle bones
DANTROLENE SODIUM (Dantrium)	Antispasticity agent	Spasticity in cerebral palsy or spinal cord injury, malignant hyperthermia prevention	*C:* 0.5 mg/kg twice daily initially; increase by 0.5 mg/kg every 4–7 days to a maximum of 3 mg/kg/dose, given two to four times daily	Weakness, drowsiness, lethargy, dizziness, tingling sensation, nausea, diarrhea; FDA warning for hepatotoxicity (liver function should be monitored); long-term side effects in children are not known
DESIPRAMINE (Norpramin)	Psychopharmacological agent	Depression, anxiety, attention-deficit/hyperactivity disorder	*T:* Not recommended in children younger than 12 years; 1–4.5 mg/kg/day; maximum 100 mg/day	Hypotension, ringing in the ears, gastrointestinal discomfort, dry mouth, blurred vision, sudden death from cardiac arrhythmia has been reported in a few cases
DEXTROAMPHETAMINE (Dexedrine, Dexadrine Spansules, DextroStat, Adderall)	Psychopharmacological agent	Attention-deficit/hyperactivity disorder	*C, L, T (5 mg):* 0.1 mg/kg, twice daily initially; increase to 0.5–1.0 mg/kg/dose, two to three times daily; sustained-release capsules are available (5, 10, and 15 mg)	Insomnia, restlessness, decreased appetite, irritability, headache, abdominal cramps, decreased appetite, irritability; FDA warning for potential for abuse; not recommended for children under 3 years of age
DIAZEPAM (Valium, Diastat)	Antispasticity agent, antiepileptic, psychopharmacological agent	Sedation, aggression, anxiety, spasticity, seizures	*C, T, L:* 0.12–0.8 mg/kg/day given three to four times daily; ***Rectal gel (Diastat):*** Not recommended for infants younger than 6 months; safety and efficacy not established in children younger than 2 years; 2–5 years, 0.5 mg/kg; 6–11 years, 0.3 mg/kg; older than 11 years, 0.2 mg/kg; not to exceed 20 mg/dose	Sedation, weakness, depression, ataxia, memory disturbance, difficulty handling secretions and chewing/swallowing foods, anxiety, hallucinations, agitation, insomnia, respiratory and cardiac depression, urinary retention or incontinence, rash, low white blood cell count; drug dependence can occur

Drug	Category	Use	Dosage/Form	Side effects
DIPHENHYDRAMINE (Benadryl)	Antihistamine	Sedation, nasal congestion, hives, extrapyramidal symptoms	**C, T, O, L:** 5 mg/kg/day given at 6–8 hour intervals to a maximum of 300 mg/day	Sedation, insomnia, dizziness, euphoria, gastrointestinal upset, paradoxical excitation
DUODERM	Skin treatment	Skin ulcers/sores, second-degree burns, and minor abrasions	Sterile occlusive dressing with hydroactive or gel formula	Allergic reaction to tape or gel formula
ERYTHROMYCIN (various brands)	Antibiotic	Used against staph, strep, and mycoplasma ("walking pneumonia") infections; used in combination with sulfisoxazole (Pediazole) for otitis media	**C, O, T, L:** 30–50 mg/kg/day, given four times daily; injection	Nausea, vomiting, interactions with other drugs
ERYTHROMYCIN (2%) (T-STAT)	Skin treatment	Acne	**Solution on pads:** Apply to clean area twice daily	Skin dryness, peeling, skin irritation
ETHOSUXIMIDE (Zarontin)	Antiepileptic	Absence seizures	**C, L:** 15–40 mg/kg/day, given twice daily to a maximum of 1.5 g/day; blood level: 40–80 mcg/l	Sedation, unsteady gait, anorexia, rash, stomach distress, low white blood count
FAMOTIDINE (Pepcid)	Gastrointestinal agent	Gastresophageal reflux; decreases stomach acidity	**C, T, L:** 1 mg/kg/day, given twice daily with meals; maximum dose: 80mg/day; injection	Headache, dizziness, constipation, diarrhea
FELBAMATE (Felbatol)	Antiepileptic	Lennox-Gastaut syndrome; also effective in generalized and secondary generalized seizures	**T, L:** 15–45 mg/kg/day	Anorexia, vomiting, insomnia, headache, rash, risk of life-threatening hepatitis and aplastic anemia; FDA recommends complete blood count and liver function tests every 1–2 weeks
FLUCONAZOLE (Fluconazole, Diflucan)	Antifungal	Treatment of susceptible fungal infections, including oral and vaginal *Candida albicans* (yeast) infections	**T, L:** 6 mg/kg once on first day of therapy, then 3 mg/kg/dose daily for 14–21 days; for vaginal candidiasis: a single 150 mg dose may be given, injection	Dizziness, headache, rash, nausea; inhibits the metabolism of many drugs, so patients must be screened for possible drug interactions

[a]Key: C, capsules; T, tablets; L, liquid suspension or elixir; O, ointment; P, powder; S, suppositories.

Medication	Category	Use(s)	Standard application[a]	Side effects
FLUOXETINE (Prozac)	Psychopharmacological agent	Depression, self-injurious behavior, Tourette syndrome, obsessive-compulsive disorder, anxiety	*C, L:* Safety and efficacy in children has not been established; adults should initially receive 20 mg/day in morning to a maximum of 80 mg/day	Anxiety, agitation, sleep disruption, decreased appetite, seizures; FDA warns of possible increased suicidal risks in children and adolescents
FOSPHENYTOIN (Cerebyx)	See PHENYTOIN	See PHENYTOIN	See PHENYTOIN	See PHENYTOIN
FUROSEMIDE (Lasix)	Diuretic	Diuresis	*T, L, injection:* 1 mg/kg/dose one to four times daily	Electrolyte abnormalities
GABAPENTIN (Neurontin)	Antiepileptic	Adjunctive therapy in partial and secondarily generalized seizures; neuropathic pain	*C, T, L:* 20–30 mg/kg/day; safety and efficacy in children younger than 12 years has not been established	Sedation, dizziness, unsteady gait, fatigue, emotional lability; do not withdraw abruptly
GLYCOPYROLATE (Robinul)	Anticholinergic	Decrease drooling in cerebral palsy	*T:* 0.05 mg/kg/dose every 3–4 hours as needed for secretions	Rapid heart rate, orthostatic hypotension, drowsiness, blurred vision, dry mouth
GUANFACINE (Tenex)	Psychopharmacological agent	Hypertension, attention-deficit/hyperactivity disorder, Tourette syndrome	*T:* Dosages of 2–4 mg/day have been reported in case reports	Dry mouth, sedation, hypotension, headache, nausea; rebound hypertension with abrupt withdrawal
HALOPERIDOL (Haldol)	Psychopharmacological agent	Self-injurious behavior, Tourette syndrome, severe agitation, psychosis	*T, L:* 0.01–0.03 mg/kg/day for agitation; 0.05–0.15 mg/kg/day, in two or three daily doses, for psychosis; and 0.05–0.075 mg/kg/day, in two or three daily doses, for Tourette syndrome	Movement disorder, hypotension, nausea, vomiting, electrocardiogram changes, neuroleptic malignant syndrome, lower seizure threshold in epilepsy
HYDROCORTISONE (e.g., Caldecort, Cort-Dome, Hytone)	Skin treatment	Eczema, dermatitis	*O, cream:* Apply thin film two to four times daily	Skin irritation, dryness, rash
HYDROCORTISONE, POLYMYXIN-B, NEOMYCIN (Cortisporin)	Skin treatment	Steroid-responsive skin conditions with secondary infection	*O, cream:* Apply sparingly and massage into skin two or three times daily.	Local irritation, kidney or ear toxicity (if neomycin is absorbed in large amounts)

Drug	Classification	Uses	Dosage	Side Effects
IBUPROFEN (Advil, Motrin)	Pain and fever, anti-inflammatory agent	Inflammatory diseases and rheumatoid disorders, including juvenile rheumatoid arthritis (JRA); mild to moderate pain; fever; dysmenorrhea; gout	**C, T, L:** Temperature: 5 mg/kg/dose; temperature >102.5°F: 10 mg/kg/dose given every 6–8 hours; maximum daily dose: 40 mg/kg/day **JRA:** 30–50 mg/kg/day in 4 divided doses; start at lower end of dosing range and titrate; maximum: 2.4 g/day **Pain:** 4–10 mg/kg/dose every 6–8 hours	Swelling, dizziness, drowsiness, fatigue, headache, rash, heartburn, nausea, vomiting, low white blood cell count
IMIPRAMINE (Tofranil, Janimine)	Psychopharmacological agent	Depression, enuresis, attention-deficit/hyperactivity disorder	**C, T:** 1.5 mg/kg/day, given in three daily doses to a maximum of 5 mg/kg/day; therapeutic blood level for depression is 150–225 nanograms/ml	Dry mouth, drowsiness, constipation, electrocardiogram abnormalities, increased blood pressure
ISOTRETINOIN (Accutane)	Skin treatment	Severe acne in adolescents (or adults)	**C:** 0.5–2 mg/kg/day, given in two daily doses for 15–20 weeks	Drying of mucous membranes, photosensitivity; FDA warning not to use in female patients who are or who may become pregnant
LAMOTRIGINE (Lamictal)	Antiepileptic	Adjunctive therapy in partial and secondarily generalized seizures; may be effective in primary generalized seizures	**T, L:** 5–15 mg/kg/day (1–5 mg/kg/day if co-administered with valproic acid); safety and efficacy in children younger than 12 years has not been established	Sedation, dizziness, ataxia, headaches, nausea, vomiting, potentially life-threatening Stevens-Johnson syndrome (allergic skin condition)
LANOLIN, PETROLATUM, VITAMINS A AND D, MINERAL OILS (A & D Ointment)	Skin treatment	Diaper rash	**O:** Apply thin film at each diaper change	Allergic reaction

aKey: C, capsules; T, tablets; L, liquid suspension or elixir; O, ointment; P, powder; S, suppositories.

Medication	Category	Use(s)	Standard application[a]	Side effects
LANSOPRAZOLE (Prevacid)	Gastrointestinal agent	Treatment for healing and symptomatic relief of active duodenal ulcer and gastroesophageal reflux disease; adjuvant therapy in the treatment of *Helicobacter pylori*-associated gastritis	**C, L, T:** Doses vary from 0.5–1.6 mg/kg/day once daily or given in divided doses twice daily; maximum dose: 60mg/day; injection (IV)	Abdominal pain, nausea, flatulence, increased appetite, headache, fatigue, rash
LEVETIRACETAM (Keppra)	Antiepileptic	Adjunctive therapy in partial seizures	**T, L:** Initially, 20 mg/kg/day divided twice daily. Dosage is increased to 40–60 mg/kg/day as tolerated; maximum daily dose: 3,000 mg/day	Somnolence, coordination difficulties, dizziness, behavior changes, irritability
LEVOTHYROXINE (Synthroid, Levothroid)	Hormone	Hypothyroidism	**T, L:** 1–5 years, 5–6 mcg/kg/day; 6–12 years, 4–5 mcg/kg/day; older than 12 years, 2–3 mcg/kg/day	Heart palpitations, nervousness, tremor, excessive sweating, diarrhea, weight loss
LINDANE (Kwell)	Skin treatment	Scabies and lice	***Cream, lotion:*** Apply thin layer and massage into body from neck down; wash off after 8–12 hours; ***shampoo:*** apply to dry hair, massage thoroughly into hair, and leave on for 4 minutes; then form lather and rinse well	None with prescribed use; risk of seizures with overuse in small children; should be reserved for patients who do not respond to other treatments
LITHIUM CARBONATE (Eskalith)	Psychopharmacologic agent	Mood stabilizer, bipolar disorder, and depression	**C, T, L:** 15–60 mg/kg/day divided in three to four doses; do not exceed 1,800 mg/day. Therapeutic range: mania, 0.6–1.5 mEq/l; bipolar disorder, 0.8–1 mEq/l	Sedation, confusion, seizures, rash, hypothyroidism, diarrhea, muscle weakness

Drug	Classification	Use	Dosage	Side effects
LORAZEPAM (Ativan)	Psychopharmacological agent	Anxiety, status epilepticus	**T, L, injection:** 0.05 mg/kg/dose every 6 hours as needed; do not exceed 4 mg/dose	Sedation, weakness, depression, unstable gait, memory disturbance, difficulty handling secretions and chewing/swallowing foods, anxiety, hallucinations, agitation, insomnia, respiratory and cardiac depression, urinary retention or incontinence, rash, low white blood count; drug dependence can develop
MAGNESIUM HYDROXIDE AND ALUMINUM HYDROXIDE (Maalox)	Gastrointestinal agent	Antacid for reflux; also helps treat constipation	**L:** 1–2 teaspoons with meals and at bedtime	Minimal
METHYLPHENIDATE (e.g., Concerta, Daytrana, Metadate, Metadate CD, Metadate ER, Methylin, Methylin ER, Ritalin)	Psychopharmacological agent	Attention-deficit/hyperactivity disorder	**T (5, 10, and 20 mg):** 0.6 mg/kg/day, given twice daily initially; increase to 1–2 mg/kg/day given two or three times daily when using regular Ritalin; **Sustained-release tablets** (Ritalin SR; 20 mg) last 5–6 hours; **Long-acting capsules** (Concerta; 18 and 36 mg) last 12 hours	Appetite suppression, insomnia, arrhythmia, hypo- or hypertension, abdominal pain, headache, irritability
METHYLPREDNISOLONE (Solu-Medrol, Medrol)	Respiratory agent	Reduction of airway inflammation during acute asthma attacks	**Injection:** 1 mg/kg/dose; **Orally:** 1 mg/kg/dose, twice daily for 3–5 days	Side effects usually mild with short-term use
METOCLOPRAMIDE (Reglan)	Gastrointestinal agent	Antireflux, increases gastric emptying	**T, L:** 0.1–0.5 mg/kg/day, given four times daily	Acute movement disorder (dystonia), drowsiness, sedation, anxiety, depression, leukopenia
MICONAZOLE (2%) (e.g., Monistat)	Skin treatment	Antifungal, *Candida albicans* (yeast) infections	**S, O, cream:** Apply twice daily for 2–4 weeks	Skin irritation, peeling, pruritis, phlebitis
MINERAL OIL (e.g., Alpha Keri)	Skin treatment	Emollient for dry skin	**Soap, oil, spray:** Add to bath or rub into wet skin as needed; rinse	Allergic reaction

aKey: C, capsules; T, tablets; L, liquid suspension or elixir; O, ointment; P, powder; S, suppositories.

Medication	Category	Use(s)	Standard application[a]	Side effects
MINERAL OIL, PETROLATUM, LANOLIN (Nivea, Lubriderm)	Skin treatment	Emollient for dry skin	**Cream, lotion, bath oil:** Apply as needed	Allergic reaction
MUPIROCIN (2%) (Bactroban)	Skin treatment	Antibiotic for impetigo, skin ulcers, burns	**O:** Apply sparingly three times daily; may cover with gauze	Burning, itching, pain at site of application
NALTREXONE (ReViA)	Psychopharmacological agent	Opiate antagonist for treatment of self-injurious behavior	**T:** 50 mg/day in adults; safety and efficacy in children younger than 18 years has not been established	None in opioid-free individuals
NORTRIPTYLINE (Pamelor, Aventyl)	Psychopharmacological agent	Depression	**C, T, L:** 10 mg three times daily and 20 mg at bedtime; not recommended for children younger than 12 years	Dry mouth, drowsiness, constipation, electrocardiogram abnormalities, increased blood pressure, mania, sudden death from cardiac arrhythmia has been reported in a few cases with overdose
NYSTATIN (Mycostatin)	Antifungal	Treatment of yeast and thrush infections in the mouth and gastrointestinal tract	**O, T, P, cream:** Apply twice daily; **Oral suspension:** 0.5–1 ml to each side of mouth four times daily; **L:** Up to 5 cubic centimeters; swish, and swallow	Diarrhea (reported with oral form), redness, skin irritation, gastrointestinal upset
OLANZAPINE (Zyprexa)	Psychopharmacological agent, Tourette syndrome, severe aggression, agitation to delirium, pervasive developmental disorders	Treatment of the manifestations of psychotic disorders	**T, C, injection (IM):** Start at 2.5 mg once daily; titrate dose weekly as required, up to a maximum of 20 mg/day	Edema, headache, somnolence, insomnia, agitation, nervousness, hostility, dizziness, dystonic reactions, Parkinsonian events, akathisia, anxiety, personality changes, fever, neuroleptic malignant syndrome, tardive dyskinesia, constipation, weight gain
OMEPRAZOLE (Prilosec)	Gastrointestinal agent	Treatment for healing and symptomatic relief of active duodenal ulcer and gastroesophageal reflux disease; adjuvant therapy in the treatment of *Helicobacter pylori*-associated gastritis	**C, T:** Doses vary from 0.2–3.5 mg/kg/day once daily or given in divided doses twice daily; maximum dose: 40 mg/day	Abdominal pain, diarrhea, nausea, flatulence, increased appetite, taste changes, headache

Drug	Classification	Use	Dosage	Side Effects
OXCARBAZEPINE (Trileptal)	Antiepileptic	Generalized tonic-clonic, complex partial, and simple partial seizures as both adjunctive and monotherapy	*T, L:* 8–10 mg/kg in two divided doses, usually not to exceed 600 mg/day; do not exceed the maximum adult dose of 2,400mg/day	Headache, drowsiness, dizziness, blurred vision or double vision, difficulty walking, speaking, or controlling body movement, abnormalities in liver function, low white blood count, hyponatremia (low blood sodium)
OXYBUTYNIN (Ditropan)	Urinary agent	Antispasmodic for neurogenic bladder	*T, L:* 0.2 mg/kg/dose 2-4 times/day or 5 mg twice daily, up to 5 mg 3 times/day, maximum: 15 mg/day, patch	Palpitations, drowsiness, dizziness, insomnia, dry mouth, nausea, vomiting, constipation, urinary hesitancy or retention, blurred vision, decreased tears, decreased sweating
PAROXETINE (Paxil)	Psychopharmacological agent	Depression, obsessive-compulsive disorder, anxiety disorders	*T, L:* 10–20 mg/day to start; increase dosage as needed by 10 mg/day weekly until a maximum of 50–60 mg/day is achieved	Heart palpitations, headache, anxiety, nausea, decreased appetite, constipation, weakness; FDA warns of possible increased suicidal risks in children and adolescents
PEMOLINE (Cylert)	Psychopharmacological agent	Attention-deficit/hyperactivity disorder	*T:* 37.5 mg/day in morning initially; increase weekly to desired dosage, but do not exceed 112.5 mg/day; not recommended for children younger than 6 years	Insomnia, anorexia, abdominal discomfort; potentially life-threatening liver toxicity has been reported
PENICILLIN (e.g., Pen V K)	Antibiotic	Drug of choice for strep throat, which in severe cases can be treated by a single intramuscular injection of Bicillin	*T, L:* 25–50 mg/kg/day, given four times daily for 7 days; injection	Allergic reactions, diarrhea

ªKey: C, capsules; T, tablets; L, liquid suspension or elixir; O, ointment; P, powder; S, suppositories.

Medication	Category	Use(s)	Standard application[a]	Side effects
PERMETHRIN (Nix, Elimite)	Skin treatment	Scabies and lice	*Cream, lotion:* Apply thin layer and message into body from neck down; wash off after 8–14 hours; *Shampoo:* Apply to dry hair, message thoroughly into hair, and leave on for 10 minutes; then form a lather and rinse well. May repeat in 1 week if live mites reappear	Pruritis, hypersensitivity, burning, stinging, rash
PETROLATUM, MINERAL OIL AND WAX, ALCOHOL (Eucerin)	Skin treatment	Emollient for dry skin, itching	*Cream, lotion, facial lotion with sunscreen, cleansing bar:* Apply as needed	Allergic reaction
PHENOBARBITAL (Luminal)	Antiepileptic	Generalized tonic-clonic, simple partial, and secondarily generalized seizures	*C, T, L:* 2–5 mg/kg/day for children; 1–2 mg/kg/day for adolescents; therapeutic blood level: 15–40 mcg/ml; injection	Paradoxical hyperactivity, sedation, learning difficulties in older children, behavioral difficulties in 50% of children younger than 10 years, rash, irritability, unsteady gait, respiratory depression, hypotension, hepatitis
PHENYTOIN (Dilantin)	Antiepileptic	Generalized tonic-clonic and complex partial seizures	*C, T, injectable, suspension:* Maintenance dosage: 4–8 mg/kg/day; blood level: 10–20 mcg/ml; free level: 1–2 mcg/ml	Swelling of gums, excessive hairiness, rash, coarsening of facial features, possible adverse effects on learning and behavior; risk of birth defects if taken during pregnancy; nystagmus and unsteady gait with toxic levels; blood dyscrasias
PREDNISOLONE (Prelone)	Respiratory agent	Reduction of airway inflammation during acute asthma attacks	*T, L:* 1 mg/kg/dose, twice daily for 3–5 days, injection	Side effects usually mild with short-term use
PREDNISONE (Deltasone)	Respiratory agent	Reduction of airway inflammation during acute asthma attacks	*T, L:* 1 mg/kg/dose, twice daily for 3–5 days	Side effects usually mild with short-term use

Drug	Classification	Use	Form/Dosage	Side effects
PRIMIDONE (Mysoline)	Antiepileptic	Generalized tonic-clonic and complex partial seizures	**T, L:** 10–25 mg/kg/day for children; 125–250 mg three times daily for adolescents; therapeutic blood level: 5–12 mcg/ml; also metabolized to phenobarbital (of which therapeutic blood level is 15–40 mcg/ml)	Drowsiness, dizziness, nausea, vomiting, leucopenia (low white blood cell count); systemic lupus-like syndrome, nystagmus (jerky eye movements), personality change (see also side effects of PHENOBARBITAL)
RANITIDINE (Zantac)	Gastrointestinal agent	Gastroesophageal reflux (decreases stomach acidity)	**C, T, L:** 2–4 mg/kg/day, given twice daily; injection	Headache, gastrointestinal upset, insomnia, sedation, rarely liver toxicity
RISPERIDONE (Risperdal)	Psychopharmacological agent	Self-injurious behavior, psychosis, Tourette syndrome, aggression, pervasive developmental disorders	**T, L:** Pediatric patients may start with 0.25–0.5 mg twice daily; slowly increase to the optimal range of 4–8 mg/day; dosages greater than 10 mg/day should be avoided.	Hypotension, sedation, dizziness, movement disorder, cessation of menses, constipation, weight gain, urinary retention, agranulocytosis
SELENIUM SULFIDE (2.5%) (Selsun Blue)	Skin treatment	Scalp conditions (dandruff or seborrhea)	**Lotion, shampoo:** Apply to wet scalp, wait 3 minutes, rinse, repeat; use twice a week for 2 weeks, and then as needed	Skin irritation, dry or oily scalp, hair loss and discoloration
SERTRALINE (Zoloft)	Psychopharmacological agent	Depression, anxiety, obsessive-compulsive disorder	**T, L:** 50 mg/day initially to a maximum of 200 mg/day in adults; safety and efficacy not established in children	Anxiety, agitation, sleep disruption, decreased appetite, nausea, diarrhea, tremors, sweating, seizures; FDA warns of possible increased suicidal risks in children and adolescents
SULFISOXAZOLE (Gantrisin; Pediazole)	Antibiotic	Prevention of otitis media	**T, L:** 50–75 mg/kg/day, given four to six times daily	Bone marrow suppression, allergic reactions

aKey: C, capsules; T, tablets; L, liquid suspension or elixir; O, ointment; P, powder; S, suppositories.

715

Medication	Category	Use(s)	Standard application[a]	Side effects
THEOPHYLLINE (Aerolate, Slo-Bid, Theo-Dur, Uniphyl)	Respiratory agent	Bronchodilator; may be used in conjunction with other treatments for acute or chronic asthma	*C, T, L:* Ages 6 weeks to 6 months: 10 mg/kg/day; children ages 6 months to 1 year: 12–18 mg/kg/day; children ages 1–9 years: 20–24 mg/kg/day; children ages 9–12 years: 20 mg/kg/day; children ages 12–16 years: 18 mg/kg/day; maximum adult dosage: 900 mg/day; injection (IV)	Nausea, vomiting, stomach pain (especially common at high blood levels), gastroesophageal reflux, anorexia, nervousness, tachypnea
THIORIDAZINE (Mellaril)	Psychopharmacological agent	Self-injurious behavior, psychosis	*T, L:* Not recommended for children younger than 2 years; children ages 2–12 years: 0.5–3 mg/kg/day; children older than 12 years with mild disorders: 10 mg, two or three times daily; children older than 12 years with severe disorders: 25 mg, two or three times daily	Drowsiness, movement disorder, electrocardiogram abnormalities, retinal abnormalities; FDA warning for QT prolongation on electrocardiogram
THIOTHIXENE (Navane)	Psychopharmacological agent	Self-injurious behavior, psychosis	*T, C, L, syrup:* 2 mg, three times daily, increase to 15 mg/day if needed; not recommended for children younger than 12 years	Movement disorder (tardive dyskinesia), neuroleptic malignant syndrome, rapid heart rate, hypotension, drowsiness, bone marrow suppression
TIAGABINE (Gabitril)	Antiepileptic	Refractory partial seizures	*T:* 12–18 years: initially 4 mg once daily for 1 week; then 8 mg/day in two divided doses for 1 week; then increase weekly by 4–8 mg/day; increase weekly by 2–4 mg/day in two to four divided doses daily; titrate dosage to response; maximum: 32 mg/day (dosages greater than 32 mg/day have been used in select adolescent patients for short periods)	Dizziness, headache, sleepiness, central nervous system depression, memory disturbance, unsteady gait, emotionality, tremors, weakness, abdominal pain

Drug	Category	Indication	Dosage	Side effects/Toxicity
TOLNAFTATE (Tinactin)	Skin	Antifungal, ringworm	**Cream, P:** Apply small amount of cream or powder to affected area 2–3 times a day for 2–4 weeks	Nontoxic
TOPIRAMATE (Topamax)	Antiepileptic	Refractory partial seizures, Lennox-Gastaut syndrome	**T, sprinkles:** Initially 0.5–1 mg/kg/day in two divided doses for 1 week, then increase by 0.5–1 mg/kg/day each week; titrate dosage to response; usual minimally effective dosage: 6 mg/kg/day in two divided doses; some children may require more than 15 mg/kg/day; dosages as high as 50 mg/kg/day have been used in select patients receiving concomitant enzyme-inducing agents (e.g., carbamazepine)	Edema (swelling), language problems, abnormal coordination, depression, difficulty concentrating, fatigue, dizziness, unsteady gait, sleepiness, constipation, weight loss, muscle pain, weakness, nystagmus; seek immediate medical attention if blurry vision occurs
TRIAMCINOLONE (Kenalog, Aristocort [skin]; Azmacort [respiratory])	Skin treatment, respiratory agent	Eczema, dermatitis; inhibition of airway inflammation in patients with chronic asthma symptoms	**T, L, O, P, cream, lotion:** Apply thin film two to four times daily; **Inhaler:** 100 mcg per spray; children ages 6–12 years: 1–2 puffs three or four times daily; adults: 2 puffs three or four times daily	Skin irritation, rash, dryness, cough, hoarseness, dry mouth, increased wheezing; rinse mouth after use to prevent thrush
TRIMETHOPRIM AND SULFAMETHOXAZOLE (TMP/SMZ) (Bactrim, Septra)	Antibiotic	Convenient dosing for otitis media and for urinary tract infections	**T, L:** 8–10 mg/kg/day, given twice daily; injection	Bone marrow suppression, allergic reactions, photosensitivity; gastrointestinal irritation, rash

[a]Key: C, capsules; T, tablets; L, liquid suspension or elixir; O, ointment; P, powder; S, suppositories.

Medication	Category	Use(s)	Standard application[a]	Side effects
VALPROIC ACID (Depakene, Depacon, Depakote)	Antiepileptic, psychopharma-cological agent	Myoclonic, simple absence, and generalized tonic-clonic seizures; Lennox-Gastaut syndrome; infantile spasms; also used to treat aggression and mood disorders, bipolar disorder, impulsive aggres-sion, intermittent explosive disorder, migraine prophylaxis	**C, syrup, sprinkle, injection:** 15–60 mg/kg/day; therapeu-tic blood level: 50–100 mcg/ml; Depakote ER may be dosed less frequently than the other preparations	Hair loss, weight loss or gain, ab-dominal distress, tremor, agranulo-cytosis, low platelet count; risk of birth defects if taken during pregnancy; FDA warning for potentially fatal liver damage (risk is 1/800 in children with develop-mental disabilities younger than 2 years who are taking more than one antiepileptic drug) and pancreatitis
ZIDOVUDINE (Retrovir)	Antiretroviral	HIV infection and prophylaxis	**C, T, syrup:** 2 mg/kg/dose every 6 hours, not to exceed 600 mg/day; injection	Malaise, dizziness, rash, nausea, vomiting diarrhea, anemia, myal-gias, tremor
ZINC OXIDE, COD LIVER OIL, LANOLIN, PETROLATUM (Caldesene ointment)	Skin	Diaper rash	**O:** Apply three or four times daily after diaper change or bath	Allergic reaction
ZONISAMIDE (Zonegran)	Antiepileptic	Adjunctive therapy in partial seizures, infantile spasms, and Lennox-Gastaut syn-drome	**O, C:** 2–4 mg/kg, gradually in-creased at 1- to 2-week inter-vals to 4–8 mg/kg; the maxi-mum daily dose is 12 mg/kg and the drug may be admin-istered as a single dose or in two or three divided doses; doses should not exceed 400 mg/day	Somnolence, dizziness, ataxia, loss of appetite, gastrointestinal dis-comfort, headache, agitation/irritability, confusion, rash, visual disturbances

[a]Key: C, capsules; T, tablets; L, liquid suspension or elixir; O, ointment; P, powder; S, suppositories.

D Childhood Disabilities Resources, Services, and Organizations

Gaetano R. Lotrecchiano

This appendix lists a number of organizations, web sources, and other resources that provide services and assist in research in the area of childhood developmental disabilities. A brief description follows each listing. The resources cited are a representative sample and are not intended to be all inclusive. We have tried to ensure that the information is as current as possible. We apologize if readers find that any information has changed. Those organizations providing Spanish-language resources and teletypewriter (TTY) are noted accordingly.

GENERAL

Libraries and Clearinghouses

Ages and Stages: Birth to 12 months
(http://www.extension.iastate.edu/Publications/PM1530A.pdf). Web site features a publication from the Iowa State University Extension program that presents information about the physical, mental, emotional, and social development of children between birth and 12 months of age. Provides ideas and tips for parents to facilitate these milestones.

Cochrane Library
Update Software, 1070 South Santa Fe Avenue, Suite 21, Vista, CA 92084 (760-631-5844; fax: 760-631-5848; e-mail: info@updateusa.com; http://www.update-software.com). Searchable, on-line database of systematic reviews of the effects of health care interventions related to pregnancy and neonatal outcomes. Also available on CD-ROM.

Disability Resources
NSNET Nova Scotia Community Organization Network, Technical Resource Centre, c/o Kings Regional Rehabilitation Centre, Post Office Box 128, Waterville, Nova Scotia, Canada B0P 1V0 (902-538-3103, ext. 112; fax: 902-538-7022; e-mail: trc@nsnet.org; http://www.nsnet.org/resource.html). Internet-based network of community organizations, information, and resources in Nova Scotia to help assist parents and families, professionals, and other agencies. Any organization or agency that supports individuals with disabilities can become an associated member at no cost.

Early Childhood Research & Practice (ECRP)
(http://www.ecrp.uiuc.edu). Web site of a peer-reviewed, bilingual electronic journal sponsored by the ERIC Clearinghouse on Elementary and Early Childhood Education (ERIC/EECE) at the University of Illinois at Urbana–Champaign. Covers topics related to the development, care, and education of children from birth to approximately age 8. Also includes articles and essays that present opinions and reflections, as well as letters to the editor.

East Tennessee Children's Hospital: Developmental Milestones
(http://www.etch.com/healthdevms.cfm). Web site presents a brief overview of typical and atypical developmental milestones from birth to 15 months. Site also provides links to information about feeding and swallowing, physical therapy and occupational therapy, and language development.

Kid Source
(http://www.kidsource.com). Web site defines early intervention and provides support for intervening as early as a disability or developmental difficulty has been identified. Site also contains a basic, although limited, reference list.

KidsHealth
(http://kidshealth.org). Sponsored by the Nemours Foundations Center for Children's Health. Web site offers a wide variety of information pertaining to child health issues. Contains helpful explanations of basic medical terminology and articles and resources for parents and professionals. Available in Spanish.

National Dissemination Center for Children with Disabilities (NDCCD)
(Post Office Box 1492, Washington, DC 20013 (800-695-0285; fax: 202-884-8441; http://www .nichcy.org). Web site contains information about specific disabilities, early intervention services for infants and toddlers, special education and related services for children in school, resources and connections in every state, individualized education programs, parent materials, disability organizations, professional associations, education rights and law requirements, and the transition to adult life. Publishes *Research Connections in Special Education* and *OSEP Digests.*

National Library of Medicine (NLM)
(8600 Rockville Pike, Bethesda, MD 20894 (888-346-3656; e-mail: publicinfo@nlm.nih .gov; http://www.nlm.nih.gov). Part of the National Institutes of Health. Is the world's largest medical library and is a national resource for all U.S. health sciences libraries. Collects materials in areas of biomedicine; health care; biomedical aspects of technology; humanities; and the physical, life, and social sciences. Medline Plus Health Information web site (http://www .medlineplus.gov) presents health information from NLM and contains extensive information for professionals and the public on diseases/ conditions and medicines, lists of hospitals, a medical encyclopedia/dictionary, information in Spanish, and links to current clinical trials. PubMed (http://www.ncbi.nlm.nih.gov/entrez/ query.fcgi) search engine allows users to research and obtain peer-reviewed articles and abstracts published by major journals of medical research.

Pediatric Development and Behavior
(http://www.dbpeds.org). Independent web site created to promote better care and outcomes for children and families affected by developmental, learning, and behavioral problems by providing access to clinically relevant information and educational material for medical providers, other service delivery professionals, and parents.

WebMD Health
(http://my.webmd.com). Provides a variety of useful information on mainstream health topics. Offers reliable information about identifying symptoms of illness and reports on highlighted topics.

Nonprofit and Philanthropic Agencies

Easter Seals
230 West Monroe Street, Suite 1800, Chicago, IL 60606 (voice: 800-221-6827; TTY: 312-726-4258; fax: 312-726-4258; e-mail: info@easter-seals.org; http://www.easter-seals.org). Nonprofit, community-based health agency dedicated to increasing the independence of people with disabilities, especially those with hearing impairments. Offers a range of quality services, research, and programs.

Federal Resource Center for Special Education (FRC)
c/o Academy for Educational Development, 1825 Connecticut Avenue NW, Washington, DC 20009 (http://www.rrfcnetwork.org). Supports a nationwide technical assistance network to respond to the needs of students with disabilities, especially those from underrepresented populations. Web site provides information and links from a variety of federally funded projects.

Healthy and Ready to Work Information Center
Maine State Title V CSHN Program (http:// www.hrtw.org). Network that works with local agencies to ensure that all youth with special health care needs receive the services necessary to make the transition to all aspects of adulthood, including adult health care, employment, and independence.

Institute for Child Health Policy
University of Florida, Post Office Box 100147, Gainesville, FL 32611 (352-265-7220; http:// www.ichp.edu). Mission is to research, evaluate, formulate, and advance health policies, programs, and systems that promote the health and well-being of children and youth through applied knowledge to health–related-systems and outcomes for children and youth.

Karolinska Institute
SE-171 77 Stockholm, Sweden (http://www .mic.ki.se/Diseases/G02.html). Contains information on many different diagnoses and conditions with specific categories for congenital,

hereditary, and neonatal diseases and abnormalities. Web site is for medical professionals and the general public, although the language is quite sophisticated. Site also has links to support sites for parents.

Kennedy Krieger Institute
707 North Broadway, Baltimore, MD 21205 (voice: 800-873-3377; TTY: 443-923-2645; fax 443-923-9405; http://www.kennedykrieger.org). Web site features information on a wide variety of diagnoses and conditions that affect young children. Also contains information about the various school and clinical programs available at the institute. News and events link is available for readers to find out about current conferences and other activities at Kennedy Krieger.

March of Dimes
1275 Mamaroneck Avenue, White Plains, NY 10605 (888-663-4637; http://www.modimes .org). Awards grants to institutions and organizations for development of genetic services, perinatal care in high-risk pregnancies, prevention of premature delivery, parent support groups, and other community programs. Campaign for Healthier Babies distributes information about birth defects and related newborn health problems. Spanish-language materials available.

**Maternal and Child
Health Bureau (MCHB)**
Parklawn Building Room 18-05, 5600 Fishers Lane, Rockville, MD 20857 (http://mchb.hrsa .gov). Established in 1912 as part of the Health Resources and Services Administration (HRSA). Provides funding and governs programs designed to ensure equal access for all to quality health care in a supportive, culturally competent, family and community setting.

**National Center for
Education in Maternal and Child Health**
2000 15th Street North, Suite 701, Arlington, VA 22201-2617 (703-524-7802; fax: 703-524-9335; e-mail: info@ncemch.org; http://www .ncemch.org). Disseminates publications and fact sheets to the public and professionals in the field and develops and maintains database of topics, agencies, and organizations related to maternal and child health.

Social Security Administration
Office of Public Inquiries, Windsor Park Building, 6401 Security Blvd. Baltimore, MD 21235 (voice: 800-772-1213; TTY: 800-325-0778;

http://www.ssa.gov). Mission is to advance the economic security of the nation's people through compassionate and vigilant leadership in shaping and managing America's Social Security programs. Provides information to the U.S. population on policy; programs and services; and, more specifically, resources for people with disabilities.

TASH
29 West Susquehanna Avenue, Suite 210, Baltimore, MD 21204 (410-828-8274; fax: 410-828-6706; e-mail: info@tash.org; http://www.tash .org). Advocates inclusive education and community opportunities for people with disabilities, disseminates research findings and practical applications for education and community living, and encourages sharing of experience and expertise. Publishes a newsletter and a journal.

ZERO TO THREE
National Center for Infants, Toddlers and Families, 2000 M Street NW, Suite 200, Washington, DC 20036 (202-638-1144; bookstore: 800-899-4301; bookstore e-mail: 0to3@presswarehouse.com; http://www.zerotothree.org). National, nonprofit organization whose mission is to promote the healthy development of infants and toddlers by supporting and strengthening families, communities, and those who work on their behalf. Web site includes various policies, research reports, and technical assistance resources for parents and professionals.

Professional Societies

American Academy of Pediatrics (AAP)
141 Northwest Point Boulevard, Elk Grove Village, IL 60007-1098 (847-434-4000; http://aap .org). The professional association of pediatricians. Committed to the optimal, physical, mental, and social health and well-being of infants, children, adolescents, and young adults. Publishes a major pediatric medical journal, *Pediatrics*.

**American Academy
of Pediatrics (AAP) Policies**
(http://aappolicy.aappublications.org). Site includes policy statements and guidelines developed by the AAP. Also offers links to printable handouts for parents that provide important health messages based on these statements.

**American College of
Obstetricians and Gynecologists (ACOG)**
409 12th Street SW, Post Office Box 96920,

Washington, DC 20090-6920 (e-mail: resources @acog.org; http://www.acog.org). Professional organization of obstetrician–gynecologists, dedicated to the advancement of women's health through education, advocacy, practice, and research. Provides on-line physician directory. Bookstore offers patient information pamphlets, professional resources, and multimedia resources.

American Medical Association (AMA)
515 North State Street, Chicago, IL 60610 (312-464-5000; http://www.ama-assn.org). Develops and promotes standards in medical practice, research, and education; advocates for patients and physicians. Publishes a leading medical journal, *JAMA: The Journal of the American Medical Association.*

Society for Disability Studies
University of Illinois at Chicago (MC 626) 1640 West Roosevelt Road, #236, Chicago, IL 60608-6904 (312-996-4664; fax: 312-996-7743; e-mail: hammel@uic.edu; http://www.uic.edu/orgs/sds). Works to explore issues of disability and chronic illness from scholarly perspectives. Publishes *Disability Studies Quarterly*; holds an annual conference that brings together scholars from a broad spectrum of fields as well as artists and community-based activists.

DEVELOPMENTAL DISABILITIES AND RELATED ILLNESSES

Acquired Immunodeficiency Syndrome (AIDS)

Centers for Disease Control and Prevention (CDC)
National Sexually Transmitted Diseases (STD) and AIDS Hotline (English: 800-342-2437; Spanish: 800-344-7432; TTY: 800-243-7889; http://www.cdc.gov). Weekday hotline that provides confidential information on transmission and prevention of human immunodeficiency virus (HIV)/AIDS and other STDs, testing, local referrals, and educational materials to the public.

Office of National AIDS Policy
The White House, 1600 Pennsylvania Avenue NW, Washington, DC 20500 (202-456-5594; http://www.whitehouse.gov/onap/aids.html). Provides broad direction for federal AIDS policy and fosters interdepartmental communication on HIV and AIDS. Works closely with the

AIDS community in the United States and around the world.

Attention-Deficit/ Hyperactivity Disorder (ADHD)

A.D.D. WareHouse
300 Northwest 70th Avenue, Suite 102, Plantation, FL 33317 (800-233-9273; fax: 954-792-8545; e-mail: sales@addwarehouse.com; http://www.addwarehouse.com). Mail-order resource for ADHD-related books, games, videotapes, and other materials for clinicians, parents, teachers, adults, and students.

Attention Deficit Disorder Association
1788 Second Street, Suite 200, Highland Park, IL 60035 (847-432-2332; fax: 847-432-5874; e-mail: mail@add.org; http://www.add.org). National organization that provides education, research, and public advocacy. Especially focused on the needs of adults and young adults with ADHD.

CHADD (Children and Adults with Attention-Deficit/Hyperactivity Disorder)
8181 Professional Place, Landover, MD 20785 (800-233-4050; fax: 301-306-7090; e-mail: national@chadd.org; http://www.chadd.org). Support group for parents of children with attention disorders. Provides continuing education for both parents and professionals, serves as a community resource for information, and advocates for appropriate educational programs.

Autism and Other Pervasive Developmental Disorders (PDDs)

American Hyperlexia Association
195 West Spangler, Suite B, Elmhurst, IL 60126 (630-415-2212; fax: 630-530-5909; e-mail: info@hyperlexia.org; http://www.hyperlexia.org). Nonprofit organization comprised of families of children, speech-language professionals, and educators dedicated to identifying hyperlexia, promoting effective teaching techniques, and educating the general public about hyperlexia.

Autism and Pervasive Developmental Disorders
(http://autism.about.com). Web site presents information on a variety of topics related to autism. Provides overview of autism, frequently asked questions, and common characteristics of children with autism. Many links to treatment options are available. Site also posts informa-

tion about current research issues related to autism.

Autism Research Institute

4182 Adams Avenue, San Diego, CA 92116 (619-281-7165; fax: 619-563-6840; http://www .autismwebsite.com/ari/index.htm). Information and referral for parents, teachers, physicians, and students working with children with autism and similar developmental disabilities. Publishes the quarterly *Autism Research Review International.*

Autism Society of America

7910 Woodmont Avenue, Suite 300, Bethesda, MD 20814-3067 (800-328-8476; fax: 301-657-0869; e-mail: info@autism-society.org; http:// www.autism-society.org). Provides information about autism, including options, approaches, methods, and systems available to parents and family members of children with autism and the professionals who work with them. Advocates for the rights and needs of individuals with autism and their families.

Autism Speaks

2 Park Avenue, 11th Floor, New York, NY 10016 (http://www.autismspeaks.org). Dedicated to helping families find answers, through funding research and education efforts and, most significantly, by spearheading the development of a national registry of individuals with autism. Web site aims to be a vital resource for anyone seeking information about autism.

AutismInfo.com

(http://www.autisminfo.com). Web site provides detailed information about autism, including current research efforts and resources about treatment options. Has the capability to be translated into Chinese, Spanish, French, Portuguese, German, Japanese, Italian, or Korean.

Bright Tots

(http://www.brighttots.com/Resourcehome.html). Web site is a resource site for parents of children with a diagnosis of an autism spectrum disorder. Contains information about developmental milestones and available intervention services. Also includes general articles about autism.

Center for the Study of Autism

Post Office Box 4538, Salem, OR 97302 (http:// www.autism.org). Provides information about autism to parents and professionals. Performs research on the efficacy of various therapeutic interventions.

International Rett Syndrome Association

9121 Piscataway Road, Clinton, MD 20735 (800-818-7388; fax: 301-856-3336; e-mail: irsa @rettsyndrome.org; http://www.rettsyndrome .org). Provides information, referral, and support to families and acts as a liaison with professionals. Also facilitates research on Rett syndrome.

National Center on Birth Defects and Developmental Disabilities (NCBDDD): Autism Information Center

1600 Clifton Road, Atlanta, GA 30333 (http:// www.cdc.gov/ncbddd/autism/index.htm). Web site has unique feature: link to the Autism Spectrum Disorders Kids' Quest, a series of informative sites provided by the NCBDDD for the purpose of educating children about developmental disabilities. Site also provides information about current research on autism spectrum disorders (ASDs) by the Centers for Disease Control and Prevention (CDC) and other federal agencies. Serves as a link for information regarding various state funding programs for ASDs.

Blindness

American Foundation for the Blind (AFB)

11 Penn Plaza, Suite 300, New York, NY 10011 (800-232-5463; fax: 212-502-7777; e-mail: afbinfo@afb.net; http://www.afb.org). Works in cooperation with other agencies, organizations, and schools to offer services to individuals who are blind or who have visual impairments; provides consultation, public education, referrals, and information; produces and distributes talking books; publishes and sells materials for professionals in the blindness field.

American Printing House for the Blind (APH)

Post Office Box 6085, Louisville, KY 40206-0085 (800-223-1839; fax: 502-899-2274; e-mail: info@aph.org; http://www.aph.org). Nonprofit publishing house for people with visual impairments. Has books in braille and large type and on audiotape and computer disk, as well as a range of aids, tools, and supplies for education and daily living. Free catalog.

National Association for Visually Handicapped

22 West 21st Street, 6th Floor, New York, NY 10010 (212-889-3141; fax: 212-727-2931;

e-mail: staff@navh.org; http://www.navh.org). Provides informational literature, guidance, and counseling in the use of visual aids, emotional support, and referral services for parents of partially sighted children and for people who work with these children. Publishes free large-print newsletter.

National Braille Association
3 Townline Circle, Rochester, NY 14623-2513 (585-427-8260; fax: 585-427-0263; e-mail: nbaoffice@compuserve.com; http://www.nation albraille.org). Produces and distributes braille reading materials for people with visual impairment. Collection consists of college-level textbooks, materials of general interest, standard technical tables, and music.

National Federation of the Blind
1800 Johnson Street, Baltimore, MD 21230 (410-659-9314; fax: 410-685-5653; e-mail: nfb@nfb.org; http://www.nfb.org). Strives for complete inclusion of people who are blind into society on the basis of equality. Offers advocacy services for these individuals in such areas as discrimination in housing and insurance. Operates a job referral and listing system for individuals to find competitive employment. Runs an aids and appliances department, a scholarship program for college students, and a loan program for people who are going into business for themselves. Publishes monthly and quarterly publications.

National Library Service for the Blind and Physically Handicapped
1291 Taylor Street NW, Washington, DC 20011 (voice: 202-707-5100; TTY: 202-707-0744; fax: 202-707-0712; e-mail: nls@loc.gov; http://www.loc.gov/nls). Administers a national library service through a network of participating public libraries to provide braille and recorded books and magazines on free loan to anyone who cannot read standard print because of visual or physical disabilities.

Prevent Blindness America
500 East Remington Road, Schaumburg, IL 60173 (800-331-2020; e-mail: info@prevent blindness.org; http://www.preventblindness.org). Committed to the reduction of preventable blindness. Provides information to people who are blind, professionals working with these individuals, and the public.

Recording for the Blind & Dyslexic (RFB&D)
20 Roszel Road, Princeton, NJ 08540 (609-452-0606; http://www.rfbd.org). Produces and distributes textbooks on audiotape, computer disk, and CD-ROM; individuals or institutions who have memberships may borrow these materials. Also provides reference librarian services for individual members.

Cerebral Palsy

American Academy for Cerebral Palsy and Developmental Medicine (AACPDM)
6300 North River Road, Suite 727, Rosemont, IL 60018-4226 (847-698-1635; fax: 847-823-0536; e-mail: woppenhe@ucla.edu; http://www .aacpdm.org/index?service=page/Home). Multidisciplinary scientific society that fosters professional education, research, and interest in the problems associated with cerebral palsy.

Cerebral Palsy, Erbs Palsy, All Types of Cerebral Palsy
(http://www.cerebralpalsy.org). Web site provides information about causes, risk factors, and types of cerebral palsy. Includes links and resources about types of help available and how to find help. Also discusses treatment interventions and special education issues.

Cerebral Palsy: Hope Through Research
(http://www.ninds.nih.gov/disorders/cerebral_palsy/detail_cerebral_palsy.htm). Web site discusses diagnostic questions related to cerebral palsy. Includes questions related to causes and treatments available. Also provides information about current research projects being conducted concerning cerebral palsy. Available in Spanish.

Cerebral Palsy—Neurology Channel
(http://www.neurologychannel.com/cerebral palsy). Web site includes information about cerebral palsy, including types, causes, treatments, risk factors, complications, and prognosis. Also provides information about orthopedic and neurological surgeries for cerebral palsy.

Children's Disabilities and Special Needs
(http://www.comeunity.com/disability/cerebral _palsy). Web site contains general articles related to cerebral palsy and articles about research concerning cerebral palsy in children born prematurely. Provides links to books and resources.

CP Resource Center

(http://www.cpparent.org). Web site provides general information about cerebral palsy, its causes, and some treatments. Contains a dictionary to help parents in understanding medical terms they may hear. Also lists books for further reading. Site speaks specifically about periventricular leukomalacia (PVL) and its relation to cerebral palsy. Hippotherapy (horseback riding therapy) discussed as a treatment option.

United Cerebral Palsy

1660 L Street NW, Suite 700, Washington, DC 20036 (voice: 800-872-5827; TTY: 202-973-7197; fax: 202-776-0414; e-mail: national@ucp.org; http://www.ucp.org). Provides direct services to children and adults with cerebral palsy that include medical diagnosis, evaluation and treatment, special education, career development, counseling, social and recreational programs, and adapted housing.

Deafness/Speech Disorders

ADARA (formerly Professional Workers with the Adult Deaf [PRWAD] and the American Deafness and Rehabilitation Association)

Post Office Box 727, Lusby, MD 20657 (e-mail: ADARAorgn@aol.com; http://www.adara.org). Serves professionals who work with deaf individuals and people interested in learning about deafness. Publishes a journal and newsletter by subscription; offers memberships.

Alexander Graham Bell Association for the Deaf

3417 Volta Place NW, Washington, DC 20007 (voice: 202-337-5220; TTY: 202-337-5221; fax: 202-337-8314; e-mail: info@agbell.org; http://www.agbell.org). Umbrella organization for the International Organization for the Education of the Hearing Impaired (IOEHI), Parents' Section (PS), and Oral Hearing Impaired Section. Provides general information and information on resources. Encourages improved communication, better public understanding, and detection of early hearing loss.

American Society for Deaf Children

Post Office Box 3355, Gettysburg, PA 17325 (voice/TTY: 717-334-7922; parent hotline: 800-942-2732; fax: 717-334-8808; e-mail: asdc1@aol.com; http://www.deafchildren.org). Provides information and support to parents and families with children who are deaf or who have hearing impairments.

American Speech-Language-Hearing Association (ASHA)

10801 Rockville Pike, Rockville, MD 20852 (voice/TTY: 800-638-8255; e-mail: actioncenter@asha.org; http://www.asha.org). Professional and scientific organization and certifying body for professionals providing speech-language and hearing therapy. Conducts research in communication disorders, publishes several journals, and provides consumer information and professional referral.

Boys Town National Research Hospital

555 North 30th Street, Omaha, NE 68131 (http://www.boystownhospital.org/home.asp). Web site provides variety of resources relating to children with hearing, language, and learning disabilities and the research currently underway at Boys Town National Research Hospital.

Collaborative Early Intervention National Training e-Resource

(http://center.uncg.edu). Target audience for web site is professionals who serve families with infants and toddlers who are deaf or hard of hearing. Provides graduate-level, web-based training for service providers. Site also offers an extensive list of resources for professionals and families.

Deafness Research Foundation

1050 17th Street NW, Suite 701, Washington, DC 20036 (e-mail: webmaster@drf.org; http://www.drf.org). Solicits funds for the support of research into the causes, treatment, and prevention of deafness and other hearing disorders.

Described and Captioned Media Program (formerly Captioned Films/Videos)

1447 East Main Street, Spartanburg, SC 29307 (800-237-6213; TTY: 800-237-6819; fax: 800-538-5636; e-mail: info@cfv.org; http://www.cfv.org). Government-sponsored distribution of open-captioned materials to eligible institutions, individuals, and families. Application sent on request.

Early Intervention Bibliography

(http://www.tr.wou.edu/dblink/lib/resources.htm). From the National Informational Clearinghouse on Children Who Are Deaf-Blind. Web site links to information about deafblindness, disability, education and technical assistance, technology, and medical and health resources. Provides bibliographic sources relevant to any disability.

**Helen Keller National Center
for Deaf-Blind Youths and Adults**
111 Middle Neck Road, Sands Point, NY 11050
(voice: 516-944-8900; TTY: 516-944-8637; fax:
516-944-7302; http://www.helenkeller.org/na
tional). Has specialists at its New York training
center and representatives in 10 regional offices
who can assist with locating assistive/adaptive
devices. Also offers technical assistance to local
agencies that are serving individuals who are
deafblind.

International Hearing Society
16880 Middlebelt Road, Livonia, MI 48154
(http://ihsinfo.org/IhsV2/Home/Index.cfm).
Provides information on how to proceed when
hearing loss is suspected. Also offers free consumer kit, facts about hearing aids, and a variety
of literature on hearing-related subjects.

**Laurent Clerc National
Deaf Education Center**
800 Florida Avenue NE, Washington, DC
20002 (http://clerccenter.gallaudet.edu/infoto
go). Web site provides information about many
topics related to deafness or hearing loss. Includes information about assistive devices and
hearing aids available for children with hearing
problems. Includes many resources regarding
where to go for information on learning sign
language or speech reading. Section of site gives
information about classroom issues related to
education of children with deafness. Information provided for children and parents about
deafness and issues surrounding the condition.

National Center for Stuttering
200 East 33rd Street, New York, NY 10016 (800-
221-2483; http://www.stuttering.com). Provides
free information for parents of young children
just starting to show symptoms of stuttering;
runs training programs in current therapeutic
approaches for speech-language professionals;
provides treatment for people older than 7 years
of age who stutter.

**National Deaf Education
Network and Clearinghouse**
Laurent Clerc National Deaf Education Center, Gallaudet University, 800 Florida Avenue
NE, Washington, DC 20002-3695 (voice/TTY:
202-651-5031; e-mail: clearinghouse.Infotogo
@gallaudet.edu; http://clerccenter.gallaudet.edu/
Clearinghouse/index.html). Provides information related to deafness; has a multitude of resources and experts available for individuals

with hearing impairments, their families, and
professionals. Collects information about resources around the country.

**Self Help for Hard of
Hearing People (SHHH)**
7910 Woodmont Avenue, Suite 1200, Bethesda,
MD 20814 (voice: 301-657-2248; TTY: 301-
657-2249; fax: 301-913-9413; e-mail: National
@shhh.org; http://www.shhh.org). Educational
organization that provides assistance to individuals with hearing impairments to participate
fully in society. Publishes journal, newsletter,
and other materials; provides advocacy and outreach programs and an extensive network of
local chapters and self-help groups; and hosts an
annual convention.

**Signing Exact English (SEE) Center
for the Advancement of Deaf Children**
Post Office Box 1181, Los Alamitos, CA 90720
(562-430-1467; fax: 562-795-6614; e-mail: seectr
@aol.com; http://www.seecenter.org). Offers information and referral services for parents of
children newly diagnosed with hearing impairments.

**Speech and Language
Development in Young Children**
(http://members.tripod.com/Caroline_Bowen/
devel1.htm). Web site presents information
about the acquisition of language in early childhood. Provides information about how language is learned and the role of the parent in
facilitating these skills. Language and communication milestones are presented along with a
section on when to seek professional help.

Speech Therapy Activities
(http://www.speechtx.com). Web site provides
free, printable speech-language activities for
speech-language pathologists and parents.

Down Syndrome

**The Association for
Children with Down Syndrome**
4 Fern Place, Plainview, NY 11803 (516-933-
4700; fax: 516-933-9524; http://www.acds.org).
Offers information and referral services, including a free list of publications.

Down Syndrome: Health Issues
(http://www.ds-health.com). For parents and
professionals. Web site includes articles concerning specific health issues related to Down
syndrome, such as gastroesophageal reflux, blood

disorders, and thyroid function. Information also provided about health guidelines and controversies in the care of children and adults with Down syndrome.

National Down Syndrome Congress (NDSC)

1370 Center Drive, Suite 102, Atlanta, GA 30338 (800-232-6372; e-mail: info@ndsccenter .org; http://ndsccenter.org). Provides information and referral materials and publishes a newsletter.

National Down Syndrome Society (NDSS)

666 Broadway, New York, NY 10012 (800-221-4602; fax: 212-979-2873; http://www.ndss.org). Provides information and publishes a newsletter and clinical care booklets.

Epilepsy

American Epilepsy Society

342 North Main Street, West Hartford, CT 06117-2507 (860-586-7505; fax: 860-586-7550; e-mail: Info@aesnet.org; http://www.aesnet.org). Promotes research and education for professionals dedicated to the prevention, treatment, and cure of epilepsy.

Epilepsy Foundation (formerly Epilepsy Foundation of America)

4351 Garden City Drive, Landover, MD 20785-7223 (800-332-1000; e-mail: webmaster@efa .org; http://www.efa.org). Provides programs of information and education, advocacy, support of research, and the delivery of needed services to people with epilepsy and their families.

International League Against Epilepsy

avenue Marcel Thiry 204, B-1200, Brussels, Belgium (e-mail: ndevolder@ilae-epilepsy.org; http://www.ilae-epilepsy.org). Global nonprofit organization that disseminates knowledge about epilepsy and fosters research, education, training, and improved services and care. Has official working relationship with the World Health Organization.

Fetal Alcohol Syndrome

Family Empowerment Network (FEN)

610 Langdon Street, Room 517, Madison, WI 53703-1195 (800-462-5254; fax: 608-265-3352; e-mail: fen@dcs.wisc.edu; http://www.fammed .wisc.edu/fen). National nonprofit organization that exists to empower families affected by fetal alcohol syndrome and other drug-related birth defects, through education and support; also publishes a newsletter, *The FEN Pen.*

National Organization on Fetal Alcohol Syndrome (NOFAS)

216 G Street NE, Washington, DC 20002 (202-785-4585; fax: 202-466-6456; e-mail: information@nofas.org; http://www.nofas.org). Nonprofit organization founded in 1990; dedicated to eliminating birth defects caused by alcohol consumption during pregnancy and to improving the quality of life for those individuals and families affected. Applies a multicultural approach in its prevention. Is the only national organization focusing solely on fetal alcohol syndrome.

PREVLINE: Prevention Online (National Clearinghouse for Alcohol and Drug Information)

11426-11428 Rockville Pike, Suite 200, Rockville, MD 20852 (800-729-6686; e-mail: info@ health.org; http://ncadi.samhsa.gov). The world's largest resource for current information and materials concerning substance abuse. Distributes brochures, offers resources for parents and teachers on prevention, and has English- and Spanish-speaking information service staff available to answer questions.

Fragile X Syndrome

FRAXA Research Foundation

45 Pleasant Street, Newburyport, MA 01950 (978-462-1866; e-mail: info@fraxa.org; http:// www.fraxa.org). Supports scientific research aimed at finding a treatment and a cure for fragile X syndrome. Funds grants and fellowships at universities worldwide. Runs an e-mail list on which individuals may post strategies and questions. Publishes *FRAXA Newsletter, Medication Guide for Fragile X Syndrome* (by Michael Tranfaglia) and *Fragile X A to Z: A Guide for Families* (edited by Wendy Dillworth; downloadable from the web site free of charge).

National Fragile X Foundation

Post Office Box 190488, San Francisco, CA 94119 (800-688-8765; fax: 925-938-9315; e-mail: natlfx@fragilex.org; http://www.fragilex.org). Promotes education concerning diagnosis of, treatment for, and research on fragile X syndrome, and provides referral to local resource centers. Sponsors a biannual conference. Offers extensive audiovisual and teaching aids.

Genetic Syndromes and Inborn Errors of Metabolism

There are many support organizations and networks for children with various syndromes and inborn errors of metabolism and their families. A representative sample is listed here. For a more complete listing, contact the National Organization for Rare Disorders (NORD [see later listing]).

The American Society of Human Genetics
9650 Rockville Pike, Bethesda, MD 20814-3998 (866-486-4363; fax: 301-530-7079; http://www.ashg.org). Organization for professionals specializing in human genetics. Publishes *The American Journal of Human Genetics* and other resources.

Arnold-Chiari Family Network
c/o Kevin and Maureen Walsh, 67 Spring Street, Weymouth, MA 02188 (617-337-2368). Informal family support network for individuals with Chiari I and Chiari II malformations and their families. Literature and occasional newsletter provided on request.

Avenues
Post Office Box 5192, Sonora, CA 95370 (209-928-3688; http://www.avenuesforamc.com). Publishes a semiannual newsletter that provides lists of parents, physicians, and experienced medical centers concerned with people with arthrogryposis multiplex congenita.

Cornelia de Lange Syndrome Foundation
302 West Main Street, #100, Avon, CT 06001 (800-223-8355; fax: 860-676-8337; e-mail: info @cdlsusa.org; http://www.cdlsusa.org). Supports parents and children affected by de Lange syndrome, encourages research, and disseminates information to increase public awareness through a newsletter and informational pamphlet.

5p-Society
Post Office Box 268, Lakewood, CA 90714 (888-970-0777; fax: 714-890-9112; e-mail: fivepminus @aol.com; http://www.fivepminus.org). Family support and information group for parents, grandparents, and guardians of individuals with 5p- (cri-du-chat) syndrome. Publishes a newsletter and sponsors an annual meeting.

GeneTests/GeneClinics
206-543-9198; e-mail: geneclinics@geneclinics .org; genetests@genetests.org; http://www.gene clinics.org; http://www.genetests.org). Free medical genetics information resource developed for physicians, other health care providers, researchers, and the public. Provides *GeneReviews*, peer-reviewed articles describing the application of genetic testing to the diagnosis, management, and genetic counseling of patients; international directories for genetic testing laboratories and genetic and prenatal diagnosis clinics; and various educational materials.

Genetic Alliance
4301 Connecticut Avenue NW, Suite 404, Washington, DC 20008-2304 (800-336-4363; fax: 202-966-8553; e-mail: info@geneticalliance .org; http://www.geneticalliance.org). International organization of families, health professionals, and genetic organizations dedicated to enhancing the lives of individuals living with genetic conditions through the provision of education, policy, and information services. Helpline staff available to address questions about genetics and to connect callers with support groups and informational resources.

Genetics Society of America
9650 Rockville Pike, Bethesda, MD 20814-3998 (866-486-4363; fax: 301-530-7079; http://www.faseb.org/genetics/gsa/gsamenu.htm). Professional organization that aims to bring together genetic investigators and provide a forum for sharing research findings. Cooperates in the organization of an international congress held every 5 years under the auspices of the International Genetics Federation. Publishes the journal *GENETICS* and other resources.

Little People of America
Post Office Box 745, Lubbock, TX 79408 (English and Spanish helpline: 888-572-2001; e-mail: LPADataBase@juno.com; http://www .lpaonline.org). Nationwide organization dedicated to helping people of short stature. Provides fellowship, moral support, and information to little people or individuals with dwarfism. The toll-free helpline provides information on organizations, products and services, and doctors in the caller's area.

National Gaucher Foundation
5410 Edson Lane, Suite 260, Rockville, MD 20852 (800-428-2437; fax: 301-816-1516; e-mail: ngf@gaucherdisease.org; http://www .gaucherdisease.org). Publishes quarterly newsletter, operates support groups and chapters, provides referrals to organizations for appropriate services, and funds research on Gaucher disease.

The National Neurofibromatosis Foundation

95 Pine Street, 16th Floor, New York, NY 10005 (800-323-7938; fax: 212-747-0004; e-mail: NNFF@nf.org; http://www.nf.org). Supplies information to lay people and professionals and offers genetic counseling and support groups throughout the United States.

National Organization for Rare Disorders (NORD)

Post Office Box 8923, New Fairfield, CT 06812-8923 (203-746-6518; fax: 203-746-6481; e-mail: orphan@rarediseases.org; http://www.rarediseases.org). Nonprofit group of voluntary health organizations serving people with rare disorders and disabilities. Dedicated to the identification, treatment, and cure of rare disorders through education, advocacy, research, and service.

National Tay-Sachs and Allied Diseases Association

2001 Beacon Street, Suite 204, Brighton, MA, 02135 (800-906-8723; fax: 617-277-0134; e-mail: NTSAD-boston@worldnet.att.net; http://www.NTSAD.org). Promotes genetic screening programs nationally, has updated listing of Tay-Sachs disease–prevention centers in a number of countries, provides educational literature to general public and professionals, and coordinates peer group support for parents.

National Urea Cycle Disorders Foundation

4841 Hill Street, La Canada, CA 91011 (e-mail: info@nucdf.org; http://www.nucdf.org). Provides information and support for families. Supports and stimulates medical research and increased awareness by the public and the legislators of issues related to urea cycle disorders.

Online Mendelian Inheritance in Man (OMIM)

(http://www.ncbi.nlm.nih.gov/entrez/query.fcgi?db=OMIM). Web site database of human genes and genetic disorders with textual information, pictures, and reference information.

Organic Acidemia Association

13210 35th Avenue North Plymouth, MN 55441 (763-559-1797; Fax: 866-539-4060; http://www.oaanews.org). A volunteer nonprofit organization whose mission is to empower families and health care professionals with knowledge in organic acidemia metabolic disorders.

Osteogenesis Imperfecta Foundation

804 West Diamond Avenue, Suite 210, Gaithersburg, MD 20878 (800-981-2663; fax: 301-947-0456; e-mail: bonelink@oif.org; http://www.oif.org). Supports research on osteogenesis imperfecta and provides information to those with this disorder, to their families, and to other interested people.

Prader-Willi Syndrome Association

5700 Midnight Pass Road, Sarasota, FL 34242 (800-926-4797; fax: 941-312-0142; e-mail: national@pwsausa.org; http://www.pwsausa.org). National organization that serves as a clearinghouse for information on Prader-Willi syndrome; shares information with parents, professionals, and other interested people.

Rare Diseases Network

Children's National Medical Center, 111 Michigan Avenue, NW Washington, DC 20010 (202-884-4679; fax: 202-884-2021; e-mail: jseminar@cnmc.org; http://rarediseasesnetwork.epi.usf.edu). National network of scientists and physicians working on cures and conducting clinical trials on a number of rare disorders. Provides study information.

Support Organization for Trisomy 18, 13, and Related Disorders (SOFT)

2982 South Union Street, Rochester, NY 14624 (English: 800-716-7638; Spanish: 631-226-3986; e-mail: barbsoft@aol.com; http://www.trisomy.org). Chapters in most states provide support and family packages with a newsletter and appropriate literature underscoring the common problems for children with trisomy 13 or trisomy 18. Holds a yearly conference for families and professionals.

Tourette Syndrome Association

42-40 Bell Boulevard, Bayside, NY 11361 (718-224-2999; fax: 718-279-9596; e-mail: ts@tsa-usa.org; http://www.tsa-usa.org). Offers information, referral, advocacy, education, research, and self-help groups for those affected by Tourette syndrome.

Treacher Collins Foundation

Post Office Box 683, Norwich, VT 05055 (e-mail: geomrf@hotmail.com; http://www.facescranio.org/Disord/Treacher.htm). Resource and referral for families, individuals, and professionals who are interested in developing and sharing knowledge and experience about Treacher Collins syndrome and related disorders. Publishes newsletter and makes print and videotape resources available by loan.

Tuberous Sclerosis Alliance

801 Roeder Road, Suite 750, Silver Spring, MD 20910 (800-225-6872; fax: 301-562-9870; e-mail: info@tsalliance.org; http://www.tsalliance .org). Offers public information about manifestations of the disease to newly diagnosed individuals, their families, and interested professionals. Referrals are made to support groups located in most states. Funds research through membership fees and donations.

Guillain-Barré Syndrome

Guillain-Barré Syndrome Foundation International

Post Office Box 262, Wynnewood, PA 19096 (610-667-0131; fax: 610-667-7036; e-mail: gbint @ix.netcom.com; http://www.gbsfi.com). Provides emotional support to individuals with Guillain-Barré syndrome and their families; fosters research; educates the public about the disorder; develops nationwide support groups; and directs people with this syndrome to resources, meetings, newsletters, and symposia.

Intellectual Disability

American Association on Intellectual and Developmental Disabilities (AAIDD) (formerly the American Association on Mental Retardation ([AAMR])

444 North Capitol Street NW, Suite 846, Washington, DC 20001 (800-424-3688; fax: 202-387-2193; http://www.aaidd.org). Professional organization that promotes cooperation among those involved in services, training, and research in intellectual disabilities. Encourages research, dissemination of information, development of appropriate community-based services, and the promotion of preventive measures designed to further reduce the incidence of intellectual disability.

The Arc of the United States

1010 Wayne Avenue, Suite 650, Silver Spring, MD 20910 (301-565-3842; fax: 301-565-5342; e-mail: info@thearc.org; http://thearc.org). National advocacy organization working on behalf of individuals with intellectual disabilities and their families; has more than 1,000 state and local chapters.

President's Committee for People with Intellectual Disabilities (PCPID)

370 L'Enfant Promenade SW, Suite 701, Washington, DC 20447-0001 (202-619-0634; fax: 202-205-9519; e-mail: pcmr@acf.dhhs.gov; http://www.acf.hhs.gov/programs/pcpid/index .html). Advises the President and the Secretary of Health and Human Services on all matters pertaining to intellectual disabilities; publishes annual reports and information on the rights of people with intellectual disabilities.

Learning Disabilities

Dyslexia Research Institute

5746 Centerville Road, Tallahassee, FL 32308 (850-893-2216; fax: 850-893-2440; e-mail: dri @dyslexia-add.org; http://www.dyslexia-add.org). Provides training, workshops, and seminars for professionals. Literature sent on request.

International Dyslexia Association (IDA) (formerly the Orton Dyslexia Society)

8600 LaSalle Road, Chester Building Suite 382, Baltimore, MD 21286-2044 (410-296-0232; fax: 410-321-5069; e-mail: info@interdys.org; http://www.interdys.org). Devoted to the study and treatment of dyslexia; provides information and referrals; sponsors conferences, seminars, and support groups; and has two regular publications and more than 40 branches in the United States and abroad.

LD Online

(e-mail: info@ldonline.org; http://www.ldonline .org). Resources on learning disabilities for parents, students, teachers, and other professionals. Interactive web site provides basic information on learning disabilities and the latest research and news; also offers e-mail consultation by experts on learning disabilities, resource lists, personal stories, bulletin boards, and materials/resources for purchase.

Learning Disabilities Association of America (LDA)

4156 Library Road, Pittsburgh, PA 15234 (412-341-1515; fax: 412-344-0224; e-mail: info@lda america.org; http://www.ldanatl.org). Encourages research and the development of early detection programs, disseminates information, serves as an advocate, and works to improve education for individuals with learning disabilities.

National Center for Learning Disabilities (NCLD)

381 Park Avenue, South, Suite 1401, New York, NY 10016 (888-575-7373; fax: 212-545-9665; http://www.ld.org). Promotes public awareness of learning disabilities and provides computerized information and referral services to consumers and professionals on learning disabilities. Publishes *Their World*, an annual magazine for parents and professionals.

Schwablearning.org

(http://www.schwablearning.org). An on-line parent's guide to helping children with learning disabilities and attention-deficit/hyperactivity disorder (ADHD), including information on identifying disabilities and on managing home, school, and learning. Site also has resources and publications for families.

Muscular Dystrophy

Muscular Dystrophy Association

3300 East Sunrise Drive, Tucson, AZ 85718 (800-572-1717; e-mail: mda@mdausa.org; http://www.mdausa.org). Health care agency that fosters research and provides direct services to individuals with muscular dystrophy; is concerned with conquering muscular dystrophy and other neuromuscular diseases.

Wellstone Muscular Dystrophy Center

Children's National Medical Center, 111 Michigan Avenue, NW Washington, DC 20010 (202-884-6029; e-mail: mpichaske@cnmc.org; http://-www.wellstone-dc.org). Description of projects underway in muscular dystrophy. Focus on Duchenne muscular dystrophy.

Scoliosis

National Scoliosis Foundation

5 Cabot Place, Stoughton, MA 02072 (800-673-6922; fax: 781-341-8333; e-mail: NSF@scoliosis.org; http://www.scoliosis.org). Nonprofit organization with state chapters; dedicated to informing the public about scoliosis and promoting early detection and treatment of scoliosis. Publishes *Spinal Connection Newsletter*.

Scoliosis Research Society

611 East Wells Street, Milwaukee, WI 53202 (414-289-9107; fax: 414-276-3349; http://www.srs.org). Sponsors and promotes research on the etiology and treatment of scoliosis and spinal disorders.

Spina Bifida and Other Neural Tube Defects (NTDs)

Spina Bifida Association of America

4590 MacArthur Boulevard NW, Suite 250, Washington, DC 20007 (800-621-3141; fax: 202-944-3295; e-mail: sbaa@sbaa.org; http://www.sbaa.org). Provides information and referral for new parents and literature on spina bifida; supports a public awareness program; advocates for individuals with spina bifida and their families; supports research; and conducts conferences for parents and professionals.

Traumatic Brain Injury (TBI)

Brain Injury Association of America (formerly National Head Injury Foundation)

105 North Alfred Street, Alexandria, VA 22314 (helpline: 800-444-6443; voice: 703-236-6000; fax: 703-236-6001; e-mail: FamilyHelpLine@biausa.org; http://www.biausa.org). Provides information to educate the public, politicians, businesses, and educators about brain injury, including effects, causes, and prevention.

Traumatic Brain Injury Resource Guide

(http://www.neuroskills.com). Web site includes educational information, books, local support groups, and research.

ACCESSIBILITY AND COMMUNITY INCLUSION

Association of University Centers on Disabilities (AUCD) (formerly American Association of University Affiliated Programs for Persons with Developmental Disabilities)

8630 Fenton Street, Suite 410, Silver Spring, MD 20910 (301-588-8252; fax: 301-588-2842; e-mail: kmusheno@aucd.org; http://www.aucd.org). Represents the professional interests of the national network of 61 university centers for excellence in developmental disabilities education, research, and service (UCEs; formerly called university affiliated programs, or UAPs) that serve people with developmental disabilities.

The Center for Universal Design

North Carolina State University College of Design, Campus Box 8613, Brooks Hall, Room 220, Pullen Road, Raleigh, NC 27695 (800-647-6777; fax: 919-515-3023; e-mail: cud@ncsu.edu;

http://www.design.ncsu.edu:8120/cud). Provides publications and information to parents and professionals concerning accessible housing design and financing issues; makes referrals to local organizations.

Center on Human Policy
Syracuse University, 805 South Crouse Avenue, Syracuse, NY 13244 (voice: 800-894-0826; TTY: 315-443-4355; fax: 315-443-4338; e-mail: thechp@sued.syr.edu; http://soeweb.syr.edu/thechp). Involved in a range of local, state, national, and international activities, including policy studies, research, information, and referral.

Job Accommodation Network (JAN)
West Virginia University, Post Office Box 6080, Morgantown, WV 26506 (in the U.S.: voice/TTY: 800-526-7234; worldwide: voice/TTY: 304-293-7186; fax: 304-293-5407; e-mail: jan@jan.icdi.wvu.edu; http://janweb.icdi.wvu.edu). Information and resources to make workplaces accessible to those with disabilities.

National Association of
Developmental Disabilities Councils
1234 Massachusetts Avenue NW, Suite 103, Washington, DC 20005 (202-347-1234; fax: 202-347-4023; e-mail: mgray@naddc.org; http://www.nacdd.org). Organization of developmental disability councils that exist in each state to provide information on and advocate for resources and services for people with developmental disabilities and their families.

National Center on Accessibility
Indiana University, 2805 East 10th Street, Suite 190, Bloomington, IN 47408-2698 (812-856-4422; TTY: 812-856-4421; fax: 812-856-4480; e-mail: nca@indiana.edu; http://www.ncaonline.org). Works with departments of parks, recreation, and tourism throughout the United States to improve accessibility. Sponsors several training sessions each year throughout the United States to educate employers on making their workplaces accessible.

National Council on Independent Living
1916 Wilson Boulevard, Suite 209, Arlington, VA 22201 (voice: 703-525-3406; TTY: 703-525-4153; fax: 703-525-3409; e-mail: ncil@ncil.org; http://www.ncil.org). A national membership association of nonprofit corporations that advances the full inclusion of people with disabilities in society and the development of centers for independent living. Provides members with technical assistance and training, publishes

a quarterly newsletter, and sponsors a national conference.

National Home of Your Own Alliance
University of New Hampshire, Institute on Disability, Center for Housing and New Community Economics (CHANCE), 7 Leavitt Lane, Suite 101, Durham, NH 03824-3522 (e-mail: drv@cisunix.unh.edu; http://alliance.unh.edu/nhoyo.html). This program is dedicated to helping people with disabilities become homeowners and in controlling their homes.

National Organization on Disability
910 16th Street NW, Suite 600, Washington, DC 20006 (voice: 202-293-5960; TTY: 202-293-5968; fax: 202-293-7999; e-mail: ability@nod.org; http://www.nod.org). Promotes the acceptance and understanding of the needs of citizens with disabilities, through a national network of communities and organizations; facilitates exchange of information regarding resources available to people with disabilities.

U.S. Access Board
1331 F Street NW, Suite 1000, Washington, DC 20004-1111 (voice: 800-872-2253; TTY: 800-993-2822; fax: 202-272-5447; e-mail: info@access-board.gov; http://www.access-board.gov). An organization created by Section 504 of the Rehabilitation Act of 1973 (PL 93-112) to enforce the Architectural Barriers Act of 1968 (PL 90-480). Offers free publications and answers to technical questions about accessibility.

ADAPTIVE
TECHNOLOGY AND EQUIPMENT

ABLEDATA
8630 Fenton Street, Suite 950, Silver Spring, MD 20910 (voice: 800-227-0216; TTY: 301-608-8912; fax: 301-608-8958; e-mail: abledata@macroint.com; http://www.abledata.com). National database of information on assistive technology and rehabilitation equipment.

Alliance for Technology Access
2175 East Francisco Boulevard, Suite L, San Rafael, CA 94901 (voice: 415-455-4575; TTY: 415-455-0491; fax: 415-455-0654; e-mail: ATAinfo@ATAccess.org; http://www.ataccess.org). A resource and demonstration center open to people with disabilities, their families, and professionals and others interested in adaptive technology.

Independent Living Aids

200 Robbins Lane, Jericho, NY 11753 (800-537-2118; fax: 516-937-3906; e-mail: can-do@independentliving.com; http://www.independliving.com). Sells aids that make daily tasks easier for those with physical disabilities; also carries clocks, calculators, magnifying lamps, and easy-to-see low-vision and talking watches for individuals with visual impairments. Free catalog.

Michigan's Assistive Technology Resource

1023 South U.S. Route 27, St. Johns, MI 48879 (voice: 800-274-7426; TTY: 989-224-0246; fax: 989-224-0330; e-mail: matr@match.org; http://www.copower.org/At/atlinks.htm). Provides free information on low-tech devices and equipment available for individuals with disabilities.

Rehabilitation Engineering and Assistive Technology Society of North America (RESNA)

1700 North Moore Street, Suite 1540, Arlington, VA 22209-1903 (voice: 703-524-6686; TTY: 703-524-6639; fax: 703-524-6630; http://www.resna.org). Multidisciplinary organization of professionals interested in the identification, development, and delivery of technology to people with disabilities. Offers numerous publications.

BEHAVIOR AND MENTAL HEALTH

American Academy of Child and Adolescent Psychiatry (AACAP)

3615 Wisconsin Avenue NW, Washington, DC 20016-3007 (202-966-7300; fax: 202-966-2891; http://www.aacap.org). National nonprofit organization comprised of child and adolescent psychiatrists. Provides information for professionals and families to aid in the understanding and treatment of childhood and adolescent developmental, behavioral, and mental health disorders. Parent and caregiver fact sheets and information on research, practice, and membership are available on the web site.

American Psychiatric Association (APA)

1400 K Street NW, Washington, DC 20005 (888-357-7924; fax: 202-682-6850; e-mail: apa@psych.org; http://www.psych.org). International organization for physicians, dedicated to the diagnosis and treatment of mental health and substance-use disorders.

American Psychological Association (APA)

750 First Street, NE, Washington, DC 20002-4242 (voice: 800-374-2721; TTY: 202-336-6123; http://www.apa.org). National scientific and professional organization that develops and promotes standards in psychological practice, research, and education. Dedicated to the dissemination of psychological knowledge to professionals, students, and the general public through meetings, reports, and publications.

Association for Behavior Analysis International (ABA International)

213 West Hall, Western Michigan University, 1903 West Michigan Avenue, Kalamazoo, MI 49008-5301 (616-387-8341; fax: 616-387-8354; e-mail: 76236.1312@compuserve.com; http://www.abainternational.org). International organization that promotes the experimental, theoretical, and applied analysis of behavior. Disseminates professional and public information. Also publishes two scholarly journals, *The Behavior Analyst* and *The Analysis of Verbal Behavior.*

Behaviour Change Consultancy

24 Rochdale, Harold Road, London SE19 3TF, England (e-mail: bcc@behaviourchange.com; http://www.behaviourchange.com). Provides advice, support, project management, policy development, and training to schools, local educational authorities, and parents on the subjects of disaffection. Also gives advice on social, emotional, and behavioral difficulties, as well as behavior management.

Bright Futures at Georgetown University

(http://www.brightfutures.org/mentalhealth). Web site explains the Bright Futures materials that help providers operationalize the guidelines for mental health promotion in children. Site also contains materials to download, including a mental health fact sheet, a listing of supporting organizations, and training tools.

Head Start/ Administration on Children and Families

(http://www.headstartinfo.org). Web site contains a wealth of information on the Head Start and Early Head Start programs. A special feature is The Mental Health Toolkit, an annotated bibliography of a variety of articles, books, and federal programs, services, and publications.

Journal of Applied Behavior Analysis

(http://seab.envmed.rochester.edu/jaba). Psychology journal that publishes research about applications of the experimental analysis of behavior to social problems. Published by The Society for the Experimental Analysis of Behavior.

Research and Training Center (RTC) on Family Support and Children's Mental Health

(http://www.rtc.pdx.edu). This federally funded RTC is dedicated to promoting effective community-based, culturally competent, family-centered services for families and their children who are or may be affected by mental health, emotional, or behavioral disorders. The center conducts collaborative research with family members, service providers, policy makers, and so forth.

PREMATURITY

BLISS

(http://www.bliss.org.uk). Web site created by parents and mainly aimed at parents and families. Provides information about causes of prematurity and levels of neonatal care. Has parent information boards with chat rooms on topics such as treatment in the neonatal intensive care unit (NICU), problems encountered by the premature infant, and discharge issues. Includes information on current research and training seminars for health professionals, primarily NICU nurses. Several informational pamphlets available for download. Photos included.

Emory Pediatrics Developmental Progress Clinic

(http://med.emory.edu/PEDIATRICS/NEON ATOLOGY/DPC/index.htm). Web site covers information regarding medical complications with implications for development, other neonatal medical complications associated with developmental problems, developmental care in the NICU, neurodevelopmental implications of neonatal trauma, developmental milestones specifically for children born prematurely, information regarding issues beyond infancy, Georgia state resources, frequently asked questions and answers, and web links.

Family Practice Notebook

(http://www.fpnotebook.com/NICCH16.htm). Web site provides information on the outcomes of infants born prematurely. Presents a formula for predicting survival and morbidity rates and examples from 23–30 weeks' gestation. Also gives neurological outcomes for 24–26 weeks' gestation and links to the references that support these outcomes.

Mayo Clinic: Premature Birth

(http://www.mayoclinic.com/health/premature-birth/DS00137). Provides information related to prematurity, such as causes of premature delivery, signs and symptoms during pregnancy, and when to seek medical help. Also includes information on the difficulties a child born prematurely may have, the course of care he or she will receive in the NICU, and what to expect upon discharge.

Medline Plus: Premature Babies

(http://www.nlm.nih.gov/medlineplus/prematur ebabies.html). Resource for health care professionals. Sections include drug information, an encyclopedia, a dictionary, news pages, and other resources. Provides links to information (e.g., car seat safety for premature infants) that can be printed out and shared with parents.

Parents of Premature Babies

(http://www.preemie-l.org). Supports families and caregivers of premature infants. Offers a discussion forum and an e-mail list. In addition to NICU and medical information, lists resources for coping and emotional support. Contains contributions from neonatologists, nurses, and other pediatric specialists. Provides essays, frequently asked questions, advice sheets for families and caregivers, booklists, and conferences. Unique feature: mentoring program for new parents of premature infants who are matched with parents of an older premature infant. Contains links to sites that may be useful.

Premature Babies: Caring for Your Baby

(http://familydoctor.org/handouts/283.html). Web site maintained by the American Academy of Family Physicians as an all-encompassing resource to address typical parent concerns. Includes discussions about the special care needed by premature babies, growth and development, feeding issues, sleep patterns, vision and hearing, immunizations, and travel concerns such as car seat placement. An excellent site for parents and for early-intervention providers. Does not provide technical information for intervention suggestions or research.

Premature Babies Guide at Keep Kids Healthy

(http://www.keepkidshealthy.com/newborn/pre mature_babies.html). General resource for parents. It defines the risk factors for having a premature baby, describes neonates at various gestational ages, and defines common medical problems that premature babies often face. Web site also answers common parent questions related to feeding, going home, and possible long-term problems. Provides links to other web sites for support and parent chats.

Premature Baby–Premature Child

(http://prematurity.org). Web site was developed by parents of children who were born prematurely and who went on to have developmental issues. Resources provided on the topics, as are discussion forums and mailing lists. Unique feature: information provided on children with special needs and the opportunities for advocacy.

Premature-infant.com

(http://premature-infant.com). Web site has touching stories and supportive information for parents, along with insights for medical personnel. Most information is parent friendly. Contains resource links to related problems/concerns. Also provides information regarding gastroesophageal reflux disease, infant massage, kangaroo care, positioning, pain, respiratory syncytial virus (RSV), and feeding issues.

The Vermont Oxford

(http://www.vtoxford.org). Web site provides information for the institutions that participate in its database. Database tracks the progress of high-risk infants within certain criteria and provides good statistical analysis and research options to those who participate.

CAREERS

Fedcap Rehabilitation Services

119 West 19th Street, New York, NY 10011 (voice: 212-727-4200; TTY: 212-727-4384; fax: 212-727-4374; e-mail: info@fedcap.org; http://www.fedcap.org). Services include vocational training and job placement for adults with severe disabilities and/or other disadvantages.

CHILD DEVELOPMENT AND PEDIATRICS

Child Development Institute

17853 Santiago Boulevard, Suite 107-328, Villa Park, CA 92861 (714-998-8617; fax: 714-637-6957; e-mail: webmaster@childdevelopmentinfo.com; http://www.childdevelopmentinfo.com). Web site for parents on child development, parenting, child psychology, teenagers, health, safety, and learning disabilities.

PEDIATRIC DEVELOPMENT AND BEHAVIOR

Society for Developmental and Behavioral Pediatrics

19 Station Lane, Philadelphia, PA 19118 (215-248-9168; e-mail: nmspota@aol.com; http://www.sdbp.org). Interdisciplinary organization that promotes research and teaching in developmental and behavioral pediatrics. Sponsors the *Journal of Developmental and Behavioral Pediatrics* and conducts annual scientific meetings.

DENTAL CARE

American Academy of Pediatric Dentistry

211 East Chicago Avenue, #700, Chicago, IL 60611-2663 (312-337-2169; fax 312-337-6329; http://www.aapd.org). National organization representing the specialty of pediatric dentistry. Dedicated to improving and maintaining the oral health of children, adolescents, and people with special health care needs. Publishes the journal *Pediatric Dentistry*.

American Society of Dentistry for Children

211 East Chicago Avenue, #710, Chicago, IL 60611-2663 (312-943-1244; fax: 312-943-5341; e-mail: asdckids@aol.com; http://www.ucsf.edu/ads/asdc.html). Professional organization for specialists in pediatric dentistry. Dedicated to improving the dental health of children through the dissemination of knowledge to professionals and the general public through educational programs, public service efforts, and research. Publishes the *Journal of Dentistry for Children*.

National Institute of Dental and Craniofacial Research

National Institutes of Health, Bethesda, MD 20892-2190 (301-496-4261; e-mail: nidcrinfo@mail.nih.gov; http://www.nidr.nih.gov). Institute dedicated to the promotion of oral, dental, and craniofacial health through study of ways to promote health, prevent diseases and conditions, and develop new diagnostics and therapeutics.

Special Care Dentistry

211 East Chicago Avenue, 5th Floor, Chicago, IL 60611 (312-440-2660; fax: 312-440-2824; e-mail: SCD@SCDonline.org; http://www.SCDonline.org). National organization of dentists, dental hygienists, dental assistants, nondental health care providers, health program administrators, hospitals, agencies that serve people

with special needs, and other advocacy and health care organizations. Publishes the journal *Special Care in Dentistry*.

EDUCATION

American Educational Research Association (AERA)

1230 17th Street NW, Washington, DC 20036-3078 (202-223-9485; fax: 202-775-1824; http://www.aera.net). International professional organization with the goal of advancing educational research and its practical education. Members are educators, counselors, evaluators, graduate students, behavioral scientists, and directors or administrators of research, testing, or evaluation.

Association for Supervision and Curriculum Development (ASCD)

1703 North Beauregard Street, Alexandria, VA 22311 (800-933-2723; fax: 703-575-5400; http://www.ascd.org). Professional membership organization for educators with interest in instruction, curriculum, and supervision. Publishes the journal *Educational Leadership*.

Association on Higher Education and Disability (AHEAD)

University of Massachusetts, 100 Morrissey Boulevard, Boston, MA 02125 (voice: 617-287-3880; TTY: 617-287-3882; fax: 617-287-3881; http://www.ahead.org). Professional organization committed to full participation in higher education for people with disabilities.

Council for Exceptional Children (CEC)

1110 North Glebe Road, Suite 300, Arlington, VA 22201 (voice: 888-232-7733; TTY: 703-264-9446; fax: 703 264 9494; e mail: service @sped.org; http://www.cec.sped.org). Provides information to teachers, administrators, and others concerned with the education of gifted children and children with disabilities. Maintains a library and database (ERIC Clearinghouse on Disabilities and Gifted Education; http://www.ericec.org) on research in special and gifted education; provides information and assistance on legislation.

National Association of Private Special Education Centers (NAPSEC) (formerly National Association of Private Schools for Exceptional Children)

1522 K Street NW, Suite 1032, Washington, DC 20005 (202-408-3338; fax: 202-408-3340; e-mail: napsec@aol.com; http://www.napsec.org). A nonprofit association that represents more than 200 schools nationally and more than 600 at the state level through its Council of Affiliated State Associations. Provides special education and therapeutic services for children in public or private educational placements. Also provides a free referral service to parents and professionals seeking appropriate placement for children with disabilities and publishes a directory of member schools.

National Information Center for Educational Media (NICEM)

Post Office Box 8640, Albuquerque, NM 87198-8640 (800-926-8328; fax: 505-998-3372; e-mail: nicem@nicem.com; http://www.nicem.com). Provides database of educational audiovisual materials, including videotapes, motion pictures, filmstrips, audiotapes, and slides.

FAMILY AND SIBLING SUPPORTS

Beach Center on Disability

The University of Kansas, 3111 Haworth Hall, Lawrence, KS 66045 (785-864-7600; fax: 785-864-7605; e-mail: beach@dole.lsi.ukans.edu; http://www.beachcenter.org). Research and training center that disseminates information about families with members who have developmental disabilities. Publishes a newsletter, and offers many other publications.

Bureau of Primary Health Care

(http://bphc.hrsa.gov/quality/Cultural.htm). Web site uses a variety of stories to illustrate values and principles one needs to appreciate and understand when providing culturally competent care to individuals with disabilities or special health care needs.

Children's Disabilities Information

(http://www.childrensdisabilities.info/prematurity/followup.html). Support site for parents that contains articles, lists of books, and web links on preemies and prematurity. Has several links for parents of children with disabilities, including parenting children with special needs, articles on several disorders, and support network links. Contains general information that is written in easily understandable terms.

The Compassionate Friends

Post Office Box 3696, Oak Brook, IL 60522-3696 (877-969-0010; fax: 630-990-0246; e-mail: nationaloffice@compassionatefriends.org; http://www.compassionatefriends.org). National and worldwide organization that supports and aids parents in the positive resolution of the grief experienced upon the death of a child; fosters the physical and emotional health of bereaved parents and siblings.

Exceptional Parent

65 East Route 4, River Edge, NJ 07661 (201-489-4111; fax: 201-489-0074 subscriptions: Post Office Box 2078, Marion, OH 43306-2178; 877-372-7368; http://www.eparent.com). Magazine published since 1971 that provides straightforward, practical information for families and professionals involved in the care of children and young adults with disabilities; many articles are written by parents.

Family Village: A Global Community of Disability-Related Resources

Waisman Center, University of Wisconsin–Madison, 1500 Highland Avenue, Madison, WI 53705-2280 (e-mail: familyvillage@waisman.wisc.edu; http://www.familyvillage.wisc.edu). Global community that integrates information, resources, and communication opportunities on the Internet for people with cognitive and other disabilities, for their families, and for people who provide services and support to these individuals.

Family Voices

2340 Alamo SE, Suite 102, Albuquerque, NM 87106 (http://www.familyvoices.org). Web site for a national, grassroots clearinghouse for information and education concerning the health care of children with special health needs. Contains links to all state chapters and the various projects the organization conducts.

Federation for Children with Special Needs

1135 Tremont Street, Suite 240, Boston, MA 02120 (800-331-0688 [in MA only]; 617-236-7210; fax: 617-572-2094; e-mail: fcsninfo@fcsn.org; http://www.fcsn.org). Offers parent-to-parent training and information; projects include Technical Assistance for Parent Programs (TAPP), Collaboration Among Parents and Health Professionals (CAPP), and Parents Engaged in Educational Reform (PEER). Part of the National Early Childhood Technical Assistance System (NEC*TAS) consortium.

PACER Center (Parent Advocacy Coalition for Educational Rights)

8161 Normandale Boulevard, Minneapolis, MN 55437 (voice: 800-537-2237 [in MN only]; voice: 952-838-9000; TTY: 952-838-0190; fax: 952-838-0199; e-mail: pacer@pacer.org; http://www.pacer.org). Provides education and training to help parents understand special education laws and to obtain appropriate school programs for their children. Workshops and program topics include early intervention, emotional disabilities, and health/medical services. Also provides a disability-awareness puppet program for schools, child abuse–prevention program services, newsletters, booklets, extensive written materials, and videotapes.

Parent Educational Advocacy Training Center (PEATC)

6320 Augusta Drive, Suite 1200, Springfield, VA 22150 (800-869-6782 [in VA only]; voice/TTY: 703-923-0010; Spanish: 703-569-6200; fax: 703-923-0030; e-mail: partners@peatc.org; http://www.peatc.org). Professionally staffed organization that helps parents to become effective advocates for their children with school personnel and the educational system.

Parent to Parent

c/o Beach Center on Families and Disability, The University of Kansas, 3111 Haworth Hall, Lawrence, KS 66045 (785-864-7600; http://www.p2pusa.org). State and local chapters provide one-to-one, parent-to-parent support by matching trained parents with newly referred parents on the basis of their children's disabilities and/or family issues they are encountering or have encountered.

Sibling Information Network

The A.J. Pappanikou Center, 249 Glenbrook Road, U-64, Storrs, CT 06269-2064 (860-486-4985; fax: 860-486-5037). Assists individuals and professionals interested in serving the needs of families of individuals with disabilities. Disseminates bibliographic material and directories, puts people in touch with each other, and publishes a newsletter written for and by siblings and parents.

The Sibling Support Project

c/o Donald Meyer, Director, the Sibling Support Project, The Arc of the United States, 6512 23rd Avenue, NW, Suite 213, Seattle, WA (206-297-6368; e-mail: donmeyer@siblingsupport.org; http://www.siblingsupport.org). National program dedicated to the interests of brothers and sisters of people with special health and developmental needs. Primary goal is to increase the availability of peer support and education programs for such siblings.

Special Child

(http://www.specialchild.com). Sponsored by the Resource Foundation for Children with Challenges (RFCC). Web site provides parent testimonials, diagnosis-related information, parent support, and a wide variety of information regarding educational and early intervention services.

Team Advocates for Special Kids (TASK)

100 Cerritos Avenue, Anaheim CA 92805 (714-533-8275; fax: 714-533-2533; e-mail: taskca@ yahoo.com; http://www.taskca.org). Offers training, education, support, information, resources, and community awareness programs to families of children with disabilities and the professionals who serve them. Conducts an advocacy training course and other workshops, and publishes a bimonthly newsletter. TASK's Tech Center (a member of the Alliance for Technology Access) conducts one-to-one guided exploration of technology to determine appropriate adapted hardware and software for people with disabilities.

Tools for Coping with Life's Stressors

(http://www.coping.org). Web site contains many links to help parents in coping with issues related to raising a child with special health care needs, such as tools for communication and tools for a balanced lifestyle. Also provides information about early identification and intervention.

DISABILITIES CULTURE

Disability Online

(http://www.disability-online.com/Detailed/214 .html). Offers a comprehensive resource center for all disability-related resources, topics, and services. Focuses on areas that relate to disability, including health, medical, social, employment, family, and personal areas. Provides a comprehensive on-line resource library for disability-related material and an interactive community for people with disabilities and their caregivers and families.

Disability Studies Quarterly (DSQ)

(http://www.dsq-sds.org). The journal of the Society for Disability Studies (SDS). A multidisciplinary, international journal of interest to social scientists, scholars in the humanities, disability rights advocates, creative writers, and others concerned with the issues of people with disabilities. Committed to developing theoreti-

cal and practical knowledge about disability and to promoting the full, equal participation of persons with disabilities in society.

National Center for Cultural Competence

(http://www.gucchd.georgetown.edu/nccc). Mission is to increase the capacity of health and mental health programs to design, implement, and evaluate culturally and linguistically competent service-delivery systems. Web site contains information on assessing culturally competent health care practices and on promoting culturally competent care. Has a Spanish-language portal specifically for families.

FEDERAL AGENCIES

Office of Disability Employment Policy

1331 F Street NW, Suite 300, Washington, DC 20004-1107 (voice: 202-376-6200; TTY: 202-376-6205; fax: 202-376-6859; e-mail: infoodep @dol.gov; http://www.dol.gov/odep). One of the oldest presidential committees in the United States. Promotes acceptance of people with physical and intellectual disabilities in the world of work, in both the public and the private sectors. Promotes the elimination of barriers, both physical and attitudinal, to the employment of people with disabilities.

Office of Special Education and Rehabilitative Services (OSERS)

U.S. Department of Education, 400 Maryland Avenue SW, Washington, DC 20202 (202-205-5465; http://www.ed.gov/about/offices/list/ osers). Part of the U.S. Department of Education. Responds to inquiries, and researches and documents information operations serving the field of disabilities. Specializes in providing information on federal funding for programs serving people with disabilities, federal legislation affecting individuals with disabilities, and federal programs benefiting people with disabilities.

FEEDING, GROWTH, AND NUTRITION

American Dietetic Association

216 West Jackson Boulevard, Chicago, IL 60606-6995 (800-877-1600; http://www.eatright .org). World's largest association of food and nutrition professionals. Web site offers healthy lifestyle and nutrition tips and referrals to registered dieticians. Publishes the *Journal of the American Dietetic Association*.

Community's Resources for Feeding and Growth of Children

(http://www.comeunity.com/premature/child/growth/resources.html). Web site contains links to recommended parent discussion lists, articles, and hospitals/institutions that offer feeding therapy.

Dysphagia Resource Center

(http://www.dysphagia.com). Web site contains links to resources on swallowing and swallowing disorders.

Food and Drug Administration (FDA)

5600 Fishers Lane, Rockville, MD 20857-0001 (888-463-6332; http://www.fda.gov). Part of the U.S. Department of Health and Human Services. Provides the latest federal warnings and updates about foods, drugs, medical devices, vaccines, animal feed, cosmetics, and radiation-emitting products. Has links for children, consumers, patients, and health care professionals.

Formula Manufacturers

The following web sites contain information about special formulas required by some infants with developmental disabilities:

- http://www.meadjohnson.com (Enfamil, Pro-Sobee, metabolic formulas)
- http://www.ross.com (Similac, Isomil, metabolic formulas)
- http://www.shsna.com (metabolic formulas)
- http://www.verybestbaby.com (Nestlé Carnation)

New Visions

1124 Roberts Mountain Road, Faber, VA 22938 (434-361-2285; fax: 434-361-1807; e-mail: sem@new-vis.com; @http://www.new-vis.com). Provides education and therapy services to professionals and parents working with children with feeding, swallowing, oral-motor, and prespeech problems. Mealtimes catalog offers therapy materials, tapes, and books.

LEGAL ISSUES

Administration for Children and Families (ACF)

(http://www.acf.dhhs.gov). Web site is from the federal agency that provides assistance to the various entities that provide family assistance, child support, child care, Head Start, child welfare, and other programs related to helping families and children.

American Bar Association Center on Children and the Law

740 15th Street NW, Washington, DC 20005-1019 (e-mail: ctrchildlaw@abanet.org; http://www.abanet.org/child). Offers information and advocacy to professionals and parents of children and adolescents with disabilities.

American Civil Liberties Union (ACLU)

125 Broad Street, New York, NY 10004-2400 (212-549-2500; to order publications: 800-775-2258; e-mail: aclu@aclu.org; http://www.aclu.org). Nonprofit organization that is the largest public-interest law firm in the United States. Offers links to disability rights topics.

Center for the Child Care Workforce

(http://www.ccw.org). Web site is maintained by a division of the American Federation of Teachers Educational Foundation that was set up to support the education of children, advocacy of early child care and education, and compensation of professionals who work with children. Site provides many resources available for teachers about educating children and a newsletter to help professionals keep current on issues of interest.

Child Development Web

(http://www.childdevelopmentweb.com/Information/EIprograms.asp). Web site offers information on early intervention for parents and families of children who might be eligible for services. Early Intervention Programs section is part of the Information Link on The Child Development Web's home page. Site contains information on obtaining services in the United States, an explanation of early intervention programs and processes, and a breakdown of the services that are available through early intervention. Provides contact information for early intervention in each state.

Children's Defense Fund (CFD)

25 E Street NW, Washington, DC 20001 (202-628-8787; e-mail: cdfinfo@childrensdefense.org; http://www.childrensdefense.org). Private non-profit organization dedicated to educating about, advocating for, and studying the needs of children, especially low-income children, minority children, and children with disabilities. Mission focuses on giving children a head start (child care), a healthy start (child health), a fair start (family income), a safe start (violence prevention, child welfare, and mental health), and a moral start (ethics, morality, and self-discipline).

Council for Exceptional Children (CEC)

(http://www.ideapractices.org). International professional organization dedicated to improving educational outcomes for individuals with exceptionalities, students with disabilities, and/or the gifted. Web site includes current governmental policies and professional standards. Targeted audience for this includes teachers, parents, administrators, students, paraprofessionals, and related support service providers.

Disabilities Rights
Education and Defense Fund (DREDF)

2212 Sixth Street, Berkeley, CA 94710 (voice/TTY: 510-644-2555; fax: 510-841-8645; e-mail: dredf@dredf.org; http://www.dredf.org). Law and policy center to protect the rights of people with disabilities. Offers referral and information regarding the rights of people with disabilities. Educates legislators and policy makers about issues affecting the rights of people with disabilities; also educates the public about the Americans with Disabilities Act (ADA) of 1990 (PL 101-336).

Do2Learn

(http://www.do2learn.com). Web site discusses the legal rights of children with special health care needs and their parents in regard to creating the individual family service plan (IFSP). Includes parent-friendly links to sites that provide information about amendments to the Individuals with Disabilities Education Act (IDEA) and other legal concerns.

Early Child Development

(http://www.worldbank.org/children). Web site is a knowledge source designed to assist policy makers, program managers, and practitioners in their efforts to promote the healthy growth and integral development of young children. Site is in Spanish, Portuguese, French, and Arabic.

Illinois Department of Human Services

(http://www.dhs.state.il.us/ei). Web site provides a library of information services to parents, providers, educators, policy makers, students, and others interested in early intervention issues. Resource library contains books, periodicals, audiovisual, and other reference materials that can be issued for use on loan. Information is for multiple audiences, but the site also offers *Early Intervention*, a quarterly newsletter directed specifically toward parents.

Indiana First Steps Early Intervention

(http://www.infirststeps.com/matrix/default.asp). Target audience includes therapists, parents, service coordinators, and other service providers for children from birth to age 3. Provides information pertaining to therapists; mainly on administrative issues, enrollment, reimbursement, and training. Parent information available for choosing a provider; also provides other early childhood links.

Information and
Referral Resource Network

http://www.acitinc.com/ir-net). Web site contains a national directory of Internet listings for medical services. Site is intended to be used by medical professionals, educators, students, and the general public. Directory includes referral information for social services, health care, drugs, doctors, hospitals, and medical services. Site also provides information on some community health and outreach programs.

Judge David L. Bazelon
Center for Mental Health Law

1101 15th Street NW, Suite 1212, Washington, DC 20005-5002 (voice: 202-467-5730; TTY: 202-467-4342; fax: 202-223-0409; e-mail: webmaster@bazelon.org; http://www.bazelon.org). Nonprofit legal advocacy program that works to define, establish, and protect the rights of children and adults with mental health disabilities, using test-case litigation, federal policy advocacy, and training and technical assistance for lawyers and other advocates nationwide.

National Association of Protection
and Advocacy Systems (NAPAS)

900 Second Street NE, Suite 211, Washington, DC 20002 (voice: 202-408-9514; TTY: 202-408-9521; fax: 202-408-9520, e-mail: napas@earthlink.net; http://www.icdri.org/legal/natpai.htm). Web site provides links to protection and advocacy agencies, located across the United States, mandated by federal law to serve and protect the rights of people with disabilities.

National Child Care
Information Center (NCCIC)

(http://www.nccic.org). An organization dedicated to linking families, providers, policy makers, researchers, and the public to information about early child care and education information. Site contains many links to information about legislation and policies affecting early childhood care, including the Administration for Children and Families Priorities, nutrition/obesity prevention, and the Bush administration's Early Childhood Initiative. Site also features links to resources for parents.

National Early Childhood Technical Assistance Center

(http://www.nectac.org). Program that provides responsive technical assistance (TA) to the programs supported under the Individuals with Disabilities Education Act (IDEA) for infants and toddlers with disabilities (Part C of IDEA) and for preschoolers with disabilities (Section 619-Part B of IDEA) in all states and participating jurisdictions, as well as to the projects funded by the Office of Special Education Programs under the Early Education Program for Children with Disabilities. Offers informational links to IDEA, publications, and other resources.

Office of Special Education Programs (OSEP)

(http://www.ed.gov/about/offices/list/osers/osep /index.html). Web site is from the division of the Department of Education that oversees IDEA. Provides information regarding IDEA and other special education initiatives.

Parents Helping Parents (PHP)

(http://www.php.com). Web site is sponsored by a California-based not-for-profit organization for parents of children with disabilities. An international consulting organization for family resources. Site provides valuable information for parents regarding laws concerning the rights of children with disability, and health care issues. Provides regional and state-specific information about support groups for parents and siblings, as well as information on topics such as special education, IDEA, the No Child Left Behind Act of 2001 (PL 107-110), and other special education initiatives.

MEDICATIONS

Drug InfoNet

(http://www.druginfonet.com). Web site that provides information about drugs, diseases, and pharmaceutical manufacturing, as well as links to related sites.

OCCUPATIONAL THERAPY

American Occupational Therapy Association (AOTA)

4720 Montgomery Lane, Post Office Box 31220, Bethesda, MD 20824 (voice: 301-652-2682; TTY: 800-377-8555; fax: 301-652-7711; http://www.aota.org). Professional organization of occupational therapists; provides such services as accreditation of educational programs, professional publications, public education, and continuing education for practitioners.

PHYSICAL THERAPY

American Physical Therapy Association (APTA)

1111 North Fairfax Street, Alexandria, VA 22314 (voice: 800-999-2782; TTY: 703-683-6748; fax: 703-684-7343; http://www.apta.org). Professional membership association of physical therapists, physical therapist assistants, and physical therapy students. Operates clearinghouse for questions on physical therapy and disabilities. Publishes bibliographies on a range of topics.

RECREATION AND SPORTS

American Alliance for Health, Physical Education, Recreation and Dance (AAHPERD)

1900 Association Drive, Reston, VA 20191 (800-213-7193; http://www.aahperd.org). National organization supporting and assisting individuals involved in physical education, recreation, dance, and health, leisure, fitness, and education. An alliance of six national associations. Offers numerous publications.

American Association of Adapted Sports Programs

Post Office Box 538, Pine Lake, GA 30072 (404-294-0070; fax 404-294-5758; e-mail: aaasp@bell south.net; http://www.aaasp.org). Mission is to enhance the health, independence, and future economic self-sufficiency of youth with physical disabilities by facilitating a national sports movement and assisting communities in creating the best member programs possible for youth with disabilities who wish to compete.

Disabled Sports USA (DS/USA)

451 Hungerford Drive, Suite 100, Rockville, MD 20850 (voice: 301-217-0960; TTY: 301-217-0963; fax: 301-217-0968; e-mail: dsusa@

dsusa.org; http://www.dsusa.org). Offers summer programs and competitions, fitness programs, "fitness is for everyone" videotapes, and winter ski programs. Local chapters offer activities (e.g., camping, hiking, biking, horseback riding, 10K runs, water skiing, whitewater rafting, rope courses, mountain climbing, sailing, yachting, canoeing, kayaking, aerobic fitness, skiing). Provides year-round sports and recreational opportunities to people with orthopedic, spinal cord, neuromuscular, and visual impairments, through a national network of local chapters.

Girl Scouts of the USA
420 5th Avenue, New York, NY 10018 (800-478-7248; e-mail: misc@girlscouts.org; http://www.girlscouts.org). Open to all girls ages 5–17 (or kindergarten through grade 12). Runs camping programs, sports and recreational activities, and service programs. Incorporates children with disabilities into general Girl Scout troop activities. Published the book *Focus on Ability: Serving Girls with Special Needs.*

International Committee of Sports for the Deaf
814 Thayer Avenue, Suite #350, Silver Spring, MD 20910 (e-mail: info@ciss.org; http://www.deaflympics.com). Gives a history of accomplishments of deaf athletes. Links to regional confederations and technical delegates throughout the world.

Little League Baseball, Challenger Division
(http://www.littleleague.org/divisions/challenger.asp). On-line resource provides information and opportunities for boys and girls with disabilities to experience the emotional development and the fun of playing Little League baseball.

National Center on Physical Activity and Disability
1640 West Roosevelt Road, Chicago, IL 60608-6904 (voice/TTY: 800-900-8086; http://www.ncpad.org). Encourages and supports people with disabilities who wish to increase their overall level of activity and participate in some form of regular physical activity. Offers searchable directories of organizations, programs, and facilities that provide opportunities for accessible physical activity, adaptive equipment vendors, conferences and meetings, and references to journal articles, books, videotapes, and more. Provides fact sheets on a variety of physical activities for people with disabilities.

The National Sports Center for the Disabled
Post Office Box 1290, Winter Park, CO 80482 (970-726-1540; fax: 970-726-4112; e-mail: info@nscd.org; http://www.nscd.org). Provides therapeutic recreation programs designed for individuals with disabilities who require adaptive equipment and/or special instruction. Offers summer and winter programs; has some scholarships.

Special Olympics International
1325 G Street NW, Suite 500, Washington, DC 20005 (202-628-3630; fax: 202-824-0200; e-mail: info@specialolympics.org; http://www.specialolympics.org). Largest organization to provide year-round sports training and athletic competition for children and adults with intellectual disabilities and certain other significant cognitive impairments. Local, state, and national games are held throughout the United States and in more than 150 countries; world games held every 4 years.

United States Association of Blind Athletes (USABA)
33 North Institute Street, Colorado Springs, CO 80903 (719-630-0422; fax: 719-630-0616; http://www.usaba.org). Aims to ensure that legally blind individuals have the same opportunities as their sighted peers in recreation and sports programs at all levels, from developmental to elite. Works to change negative stereotypes related to the abilities of individuals who are blind and other people with disabilities. Publishes a newsletter (also available on cassette). Web site has links to related sites and event calendars with sport descriptions.

Wheelchair Sports, USA
3595 East Fountain Boulevard, Suite L-1, Colorado Springs, CO 80910 (719-574-1150; fax: 719-574-9840; e-mail: wsusa@aol.com; http://www.wsusa.org). Governing body of various sports of wheelchair athletics, including swimming, archery, weightlifting, track and field, table tennis, and air weapons. Publishes a newsletter.

Yoga for the Special Child
1521 Chicago Avenue, Evanston, IL 60201 (888-900-9642; fax: 847-869-8329; http://www .specialyoga.com). A comprehensive program of yoga techniques designed to enhance the natural development of children with special needs.

REHABILITATION

**Healthy and Ready to
Work Information Center**
Maine State Title V CSHN Program (http:// www.hrtw.org). Network that works with local agencies to ensure that all youth with special health care needs receive the services necessary to make the transition to all aspects of adulthood, including adult health care, employment, and independence.

Institute for Child Health Policy
University of Florida, Post Office Box 100147, Gainesville, FL 32610 (352-265-7220; http:// www.ichp.edu). Mission is to research, evaluate, formulate, and advance health policies, programs, and systems that promote the health and well-being of children and youth through applied knowledge to health related-systems and outcomes for children and youth.

**National Center on
Physical Activity and Disability**
1640 West Roosevelt Road, Chicago, IL 60608 (800-900-8086; fax: 312-355-4058; http://www .ncpad.org). Mission of the National Center on Physical Activity and Disability (NCPAD) is to promote substantial health benefits that can be gained from participating in regular physical activity.

**National Institute on Disability
and Rehabilitation Research (NIDRR)**
400 Maryland Avenue SW, Washington, DC 20202-2572 (voice: 202-205-8134; TTY: 202-205-4475; http://www.ed.gov/about/offices/ list/osers/nidrr). Provides leadership and support for a comprehensive program of research related to the rehabilitation of individuals with disabilities.

**National Rehabilitation
Information Center (NARIC)**
4200 Forbes Boulevard, Suite 202, Lanham, MD 20706 (800-346-2742; fax: 301-562-2401; e-mail: naric@heitechservices.com; http://www .naric.com). Rehabilitation information service and research library; provides quick-reference and referral information, bibliographic searches, and photocopies of documents. Publishes several directories and resource guides.

E | Cognitive Testing and Screening Testing

Nancy J. Roizen

Instrument (author, year; publisher)	Age/grade Administration time (if available)	Purpose/description
Academic Achievement Tests		
Bracken School Readiness Assessment (Bracken, 2002; Harcourt Assessment)	2 years 6 months through 7 years 11 months 10–15 minutes	Assesses academic readiness by evaluating a child's understanding of important fundamental concepts in the categories of colors, letters, numbers/counting, sizes, comparisons, and shapes
Brigance Diagnostic Comprehensive Inventory of Basic Skills–Revised (Brigance & Glascoe, 1999; Curriculum Associates)	5–13 years	Designed for diagnostic and classroom assessment in basic reading skills, reading comprehension, math calculation, math reasoning, written language, listening comprehension, and information processing
Kaufman Test of Educational Achievement–Second Edition (KTEA-II; Kaufman & Kaufman, 2003; AGS Publishing)	4 years, 6 months through 25 years 90+ minutes	Measures reading, reading-related skills, math, written language, and oral language
Peabody Individual Achievement Test–Revised (PIAT-R; Markwardt, 1998; AGS Publishing)	K–12 60 minutes	Designed to measure academic achievement
Wechsler Individual Achievement Test–Second Edition (WIAT-II; Wechsler, 2001; Harcourt Assessment)	4–85 years 45–120 minutes (abbreviated version: 12–25 minutes)	Measurement tool useful for achievement skills assessment, learning disability diagnosis, special education placement, curriculum planning, and clinical appraisal
Wide Range Achievement Test–Fourth Edition (WRAT4; Wilkinson & Robertson, 2006; PAR)	5–94 years 15–45 minutes	Examines development of reading, spelling, and arithmetic skills
Woodcock-Johnson III Tests of Achievement (WJIII; Woodcock, McGrew, & Mather, 2001; Riverside Publishing)	2–90 years	Word recognition, reading fluency, reading comprehension, calculation, math fluency, applied math reasoning, spelling, writing fluency, written expression, oral expression, and listening comprehension
Cognitive Assessment		
Bayley Scales of Infant and Toddler Development–Third Edition (Bayley III; Bayley, 2006; Harcourt Assessment)	1–42 months 50–90 minutes	Assessment of current developmental function including cognitive, language (receptive and expressive communication), motor (fine and gross), social-emotional, and adaptive behavior

A Developmental Neuropsychological Assessment (NEPSY; Korkman, Kirk, & Kemp, 1997; Harcourt Assessment)	3–12 years 45–120 minutes	Designed to assess neuropsychological development
Differential Ability Scales (DAS; Elliott, 1990; Harcourt Assessment)	2.5 years through 17 years 11 months 25–65 minutes	Measure of overall cognitive ability and specific abilities
Kaufman Assessment Battery for Children, Second Edition (KABC-II; Kaufman & Kaufman, 2004; AGS Publishing)	3–18 years 25–70 minutes	Measure of intelligence that focuses on the assessment of processing styles—sequential and simultaneous processing, planning, learning, and crystallized abilities, with a mental processing index and a nonverbal index
Leiter International Performance Scale–Revised (Leiter-R; Roid & Miller, 1998; Stoelting Co.)	2.0–20.11 years 90 minutes	Constructed as a "nonverbal cognitive assessment"
Reynolds Intellectual Assessment Scales (RIAS; Reynolds & Kamphaus, 2005; Psychological Assessment Resources)	3–94 years 20–25 minutes	Individually administered test of intelligence
Stanford-Binet Intelligence Scales, Fifth Edition (SB5; Terman & Merrill, 2003; Riverside Publishing)	2 years to adult	Designed for measuring verbal reasoning, abstract visual reasoning, quantitative skills, and short-term memory skills
Wechsler Abbreviated Scale of Intelligence (WASI; Wechsler, 1999; Harcourt Assessment)	6–89 years 30 minutes	Designed as a "short and reliable measure of intelligence"
Wechsler Intelligence Scale for Children–Fourth Edition (WISC-IV; Wechsler, 2003; Harcourt Assessment)	6–17 years	Standard measure of intelligence in children; focuses on approach to problem solving
Wechsler Preschool and Primary Scale of Intelligence–Third Edition (WPPSI-III; Wechsler, 2002; Harcourt Assessment)	3–7 years	General intelligence scale for young children
Language Tests		
Clinical Evaluation of Language Fundamentals, Fourth Edition (CELF-4; Semel, Wiig, & Secord, 2003; Harcourt Assessment)	5–21 years 30–60 minutes	Quickly and accurately identify and diagnose language disorders
Clinical Evaluation of Language Fundamentals, Preschool (CELF-P; Semel, Wiig, & Secord, 2004; Harcourt Assessment)	3–6 years 30–45 minutes	Quickly and accurately identify and diagnose language disorders
Comprehensive Assessment of Spoken Language (CASL; Carrow-Woolfolk, 1999; AGS Publishing)	3–21 years 30–45 minutes	Fifteen tests measure language-processing skills—comprehension, expression, and retrieval—in four language structure categories: lexical/semantic, syntactic, supralinguistic, and pragmatic

Expressive One-Word Picture Vocabulary Test–2000 Edition (EOWPVT-2000; Brownell, 2000; Academic Therapy Publications)	2–18 years 10–15 minutes	Designed to measure an individual's English-speaking vocabulary
Goldman Firstoe Test of Articulation–Second Edition (GFTA-2; Goldman & Firstoe, 2000; AGS Publishing)	2–21 years 5–15 minutes	Designed as "a systematic means of assessing an individual's articulation of the consonant sounds of Standard American English"
MacArthur-Bates Communication Development Inventories (CDIs), Second Edition (Fenson, Marchman, Thal, et al., 2007; Paul H. Brookes Publishing Co.)	8–30 months 23–30 minutes	Evaluates young children's communication skills with norm-referenced parent checklists
Peabody Picture Vocabulary Test–Third Edition (PPVT-III; Dunn, Williams, & Wang, 1997; AGS Publishing)	2.5–90 years 11–12 minutes	Measure receptive vocabulary—used as a screening test for verbal ability
Test of Pragmatic Language (TOPL; Phelps-Terasaki & Phelps-Gunn, 1992; PRO-ED)	5 years to 13 years 11 months 20–30 minutes	Designed to provide an in-depth screening of the effectiveness and appropriateness of a student's pragmatic, or social, language skills

Screening Tests

Ages & Stages Questionnaires® (ASQ), Second Edition (Bricker, Squires, & Mounts, 1999; Paul H. Brookes Publishing Co.)	4–60 months	Each questionnaire assesses communication, fine- and gross-motor, problem-solving, and personal-social skills.
Battelle Developmental Inventory Screening Test (BDIST; Svinicki, 1984; Riverside Publishing)	Birth through 8 years 15–35 minutes	Assesses developmental skills in motor, language, cognitive, and personal-social area
Bayley Infant Neurodevelopmental Screener (BINS; Aylward, 1995; Harcourt Assessment)	3–24 months 10–15 minutes	Screens receptive and expressive functions, cognitive processes, and neurologic integrity
Child Development Inventory (Ireton, 1992; Behavior Science Systems)	18 months through 5 years	Parent questionnaire that screens social, self-help, gross-motor, fine-motor, and language areas of development
Early Language Milestone Scale–Second Edition (ELM Scale-2; Coplan, 1993; PRO-ED)	1–36 months 1–10 minutes	Assesses language in a format similar to DDST: auditory expressive and receptive; visual and global language
Parent Evaluations of Developmental Status (PEDS; Glascoe, 1997; Ellsworth & Vandermeer Press)	Birth through 9 years 2 minutes	Determines when to refer, provide parent education, or monitor developmental, behavioral/emotional, and academic progress

Other Tests

Adaptive Behavior Assessment System–Second Edition (ABAS-II; Harrison & Oakland, 2003; Harcourt Assessment)	0–89 years 15–20 minutes	Provides a complete assessment of adaptive skills functioning

Developmental Test of Visual-Motor Integration–Revised Fourth Edition (VMI-R; Berry & Buktenica, 2004; Modern Curriculum Press)	3 years to 17 years, 11 months	Designed to assess the extent to which individuals can integrate their visual and motor abilities (three scores: VMI, visual, and motor)
Peabody Developmental Motor Scales–Second Edition (PDMS-2; Folio & Fewell, 2000; PRO-ED)	Birth through 72 months 30–45 minutes	Designed to assess gross-motor skills
Scales of Independent Behavior-Revised (SIB-R; Bruininks, Woodcock, Weatherman, & Hill, 1996; Riverside Publishing)	0 years to adult 45–60 minutes	Provides a comprehensive assessment of 14 areas of adaptive behavior and eight areas of problem behavior
Vineland Adaptive Behavior Scales, Second Edition, (Vineland II; Sparrow, Cicchetti, & Balla, 2005; AGS Publishing)	birth–90 years (parent/caregiver interview and self completed forms and teacher completed questionnaires) 3 years to 21 years, 11 months (teacher) 20–60 minutes	A measure of personal and social skills (self-sufficiency) in four domains: communication, daily living skills, socialization, and motor skills

REFERENCES

Conoley, J.C., & Impara, J.C. (Eds.). (1995). *The Twelfth Mental Measurements Yearbook.* Lincoln: University of Nebraska Press.

Conoley, J.C., & Kramer, J.J. (Eds.). (1989). *The Tenth Mental Measurements Yearbook.* Lincoln: University of Nebraska Press.

Impara, J.C., & Plake, B.S. (Eds.). (1998). *The Thirteenth Mental Measurements Yearbook.* Lincoln: University of Nebraska Press.

Mitchell, J.V., Jr. (Ed.). (1985). *The Ninth Mental Measurements Yearbook.* Lincoln: University of Nebraska Press.

Plake, B.S., & Impara, J.C. (Eds.). (2001). *The Fourteenth Mental Measurements Yearbook.* Lincoln: University of Nebraska Press.

Plake, B.S., Impara, J.C., & Spies, R.A. (Eds.). (2003). *The Fifteenth Mental Measurements Yearbook.* Lincoln: University of Nebraska Press.

Index

Page references to figures, tables, and notes are indicated by *f*, *t*, and *n* respectively.